Cells, Tissues, and Disease:

PRINCIPLES OF GENERAL PATHOLOGY

COVER ILLUSTRATION

This illustration is a pun on the title of the book. It shows an *en face* view of the inner surface of the aorta of a hypercholesterolemic rat (experimental atherosclerosis), stained with silver nitrate (which outlines each endothelial cell in black) and with Oil red O (which stains fat droplets in red). Each unit of the flagstone pattern is a *cell*; the overall flagstone pattern of endothelium is a *tissue*; and the red droplets of fat represent *disease*.

Cells, Tissues, and Disease:

PRINCIPLES OF GENERAL PATHOLOGY

Guido Majno, MD
Isabelle Joris, PhD

Department of Pathology
University of Massachusetts Medical School
Worcester, Massachusetts

b

**Blackwell
Science**

BLACKWELL SCIENCE

EDITORIAL OFFICES: 238 Main Street, Cambridge, Massachusetts 02142, USA
Osney Mead, Oxford OX2 0EL, England
25 John Street, London WC1N 2BL, England
23 Ainslie Place, Edinburgh EH3 6AJ, Scotland
54 University Street, Carlton, Victoria 3053, Australia
Arnette Blackwell SA, 224, Boulevard Saint Germain, 75007 Paris, France
Blackwell Wissenschafts-Verlag GmbH
Kurfüurstendamm 57, 10707 Berlin, Germany
Zehetnergasse 6, A-1140 Vienna, Austria

DISTRIBUTORS: Marston Book Services, Ltd.
P.O. Box 269
Abingdon
Oxon OX14 4YN
(*Orders*: Tel: 01235465500 Fax: 01235465555)

USA
Blackwell Science, Inc., 238 Main Street, Cambridge, Massachusetts 02142
(*Orders*: Tel: 800-215-1000 or 617-876-7000 Fax: 617-492-5263)

Canada
Copp Clark, Ltd
2775 Matheson Blvd East
Mississauga, Ontario L4W 4P7
(*Orders*: Tel: 800-263-4374 Fax: 905-238-6074)

Australia
Blackwell Science Pty Ltd, 54 University Street, Carlton, Victoria 3053
(*Orders*: Tel: 03 9347 0300 Fax: 03 9349 3016)

Outside North America and Australia
Blackwell Science, Ltd., c/o Marston Book Services, Ltd.
P.O. Box 87, Oxford OX2 0DT, England   (*Orders*: Tel: 4-865-791155)

Production: Karen Feeney, Ellen Samia
Design: Leslie Haimes
Typesetter: Huron Valley Graphics
Printed and bound by Braun-Brumfield, Inc.
© 1996 by Guido Majno and Isabelle Joris
Printed in the United States of America
96 97 98 99 5 4 3 2 1

Notice: The indications and dosages of all drugs in this
book have been recommended in the medical literature
and conform to the practices of the general medical community. The medications described do not necessarily
have specific approval by the Food and Drug Administration for use in the diseases and dosages for which they
are recommended. The package insert for each drug
should be consulted for use and dosage as approved by the
FDA. Because standards of usage change, it is advisable to
keep abreast of revised recommendations, particularly
those concerning new drugs.

Library of Congress Cataloging in Publication Data

Majno, Guido.
    Cells, tissues, and disease : principles of general pathology /
Guido Majno, Isabelle Joris.
            p.   cm.
    Includes bibliographical references and index.
    ISBN 0-86542-372-5
    1. Pathology. I. Joris, Isabelle. II. Title.
    [DNLM: 1. Histology. 2. Pathology. QZ 4 M233c 1994]
RB111.M265   1994
616.07′1—dc20
DNLM/DLC
for Library of Congress   94-44912
                                                CIP

This book is dedicated
to all patients
in all times and places
and to all those who helped us understand
the primal patient—
the cell

CONTENTS

Contents

CONTENTS

Wherever there is life there is function—and malfunction. The science of life (function) is biology; the science of malfunction (disease) is pathology. By its very nature, modern pathology is a colorful quilt of all the basic sciences. Its sources range from anatomy and cell biology to biophysics and the laws of atomic structure; it can be studied at no less than eight levels of complexity (Figure P-1).

Although contributions to this body of knowledge come from dozens of different professions, the task of coordinating them has always fallen to pathologists. As a result, it was learned that all disease processes have some principles in common: these are collected under the heading of *general pathology*. This is the subject of this book. Because general pathology is best understood in relation to cells and tissues, we chose to focus our book primarily at this level.

Who, then, should study general pathology?

Half of the answer is easy: *physicians*. Nobody can practice medicine in the "Western" style without a solid background in general pathology.

The other half of the answer is less obvious: *scientists (non-physicians) who work in fields relevant to Medicine*, and they are numerous indeed. We have in mind all biologists in the broadest sense; the prototype are the molecular biologists who generate fascinating new models of pathology, such as transgenic mice, but can not fully enjoy their discoveries because they lack the necessary background in general pathology. As regards the bacteriologists and immunologists, their specialties were taught as part of pathology only a few decades ago. When they branched off, they also sawed themselves off from the main trunk and dropped all connections with the study of disease. It is, in our opinion, an aberration that most graduate school curricula continue to ignore pathology, when much of the laboratory work actually deals with the abnormal. Because one of us is a Ph.D., we can take the liberty of adding that these colleagues can not know what they are missing, because they were taught with that blind spot. Years ago one of us tried to fill the gap by offering a three-week summer course entitled "Pathology for Non-MDs" (5); this book is meant to include that approach.

So we have written this book for two sets of readers. In the medical field, we hope to reach *all pathologists, as well as physicians*, be they involved

Populations

Individuals

Isolated organs

Tissues

Cells

Cellular organelles

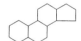

Molecules

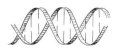

Genes

FIGURE P-1. *Disease can be studied at many levels: whole populations (epidemiology), individual patients (clinical medicine), individual organs (pathophysiology), tissues (histopathology), cells (cytology), single organelles (biochemistry), molecules (biophysics), and genes (molecular biology).*

in medical practice or in research, who may be curious to know what happened to these basic principles since graduation; *all teachers of pathology*, who need background and synthesis as well as a source of illustrations and references; *pathology residents*, who face general pathology every day in their diagnostic work, and should therefore know it a lot better than the average medical student; and last but not least, *inquisitive medical students,* who want to know more than what is necessary to pass an exam. In the scientific fields we hope to reach *biologists, including college teachers; molecular biologists, immunologists, bacteriologists, physiologists, researchers, and graduate students in the basic sciences,* none of whom had access to a general pathology book—let alone a general pathology course.

Both sets of readers should find their place in the Tree of Medicine (Figure P-2).

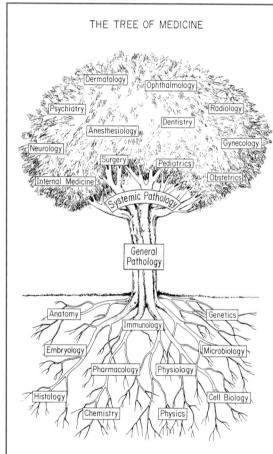

FIGURE P-2. *The Tree of Medicine: the trunk is General Pathology, which draws from all the basic sciences, and divides into the many branches of Special Pathology; each one of these supports a specialized field of Medicine. (Courtesy of Dr. George Th. Diamandopoulos, Harvard Medical School, Boston, MA.).*

Why another General Pathology textbook? First of all because we want to share our enthusiasm for the topic. Both our careers were influenced and possibly determined by a British classic: Payling Wright (7) for G.M. and Florey (2) for I.J. It is also true that many distinguished textbooks are currently available (see 1,4,6,8,9—just to mention a few in the English language). However we were driven by the reasons that all authors give: we had something different in mind.

• *We tried to produce a book suitable for medical and non-medical readers.* The language and the content were chosen accordingly. In this regard we were helped by circumstances: one of us is an M.D. (pathologist), the other a Ph.D. in biology and pathology. Because we each enjoy our chosen field, we also tried to convey our enthusiasm to the readers.

• *We chose to focus on the cell as the elementary patient* and on the interactions of cells in tissues; this is primarily the task of microscopy. We are living in an era so fascinated by the genes and their molecular products that their ultimate products—the cell and the individual—tend to be overlooked.

• *We emphasized principles rather than the latest fact.* In our era of overwhelming "fact overload" this was a prime concern. Principles have a longer half-life than details, and readers who may need more detail can always find it in hundreds of specialized monographs, which we cited, but which will continue to come and go every year or two. Detail, of course, is essential, but we tried to be sparing.

• *We used the historical approach* in many instances, because the path to a discovery helps to understand it. We even included, for fear that it might be lost, the historical origin of the name *endoplasmic reticulum* (a structure that is neither endoplasmic nor reticular). We recounted some of the investigators' meanderings and mistakes, especially the useful mistakes, and some fascinating sparks of insight, be they due to a dead horseshoe crab or to a piece of stained laboratory tubing. We also described some of the most imaginative experimental models, such as the admirable chicken-quail chimeras of Nicole LeDourarin.

• *Illustrations are an integral part of our message:* not only because we live in an era of visual communication, but also because morphologic documents may not be easily accessible to our non-medical readers. Furthermore, a beautiful landscape is better seen than described. In the study of disease a large portion of the data is visual, and a well-chosen picture (we borrowed many) conveys more credibility and sometimes more information than a graph. For schemes and drawings we had the benefit of three artists, each specializing in a given area.

• *We tried to underscore that disease (and the elementary patient) can be found in all walks of life;* hence the reader will meet with references to fish markets, deer antlers, cooked meat, autumn leaves, oranges, wounded trees, branded cattle, linoleum, irises (the flowers), nettles and wasps, pâté de foie gras, sky and snow, dried insects, and Japanese pearls, not to mention Buddha and many other subjects not usually encountered in this academic setting. In the same vein, we also pointed out that some pathologic findings eventually had an impact on industry: dead cells, for example, produce the so-called myelin figures; myelin figures led to liposomes, and liposomes rocketed to fame. They are now to be found even in the ads of the cosmetic industry. Free radicals, on the other hand, came to be appreciated largely through studies by the food industry, and found their way into pathology much later.

• *We tried to tell a single story from beginning to end.* This internal coherence (including planned repetition) is best achieved by a single-author book, and since we are a married couple we should qualify as a single author. Our joint experience in general pathology, as researchers and teachers, adds up to 60 years. We are fully aware that single authorship comes at the expense of firsthand competence in many areas, but we believe the trade is worthwhile. We have tried to offset this obvious criticism by asking experts to read and criticize specific sections.

• Finally, *we tried to cope constructively with the literature explosion.* This had been a major concern. We did consult thousands of papers and hundreds of books and monographs, but we always kept an eye on the general principle if one seemed to emerge. Many simple nouns in this book, such as *calcium, leukocyte, shock,* and *membrane,* are also the names of large volumes as well as of monthly journals that make the volumes obsolete. The output of scientific facts is torrential, but anyone looking for synthesis finds just a trickle.

This distillation process meant that day after day, year after year, we had to drag home (and back) suitcases full of books and papers, while onlookers envied us for going once again on vacation. Hopefully this muscular and synthetic effort will spare our readers some effort and help them reach their own syntheses. One of our safeguards has been to write letters all over the world asking for advice, reprints, and illustrations. We are indebted to hundreds of generous colleagues who graciously complied.

A note on the subject matter: *We assumed that the reader would be familiar with basic cell biology and histology. The five parts of our text deal with what we consider the five main subdivisions of general pathology: cellular pathology, injury and inflammation, vascular disturbances, immunopathology, and tumors. We omitted immunology per se, because every school usually has its own immunology bible; thus, even if we were card-carrying immunologists, our text would be second choice. Genetics was also omitted, because it is usually the subject of a separate course.*

The title was composed after a great deal of thinking; it had to emphasize the cell as the "elemen-

tary patient," and tissues as the context of cells. We later discovered quite accidentally that a British pathologist had published in 1977 a small book entitled Cell, tissue, and disease *(10). We apologized in writing to Dr. Woolf.*

As regards references: Our policy has been to cite the source of every significant statement, unless it represented common knowledge or current textbook material. Where a string of references might have been used, we often chose the most recent as a key to the earlier publications.

Wherever we went wrong, we will appreciate being corrected; wherever we missed the key concept, the best example, the best reference, or the best illustration, we will equally appreciate the reader's help. We are acutely aware that every paragraph could be improved. Despite its inevitable shortcomings, we hope this book will help many readers appreciate the wondrous ways of the body challenged by disease.

Guido Majno
Isabelle Joris

∽

REFERENCES

1. Damjanov I. *General Pathology, 2nd ed.* New York: Medical Examination Publishing Co. Inc., 1983.

2. Florey HW. *General Pathology, 4th ed.* Philadelphia: WB Saunders Company, 1970.

3. Hill RB Jr, La Via MF. *Principles of Pathobiology, 3rd ed.* New York: Oxford University Press, 1980.

4. King DW, Fenoglio CM, Lefkowitch JH. *General Pathology: Principles and Dynamics.* Philadelphia: Lea & Febiger, 1983.

5. Majno G. *A course in pathology for non-medical students.* J Med Educ 1962; 37:421-428.

6. McGee JO'D, Isaacson PG, Wright NA. *Oxford Textbook of Pathology.* Oxford: Oxford University Press, 1992.

7. Payling Wright G. *An Introduction to Pathology, 3rd ed.* Boston: Little, Brown and Company, 1958.

8. Pérez Tamayo R. *Mechanisms of Disease. An Introduction to Pathology, 2nd ed.* Chicago: Year Book Medical Publishers Inc., 1985.

9. Walter JB, Israel MS. *General Pathology, 6th ed.* Edinburgh: Churchill Livingstone, 1987.

10. Woolf N. *Cell, Tissue and Disease. The Basis of Pathology.* London: Baillière Tindall, 1977.

ACKNOWLEDGEMENTS

One day, as we were attempting to calculate how many letters had been written for this book, Mrs. Linda Johnston, our precious secretary, quietly commented: "This book should have thousands of authors." She was absolutely right, and we should begin by acknowledging our secretarial help.

Secretaries. The roots of this book go back at least 20 years, when we enjoyed the assistance of Lise Karageorge and Karen Melia. Then, during 11 years, we were fortunate to have the extraordinary help of Jane M. Manzi, who typed as fast as we could speak, and took us from the age of the typewriter through that of the word processor to that of the computer. It is absurd to thank her in only a few words. Jane Manzi's tenure overlapped with that of Linda Johnston, who also helped us collect and file thousands of photographs, not to mention endless references and scores of bibliographic searches, and never lost her smile even when a key reference disappeared. Without her sense of perfection, her care, and her unfailing memory, this book would never have come to completion. Paula Dadian did a masterly job in gathering and keeping track of hundreds of permissions. Finally, we are indebted to Berul Edney who took over with great enthusiasm and competence in the last, critical and very demanding phase.

Illustrations. Most of our 1074 illustrations were obtained from all over the world, including Moscow when it was still behind the Iron Curtain. Many colleagues took the trouble of preparing new figures or sending us microscopic sections to photograph. Our warmest thanks go to all.

Having overheard the words "medical illustrator" in the crowd of a concert hall, we were fortunate to discover and then acquire the help of Anne B. Greene, whose exceptional skill is matched by her knowledge of biology and her sense of accuracy. On many occasions Anne Greene pointed out inaccuracies in our sketches and miraculously turned our scribbles into beautiful drawings. The inimitable skills of Mr. J.B. Clark are also reflected in many illustrations. Beth H. Maynard of the Biomedical Media Service of this Medical Center designed almost all of our graphs and helped us assemble some of our most demanding illustrations, kindly and gracefully even in times of great pressure. In some of her drawings Beth was assisted by Themia A. Pappas-Fillmore and by George W. Jamieson. Credits for individual illustrations are listed below.

Photographers. Peter W. Healey was our first departmental photographer, and prepared gross and microscopic photographs in large numbers, while also setting the standards of excellence that were picked up by his followers. Christopher D. Hebert, aided by his background in biology, was a master in producing top-notch electron micrographs; he was also instrumental in setting up the messy but extremely effective technique of photographing gross specimens under water. We will never forget his patience while waiting until the last little bubble had disappeared, and the last floater had stopped moving. He was followed by Marie Picard-Craig; we especially appreciated her understanding of electron micrographs and her skill in converting color slides to black and white prints. Some of our earlier photographs were taken by Jean-Claude Rumbeli in Geneva. The patience and dedication of these wonderful artists is reflected throughout this volume. We are equally indebted to Jean M. Underwood and John J. Nunnari, who—in addition to their ordinary duties—laboriously navigated through our files, trimmed illustrations, calculated enlargements, and lettered photographs, while often pointing out to us ways to improve the final result.

Medical Students. Many medical students, mostly from the second year, worked with us during summers to collect references and prepare summaries on specific subjects. Their input contributed a great deal to our overall effort of synthesis. The list includes Jim A. Goldman, Rick J. Evans, Joseph E. Fuller, Reynaldo Cordero, Diane M. Pingeton (who drew also from her background as a nurse), Subhash C. Gumber (whose background in biochemistry allowed him to tackle some of the most intricate topics), Leslie A. O'Meara, a true expert in library research, Judy E. Tapper, who convinced us that matrix vesicles really exist, Stephen J. Barr, who provided some masterful orthopedic summaries, Matthew E. Cohen, who also produced some masterful summaries, and Deborah A. Vatcher who researched the history of oncogenes. A special place must be reserved for Charles R. Taylor, who spent a summer at the thankless task of counting the number of diseases (published here for the first time). To all these generous young people, and to any others whose names may have remained buried in our files, go our warmest thanks.

We should extend these thanks to include all the medical students who asked questions in class and in the lab—and forced us to think WHY.

Libraries. We are profoundly indebted to the staff of the Lamar Soutter Library at the University of Massachusetts Medical Center, especially to Dr. Donald J. Morton, Annanaomi Sams, Karen R. Cangello, Gael A. Evans, Linda M. Hayes, Paul H. Julian, Mary J. Markland, and Eileen M. Ritchie; once again, without them, this book could not have existed. Although we were perennially delinquent in returning books we were treated with great understanding, even when the computer coughed up threatening letters. Mme Muriel Serodino, Director of the Library of the Faculty of Medicine in Geneva, kindly helped us track down the papers of Wilhelm Zahn; and as always, Richard Wolfe of the Rare Books division of Harvard's Countway Library stood by to help us solve historical problems.

Help on Specific Topics. The input of experts has been essential in preventing us from making major blunders. However, let it be clear that we are entirely responsible for whatever blunders have slipped through the filter. One of the sections on Cellular Pathology returned from an expert consultant with an entire page crossed out, and the following notation in huge capital letters: **NO WAY**. We were a little shaken up, but to the horror of Linda Johnston we decided to keep that page anyway. This goes to say that our generous readers can be in "no way" responsible for whatever mistakes slipped through.

The section on Cellular Pathology was carefully read and annotated by Dr. George E. Palade, who took his precious time to make wonderful suggestions typically ranging from ATP to Zeus. The same section was also checked by Maya and Nicolae Simionescu in Bucharest, who remained our friends even after the arrival of a 40-pound package of manuscript and illustrations. The section on immunopathology was reviewed by Dr. Peter C. Kolbeck of the University of Nebraska. The section on vascular disturbances was reviewed by Dr. Henri F. Cuénoud, whose criticisms and contributions—including several illustrations—were absolutely essential. The section on tumors was read and criticized by Dr. Samuel M. Cohen of the University of Nebraska. Specific chapters or segments were further reviewed by specialists: the chapter on free radicals was reviewed by Dr. Steven D. Aust of Utah State University, the topic of molecular pathology was checked by Dr.

James M. Pullman of our institution, the chapter on amyloid by Dr. Alan S. Cohen of Boston University, the chapter on calcification by Dr. Adele L. Boskey of Cornell University. Dr. Marie-Claude Badonnel was very helpful in guiding us through the HLA maze, and Dr. Parker A. Small, Jr. of the University of Florida checked our rendition of his influenza story.

We are also indebted to countless others whom we consulted on specific topics, often with the excuse of having lunch together. Here is a partial list, beginning with our Medical Center: Dr. Thomas W. Smith (an inexhaustible source of advice, slides and illustrations on the biology and pathology of nervous tissue), Dr. David A. Drachman (our wise neurologic consultant), Dr. Ashley Davidoff (a patient and thorough source of help on radiologic problems), Drs. Jag Bhawan, Rajwant Malhotra and Jeffrey D. Bernhard (our key consultants in matters of skin diseases), Dr. Thomas Zand (who stood by year after year and generously provided us with input on pediatric problems as well as on a variety of practical and philosophical problems), Dr. Armando Fraire (lung dilemmas), Dr. Bruce A. Woda and Marcia L. McFadden (lymphocyte dilemmas, cell sorting, lymphomas and immunology), Dr. Aldo A. Rossini (our guide through the complications of diabetes), Dr. Frank R. Reale and Joyce M. Compton (cytology, gynecologic pathology), Dr. Umberto De Girolami (muscle and nervous tissue), Dr. Arthur A. Like (experimental diabetes), Dr. Barbara F. Banner (kidney pathology), Dr. Ray M. Welsh (immunology), Dr. John J. Monahan (orthopedic problems), Dr. Gary V. Doern (bacterial problems), Dr. Irma O. Szymanski (red blood cells), Dr. H. Brownell Wheeler (wound healing), Dr. Harriet L. Robinson (viral infection). From other medical centers we should mention at least Dr. John W. Harshbarger of the Smithsonian Institution, who went to a great deal of trouble to provide us with information and illustrations on tumors in fish, oysters and other "lower animals", Dr. Bernie A. Ackerman (for cutaneous puzzles), Dr. Stephen J. Galli (mast cells), Dr. Abul Abbas (delayed hypersensitivity), Dr. Victor E. Gould (neuroendocrine tumors and much else), Dr. Yusuf Kapanci (oxygen damage to the lungs, metastatic calcification), Drs. Linda M. McManus and R. Neal Pinckard (platelet activating factor), Dr. Michael A. Gimbrone (thrombosis), Dr. Pietro Gullino (experimental tumors), Dr. Henry C. Pitot ("what is a benign tumor?"), Dr. Gerald Nash (lung pathology), Dr. David L. Gang (gastroenterology), Dr. G. Fiore-Donno of Geneva (who should be an oral pathologist *honoris causa*), Dr. Lelio Orci of Geneva and his pioneering team for various topics of cell biology. The friendship of Dr. Ruy Pérez Tamayo was always a stimulus and a source of wisdom. Special thanks are due to colleagues who wrote us personal accounts of their discoveries, such as a wonderful two-page letter from Dr. Björn Afzelius on the discovery of the immotile cilia syndrome, and a similar message from the late David Th. Purtilo on the discovery of XLP disease.

The pathogenesis of Japanese cultured pearls was unveiled to us thanks to Dr. Makoto Katori of Tokyo, who took us to the National Aquaculture Research Institute in Nansei, where Dr. Koji Wada guided us through that amazing biological process.

The title of this book is largely due to a conversation with a microbiologist, Dr. Jon D. Goguen, who told us that he would certainly buy a book on cellular disease—but not a book entitled "Pathology."

Former Collaborators, Friends, and Family. Much of the information presented in this book was derived from research that we accomplished with many collaborators. The first place must be reserved for Dr. Ramzi S. Cotran, who contributed in a major way not only as an investigator but also as a constant advisor; it was very important for us to have his blessing for our choice of an unusual title. Among our former collaborators we should also thank Dr. Gutta I. Schoefl, Dr. Renate Müller, Dr. Kaethe Kretchmer, Dr. Graeme B. Ryan (with whom the first few pages of this book were written), Dr. Giulio Gabbiani, Dr. Mark C. Kowala, Dr. Carl A. Boswell, Dr. John T. Doukas, as well as Monica Clowes and other marvelous research technicians including Geneviève Leyvraz of Geneva, Claudia Froesch, Suzie Edwards, Jean M. Underwood, John J. Nunnari, and Anne H. Cutler. For our choice histologic sections we are indebted to Eva Moring, Laura S. Rooney and Gail L. Bouliane.

Our friends and families also contributed in another way. A book such as this one should be the product of full-time work; because we could only give it part-time attention, we had to expand the work into nights and week-ends, thus stealing time from all those dear to us, who had to wait year after year for the completion of "The Book," and accept the fact that Inflammation could take priority over Christmas. They deserve special thanks for their patience, which amounted to a substantial and needed support.

Publishers. We are especially grateful to the team at Blackwell Science, Inc. for the enthusiasm with which our book was adopted after it had been dropped by another publisher. Rather than trying to explain why publication took the better part of 3 years, we prefer to thank the President, William L. Gibson, for taking the matter in his own hands and assigning to us the precious help of Karen M. Feeney, Ellen D. Samia, Heather Garrison, Irene Herlihy, and Lisa Flanagan. For the wise editing of the text we are indebted to Penny Hull, Yvonne Howell and Charlie Cochran.

Last, in the process of physically handling several tons of books, reprints, photocopies, and manuscript pages—just our first mailing to the publisher weighed 200 pounds—we are acutely aware that we have consumed vast amounts of cellulose. As a token of gratitude, upon the completion of this book, we planted 101 trees.

Guido Majno, M.D.
Isabelle Joris, Ph.D.

Credits for individual illustrations:

Anne B. Greene: 1.1, 2.9, 2.35, 2.58, 2.59, 2.63, 3.1, 3.7, 3.59, 3.60, 4.6, 4.18, 4.24, 4.33, 5.8, 5.11, 5.13, 5.29, 6.11, 8.1, 8.2, 8.15, 9.10, 9.15, 9.20, 9.28, 9.29, 10.5, 11.6, 11.7, 11.16, 11.24, 12.14, 13.16, 13.22, 13.42, 14.1, 14.2, 16.2, 17.1, 17.6, 17.13, 17.17, 17.22, 17.27, 17.39, 17.41, 17.45, 19.14, 21.15, 22.1, 22.23, 22.28, 22.34, 23.1, 23.5, 23.8, 23.31, 23.32, 23.36, 23.37, 23.42, 24.9, 24.29, 24.31, 26.51, 26.56, 26.71, 27.9, 27.16, 27.18, 27.19, 27.20, 27.28, 27.31, 27.33, 27.35, 27.41, 28.17, 28.44, 28.46, 31.6, 31.11, 33.3

Joshua B. Clark: I.6, 2.11, 2.34, 3.17, 4.50, 7.9, 7.45, 22.13, 24.5

Dr. H.F. Cuénoud: I.4, 2.28, 21.15, 21.16, 23.20, 30.2

Beth H. Maynard prepared the 204 remaining original charts and drawings.

INTRODUCTION

What is Disease?

Life, Death, and
Suspended Life

The Scope of General
Pathology

The Jargon of Pathology

What is Disease?

As seen through the microscope or in a test tube, disease is fairly easy to define. For every tissue there are standards of form and function, with some allowance for acceptable variance; any deviation from those limits implies disease. Normal bronchi, for example, are lined by ciliated, mucus-secreting epithelium. If this is replaced by squamous stratified epithelium—as is often the case in smokers—the bronchus becomes pathologic; not only structurally, but also functionally, because ciliary motion and mucus secretion are lost.

Disease at the level of the individual is much more difficult to define because the boundaries are vague and shifting. But here is an old definition that we can use as a starting point:

Disease is any condition of the body or mind that decreases the chances of survival of the individual or of the species.

This definition has some merit, but it can be challenged in many ways. It suggests that the discovery of the atomic bomb should be a disease (perhaps it is, in the big picture). Furthermore, the threatening condition must be qualified as intrinsic to the body or mind; otherwise flying in an airplane would be a disease. More important, if we base our definition of disease on the threat to survival, it will include two threatening conditions that seem perfectly normal: old age and childbirth. In fact, these two conditions do lie in a gray area. Old age does predispose to disease and death; and childbirth, even though it is the very mechanism for preserving the species, does imply a certain threat to the mother. There are lying-in *hospitals* where mothers are routinely referred to as *patients*.

Another flaw in this definition is that *some diseases can be assets and actually increase the chances of survival.* The best-known example is sickle cell anemia, which confers some protection against malaria (11). Then there is the peculiar case of the basset hound, which owes its existence to a congenital disease, **achondroplasia.** Dog fanciers decided thousands of years ago to perpetuate this defect, which must have sprung up in a family of hounds. In this condition, the growth of long bones is stopped prematurely, whereas flat bones such as those of the head are unaffected; this is why bassets are small but bright (Figure I.1). So were

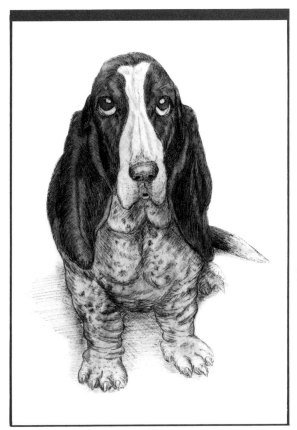

FIGURE I.1
A disease that favored propagation: the short legs of the basset hound are the result of an inborn defect, achondroplasia. (Etching by Martha Hinson.)

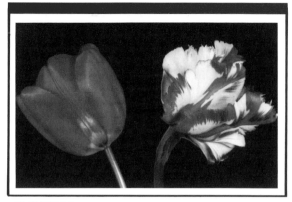

FIGURE I.2
See color plate 1. Another disease that favored propagation: the tulip at the right is infected with a virus of the mosaic type. These Rembrandt or broken tulips are less hardy but much coveted; in Holland in the early 1600s they caused an outbreak of social tulipomania. Tiger lilies are a similar example of "beautiful disease."

the medieval court jesters, history's most famous achondroplastics. Horticulturists have provided another example of selected disease: the attractive splotchy color of the so-called Rembrandt tulips is due to a viral infection (10) (Figure I.2).

Not all conditions that suppress reproduction (survival of the species) are diseases: consider celibacy. The case of homosexuality is more complex. For the ancient Greeks it was a godly way of life (Zeus himself fell in love with a human male, Ganymede, snatched him up and gave him a place among the gods). In the Christian world it became a crime, and later a disease, which it still is in many countries. Then, in 1973, the American Psychiatric Association eliminated homosexuality from its roster of diseases (25) for reasons far more political than scientific (we are reminded of the distinction between weeds and plants: a weed is a plant that you don't want at a particular time and place). And now there is some evidence that homosexuality may be a matter of genes (2, 13, 20). If we consider homosexuality just from the standpoint of a "threat to the survival of the species," we should recall that in the most successful insect societies—ants and bees—some individuals are programmed to be sterile, and the species still thrive. It has also been argued that, in human evolution, putative "homosexuality genes" could have been preserved because certain societal roles of homosexuals may have outweighed their weak or negative role in reproduction (28).

Last, it can be argued that *disease in general helps the survival of species by eliminating the unfit*. In this

view, disease is not just a curse; it is also a major driving force of evolution (29).

We must conclude that tying the definition of clinical disease to the notion of survival can be misleading. Perhaps we should side with the pessimists who argue that no final definition is possible and that *the clinical notion of disease is colored by the cultural, social, and political climate* (15, 16, 19). There is a great deal of truth in this statement. In our culture the loss of a tooth calls for medical attention; in other cultures teeth are knocked out for beauty. For a Navajo, the fact of having a car accident is the result of a hidden disease (18). In the Soviet Union, opposition to the government was treated as a disease. If we look back into our own not-too-distant history, there are many examples of "diseases" related to the prevailing social climate. In the Napoleonic armies, *nostalgia* was listed as a dangerous contagious disease, and was treated by burying alive the first case to appear (23); during the American Civil War nostalgia was an accepted complication of wounds. In 1851 the New Orleans Medical and Surgical Journal published a *Report on the Diseases of the Negro Race* (5); one of these diseases was the tendency to run away. It was actually given a scientific name, *drapetomania* (from the Greek *drapetéuein*, "to run away"). Up to the late 1800s, masturbation was considered a dangerous disease; the appropriate therapy was thought to be "preventive" circumcision. Later, the purpose was forgotten but the operation persisted, which is how the United States has become the only country in the world in which nonreligious circumcision is still routinely practiced (27). So here is a supposed mental disease that has left millions of physical scars.

There is much to be learned from diseases that have disappeared. Some, such as smallpox, vanished because they were truly eradicated; others vanished because they were a product of erroneous medical theories and faded away as knowledge advanced.

Just before World War II, one of us (GM) received elaborate therapy for a disease that was very common at that time, "dropped stomach," also known as gastroptosis or Glénard's disease. The diagnosis was based on the radiologic misconception that the normal stomach was supposed to be in the same horizontal position as seen at autopsy. Now: if a patient standing behind a fluoroscopic screen is asked to swallow a cup of barium sulfate (barium means "heavy"), his or her stomach will tend to sag. This means that most people in a radiologist's clinic would be diagnosed as suffering from dropped stomach. As radiologic knowledge advanced, gastroptosis quietly disappeared, but it is a fair guess that we are still living with "diseases" of this kind.

All in all, we are obliged to conclude that the microcosm of individual diseases is related to the macrocosm of society: it depends on time, place, and culture. The same correlation is recognized in the definition of health adopted in 1946 by the World Health Organization (30):

"Health is the state of complete physical, mental, and social well-being, and not only the absence of disease or ailment."

If this is health, the World Health Organization is telling us that poverty, poor housing, and poor education are part of disease.

Let all this be food for thought. This book will deal, more modestly, with mechanisms of physical disease within the microcosm of cells and tissues.

Life, Death, and Suspended Life

Anyone interested in disease would also want to know the meaning of life and death (4). We have no final answer, but we can offer a few facts and a few thoughts drawn from biology.

Thirty years ago it was safe to define death as prolonged cessation of respiration and circulation. But then, heart pumps and respirators made these criteria obsolete and complicated the issue by making it possible to postpone the time of "death" almost indefinitely. So the focus shifted to the brain, and it is now generally agreed that when the electroencephalogram is irreversibly flat, brain death has occurred (Figure I.3). However, does brain death correspond to death of the individual? In the Japanese view the answer is no (4). In the USA, most states leave that decision to the parents or guardians, but some do not. As of 1990 the Supreme Court rule 5 to 4 that Nancy Cruzan, brain-dead for seven years, should be kept alive artificially if the State of Missouri so required (1); in that same year, it was estimated that 10,000 Americans were being maintained in irreversible coma because they had not left any clear instructions such as a "living will" (12).

At a purely biological level, one fact is clear: cells can continue to live in the absence of both heart and brain, indeed in the absence of the entire body. This is the very principle of cell

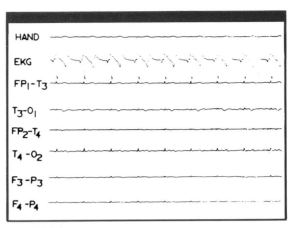

FIGURE I.3
Brain death ("electrocerebral silence") in a head-injured man. The first channel, taken from the back of the hand, is a control to show the baseline noise. The second is the electrocardiogram; the others refer to the brain and show no activity except artifacts correlated with the electrocardiogram. (From Walker, A.E.: *Cerebral Death*, 3rd ed. Baltimore, Urban & Schwarzenberg, 1985). (Reproduced by permission from [26]).

culture *in vitro*. Should we then accept the cell as the ultimate level of organized life? Probably so, because a key attribute of life as we know it is self-replication, and the cell is the smallest unit that can replicate independently. It is true that biochemists break up cells and study "surviving" mitochondria (until they, too, eventually die); however, mitochondria that are breathing oxygen in a test tube are alive only in a limited way, because they are unable to self-replicate (mitochondria do replicate *in vivo*, perhaps because they derive from archaic bacterial cells, but they are not known to replicate *in vitro*). So, for the time being, we can assume that there is no life below the level of cells.

While society struggles to fit all this into a new and acceptable definition of somatic death, we must tentatively conclude that *life can exist at several levels*, from the whole body to isolated organs to cells, and perhaps—in part—to subcellular particles. The next question, then, should be: what is the intrinsic difference between a live being and an inanimate object?

One answer could be metabolic processes. This is a defensible proposition, except that *metabolism can be stopped without compromising life*. Scientists who use tissue cultures freeze their cells routinely and store them for as long as 20 years until they are ready to thaw them out and use them. This suggests that life, whatever it may be, can be

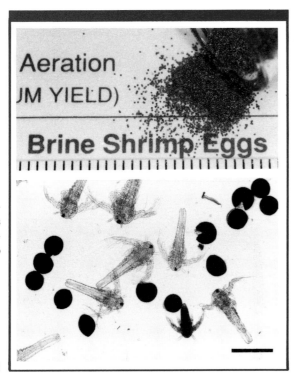

FIGURE I.4
Example of suspended life. *Top:* Commercial dried brine shrimp eggs. Scale in mm. *Bottom:* After 3 days in a suitable medium, the shrimp have hatched. **Bar** = 500 μm. (Courtesy of Dr. H.F. Cuénoud, University of Massachusetts Medical Center, Worcester, MA.)

suspended. So what are the mechanisms of suspended life?

One of the best models of suspended life is the dried food you buy in a pet store to feed aquarium fish: eggs of brine shrimp (Figure I.4). These microscopic eggs can be stored in the dry state for months or years. Placed in water they swell, and 16 hours later they hatch: instant shrimp. A variety of small animals are capable of suspended life in the dry state, including rotifers, nematodes and insects. "Instant insects" wait for the next flood in parched African soils (14). Some are endowed with a nervous system, a digestive tract, and muscle—all it takes to make a respectable multicellular creature, although usually smaller than one millimeter (6–9).

The first to marvel at "animalcules" that could survive drying was Leeuwenhoek in 1702, but his letter to the Royal Society of London was soon forgotten (7). In 1743 an English Jesuit working in France, John Turberville Needham, rediscovered them in the microscopic eelworms of blighted wheat. He sent a little package of eelworms to the Royal Society, and his discovery was confirmed by Henry Baker, who wrote:

> We find an instance here that life may be suspended and seemingly destroyed; that by an Exhalation of the Fluids necessary to a living Animal, the Circulations

may cease, all the Organs and Vessels of the Body may be shrunk up, dried and hardened, and yet, after a long while, Life may begin anew to actuate the same Body and all the animal Motions and Faculties may be restored, merely by replenishing the Organs and Vessels with a fresh supply of Fluid. . . . What life really is, seems as much too subtle for our Understanding to conceive or define, as for our senses to discern and examine. (7)

Needham's discovery was sensational. Was it resurrection? Voltaire attacked it viciously in prose and verse, as "providing weapons for atheistic philosophy" (22). In Italy, Lazzaro Spallanzani (1729–1799), an abbot and one of the greatest biologists of all time, joined Needham's camp. "The phenomenon," he wrote, "confounds the most accepted ideas of animality." While the "admirable resurrections" of nematodes became a form of entertainment in French society, the debate went on and flared up acrimoniously in the 1850s between two sharply divided camps, the resurrectionists and antiresurrectionists. The prestigious French Society of Biology was asked to arbitrate; it did so by nominating a Commission of Seven, presided over by no less than Paul Broca, the physician and anthropologist who discovered the speech center of the brain. The learned men spoke to both parties, met 42 times, dried rotifers as best they could (82 days in a vacuum, plus 30 minutes at 100°C at atmospheric pressure), and yet the creatures "revived in contact with water." Such was the essence of the 60,000-word report published in 1860. However, the group wisely refrained from discussing the metaphysical point: resurrection (5).

Today the argument is avoided by using the new and conveniently ambiguous word *cryptobiosis* (hidden life). There are four subtypes, depending on the mechanism that suspends life: anhydrobiosis (dehydration), cryobiosis (cooling), anoxybiosis (lack of oxygen), and osmobiosis (high salt concentration) (7). As a prototype of cryptobiotic animals we propose the so-called water bears, or tardigrades (slow walkers) (Figure I.5), a name chosen by Spallanzani. These creatures can survive a vacuum of a millionth of a millimeter, heating to 151°C, cooling to near absolute zero (conditions not unlike those of outer space). The record is 120 years of suspended life in the moss of a museum collection; however, in the tardigrades recovered from this specimen, the revival lasted only a few minutes (21).

Cryptobiotic animals exist in all habitats, from the poles to the deserts to anybody's back yard.

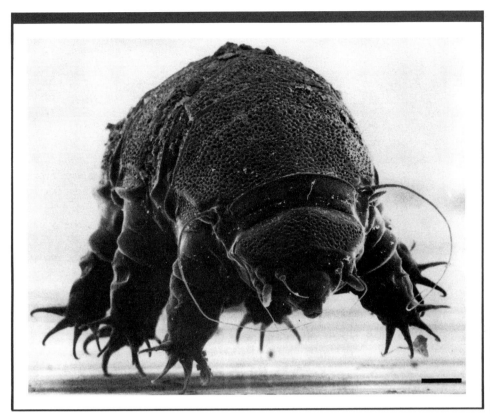

FIGURE I.5
One of the creatures that share the secret of death and resuscitation: a tardigrade, as seen by scanning electron microscopy. The name means "slow walker." **Bar** = 100 μm. (Reproduced by permission from [8]).

Leeuwenhoek took them from the lead gutter of his roof. Clearly they have developed their physiology as an adaptive strategy to favor dissemination, to survive hostile environments, and to time their existence with "good days." Their normal life span of a couple of months can be prolonged to something on the order of a century.

The secret of resuscitation from dryness, it is now clear, lies in drying slowly. As the creature on its way to cryptobiosis begins to lose water, it produces two chemicals that it does not contain in its normal state: trehalose (made of two molecules of glucose) and glycerol (another small molecule). As the cellular organelles dry up and collapse, these molecules insert themselves between the layers of folding structures, keeping them separate and ready to reexpand (9). It is surely no coincidence that glycerol also protects cells against another type of dehydration: freezing. We use it today to preserve frozen red blood cells.

For our purposes, *the most important aspect of cryptobiosis is that metabolism comes to a complete standstill (7).* It was once found that a small amount of oxygen is taken up by cryptobiotic animals kept in air (7), but it then turned out that this uptake indicates damage, not respiration. It is the equivalent of turning rancid by oxidation (8) (free radical injury, p. 184), which has nothing to do with metabolism. Potato chips can do it too (21).

What does this tell us about life? The resuscitation of cryptobiotic animals suggests that *the critical requirement for life as we know it is a molecular arrangement; a structure that—in the presence of water—behaves like a machine.* Its function is called metabolism. If water is removed or frozen the machine can stop for a limited time; otherwise it grinds forth toward its basic goal, replication.

In essence, then, the message whispered by the tardigrades seems to be—*life is a molecular machine.*

The Scope of General Pathology

The number of possible diseases is enormous. Internal mechanisms can go wrong in countless ways. There are thousands of bacteria, viruses, protozoans, worms, insects, and other creatures that are pathogenic (capable of causing disease); toxic agents defy counting.

If each of these agents caused a special type of disease, different from all others, learning pathology or medicine would be a hopeless task.

Fortunately, this is not the case. Bacteria, for example, are of many types, but their ways of producing disease fall into a few categories: they all tend to elicit reactions known as **inflammation** and **immune response,** and they all produce fever by a similar mechanism. *The purpose of general pathology is to work out these common pathways.*

Although the number of diseases, at the latest count, is 8294 (24) (Table I.1), the basic processes that are always at work can be grouped under five main headings, which we cover in the five parts of this books.

The Jargon of Pathology: A Few Key Terms

The reader will be well advised to absorb in advance the following few basic terms. They may sound empirical and imprecise, and so they are: many are at least 2500 years old. But they are practical.

THE TOPOGRAPHY OF DISEASE

The following terms are illustrated in Figure I.6.

- **Focal** is said of a disease limited to a discrete, well-limited *focus* (e.g., a boil); the plural is *foci*. It is similar to **localized,** which means limited to a given part (e.g., a hand, a lobe of the lung).
- **Diffuse** means that the disease affects a large area (e.g., pneumonia can diffusely affect a whole lung) rather than forming discrete foci.
- **Disseminated** means scattered in many small foci.

Table I.1

Diseases Listed in the International Classification of Diseases (US PHS 1980)

CATEGORY[a]	NUMBER OF DISEASES
1 Blood	71
2 Skin	143
3 Perinatal conditions	162
4 Respiratory	174
5 Ill-defined	195
6 Endocrine, nutritional, metabolic; immunity	228
7 Mental	293
8 Circulatory	300
9 Genitourinary	311
10 Digestive	332
11 Congenital	357
12 Neoplasms	579
13 Infectious and parasitic	691
14 Muscle, skeleton, connective tissue	858
15 Pregnancy, childbirth, and puerperium	917
16 Nervous system	1167
17 Injury and poisons	1516
TOTAL	8294

[a]Categories are listed in order of increasing size.

Data collected by Dr. C. Taylor when he was a medical student.

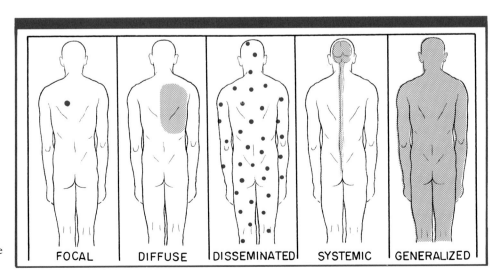

FIGURE I.6
Five terms referring to the topographic distribution of disease in the body.

FOCAL   DIFFUSE   DISSEMINATED   SYSTEMIC   GENERALIZED

- **Systemic** should be used to mean spread throughout a single system (like the nervous system). It is sometimes used loosely and improperly as a synonym of *generalized.*
- **Generalized** means spread through the entire body (e.g., an infection spread by the blood stream).

THE TIME COURSE OF DISEASE

- **Acute** means "coming sharply to a climax"; changes (good or bad) are occurring rapidly. It does not mean severe, although many acute diseases are severe. In terms of real time, acute can mean anything from minutes to a few days (e.g., acute appendicitis).
- **Chronic** means long-lasting. It usually refers to weeks, months, or years.
- **Subacute** means "not very acute," and **Subchronic** means "not very chronic" (imprecision compounded by imprecision, but again very handy to describe clinical situations).

* * *

- **Pathogenesis** refers to the steps whereby an agent brings about disease. It concerns the mechanisms rather than the causes. For example, pollen is the single cause of hay fever, but the pathogenesis of hay fever requires many steps: pollen proteins are picked up by macrophages, which pass them on to appropriate lymphocytes, which produce antibodies, which sensitize mast cells, which respond to the pollen antigens by releasing inflammatory agents.
- **Differential diagnosis** is the exercise of listing in orderly fashion all possible diagnoses of a given condition, usually from the most likely to the least likely (e.g., a lump on the head could be a mass of spilled blood, a tumor of the skin, a tumor of the skull, a metastatic tumor of an internal organ, an abscess, or a congenital defect).

Armed with these basic means of communication, we can now begin our trek through the world of disease.

References

1. Annas GJ. Nancy Cruzan and the right to die. N Engl J Med 1990;323:670–673.
2. Barinaga M. Is homosexuality biological? Science 1991;253:956–957.
3. Bayer R. Homosexuality and American Psychiatry. The Politics of Diagnosis. Princeton: Princeton University Press, 1987.
4. Botkin JR, and Post SG. Confusion in the determination of death: distinguishing philosophy from physiology. Perspect Biol Med 1992;36:129–138.
5. Cartwright SA. Report on the diseases and physical peculiarities of the Negro race. In: Caplan AL, Engelhardt HT Jr, McCartney JJ. (eds.), Concepts of Health and Disease. Interdisciplinary Perspectives. Reading, MA: Addison-Wesley Publishing Company, 1981, pp. 305–325.
6. Clegg JS. Interrelationships between water and cellular metabolism in Artemia cysts. XI. Density measurements. Cell Biophys 1984;6:153–169.
7. Crowe, JH, Clegg, JS. (eds). Anhydrobiosis. Stroudsberg: Dowden, Hutchinson & Ross, Inc., 1973.
8. Crowe JH, Cooper AF Jr. Cryptobiosis. Sci Am 1971;225:30–36.
9. Crowe JH, Crowe LM. Induction of anhydrobiosis: membrane changes during drying. Cryobiology 1982;19:317–328.
10. Dubos RJ. Tulipomania and the benevolent virus. Perspect Virol 1959;1:291–299.
11. Eaton JW, Wood, PA. Antimalarial red cells. Prog Clin Biol Res 1984;165:395–412.
12. Friedrich O. A limited right to die. Time, July 9, 1990, p. 59.
13. Hamer DH, Hu S, Magnuson VL, Hu N, Pattatucci AM. A linkage between DNA markers on the X chromosome and male sexual orientation. Science 1993;261:321–327.
14. Hinton HE. A new Chironomid from Africa. Proc Zool Soc 1951;121:371–380.
15. King LS. What is disease? Phil Sci 1954;21:193–203.
16. King LS. Medical Thinking. A Historical Preface. Princeton: Princeton University Press, 1982.
17. LeVay S. A difference in hypothalamic structure between heterosexual and homosexual men. Science 1991;253:1035–1037.
18. Majno G. The lost secret of ancient medicine. In: Bulger RJ. (ed.), In search of the modern Hippocrates. Iowa City: University of Iowa Press, 1987, pp. 146–155.
19. Pérez Tamayo R. El concepto de enfermedad. 2 volumes. Mexico: Fondo de Cultura Económica, 1988.
20. Pool R. Evidence for homosexuality gene. Science 1993;261:291–292.
21. Rensberger B. Life in limbo. Science 1980;1:36–43.
22. Roe S. Voltaire versus Needham: atheism, materialism, and the generation of life. J Hist Ideas 1985;46:65–87.
23. Starobinski J. The idea of nostalgia. Diogenes 1966;54:92–115.
24. Taylor C, Majno G. Unpublished data.
25. U.S. Dept. of Health and Human Services. The international classification of diseases, 9th revision. Clinical modification, volume I, diseases tabular list, 2nd edition, September 1980. DHHS Publication No (PHS) 80-1260, Washington, D.C.
26. Walker AE. Cerebral Death, 3rd ed. Baltimore: Urban & Schwarzenberg, 1985.
27. Wallerstein E. Circumcision: An American Health Fallacy. New York: Springer Publishing Company, 1980.
28. Wilson EO. Sociobiology. The New Synthesis. Cambridge: Harvard University Press, 1975.
29. Wolbach SB. The glorious past, the doleful present and the uncertain future of pathology. Harvard Medical Alumni Bulletin June, 1954, pp. 45–48.
30. World Health Organization. Constitution of the World Health Organization. New York: WHO Interim Commission, 1946.

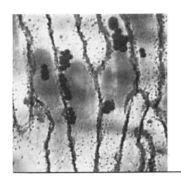

CELLULAR PATHOLOGY

The Long Road to the Elementary Patient

E very branch of science has its elementary unit; for physics it is the atom, for chemistry the molecule. *Medicine is both art and science; as an art, its elementary unit has always been the patient; as a science, its unit is the cell.* Indeed, modern medicine is largely a gift of the microscope.

Because they lacked this basic unit, our ancestors were obliged for thousands of years to struggle for some other way to explain disease. Primal people blame several mechanisms; the most common are magic curses, intrusion of some extraneous object into the body, punishment, or even loss of the soul (Figure 1.1): the specific function of the shaman (a word of Siberian origin) is precisely to go and retrieve the soul.

The ancient Greeks broke away from this pattern. Although they were a very religious people, they felt that the gods were not necessarily involved in disease. They blamed natural causes, such as a "breath" or "wind" (a similar thought also prevailed in China). Another Greek theory, adopted by Hippocrates, was that the body was composed of four humors that were normally blended in a delicate fashion; any imbalance of the humors caused disease. The four humors were blood, phlegm, yellow bile, and black bile; exactly how they were chosen is not clear. Note that this theory focuses entirely on internal causes and leaves no space for infection. In fact, the ancient Greeks ignored infection entirely; they did not even have a word for it (*infection* comes from Latin).

The theory of the four humors was especially convenient because it implies that there is only one disease—an imbalance of humors—and correspondingly only one therapy: removing fluids in any possible way—by bleeding, purging, emptying the stomach by vomiting, and even sweating—in the hope of giving the humors a fresh start. The theory was so successful that it lasted into our own days: in his childhood, the senior author of this book was purged for every minor ailment (bleeding was already frowned upon); the younger author was treated for bronchitis with suction cups that were supposed to draw out bad humors. Even now we refer to the four humors when we speak of someone being phlegmatic, sanguine, choleric, or melancholic (from *mélas*, "black," and *cholé*, "bile").

The peoples of antiquity did discover a number of deadly poisons and used them as drugs, but they knew little anatomy and physiology. Progress in medicine was limited because it is very nearly impossible to repair an ailing machine without knowing how it is made and how it works. The first systematic approach to dissection in the Western world occurred at that magnificent, state-supported institution called the Museum ("Place of the Muses") in Alexandria of Egypt, around 300 B.C.; the names *prostate* and *duodenum* come from that time. Those Greeks working at Alexandria had no microscope, but they had the "eye of the mind": they used it so well that two of our key

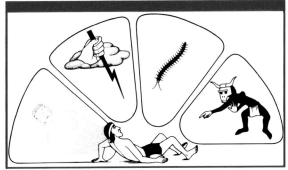

FIGURE 1.1
Four primal concepts of disease: loss of the soul, divine punishment, intrusion of a foreign body or creature, and a spell cast by a witch.

microscopic concepts, **tissue** and **parenchyma,** were created then and there (4).

After these and many other great achievements, such as measuring the diameter of the earth, the flame of the Museum flickered out. Experimentation was revived in the second century A.D. by another Greek, Galen, who was born in Pergamon (Asia Minor) but worked in Rome and also studied at Alexandria. Galen dissected animals, both dead and alive; it was by dissecting a live pig that he discovered the function of Galen's nerve, the recurrent laryngeal nerve (when he cut it, the squeal of the unfortunate pig became inaudible). Galen also observed the effects of partial and total section of the spinal cord and went as far as refuting one of the pet notions of antiquity: that arteries contain air. Again using a live animal, Galen proved beyond a doubt that arteries contained blood.

Later, the western Roman Empire collapsed and the turbulent conditions of Europe were no climate for scholarly efforts. Social conditions favorable to dissection finally appeared in Italy in the late thirteenth century; the first small textbook of anatomy was written around 1316 by

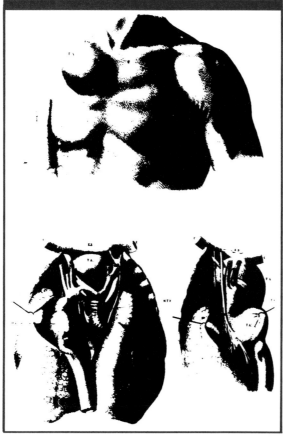

FIGURE 1.2
From the golden age of gross pathology, a syphilitic aneurysm of the aortic arch, illustrated in the famous atlas of Cruveilhier (1829–1842) (2). The patient was a 42-year-old man said to have indulged in "all manner of excesses." The bulge under the skin demonstrates that constant pressure against bony structures (in this case the first ribs and the clavicle) causes them to be reabsorbed.

Mondino de' Luzzi in Bologna (it had 39 editions). In those days it was a heroic enterprise to dissect a human corpse. Consider the realities of performing an autopsy on a partially decomposed body without rubber gloves, antiseptics, fixatives, running water, or notions of infection. Many an early dissector must have died of tuberculosis contracted at an autopsy. Furthermore, religion took a dim view of any such intrusion into the dead body. One of the Church's concerns was the removal of bodily parts, in view of future resurrection. Mondino himself felt that he would have better understood the inner ear if he could have boiled the temporal bone, but he refrained from doing so because it was a sin (*peccatum*).

As the first universities were born in the late Middle Ages, dissection became a major part of the medical curriculum, and chairs of anatomy were established. This means that the anatomists were also the first pathologists: inevitably, during their dissections, anatomists encountered diseased organs and provided us with the first descriptions of internal disease.

As the practice of "anatomies" continued—today we prefer to say autopsies—better and better descriptions of diseased organs were given. The most systematic came from the pen of Giovanni Battista Morgagni, Professor of Anatomy in Padua (1682–1771). His book, *On the Seats and Causes of Disease Investigated by Anatomy*, was published after his death. For each case, Morgagni considered first the clinical history and then attempted to explain it by the autopsy, pioneering work in what we now call clinicopathologic correlations. He used no illustrations, but as soon as color printing was invented, medical illustrations became a form of art. A spectacular collection of such illustrations is the huge atlas published in Paris by G. B. Cruveilhier (1829–1842). Torn out of their context, many of its plates now decorate the walls of pathologists' offices (Figure 1.2).

These masterpieces show both the achievements and the limitations of dissection. Some basic correlations could be established beyond a doubt. Perforations or obstructions of the intestine could easily explain disease and death; compression of the main bile duct by a tumor could easily be correlated with jaundice. But the ultimate mechanism of disease could not be worked out: it was fine to describe an internal abscess, but nobody knew what an abscess really was.

Without such basic data, therapy could make

no progress. By 1850, European medicine was grinding to a halt. Even surgery, potentially improved by a much better knowledge of anatomy, was paralyzed by infection. Internal medicine could offer some diagnoses, thanks to knowledge gained from autopsies, but practically no cures. It was clear to many that a new approach was needed. But what approach?

The answer was at hand. Today it seems obvious, but in the darkness nothing is obvious. The first clue came from botany: a whole new Promised Land could be reached through the microscope. The basic structure of plants (compared with that of the brain or the liver) is starkly simple: each cell is individually packaged in a box that retains its walls even after the cell is dead. In fact, the term **cell** was originally applied to the "empty boxes" of cork (Figure 1.3). In 1838, Matthias Jacob Schleiden (lawyer, botanist, and physician), published a momentous paper stating that plants are made of microscopic units, or cells. Then, one evening after dinner, Schleiden had a chat with a younger colleague named Theodor Schwann (1810–1882). Schwann, a creative anatomist and physiologist, had recently discovered nucleated cells in animal tissues. As an anatomist he had just described what we now call the Schwann sheath of nerves; as a physiologist he had discovered pepsin and recognized that yeast is a living creature (i.e., a cell). Instantly, thanks to that after-dinner conversation, Schwann saw the light: *all plant and animal tissues are made of individual microscopic units.* The result was his famous book, published in 1839, entitled *Microscopic Researches on the Similarity in Structure and Function of Animals and Plants.* He was made professor of anatomy and physiology in Louvain (Belgium) and did little else thereafter, but he had hit on one of the most important generalizations in the history of biology. At long last biology had its elementary unit, the cell.

Plant and animal tissues could now be seen in a new light, and it became immediately obvious that the entire field of disease had to be restudied in the context of the cell. All revolutions have a hero, and the hero of cellular pathology is Rudolf Virchow, Professor of Pathology and Therapy in Berlin (1821–1902). He was a man of gigantic intellect, a statesman and an anthropologist as well as a physician and scientist (1). Despite his overwhelming professional and political commitments, he found time to help Schliemann discover the treasures of ancient Troy and to edit three journals of anthropology as well as the prestigious

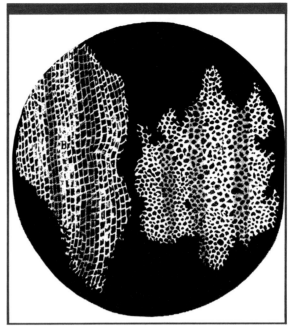

FIGURE 1.3
First illustration of cells by Robert Hooke in 1665. The drawing represents a longitudinal and transversal section of cork. Writes Hooke (3, p. 116): "In several . . . Vegetables, . . . I have with my *Microscope,* plainly enough discover'd these Cells . . . [But regarding tissues of] Animals I have not hitherto been able to say anything positive. . . . Though, me thinks, it seems very probable, that Nature has in these passages, as well as in those of Animal bodies, very many appropriated Instruments and contrivances, whereby to bring her designs and end to pass, which 'tis not improbable, but that some diligent Observer, if help'd with better *Microscopes,* may in time detect."

Archiv für pathologische Anatomie und Physiologie (1847), now known as *Virchow's Archiv.* Few medical journals can match its record of continuous publication. Virchow also realized that social conditions can create disease, fought for the rights of the underprivileged, even took to the barricades in 1848, lost his academic position, and had to leave Berlin. Eight years later, however, he was recalled with full honors, including the directorship of a "Pathological Institute" built for him. Eventually he became a member of the Prussian parliament, and as such he continued to press for social reform.

In 1858, just 19 years after the birth of the cell theory, Virchow gave a set of 20 lectures that changed the face of medicine. Collected in a small book entitled (in translation) *Cellular Pathology as Based upon Physiological and Pathological Histology* (5), these lectures conveyed a new point of view:

disease cannot be understood unless it is realized that the ultimate abnormality must lie in the cell. The body, therefore, had to be understood as a cell-state in which every cell is a citizen; "a society of living cells, a tiny well-ordered state, with all the accessories—high officials and underlings, servants and masters. . . . The human individual is also a commonwealth" (6, pp. 130, 138). It was a revelation. So forceful was its impact that by the end of the century Virchow's word was gospel.

Virchow used the microscope but also drew the best he could from the chemistry and physiology of his time. As a matter of fact, we owe him a marvelous, functional definition of pathology: *pathology is physiology with obstacles* (6, p. 81).

Many of the terms we use today—thrombosis, leukemia, atrophy, hypertrophy, amyloid, myelin, teratoma—were created by Virchow. His feats are all the more astounding if we consider that in 1858 methods for embedding and for cutting thin sections of tissues were not available. His drawings show the effort of reproducing thick, three-dimensional structures as he saw them in slivers of fresh tissue cut by hand (Figure 1.4).

In essence, modern pathology is based squarely on Virchow's cellular pathology: this is why Part One of this book deals with the cell as the elementary patient. Modern cell biology makes this concept even more fitting because it portrays the cell as an individual little creature with a skeleton, a musculature, digestive organs, respiratory organs, a synthetic apparatus that functions like a microscopic liver, and of course a skin. Clinicians now think in terms of cellular receptors and organelles, and they treat with drugs that select specific cellular targets. Even shock, the

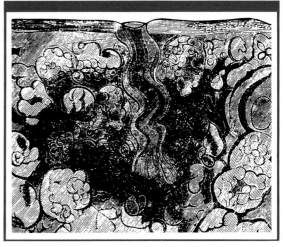

FIGURE 1.4

Illustration from Virchow's *Cellular Pathology* (1858) (5). It shows that microscope sections at that time were really slabs of tissue sliced with a razor and examined unstained; the thickness of the slice is clearly indicated by the perspective at the top. Shown here is a lymph node from the axilla of a tattooed sailor; the black mass in the center represents red pigment (cinnabar). The winding vessel is the lymphatic—actually seen more clearly here than in modern thin sections.

ultimate "total" disease, is now recognized as a generalized cellular disease.

The last two decades have produced an even finer, molecular pathology, capable of revealing faults in the molecule of DNA. And yet, although we now can study disease at no less than eight levels of complexity, from populations to single genes (Figure P-1), at each level, disease ultimately makes sense only in the context of the elementary patient—the cell.

References

1. Ackerknecht EH. Rudolf Virchow. doctor, statesman, anthropologist. Madison: University of Wisconsin Press, 1953.
2. Cruveilhier J. Anatomie pathologique du corps humain, 2 vols. Paris: J.B. Baillière, 1829–1842.
3. Hooke R. Micrographia. London: John Martyn and Alleftry, 1665.
4. Majno G. The healing hand. man and wound in the ancient world. Cambridge: Harvard University Press, 1975.
5. Virchow R. Cellular pathology as based upon physiological and pathological histology. (Translated from 2nd German ed. by B. Chance, 1859, reproduced by Dover Publications, New York, 1971.)
6. Virchow R. Disease, life and man. (Translated by L.J. Rather.) Stanford: Stanford University Press, 1958.

Cellular Adaptations

CHAPTER 2

Regeneration

Hypertrophy,
Hyperplasia

Atrophy

Phenotypic Changes
(Modulation,
Metaplasia)

Cell Activation and
Priming

Disease affects individual cells as it affects individual human beings: it causes changes in structure, function, and social behavior. The problem of diagnosing cellular disease is not as difficult as it may seem because, fortunately for pathologists, most cellular malfunctions are accompanied by structural changes, which are easier to identify. Furthermore, *structural changes guide us to the underlying functional problems.* For example, unusual droplets of triglyceride point to a metabolic problem affecting lipids; hemoglobin escaping from red blood cells points to a defect in the red cell membrane.

Quite a few cellular changes are visible to the naked eye. Hypertrophic muscles in body builders can be seen without a microscope; droplets of fat in liver cells change that organ's color from deep red to yellow, and grains of hemosiderin (a form of stored iron) change it to a rusty brown. For this reason, *the naked eye is an important guide in choosing areas to be studied microscopically.* After the microscope has provided its answers, the path is clear to countless histochemical, biochemical, and functional tests.

A powerful tool for cellular diagnosis is a computer-assisted machine called **fluorescence-activated cell sorter** (FACS) (Figure 2.1), which can provide almost instantly quantitative answers regarding size, shape, and specific qualities of as few as 10,000 cells. The FACS is fast becoming an essential tool, especially for diagnosing tumors.

For cells, as for human beings, there are degrees or "shades" of normality. An athlete may weigh three or four times as much as an ascetic monk, yet both are normal; they just differ in their adaptations to the calls of life, and both face certain hazards due to their adaptations. Similarly, cells can respond to challenges that are not severe enough to cause injury by adaptations that are not truly pathologic, although they may open the door to disease. Cells adapt in many ways. They may

- multiply to replace losses (regeneration)
- increase in number above normal (hyperplasia)
- increase in size (hypertrophy, polyploidy)
- become smaller (atrophy)
- modify their phenotype reversibly (modulation)
- be replaced by different types of cells (metaplasia)
- adapt their organelles (subcellular adaptations)

On this tremendous span of cellular adaptability hinges our capacity to meet the challenges of this dangerous world. We begin our trek through cellular pathology with these adaptations.

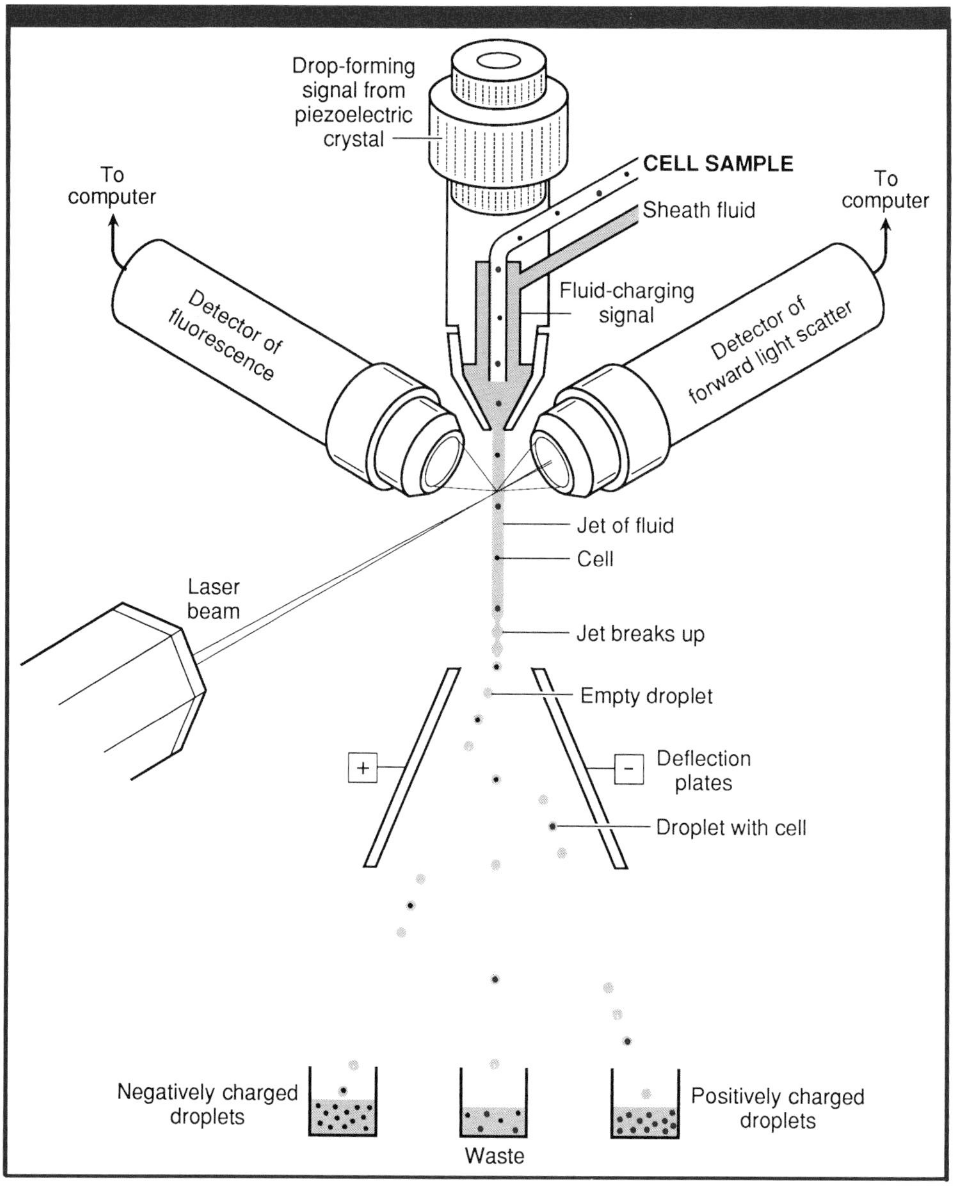

FIGURE 2.1
The principle of fluorescence-activated flow cytometry. In this example, two types of cells are fed into the cytometer (e.g., fluorescent and nonfluorescent, which will have to be sorted out by being assigned either a positive or a negative charge). The cells emerge from the nozzle in a threadlike stream; single cells flow in the axis of the stream, surrounded by a sheath of fluid. As each cell is individually hit by the laser beam, the cytometer senses whether it is fluorescent or not and advises the computer, which will then decide whether the cell should be charged positively or negatively. The charge is instantly applied to the stream, and as the stream breaks up into droplets, each droplet maintains the charge that the stream had. The droplets then pass between two charged plates, which deflect the droplets right or left depending on their charge. The flow is adjusted in such a manner that (ideally) one droplet containing a single cell is flanked by two empty droplets with the same charge. In some cases the computer's decision is aborted, and these droplets are collected as waste. (Adapted from [61].)

Regeneration

Tissues can be destroyed by trauma and infection, killed by infarction, cut or removed by surgeons. Will they regenerate? It depends on their cells. We must learn the rules of the game.

Regeneration Versus Reconstitution *Regeneration* refers to *the replacement of lost cells by cells of the same kind.* This can be a normal event; the bone marrow, for instance, continues to replace obsolete red and white blood cells. It is useful, though no longer customary, to distinguish regeneration from **reconstitution,** which *refers to the replacement of a lost part of the body, requiring the*

coordinated regeneration of several types of cells (88), such as, for example, the regrowth of a lizard's tail. In mammals, many types of cells regenerate very well, but the power to reconstitute lost parts is minimal. Most mammals cannot reconstitute even a lost nail or the root of a hair; if you have a scar, you may have noticed that it is hairless (37, 47).

This being said, there are some partial exceptions. There is one set of microscopic organs that even human beings unfailingly reconstitute: small blood vessels (capillaries, small arteries, and veins). Without this exception wound healing would be virtually impossible.

It has also been reported that children under the age of 4½ years can reconstitute the tip of a finger if it has been cleanly severed and if the amputation falls beyond the distal phalangeal joint (36, 59, 60, 113). Similar findings have been reported in mice (16). The published documents are not very convincing; they do show, however, that repair in young age is excellent; the most interesting conclusion of these studies is that optimal regeneration occurs if the raw surface is not occluded by a dressing, which inhibits growth.

Whatever regrowth does occur in these childrens' fingers, the average male deer would not be impressed. He is able to regrow a new set of antlers each year, a startling example of reconstitution (48) (Figure 2.2); antlers are complex organs made of bone, skin, nerves, and a large supply of blood vessels. There are other minor examples among mammals: rabbits and cats can repair holes punched into their ears, but only up to a point; in fact the expression ear-marking proves that notches or holes in mammalian ears tend to be permanent (49). It has been speculated that reconstitution in mammals never developed because it could not confer a selective advantage. By the time a mammal could have regenerated a whole limb it would have succumbed to predators or to starvation (49).

The Spectrum of Regeneration: Labile, Stable, and Permanent Cells In 1894 a pathologist named

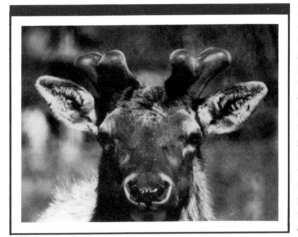

FIGURE 2.2 Antler buds are among the fastest-growing mammalian tissues. This wapiti's buds will elongate at the rate of about 17.5 mm/day. The regeneration of antlers is a rare example of reconstitution (as opposed to regeneration) in mammals. (Reproduced from [45].)

Giulio Bizzozero (one of Golgi's teachers and the man who named the platelets) proposed that cells be classified into three categories, depending on their capacity to multiply (14): **labile** (those that continue to multiply throughout life), **stable** (those that can multiply but are normally quiescent), and **permanent** (those that cannot proliferate). This classification is still valuable as a framework, but it is now clear that *the capacities of cells to multiply are scattered over a continuous spectrum from labile to permanent* (22) (Table 2.1).

Table 2.1

Regenerating Potential of Various Cell Types

	CELL TYPE	COMMENTS
PERMANENT CELLS		
Not known to replicate DNA	Neurons Sertoli cells Fat cells(?) Lens cells	Neurons: DNA does not replicate in postneonatal life (exceptions: the "song center" in canary brain, mouse cortex *in vitro*). Fat cells do not multiply but can revert to a fibroblast-like phenotype that can perhaps multiply.
With capability to duplicate DNA	Striated muscle Myocardium Glomerular podocytes	Nuclei retain the capability to multiply (muscle) or to become polyploid (myocardium) or to multiply *in vitro* (podocytes).
STABLE CELLS	Hepatocytes Fibroblasts Endothelium Smooth muscle (and so on)	Normal mitotic rate is very low but a regenerative burst can occur.
LABILE CELLS	Bone marrow Most epithelia	Continue to replicate throughout life

For example, consider the category of permanent cells. The neurons of vertebrates are traditionally called permanent, but those of birds and mice, as we will see, offer a partial exception; myocardial and striated muscle fibers can certainly duplicate their DNA under certain conditions. The glomerular podocytes are said not to regenerate in vivo (86), but they certainly can regenerate in vitro (111).

REGENERATION OF CONNECTIVE TISSUES

All varieties of connective tissue can regenerate, but to different degrees.

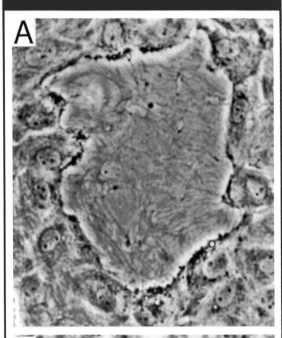

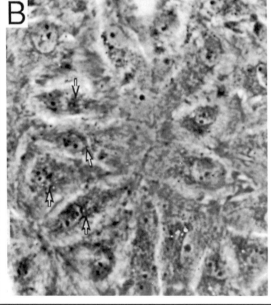

FIGURE 2.3 Healing of a microscopic wound in a sheet of endothelial cells growing *in vitro.* **A:** Phase-contrast micrograph of a nine-cell wound immediately after microsurgery. **B:** The wound has become reendothelialized 150 minutes later by expanded cells, without duplication. (Reproduced from [123].)

Fibroblasts and Endothelial Cells These cells regenerate beautifully; in fact, nature has assigned them the principal role in wound healing. (Vascular regeneration, or **angiogenesis,** is a key feature of wound healing and tumors, and will be discussed in the sections on those subjects.)

Much has been learned by studying the repair of microscopic wounds in sheets of endothelium. For the cells surrounding a wound, the most urgent requirement is to close the gap, and because regeneration takes time, they go about repair in two phases: *first they spread out to cover the open space, then they multiply.* For example, if a cell is plucked out of a sheet of endothelial cells grown *in vitro,* its neighbors spread over the gap in 30–45 minutes (126, 127); nine-cell wounds begin to heal in the same way (Figure 2.3). Similarly, if the aortic intima of a live rat is scratched transversely with a fine thread, the wound, about 50 micrometers (μm) wide, is healed in 8 hours, again by cellular spreading without multiplication (94) (Figure 2.4). This two-phase repair mechanism speeds up the healing process. Epithelia use it as well. This is how corneal scratches can heal within a day and gastric erosions can be covered in minutes, as we will see shortly.

Bone Tissue Stone hard as it is, bone tissue also regenerates beautifully, as might be predicted from the fact that osteoblasts and osteoclasts continue to perform their contrasting jobs throughout life. It is amazing that bone regenerates as fast as it does because its cells face two problems: they must regenerate themselves while also rebuilding a complex extracellular scaffolding. Like a well-trained emergency repair team, they perform their task in two phases. First *the cells hurriedly make temporary bone* of immature-looking trabeculae in which the collagen fibers are woven haphazardly; this is **woven bone,** which is very similar to fetal bone (Figure 2.5). Later, *swarms of osteoclasts slowly remove this provisional bone and then osteoblasts replace it with better built,* orderly **lamellar bone.**

Bone contains more polypeptide growth factors than any other tissue (55). One of these factors, bone morphogenetic protein (BMP), causes connective tissue cells to differentiate into bone-forming cells (119).

Tendons If severed, tendons heal very slowly, which is understandable because they have few cells and few blood vessels. The tendon sheath sometimes participates in the healing process (65,

90), but at the price of adhesions that impair the function of the tendon (3). Secondary rupture at the injured site is not uncommon.

Articular Cartilage This cartilage regenerates poorly, in line with the fact that its cells practically never show mitoses in adults. Note, however, that *the difficulty of regeneration does not lie with hyaline cartilage itself;* foci of newly formed hyaline cartilage are common in healing fractures, especially if motion is allowed. In the context of a joint, the obstacle to cartilage regeneration must be partly mechanical. Suppose that constant rubbing of an articular surface would wear down the matrix and expose chondrocytes. Those cells might well multiply and attempt to create more cartilage, but they would probably be rubbed off before they could accomplish that goal. Foci of regeneration (although ineffective) do not occur in degenerating cartilage, and fragments of articular cartilage maintained *in vitro* produce excellent outgrowths (Figure 2.6); in fact, human knee cartilage has been grown *in vitro* and the resulting cells were used to treat defects of the knee joint (18). We conclude that *articular cartilage can regenerate, but not well enough to ensure the spontaneous repair of a joint.* If an injury removes the superficial layer of the cartilage, leaving the deep, calcified layer intact, the chondrocytes respond ineffectually and do not replace the loss. However, if the injury extends into the subchondral bone, some repair does occur by metaplasia. A hole drilled through the articular surface into the bone is filled by fibrocartilage but not by mature cartilage (27) (Figure 2.7) Interestingly, the chondrocytes, which ordinarily synthesize the special Type II collagen, can switch to Type I; this happens, for example, in osteoarthritis (42).

If a piece of cartilage and bone is chipped off accidentally and allowed to move about in the joint, it behaves as if it were in tissue culture (10); it grows and gives rise to a rounded body consisting of a crust of cartilage over a core of dead bone tissue (the cartilage survives because it is nourished by diffusion). The chip survives even better if it becomes attached to the synovium. The free bodies are called **joint mice** *and can cause sudden blockage of the joint, especially in the knee.*

Adult Fat Cells (Adipocytes) This type of connective tissue cell cannot duplicate itself at all, so we have listed it among the permanent cells. Actually, it is hard to imagine how a fat cell could partition its fat droplet between two daughter cells. However,

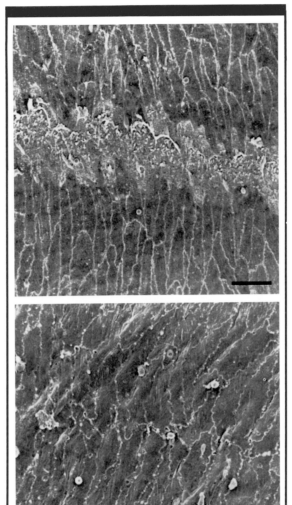

FIGURE 2.4 Regenerative efficiency of rat aortic endothelium. *Top:* Scanning electron micrograph showing a transverse scratch produced *in vivo* with a nylon filament. The irregular white dots on the denuded surface are platelets. *Bottom:* Eight hours later, endothelial cells have migrated into the site of the scratch, without replication. **Bars** = 25 μm. (Reproduced from [90]. © by the U.S. and Canadian Academy of Pathology, Inc.)

everyone knows that fat tissue can very definitely expand; this happens because new fat cells are formed by the few undifferentiated but committed cells that lie among adipocytes; they look like fibroblasts (adipoblasts and preadipocytes) (15). We will discuss these in relation to hypertrophy.

REGENERATION OF EPITHELIA
Epithelia regenerate very well, but again with exceptions. The black sheep are the cells of the lens and the renal podocytes.

Liver Hepatic cells have great powers of regeneration, although not quite as great as the ancient Greeks assumed (Figure 2.8). Experimentally, it is

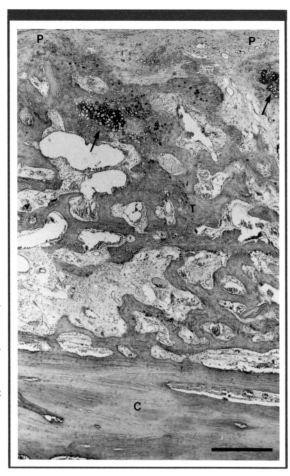

FIGURE 2.5
Regenerating
bone (callus)
near a tibial frac-
ture in a rabbit.
A network of
newly formed tra-
beculae (**T**) has
appeared be-
tween the cortex
(**C**) and the
periosteum (**P**).
Arrows: Islands
of cartilage. **Bar**
= 500 μm.

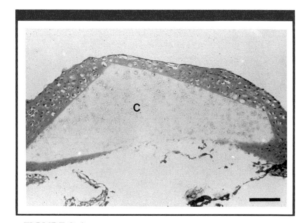

FIGURE 2.6
Regeneration of cartilage *in vitro*. **C:** Sliver of articular cartilage taken from an adult rabbit and placed in culture; 32 days
later it is surrounded by a rim of regenerating chondrocytes 5
to 6 cells deep, which are emphasized by the stain (Safranin
O-fast green). **Bar** = 250 μm. (Reproduced from [74], by
permission of Grodon and Breach, Science Publishers.)

easy to remove about 70 percent of a rat's liver; it
will promptly regrow (but note that if a liver lobe
is cut off, no new lobe grows outward like the tail
of a lizard; rather, new cells are added throughout
the organ until the volume is restored). The quest
for a circulating liver regeneration factor has
produced a long list of candidates, including liver-
specific mitogens (40, 43, 70, 82). Liver regeneration may be triggered by metabolic overload, after
which regenerating liver cells appear to come
under the double control of a stimulator, transforming growth factor (TGF)-alpha (produced by the
liver cells themselves), and an inhibitor, TGF-
beta (produced by endothelial cells) (38, 39). A
powerful, blood-borne hepatocyte growth factor is
also involved (4). The fine-tuning of liver regeneration is beautifully demonstrated by the fact that
transplanted livers adjust their size to the body size
of the recipient (38).

*After partial hepatectomy in rats, minimal cellular
changes are visible in 1–3 hours; after 6–12 hours the
cells, nuclei, and nucleoli enlarge; mitoses begin after
about 12 hours and peak at 30 hours. In 7 days, the
original weight is restored. When partial hepatectomy
is performed in humans to remove tumors, the
response is more sluggish than in rats; original weight is
restored in about 6 months (20, p. 19).*

Surface Epithelia All surface epithelia are programmed to regenerate over denuded areas. They
do so by an efficient two-phase operation as described for the endothelium. The most urgent
task is to cover the exposed connective tissue
surface, no matter how. Thus, a sheet of cells
emerges from the edge of the epithelium and
glides over the denuded surface while new cells
are produced a millimeter or two behind the
edge; it seems that cells will *either* move or
multiply (110). Currently, two theories attempt
to explain the gliding of the new epithelial sheet:
caterpillar motion for single-cell epithelia and
leap-frog motion for stratified epithelia. These
mechanisms are best explained in diagrams (Figure 2.9). After they have covered the gap, the
undifferentiated cells eventually mature into the
required types, such as ciliated or mucus-secreting
cells (46, 117, 124). Maturation may take a week
or two, sometimes less. The gastric lining of the
rat stomach repairs itself with incredible speed;
after absolute alcohol has destroyed over 90
percent of the surface cells, 45 percent of the
denuded surface is covered within *7 minutes* by
flat cells emerging from the gastric pits and

moving at the rate of 1–2 μm per minute; within one hour 95 percent of the damage is repaired with near-normal columnar cells (71). It must be an urgent matter to reline the stomach.

Mesothelia The sheets of flat cells that line the serosal cavities are definitely epithelial: they contain cytokeratin as well as—surprisingly—a surfactant similar to that produced by pulmonary alveolar epithelium (35). They regenerate quickly, but how they do so is not well established. If the peritoneal lining of a rat is destroyed by drying with a jet of air, a new mesothelium reappears within 3–5 days; much evidence suggests that the new lining is formed by the free "monocytes" that live in the peritoneal cavity and settle on the denuded surface, flattening out and turning into epithelial cells (100). This is biologically possible and experimentally well supported, but it is heresy to the current monocyte experts. Others believe that new mesothelial cells are supplied by subperitoneal precursors or by free-floating mesothelial cells. Whatever the mechanism(s) may be, this topic is practically important: the loss of peritoneal lining can lead to the fusion (adhesion) of two apposed viscera, such as intestinal loops. Adhesions can develop

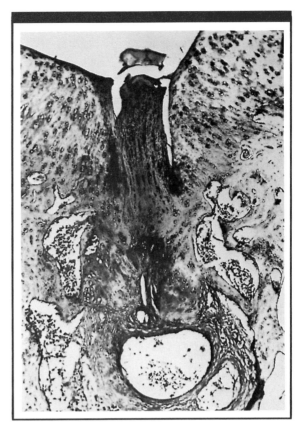

FIGURE 2.7 Repair of articular cartilage. Two months after it was drilled, this 1-mm hole is filled with a tissue that resembles hyalin cartilage, but perfect regeneration is not achieved. Low-power view. (Reproduced from [24].)

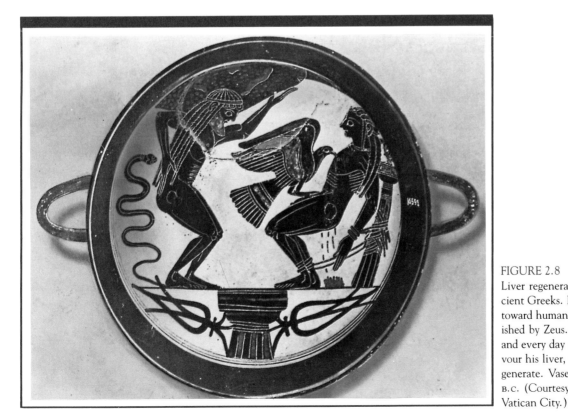

FIGURE 2.8 Liver regeneration as seen by the ancient Greeks. For being too friendly toward humans, Prometheus was punished by Zeus. He was tied to a pole, and every day an eagle came to devour his liver, which continued to regenerate. Vase (Kylix) from 575–550 B.C. (Courtesy of the Museo Etrusco, Vatican City.)

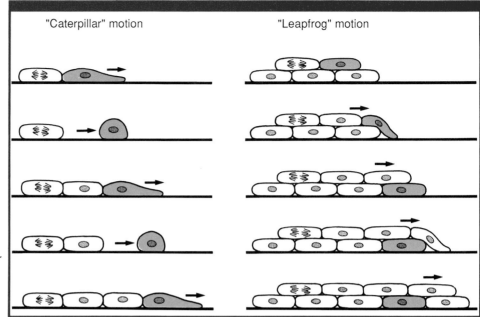

FIGURE 2.9
How epithelia cover a gap. *Left:* caterpillar motion concept proposed for simple epithelia. *Right:* leapfrog motion concept proposed for stratified epithelia.

after abdominal surgery or after repeated peritoneal dialysis; they can be a hazard (p. 435).

Melanocytes These cells of neuroepithelial origin regenerate rather capriciously—too little or too much. Often, especially after freezing (115), they fail to regenerate altogether, which is why most scars in pigmented skin are pale. This property is currently exploited for "freeze branding" cattle, a more humane procedure than fire branding (Figure 2.10).

Role of the Basement Membrane in Epithelial Repair The gliding motion of epithelial cells can occur only over a suitable surface, which in most cases is the basement membrane. For example,

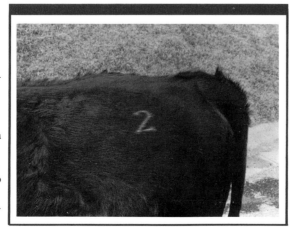

FIGURE 2.10
Freeze-branding of a cow: the procedure exploits the failure of melanocytes to regenerate after a freezing injury. (Courtesy of T. J. Steinhaus, Nasco International, Inc., Fort Atkinson, WI.)

imagine that a kidney tubule has lost some cells as a result of bacterial injury. If the basement membrane is spared, it will railroad the regenerating cells to their proper place, and the tubule will be neatly reconstructed; but if the basement membrane is destroyed, the epithelial cells will pile up in disorderly fashion and the continuity of the tubule will be lost (Figure 2.11). A similar sequence occurs in the liver lobule (Figure 2.12). *This guiding role of the basement membrane is a common theme in the repair of injury* (121). However, it has been overemphasized. When epidermis regenerates over a wound, it has no shred of basement membrane to guide it, and the advancing cells find a surface of collagen, fibrin, and fibronectin acceptable. They probably lay down some of it as they move along (p. 468).

Basement membranes are also reservoirs of growth factors, which have been adsorbed to its heparin-like components. It is thought that these growth factors, which are usually inactive, may somehow be drafted when need arises, for example, in the course of muscle regeneration (129).

It is remarkable that many surface epithelia regenerate well in heavily infected environments, such as the mouth or intestine. In fact, it has been shown that the physiologic renewal of intestinal lining cells takes place twice as fast in normal mice (2 days) as in germ-free mice (1) (Figure 2.13). In this case the bacteria seem to provide a useful stimulus.

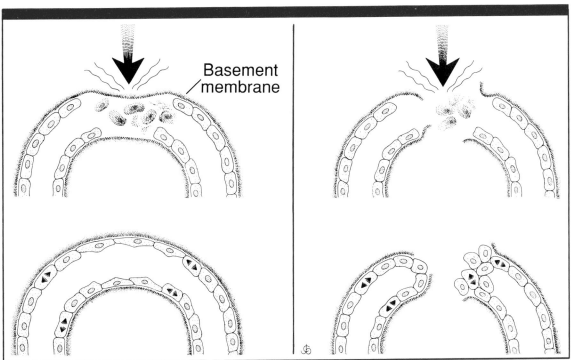

FIGURE 2.11
Guiding role of the basement membrane illustrated in a hypothetical epithelial tubule. *Left:* Mild injury to the tubule destroys some epithelial cells but not the basement membrane; the basement membrane remains as a guide to the regenerating epithelial cells, which crawl along it. *Right:* If the endothelial membrane is destroyed together with the epithelial cells, the latter regenerate at random, and the continuity of the tubule is lost.

This raises a philosophical question: is the intestinal mucosa ever "normal"? In germfree mice, the lamina propria is very thin and lacks the usual complement of mononuclear cells; it simply looks atrophic (Figure 2.13). We must conclude that the normal appearance of the intestinal mucosa is due to its bacterial content. Bacterial antigens are constantly carried across the intestinal epithelium. We will discuss this topic in relation to intestinal allergies (p. 523).

REGENERATION OF MUSCULAR TISSUES

Smooth muscle cells belong to the stable family and regenerate very well (30, 81); for example, during would healing, when new microscopic blood vessels develop, the arteries acquire a new coat of smooth muscle cells supplied by the media of the preexisting vessels. The so-called plaques on the intima of atherosclerotic arteries consist largely of medial smooth muscle cells that have migrated to the intima and multiplied there, presumably in response to chemotactic and mitogenic factors.

Striated muscle has been traditionally maligned

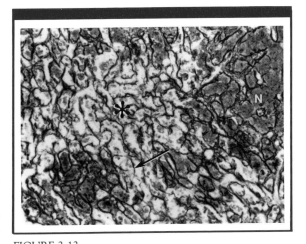

FIGURE 2.12
Liver tissue: Basement membranes remain in place after the death of parenchymal cells and provide a framework for regeneration. Anoxia due to congestion has caused the liver cells in the center of the lobule to disappear, but the reticular framework has remained (**arrow**) and later guides regenerating liver cells to repopulate the center of the lobule. **N:** normal liver parenchyma; **∗:** central part of a congested liver lobule. Silver stain.

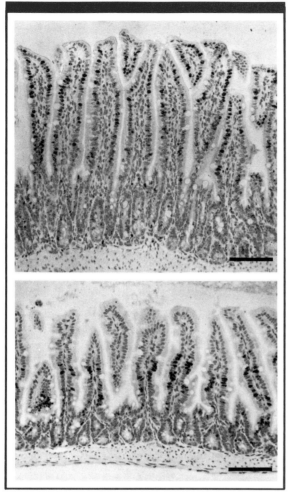

FIGURE 2.13
The structure and function of the normal intestinal mucosa depend in part on the presence of bacteria in the lumen. *Top:* Ileum of a normal mouse 48 hours after administration of tritiated thymidine. The regenerating, labeled epithelial cells (black) have almost reached the tip of the villi. *Bottom:* Ileum of a germ-free mouse under similar conditions. The villi are shorter and thinner, and the crypts are shallow. The labeled epithelium extends only halfway up the villi. Autoradiographs; hematoxylin. **Bars** = 100 μm. (Reproduced from [1]. © by the U.S. and Canadian Academy of Pathology, Inc.)

as a permanent tissue, incapable of regeneration. It is true that a muscle surgically amputated does not grow back, but at the biological level some potential for regeneration is certainly present (23–25). If striated muscle cells, which are several centimeters long, are cut in two, the ends retract immediately and form **retraction clots,** masses of tangled filaments that probably protect the cell from the influx of extracellular calcium (80).

Then a mass of nuclei and cytoplasm slowly sprouts from each stump (Figure 2.14). Within 2 or 3 days, streaks of nuclei with little cytoplasm (called **myotubes**) appear at the tip of the sprout and also beyond it (Figure 2.15).

Where do all these nuclei come from? The question has profound practical implications. The first thought—from muscle nuclei—is probably wrong (80). It now seems certain that major contributors to muscle regeneration are the **satellite cells,** flat stem cells that normally lie dormant within the basement membrane (6) (Figure 2.16). Elegant experiments *in vitro* show that a gap in a muscle fiber is indeed rebuilt by satellite cells as long as the tube of basement membrane is intact (Figure 2.17) (13). After injury *in vivo,* the sequence seems to be the following: the satellite cells "wake up," turn into myoblasts, which fuse to form myotubes, which fuse with the stump and differentiate into mature fibers. It may be that satellite cells from neighboring fibers join the effort.

A third possible source of regenerating cells are **muscle precursor cells,** which are thought to lie in the interstitium waiting for their chance, like substitute singers during an opera. After an injury, these cells are supposed to switch on different genes, turn into myoblasts and myotubes, fuse with the sprout, and play the role of striated muscle (50–53, 98).

What are the practical implications of striated muscle regeneration? Because myotubes and single myoblasts "know" the secret of fusing with striated muscle cells, creative scientists thought of injecting cultured, genetically engineered myoblasts into striated muscle as a way to introduce gene products into muscle cells and thereby into the body as a whole. The plan is to deliver dystrophin into muscles suffering from lack of dystrophin, in Duchenne's muscular dystrophy (87), and even to deliver hormones such as human growth hormone (9). Early results are encouraging (80a).

In the real world, the attempt of striated muscle to regenerate usually fails because the stumps retract too far apart, and the gap is filled by clotted blood and eventually by a scar. However, if the gap between the stumps is bridged by a graft of striated muscle, the cells of the graft die but their cylindrical wrappings of basal lamina remain as guides for the regenerating muscle fibers (26). Similarly, if part of a striated muscle is not

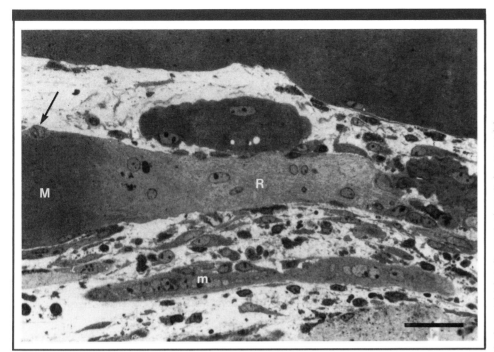

FIGURE 2.14
Regenerating striated muscle of an adult mouse 10 days after a crush injury. **M:** striated muscle fiber; **arrow:** satellite cell; **R:** regenerating sprout (most of its nuclei probably derive from satellite cells); **m:** "myotube," which may later fuse with a regenerating sprout. Myotubes derive from sprouts and perhaps also from interstitial cells with myogenic potential. **Bar** = 25 μm. (Courtesy of Mr. T.A. Robertson and Dr. M.D. Grounds, Department of Pathology, University of Western Australia, Nedlands, Western Australia.)

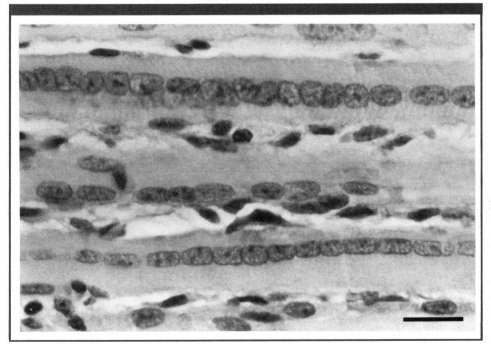

FIGURE 2.15
Longitudinal section of several myotubes containing arrays of centrally placed nuclei. From a striated muscle of an adult mouse, 10 days after a crush injury. **Bar** = 25 μm. (Courtesy of Dr. M.D. Grounds, Department of Pathology, University of Western Australia, Nedlands, Western Australia.)

cut, but crushed or frozen, the remaining basal laminae guide the young sprouts to successful regeneration (105). The same is true when the muscle cells are killed by injection of a local anesthetic (11). *These examples show once again the importance of the basement membrane as a guide for regenerating cells.*

REGENERATION OF NERVOUS TISSUES

PERIPHERAL NERVES

Nerves regenerate quite predictably. If a nerve is cut, the axons in the distal part break down; the Schwann cells, still wrapped around them, phagocytize the debris but, thanks to their basement

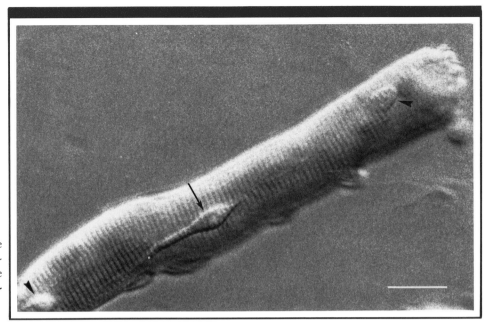

FIGURE 2.16
Satellite cell (**arrow**), attached to a dissociated striated muscle fiber of a rat. Satellite cells are included in the basement membrane wrapping of muscle cells; they are responsible for the regeneration of damaged muscle. **Arrowheads:** muscle nuclei. **Bar** = 50 μm. (Reproduced from [4].)

membrane, remain connected in long chains (**Büngner bands**). The overall process is known since 1850 as **Wallerian degeneration** (Figure 2.18). In the meantime, sprouts arise from the severed axon, presumably as a response to growth factors: if the sciatic nerve of a rat is severed, insulinlike growth factor I (IGF-I) accumulates in and around the Schwann cells of the proximal stump, and local infusion of additional IGF-I speeds up the process (83). If the sprouts manage to bridge the gap and penetrate the distal stump, they grow about 1–3 mm per day (116), which amounts to advancing the width of 1–3 red blood cells every 10 minutes (Figure 2.19). So goes the theory; in practice, when severed nerve filaments in the hand are resutured, years may pass before complete sensitivity is restored. If the gap is too wide, they form a disorderly tangle, which can become clinically evident as a painful **amputation neuroma** (107) (Figure 2.20). It is not known why amputation neuromas develop in some patients and not in others, why they may recur after removal, or why they eventually stop growing.

CENTRAL NERVOUS SYSTEM

In humans, lost neurons cannot be replaced (they cease to multiply before birth), and severed axons of the central nervous system do not grow back effectively. This is baffling because most axons—be they in peripheral nerves or in the central white matter—arise from cells located in the central

nervous system. Abortive attempts to regenerate have long been observed in severed central neurons, but they are functionally ineffective. Because injuries of the central nervous system play such a large part in human disease (10,000 new paraplegics per year in the United States), great efforts are being concentrated on this puzzle. The traditional view has been that regenerating axons in the central nervous system are mechanically intercepted by a tangle of regenerating glial cells (i.e., a scar); perhaps the glia acts also in a more subtle fashion by giving the axons a biological signal that "turns them off" (74). Current thinking is that the obstacle encountered by the axons, whatever it may be, might be removable (102), and imaginative experiments over the past two decades give some hope (54, 64, 95, 101, 120).

Here are some enticing bits of information.
- In small fish, the entire spinal cord, if severed, can regenerate (118).
- In the hamster, pyramidal tracts (63) or the lateral olfactory tract (7, 50) if severed during the first week of life, regenerate with full recovery of function; here the secret is young age.
- In the adult rat, if the iris (which is rich in parasympathetic fibers) is implanted into the brain, it becomes recolonized by new cholinergic fibers that obviously sprout from the white or gray matter (113).

- In the adult rat, if the spinal cord is transsected and the two stumps are connected by a bridge of peripheral nerve, some fibers cross the bridge. Similarly, an 8-mm piece of autologous sciatic nerve implanted into the brain of a rat becomes inhabited by new axons (2, 28, 97).

These findings suggest that *the central nervous system axons are intrinsically able to regenerate, and that the microenvironment of the peripheral nerve is somehow more conducive to their effective regrowth* (Figure 2.21).

All these facts are established, but beware. Nobody has any doubt that axons—by clever experimental tricks—can be coaxed to grow out of the central nervous system; but nobody, to this day, has found a way to make them grow back into it. *Most of the axons that grow into a bridge stop as soon as they confront central nervous tissue.* This remains a great challenge.

Remyelination Remyelination means the rewrapping of a myelin sheath around a living axon that has lost it, which amounts to a partial regeneration. In peripheral nerves, remyelination is prompt and effective; the Schwann cells perform it beautifully (77). In the central nervous system, the oligodendrocytes (homologous to the Schwann cells as "nurse cells" in charge of the myelin sheath) are more sluggish, but some remyelination does occur. This is another reason to be optimistic about the future of regeneration in the central nervous system, which is the main target of demyelinating diseases such as multiple sclerosis.

Regeneration of Neurons Neuron regeneration was traditionally regarded as impossible, with the bright side being that these cells also fail to produce tumors. Exceptions to the rule, however, are worthy of notice. The first startling news came in the 1700s, when J. T. Needham and L. Spallanzani (106) showed that decapitated snails could survive and regenerate new heads (Figure 2.22). This caused "from novelty and singularity, a great noise" (106) because survival after decapitation was not compatible with the notion that the soul is in the head. In retrospect, we note that Spallanzani's 745 decapitated snails must have been cut rather high up because it is now known that they can regenerate only half of their brain (92).

At least as startling was news from Rockefeller

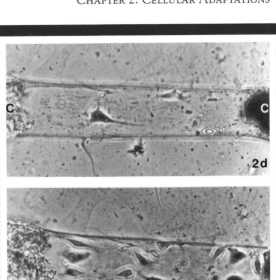
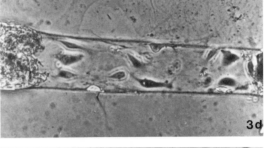
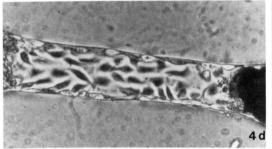
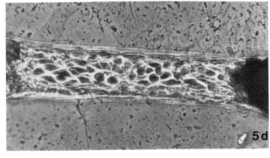
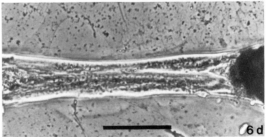

FIGURE 2.17 Regeneration of a striated fiber *in vitro*. *Top:* Muscle fiber that broke accidentally during dissection; the two stumps retracted within the basement membrane to form "retraction clots" (**C**). A satellite cell is present in the intervening space. The subsequent stages show that this space becomes filled with myoblasts, which may have derived from one or more satellite cells. *Bottom:* After 6 days most of the myoblasts have fused to form striated myotubes. **Bar** = 50 μm. (Reproduced from [10]. Copyright © 1975 by the Wistar Institute Press. Reprinted by permission of Wiley-Liss, a division of John Wiley and Sons, Inc.)

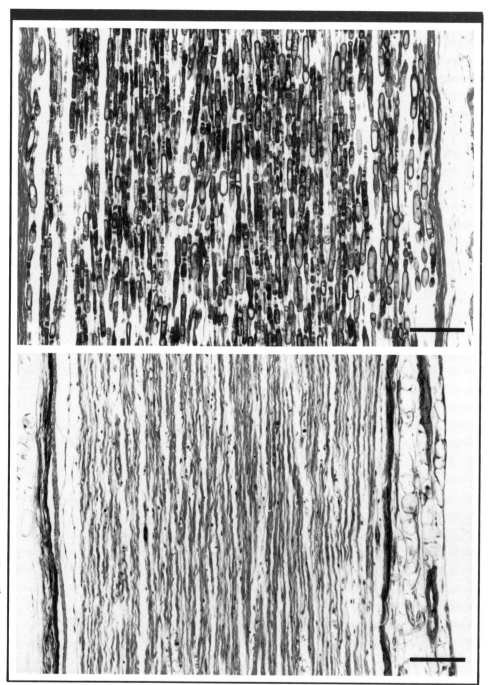

FIGURE 2.18
Two stages of Wallerian degeneration in the severed sciatic nerve of the rat. *Top:* After 4 days the myelin sheaths have broken down into oval bodies. *Bottom:* After 49 days the debris of myelin sheaths has been removed; all that remains is a bundle of cords representing interconnected Schwann cells. **Bars** = 100 μm.

University in 1984. F. Nottebohm had chosen a topic that might appear frivolous: bird songs. Having taped the songs of male canaries, he identified the part of the brain from which they originated. He then discovered that this lobe swells and shrinks with the coming and going of the singing season (Figure 2.23). The swelling is due to the formation of 30,000 to 40,000 new neurons, which are destroyed when the season is over. The stimulus is testosterone. Female canaries

do not sing but their brain undergoes the same cycle, presumably because they have to recognize the songs (45, 69, 84, 88). There are several morals to this amazing discovery; we leave them to the reader's imagination.

Another stunning blow to the "no new neurons" dogma has come from Alberta, Canada (8): cultures of adult mouse brain treated with epidermal growth factor (EGF) produce new astrocytes *and new neurons.* These miraculous cells apparently derive from dormant, undifferentiated stem cells that persist in the brain of the adult mouse (96). Is this the beginning of a new era? Time will tell.

"Plasticity" and Regeneration in the Nervous System The dismal performance of regeneration in the central nervous system (as we just described it) might lead us to conclude that recovery from massive brain lesions should be practically impossible. The facts speak otherwise. Patients who have suffered from hemiplegia due to a stroke can—over months—make spectacular recoveries. What is the mechanism if axon regeneration is not possible? The answer is **plasticity,** a vague term denoting *the ability of the central nervous system to establish alternative pathways.* Axonal sprouting could lead to the formation of new circuits. Morphologic proof of this mechanism is very difficult to obtain, but some evidence exists (12, 44, 93). For example, injury to a peripheral nerve causes sprouting in the central nervous system (128). Plasticity seems to be the central nervous system's secret way of regenerating.

THREE CRITICAL QUESTIONS ABOUT CELL REGENERATION

In the last few pages we have reviewed many types of regenerating cells; this leads us to ask three critical questions.

ARE THE REGENERATED CELLS AS GOOD AS THE OLD ONES?

The answer is *usually yes, but not always and not immediately.* In general, the new cells look undifferentiated and take some time to reach full maturity, as shown by their enzymatic activities (5, 41). For example, if the kidneys of a rat are acutely poisoned with mercuric chloride, the epithelial cells quickly regenerate and reline the tubules, but they are low, almost flat, and partly undifferentiated. The functional result is an excess of urine outflow (**polyuria**) because the cells are still unable to reabsorb water and solutes as they should. Biochemically, there is a return to anaerobic glycolysis (5), which is, interestingly, a characteristic of embryonic cells. A return to normal metabolism requires 2–3 weeks. The same shift occurs in the regenerating liver, perhaps explaining the accumulation of unoxidized triglycerides in this condition (p. 86). It has been reported that regenerated endothelium in pig coronary arteries gives inappropriate functional responses for up to 6 months (103) and that

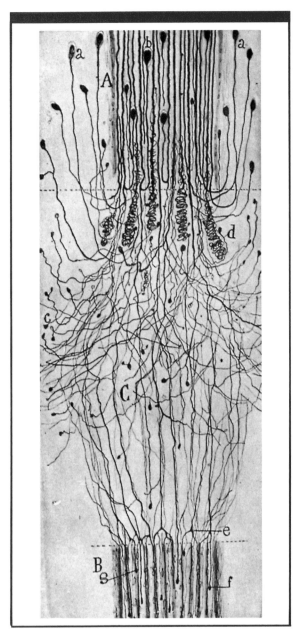

FIGURE 2.19 Pattern of axonal regeneration when a nerve is transsected and the stumps are only slightly separated. Some axons reach the distal stump and grow into it, others wander at random and eventually form a purposeless tangle—an extreme case being the "amputation neuroma." (Reproduced from [18].)

regenerated axons may show abnormal reactions for as long as 2 years (68).

Sometimes this slow recovery is an advantage. Precisely *because regenerating cells are immature, they may be insensitive to certain toxic effects* (p. 137). Similarly, influenza virus kills the epithelial cells of the upper respiratory tract but spares the regenerating cells that follow because they do not yet have receptors for influenza virus (p. 589).

IS THERE A LIMIT TO REGENERATION?

The unfortunate lizards whose tails Spallanzani amputated over and over again two centuries ago

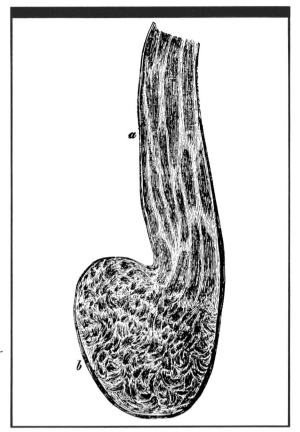

FIGURE 2.20
Amputation
neuroma of the
sciatic nerve, 9
years after amputation. **a:** nerve;
b: neuroma. Enlarged 3–4 ×.
(Reproduced
from [126].)

provided part of the answer: *cells can regenerate many times.* But how many? In 1961, Hayflick and Moorhead asked the question *in vitro* and discovered that cultured human fibroblasts can replicate 50 ± 10 times, and no more (56, 57). In other animals the "Hayflick number" is larger or smaller, depending on the maximum life-span of the species (91) (Table 2.2). The mechanism for these limits is not yet clear.

Personally, we must confess that at first we found it difficult to reconcile the Hayflick number with the kinetics of labile cells that continue to replicate throughout life, such as the hematopoietic cells of the bone marrow or the epithelial cells of the intestinal lining, which have a lifespan of about 2 days. So we wrote to Dr. Hayflick. Here is his definitive reply:

> *The limit of 50 population doublings is 2^{50}. That number translates to 20,000,000 metric tons of cells. That quantity of cells is ample by several orders of magnitude to account for all the cells that are sloughed from the tissues that you mentioned throughout a single lifetime.*

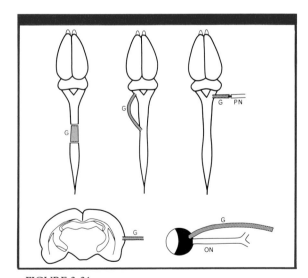

FIGURE 2.21
Experiments on rats proving that axons can be made to grow out of the central nervous system into peripheral nerve tissue. The basic method is to insert a free segment of rat peripheral nerve (stippled, **G**) into central nervous tissue; axons grow into it. **ON:** optic nerve; **PN:** peripheral nerve. (Reproduced from [2].)

Table 2.2

Correlation Between Life-Span of Species and Hayflick Number[a]

SPECIES	MAXIMUM LIFE-SPAN (YEARS)	MEAN NUMBER OF CELL POPULATION DOUBLINGS
Mouse	2	9.2
Rat	3.5	12.8
Rat kangaroo	7	12.8
Mink	10	25.0
Rabbit	13	22.5
Bat	14	18.0
Chicken	30	25
Horse	46	28.8
Human	110	61.3
Galapagos tortoise	150+	120

Adapted from Kirkwood TBL. In vitro ageing of animal cells. In: Davies I, and Sigee DC, eds. Cell ageing and cell death. Cambridge: Cambridge University Press, 1984: 55–72.
[a]*Number of potential fibroblast divisions (in vitro).*

Will it ever be possible to escape from this fatal number? Recent work has shown that cholera toxin (a mitogen) temporarily rejuvenates senescent mouse mammary epithelium grown *in vitro*. Perhaps the limit to mitosis is due not to cellular deterioration but to specific changes in cell regulation (32). There are other pieces of the puzzle. *Malignant cells grow indefinitely.* Also it is possible to immortalize cultured cells without conferring malignant characteristics to them; this is the nature of the so-called cell lines. And *many plant cells can grow* in vitro *without limit*, like cancer cells (99). Even more intriguing: *mouse embryo cells grown in the absence of serum do not undergo senescence*, which suggests that the standard conditions of cell culture are the limiting factor (75, 76). *Senescence of human cell cultures is prevented by the loss of chromosome 1; is it a genetic phenomenon* (112)?

Given the reality of the Hayflick number, we must wonder in retrospect how to account for the phenomenon of Dr. Carrel's much publicized culture of (normal) immortal cells. In 1912, Alexis Carrel, Nobel laureate and pioneer of cell culture, established a culture of embryonic chick heart that was discontinued after 34 years. His culture played an important role in the development of theories of cell aging. Alas, it now seems that overzealous attendants piously replenished the cultures whenever they appeared ready to fail (125).

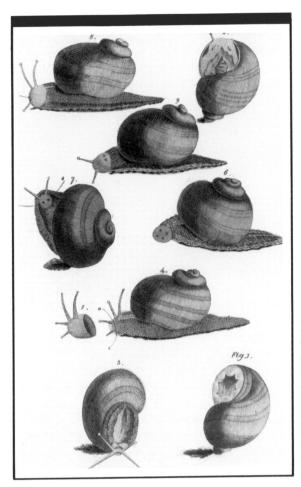

FIGURE 2.22
Some of the 745 snails that Spallanzani decapitated, fully or partially, around 1766; heads regenerated in 219 snails. (Reproduced from [28].)

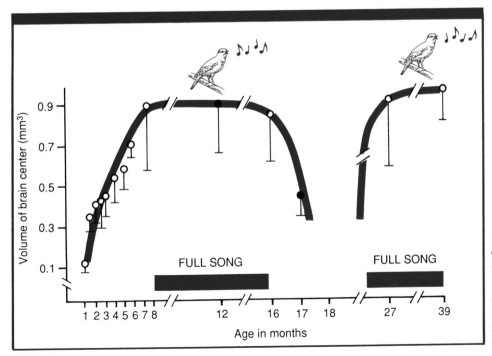

FIGURE 2.23
Correlation—in canaries—between the season of "full song" and the volume of the brain nucleus where the song originates. The fall and rise of the curve corresponds to death and regeneration of nerve cells. (Reproduced from [80].)

WHAT MAKES CELLS REGENERATE?

Something must be telling cells that new cells are needed and making them turn on their replication program. As far as we know, the news could reach the cells in four ways: (a) principally by growth factors diffusing in the microenvironment, a well-established mechanism, and to a lesser extent by (b) electric currents, (c) cell-to-cell communication, and (d) nervous stimuli.

Growth Factors The study of growth factors is now one of the busiest fields of research (29, 33, 123), not only because of their enormous therapeutic potential but also because it turns out that the same genes (protooncogenes) that are responsible for cell proliferation are also involved in carcinogenesis (p. 843). There are so many growth factors and they are so varied in their effects that we cannot begin to describe them here; we will limit ourselves to a few generalizations and discuss individual growth factors in more detail later on.

Growth factors are polypeptides with a molecular weight between 5,000 and 30,000 kD that act on specific surface receptors. Unlike the hormones of the endocrine organs, which reach their targets via the blood stream, growth factors behave as local hormones, acting over a short distance or on the secreting cell itself (**paracrine, autocrine, and intracrine secretion**) (Figure 2.24). They have been extracted not only from growing tissues and from tumors but also from normal tissues. Some growth factors become attached to extracellular materials such as basement membranes, where they are probably stored but are not necessarily active.

Growth factors are multifunctional (Table 2.3); they can inhibit as well as stimulate. *They modulate each other,* which means that their effects depend on the presence or absence of other factors. It has been suggested that they function together like letters of an alphabet, from which the cells synthesize the ultimate message (108).

The biology of the growth factors puts a severe strain on the memory of the nonexpert, who is endowed with a brain and not with a computer. Here is a partial list of effects:
- cell growth
- cell proliferation or inhibition
- cell differentiation
- cell maintenance (viability)
- cell activation (in inflammation)
- chemotaxis
- other effects, such as vasoconstriction by platelet-derived growth factor (PDGF)

A further strain for the nonexpert is that the growth factors are plagued by names that are either obsolete or misleading. We are particularly distressed by the "transforming growth factors," which do not really transform (p. 728). Appropriate names would be hard to find anyway because each factor has so many effects. It would be like naming Harlequin from a single one of his colors.

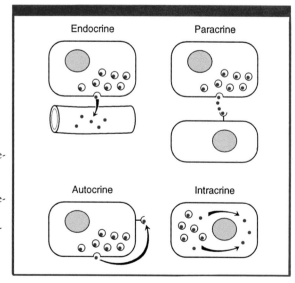

FIGURE 2.24 What was once called internal secretion is now subdivided into four subtypes, depending on the location and distance of the target. (Adapted from [29a].)

The first growth factor to be discovered was nerve growth factor (NGF). Rita Levi-Montalcini noticed in 1948 that fragments of a mouse sarcoma, implanted into the body wall of a 3-day-old chick embryo, caused an outgrowth of sensory and sympathetic fibers; a similar effect was produced (an accidental discovery) by snake venom and by an extract of mouse salivary glands, tested as potentially homologous to snake venom glands (73). NGF was then extracted with the help of chemist Stanley Cohen. Tested in vitro on sympathetic ganglia, it produced the now-classic halo of sprouting fibers (Figure 2.25). Later, Cohen tested the effect of crude preparations of NGF injected into newborn mice. A sharp biologist as well as a chemist, he noticed two epithelium-related events that pure NGF did not produce: the teeth erupted faster, and the eyelids, normally closed at birth, separated earlier. The active agent turned out to be an impurity, which was named epithelial growth

Table 2.3

Peptide Growth Factors Are Multifunctional

GROWTH FACTOR	PROLIFERATIVE EFFECTS	ANTI-PROLIFERATIVE EFFECTS	EFFECTS UNRELATED TO PROLIFERATION
Epidermal growth factor	Keratinocytes, fibroblasts	Hair follicle cells	Suppression of gastric acid secretion
Fibroblast growth factor (basic)	Many mesenchymal cells, especially endothelial cells	Ewing's sarcoma cells, other tumor cells	Regulation of pituitary and ovarian cell function
Transforming growth factor-beta	Fibroblasts, osteoblasts	Fibroblasts, epithelial cells, T-lymphocytes, osteoblasts	Suppression of immunoglobulin secretion and adrenal steroidogenesis
Interleukin-1	Lymphocytes, keratinocytes, fibroblasts	Breast cancer cells	Endogenous pyrogen, bone resorption
Interleukin-2	T- and B-lymphocytes, oligodendrocytes	T-lymphocytes, oligodendrocytes	Increased cytotoxic activity of monocytes
Interleukin-6	Hybridoma, plasmacytoma cell lines	Breast cancer cells	Increased expression of cell surface antigens and secretion of immunoglobulins
Tumor necrosis factor-alpha	Diploid fibroblasts, epithelial cells	Many tumor cells	Inhibition of lipoprotein lipase, stimulation of collagenase

Adapted from Sporn MB and Roberts AB. Peptide growth factors are multifunctional. Nature 1988; 332:217–219.

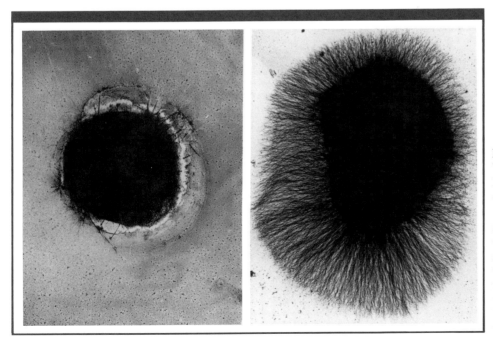

FIGURE 2.25
The famous halo effect that enabled Rita Levi-Montalcini to confirm the existence of the nerve growth factor (NGF). Low-power photomicrographs of two sensory ganglia from an 8-day chick embryo. *Left:* Ganglion grown in ordinary medium. *Right:* Ganglion grown in a medium enriched with NGF. The halo is due to the outgrowth of axons. (Courtesy of Dr. R. Levi-Montalcini, Istituto Superiore di Sanità, Rome, Italy.)

factor (EGF). Rita Levi-Montalcini and Stanley Cohen shared the Nobel prize in 1986.

We now return to the other factors that may be involved in regeneration.

Electric Currents Electric currents are generated by injury (p. 182, 355). Could they be a stimulus to regeneration? Indeed, mild currents have been used successfully for many years to encourage bone healing (17); new bone forms at the anode, whereas osteoclasts get to work at the cathode. There are good data to show that electric currents play a role in the regeneration of limbs in amphibians. Beyond these encouraging facts and a few others on wound healing, the literature is meager (18).

Cell-to-Cell Communication Cells connected by communicating junctions (also called gap junctions) should be able to pass along the news of a local injury; some do so *in vitro* (72), but the importance of this mechanism is not yet known.

Nervous Stimuli Nerves assist the regeneration of limbs in amphibians and of fins in fish (104), perhaps by supplying mitogenic factors (19). Nothing similar is known in mammals with one peculiar exception. In rats, the submandibular salivary gland fails to grow if the corresponding sympathetic ganglion is removed; it shrinks with adrenergic blocking agents and swells with sympathicomimetics (122).

TO SUM UP: There have been enormous advances in our knowledge regarding growth factors; some of these are already used in clinical medicine, especially to whip up a reluctant or exhausted bone marrow, and there is hope for many more applications, such as accelerating repair after injury (59). However, the field of regeneration *per se* has not seen great progress in recent years (66) except for the recent breakthrough regarding mouse neurons. To those readers who regret especially the lack of regeneration of human neurons, we can offer a consoling thought by Nottebohm: "Humans thrive in the recollection of events long past, and neuronal replacement would disrupt such memories" (85).

Hypertrophy, Hyperplasia

Regeneration, as we have described it, refers to the replacement of lost parts. Now we are about to see how cells and organs adapt by enlarging beyond their normal sizes.

Hypertrophy means acquired increase in the size of a cell, tissue, or organ. When a part of the body is called upon to increase its size, it can do so by increasing the volume of its cells (cellular hypertrophy), their number (hyperplasia), and often both. *Knowing the regenerating capacity of each cell type makes it easy to predict the type of response to the need for increased size:* cells that cannot multiply have no option but to become larger. **Hyperplasia** is biologically similar to regeneration, but it leads to an increase in size of the organ.

Cells that are undergoing either hypertrophy or hyperplasia are synthesizing more cytoplasm (i.e., more protein). Consequently, we can expect that this cytoplasm, seen by light microscopy, will be more basophilic than in ordinary cells because the number of ribosomes is increased. The nucleolus will be enlarged because it is synthesizing more ribosomes; as for the nucleus, it will also be enlarged but *less* basophilic(!) because its chromatin is dispersed, reflecting enhanced DNA transcription.

Note: If a cell appears much larger than normal and its nucleus is also very large, it is reasonable to suspect more than hypertrophy, namely **polyploidy,** an increased number of chromosomes (p. 39).

EXAMPLES OF HYPERTROPHY AND HYPERPLASIA

The following typical examples are listed according to the stimulus (Table 2.4).

INCREASED FUNCTIONAL DEMAND

A simple way to study the effects of functional overstrain is to remove one of two paired organs; if one kidney is removed (nephrectomy) the other enlarges. This is called **compensatory hypertrophy.**

Kidney Hypertrophy can be induced in the kidney by many stimuli (Figure 2.26), and the basic mechanism of enlargement is a combination of diffuse hypertrophy

Table 2.4

Causes of Hypertrophy and Hyperplasia

CAUSE	EXAMPLE
Increased functional demand	High blood pressure → myocardial hypertrophy
Endocrine stimulation	Estrogen → uterine hypertrophy
Local hormones or mitogens	Lymphokines → macrophage hypertrophy/hyperplasia
Increased nutrition	Extra calories → adipose tissue and muscle hypertrophy
Increased blood flow	Arterio-venous fistula → accelerated limb growth
Mechanical factors	Traction on skin → skin hypertrophy
Imbalance between tissue anabolism and catabolism	Bone → osteopetrosis
Pharmacologic agents	Isoproterenol → salivary gland hypertrophy

and hyperplasia (20, 167) (Figure 2.27). The glomeruli enlarge and their capillaries become longer (195), but there are no new glomeruli or new tubules; this would be reconstitution. The podocytes, remember, behave *in vivo* as permanent cells, which further limits glomerular enlargement. The cellular response to unilateral nephrectomy is somewhat sluggish because the remaining kidney can increase its function almost instantly by vascular adjustments (155). In dogs, the glomerular filtration rate can increase up to 100 percent within minutes. In rats, the weight of the remaining kidney increases by 30 percent in one week; it never doubles.

Striated Muscle Increased functional demand on striated muscles has dramatic cellular effects. Clearly, the cells know what they are doing because they adapt their response to the type of challenge. *In response to endurance exercise they increase the number and volume of the mitochondria, whereas heavy resistance training induces mainly hypertrophy of the contractile apparatus* (135) and probably also an increase in fiber number (134). The capillary network increases too (171).

Smooth Muscle *Enlargements of smooth muscle tissue are usually due to a combination of hypertrophy, polyploidy, and hyperplasia* (166, 188). For instance, in pregnancy the body of the uterus enlarges about 70-fold by these mechanisms. It is

common to observe smooth muscle thickening above an intestinal stenosis due to the effort of pumping the content through the stricture; a 10-fold increase in mass can be measured experimentally in 3–5 weeks (157, 166). In hypertensive rats, the aortic media acquires more cells, larger cells, thicker elastic fibers, and more collagen—changes that are only partly reversible (188).

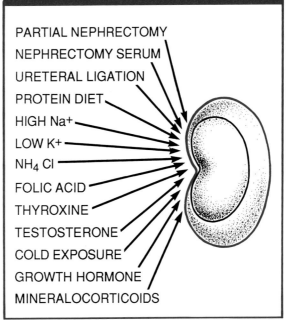

FIGURE 2.26 Experimental methods for inducing kidney hypertrophy. (Adapted from [30].)

FIGURE 2.27
Relative extents
of hyperplasia
and hypertrophy
of a mouse kid-
ney after contra-
lateral nephrec-
tomy. The space
between the two
curves (dry
weight, number
of cells) reflects
cellular hypertro-
phy. (Adapted
from Johnson,
H.A., and Vera
Roman, J.M.
Compensatory re-
nal enlargement.
Hypertrophy ver-
sus hyperplasia.
Am. J. Pathol.,
49:1–13, 1966.)

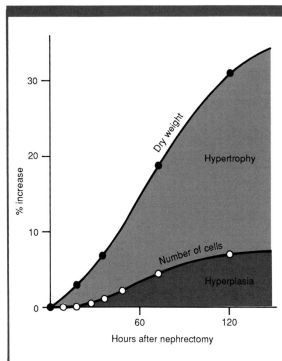

FIGURE 2.28
New sarcomeres
can develop (dur-
ing myocardial
hypertrophy) by
broadening and
splitting of the Z
lines. (Courtesy
of Dr. H.F.
Cuénoud, Uni-
versity of Massa-
chusetts Medical
Center, Worces-
ter, MA.)

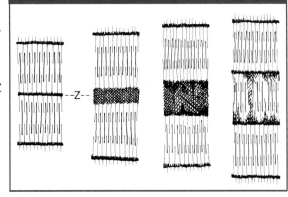

FIGURE 2.29
With increasing
heart weight
there is a progres-
sive increase in
ploidy of myocar-
dial cells (indi-
cated by the fig-
ures on the
bars). The 125-g
heart came from
an 8-year-old
child. (Adapted
from [2].)

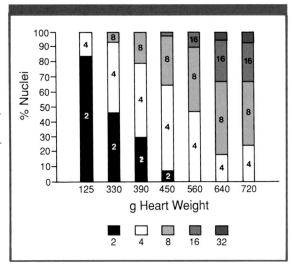

Heart Increased effort due to exercise, hypertension, or a valvular defect translates into increased
mass of the heart. Athletic exertion alone can
increase the human heart weight to 500 g (300 g is
normal for men and 250 g for women) (165). Up
to this point *the increase is based on hypertrophy*
only; thereafter *there is also an increase in cell
number*. Occasionally, the heart of a patient with
long-standing valvular disease can exceed 1 kg;
such enormous increases are not seen in other
animals (153). The cells increase their contractile
machinery not by stretching the sarcomeres but by
adding new ones, end to end, side by side, and also
by the peculiar mechanism of **Z-band splitting**
(153, 177) (Figure 2.28).

Myocardial hypertrophy is clinically so important that it has created a huge literature. Although
the heart cells (**myocardiocytes**) are often said to
be incapable of dividing, the facts are different.
Shortly after birth, human myocardiocytes cease
to multiply and then enlarge 30–40 times (**hypertrophic growth**) (187). Later, between 5 and 9
years of age, they begin to become polyploid and
continue to do so through life; in adults two-thirds
of these cells are polyploid (up to 16N) and about
one-fifth of them are binucleated (153, 191). If
the heart is submitted to functional strain,
polyploidization increases (132) (Figure 2.29), and
in humans, gigantic nuclei appear (Figure 2.30).
Because the size of the cells ceases to increase after
a critical heart weight is reached, an increase in
numbers must take place; on the assumption that
mitoses are unlikely to occur in the adult (153) it
is hypothesized that the polyploid nuclei somehow
split and the cell then divides. However, it seems
that mammalian atrial myocardium retains the
ability to perform mitosis (198).

As myocardial hypertrophy progresses, ominous
developments occur in the extracellular spaces.
The connective tissue stroma increases (which is
understandable), but it does so in excess of the
apparent need (131) (Figure 2.31). This **fibrosis**
stiffens the myocardium and decreases its compli-
ance. Why fibrosis develops is unclear; perhaps it is
a response to cellular damage (196). To this day it is
not treatable. At the same time, the number of
capillaries increases but does not keep pace with the
muscular mass, leading to relative anoxia (137,
138, 174, 193). Furthermore, as the myocardial
cells continue to enlarge, they develop pathologic
features (153, 177) such as abnormal aggregates of
sarcotubules, masses of abnormal mitochondria and
myelin figures, excessive amounts of glycogen

(including intramitochondrial glycogen), bizarre nuclear infoldings (154), and eventually loss of contractile elements and specialized intercellular junctions.

We have now partially answered a critical question: is myocardial hypertrophy pathologic? *The many structural changes that occur in progressive hypertrophy lead eventually to myocardial "exhaustion."* It should be clear, however, that an athlete's heart does not fit this category; it may have a reduced reserve, but it is not intrinsically diseased (165). Notice also that an athlete's heart (unlike that of a patient with a valvular defect) is placed under strain for a few hours at a time, after which it has the rest of the day to recover.

Is myocardial hypertrophy reversible? Initially, it is. However, it has been shown experimentally that *if the cause of the hypertrophy is removed, the muscle mass and the RNA return to normal, but the DNA and the interstitial collagen do not* (149). This leads to the bizarre situation of huge polyploid nuclei in fibers of normal size.

ENDOCRINE AND PARACRINE STIMULATION

The enlargement of the uterus due to estrogen (162) is a classic example of **endocrine stimulation**. The result is hypertrophy as well as hyperplasia. Another example is the estrogen-induced hypertrophy of bone in egg-laying hens (201) (Figure 2.32).

Local hormones (paracrine stimulation) act within a very short range and usually also for a very short time (e.g., prostaglandins, lymphokines); however, before they fade away they have time to leave their mark. An example is the hypertrophy ("activation") and hyperplasia of macrophages in response to a host of inflammatory mediators, especially interferon gamma (IFNγ) (p. 326).

EXCESSIVE NUTRITION

Excess nutrition leads to an increase, as everyone knows, of fat tissue. It is less known that it also leads to a 50 percent increase in protein synthesis throughout the body (178). In other words, the overfed Sumo wrestlers do not accumulate fat only.

The interplay between hypertrophy and hyperplasia in fat is still controversial but fascinating. There is some consensus, as follows (136, 141, 185). During the first year of life, fat cells increase in size and by 12 months the adipocytes reach adult size; from then on, increase in adipose tissue mass is mainly due to an increase in cell number. In adults, excess calories are stored at first in

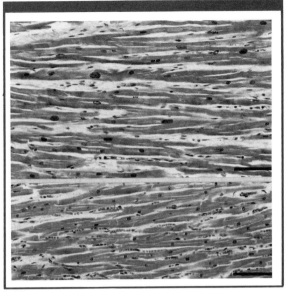

FIGURE 2.30
Top: Hypertrophic myocardium. Note the enlarged, polyploid nuclei. *Bottom*: Normal myocardial fibers. **Bars** = 50 μm.

preexisting fat cells, which become larger (hypertrophy), but prolonged overnutrition can eventually induce an increase in fat cell number. This means that obese individuals have more *and* bigger fat cells (141) (Figure 2.33).

It seems that fat cells can enlarge up to a certain critical size; at that point they transmit a signal to the preadipocytes, which differentiate into new fat

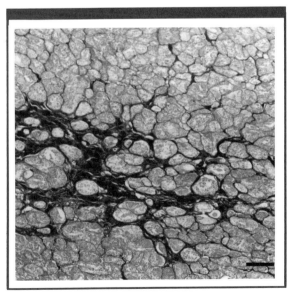

FIGURE 2.31
Fibrosis tends to develop in hypertrophic human hearts. Note the infiltration of connective tissue strands between individual myocardial fibers. Trichrome stain: the connective tissue (blue in the original) appears black. **Bar** = 50 μm. (Preparation courtesy of Dr. F.J. Schoen, Brigham and Women's Hospital, Boston, MA.)

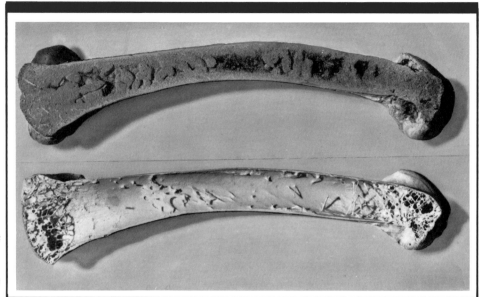

FIGURE 2.32
Physiologic hypertrophy and atrophy of the femur in hens. *Top:* The bone of a laying bird is filled with medullary bone as a source of calcium. *Bottom:* In a nonlaying bird the bone is hollow. (Reproduced from [70].)

cells. It is thought that once new fat cells are formed, they can be made to shrink, but they never disappear (152, p. 44). We just said *never,* a word *never* to be used in a medical context. The fact is that *under conditions of extreme starvation, all traces of adipose tissue do disappear.*

Because getting rid of fat cells is nearly impossible, it is particularly bad for obesity to develop in children. *Fat cells acquired at an early age will be there for life.* Adult-onset obesity seems to imply mainly hypertrophy, which can be reversible. In this regard we can only wish that we could be more like the woodchuck (152, p. 45). Before hibernation the woodchuck goes through a phase of overeating in order to store fat; if its fat cells had to undergo a wave of hyperplasia every year, it would soon become obese and unfit to survive. Thus, the woodchuck has a built-in mechanism that allows fat cells to undergo hypertrophy but not hyperplasia.

There seems to be a peculiar correlation between fat-cell size and the brain. If adult rats are submitted to lipectomy (removal of about 25 percent of their adipose tissue, which reduces the fat storage capacity) (151), their appetite drops (151). Also, if fat cells are depleted beyond a certain point by a severely restricted diet, symptoms of depression and hormonal changes ensue (152, p. 41), as if the fat cells were signaling that fat reserves are too low. This is another reason that makes it very difficult for obese people to return to normal weight.

We can now ask the same question we asked about hypertrophy of the the heart: is excess fat a disease? Obesity was indeed declared a disease in 1985 (170). To be precise, obesity is a symptom *that becomes a hazard in itself,* leading to hypertension, increased mortality, and a number of other complications. For example, enlarged fat cells are not just larger. They have fewer insulin receptors on their surface, so their sensitivity to insulin is decreased. This may explain the hyperinsulinemia of obese patients, a condition that may lead to exhaustion of the pancreatic beta cells and therefore to diabetes (152, p. 49). Overweight adolescents face a higher risk of coronary heart disease, atherosclerosis, stroke, colorectal cancer, gout (181) osteoarthritis, and even poverty (160).

There are other cellular problems with obesity. *Fat cells are also depots of cholesterol* (for each kilogram of fat there are 20 milligrams of cholesterol). Cholesterol is excreted through the bile, and a chain of events correlates obesity and gall stone formation (143, p. 22). More ominously, fat

FIGURE 2.33
Microphotograph of fat cells from a normal child (*left*) and from an obese child (*right*). The cells are black because they have been fixed with osmium tetroxide. (11)

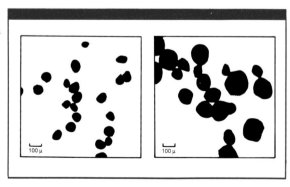

cells are able to aromatize androgens to estrogens; in fact they are the major source of extragenital estrogen synthesis in postmenopausal women. There are also established correlations among obesity, estrone secretion, and cancer of the endometrium (150, 200).

If the genes linked to obesity are so detrimental, why have they been conserved against strong evolutionary pressure? One theory, too complex to discuss here, is that they may have been an asset under primal conditions when humans were foraging for limited food supplies and periods of abundance alternated with periods of starvation (148).

INCREASED BLOOD FLOW

Vascular tumors of a limb can cause that limb to become longer. A similar overgrowth is sometimes seen in children after fracture or infection of a long bone (**osteomyelitis**). These effects are usually attributed to increased blood flow, but a local flooding with growth factors should also be considered.

MECHANICAL FACTORS

When plastic surgeons need to cover a skin defect but the surrounding skin cannot be stretched over it, they use a method known as **tissue expansion.** A balloonlike device is slipped under the skin and slowly inflated over several weeks, until the overlying skin expands enough for the purpose (144). This stretching mechanism was known thousands of years ago and exploited for cosmetic and even surgical purposes. Even today, in several parts of the world, earlobes and lips are elongated with weights or other devices; Buddha is usually represented with stretched earlobes (176). How the cells transduce a pull to hyperplasia, nobody knows.

IMBALANCE BETWEEN TISSUE ANABOLISM AND CATABOLISM

This odd mechanism is known only in bone tissue, which is unique in that it is constantly built and destroyed. Therefore, an excess of bone formation can be due to hyperactive osteoblasts or to ineffective osteoclasts. **Osteopetrosis,** or marble bone disease, in which the metaphyses of growing bones become filled with dense marblelike bone tissue, is due to inadequate osteoclastic removal (203).

MISCELLANEOUS CAUSES

A pharmacologic agent occasionally induces a specific target tissue to increase (or decrease) in size; for instance, **isoproterenol,** a beta-adrenergic agonist, mysteriously induces hypertrophy of the salivary glands in rats and mice (139).

Any unexplained hypertrophy is qualified in medical jargon as **idiopathic.** An example is the so-called idiopathic hypertrophic cardiomyopathy, in which there is no apparent hydraulic problem to justify the hypertrophy; the myocardium may be responding by hypertrophy to a congenital anomaly of the fibers, which form a network-pattern rather than the normal bundles.

Can any cell be stimulated to exhaustion? Certainly there is a limit to hypertrophy. Cells do not enlarge beyond certain sizes, and if a hypertrophic myocardium is subjected to excessive demands, it fails. We have already mentioned the supposed "metabolic exhaustion" of pancreatic beta cells coping with chronic hyperglycemia (173). There are hints that exhaustion can occur in other systems; renal glomeruli, for example, can be overstrained. By removing five-sixths of a rat's kidney tissue, the remaining portion (called remnant kidney) shows glomerular damage that has been ascribed to hyperfiltration (156, 164, 179, 183, 186, 192, 195, 199), and the damage is more severe if the rat is kept on a high protein diet (164), which is itself a stimulus to renal hypertrophy. The glomerular exhaustion may be due to the fact that the glomerular epithelial cells (podocytes) do not regenerate and therefore cannot keep up with the increased functional demands (156). Finally, we offer two teasers.

- High-altitude anoxia causes hypertrophy of the myocardium. How could lack of oxygen increase the size of the heart? If the supply of atmospheric oxygen is low, the heart has to pump harder to maintain a normal oxygen supply to all the tissues (175). However, there is an additional factor: the heart must also pump harder because anoxia, strangely enough, causes the pulmonary arteries to constrict (180).
- Why is myocardial hypertrophy sometimes seen after a large myocardial infarct? Infarcts leave scars that do not contract and therefore oblige the rest of the ventricular myocardium to undergo compensatory hypertrophy.

THE BIOLOGY OF POLYPLOIDY

In discussing hypertrophy and hyperplasia, we mentioned several circumstances in which polyploid cells may develop. As a matter of fact, polyploid cells—recognized by their large nuclei

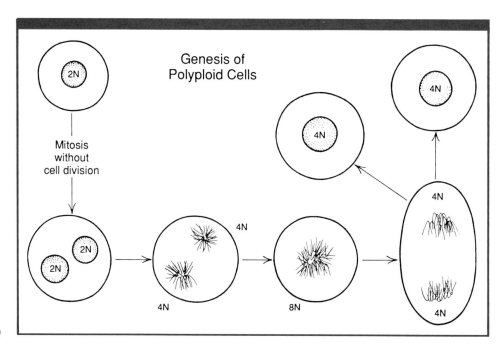

FIGURE 2.34
Steps leading from a diploid to a
polyploid cell. (Adapted from [51].)

and overall large size—are also found in normal
tissues, including the uterus, salivary glands,
pancreas, epidermis, and other organs (140, 142,
145); *the number of polyploid cells increases with age*
(159). In the normal liver, polyploidy (reflected by
nuclear size) is especially striking. If it is true that
some brain cells are polyploid, a relatively old
observation (172), it would be very interesting to
find out at what stage of development these
usually permanent cells have duplicated their
DNA.

The mechanism leading to polyploidy seems
fairly straightforward (Figure 2.34), but why it
should occur in animal tissues is not at all clear.
One cell that should know the answer is the
megakaryocyte, which qualifies as a truly professional polyploid in that its complement of DNA
ranges from 4N to 64N (184, 189, 190). Especially
intriguing is the fact that *the megakaryocyte does not
begin to make platelets until it is octoploid* (145), and
then the platelets differ slightly depending on the
degree of ploidy of the parent cell.

What function might be served by polyploidy?
The likeliest advantage of polyploid cells seems to
be that *having several copies of the same gene is
insurance against gene damage* (e.g., by radiation);
thus, it might counteract aging (158). There is
actually some evidence that polyploid cells are
more resistant to radiation. There is a species of
wasp, *Habrobracon*, that comes in two variants:

haploid and diploid. Radiation damage, as measured by survival, is markedly more severe in
haploids (147).

The significance of polyploidy is much more
obvious in the world of botany, in which
polyploidy is a major mechanism for the development of new species. Almost half of the existing
300,000 plant species have a polyploid origin
(194). Famous polyploids include the chrysanthemum, the potato (here the advantage of larger cell
size is obvious at least for the farmer), wheat,
tobacco, and sugar cane. In plants, at least,
polyploidy is a major evolutionary mechanism.
The effect of polyploidy on the plant varies, but it
is often associated with greater size and vigor
(169). Because polyploid plants usually cannot
produce fertile offspring with diploid plants, the
new hybrids are reproductively isolated from the
parental strains and become new species. Polyploid animals are very rare (202).

*Unlike animals, plants live in a cloud of potentially
fertilizing pollen. In most cases nothing comes of it,
but if hybridization does occur, the two sets of
chromosomes may be so different that at the time of
meiosis the chromosomes cannot pair off acceptably
and no fertile gamete develops. However, if a
"mistake" occurs at meiosis, such that the chromosomes double but the cell fails to divide, a tetraploid
cell results. Meiosis at this stage can produce two
fertile tetraploid gametes (197).*

MECHANISMS OF ATROPHY

Two options are available to an organ that must shrink; it can reduce the number of its cells by cell deletion or the size of its cells by shrinkage. The modality depends mainly on the type of tissue.

CELL DELETION

Deletion is indeed a peculiar phenomenon. Certain cells are somehow picked out as obsolete and are induced to commit suicide. Virchow, who considered the body as a democratic cell-state in which each individual has its function, might have had some difficulty in justifying this ruthless arrangement, which occurs also physiologically as **programmed cell death** (p. 205). Histologically, in an organ undergoing atrophy, cell deletion requires attentive searching because the cells disap-

Table 2.5
Causes of Atrophy
Decreased function
Starvation
Reduced blood flow
Local pressure
Occlusion of secretory ducts
Hormonal effects
Old age
Denervation
Toxic agents, drugs
X-rays
Immunologic mechanisms

TO SUM UP: We have learned that cells respond to a variety of stimuli by becoming larger; when these stimuli disappear the cells return to their standard size, but in some cases they can make the enlargement permanent by becoming polyploid. We have also learned that hypertrophic cells, tissues, and organs may have built-in liabilities: bigger is not necessarily better.

Atrophy

Atrophy is an acquired decrease in size of cells, tissues, or organs. In ancient Greece *a-trophía* meant lack of food. Starvation is indeed the most obvious cause of atrophy, but there are at least 10 others (Table 2.5).

A few bits of necessary jargon: if an organ or tissue is congenitally underdeveloped the proper term is **hypoplasia. Aplasia** means that an organ has never developed at all (e.g., aplasia of the left kidney) or that its cells have ceased to multiply (e.g., aplasia of the bone marrow in aplastic anemia). **Involution** overlaps atrophy; it applies to the normal, programmed shrinkage of certain organs such as the uterus after childbirth, the thymus in early life, and temporary fetal organs such as the pro- and mesonephros. Do not confuse atrophy with **atresia,** literally translated as "no-orifice," which refers to congenital imperforation (e.g., atresia of the anus or vagina).

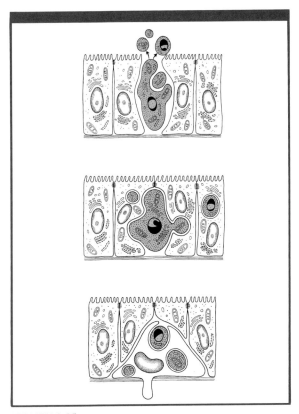

FIGURE 2.35
Apoptosis in an epithelium: a single cell dies and becomes detached from its neighbors; its rounded fragments (apoptotic bodies) can be extruded to the lumen (*top*), phagocytized by neighboring cells (*center*), or phagocytized by a marauding macrophage (*bottom*). How the macrophage is attracted to this site is not known; in some mucosae, occasional macrophages are found lying among the epithelial cells on the basement membrane. (Adapted from [92].)

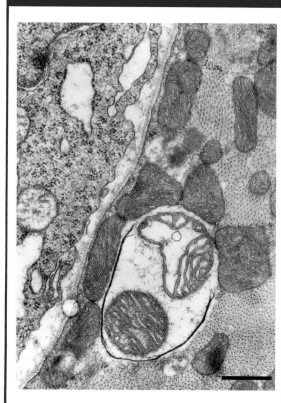

FIGURE 2.36
Autophagic vacuole in the leg muscle of a mouse 5 days after strenuous exercise (9 hours of running). **Bar** = 0.5 μm. (Reproduced from [70].)

pear quickly and without fanfare. They shrink and break up, and so do their nuclei, according to a ritual known as **apoptosis** (p. 200). If they line a free surface, their remains are cast off as apoptotic bodies; otherwise they are swiftly removed by macrophages or by the very cells that hours before were friendly neighbors (Figure 2.35).

The death sentence—more correctly, the order to commit suicide—is somehow delivered to the various types of cells within a given organ in hierarchical order: the most specialized disappear first (e.g., secretory cells disappear before duct cells). The stroma, however, is spared, relatively, so in the end an atrophic organ may appear to contain too much connective tissue.

CELL SHRINKAGE

The second option available to an organ that must decrease its size is to make each of its cells shrink. This mechanism works, but it has limits because most cellular organelles are essential for survival; however, some can be trimmed down, at least those that do not perform a function essential to the cell itself. This is best seen in striated muscle; its cells are huge because they contain a vast amount of fibrillar material, which they can lose

without dying, although their specific function, of course, will be affected.

A cell can shrink by **self-digestion;** that is, it accelerates its normal catabolic mechanisms, of which two are known: (a) chunks of cytoplasm including membrane-bound organelles are removed by autophagocytosis and digested in vacuoles by lysosomal enzymes; (b) proteins and other macromolecules are digested diffusely throughout the cell by free, nonlysosomal hydrolases. The latter process is thought to be the most important pathway.

Autophagic vacuoles These busy and still rather mysterious little bodies were discovered in 1962 (206) in liver cells, where they are prominent also under normal circumstances. They are membrane bound and usually contain one or more semidigested cellular organelles. They can form amazingly fast, within 5 minutes or so (264). A tongue-shaped process seems to arise out of nowhere (but probably from the endoplasmic reticulum) (259, 271), curves spoonlike around a little island of cytoplasm, surrounding it completely, and imprisons whatever organelles happen to be within (230, 279, 289) (Figure 2.36). Primary lysosomes are sometimes seen fusing with autophagic vacuoles (Figure 2.37).

As autodigestion advances, the content of the vacuole is dissolved and presumably reutilized. However, some of the lipid seems to be difficult to digest; it becomes denser and darker and eventu-

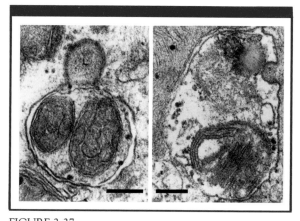

FIGURE 2.37
Autophagic vacuoles in rat myocardium. *Left:* Two mitochondria have been segregated for destruction; at the top, a lysosome (**L**) seems to be fusing with the autophagosome. *Right:* More advanced stage of digestion. The content includes a semidigested mitochondrion. **Bars** = 0.2 μm. (Reproduced from [23], by permission of Dr. U. Pfeifer.)

ally forms brownish granules called **lipofuscin** (p. 97). The few autophagic vacuoles that are condemned to remain stuffed with this undigestible material are called **residual bodies,** spent autophagosomes containing the remains of spent organelles. Residual bodies seem to be the internal garbage cans in which cells dump all the material that they are unable to digest or excrete (Figure 2.38). They can be numerous enough to give an atrophic organ a brownish hue, especially in the liver and heart, hence the term **brown atrophy.** The same discoloration can be induced at a slower rate by the normal process of aging.

Single electron micrographs cannot do justice to the extraordinarily active behavior of autophagic vacuoles in their normal task of organelle turnover. They may account for as much as 50 percent of mitochondrial turnover in the liver. Considering that a liver cell has some 2000 mitochondria and that about 5 percent per day are taken in by autophagic vacuoles, we can say that about four mitochondria have to be digested per cell per hour. The job is performed very fast: the half-life of the autophagic vacuoles is of the order of 8 or 9 minutes, with some difference according to the organelle engulfed (261, 265). Clearly there is plenty of work for the autophagic vacuoles even in the absence of atrophy.

Several mysteries remain about autophagic vacuoles. For example, what makes them entrap this or that organelle and never the nucleus? They certainly have no horror of DNA because there is some in the mitochondria that they happily devour. Incidentally, no genetic harm is done by destroying some of the mitochondria, because the DNA is identical in each mitochondrion, as it is in each bacterium of a given species.

Autophagic vacuoles increase in number in muscle after strenuous exercise (276) (Figure 2.36). Experimentally they can be rapidly induced in the liver by glucagon, a catabolic agent (206, 279); by isoproterenol, a beta-adrenergic stimulant (265); and by antimicrotubule agents such as vinblastine and colchicine (271). In the liver they can be produced in such numbers that they can be isolated by cell fractionation (214). Their number is reduced by insulin, an anticatabolic hormone (264, 265), and during hypertrophy (226). For reasons unknown, they have a circadian rhythm (262).

The other mechanism of cell shrinkage, working side-by-side with the autophagic vacuoles, is provided by several **nonlysosomal, cytosolic proteolytic systems** (209, 223, 235, 238, 252,

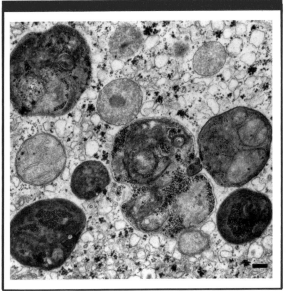

FIGURE 2.38 Autophagic vacuoles and residual bodies rapidly forming in a liver cell during acute atrophy induced by ligation of a branch of the portal vein. The recognizable content of the vacuoles includes glycogen and mitochondria. **Bar** = 0.2 μm. (Reproduced from [38], by permission of Dr. U. Pfeifer.)

253). The existence of these systems can be inferred just by looking at the electron micrograph of a muscle undergoing atrophy as bundles of fibrils break up and disappear without any evidence of lysosomal attack. The best known of these systems depends on a marvelous 76-residue polypeptide so widespread in nature that it is called **ubiquitin** (p. 177, 195). Ubiquitin combines covalently with proteins that are to be removed and targets them for destruction by free proteases. *The mechanism requires ATP and probably accounts for most of the intracellular protein turnover.*

Among the structures that can be disassembled without lysosomal intervention are the microtubules; this is how cilia are dismantled. The disappearance of cilia has been studied extensively in protozoa and other lower organisms, but little is known for humans, although the loss of cilia from bronchial epithelium affects millions of smokers. Figure 2.39 illustrates the surprising variety of mechanisms whereby cilia are lost in lower organisms (216).

Generally, the enzymes of an atrophic cell tend to decrease (Figure 2.40) (292); however, while striated muscle undergoes atrophy, acid phosphatase increases (273). This is not a contradiction. Acid phosphatase is the hallmark of lysosomes, which become temporarily more active in a self-digesting cell.

ATROPHY AND THE EXTRACELLULAR MATERIALS

Although not alive, *extracellular materials are not spared by atrophy because they depend in part on*

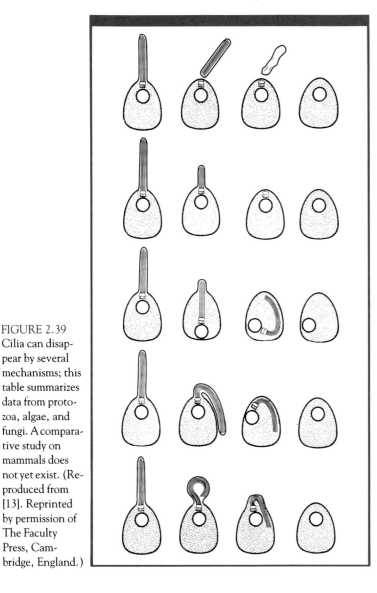

FIGURE 2.39
Cilia can disappear by several mechanisms; this table summarizes data from protozoa, algae, and fungi. A comparative study on mammals does not yet exist. (Reproduced from [13]. Reprinted by permission of The Faculty Press, Cambridge, England.)

cellular metabolism. Thus, in immobilized limbs the articular cartilage tends to lose its proteoglycans (p. 265), and even the ligaments lose strength and may take months to recover (204, 260). The most dramatic changes occur in bone because its extracellular materials are perpetually remodeling. If the balance between osteogenesis and osteoclasis is upset, the amount of tissue can increase or decrease strikingly.

Bone atrophy, commonly known as **osteoporosis** or **osteopenia,** is an enormous public health problem in the United States (at least 1.2 million fractures per year) (Figure 2.41). The slow, age-related osteoporosis is due to reduced bone formation, and the postmenopausal accelerated osteoporosis to an increase in osteoclasts. Because a major stimulus to bone formation is mechanical stress, bone atrophy is a problem for bedridden patients and astronauts (245). In a heroic 36-week experiment on bedridden volunteers, the total calcium loss amounted to 4.2 percent of the body's store (229).

Remember, however, that there is no such thing as bone decalcification, though the expression still recurs in clinical settings. No matter how atrophic, bone never loses its calcium; the loss of opacity to X-rays represents loss of bone mass.

CAUSES OF ATROPHY

Cells and tissues can be induced to shrink by a surprising variety of agents; eleven are discussed here.

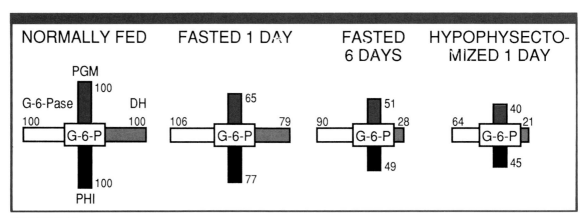

FIGURE 2.40
Atrophy at the level of enzymes: reduced activity of four enzymes involved in the utilization of glucose-6-phosphate (G-6-P) under various conditions (expressed as percent of normal). **G-6-Pase:** Glucose-6-phosphatase; **PHI:** phospho-hexose-isomerase; **DH:** glucose-6-phosphate dehydrogenase; **PGM:** phosphoglucomutase. (From Weber, G. Pathology of glucose-6-phosphate metabolism. A study in enzyme pathology. *Rev. Can. Biol.*, 18:245–282, 1959.)

(1) Decreased Function As everyone knows, decreased function causes organs to atrophy. The process can occur very fast. When a fractured limb is placed in a plaster cast, for example, the muscles shrink in a matter of days. However, this atrophy has two components: inactivity and trauma (207). **Inactivity** accelerates protein catabolism; in a striated muscle isolated *in vitro*, protein breakdown can be reduced by passive mechanical stretching and by electrical stimulation (234)—facts that are clinically applied in physiotherapy. The **trauma** itself—more precisely, *the very fact of having sustained an injury— brings about a general reaction that speeds up the catabolism of muscle* (p. 491).

Experiments on three volunteers with both lower limbs immobilized in plaster casts showed that a negative nitrogen balance appeared (despite an adequate diet) after 5 days (277). The data suggest that protein synthesis was reduced while breakdown continued.

The popular notion that the function makes the organ is strikingly illustrated by experiments on the eye. If one eyelid of a kitten is kept closed for the first 3–4 months of its life, the central visual pathways do not develop properly (in this case, however, we are dealing with hypoplasia rather than atrophy) (280, 282). That darkness should affect the visual cortex is perhaps not too surprising, but it is somewhat startling that in hamsters it should cause atrophy of the *testes*. The mechanism is hormonal and operates through the hypophysis. But male readers need not worry. This happens, it seems, in hamsters only (237).

(2) Starvation This topic echoes grim circumstances (Table 2.6). Compared with other organs the brain is the least susceptible of all organs to atrophy, as measured by changes in weight (285, 297). This means only that the nutritionally starved adult brain is protected from gross atrophy; however, biochemical changes do occur (283), and *starvation during growth can lead to permanent brain damage* (210, 267, 270).

In contrast, the effects of starvation on the adipocytes (energy-storing cells) are great. As triglycerides are depleted, the cells shrink drastically (296); the same can happen during the ketotic phase of diabetes (219, 221) (Figure 2.42). Oddly enough, the fat cells in some areas are affected more than others; the mechanism is not

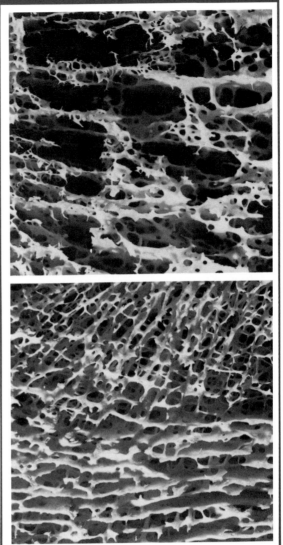

FIGURE 2.41 Atrophic (osteopenic) and normal human bone. Slices of vertebrae, washed clean of bone marrow, were bleached and dried. (Courtesy of Dr. C. Hedinger, Kantonsspital, Zurich, Switzerland.)

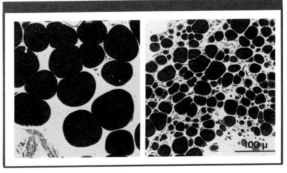

FIGURE 2.42
Atrophy of fat cells in acute experimental diabetes. *Left:* Control adipose tissue, blackened with osmium tetroxide (OsO_4). *Right:* 6 days after an intravenous injection of streptozotocin, which destroys the pancreatic beta cells: dramatic atrophy of the adipocytes. A similar result is produced by fasting. (Reproduced from [18], the *Journal of Cell Biology*, 1977, 104–117, by copyright permission of the Rockefeller University Press.)

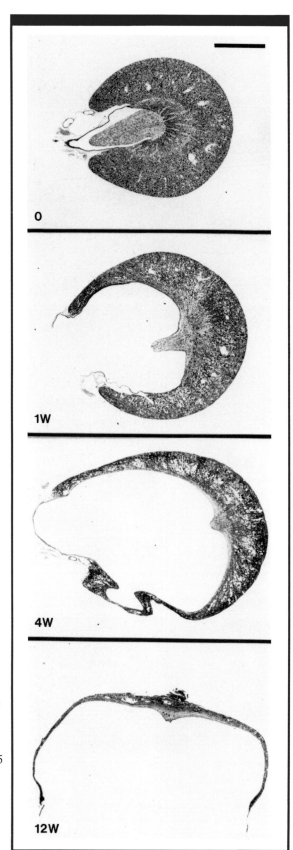

Table 2.6

Human Hunger Disease

ORGAN	WEIGHT RECORDED[a]	NORMAL VALUE[b]
Brain	1309	1310
Heart	220	275
Liver	865	1500–2000
Kidneys	226	305
Spleen	103	150–250

[a]Values in grams from 492 autopsies recorded at the Jewish Hospital in Warsaw during the 2½ years before the ghetto was overrun. The work was performed under heroic conditions; the manuscript survived because it was buried.
[b]Normal values quoted by the authors refer to a contemporary source; present values in grams would be heart 300–350, liver 1500, and spleen 150.
Slightly simplified from Stein, J., and Fenigstein, H. Pathological anatomy of hunger disease. In Winick, M. (ed.), Hunger Disease. New York, John Wiley & Sons, 1979, p. 220.

known, but this is merely one of many examples showing that cells of a given type are not identical throughout the body. Regional differences in the lipid content and behavior of adipocytes are well known (205).

(3) Prolonged Inadequacy of Blood Flow Chronic ischemia leads to atrophy of the blood-starved areas. Note the difference between a sudden stoppage of flow, which promptly kills the blood-starved tissue, and a partial but prolonged inadequacy of flow, which leads to tissue atrophy. A classic example is the kidneys of people who suffer from sclerosis (hardening) of the renal arterioles. The nephrons supplied by these arterioles slowly shrink, leaving a shallow depression on the surface of the kidney; the presence of many such areas gives the surface a granular aspect.

(4) Local Pressure Growing tumors or other swellings can cause local pressure. The surface of a cerebral hemisphere may become deeply indented by a slow-growing meningeal tumor, leading to the atrophy of a large mass of brain tissue. The mechanism is certainly due (in part) to reduced blood flow. Mild, persistent pressure on a bone surface can cause the surface to recede as if it were made of a plastic material. Before the days of thoracic surgery, an aneurysm of the thoracic aorta (an outpouching that develops when the aortic wall is weakened) could press against the sternum, gnaw its way through it, and appear beneath the skin as a pulsating mass (see Figure 1.2).

Bone does behave like a malleable material, but this plasticity must be understood in a biological, rather than physical sense; it occurs over weeks and months by a slow process of remodeling. Constant local pressure somehow stimulates the osteoclasts. Pressure from a tumor acts in this fashion; prostaglandin E_2 secreted by tumor cells may be the stimulant (269).

(5) Occlusion of a Duct In exocrine glands, occlusion causes the glandular cells to stop secreting; ultimately they commit suicide and disappear by apoptosis. For example, if one ureter is occluded, the kidney continues to produce urine for a short time; urinary pressure rises, and there is a great dilatation of the urinary pathways above the occlusion, while the kidney itself becomes atrophic and eventually becomes almost paper-thin (233) (Figure 2.43). In mouse kidneys, the tubules may disappear in 12 weeks (218). The tubular epithelial cells disappear by apoptosis (Figure 2.44). In general, the pressure within occluded ducts rises, then falls; the longer the period of obstruction, the greater the effects. *The testis seems to be a partial exception.* After ligation of the vas deferens, the pressure within the seminiferous tubules rises little or not at all. Correspondingly, atrophy is not progressive, which is why vasectomy can be successfully reversed after 10 years (243) (Figure 2.45).

Exocrine glands in general are very sensitive to duct ligation (Figure 2.46). In the rat, 31 days after the duct of the submaxillary gland is occluded, the secretory cells have become atrophic and stop secreting; they retain the capacity to regenerate if the occlusion is removed, although after 180 days they have not yet fully recovered (286). In this model, the changes induced by ligation resemble those brought on by starvation. In the pancreas, ligation of the main duct leads to the slow disappearance of the exocrine component alone, by cell deletion (290); in the end the pancreas becomes a mass of connective tissue containing the larger ducts and intact islets of Langerhans (Figure 2.47). This principle led to the discovery of insulin.

One evening in 1920 in London, Ontario, while preparing a lecture for medical students, F.G. Banting came across a paper reporting that a pancreatic stone in a patient had blocked the main duct, causing atrophy of the exocrine pancreas but

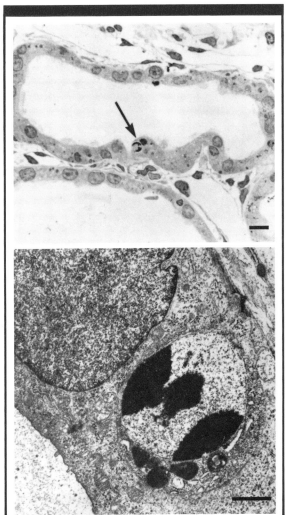

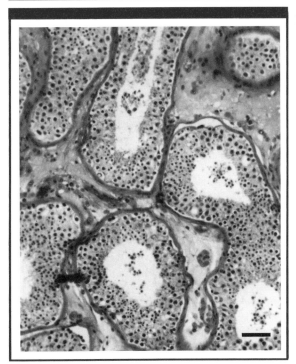

FIGURE 2.44 *Top:* Cell deletion by apoptosis in the tubular epithelium of a kidney undergoing atrophy 7 days after ligation of the ureter. Arrow points to the typical condensation and margination of the nuclear chromatin. **Bar** = 10 μm. *Bottom:* Electron microscopic aspect of a typical apoptotic body: a fragment of condensed nuclear material phagocytized by a neighboring, viable epithelial cell. **Bar** = 1 μm. (Reproduced from [29], © by the U.S. and Canadian Academy of Pathology, Inc.)

FIGURE 2.45 Biopsy of a human testis 10 years after vasectomy in a 35-year-old man. Spermatogenesis is reduced, but all the various cellular elements in the tubular wall are preserved. This lack of atrophy after ligation of the secretory duct is characteristic of the testes. **Bar** = 50 μm. (Reproduced from [39]. Reprinted by permission of *The New England Journal of Medicine,* 313:1252–1256, 1985.)

FIGURE 2.46
Effect of obstructing the duct of a parotid gland in the rat. *Left:* Normal control. *Center:* One week after obstruction there is significant loss of acinar cells. *Right:* Four weeks after obstruction, the acini have disappeared; the gland is reduced to collecting ducts in a bed of connective tissue. These changes are accompanied by a reduction in the capillary bed. (Reproduced from [85]. Reprinted by permission of John Wiley & Sons, Ltd.)

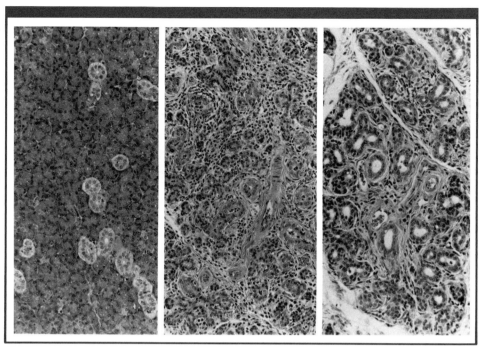

sparing the islets. Suddenly he saw an answer to his problem: he was trying to obtain a pure preparation of islets, to extract their endocrine secretion. He promptly tried ligating the pancreatic duct in dogs, and it worked. Later it turned out that the ligation was unnecessary, but he and his student assistant, Charles Best, won the Nobel prize anyway (215).

(6) Hormones Hormones are a common cause of atrophy, despite their name, which means "stimulators." Common targets of hormonal atrophy are the endocrine glands themselves. *The best way to shut down and to atrophy an endocrine gland is to supply it with its own hormone.* This fact can be put to practical use. For example, some people are at an increased risk of developing cancer of the thyroid because their thyroid was irradiated "incidentally" in childhood. It was fashionable at one time to prescribe X-rays on the neck for enlarged tonsils, whooping cough, and other conditions. The best way to reduce the proliferative activity of the thyroid follicles in such cases is to administer small doses of L-thyroxine (257).

Another mechanism of endocrine-induced atrophy is absence of a trophic hormone. Hypophysectomy leads to adrenal atrophy, which can be reversed, up to a point, with ACTH (288).

(7) Old Age Aging is, of course, a much broader problem than atrophy, but it does include atrophy at many levels. There is a total decrease in body mass after the age of 45–55, with a relative increase of body fat and a well-documented decrease in weight of the brain, liver, kidneys, and spleen (217). The immune system becomes less responsive (293).

The mechanism of senescence is being studied intensively but is still far from being understood (224, 227, 240, 250, 255). The notion of a limit to life brings the Hayflick number to mind (p. 30), but senescence is probably much more complex a problem than running out of mitoses. One way to look at senescence would be to consider it the ultimate step in differentiation (241). Among the many other theories of aging, a popular one blames somatic mutations that result in a progressive accumulation of errors in informational macromolecules until the system can no longer function (247). The errors could be due to free radical damage. The free radical hypothesis (239) is supported by many facts; for example, antioxidants increase the life-spans of many species—from yeast, worms, and mosquitoes (272) to mice, rats, and guinea pigs (256). Recent studies on senescent human fibroblasts showed a progressive shift in gene expression, including the repression of c-*fos*, which is essential for proliferation; it follows that cellular senescence could be a process of terminal differentiation (278). In other words, senescence would not be the result of accidents or errors but of programming. Which sounds very likely.

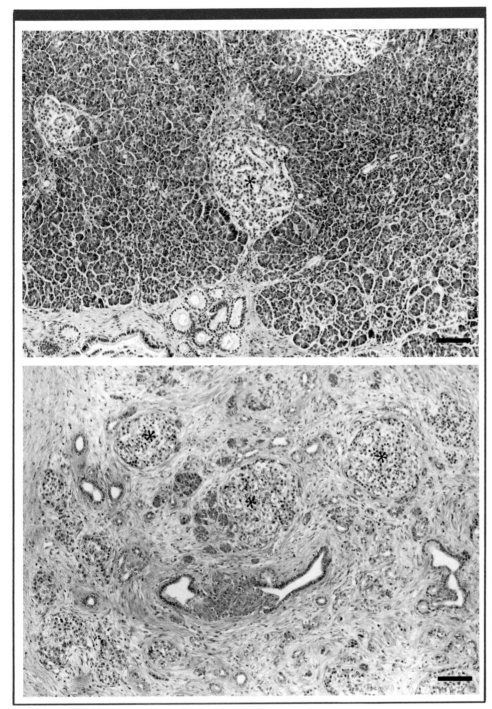

FIGURE 2.47
Top: Normal human pancreas. •: Islet of Langerhans. *Bottom:* Atrophic human pancreas after long-standing obliteration of the main duct. The exocrine pancreas has largely disappeared; the islets (•) have survived and appear closer together. **Bars =** 100 μm.

Senescence is inevitable, and the life-span is fixed. However, at the end of this section on atrophy the reader will find some good news: there *is* a way to prolong life. Quite a simple way.

(8) Denervation Removal of the nerve supply has different effects depending on the type of nerve and end organ. **Motor nerve denervation** has drastic effects on striated muscle (Figure 2.48).

Apparently the nerves supply their target organs with some trophic material; its nature is not clear, but the trophic interaction may be mutual (268). As to **sensory nerve denervation,** for reasons unknown the effects are pronounced only on the hand and to a lesser degree on the foot; the mitotic rate of the epidermis drops, the skin becomes thinner (atrophic) and scaly, and the nails become coarse and brittle (281). An

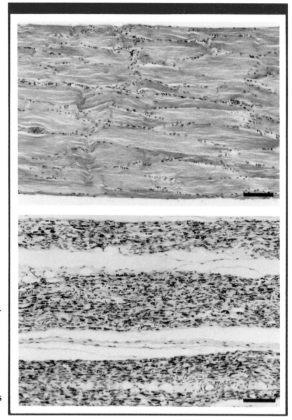

FIGURE 2.48 *Top:* Single bundle of normal human striated muscle fibers (control). *Bottom:* Extreme atrophy of striated muscle in a long-standing paraplegic. Each of the 3 bundles shown was originally about the size of the control. **Bars** = 100 μm.

(9) Toxic Agents and Drugs Specific tissues, such as the testis, are induced to atrophy by specific substances (244). Bone marrow is a sensitive and frequent target (249). Some drugs induce atrophy by causing selected cells to undergo apoptosis.

For readers who enjoy puzzles: chronic intoxication of rats with selenium was said to cause atrophy of the left liver lobe and hypertrophy of the right liver lobe (220). Bizarre as this may be, there is a plausible explanation. Selenium is absorbed by the gut in such a way that it drains preferentially into the left lobe, which shrinks, while the right lobe increases by compensatory hypertrophy.

(10) X-Rays X-rays induce atrophy of many tissues, but at the level of cells their effects are complicated, a mixture of direct cellular damage, including cell death, and indirect effects by microcirculatory damage (202, 242, 284) (Figure 2.49). Another peculiar effect has been called reproductive cell death, in which the cells survive but lose their ability to divide; sometimes they form multinucleated giant cells (p. 207).

(11) Immunologic Mechanisms In pernicious anemia, the gastric mucosa becomes atrophic. The loss of parietal cells in this typical atrophic gastritis is attributed to an autoimmune attack, and autoantibodies against parietal cells can often be demonstrated. Another mechanism of immunologic atrophy is the overactivation of suppressor T lymphocytes; aplastic anemia can arise in this manner (300).

IS ATROPHY REVERSIBLE?

Atrophy is reversible up to a point, but as months and years go by hopes of recovery fade. Muscle fibers can recover from denervation atrophy if the nerve is repaired within 3–5 weeks; longer intervals imply loss of function, and after 20–24 months nerve repair is useless because the fibers are atrophied almost beyond recognition (Figure 2.48). Ultimately, in advanced atrophy, the parenchymal cells tend to disappear and to be replaced by connective tissue (or by astrocytes in the brain).

Is Atrophy Treatable? *Atrophy is best treated by early removal of its cause.* It has been suggested that protease inhibitors, by decreasing protein catabolism, might slow down the pace of atrophy (248). Seemingly hopeless cases of atrophy may be

intriguing observation is that in paraplegic and tetraplegic patients, wounds below the level of spinal denervation do have more complications than expected (212).

Complete sympathetic denervation can be obtained by chemically treating newborn animals with 6-hydroxydopamine. It has been said that such denervation has metabolic effects on arteries (231). The surgical sympathetic denervation of arteries, a procedure used to obtain vasodilatation and thus increased flow, leads to structural changes in the arterial wall that mimic, interestingly, those of old age (232). Sympathetic denervation of the major salivary glands induces atrophy; in perirenal fat it does not cause atrophy but leads, surprisingly, to metaplasia from yellow to brown fat (p. 55). The paradox of bladder hypertrophy by denervation (neurogenic bladder) occurs in paraplegics because the connections between the bladder and the brain are interrupted; the bladder becomes overfilled, but the sphincter receives no message to relax. Evacuation occurs only by overflow. Under such conditions the smooth muscle is stretched and becomes hypertrophic.

retrievable some day. Baldness in adult males is due to atrophy of hair follicles (246), which until recently had eluded all cures. Accidentally, it was found that an antihypertensive agent, minoxidil, has the side effect of causing the hair to grow back—sometimes.

STARVATION AND THE PROLONGATION OF LIFE

Here comes the really good news: *a moderate degree of food restriction can increase the life-span by about 50 percent* (294). This is the only known method for extending the life-span of warm-blooded animals (225, 299). It works even for spiders (208) (Figure 2.50), for paramecia (274), and in fact for all the animals that have been tested (266). Experimentally it delays many conditions associated with aging, such as skin problems, loss of fertility (213), many chronic diseases (254), senile cataracts (287), cancers, and the decline of T-lymphocyte function (295). It even protects rats against kidney damage (251) and rabbits against myocardial infarcts (228). The basic premise, let this be clear, is *undernutrition but without malnutrition.*

Why undernutrition should be so beneficial is not clear. Whatever the mechanism may be, it must be important for survival because evolution has preserved it in animals from single cells up. "Reduced use of the genetic code" has been suggested (211).

Primates have not yet been tested, but all indications are that the principle should work also for humans (294). The path has been shown. Who will take the first step?

The argument in favor of undernutrition can be stretched even further. It has been reported that famine can have protective effects, which are abolished by feeding (258). This paradox has been observed for centuries; in recent times, a study among natives of Niger has shown that cerebral malaria selected undernourished children *after they were refed.* The protective mechanism of starvation may be related to iron deficiency since many parasites, including those of malaria, thrive in an excess of free iron (236). We will see later that one of the body's standard responses to injury is to make iron *less* available (p. 492). Evolution may have preserved this response to starvation as a protection during hard times.

TO SUM UP: Atrophy, more often than hypertrophy, is linked with disease; it is also linked with

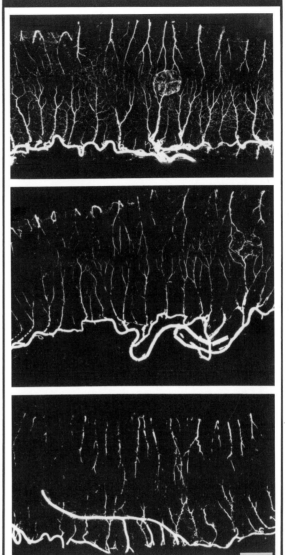

FIGURE 2.49 Effect of X-rays on the microcirculation. Microangiographs of rat duodenum 1 day after various X-ray exposures. *Top:* No exposure, normal. *Center:* After exposure to 1000 R. *Bottom:* After exposure to 1460 R. Note the progressively decreased filling of the finer vessels. **Bar** = 100 μm. (Reprinted from Casarett, G.W. *Radiation Histopathology*, vol. I. Copyright © 1981 CRC Press, Inc., Boca Raton, FL.)

senescence. In recent times the study of atrophy has taught us three valuable lessons. At the whole-body level it has revealed that leanness is an excellent survival formula, as the Spartans seem to have known (258). At the cellular level, it taught us that cells can shrink by the strange phenomenon of autophagocytosis. It also taught us that organs forced to shrink beyond a certain point do so by deleting some of their cells, and this led to the discovery of apoptosis, a modality of cell death not previously recognized, which is now hailed as a biological event of major significance (p. 200). One wonders why this very obvious phenomenon was not discovered before; presumably because

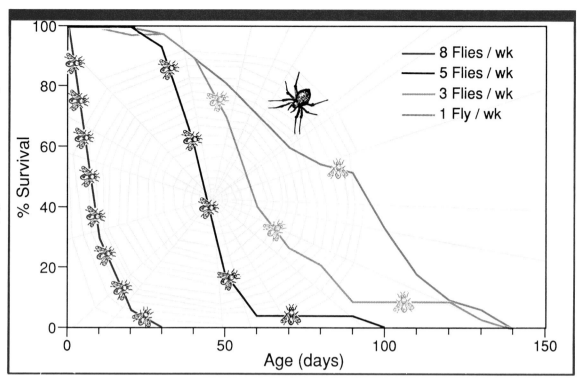

FIGURE 2.50 The prolongation of life by dietary restriction applies also to the spider *Frontinella pyramitela.* In free-living spiders on a rich diet of eight flies per week, the average life-span is 30 days. In captured spiders on an austerity diet of one to three flies per week, the life-span increases to 140 days. (Adapted from [24].)

atrophy seemed like a very dull subject for study— not likely to be funded.

Phenotypic Changes

Phenotypic changes in response to the environment are common in people as well as in cells. Human beings can adapt reversibly by developing a suntan, growing a beard, or changing profession; cells can switch genes on and off, change shape, alter their function. These cellular adaptations are important; they are just beginning to be studied at the level of gene expression.

What types of changes can occur and how do they occur? The terminology in this field is still in a state of flux (303, 304, 325). Pathologists have long used *metaplasia* to mean the replacement of one cell type by another of a different type. Cell biologists added *modulation* for mild changes observed in cultures; recently they added *transdifferentiation*, which overlaps metaplasia (332). There was little need for this new seven-syllable monster; wherever it is used, metaplasia will do just as well. While the biologists work at better definitions, we will use our own working terminology, which will enable readers to communicate with all persons involved:

- **Modulation** refers to mild, reversible phenotypic changes often observed in cell cultures (somewhat reminiscent of a chameleon changing from green to brown).
- **Indirect metaplasia** means that cells of one phenotype are eliminated and replaced by cells of a different phenotype. This can happen when precursor cells switch to producing a different type of progeny. This sequence is well proven in epithelia.
- **Direct metaplasia (transdifferentiation)** implies that a differentiated cell turns into a wholly different type of cell (as if a chameleon started to croak and turned into a frog). In adult vertebrates this mechanism is at most very rare.

MODULATION

Modulation as we have defined it can probably occur in any kind of cell in a matter of hours and does not require cell division. Modulated cells are not pathologic; they are temporarily adapted to different needs or to different stimuli, and *they remain recognizable as members of their cell type.* A smooth muscle cell, for instance, may modulate by increasing its synthetic apparatus and decreasing its contractile machinery, but it remains recognizable as a smooth muscle cell (340).

Modulation is the daily concern of tissue culture experts, who are constantly bewildered by the variations of their favorite cells when the conditions are slightly altered. Thus, the best-documented modulations occur to cells in culture, which can be monitored hour by hour. Endothelial cells, for example, are naturally programmed either to cover large surfaces (as in the aorta) or to form little tubes (as in capillaries). If they are grown *in vitro* on a surface coated with collagen, they form a continuous sheet; if at that point they are sandwiched beneath another layer of collagen, they modulate into little tubes (Figure 2.51) (338). Studies of this kind are teaching a great deal about the mechanisms of morphogenesis: *cells modulate in response to soluble factors (e.g., vitamins and cytokines) (324) or to the nature of the substrate* (312, 333, 337).

Other examples of modulation are offered by smooth muscle cells and fibroblasts; both cells have contractile as well as synthetic functions and can be modulated to express one or the other to a greater degree. **Fibroblasts** are in some respects the mirror image of smooth muscle cells. They are equipped mainly for synthesis, but they also possess contractile machinery, which tends to hypertrophy in culture. They can also be induced to increase their contractile machinery *in vivo* and to modulate into myofibroblasts, which explains the once mysterious phenomenon of connective tissue contraction in wounds and other pathologic conditions (p. 472). Myofibroblasts can modulate further into subtypes, probably under the influence of cytokines (349). **Smooth muscle cells** are specialized for contraction, but they also manufacture collagen, elastin, and glycosaminoglycans. In culture they can be made to emphasize reversibly either their synthetic or their contractile apparatus—for example, by adding heparin (308, 328). These two conditions of smooth muscle cells have been called **synthetic mode** and **contractile mode;** however, there is no evidence that the contractility is lost and regained in the process. Endothelial cells can modulate from the continuous to the fenestrated variety in many pathologic conditions (323, 329).

METAPLASIA

Metaplasia is recognized under the microscope when *a differentiated tissue of one kind is replaced by a differentiated tissue of another kind.*

Theoretically, the possibilities of metaplasia

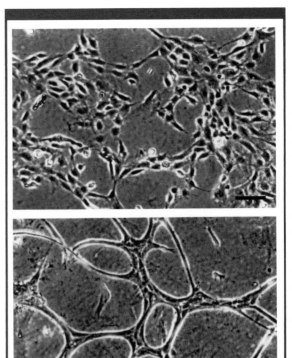

FIGURE 2.51 Example of modulation. *Top:* Capillary endothelial cells grown on a collagen gel. *Bottom:* The same culture, 2 days after it has been overlaid with a second layer of collagen. The cells have now formed a network of cords; some of these are hollow and represent early capillary formation. **Bars** = 100 μm. (37, reproduced from the *Journal of Cell Biology,* 1983, 97:1648–1652, by copyright permission of the Rockefeller University Press.)

may seem almost infinite because each cell has a full complement of genetic information, and any repressed gene might conceivably be derepressed (311). In practice, the rules of the game are more strict. In adult mammals *metaplasia occurs within varieties of epithelium and within varieties of mesenchyme;* there is no proven metaplasia across germ layers (e.g., from bone to nerve) or from a connective tissue (mesenchyme) to epithelium. However, embryonic cells have greater possibilities, as we will see, and so do the amphibians. Future progress in the manipulation of gene expression may hold some surprises.

Could there ever be metaplasia from epithelium to connective tissue or vice versa? The evidence is minimal; it is said that retinal pigment epithelium can give rise to fibroblasts as a result of injury (339). Remember also that the epithelium of the kidney tubules does derive from embryonic mesenchyme (312). In the plant kingdom, instances of major genetic reprogramming are routine: a somatic cell can be coaxed into reproducing a whole tree. In mammals, there is one well-documented case of

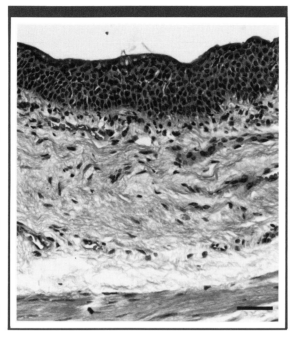

FIGURE 2.52
Squamous metaplasia in the bronchus of a smoker: the normal cylindrical, ciliated epithelium is replaced by a multilayered epithelium resembling the epidermis. The lack of cilia interrupts the outflow of mucus. **Bar** = 50 μm.

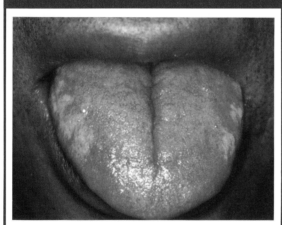

FIGURE 2.53
Patches of leukoplakia on the margin of the tongue in a heavy smoker. (Courtesy of Dr. R. Johnson, Department of Dermatology, Harvard Community Health Plan, Cambridge, MA.)

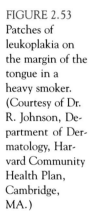

FIGURE 2.54
Histological aspect of leukoplakia. The superficial cells have become keratinized but retain their nuclei, a phenomenon called *parakeratosis*. (Courtesy of M.J. Imber, Dermatopathology Division, Massachusetts General Hospital, Boston, MA.)

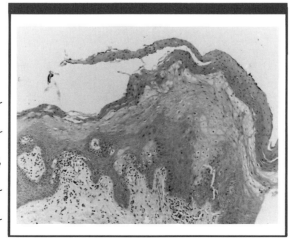

metaplasia from embryonic striated muscle into cartilage, induced in vitro by demineralized bone (341).

EXAMPLES OF METAPLASIA

Metaplasia occurs in cells that can replicate; it is not known to occur in adult striated muscle cells and in neurons.

Epithelial Metaplasia Epithelial metaplasia is common on surface linings, presumably because they are more exposed to insults. For example, in the bronchi of a smoker, patches of the normal columnar ciliated epithelium may be replaced by a squamous stratified epithelium (**squamous metaplasia**), sometimes even keratinized (**epidermoid metaplasia**) (331) (Figure 2.52). If the left nostril of a rabbit is closed by a suture, the respiratory epithelium on the right side will undergo metaplasia to stratified squamous; on the left it becomes mucus-secreting (316). Gland ducts can also undergo epidermoid metaplasia, especially in the pancreas; the stimulus may be chronic inflammation or vitamin A deficiency. On the tongue and in the esophagus of a smoker, the epithelium may become thicker and excessively keratinized, forming whitish plaques quite obvious to the naked eye; this is **leukoplakia,** equivalent to the smoker's patches described in 1870 by James Paget (350) (Figure 2.53). Similar patches—but not related to smoking—are common in the cervix. The histology of leukoplakia is shown in Figure 2.54.

Glandular Metaplasia In grandular metaplasia, a flat, nonsecreting epithelium is replaced by secretory epithelium or by glands. This is sometimes seen in the ureters and bladder (325), but the commonest example is found in the lower esophagus: through a malfunction of the cardia, gastric juice may flow back into the esophagus. In the long run, erosions develop and become lined by metaplastic epithelium of the gastric or intestinal type. These metaplastic patches are commonly known as Barrett's epithelium (314) (p. 875).

The digestive tract, with its many varieties of epithelium and its propensity to become eroded and to regenerate quickly, is a favorite site of metaplasia. In the stomach, patches of epithelium with the features of intestinal lining (**intestinal metaplasia**) are common (327); they include endocrine cells typical of the small intestine (305).

Connective Tissue Metaplasia This type of metaplasia is little understood but offers some striking examples:

- **Metaplasia of connective tissue to bone.** This is commonplace in atherosclerotic arteries as part of a sequence: calcification → ossification → bone marrow formation, truly a chain metaplasia. Metaplastic bone often develops in the connective tissue of muscles as a result of trauma (traumatic *myositis ossificans*), especially in young people, as athletes well know. A classic setting is that of a muscle bruised, for example, by the kick of a horse; a stone-hard mass develops under the bruise, visible in X-ray. Fortunately, such masses tend to disappear spontaneously by metaplasia in the reverse direction. For reasons totally unknown, metaplastic bone tends to form around the joints of some paraplegic patients (320); a bony shell can form around the knees in a few weeks. Metaplastic bone is sometimes found in scars, especially after abdominal operations.

- **Chondroid metaplasia.** Where metaplastic bone is formed, cartilage also tends to appear. Typically, when a long bone is broken and immobilized, it heals by means of a bony callus, but if the two ends are not properly immobilized, motion induces the formation of cartilage (Figure 2.55).

- **Myxoid metaplasia.** In the heart valves, the fibrous tissue can turn into myxoid (meaning mucoid) connective tissue of the embryonic type. This is usually and incorrectly referred to as myxoid degeneration: nothing at all is degenerating: there is just a change in cell type and cell secretion. This may be, in fact, an adaptive response to abnormal shear forces in the valve: we have seen myxoid metaplasia also in the so-called singer's nodules, which arise on vocal cords perhaps as a result of another type of shear: forced vibration. Heart valves with myxoid metaplasia tend to expand, so the cusps come to be shaped like parachutes (Figure 2.56).

- **Adipose tissue metaplasia.** The metaplasia of adipose tissue into brown fat may be hiding a jackpot of enormous dimensions. Here is a tale for entrepreneurial biologists.

The type of adipose tissue called brown fat is made of cells filled with a special variety of mitochondria (plus small droplets of fat); these mitochondria are able to consume energy to produce heat. They can do this thanks to a specific mitochondrial uncoupling protein (346), which uncouples oxidative phosphorylation and allows the respiring brown fat to become a "heat gland" (322). As may be expected in rats, this protein is produced in greater amount by exposure to the cold (306) (Figure 2.57). Now, brown fat is richly supplied with sympathetic nerves. If these nerves are severed, the brown fat turns into white fat (315); conversely, in patients bearing a pheochromo-

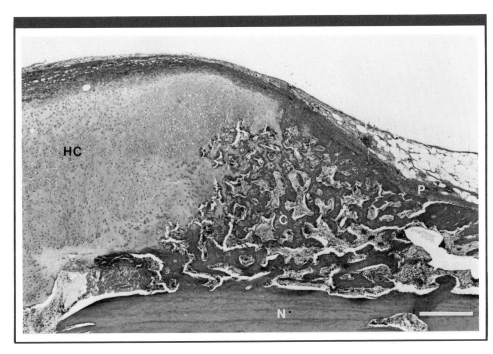

FIGURE 2.55
In a rabbit 21 days after a tibial fracture (not immobilized), a large callus (**C**) has developed over the necrotic tibial cortex (**N**). Most of the callus consists of bony trabeculae; however, a large mass of hyalin cartilage (**HC**) has also developed, probably in response to motion of the stumps. **P:** Periosteum. **Bar** = 500 μm.

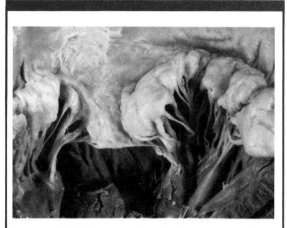

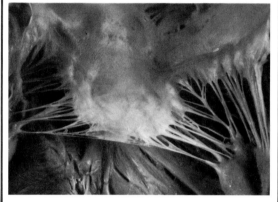

FIGURE 2.56
Result of myxoid metaplasia (usually called myxoid degeneration) of the mitral valve. *Top:* The leaflets of the valve give way under functional strain and tend to protrude, recalling the shape of a parachute (floppy valve syndrome). This anatomical prolapse of the valve results in functional insufficiency. *Bottom:* Normal mitral valve of a 22-year-old man. (Courtesy of Dr. W.D. Edwards, Mayo Clinic, Rochester, MN.)

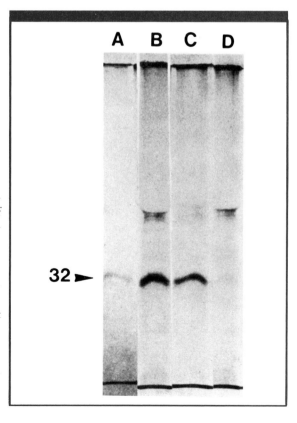

FIGURE 2.57
Gel demonstrating the presence of the 32-kD *uncoupling protein* of brown adipose tissue in control rats (lane **A**), in the brown fat of cold-exposed animals (lane **B**), and in brown fat of animals bearing a pheochromocytoma (lane **C**). Lane **D**: control. (Reproduced from [6].)

cytoma (*a tumor that secretes epinephrine and other catecholamines*), the perirenal fat may turn from white to brown (334). The same effects have been observed in rats (347). The change from white to brown fat is accompanied by the appearance of the typical uncoupling protein in the inner mitochondrial membrane. This seemingly academic observation is currently the object of intense interest. Imagine what would happen in overfed countries if someone discovered a harmless analog of epinephrine that would cause excess dietary calories to be burned up and released as heat rather than stored as fat.

MECHANISMS OF METAPLASIA

The basic event in metaplasia is that one cell type—we will call it Type A—is replaced by Type B. This can happen in two ways.

(1) Type A Turns Directly into Type B Actually, this is what Virchow thought when he chose the name metaplasia, which comes from the Greek verb *metaplássein*, "to cast into a new mold, to counterfeit" (303, 326). In the terminology we have adopted, we would call this *direct metaplasia* (Figure 2.58). Among mammalian cells this mechanism is thought to be extremely rare, but a couple of examples do exist. Aloe and Levi-Montalcini have shown that chromaffin cells of the neonatal rat adrenal medulla can be induced to sprout axons and to turn into neural cells; this was done by injecting nerve growth factor into pregnant rats, and then again for 10 days into the newborn rats (301). The same result was obtained *in vitro* (342). There may be another example of direct metaplasia *in vivo*: in the rat, if the aorta is partially constricted, the smooth muscle cells in the small arteries of the kidney were said to turn into endocrine cells of the juxtaglomerular type (304, 309).

Clear-cut examples of direct metaplasia occur among "lower" animals (which cannot be very low if they can do more than the higher ones). In the silk moth, during metamorphosis, cells that produced cuticle turn to secreting salt (343). In humans, some believe that fully differentiated bronchial mucus-secreting cells can turn into epidermoid cells, as Virchow suggested (354). It has also been pointed out that mammalian striated muscle fibers can easily change from the fast to the slow type (304), but we would call this a modulation.

A variant of direct metaplasia is that Type A undergoes one or more rounds of division and eventually turns into B. This process can be seen as a dedifferentiation of Type A followed by a

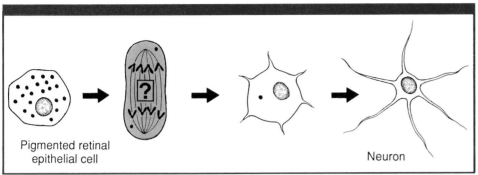

FIGURE 2.58
A rare mechanism of metaplasia, not proven beyond doubt in adult mammals. A mature cell is directly transformed into a totally different type of cell with or without an intervening mitosis.

reprogramming to Type B (343, 357). The propensity to follow this path (*in vitro*) is typical of eye tissues in amphibians and of eye tissues of vertebrate embryos (including humans). When cultured long enough, tissues as diverse as neural retina, pigmented epithelium, and lens cells can change into each other (343, 345). Why all this should happen in eye tissues is not known.

(2) Type A is Eliminated, and its Progenitors Produce Type B This reprogramming of stem cells is an accepted mechanism for epithelial metaplasia (Figure 2.59) (356). Basal, undifferentiated cells are known to exist in all epithelia. As for connective tissues, this line of thinking would suggest that bone metaplasia starts from (putative) undifferentiated connective tissue cells. Seen in this light, *metaplasia amounts to abnormal regeneration*, which fits with the fact that *metaplasia is often induced by stimuli that cause cell proliferation*, such as chemical or mechanical irritants (smoke, a dental prosthesis), hormones (335), or vitamins.

An example of metaplasia as abnormal regeneration is that in rats and hamsters, the pancreas can be

induced to regenerate by toxic agents, and some ductular cells give rise to liver cells (330).

SIGNALS THAT INDUCE METAPLASIA

Cells can be coaxed into metaplasia by the same two sets of signals that induce modulation: **soluble chemicals** *(hormones, vitamins, drugs) and the* **substrate** *on which the cells are growing* (318, 345). A role for vitamin A (retinoic acid) in epithelial metaplasia was demonstrated in 1928 by Wolbach and Howe (355) in their classic experiments on vitamin-A–deficient guinea pigs (Figure 2.60). Then, in 1953, metaplasia by vitamin A was produced *in vitro*. This experiment too became a classic because it explained the cellular mechanism of metaplastic cell replacement. In Cambridge, England, Dame Honor B. Fell and E. Mellanby (313) found that chick embryo ectoderm, maintained in organ culture with normal medium, produces normal skin epithelium (stratified, squamous, keratinizing). If excess vitamin A is added, keratinization is suppressed, and the basal cells give rise to a layer of mucus-secreting or ciliated cells. If the medium is changed again to normal, the basal cells produce a new layer of flat cells that undermine the

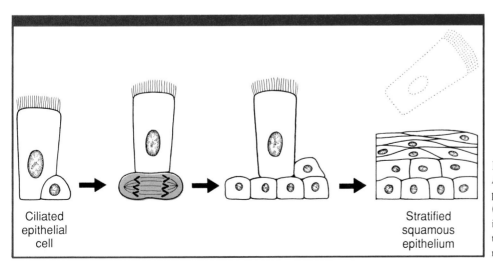

Ciliated epithelial cell

Stratified squamous epithelium

FIGURE 2.59
A mechanism of metaplasia well proven in epithelia. Reserve cells (stem cells) multiply, differentiate into a new phenotype, and displace the old cells. In essence, this is "abnormal regeneration."

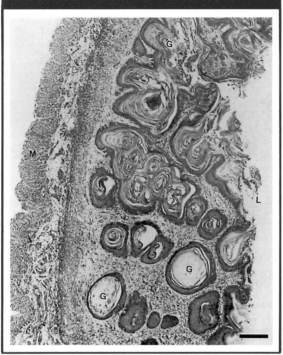

FIGURE 2.60
Severe squamous stratified metaplasia of the guinea pig uterus due to vitamin A deficiency. **M:** Muscular layer; **L:** lumen. The endometrial glands (**G**) are altered beyond recognition. Such uteri may be filled with a white pasty mass of desquamated cornified cells, just as in an epidermal cyst. **Bar** = 250 μm. (354)

columnar cells and eventually replace them. This has been confirmed many times (310, 318). Correspondingly, *in vivo*, vitamin A deficiency causes diffuse squamous metaplasia (348). Estrogen induces epidermoid metaplasia in the prostate (335). In the field of connective tissue metaplasia, bone can be induced in connective tissue by injecting bone extracts.

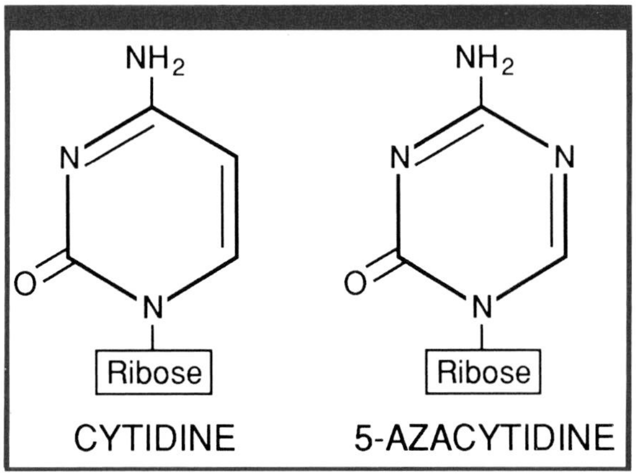

FIGURE 2.61
The chemical 5-azacytidine, an analog of cytidine, which affects gene expression. (Reproduced from [19]. Copyright © 1980 by Cell Press.)

NH₂ ... CYTIDINE ... 5-AZACYTIDINE

At the level of genes, the secret of modulation and metaplasia must lie in the expression of a new genetic program. The curtain over this field is beginning to rise, thanks to advances in the understanding of gene expression. Telling experiments were performed with an analog of the nucleoside cytidine, a powerful cytostatic (Figure 2.61); cultures of fibroblasts treated with 5-azacytidine turn into fat cells, muscle cells, or cartilage (Figure 2.62).

The premise of these experiments was that DNA methylation is involved in the control of gene expression and that specific patterns of cytosine methylation are associated with differentiation. An analog modified in the 5 position such as 5-azacytidine should disrupt these methylation patterns, and it does (319, 321, 352, 353).

BIOLOGICAL SIGNIFICANCE OF METAPLASIA

Sometimes metaplasia is clearly adaptive and useful. When bone marrow is destroyed by disease, the metaplasia of spleen tissue to bone marrow (myeloid metaplasia) is a helpful response. Similarly, the squamous stratified epithelium that forms in the renal pelvis around a ragged stone is presumably more resistant to mechanical abrasion.

In other situations, metaplasia is of no apparent use and may even be obnoxious. Epidermoid metaplasia of the pancreatic ducts has been listed among the possible causes of obstruction, because the new epithelium is much thicker. In the bronchi of smokers, squamous metaplasia interrupts the cleansing flow of mucus, which is produced by mucus-secreting cells and whipped along by ciliated cells (epidermal cells produce no mucus and have no cilia). Worse yet, it is well established that several types of epithelial metaplasia predispose to malignant epithelial tumors; leukoplakia (350), Barrett's epithelium (307, 351), and intestinal metaplasia of the stomach (336) are classic examples. Why epithelial metaplasia should progress to dysplasia (344) and finally to neoplasia is not understood.

Now here is a peculiar contrast. *Connective tissue metaplasia in its many forms is not known to predispose, in any of its varieties, to malignant evolution.*

Metaplasia is always reversible, at least potentially, but little is known about the mechanisms. As might be expected, vitamin A (retinoic acid) is used with success in the treatment of oral leukoplakia (317), but the mechanism is not understood (350).

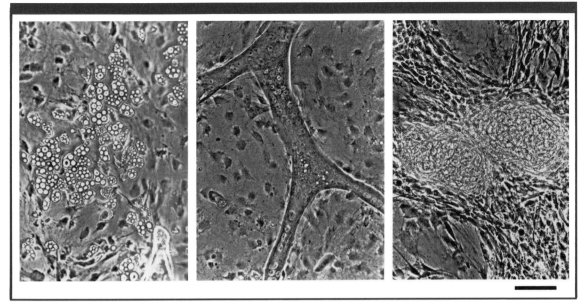

FIGURE 2.62 Different phenotypes induced in cultured embryonic fibroblasts by a nucleoside analog, 5-azacytidine. Within 2–4 weeks these embryonic fibroblasts give rise to adipocytes, striated muscle myotubes, and islands of cartilage. **Bar** = 100 μm. (Reproduced from [19]. Copyright © 1979 by Cell Press.)

TO SUM UP: *Modulation and metaplasia are useful concepts, but it must be kept in mind that they represent a series of partially overlapping notions that include differentiation, activation, and hypertrophy.* The basic fact is that a cell can assume a different structure and a different function by turning certain genes on and off. Experiments of transfection with selected genes will teach us more; for example, fibroblasts transfected with *ras* oncogenes have turned into fat cells (302).

Cell Activation and Priming

It may seem obvious now that cells, like people, can exist at several levels of activity, but this concept emerged very slowly, through studies of leukocytes. Metchnikoff himself, who discovered and named the macrophages, noticed that those from an infected animal were better able to phagocytize bacteria (365). Almost a century later the "angry macrophage" was described (p. 326). All the cells involved in inflammation need to be activated before they can perform their defensive functions (Figure 2.63). *Activation means that the cell acquires the ability to perform one or more new functions or to perform normal function(s) at a higher rate* (358). For example, a macrophage can be induced to secrete a given protein in quantities 800 times greater than normal; a mast cell will release most of its histamine.

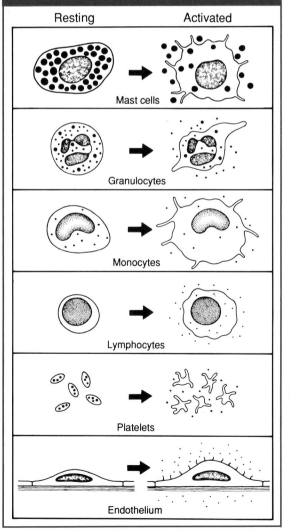

FIGURE 2.63 Six cell types that can be activated from their resting state. Note that they are all participants of the inflammatory reaction.

An activated cell undergoes subtle changes in structure and function that may require seconds, minutes, or days. Neurons are activated faster than any other cell type. Recent studies by positron emission tomography show that individuals asked to think sad thoughts activate almost instantly a certain center in the left frontal lobe; in clinically depressed individuals the same center is chronically activated (364) (Figure 2.64). In some cells activation is a multistep process that begins with priming, a condition recalling a state of alert with no visible changes. For those who study cells *in vitro*, it is important to make sure whether the properties they describe represent the cells' baseline condition or are the result of priming and activation induced by the experimental procedure.

We will discuss the activation of individual cells further on. Here we want to make one general point: *research on cell activation owes a great deal to*

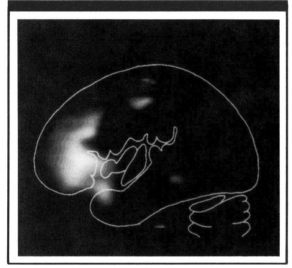

FIGURE 2.64

Evidence of activation in brain cells, as a mechanism of disease (depression). This type of image is obtained by positron emission tomography, which actually measures the blood flow in specific areas of the brain after an intravenous injection of radioactive water ($H_2{}^{15}O$). The area shown in graded white in the left ventrolateral prefrontal cortex shows the computed *difference* in regional blood flow between a normal series of individuals ($n = 33$) and a series affected by familial depressive disease ($n = 13$). Although the method reveals blood flow rather than neuronal activity, it is safe to assume that increased flow reflects increased local activity of neurons. (Courtesy of Dr. M. E. Raichle, Mallinckrodt Institute of Radiology, Washington University School of Medicine, St. Louis, MO.)

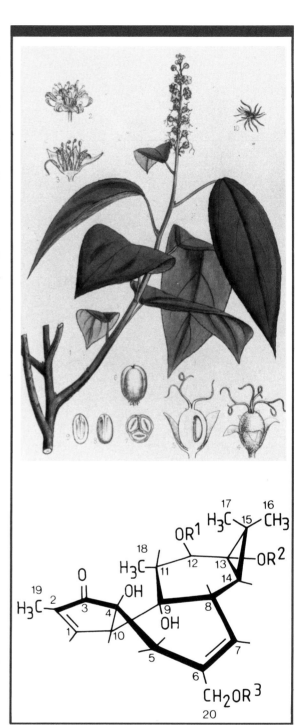

FIGURE 2.65

Top: Croton tiglium, the source of croton oil and of phorbol esters. (Reproduced from [5].) *Bottom:* Chemical formula of phorbol. ([358] Copyright © 1986 CRC Press, Inc., Boca Raton, FL.)

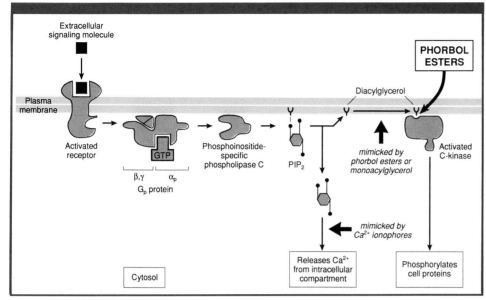

FIGURE 2.66
The secret of phorbol esters as cell activators: they activate protein kinase C (C-kinase) in the place of diacylglycerol. (Reproduced from [3].)

ancient medicine. For thousands of years, on the eastern coast of India, an irritating oil of incredible potency was extracted from the seeds of *Croton tiglium* (Figure 2.65). Tiny amounts on the skin produced blisters, and taken by mouth they induced vomiting and a bloody diarrhea. Because the effects were so drastic, medical uses faded away in the 1800s, but the oil remained in use for producing experimental inflammation; then it also became the standard tumor promotor (p. 409).

Eventually, its active principle was isolated. It is a derivative of phorbol (Figure 2.66), phorbol myristate acetate (PMA), now widely used as a an all-purpose cellular activator. The secret of its power is now known: PMA activates protein kinase C, for which the physiologic activators are diacylglycerols; in this way, PMA inserts itself as a link in the transduction of signals from the cell surface to effectors in the cytoplasm (361, 363). Modern cell biologists stand on the shoulders of ancient healers.

References

Regeneration

1. Abrams GD, Bauer H, Sprinz H. Influence of the normal flora on mucosal morphology and cellular renewal in the ileum. A comparison of germ-free and conventional mice. Lab Invest 1963; 12:355–364.

2. Aguayo AJ. Axonal regeneration from injured neurons in the adult mammalian central nervous system. In: Cotman CW (ed). Synaptic Plasticity. New York: Guilford Press, 1985, pp. 457–484.

3. Amadio PC. Tendon and ligament. In: Cohen IK, Diegelmann RF, Lindblad WJ (eds). Wound healing: biochemical & clinical aspects. Philadelphia: WB Saunders Company, 1992, pp. 384–395.

4. Appasamy R, Tanabe M, Murase N, Zarnegar R, Venkataramanan R, Van Thiel DH, Michalopoulos GK. Hepatocyte growth factor, blood clearance, organ uptake, and biliary excretion in normal and partially hepatectomized rats. Lab Invest 1993; 68:270–276.

5. Ash SR, Cuppage FE. Shift toward anaerobic glycolysis in the regenerating rat kidney. Am J Pathol 1970; 60:385–402.

6. Bader CR, Bertrand D, Cooper E, Mauro A. Membrane currents of rat satellite cells attached to intact skeletal muscle fibers. Neuron 1988; 1:237–240.

7. Barber PC. Neurogenesis and regeneration in the primary olfactory pathway of mammals. Bibl Anat 1982; 23:12–25.

8. Barinaga M. Challenging the "no new neurons" dogma. Science 1992; 255:1646.

9. Barr E, Leiden JM. Systemic delivery of recombinant proteins by genetically modified myoblasts. Science 1991; 254:1507–1509.

10. Barrie HJ. Intra-articular loose bodies regarded as organ cultures in vivo. J Pathol 1978; 125:163–169.

11. Basson MC, Carlson BM. Myotoxicity of single and repeated injections of mepivacaine (carbocaine) in the rat. Anesth Analg 1980; 59:275–282.

12. Bernstein JJ, Bernstein ME. Plasticity in the damaged spinal cord. In: Windle WF (ed). The spinal cord and its reaction to traumatic injury. New York-Basel: Marcel Dekker, Inc., 1980, pp.237–247.

13. Bischoff R. Regeneration of single skeletal muscle fibers in vitro. Anat Rec 1975; 182:215–236.

14. Bizzozero G. An address on the growth and regeneration of the organism. Br Med J 1894; 1:728–732.

15. Björntorp P. Adipocyte precursor cells. In: Björntorp P Cairella M, Howard AN (eds). Recent advances in obesity research:III. London: John Libbey, 1981, pp. 58–69.

16. Borgens RB. Mice regrow the tips of their foretoes. Science 1982a; 217:747–750.

17. Borgens RB. What is the role of naturally produced electric current in vertebrate regeneration and healing? Int Rev Cytol 1982b; 76:245–298.

18. Borgens RB, Robinson KR, Vanable JW Jr, McGinnis ME, McCaig CD. Electric fields in vertebrate repair. New York: Alan R. Liss, Inc., 1989.

18a. Matts B, Anders L, Anders N, et al. Treatment of deep cartilage defects in the knee with autologous chondrocyte transplantation. N Engl J Med 1984; 331:889–895.

19. Brockes JP. Mitogenic growth factors and nerve dependence of limb regeneration. Science 1984; 225:1280–1287.

20. Bucher NLR, Malt RA. Regeneration of liver and kidney. Boston: Little, Brown & Co., 1971.

21. Cajal SR. Degeneration and regeneration of the nervous system, Vol. 1. London: Oxford University Press, 1928.

22. Cameron IL, Thrasher JD (eds). Cellular and molecular renewal in the mammalian body. New York: Academic Press, 1971.

23. Carlson BM. The regeneration of minced muscles. Monogr Dev Biol 1972; 4:3–128.

24. Carlson BM. The regeneration of skeletal muscle—A review. Am J Anat 1973; 137:119–150.

25. Carlson BM. Regeneration of entire skeletal muscles. Fed Proc 1986; 45:1456–1460.

26. Carlson BM, Gutmann E. Regeneration in grafts of normal and denervated rat muscles. Pflügers Arch 1975; 353:215–225.

27. Cheung HS, Cottrell WH, Stephenson K, Nimni ME. In vitro collagen biosynthesis in healing and normal rabbit articular cartilage. J Bone Joint Surg 1978; 60-A:1076–1081.

28. Chi NH, Dahl D. Autologous peripheral nerve grafting into murine brain as a model for studies of regeneration in the central nervous system. Exp Neurol 1983;79:245–264.

29. Ciba Foundation Symposium 116. Growth factors in biology and medicine. London: Pitman, 1985.

29a. Cohen IK, Diegelmann RF, Crossland, MC. Wound care and wound healing. In: Swartz SI. Principles of Surgery. New York: McGraw Hill, Inc., 1994, pp. 279–303.

30. Dalley BK, Bartone FF, Gardner PJ. Smooth muscle regeneration in swine ureters. A light and electron microscopic study. Invest Urol 1976; 14:104–110.

31. Dalyell JG. Tracts on the natural history of animals and vegetables. Edinburgh: William Creech and Archd Constable, 1803.

32. Daniel CW, Silberstein GB, Strickland P. Reinitiation of growth in senescent mouse mammary epithelium in response to cholera toxin. Science 1984; 224:1245–1247.

33. Deuel TF. Polypeptide growth factors: roles in normal and abnormal cell growth. Annu Rev Cell Biol 1987; 3:443–492.

34. Dhawan J, Pan LC, Pavlath GK, Travis MA, Lanctot AM, Blau HM. Systemic delivery of human growth hormone by injection of genetically engineered myoblasts. Science 1991; 254:1509–1512.

35. Dobbie JW. New concepts in molecular biology and ultrastructural pathology of the peritoneum: their significance for peritoneal dialysis. Am J Kidney Dis 1990; 15:97–109.

36. Douglas BS. Conservative management of guillotine amputation of the finger in children. Aust Paediatr J 1972; 8:86–89.

37. Elder D. Why is regenerative capacity restricted in higher organisms? J Theor Biol 1979; 81:563–568.

38. Fausto N. Hepatic regeneration. In: Zakim D, Boyer T, (eds). Hepatology: A textbook of liver disease, 2nd ed., vol. 1. Philadelphia: WB Saunders, 1990, pp. 49–65.

39. Fausto N, Mead JE. Regulation of liver growth: protooncogenes and transforming growth factors. Lab Invest 1989; 60:4–13.

40. Francavilla A, Ove P, Polimeno L, Coetzee M, Makowka L, Barone M, Van Thiel DH, Starzl TE. Regulation of liver size and regeneration: importance in liver transplantation. Transplant Proc 1988; 20:494–497.

41. Galjaard H, Bootsma D. The regulation of cell proliferation and differentiation in intestinal epithelium. Exp Cell Res 1969; 58:79–92.

42. Gay S, Rhodes RK. Immunohistologic demonstration of distinct collagens in normal and osteoarthritic joints. Semin Arthritis Rheum 1982; 11:43–44.

43. Gohda E, Tsubouchi H, Nakayama H, Hirono S, Sakiyama O, Takahashi K, Miyazaki H, Hashimoto S, Daikuhara Y. Purification and partial characterization of hepatocyte growth factor from plasma of a patient with fulminant hepatic failure. J Clin Invest 1988; 81:414–419.

44. Goldberger ME, Murray M. Patterns of sprouting and implications for recovery of function. Adv Neurol 1988; 47:361–385.

45. Goldman SA, Nottebohm F. Neuronal production, migration, and differentiation in a vocal control nucleus of the adult female canary brain. Proc Natl Acad Sci USA 1983; 80:2390–2394.

46. Gordon RE, Lane BP. Wound repair in rat tracheal epithelium. Lab Invest 1980; 42:616–621.

47. Goss RJ. Prospects for regeneration in man. Clin Orthop 1980; 151:270–282.

48. Goss RJ. Deer antlers. Regeneration, function, and evolution. New York: Academic Press, 1983.

49. Goss, RJ. Why mammals don't regenerate—or do they? News Physiol Sci 1987; 2:112–115.

50. Grafe MR. Developmental factors affecting regeneration in the central nervous system: Early but not late formed mitral cells reinnervate olfactory cortex after neonatal tract section. J Neurosci 1983; 3:617–630.

51. Grounds MD. Factors controlling skeletal muscle regeneration in vivo. In: Kakulas BA, Mastaglia FL (eds). Pathogenesis and therapy of Duchenne and Becker muscular dystrophy. New York: Raven Press Ltd. 1990, pp. 171–185.

52. Grounds MD. Towards understanding skeletal muscle regeneration. Pathol Res Pract 1991; 187:1–22.

53. Grounds MD, Garrett KL, Lai MC, Wright WE, Beilharz MW. Identification of skeletal muscle precursor cells in vivo by use of MyoD1 and myogenin probes. Cell Tissue Res 1992; 267:99–104.

54. Guth L. History of central nervous system regeneration research. Exp Neurol 1975; 48:3–15.

55. Hauschka PV, Mavrakos AE, Iafrati MD, Doleman SE, Klagsbrun M. Growth factors in bone matrix. J Biol Chem 1986; 261:12665–12674.

56. Hayflick L. The biology of human aging. Am J Med Sci 1973; 265:432–445.

57. Hayflick L. Recent advances in the cell biology of aging. Mech Aging Dev 1980; 14:59–79.

58. Humes HD, Beals TF, Cieslinski DA, Sanchez IO, Page TP. Effects of transforming growth factor-β, transforming growth factor-α, and other growth factors on renal proximal tubule cells. Lab Invest 1991; 64:538–545.

59. Illingworth CM. Trapped fingers and amputated finger tips in children. J Pediatr Surg 1974; 9:853–857.

60. Illingworth CM, Barker AT. Measurement of electrical currents emerging during the regeneration of amputated finger tips in children. Clin Phys Physiol Meas 1980; 1:87–89.

61. Jones S. Flow cytometry: applications in research and medicine. Immunochemica 1989; 3:1–4.

62. Kalil K, Reh T. Regrowth of severed axons in the neonatal central nervous system: establishment of normal connections. Science 1979; 205:1158–1160.

63. Kerr FWL. Structural and functional evidence of plasticity in the central nervous system. Exp Neurol 1975; 48:16–31.

64. Ketchum LD. Tendon healing. In: Hunt TK, Dunphy JE. (eds). Fundamentals of wound management. New York:Appleton-Century-Crofts 1979, pp. 500–523.

65. Kiortsis V, Koussoulakos S, Wallace H. Recent trends in regeneration research. New York: Plenum Press 1989.

66. Kirkwood TBL. In vitro ageing of animal cells. In: Davies I, Sigee DC (eds). Cell ageing and cell death. Cambridge: Cambridge University Press, 1984, pp. 55–72.

67. Kocsis JD, Waxman SG. Membrane organization and myelin remodeling in regenerating axons. Adv Neurol 1988; 47:31–50.

68. Kolata G. New neurons form in adulthood. Science 1984; 224:1325–1326.

69. Kubo S, Matsui-Yuasa I, Otani S, Morisawa S, Kinoshita H, Sakai K. Liver regeneration factor detected in human serum after partial hepatectomy. Am J Gastroenterol 1987; 82:1120–1126.

70. Lacy ER, Ito S. Rapid epithelial restitution of the rat gastric mucosa after ethanol injury. Lab Invest 1984; 51:573–583.

71. Larson DM, Haudenschild CC. Junctional transfer in wounded cultures of bovine aortic endothelial cells. Lab Invest 1988; 59:373–379.

72. Levi-Montalcini R. The nerve growth factor 35 years later. Science 1987; 237:1154–1162.

73. Liuzzi FJ, Lasek RJ. Astrocytes block axonal regeneration in mammals by activating the physiological stop pathway. Science 1987; 237:642–645.

74. Loo DT, Fuquay JI, Rawson CL, Barnes DW. Extended culture of mouse embryo cells without senescence: inhibition by serum. Science 1987; 236:200–202.

75. Loo D, Rawson C, Schmitt M, Lindburg K, Barnes D. Glucocorticoid and thyroid hormones inhibit proliferation of serum-free mouse embryo (SFME) cells. J Cell Physiol 1990; 142:210–217.

76. Ludwin SK. Remyelination in the central nervous system and the peripheral nervous system. Adv Neurol 1988; 47:215–254.

77. Malemud CJ, Norby DP, Sokoloff L. Explant culture of human and rabbit articular chondrocytes. Connect Tissue Res 1978; 6:171–179.

78. Mauro A. Satellite cell of skeletal muscle fibers. J Biophys Biochem Cytol 1961; 9:493–495.

79. Mazanet R, Franzini-Armstrong C. The satellite cell. In: Engel AG, Banker BQ (eds). Myology: basic and clinical. New York: McGraw-Hill Book Company, 1986 pp. 285–307.

80. McGeachie JK. Smooth muscle regeneration. Monogr Dev Biol 1975; 9:1–90.

80a. Mendell JR, Kissel JT, Amato AA, King W, Signore L, Prior TW, Sahenk Z, Benson S, McAndrew PE, Rice R, Nagaraja H, Stephens R, Lantry L, Morris GE, Burghes AHM. Myoblast transfer in the treatment of Duchenne's muscular dystrophy. N Engl J Med 1995; 333:832–838.

81. Michalopoulos GK. Liver regeneration: molecular mechanisms of growth control. FASEB J 1990; 4:176–187.

82. Nachemson AK, Lundborg G, Hansson H-A. Insulin-like growth factor I promotes nerve regeneration: an experimental study on rat sciatic nerve. Growth Factors 1990; 3:309–314.

83. Nottebohm F. Birdsong as a model in which to study brain processes related to learning. The Condor 1984a; 86:227–236.

84. Nottebohm F. From bird song to neurogenesis. Sci Am 1989; 260:74–79.

85. Pabst R, Sterzel RB. Cell renewal of glomerular cell types in normal rats. An autoradiographic analysis. Kidney Int 1983; 24:626–631.

86. Partridge TA. Invited review: myoblast transfer: a possible therapy for inherited myopathies? Muscle Nerve 1991; 14:197–212.

87. Paton JA, Nottebohm F. Neurons generated in the adult brain are recruited into functional circuits. Science 1984; 225:1046–1048.

88. Payling Wright G. Introduction to pathology. Boston: Little, Brown, & Co., 1958.

89. Peacock EE, Van Winkle W. Surgery and biology of wound repair. Philadelphia: WB Saunders Company, 1970.

90. Phillips PD, Cristofalo VJ. A review of recent cellular aging research: the regulation of cell proliferation. Rev Biol Res Aging 1985; 2:339–357.

91. Price CH. Regeneration in the central nervous system of a pulmonate mollusc, Melampus. Cell Tissue Res 1977; 180:529–536.

92. Raisman G. Neuronal plasticity in the septal nuclei of the adult rat. Brain Res 1969; 14:25–48.

93. Reidy MA, Schwartz SM. Endothelial regeneration. III. Time course of intimal changes after small defined injury to rat aortic endothelium. Lab Invest 1981; 44:301–308.

94. Reier PJ, Houle JD. The glial scar: its bearing on axonal elongation and transplantation approaches to CNS repair. Adv Neurol 1988; 47:87–138.

95. Reynolds BA, Weiss S. Generation of neurons and astrocytes from isolated cells of the adult mammalian central nervous system. Science 1992; 255:1707–1710.

96. Richardson PM, McGuinness UM, Aguayo AJ. Axons from CNS neurones regenerate into PNS grafts. Nature 1980; 284:264–265.

97. Robertson TA, Grounds MD, Mitchell CA, Papadimitriou JM. Fusion between myogenic cells in vivo: an ultrastructural study in regenerating murine skeletal muscle. J Struct Biol 1990; 105:170–182.

98. Romberger JA. An appraisal of prospects for research on juvenility in woody perennials. Acta Horticulturae 1976; 56:301–317.

99. Ryan GB, Grobéty J, Majno G. Mesothelial injury and recovery. Am J Pathol 1973; 71:93–112.

100. Schnell L, Schwab ME. Axonal regeneration in the rat spinal cord produced by an antibody against myelin-associated neurite growth inhibitors. Nature 1990; 343:269–272.

101. Schwartz M, Cohen A, Stein-Izsak C, Belkin M. Dichotomy of the glial cell response to axonal injury and regeneration. FASEB J 1989; 3:2371–2378.

102. Shimokawa H, Flavahan NA, Vanhoutte PM. Natural course of the impairment of endothelium-dependent relaxations after balloon endothelium removal in porcine coronary arteries. Possible dysfunction of a pertussis toxin-sensitive G protein. Circ Res 1989; 65:740–753.

103. Singer M, Géraudie J. An overview of the historical origin of the nerve influence on limb regeneration. In: Kiortsis V, Koussoulakos S, Wallace H (eds). Recent trends in regeneration research. New York: Plenum Press, 1989, pp. 1–5.

104. Sloper JC, Pegrum GD. Regeneration of crushed mammalian skeletal muscle and effects of steroids. J Pathol Bacteriol 1967; 93:47–63.

105. Spallanzani L. Tracts on the natural history of animals and vegetables, 2nd ed., vol. II. (Translated from the

original Italian edition by John Graham Dalyell.) Edinburgh: W. Creech and A. Constable, 1803.

106. Spencer PS. The traumatic neuroma and proximal stump. Bull Hosp Joint Dis 1974; 35:85–102.

107. Sporn MB, Roberts AB. Peptide growth factors are multifunctional. Nature 1988; 332:217–219.

108. Sporn MB, Todaro GJ. Autocrine secretion and malignant transformation of cells. N Engl J Med 1980; 303:878–880.

109. Stenn KS, DePalma L. Re-epithelialization. In: Clark RAF, Henson PM (eds). The molecular and cellular biology of wound repair. New York: Plenum Press, 1988, pp. 321–335.

110. Striker LJ, Tannen RL, Lange MA, Striker GE. The contribution of cell culture to the study of renal diseases. Int Rev Exp Pathol 1988; 30:55–105.

111. Sugawara O, Oshimura M, Koi M, Annab LA, Barrett JC. Induction of cellular senescence in immortalized cells by human chromosome 1. Science 1990; 247:707–710.

112. Svendgaard N-A, Björklund A, Stenevi U. Regeneration of central cholingergic neurones in the adult rat brain. Brain Res 1976; 102:1–22.

113. Tassava RA, Olsen CL. Higher vertebrates do not regenerate digits and legs because the wound epidermis is not functional. Differentiation 1982; 22:151–155.

114. Taylor AC. Survival of rat skin and changes in hair pigmentation following freezing. J Exp Zool 1949; 110:77–111.

115. Thomas PK. Clinical aspects of PNS regeneration. Adv Neurol 1988; 47:9–29.

116. Trudinger BJ, Wilhelm DL. Regeneration of gastric mucosa at the squamo-columnar junction in the rat. J Pathol 1969; 97:127–135.

117. Tuge H, Hanzawa S. Physiological and morphological regeneration of the sectioned spinal cord in adult teleosts. J Comp Neurol 1937; 67:343–365.

118. Urist MR, DeLange RJ, Finerman GAM. Bone cell differentiation and growth factors. Science 1983; 220:680–686.

119. Veraa RP, Grafstein B. Cellular mechanisms for recovery from nervous system injury: A conference report. Exp Neurol 1981; 71:6–75.

120. Vracko R, Benditt EP. Basal lamina: the scaffold for orderly cell replacement. Observations on regeneration of injured skeletal muscle fibers and capillaries. J Cell Biol 1972; 55:406–419.

121. Wells H, Handelman C, Milgram E. Regulation by sympathetic nervous system of accelerated growth of salivary glands of rats. Am J Physiol 1961; 201:707–710.

122. Westermark B, Betsholtz C, Hookfelt B (eds). Growth factors in health and disease: basic and clinical Aspects (International Congress Series No. 925). Amsterdam: Excerpta Medica, 1990.

123. Wilhelm DL. Regeneration of tracheal epithelium. J Pathol Bacteriol 1953; 75:543–550.

124. Witkowski JA. Dr. Carrel's immortal cells. Med Hist 1980; 24:129–142.

125. Wong MKK, Gotlieb AI. In vitro reendothelialization of a single-cell wound. Role of microfilament bundles in rapid lamellipodia-mediated wound closure. Lab Invest 1984; 51:75–81.

126. Wong MKK, Gotlieb AI. The reorganization of microfilaments, centrosomes, and microtubules during in vitro small would reendothelialization. J Cell Biol 1988; 107:1777–1783.

127. Woolf CJ, Shortland P, Coggeshall RE. Peripheral nerve injury triggers central sprouting of myelinated afferents. Nature 1992; 355:75–78.

128. Yamada S, Buffinger N, Dimario J, Strohman RC. Fibroblast growth factor is stored in fiber extracellular matrix and plays a role in regulating muscle hypertrophy. Med Sci Sports Exerc 1989; 21 (No. 5 suppl.):S173–S180.

129. Ziegler E. General pathology. New York: William Wood and Company, 1908.

Hypertrophy and Hyperplasia

130. Abrahams C, Janicki JS, Weber KT. Myocardial hypertrophy in Macaca fascicularis. Structural remodeling of the collagen matrix. Lab Invest 1987; 56:676–683.

131. Adler CP, Sandritter W. Numerische Hyperplasie der Herzmuskelzellen bei Herzhypertrophie. Dtsch Med Wochenschr 1971; 48:1895–1897.

132. Alberts B, Bray D, Lewis J, Raff M, Roberts K., Watson JD. Molecular biology of the cell, 2nd ed. New York: Garland Publishing, Inc., 1989.

133. Alway SE, Grumbt WH, Gonyea WJ, Stray-Gundersen J. Contrasts in muscle and myofibers of elite male and female bodybuilders. J Appl Physiol 1989; 67:24–31.

134. Alway SE, MacDougall JD, Sale DG, Sutton JR, McComas AJ. Functional and structural adaptations in skeletal muscle of trained athletes. J Appl Physiol 1988; 64:1114–1120.

135. Angel A, Hollenberg CH, Roncari DAK. The Adipocyte and obesity: cellular and molecular mechanisms. New York: Raven Press, 1983.

136. Anversa P, Beghi C, McDonald SL, Levicky V, Kikkawa Y, Olivetti G. Morphometry of right ventricular hypertrophy induced by myocardial infarction in the rat. Am J Pathol 1984; 116:504–513.

137. Astorri E, Bolognesi R, Colla B, Chizzola A, Visioli O. Left ventricular hypertrophy: a cytometric study on 42 human hearts. J Mol Cell Cardiol 1977; 9:763–775.

138. Barka T, Yagil C, van der Noen H, Naito Y. Induction of the synthesis of a specific protein in rat submandibular gland by isoproterenol. Lab Invest 1986; 54:165–171.

139. Barrett TB, Sampson P, Owens GK, Schwartz SM, Benditt EP. Polyploid nuclei in human artery wall smooth muscle cells. Proc Natl Acad Sci USA 1983; 80:882–885.

140. Bonnet F, Gosselin L, Chantraine J, Senteree J. Adipose cell number and size in normal and obese children. Rev Eur Etud Clin Biol 1970; 25:1101–1104.

141. Bowen RE, Swartz FJ. The ultrastructure of polyploid B-cells in the islets of normal mice. Diabetologia 1976; 12:171–180.

142. Bray GA. Obesity: what comes first. In: Angel A, Hollenberg, CH, Roncari DAK (eds). The adipocyte and obesity: cellular and molecular mechanisms. New York: Raven Press, 1983, pp. 19–27.

143. Brent B, Brent BP. The artistry of reconstructive surgery. St. Louis: The CV Mosby Company, 1987.

144. Brodsky WY, Uryvaeva IV. Cell polyploidy: its relation to tissue growth and function. Int Rev Cytol 1977; 50:275–332.

145. Bucher NLR, Malt RA. Regeneration of liver and kidney. Boston: Little Brown and Company, 1971.

146. Clark AM, Rubin MA. The modification by X-irradiation of the life span of haploids and diploids of the wasp, Habrobracon SP. Radiat Res 1961; 15:244–253.

147. Coleman DL. Obesity genes: beneficial effects in heterozygous mice. Science 1979; 203:663–665.

148. Cutilletta AF, Dowell RT, Rudnik M, Arcilla RA, Zak R. Regression of myocardial hypertrophy. I. Experimental model, changes in heart weight, nucleic acids and collagen. J Mol Cell Cardiol 1975; 7:767–781.

149. Enriori CL, Reforzo-Membrives J. Peripheral aromatization as a risk factor for breast and endometrial cancer in postmenopausal women: a review. Gynecol Oncol 1984; 17:1–21.

150. Faust IM, Johnson PR, Hirsch J. Surgical removal of adipose tissue alters feeding behavior and the development of obesity in rats. Science 1977; 197:393–396.

151. Faust IM, Miller WH Jr. Hyperplastic growth of adipose tissue in obesity. In: Angel A, Hollenberg CH, Roncari DAK (eds). The adipocyte and obesity: cellular and molecular mechanisms. New York: Raven Press, 1983, pp. 41–51.

152. Ferrans VJ. Cardiac hypertrophy: morphological aspects. In: Zak R (ed). Growth of the heart in health and disease. New York: Raven Press, 1984, pp. 187–239.

153. Ferrans VJ, Jones M, Maron BJ, Roberts WC. The nuclear membranes in hypertrophied human cardiac muscle cells. Am J Pathol 1975; 78:427–446.

154. Fleck C, Bräunlich H. Kidney function after unilateral nephrectomy. Exp Pathol 1984; 25:3–18.

155. Fries JWU, Sandstrom DJ, Meyer TW, Rennke HG. Glomerular hypertrophy and epithelial cell injury modulate progressive glomerulosclerosis in the rat. Lab Invest 1989; 60:205–218.

156. Gabella G. Hypertrophic smooth muscle. Cell Tissue Res 1979; 201:63–78.

157. Gahan PB. Increased levels of euploidy as a strategy against rapid ageing in diploid mammalian systems: an hypothesis. Exp Gerontol 1977; 12:133–136.

158. Goldberg ID, Shapiro H, Stemerman MB, Wei J, Hardin D, Christenson L. Frequency of tetraploid nuclei in the rat aorta increases with age. Ann N Y Acad Sci 1984; 435:422–424.

159. Gortmaker SL, Must A, Perrin JM, Sobol AM, Dietz WH. Social and economic consequences of overweight in adolescence and young adulthood. N Engl J Med 1993; 329:1008–1012.

160. Goss RJ, Dittmer JE. Compensatory renal hypertrophy: problems and prospects. In: Nowinski WW, Goss RJ (eds). Compensatory renal hypertrophy. New York: Academic Press, 1969, pp. 299–307.

161. Greene GL, Press MF: I. Steroid receptor structure (including monoclonal antibodies and new methods of determination). Structure and dynamics of the estrogen receptor. J Steroid Biochem 1986; 24:1–7.

162. Hostetter TH, Meyer TW, Rennke HG, Brenner BM, Noddin JA, Sandstrom DJ. Chronic effects of dietary protein in the rat with intact and reduced renal mass. Kidney Int 1986; 30:509–517.

163. Hostetter TH, Olson JL, Rennke HG, Venkatachalam MA, Brenner BM. Hyperfiltration in remnant nephrons: a potentially adverse response to renal ablation. Am J Physiol 1981; 241:F85–F93.

164. Huston TP, Puffer JC, Rodney WM. The athletic heart syndrome. N Engl J Med 1985; 313:24–32.

165. Johansson B. Different types of smooth muscle hypertrophy. Hypertension 1984; 6(suppl.III):64–68.

166. Johnson HA. Cytoplasmic response to overwork. In: Nowinski WW, Goss RJ (eds). Compensatory renal hypertrophy. New York: Academic Press, 1969, pp. 9–26.

167. Johnson HA, Vera Roman JM. Compensatory renal enlargement. Hypertrophy versus hyperplasia. Am J Pathol 1966; 49:1–13.

168. Kimball JW. Biology. Reading, Mass: Addison-Wesley Publishing Company, Inc., 1965.

169. Kolata G. Obesity declared a disease. Science 1985; 227:1019–1020.

170. Kuzon WM Jr, Rosenblatt JD, Huebel SC, et al. Skeletal muscle fiber type, fiber size, and capillary supply in elite soccer players. Int J Sports Med 1990; 11:99–102.

171. Lapham LW. Tetraploid DNA content of Purkinje neurons of human cerebellar cortex. Science 1968; 159:310–312.

172. Leiter EH. Genetics of ß-cell abnormalities in rodents. In: Hanahan D, McDevitt HO, Cahill GF Jr (eds). Perspectives on the molecular biology and immunology of the pancreatic ß cell. Cold Spring Harbor: Cold Spring Harbor Laboratory, 1989, pp. 69–79.

173. Loud AV, Beghi C, Olivetti G, Anversa P. Morphometry of right and left ventricular myocardium after strenuous exercise in preconditioned rats. Lab Invest 1984;51:104–111.

174. Lund DD, Tomanek RJ. The effects of chronic hypoxia on the myocardial cell of normotensive and hypertensive rats. Anat Rec 1980; 196:421–430.

175. Majno G. The healing hand: man and wound in the ancient world. Cambridge: Harvard University Press 1975.

176. Maron BJ, Ferrans VJ. Ultrastructural features of hypertrophied human ventricular myocardium. Prog Cardiovasc Dis 1978; 21:207–238.

177. McNurlan MA, McHardy KC, Broom J, Milne E, Fearns LM, Reeds PJ, Garlick PJ. The effect of indomethacin on the response of protein synthesis to feeding in rats and man. Clin Sci 1987; 73:69–75.

178. Meyer TW, Brenner BM. The contribution of glomerular hemodynamic alterations to progressive renal disease. In: Mitch WE, Brenner BM, Stein JH (eds). The progressive nature of renal disease. New York: Churchill Livingstone, 1986, pp. 1–16.

179. Meyrick B, Reid L. The effect of continued hypoxia on rat pulmonary arterial circulation. An ultrastructural study. Lab Invest 1978; 38:188–200.

180. Must A, Jacques PF, Dallal GE, Bajema CJ, Dietz WH. Long-term morbidity and mortality of overweight adolescents. N Engl J Med 1992; 327:1350–1355.

181. Nadal C, Zajdela F. Polyploïdie somatique dans le foie de rat. I. Le rôle des cellules binucléées dans la genèse des cellules polyploïdes. Exp Cell Res 1966; 42:99–116.

182. Novick AC, Gephardt G, Guz B, Steinmuller D, Tubbs RR. Long-term follow-up after partial removal of a solitary kidney. N Engl J Med 1991; 325:1058–1062.

183. Odell TT Jr, Jackson CW, Friday TJ. Megakaryocytopoiesis in rats with special reference to polyploidy. Blood 1970; 35:775–782.

184. Olivecrona T, Bengtsson G. Lipoprotein lipase. In: Angel A, Hollenberg CH, Roncari DAK (eds). The adipocyte and obesity: cellular and molecular mechanisms. New York: Raven Press, 1983, pp. 117–126.

185. Olson JL, Gaskin de Urdaneta A, Heptinstall RH. Glomerular hyalinosis and its relation to hyperfiltration. Lab Invest 1985; 52:387–398.

186. Oparil S, Bishop SP, Clubb FJ. Myocardial cell hypertrophy or hyperplasia. Hypertension 1984; 6(suppl. III):38–43.

187. Owens GK. Growth response of aortic smooth muscle cells in hypertension. In: Lee RMKW (ed). Blood vessel changes in hypertension: structure and function, vol. 1. Boca Raton: CRC Press, Inc., 1989, pp. 45–63.

188. Penington DG. The cellular biology of megakaryocytes. Blood Cells 1979; 5:5–10.

189. Penington DG, Streatfield K, Roxburgh AE. Megakaryocytes and the heterogeneity of circulating platelets. Br J Haematol 1976; 34:639–653.

190. Pfitzer P, Capurso A. Der DNS-Gehalt der Zellkerne im Herzohr des Menschen. Virchows Arch B Zellpathol 1970; 5:254–267.

191. Polzin DJ, Leininger JR, Osborne CA, Jeraj K. Development of renal lesions in dogs after 11/12 reduction of renal mass. Influences of dietary protein intake. Lab Invest 1988; 58:172–183.

192. Rakusan K, Moravec J, Hatt P-Y. Regional capillary supply in the normal and hypertrophied rat heart. Microvasc Res 1980; 20:319–326.

193. Raven PH, Curtis H. Biology of plants. New York: Worth Publishers, Inc., 1971.

194. Rennke HG. Glomerular adaptations to renal injury or ablation. Blood Purif 1988; 6:230–239.

195. Revis NW, Cameron AJV. Association of myocardial cell necrosis with experimental cardiac hypertrophy. J Pathol 1979; 128:193–202.

196. Rost TL, Barbour MG, Thornton RM, Weier TE, Stocking CR. Botany. 2nd ed. New York: John Wiley & Sons, 1984.

197. Rumyantsev PP. Interrelations of the proliferation and differentiation processes during cardiac myogenesis and regeneration. Int Rev Cytol 1977; 51:187–273.

198. Schwartz MM, Bidani AK, Lewis EJ. Glomerular epithelial cell function and pathology following extreme ablation of renal mass. Am J Pathol 1987; 126:315–324.

199. Siiteri PK, Schwarz BE, MacDonald PC. Estrogen receptors and the estrone hypothesis in relation to endometrial and breast cancer. Gynecol Oncol 1974; 2:228–238.

200. Taylor TG. How an eggshell is made. Sci Am 1970; 222:89–95.

201. Weisz PB, Keogh RN. The Science of Biology, 5th ed. New York: McGraw-Hill Book Company, 1982.

202. Yoshida H, Hayashi S-I, Kunisada T, et al. The murine mutation osteopetrosis is in the coding region of the macrophage colony stimulating factor gene. Nature 1990; 345:442–444.

Atrophy

203. Amiel D, Woo S L-Y, Harwood FL, Akeson WH. The effect of immobilization on collagen turnover in connective tissue: a biochemical-biomechanical correlation. Acta Orthop Scand 1982; 53:325–332.

204. Angel A, Hollenberg CH, Roncari DAK (eds). The adipocyte and obesity: cellular and molecular mechanisms. New York: Raven Press, 1983.

205. Ashford TP, Porter KR. Cytoplasmic components in hepatic cell lysosomes. J Cell Biol 1962; 12:198–202.

206. Askanazi J, Elwyn DH, Kinney JM, Gump FE, Michelsen CB, Stinchfield FE. Muscle and plasma amino acids after injury: the role of inactivity. Ann Surg 1978; 188:797–803.

207. Austad SN. Life extension by dietary restriction in the bowl and doily spider, Frontinella pyramitela. Exp Gerontol 1989; 24:83–92.

208. Bachmair A, Finley D, Varshavsky A. In vivo half-life of a protein is a function of its amino-terminal residue. Science 1986; 234:179–186.

209. Barnes RH. Nutrition and man's intellect and behavior. Fed Proc 1971; 30:1429–1433.

210. Barrows CH Jr, Kokkonen GC. Diet and life extension in animal model systems. Age 1978; 1:131–143.

211. Basson MD, Burney RE. Defective wound healing in patients with paraplegia and quadriplegia. Surg Gynecol Obstet 1982; 155:9–12.

212. Bellamy D. Cell death in the context of ageing. In: Davies I, Sigee DC (eds). Cell ageing and cell death. Cambridge: Cambridge University Press, 1984, pp. 105–121.

213. Berkenstam A, Ahlberg J, Glaumann H. Isolation and characterization of autophagic vacuoles from rat kidney cortex. Virchows Arch B Cell Pathol 1983; 44:275–286.

214. Bliss M. The discovery of insulin: how it really happened. In: Hollenberg MD (ed). Insulin: its receptor and diabetes. New York: Marcel Dekker, Inc., 1985, pp. 7–19.

215. Bloodgood RA. Resorption of organelles containing microtubules. Cytobios 1974; 9:143–161.

216. Buetow DE. Cell numbers vs. age in mammalian tissues and organs. In: Cristofalo VJ (ed). CRC handbook of cell biology of aging. Boca Raton: CRC Press, Inc., 1985, pp. 1–115.

217. Bührle CP, Hackenthal E, Helmchen U, et al. The hydronephrotic kidney of the mouse as a tool for intravital microscopy and in vitro electrophysiological studies of renin-containing cells. Lab Invest 1986; 54:462–472.

218. Cahill GF. President's address: starvation. Trans Am Clin Climatol Assoc 1982; 94:1–21.

219. Cameron GR. Liver atrophy produced by chronic selenium intoxication. J Pathol Bacteriol 1947; 59:539–545.

220. Carpentier J-L, Perrelet A, Orci L. Morphological changes of the adipose cell plasma membrane during lipolysis. J Cell Biol 1977; 72:104–117.

221. Casarett GW. Radiation histopathology, vol. I. Boca Raton: CRC Press, Inc., 1981.

222. Ciechanover A, Finley D, Varshavsky A. The ubiquitin-mediated proteolytic pathway and mechanisms of energy-dependent intracellular protein degradation. J Cell Biochem 1984; 24:27–53.

223. Cristofalo VJ (ed). CRC handbook of cell biology of aging. Boca Raton: CRC Press, Inc., 1985.

224. Cristofalo VJ. Perspectives in the biology of aging. In: Bates SR, Gangloff EC (eds). Atherogenesis and aging. New York: Springer-Verlag, 1987, pp. 48–56.

225. Dämmrich J, Pfeifer U. Cardiac hypertrophy in rats after supravalvular aortic constriction. II. Inhibition of cellular autophagy in hypertrophying cardiomyocytes. Virchows Arch B Cell Pathol 1983; 43:287–307.

226. Davies I, Sigee DC (eds). Cell ageing and cell death. Cambridge: Cambridge University Press, 1984.

227. Decker RS, Crie JS, Poole AR, Dingle JT, Wildenthal K. Resistance to ischemic damage in hearts of starved rabbits. Correlation with lysosomal alterations and delayed release of cathepsin d. Lab Invest 1980; 43:197–207.

228. Donaldson CL, Hulley SB, Vogel JM, Hattner R, Bayers JH, McMillan DE. Effect of prolonged bed rest on bone mineral. Metabolism 1970; 19:1071–1084.

229. Ericsson JLE, Trump BF, Weibel J. Electron microscopic studies of the proximal tubule of the rat kidney. II. Cytosegresomes and cytosomes: their relationship to each other and to the lysosome concept. Lab Invest 1965; 14:1341–1365.

230. Fronek K. Trophic influence of the sympathetic nervous system on the arterial wall. In: Gaehtgens P (ed). Bibliotheca anatomica, No. 20, Basel S. Karger, 1981, p. 414–417.

231. Fronek K, Bloor CM, Amiel D, Chvapil M. Effect of long-term sympathectomy on the arterial wall in rabbits and rats. Exp Mol Pathol 1978; 28:279–289.

232. Gobé GC, Axelsen RA. Genesis of renal tubular atrophy in experimental hydronephrosis in the rat. Role of apoptosis. Lab Invest 1987; 56:273–281.

233. Goldberg AL, Etlinger JD, Goldspink DF, Jablecki C. Mechanism of work-induced hypertrophy of skeletal muscle. Med Sci Sports 1975; 7:248–261.

234. Goldberg AL, Strnad NP, Swamy KHS. Studies of the ATP dependence of protein degradation in cells and cell extracts. Ciba Found Symp 1980;75:227–251.

235. Gordeuk V, Thuma P, Brittenham G, McLaren C, Parry D, Backenstose A, et al. Effect of iron chelation therapy on recovery from deep coma in children with cerebral malaria. N Engl J Med 1992; 327:1473–1477.

236. Gravis CJ, Weaker FJ. Testicular involution following optic enucleation. An ultrastructural and cytochemical study. Cell Tissue Res 1977; 184:67–77.

237. Griffin WST, Wildenthal K. Myofibrillar alkaline protease activity in rat heart and its responses to some interventions that alter cardiac size. J Mol Cell Cardiol 1978; 10:669–676.

238. Harman D. Free radical theory of aging: the "free radical" diseases. Age 1984; 7:111–131.

239. Hart RW, Turturro A. Review of recent biological research on theories of aging. Rev Biol Res Aging 1985; 2:3–12.

240. Hayflick L. Recent advances in the cell biology of aging. Mech Ageing Dev 1980; 14:59–79.

241. Hopewell JW, Young CMA. Changes in the microcirculation of normal tissues after irradiation. Int J Radiat Oncol Biol Phys 1978; 4:53–58.

242. Jarow JP, Budin RE, Dym M, Zirkin BR, Noren S, Marshall FF. Quantitative pathologic changes in the human testis after vasectomy. A controlled study. N Engl J Med 1985; 313:1252–1256.

243. Jaweed MM, Alleva FR, Herbison GJ, Ditunno JF, Balazs T. Muscle atrophy and histopathology of the soleus in 6-mercaptopurine-treated rats. Exp Mol Pathol 1985; 43:74–81.

244. Johnston RS, Dietlein LF (eds). Biomedical results from Skylab. Washington, DC: National Aeronautics and Space Administration, 1977.

245. Lattanand A, Johnson WC. Male pattern alopecia. A histopathological and histochemical study. J Cutan Pathol 1975; 2:58–70.

246. Lewis CM, Tarrant GM. Error theory and ageing in human diploid fibroblasts. Nature 1972; 239:316–318.

247. Libby P, Goldberg AL. Leupeptin, a protease inhibitor, decreases protein degradation in normal and diseases muscles. Science 1978; 199:534–536.

248. Mamus SW, Burton JD, Groat JD, Schulte DA, Lobell M, Zanjani ED. Ibuprofen-associated pure white-cell aplasia. N Engl J Med 1986; 314:624–625.

249. Masoro EJ. Biology of aging: facts, thoughts, and experimental approaches. Lab Invest 1991; 65:500–510.

250. Masoro EJ, Yu BP. Diet and nephropathy. Lab Invest 1989; 60:165–167.

251. Mayer M, Amin R, Shafrir E. Rat myofibrillar protease: enzyme properties and adaptive changes in conditions of muscle protein degradation. Arch Pathol Biophys 1974; 161:20–25.

252. Mellgren RL. Calcium-dependent proteases: an enzyme system active at cellular membranes? FASEB J 1987; 1:110–115.

253. Merry BJ, Holehan AM. Serum profiles of LH, FSH, testosterone and 5α-DHT from 21 to 1000 days of age in ad libitum fed and dietary restricted rats. Exp Gerontol 1981; 16:431–444.

254. Miquel J, Economos AC, Johnson JE. A systems analysis—thermodynamic view of cellular and organismic aging. In: Johnson JE (ed). Aging and cell function. New York: Plenum Press, 1984, pp. 247–280.

255. Munkres KD. Biochemical genetics of aging of Neurospora crassa and Podospora anserina: a review. In: Sohal RS (ed). Age pigments. Amsterdam: Elsevier/North-Holland Biomedical Press, 1981, pp. 83–100.

256. Murphy ED, Scanlon EF, Garces RM, Khandekar JD, Bailey L. Thyroid hormone administration in irradiated patients. J Surg Oncol 1986; 31:214–217.

257. Murray J, Murray A. Suppression of infection by famine and its activation by refeeding — a paradox? Perspect Biol Med 1977; 20:471–483.

258. Novikoff AB, Shin WY. Endoplasmic reticulum and autophagy in rat hepatocytes. Proc Natl Acad Sci USA 1978; 75:5039–5042.

259. Noyes FR. Functional properties of knee ligaments and alterations induced by immobilization. Clin Orthop 1977; 123:210–242.

260. Papadopoulos T, Pfeifer U. Regression of rat liver autophagic vacuoles by locally applied cycloheximide. Lab Invest 1986; 54:100–107.

261. Pfeifer U. Cellular autophagy and cell atrophy in the rat liver during long-term starvation. A quantitative morphological study with regard to diurnal variations. Virchows Arch Abt B Zellpathol 1973; 12:195–211.

262. Pfeifer U. Kinetic and subcellular aspects of hypertrophy and atrophy. Int Rev Exp Pathol 1982; 23:1–45.

263. Pfeifer U. Application of test substances to the surface of rat liver in situ: opposite effects of insulin and isoproterenol on cellular autophagy. Lab Invest 1984; 50:348–354.

264. Pfeifer U, Werder E, Bergeest H. Inhibition by insulin of the formation of autophagic vacuoles in rat liver. A morphometric approach to the kinetics of intracellular degradation by autophagy. J Cell Biol 1978; 78:152–167.

265. Pierpaoli W, Fabris N. Physiological senescence and its postponement: Theoretical approaches and rational interventions. (Ann N Y Acad Sci, vol. 621). New York: The New York Academy of Sciences, 1991.

266. Pryor G. Malnutrition and the "critical period" hypothesis. In: Prescott JW, Read MS, Coursin DB (eds). Brain function and malnutrition. New York: John Wiley & Sons, 1975, pp. 103–112.

267. Purves D, Snider WD, Voyvodic JT. Trophic regulation of nerve cell morphology and innervation in the autonomic nervous system. Nature 1988; 336:123–128.

268. Raisz LG. What marrow does to bone. N Engl J Med 1981; 304:1485–1486.

269. Read MS. Malnutrition and behavior. Appl Res Mental Retard 1982; 3:279–291.

270. Reunanen H, Hirsimaki P. Studies on vinblastine-induced autophagocytosis in mouse liver. IV. Origin of membranes. Histochemistry 1983; 79:59–67.

271. Richie JP Jr, Mills BJ, Lang CA. Dietary nordihydroguaiaretic acid increases the life span of the mosquito. Proc Soc Exp Biol Med 1986; 183:81–85.

272. Romanul FCA, Hogan EL. Enzymatic changes in denervated muscle. I. Histochemical studies. Arch Neurol 1965; 13:263–273.

273. Rudzinska MA. The use of a protozoan for studies on ageing. III. Similarities between young overfed and old normally fed Tokophrya infusionum: A light and electron microscope study. Gerontologia 1962; 6:206–226.

274. Rusting RL. Why do we age? Sci Am 1992; 267:130–141.

275. Salminen A, Vihko V. Autophagic response to strenuous exercise in mouse skeletal muscle fibers. Virchows Arch B Cell Pathol 1984; 45:97–106.

276. Schonheyder F, Heilskov NSC, Olesen K. Isotopic studies on the mechanism of negative nitrogen balance

produced by immobilization. Scand J Clin Lab Invest 1954; 6:178–188.

277. Seshadri T, Campisi J. Repression of c-fos transcription and an altered genetic program in senescent human fibroblasts. Science 1990; 247:205–209.

278. Shelburne JD, Arstila AU, Trump BF. Studies on cellular autophagocytosis. The relationship of autophagocytosis to protein synthesis and to energy metabolism in rat liver and flounder kidney tubules in vitro. Am J Pathol 1973; 73:641–662.

279. Sherman SM, Spear PD. Neural development of cats raised with deprivation of visual patterns. In: Rosenberg RN (ed). The clinical neurosciences. New York: Churchill Livingstone, 1983, pp. V:385–V:434.

280. Sinclair D. Motor nerves and reflexes. In: Jarrett A (ed). The physiology and pathophysiology of the skin. New York: Academic Press, 1973, p. 475–573.

281. Smith DC. Functional restoration of vision in the cat after long-term monocular deprivation. Science 1981; 213:1137–1139.

282. Smith ME. The effect of fasting on lipid metabolism of the central nervous system of the rat. J Neurochem 1963; 10:531–536.

283. Stearner SP, Christian EJB. Long-term vascular effects of ionizing radiations in the mouse: capillary blood flow. Radiat Res 1978; 73:553–567.

284. Stein J, Fenigstein H. Pathological anatomy of hunger disease. In: Winick M (ed). Hunger disease. New York: John Wiley & Sons, 1979, p. 220.

285. Tamarin A. Submaxillary gland recovery from obstruction. I. Overall changes and electron microscopic alterations of granular duct cells. J Ultrastruct Res 1971; 34:276–287.

286. Taylor A, Zuliani AM, Hopkins RE, et al. Moderate caloric restriction delays cataract formation in the Emory mouse. FASEB J 1989; 3:1741–1746.

287. Tchen TT, Chan SW, Kuo TH, Mostafapour KM, Dezewiecki VH. Studies on the adrenal cortex of hypophysectomized rats: A model for abnormal cellular atrophy and death. Mol Cell Biochem 1977; 15:79–87.

288. Trump BF, Bulger RE. Studies of cellular injury in isolated flounder tubules. I. Correlation between morphology and function of control tubules and observations of autophagocytosis and mechanical cell damage. Lab Invest 1967; 16:453–482.

289. Walker NI. Ultrastructure of the rat pancreas after experimental duct ligation. I. The role of apoptosis and intraepithelial macrophages in acinar cell deletion. Am J Pathol 1987; 126:439–451.

290. Walker NI, Gobé GC. Cell death and cell proliferation during atrophy of the rat parotid gland induced by duct obstruction. J Pathol 1987; 153:333–344.

291. Weber G. Pathology of glucose-6-phosphate metabolism. A study in enzyme pathology. Rev Can Biol 1959; 18:245–282.

292. Weindruch RH, Walford RL. Aging and functions of the RES. In: Cohen N, Sigel MM (eds). The reticuloendothelial system: a comprehensive treatise, vol. 3. New York: Plenum Press, 1982, pp. 713–748.

293. Weindruch R, Walford RL. The retardation of aging and disease by dietary restriction. Springfield: Charles C Thomas, 1988.

294. Weindruch R, Walford RL, Fligiel S, Guthrie D. The retardation of aging in mice by dietary restriction: longevity, cancer, immunity and lifetime energy intake. J Nutrition 1986; 116:641–654.

295. Williamson JR. Adipose tissue. Morphological changes associated with lipid mobilization. J Cell Biol 1964; 20:57–74.

296. Winick M (ed). Hunger disease. New York: John Wiley & Sons, 1979.

297. Wyllie AH, Kerr JFR, Currie AR. Cell death: the significance of apoptosis. Int Rev Cytol 1980; 68:251–306.

298. Yu BP. Recent advances in dietary restriction and aging. In: Rothstein M (ed). Review of biological research in aging, vol. 2. New York: Alan R. Liss, Inc., 1985, pp. 435–443.

299. Zoumbos NC, Gascón P, Djeu JY, Trost SR, Young NS. Circulating activated suppressor T lymphocytes in aplastic anemia. N Engl J Med 1985; 312:257–265.

Phenotypic Changes

300. Aloe L, Levi-Montalcini R. Nerve growth factor-induced transformation of immature chromaffin cells in vivo into sympathetic neurons: effect of antiserum to nerve growth factor. Proc Natl Acad Sci USA 1979; 76:1246–1250.

301. Benito M, Porras A, Nebreda AR, Santos E. Differentiation of 3T3-L1 fibroblasts to adipocytes induced by transfection of ras oncogenes. Science 1991; 253:565–568.

302. Beresford WA. Chondroid bone, secondary cartilage and metaplasia. Baltimore-Munich: Urban & Schwarzenberg, 1981.

303. Beresford WA. Direct transdifferentiation: can cells change their phenotype without dividing? Cell Differ Dev 1990; 29:81–93.

304. Bordi C, Ravazzola M. Endocrine cells in the intestinal metaplasia of gastric mucosa. Am J Pathol 1979; 96:391–398.

305. Bouillaud F, Ricquier D, Mory G, Thibault J. Increased level of mRNA for the uncoupling protein in brown adipose tissue of rats during thermogenesis induced by cold exposure or norepinephrine infusion. J Biol Chem 1984; 259:11583–11586.

306. Cameron AJ, Ott BJ, Payne WS. The incidence of adenocarcinoma in columnar-lined (Barrett's) esophagus. N Engl J Med 1985; 313:857–859.

307. Campbell GR, Campbell JH. Smooth muscle phenotypic changes in arterial wall homeostasis: implications for the pathogenesis of atherosclerosis. Exp Mol Pathol 1985; 42:139–162.

308. Cantin M, Araujo-Nascimento Mdef, Benchimol S, Desormeaux Y. Metaplasia of smooth muscle cells into juxtaglomerular cells in the juxtaglomerular apparatus, arteries, and arterioles of the ischemic (endocrine) kidney. Am J Pathol 1977; 87:581–602.

309. Chopra DP. Squamous metaplasia in organ cultures of vitamin A-deficient hamster trachea: cytokinetic and ultrastructural alterations. J Natl Cancer Inst 1982; 69:895–905.

310. DiBerardino MA, Hoffner NJ, Etkin LD. Activation of dormant genes in specialized cells. Science 1984; 224:946–952.

311. Ekblom P. Developmentally regulated conversion of mesenchyme to epithelium. FASEB J 1989; 3:2141–2150.

312. Fell HB, Mellanby E. Metaplasia produced in cultures of chick ectoderm by high vitamin A. J Physiol 1953; 119:470–488.

313. Hamilton SR. Pathogenesis of columnar cell-lined (Barrett's) esophagus. In: Spechler SJ, Goyal RK (eds). Barrett's esophagus: pathophysiology, diagnosis and management. New York: Elsevier, 1985, pp. 29–37.

314. Hausberger FX. Über die nervöse Regulation des Fettstoffwechsels. Klin Wochenschr 1935; 14:77–79.

315. Hilding A. Experimental surgery of the nose and sinuses. I. Changes in the morphology of the epithelium following variations in ventilation. Arch Otolaryngol 1932; 15:9–18.

316. Hong WK, Endicott J, Itri LM, et al. 13-cis-retinoic acid in the treatment of oral leukoplakia. N Engl J Med 1986; 315:1501–1505.

317. Jetten AM, Brody AR, Deas MA, Hook GER, Rearick JI, Thacher SM. Retinoic acid and substratum regulate the differentiation of rabbit tracheal epithelial cells into squamous and secretory phenotype. Morphological and biochemical characterization. Lab Invest 1987; 56:654–664.

318. Jones PA, Taylor SM. Cellular differentiation, cytidine analogs and DNA methylation. Cell 1980; 20:85–93.

319. Kim SW, Charter RA, Chai CJ, Kim SK, Kim ES. Serum alkaline phosphatase and inorganic phosphorus values in spinal cord injury patients with heterotopic ossification. Paraplegia 1990; 28:441–447.

320. Konieczny SF, Emerson CP Jr. 5-Azacytidine induction of stable mesodermal stem cell lineages from 10T1/2 cells: evidence for regulatory genes controlling determination. Cell 1984; 38:791–800.

321. Lean MEJ, James WPT, Jennings G, Trayhurn P. Brown adipose tissue in patients with phaeochromocytoma. Int J Obesity 1986; 10:219–227.

322. Lombardi T, Montesano R, Furie MB, Silverstein SC, Orci L. Endothelial diaphragmed fenestrae: In vitro modulation by phorbol myristate acetate. J Cell Biol 1986; 102:1965–1970.

323. Lombardi T, Montesano R, Furie MB, Silverstein SC, Orci L. In vitro modulation of endothelial fenestrae: opposing effects of retinoic acid and transforming growth factor ß. J Cell Sci 1988; 91:313–318.

324. Lugo M, Petersen RO, Elfenbein IB, Stein BS, Duker NJ. Nephrogenic metaplasia of the ureter. Am J Clin Pathol 1983; 80:92–97.

325. Lugo M, Putong PB. Metaplasia. An overview. Arch Pathol Lab Med 1984; 108:185–189.

326. Ma J, De Boer WGRM, Nayman J. Intestinal mucinous substances in gastric intestinal metaplasia and carcinoma studied by immunofluorescence. Cancer 1982; 49:1664–1667.

327. Majack RA, Bornstein P. Heparin regulates the collagen phenotype of vascular smooth muscle cells: Induced synthesis of an M_r 60,000 collagen. J Cell Biol 1985; 100:613–619.

328. Majno G, Joris I. Endothelium 1977: a review. Adv Exp Med Biol 1978; 104:169–225; 481–526.

329. Makino T, Usuda N, Rao S, Reddy JK, Scarpelli DG. Transdifferentiation of ductular cells into hepatocytes in regenerating hamster pancreas. Lab Invest 1990; 62:552–561.

330. McCarthy PL, Shklar G. Diseases of the oral mucosa, 2nd ed. Philadelphia: Lea & Febiger, 1980.

331. McDevitt DS. Transdifferentiation in animals. A model for differentiation control. Dev Biol (NY 1985) 1989; 6:149–173.

332. McGuire PG, Orkin RW. Isolation of rat aortic endothelial cells by primary explant techniques and their phenotypic modulation by defined substrata. Lab Invest 1987; 57:94–105.

333. Melicow MM. Hibernating fat and pheochromocytoma. Arch Pathol 1957; 63:367–372.

334. Merk FB, Warhol MJ, Kwan PW-L, et al. Multiple phenotypes of prostatic glandular cells in castrated dogs after individual or combined treatment with androgen and estrogen. Morphometric, ultrastructural, and cytochemical distinctions. Lab Invest 1986; 54:442–456.

335. Ming S-C, Goldman H, Freiman DG. Intestinal metaplasia and histogenesis of carcinoma in human stomach. Light and electron microscopic study. Cancer 1967; 20:1418–1429.

336. Montesano R, Orci L, Vassalli P. In vitro rapid organization of endothelial cells into capillary-like networks is promoted by collagen matrices. J Cell Biol 1983; 97:1648–1652.

337. Montesano R, Orci L, Vassalli P. Human endothelial cell cultures: phenotypic modulation by leukocyte interleukins. J Cell Physiol 1985; 122:424–434.

338. Morris DA, Henkind P. Pathological responses of the human retinal pigment epithelium. In: Zinn KM, Marmor MF (eds). The retinal pigment epithelium. Cambridge: Harvard University Press, 1979, p. 247–266.

339. Mosse PRL, Campbell GR, Wang ZL, Campbell JH. Smooth muscle phenotypic expression in human carotid arteries. I. Comparison of cells from diffuse intimal thickenings adjacent to atheromatous plaques with those of the media. Lab Invest 1985; 53:556–562.

340. Nathanson MA. Transdifferentiation of skeletal muscle into cartilage: transformation or differentiation? Curr Top Dev Biol 1986; 20:39–62.

341. Ogawa M, Ishikawa T, Ohta H. Transdifferentiation of endocrine chromaffin cells into neuronal cells. Curr Top Dev Biol 1986; 20:99–110.

342. Okada TS. Cellular metaplasia or transdifferentiation as a model for retinal cell differentiation. Curr Top Dev Biol 1980; 16:349–380.

343. Rabinovitch PS, Reid BJ, Haggitt RC, Norwood TH, Rubin CE. Progression to cancer in Barrett's esophagus is associated with genomic instability. Lab Invest 1988; 60:65–71.

344. Reh TA, Nagy T, Gretton H. Retinal pigmented epithelial cells induced to transdifferentiate to neurons by laminin. Nature 1987; 330:68–71.

345. Ricquier D, Mory G, Bouillaud F, Combes-George M, Thibault J. Factors controlling brown adipose tissue development. Reprod Nutr Dev 1985; 25:175–181.

346. Ricquier D, Mory G, Nechad M, Combes-George M, Thibault J. Development and activation of brown fat in rats with pheochromocytoma PC 12 tumors. Am J Physiol 1983; 245:C172–C177.

347. Salley JJ, Bryson WF. Vitamin A deficiency in the hamster. J Dent Res 1957; 36:935–944.

348. Sappino AP, Schürch W, Gabbiani G. Differentiation repertoire of fibroblastic cells: expression of cytoskeletal proteins as marker of phenotypic molulations. Lab Invest 1990; 63:144–161.

349. Shklar G. Oral leukoplakia. N Engl J Med 1986; 315:1544–1546.

350. Spechler SJ. The risk of cancer in Barrett's esophagus. In: Spechler SJ, Goyal RK (eds). Barrett's esophagus: pathophysiology, diagnosis, and management. New York: Elsevier, 1985, pp. 189–197.

351. Tapscott SJ, Davis RL, Thayer MJ, Cheng P-F, Weintraub H, Lassar AB. MyoD1: A nuclear phosphoprotein requiring a Myc homology region to convert fibroblasts to myoblasts. Science 1988; 242:405–411.

352. Taylor SM, Jones PA. Multiple new phenotypes induced in 10T1/2 and 3T3 cells treated with 5-Azacytidine. Cell 1979; 17:771–779.

353. Trump BF, McDowell EM, Glavin F, et al. The respiratory epithelium. III. Histogenesis of epidermoid metaplasia and carcinoma in situ in the human. J Natl Cancer Inst 1978; 61:563–575.

354. Wolbach SB, Howe PR. Vitamin A deficiency in the guinea-pig. Arch Pathol 1928; 5:239–253.

355. Wong Y-C, Buck RC. An electron microscopic study of

metaplasia of the rat tracheal epithelium in Vitamin A deficiency. Lab Invest 1971; 24:55–66.

356. Yamada T. Transdifferentiation of lens cells and its regulation. In: McDevitt DS (ed). Cell biology of the eye. New York: Academic Press, 1982, pp. 193–242.

Cell Activation and Priming

357. Adams DO, Hamilton TA. The cell biology of macrophage activation. Annu Rev Immunol 1984; 2:283–318.

358. Aitken A. The biochemical mechanism of action of phorbol esters. In: Evans FJ (ed). Naturally occurring phorbol esters. Boca Raton: CRC Press, Inc., 1986, pp. 271–288.

359. Alberts B, Bray D, Lewis J, Raff M, Roberts K, Watson JD. Molecular biology of the cell, 2nd ed. New York: Garland Publishing, Inc., 1989.

360. Altman J. Ins and outs of cell signalling. Nature 1988; 331:119–120.

361. Bentley R, Trimen H. Medicinal plants, vol. 4. London: Churchill, 1880.

362. Chiu R, Imagawa M, Imbra RJ, Bockoven JR, Karin M. Multiple cis- and trans-acting elements mediate the transcriptional response to phorbol esters. Nature 1987; 329:648–651.

363. Drevets WC, Videen TO, Price JL, Preskorn SH, Carmichael ST, Raichle ME. A functional anatomical study of unipolar depression. J Neurosci 1992; 12:3628–3641.

364. Metchnikoff E. L'immunité dans les maladies infectieuses. Paris: Masson & Co., 1901.

Symptoms of Cellular Disease: Intracellular Accumulations

CHAPTER 3

Accumulation of Fluid

Accumulation of Lipids

Accumulation of Glycogen and Related Materials

Accumulation of Pigments

Up to this point we have discussed cellular adaptations such as increases or decreases in cell size or number. Now we can proceed to examine true symptoms of cellular disease. To begin, we can assume that something is wrong with a cell if it contains unusual intracellular granules or droplets (vacuoles). The hoarded material may be derived from the cell's own metabolism, from the extracellular space (such as spilled blood), or from the outer environment (such as dust). Whatever its nature, this material always carries a message, which may be good, bad, or indifferent regarding the health of the cell. Some cell types are especially prone to hoard certain types of material, such as triglycerides in liver cells.

It is convenient to classify abnormal intracellular content by its chemical nature. If we exclude rare congenital storage diseases, in which special macromolecules are hoarded (p. 142), there are five main groups:

- water and electrolytes
- lipids
- carbohydrates
- proteins
- a motley group of "pigments"

The ultimate fate of any of these materials depends on its digestibility: *if the cell is unable to metabolize a substance, it is condemned to live with it.*

Accumulation of Fluid

Excess fluid can appear in the cell as discrete droplets (*vacuoles*) or as diffuse waterlogging of the entire cell, which results in cellular swelling, sometimes called **hydropic swelling.**

VACUOLES

Droplets of fluid in cells are very common; under the microscope they appear as empty little spheres, hence their name (*vacu-olus* is Latin for "empty-small"). In plant cells, but not in animal cells, a large vacuole called a **tonoplast** is a normal and important cellular oganelle that contributes to the cell's turgor (9, 28). If the tonoplasts of a leaf collapse, the whole leaf collapses; this is why plants wilt and animals do not—we have no tonoplasts.

Simple as they may look, vacuoles can form in at least four different ways: by pinocytosis, by swelling of one organelle or another, and by herniation—plus a bizarre type of extracellular vacuole specific to the kidney tubules. One cell may contain vacuoles of different kinds.

VACUOLES DUE TO PINOCYTOSIS

Some cells drink more than others. The champions are the activated macrophages, which pinocytize so

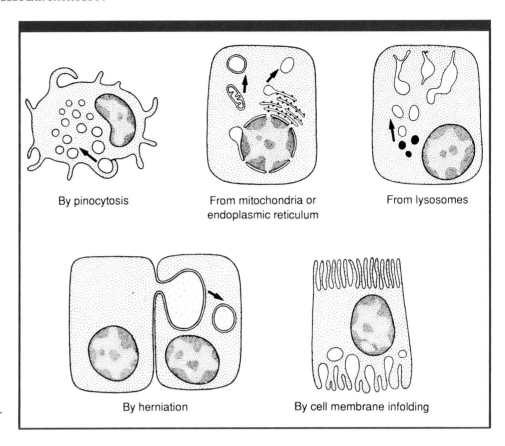

By pinocytosis

From mitochondria or
endoplasmic reticulum

From lysosomes

By herniation

By cell membrane infolding

FIGURE 3.1
Mechanisms that lead to the formation of vacuoles.

frantically that every hour they can take in one quarter of their volume of fluid (12, 31). Of course, most of the fluid taken in is promptly returned to the outside. Vacuoles generated in this manner are of little or no pathologic significance, except that they point to heavy drinking. Now, *if the medium happens to contain a soluble molecule that the macrophages cannot digest, such as sucrose, they can still expel the fluid—but not the sucrose, which is retained.* If this is happening *in vitro*, the overloaded macrophage can be put out of its misery by adding the missing enzyme to the medium (Figure 3.2) (13).

Osmotic nephrosis. There is an *in vivo* counterpart to this sucrose indigestion. In the 1940s it was noticed that patients who had been given intravenous injections of hypertonic sucrose solutions developed extensive vacuolization of the renal convoluted tubules (27). The tubular epithelium had reabsorbed tubular fluid loaded with sucrose. The resulting vacuoles correspond to enlarged lysosomes, and the tubular change that follows is known as **sucrose nephrosis** or **osmotic nephrosis** (23, 24, 33).

VACUOLES DUE TO ORGANELLE SWELLING

Three organelles are prone to pathologic swelling: *the mitochondria, the endoplasmic reticulum, and the lysosomes.* The mechanisms are not understood, nor

is it clear why the other ten or twelve membrane-bound intracellular compartments are relatively spared. Even with the electron microscope it can be difficult to find out how a vacuole developed; however, if a vacuole contains acid phosphatase, it can be assumed to derive from a lysosome.

In suffering cells, *one or more mitochondria are apt to swell to the point of appearing like vacuoles;* this change is extremely common and extremely fast (minutes), and almost unfailingly develops as an artefact in tissue samples if fixation is not immediate, because cells have time to suffer from asphyxia or from slow poisoning by the fixative. Mitochondrial swelling is therefore a curse for the electron microscopist; it is not always easy to decide whether it represents an artefact or disease.

Other vacuoles represent expanded cisternae of the endoplasmic reticulum (4, 5). For reasons unknown, the perinuclear cisterna is especially prone to swell; and when it does so, this is a reliable sign of cellular distress.

Genesis of vacuoles from cisternae of the endoplasmic reticulum was proven by a technical tour de force by a determined Australian pathologist, Ian Buckley (5). Although single cisternae should not be visible by light microscopy, Buckley (working in the laboratory of Keith Porter) managed to see them in very thin expansions of cell grown in vitro, the same biological model that had allowed Porter to discover the endoplasmic reticulum (p. 138). In asphyxiated fibroblasts, Buckley saw swellings appear here and there in the endoplasmic reticulum, running up and down a cisterna like beads on a string, as documented by an excellent movie (Figure 3.3).

The third organelle that is prone to swell is the lysosome. The primal studies are due again to Ian Buckley (6), who examined living cultured cells that either were undergoing spontaneous aging or were mildly injured by cooling to 25°C. The lysosomes swelled into vacuoles; then their membranes began to emit and retract thin tubular extensions, which could also anastomose and form a network that was very difficult to distinguish from the endoplasmic reticulum network just described. The tentacles of the swollen lysosomes seemed to be probing the cytoplasm for material to digest. If this optimistic interpretation is correct, we would have an instance of "helpful" vacuoles.

Nerve fibers can form vacuoles due to localized swelling of the myelin, as if fluid were being pumped between the membrane layers; the mechanism is not understood. A change of this kind explains the vacuolar myelopathy of nervous tissue typical of AIDS (2).

VACUOLES THAT REPRESENT CELLULAR HERNIAE

This strange microscopic accident happens when a cell gives rise to a mushroom-shaped process—a

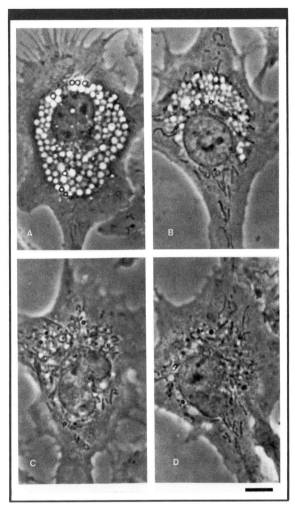

FIGURE 3.2
Cellular indigestion and its treatment. **A.** Vacuolization of a mouse macrophage *in vitro* after 24-hour exposure to an undigestible sugar (sucrose). **B:** 30 minutes after the addition of invertase. **C:** 75 minutes after the addition. **D:** 120 minutes after the addition. The vacuoles disappear, leaving a residue of small dense granules. **Bar** = 5 μm. (Reproduced with permission from [13].)

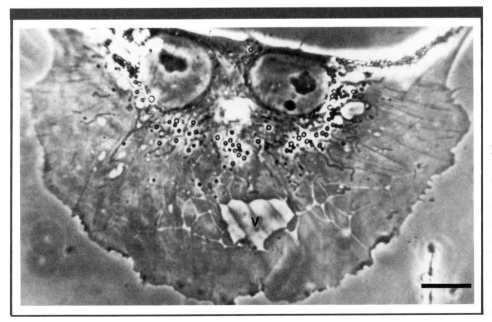

FIGURE 3.3
Development of vacuoles from the endoplasmic reticulum. This live, cultured chick embryo cell contains a reticular network that appears white by phase contrast microscopy: the endoplasmic reticulum (ER). **V:** vacuole arising within it. As seen *in vivo* the size and shape of such ER vacuoles continue to change. **Bar** = 10 μm. (Reproduced with permission from [4]).

hernia—that pokes into a neighboring cell (19) (Figure 3.4). Dictionaries define hernia as *the protrusion of a bodily structure through the wall that normally contains it.* It must be understood that the retaining wall of a hernia is weakened but not broken, so that the herniating structure becomes contained in a thin sac called a hernia sac.

Most commonly cellular herniation occurs between smooth muscle cells. As they contract, their surface gives rise to bulges that can be firm enough to push their way into the nearest cell, usually at points of close contact where the basement membrane is absent. During relaxation the bulges can retract, but some break off and remain inside the "host" cell, where they tend to swell and become vacuoles. We call these structures **cell-to-cell herniae.** They are interesting because, in the media of arteries, they tell us that an intense contraction (spasm) has occurred (19) and because, in a more general way, they mean that a smooth muscle cell can be damaged in the course of its physiologic function. The hallmark of these special vacuoles, as shown by electron microscopy, is that they are limited by two cell membranes: the inner from the herniating cell and the outer (hernia sac) from the host cell.

Similar herniae can occur when a medial smooth muscle cell pokes into an endothelial cell (myoendothelial herniae) (32) or when a myocardial cell protrudes into its neighbor across the intercalated disc. Why the cell-to-cell herniae tend to swell is not clear. Perhaps they do so because they are lined with two cell membranes facing each other, both endowed with sodium pumps. It is conceivable that the pump in the inner membrane fails because it is cut off from its cell, while the outer one continues to pump water and sodium into the enclosed space.

*The term **extracellular vacuoles** sounds like a contradiction, but in renal convoluted tubules the following can happen, thanks to the unique arrangement of the basal part of the cells. Deep infoldings of the basal cell membrane create a succession of thin cytoplasmic sheets and virtual extracellular spaces. If the latter swell, the fluid is anatomically outside the cell wall, but with the light microscope it appears as a basal vacuole (subbasilar vacuolation) (Figure 3.1) (3). This lesion was once thought to be specific for low-plasma potassium (hypokalemia), such as may occur with chronic diarrhea or vomiting; actually it has a variety of causes that presumably affect the function of the basilar cell membrane. Even an overload of intravenous saline can produce it (26).*

CELLULAR SWELLING

Besides suffering from fluid-filled vacuoles, cells can also become waterlogged as a whole, as a result of an osmotic disturbance. In this condition they are enlarged but not hypertrophic. Typically, this disturbance occurs in an acute setting, in a matter of minutes and hours. There is also a chronic form of osmotic swelling that occurs in diabetes, over weeks, months, and years. Whether chronically swollen cells may adapt by becoming hypertrophic is not known.

ACUTE CELLULAR SWELLING

Some cells rapidly become bloated—**hydropic** is the traditional term—if the ionic pumps in the cell membrane fail (23a). This happens when the cell's energy supplies are cut off, either by failure of the blood supply or by a metabolic poison. Sodium ions seep in, taking water with them, and the cell swells. We will return to this topic in discussing cellular injury (p. 191).

Acute cellular swelling is an indication of severe cellular distress, but it may become the cause of further problems by the very fact that it takes up space and may therefore impair blood flow. This is especially critical in the brain, where there is no room for expansion. The impairment of blood flow by acute

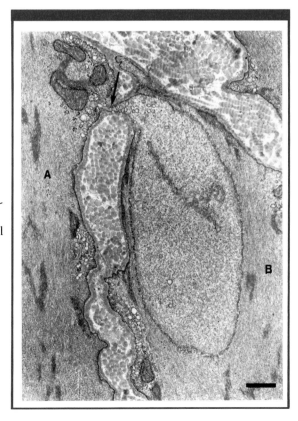

FIGURE 3.4 Special type of vacuole, caused by herniation of one smooth muscle cell into another in the wall of a contracting artery. Cell **A** is herniating into its neighbor **B**. The stalk of the hernia is indicated by the **arrow. Bar** = 0.5 μm. (Reproduced with permission from [19].)

cellular swelling was first demonstrated in rat liver by a simple experiment. The liver is acutely poisoned by means of carbon tetrachloride; four hours later it has become so swollen that India ink injected into the portal blood cannot flow through the lobules (Figure 3.5) (16). We will see shortly that a similar circulatory problem arises if the liver cells are bloated with fat.

Another example of flow impaired by swollen cells is provided by the toxemia of pregnancy, or **eclampsia,** a serious complication of pregnancy characterized by hypertension, proteinuria, and edema. In this case the endothelial cells of the glomeruli swell and reduce blood flow through the kidney (ischemia); this may be responsible for the hypertension.

> *Renal ischemia causes hypertension because it stimulates the juxtaglomerular cells to secrete more renin, which acts on angiotensinogen to produce angiotensin I, which is converted in the lung to the potent vasoconstrictor angiotensin II. Why, in eclampsia, the endothelial cells swell only in the glomeruli is not understood, but the plasma of these patients does contain a material that is toxic for cultured endothelial cells (29).*

CHRONIC CELLULAR SWELLING: A MISDEED OF SUGARS

Chronic cellular swelling was discovered by studying the complications of diabetes, especially the cataract and the nerve changes (neuropathies).

Despite many open ends, the basic mechanism is clear. Some types of cells, such as those of the lens and the Schwann cells of nerve sheaths, allow glucose to penetrate the cell membrane independent of insulin control (by contrast with fat and muscle cells, in which the entry of glucose is regulated by insulin). This means that if the blood glucose rises, the cells become overloaded with glucose. Then the trouble begins: some of the excess glucose is reduced to sorbitol by the enzyme aldose reductase, and some of the sorbitol is converted to fructose. Both sorbitol and fructose are retained within the cell, and being osmotically active, they cause the cell to swell. *The lens is especially vulnerable because its ability to metabolize glucose is very low* (34). Eventually the plasma membranes become leaky and the cells die: for the lens, this means developing a cataract (p. 195). The crowning proof of this mechanism is that, in hyperglycemic animals, inhibitors of aldose reductase prevent the cataract (21).

> *As related to experimental cataracts the sorbitol mechanism seems to fit like a glove, but when applied to other tissues and to human diabetes the fit is not as good (7, 8, 11, 14, 22). In diabetic neuropathies, for example, sorbitol in degenerated nerves is not always increased. The preventive or curative effect of aldose reductase (20) has many exceptions, and besides, in humans both cataract and neuropathies develop so slowly that the effects of therapy are*

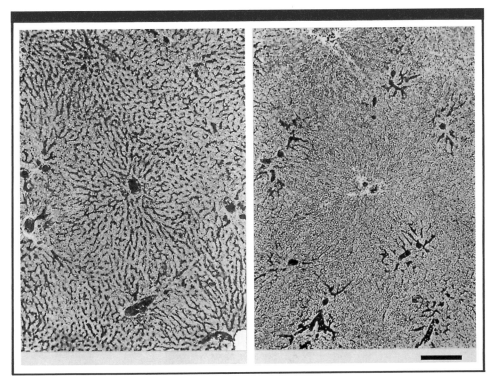

FIGURE 3.5
Impaired circulation in the liver lobule due to cellular swelling. India ink was injected into the portal circulation just prior to sacrifice. *Left:* Normal rat liver; the sinusoids are completely filled with India ink. *Right:* 2 hours after carbon tetrachloride injection (0.2 ml/100 g) the India ink is present at the periphery of the lobule but has difficulty in penetrating toward the central vein. **Bar** = 200 μm. (Reproduced with permission from [16].)

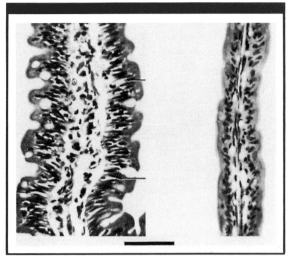

FIGURE 3.6
Effect of dehydration on the intestinal mucosa. *Left:*
Control; normal villus incubated for one minute with 150
mM saline solution. Some dilatation of intercellular spaces
(**arrows**) appears in the epithelium. *Right:* Villus of the
same animal after one minute exposure to 780 mOsm/kg
solution (a 50% solution of the hypertonic radiographic
contrast medium Hypaque). **Bar** = 50 μm. (Reproduced
with permission from [25].)

*difficult to evaluate. Furthermore, another metabolic
mechanism seems to intervene, namely a drop in
myo-inositol. This is a six-carbon cyclic hexanol
sterically similar to glucose that is ubiquitous in
animal and plant cells, often in millimolar
concentrations—yet its functions are not well understood (17). Cells obtain it from nutritional sources
and by synthesis. Somehow, in hyperglycemia the
intracellular myo-inositol drops; this leads to metabolic disturbances in the membrane phospholipids
(phosphoinositides) and thereby to defects in membrane functions, including signal transduction, leading to cell death. Alas, the neat sorbitol-related cell
swelling has grown into a gigantic puzzle—but one
that promises to be very important for understanding
some of the complications of diabetes.*

*Cellular shrinkage may also occur. Whereas
tardigrades and other small creatures can survive the
loss of virtually all their water, animal cells cannot
afford to lose more than roughly 50 percent (10).
Possible causes of cell death by dehydration include
damage to the plasma membrane, to the cytoplasmic
proteins, to the cytoskeleton, and even to the
microtrabecular lattice (MTL; p. 158) (10, 18). To
our knowledge, this is the only suggested role for the
MTL in cellular pathology. Dehydration of the
intestinal mucosa for one minute with a hypertonic
solution produces severe changes (Figure 3.6) (25),
and dehydration of the body as a whole leads to
damage to the renal medulla (30), where—
interestingly—the interstitium is normally hypertonic. This topic needs further study.*

Accumulation of Lipids

Lipid droplets and phospholipid membranes are
part of life, but when they are in the wrong place
or in the wrong amount, they mean cellular
disease. Microscopically they can be identified as
lipid by means of lipid-soluble stains. Three types
of lipid that tend to form abnormal deposits belong
to the three main groups of lipids that are found in
the body; to these we must add a group of oxidized
lipids (Figure 3.7).

- **Triglycerides** (the main lipids of fat cells,
  also called **triacylglycerols**) are such frequent offenders in liver cells that this cellular storage has earned its own special name,
  steatosis (from the Greek *stéar*, "fat").
- **Cholesterol** and its esters are chemically
  ubiquitous, but they are typically hoarded
  by a few cell types that are especially at risk
  because they can be exposed to a high cholesterol "diet." Most prone are macrophages, whose scavenger habits often lead
  to cholesterol overload, and arterial smooth

FIGURE 3.7
Abnormal deposits of intracellular
lipid can take these principal forms.
Droplets of **triglycerides** are usually
non membrane-bound. **Cholesteryl
esters** are mainly intralysosomal. **Myelin figures** can be intracellular and
extracellular. **Lipofuscin** which can
be classified as a lipid or as a pigment, is present in residual bodies, together with other materials.

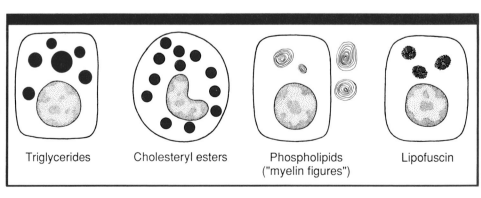

Triglycerides   Cholesteryl esters   Phospholipids   Lipofuscin
                                       ("myelin figures")

muscle cells in atherosclerosis. In the latter case the risk factor is the location within the arterial wall; plasma, unlike other body fluids, is loaded with cholesterol, and the endothelium (in atherosclerosis) may let some through.

- **Phospholipids,** the ubiquitous components of cell membranes, tend to form abnormal membranous structures called **myelin figures,** either within the cells or in the tissue spaces (p. 211).
- **Lipofuscin,** a special category of heavily oxidized, indigestible, brownish, leftover intracellular lipids, will be considered among the pigments (p. 97).

A technical parenthesis: how are lipids identified? This is not a small problem because lipids are microscopically elusive, at least compared with the thousands of different proteins that can be identified by antibody methods. In fact, some lipids may be gone by the time we would like to see them. Triglycerides and cholesteryl esters (collectively known as **neutral fats**) are lost forever during paraffin embedding, which requires soaking the tissues in fat solvents (alcohol, xylene). Therefore, to search for neutral fats, unprocessed tissue must be cut in the frozen state (with or without previous fixation) using a special type of microtome; the sections are then treated with a fat stain. Fat stains are simply dyes that are indiscriminately soluble in neutral fats. Thus, a stained droplet tells us, "This is triglyceride, cholesteryl ester, or a mixture of both," which enables us to rule out proteins and water-soluble materials; but we still do not know which type of neutral fat is present. There are no specific stains for triglycerides, so the best approach is to rule out cholesterol ester by study in polarized light. If the droplet is birefringent—that is, it produces the typical "maltese cross"—it should contain cholesteryl ester. In highly specialized laboratories the lipid droplet can be diagnosed by studying its melting point on a heating stage (87). However, remember that lipids tend to dissolve into each other; thus, in practice, *all lipid droplets are likely to contain a mixture of lipids.* Definitive identification of triglyceride must always rest on chemical analysis of the tissue. This means that the light microscopic diagnosis of steatosis, strictly speaking, is always circumstantial even for frozen sections.

On paraffin-embedded tissue, neutral fats cannot be identified at all because the droplets have disappeared altogether, leaving a hole. The mean-

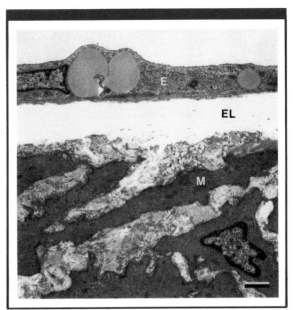

FIGURE 3.8 Droplets of lipid (cholesterol esters) in the aortic endothelium of a hypercholesterolemic rat. **E:** endothelium. **EL:** internal elastic lamina. **M:** smooth muscle cells. **Bar** = 1 μm.

ing of this hole can only be a guess based on cell type, circumstances, size and number of droplets, and experience. Phospholipids are not extracted by histologic processing, in part because they are bound to cell proteins as structural components of all membranes.

In tissues processed for electron microscopy and fixed with osmium tetroxide, small droplets of neutral fats are usually preserved as a homogeneous mass (Figure 3.8). In any case, the diagnosis of lipid is again circumstantial.

ACCUMULATION OF TRIGLYCERIDES (STEATOSIS)

Droplets of triglycerides are normally present in a few types of cells, especially in the liver, heart, and muscle, and strangely enough, in the chondrocytes (77). When the number or size of these droplets is excessive or when the droplets appear in cells usually devoid of triglycerides, we are dealing with **steatosis,** a reversible process. This cellular anomaly has long been in the limelight because it can be diagnosed—note!—with the naked eye: the color of the liver changes from red to golden yellow (Figure 3.9). Furthermore, steatosis has the singular privilege of being one of the few diseases that are eaten; foie gras is the sick, fatty liver of artificially overfed geese.

Steatosis is also called fatty change; this awkward name was created as a reaction against the ancient term fatty degeneration, which implied, wrongly, that

FIGURE 3.9 **See color plate 2.** Close-up view of two livers, placed next to each other and reproduced here in natural size. *Left:* Fatty liver with early cirrhosis in an alcoholic. *Right:* Normal liver as a control.

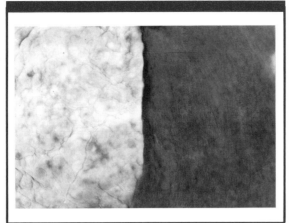

the fat appeared as a result of some obscure degenerative process.

ORGANS AFFECTED BY STEATOSIS

Steatosis is most common in the liver, which is, after adipose tissue, the principal organ of triglyceride synthesis. *Steatosis has been chemically confirmed in only four organs: liver, heart, muscle, and kidney cortex.* It is surely no accident that these four organs can derive all or almost all their energy from the oxidation of fatty acids (39, 66, 87), the principal building blocks of triglycerides. It was once believed that steatosis can occur in any cell, which may well be true, but we found no chemical proof that steatosis occurs in cells other than those mentioned. Electron microscopy suggests that it also occurs in the pancreas of starved animals (72). The presence of stained lipid droplets is all to often labeled uncritically as steatosis without ruling out cholesteryl esters.

GROSS FEATURES OF STEATOSIS

To the naked eye, a pale liver, heart, or kidney always suggests steatosis, especially *if the organ has a yellowish hue* (paleness alone can also mean reduced blood content). It is surprising that tiny intracellular droplets of lipid can lead to such a difference in the gross color (Figure 3.9). Triglycerides are actually white; the pigmentation is due to the nutritionally derived carotenoids that are dissolved in the droplets (74).

There has been a language mixup about cirrhosis. It was the yellowness of the liver in chronic alcoholics that first impressed Laennec in 1819, when he coined the name cirrhosis from the Greek kirrhós, "yellow." Posterity then decided that the fibrosis of these livers is more impressive than the color, and so we now use the name cirrhosis to mean "severe fibrosis." Cirrhosis has therefore lost all connections with yellowness. Laennec would probably be horrified.

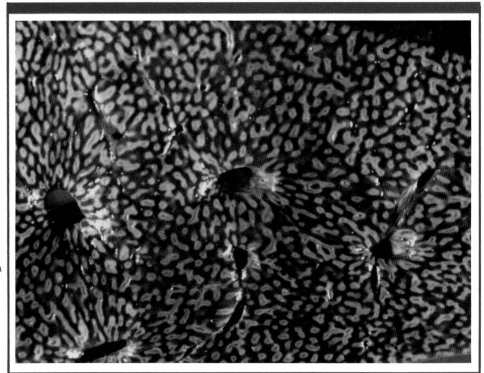

FIGURE 3.10
Centrolobular fatty change from anoxia in the liver of a horse, which died of a methemoglobinemia from eating red maple leaves off the ground in the fall. The central cells of each liver lobule are oxygen-starved because methemoglobin does not carry oxygen. (Reproduced with permission from [84].)

Advanced steatosis increases the size of the organ; the liver can double its normal weight of 1500 g. The change in liver texture can be great enough to be picked up as decreased density by computer tomography (CT scan), ultrasonography, and magnetic resonance imaging; radiologists use the density of the spleen for comparison. At autopsy, organs with severe steatosis feel softer, and the knife that cuts them becomes greasy.

Steatosis in a given organ can be focal. Because anoxia is a major cause of steatosis, local differences in oxygen supply are reflected in lipid deposition. For example, in cases of severe anemia, fatty hepatocytes prevail in the centrolobular zone, where oxygen supply is poorest. The same pattern is produced if the oxygen-carrying capacity of hemoglobin is impaired (toxic anoxia) (Figure 3.10). Steatosis is common around myocardial infarcts; we can rationalize that the bulk of the infarct consists of cells that received no oxygen, whereas the cells at the periphery are surviving on a minimal supply (40). Severely anemic hearts sometimes show a strange patch of fine, parallel, yellowish stripes known as **thrush-breast heart** or **tabby-cat heart** (*coeur tigré*, in French). Despite the zoological flurry no study has been made, but the yellow stripes probably represent perivenular zones of poor oxygenation.

MICROSCOPIC FEATURES OF STEATOSIS

In the liver, steatosis can assume two aspects. In some forms of toxic steatosis, such as by tetracycline treatment (41), the droplets of fat are many, small, and membrane-bound; this is called **microvesicular steatosis** (Figure 3.11). In all other forms of steatosis, such as in the alcoholic liver, the droplets are free in the cytoplasm, are larger, and tend to coalesce into a single large drop (Figure 3.12). The cells can become so distended with fat that they resemble adipocytes. In extreme cases the droplets can burst free, find their way into the bloodstream, and be carried to the lung, where they remain impacted (64). In the fatty livers of choline-deficient rats, microscopic "cysts" of free fat can develop by the rupture of fat-laden hepatocytes (51). In muscle cells, where the cytoplasm is crowded with fibrils, the lipid droplets remain quite small; they are neatly strung like beads along the rows of mitochondria (Figure 3.13).

Seen by electron microscopy, in normal liver small triglyceride droplets lie free in the cytoplasm and have no limiting membrane, even though their outer rim may appear slightly darker (69). In most

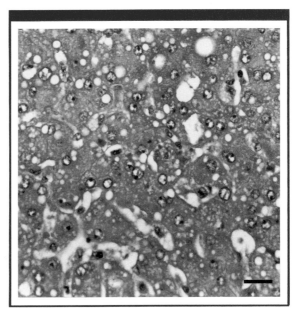

FIGURE 3.11 Human liver biopsy showing steatosis of the "microvesicular" type, usually associated with toxic agents. In this case the change was attributed to sepsis. **Bar** = 25 μm.

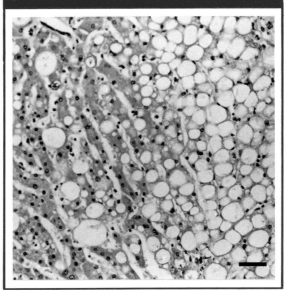

FIGURE 3.12 Steatosis of liver cells in an alcoholic. Many liver cells are distended by large, single droplets of triglyceride. Where the change is most severe (*right*), the liver tissue resembles adipose tissue. **Bar** = 50 μm.

cases of steatosis the droplets are of this same kind, only larger than normal. That fat droplets may grow or shrink while free in the cytosol should not surprise because, presumably, the enzymes that assemble and break down the triglycerides are also available in the cytosol. The same is true for glycogen; it makes sense that fuels such as fat or glycogen should be freely available and not barricaded behind membranes. *The lack of a limiting membrane probably explains the tendency of the droplets to coalesce,* like drops of fat floating on a broth. Mitochondria are often apposed to the droplets, which they are probably oxidizing (Figure 3.13) (65, 72).

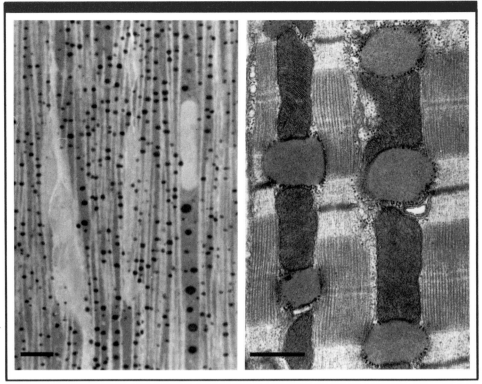

FIGURE 3.13
Steatosis of the myocardium in a rat, after treatment with clofibrate (clinically used as a hypolipemic agent). *Left:* Staining with Sudan black to demonstrate lipid. **Bar** = 10 μm. *Right:* Electron microscopy shows the close association between lipid droplets and mitochondria. This steatosis may be due to an inhibitory effect of the drug on mitochondrial oxidation. **Bar** = 0.5 μm. (Reproduced with permission from [45].)

Electron microscopy shows that the fat droplets in microvesicular steatosis of the liver are membrane-bound. An example is experimental poisoning with ethionine. These droplets are born in small expansions of the endoplasmic reticulum (Figure 3.14) (62, 69, 70, 83), which tends to break up or "vesiculate" in response to many chemical insults (68). Again in the liver, peroxisomes, endoplasmic reticulum, and fat droplets tend to aggregate and

form intracellular "constellations" (67). We will see later that peroxisomes are involved in lipid metabolism.

BIOCHEMICAL MECHANISMS OF STEATOSIS

The biochemical mechanisms of steatosis have been studied almost exclusively in the liver (42), not only because this organ is so well suited for chemical analysis but also because, historically, many of the toxic agents that were in vogue at a given time—for reasons industrial, medical, or cultural—were found to induce a fatty liver (remember that the liver is the principal site of detoxification). Classic examples are chloroform in the early days of anesthesia; yellow phosphorus, once used in matches and also for suicidal purposes; and especially carbon tetrachloride, a deadly fat solvent used until recently for many industrial and household purposes, for cleaning fluids, paints, and detergents, and even in bulk in fire extinguishers, which were about as dangerous as the fire itself (63). Today fatty liver is still a social problem, being the first stage of the liver disease induced by the most common poison of our day, alcohol.

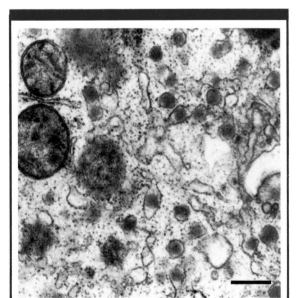

FIGURE 3.14
The early phase of steatosis in some cases occurs in this manner: ultramicroscopic lipid droplets appear inside the endoplasmic reticulum. **Bar** = 0.5 μm. (Reproduced with permission from [83].)

Steatosis requires a supply of fatty acids from other tissues, so it will be useful to summarize the key facts

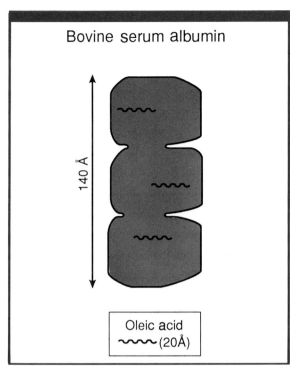

Bovine serum albumin

140 Å

Oleic acid
~~~(20Å)

FIGURE 3.15
Serum albumin acts as a carrier for fatty acids and for many other small molecules that have a low water solubility. It can carry up to 10 fatty acid molecules (J. A. Hamilton, personal communication) and in this sense it can be considered as a lipoprotein. (Adapted from Spector, A.A.: Plasma albumin as a lipoprotein. *In* Scanu, A.M., spector, A.A. (eds.): Biochemistry and Biology of Plasma Lipoproteins. New York, Marcel Dekker, Inc., 1986, pp. 247–280.).

about fatty acid physiology. Fatty acids can arise from three sources.
- ***Dietary fat,** which enters the circulation packaged into droplets of triglycerides (chylomicrons).*
- ***Fat mobilized** from stores in adipose tissue. Here the triglycerides are broken down and reach the bloodstream as free fatty acids (FFA) transported by albumin molecules, which have special hydrophobic domains for this purpose (Figure 3.15). The release of fatty acids from fat cells is induced by hormones (epinephrine, norepinephrine, cortisol, ACTH, some prostaglandins) and drugs (caffeine, theophylline) (42). Steatosis of liver and muscles has been induced experimentally with some of these agents (60) (Figure 3.16).*
- ***New synthesis** from acetate, a lesser source. Circulating free fatty acids (FFA) are taken up mainly by the liver (30 percent) and by muscle; chylomicrons are taken up by the liver (30 percent), adipose tissue (40 percent), and other tissues. Chylomicrons in the liver cell are hydrolyzed by*

lysosomes, and the resulting fatty acids join the FFA intracellular pool.

The simplified metabolic scheme of Figure 3.17 was conceived for the liver and therefore includes lipoprotein synthesis; but if the latter part of the scheme is left out, the remaining pathways should be applicable to other cell types. The scheme shows that free fatty acids supplied by the bloodstream find their way to a FFA pool inside the liver cell. The main point for our purpose is that *fatty acids are used to form triglycerides, but they can also be processed in at least two other ways:*
- They can combine with glycerol and give rise to triglycerides.
- They can be oxidized by mitochondria and/ or burned as fuel.
- They can be combined with glycerol, plus choline and phosphate, giving rise to phospholipids.

To be exported out of the liver cell, the triglycerides need to be assembled into a particle summarily called a **lipoprotein,** actually a globule filled with molecules of cholesteryl esters and free cholesterol, wrapped in a membrane of phospholipids and held together by a winding molecule of apoprotein (Figure 3.18). *The key point is that without the apoprotein, the lipoprotein cannot be built and its lipid components cannot be exported from the cell.* This helps to understand why steatosis can be induced by inhibitors of protein synthesis. One of the favorite experimental models of fatty liver (ethionine poisoning) exploits this mechanism.

With the preceding facts in mind we can begin to unravel what happens in individual situations. The innumerable causes of steatosis fall into three groups: lack of oxygen, nutritional disturbances, and toxic and hormonal effects.

Lack of Oxygen If fewer molecules of fatty acids are oxidized, more should remain available for triglyceride synthesis. In practice, this is seen in anemia and in some intoxications; data are available only for the liver.

Regarding failure of oxygen supply, consider the long path that atmospheric oxygen must travel to reach the mitochondria where it will be used. This means that there must also be a long list of possible mechanisms for causing the supply to run short:
- *drop in atmospheric oxygen (**anoxic anoxia**) (thus high altitude can cause steatosis, and so can hypoxia in tissue cultures) (48)*

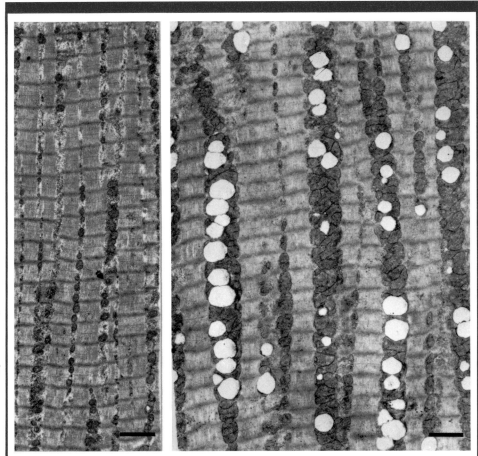

FIGURE 3.16
Catecholamines increase the mobilization of free fatty acids. *Right:* Lipid droplets are packed between the mitochondria in a striated muscle fiber of a dog, 8 hours after infusion of noradrenaline. *Left:* An adjacent fiber is completely spared, presumably reflecting functional differences between muscle fibers. **Bars** = 2 μm. (Reproduced with permission from [65]).

FIGURE 3.17
Fatty acid metabolism in a liver cell. The diagram can be used as a basis for understanding triglyceride deposition (steatosis). Steatosis develops if (a) fatty acid intake is increased; (b) fatty acid oxidation is reduced, leaving more substrate for the synthesis of triglycerides; (c) when protein (apoprotein) synthesis is reduced, whereby the packaging of different types of lipids into the lipoprotein molecule is impaired. In experimental animals, choline deficiency also produces steatosis by limiting phospholipid synthesis; it makes more substrate available for the triglyceride pathway.

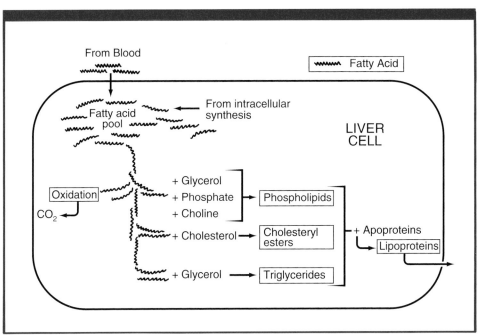

- *obstacle in the bronchial tree*
- *defect in the alveolar membrane*
- *defect in the transport system due to inadequate blood flow, inadequate number of red blood cells (**anemic anoxia**), or a defect in the hemoglobin (carboxyhemoglobin—hemoglobin combined with CO—can no longer carry oxygen)*
- *toxic effect on the cell's oxidative metabolism, called **toxic anoxia** (when diphtheria was prevalent, steatosis of the heart was an expected finding: diphtheria toxin depresses the oxidation of long-chain fatty acids by inducing a deficiency of carnitine, which is required for that step) (90, 91)*
- *vitamin deficiencies affecting the respiratory chain (niacin, riboflavin, etc.)*

Nutritional Disturbances Before the 1960s, malnutrition was thought to be the main cause of steatosis, hence the persistent and complacent legend that a hearty meal could prevent liver damage by alcohol.

This legend, which maintained that alcoholics developed fatty livers simply because they were malnourished, was hard to extirpate even after the evidence of alcohol toxicity became overwhelming in 1974 (82). The belief stemmed in part from experiments with rodents kept on a diet deficient in choline and methionine, ingredients essential for phospholipid synthesis; the animals acquired typical fatty livers. However, this mechanism appears to have little or no relevance for humans.

Imbalanced nutrition can work in several ways. *Overfeeding* causes liver steatosis (including the commercial foie gras) by oversupplying the cells with fatty acids. Paradoxically, *starvation* also causes a steatosis of the liver and heart (90, 91). This is not so surprising when it is realized that in laboratory rodents starved for 2–3 days the peripheral fat stores (adipose tissue) are mobilized so rapidly that the plasma appears milky. A sorry example of chronic starvation is offered by **kwashiorkor,** a Ghanian name that means "the-disease-that-the-older-one-gets-when-the-second-one-is-born" (86, 87). When the second child is born, the older one is taken off the breast and fed a meager cereal diet that leads to protein-calorie starvation; despite emaciation the liver is usually enlarged and fatty (Figures 3.19, 3.20). Presumably, *lack of protein synthesis blocks the synthesis and export of lipoproteins, with retention of the lipid components as shown in Figure 3.17.*

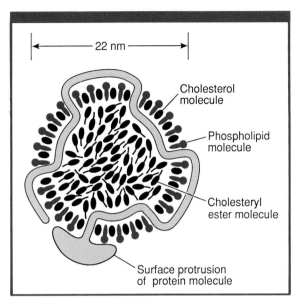

FIGURE 3.18
Cross section of a low-density lipoprotein (LDL) particle. A core of about 1500 cholesterol molecules, esterified to long-chain fatty acids, is surrounded by a lipid monolayer. A single large protein molecule organizes the particle. (Adapted from [1].)

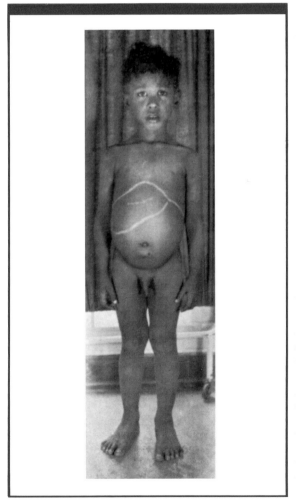

FIGURE 3.19
Kwashiorkor in a $5\frac{1}{2}$-year-old child. Note the distended abdomen and enlarged liver (margin outlined with chalk) contrasting with an otherwise fair nutritional state. (Reproduced with permission from [87].)

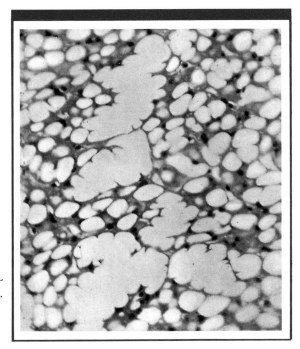

FIGURE 3.20
Fatty liver in a case of kwash-iorkor. Note the confluence of fat droplets from adjacent liver cells. (Reproduced with permission from [87].)

In birds, malnutrition can produce a severe steatosis of the liver and kidney known as fatty liver and kidney syndrome (FLKS), which has troubled not only wild birds but also the poultry industry (36, 73).

Toxic and Hormonal Effects Toxic agents can induce steatosis by a bewildering variety of mechanisms (46) because they may disrupt any conceivable link in lipid, protein, and energy metabolism. In the liver, the most common mechanism by far is decreased synthesis of lipoproteins. This can be proven experimentally with inhibitors of protein synthesis.

Ethionine depresses protein synthesis primarily by sequestering ATP and thus preventing the activation of amino acids (42). Puromycin is another inhibitor, so is tetracycline (41), and so is a toxin of the highly poisonous mushroom Amanita phalloides *(Figure 3.21), alpha-amanitin, a specific inhibitor of RNA polymerase II, the enzyme-synthesizing RNA (42).*

It is satisfying to pinpoint simple biochemical mechanisms, but beware: *a toxic agent can act in many different ways by disrupting different metabolic pathways (81).*

So goes the standard theory, but the picture is probably more complicated. Some children affected by kwashiorkor are breast-fed and even well nourished: aflatoxin intoxication seems to be a complicating factor (52, 53).

Nutritional imbalance is well demonstrated in genetically obese Zucker rats, which are also hyperlipemic, hyperinsulinemic, but normoglycemic: a diet enriched in sucrose rapidly induces a fatty liver (70). A similar mechanism probably underlies the fatty livers typical of very obese humans consuming a low-protein, high-carbohydrate diet (55); however, morbid obesity and fatty liver are not always associated (35).

Anyone who needs to be cured of wanting to know the mechanism of toxic steatosis should look into carbon tetrachloride intoxication of the liver, which has been studied for decades because industrial and household exposure to inhalation of CCl$_4$ vapors was a common accident. The principal effect is decreased export of lipoproteins from the liver, but a variety of mechanisms are possible: a decrease of lipoprotein export by blockage of tubulin and possibly by a direct denaturation of lipoproteins; a block in protein synthesis by free radical damage to the ER membranes (p. 187); a decrease of FFA oxidation by the mitochondria; and stress, which increases lipolysis (p. 81) and thus leads to an increased supply of FFA (42).

Ethanol intoxication is just as complicated as CCl$_4$ intoxication (61, 47, 85): the mechanisms of steatosis include increased synthesis of glycerol as well as of fatty acids, decreased oxidation of FFA due to mitochondrial damage, possibly decreased lipoprotein secretion, and increased lipolysis in adipose tissue (61, 82). An interesting point—more important to remember—is that ethanol can lead to steatosis after a weekend of heavy social drinking without drunkenness (Figure 3.22) (82). However, it should not be forgotten that liver damage by ethanol includes much more than steatosis (61).

Steatosis is reversible. It is common clinical experience that an alcoholic fatty liver that is

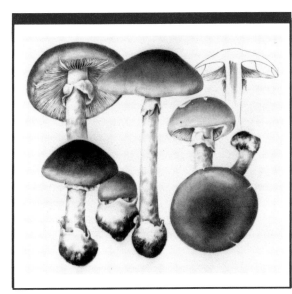

FIGURE 3.21
Phalloidin is obtained from *Amanita phalloides*, a mushroom that is deadly even when cooked. (Reproduced with permission from [79].)

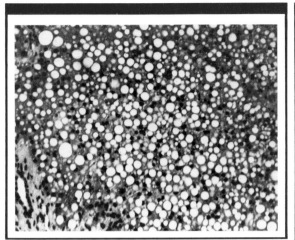

FIGURE 3.22

Alcoholic fatty liver without drunkenness. This patient (an alcoholic) was hospitalized long enough to develop a histologically normal liver. She then received alcohol in fruit juice, about half the daily amount she would previously absorb (86 proof whiskey, 8 oz/day for 2 days; then 12 oz/day for 2 days; then 16 oz/day for 3 days). The patient was never drunk. (Courtesy of Dr. E. Rubin, Thomas Jefferson University Medical Center, Philadelphia, Penn..)

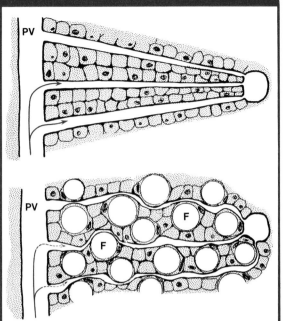

FIGURE 3.23

Compression of sinusoids in liver lobules in severe steatosis. Blood flow is from left to right (**PV**: portal vein). *Top:* Normal liver. *Bottom:* Liver cells bloated with fat (**F**) impair flow and can lead to increased pressure in the portal vein (portal hypertension). (Modified from [75].)

proven by biopsy can be reversed in about 10 days (1–6 weeks) provided that alcohol supplies are out of reach.

Does steatosis cause any damage? *Mild steatosis is clinically asymptomatic and has no significant effect on the cell's metabolism.* Persistent steatosis of the liver in alcoholics leads to fibrosis (cirrhosis), but this is more likely due to the alcohol itself. However, it is difficult to believe that a liver cell bloated with lipid can function properly (42). Some liver tests can show abnormal function (low albumin from decreased synthesis, increased plasma transaminases because these enzymes are released by damaged cells), but correlation with the biopsy findings is poor. The effects of toxic agents have not been clearly separated from steatosis per se. Perhaps some liver-function tests on the geese used to produce foie gras could be illuminating. On the other hand, *steatosis might cause damage indirectly*, at least in the liver: bloated cells expand into the sinusoids and should therefore restrict blood flow, as we have shown for acute cellular swelling (p. 74) (Figure 3.23) (75). Consider that blood flow in the lobule is from the periphery to the center; this means that under normal conditions the central cells receive less oxygen than those at the periphery. If the peripheral cells swell and reduce blood flow, the central cells will be in double jeopardy;

the result can be anoxic steatosis, cell atrophy, or cell death (see p. 681).

ACUTE FATTY LIVER OF PREGNANCY: A TOXIC ROLE FOR FATTY ACIDS?

This topic is still unclear but it may contain an important lead. Acute fatty liver developing during pregnancy was long feared as a rare but usually fatal condition; a recent survey finds it to be more common than once believed but not as fatal (78). In this study, nine of nine women survived, and all suffered from toxemia of pregnancy (preeclampsia). Clinically the syndrome is one of hypertension, proteinuria, and edema (preeclampsia) complicated by acute liver failure with jaundice; the liver shows steatosis with a microvesicular pattern (Figure 3.24) (43, 54, 56). Most surprisingly, chemical analysis shows a high percentage of free fatty acids along with the triglycerides (43, 71). Fatty acids are toxic (43). Why do they accumulate? Are they responsible for the toxic effects on the liver? They also accumulate (43) in another acute toxic condition, **Reye's syndrome,** a pediatric disorder of uncertain origin that presents as an encephalopathy with deposition of lipid droplets in both liver and brain (76). *A hypothesis worth investigating is that the so-called microvesicular pattern of steatosis may have something to do with storage of fatty acids.*

Steatosis can occur by congenital mechanisms.
 • *Triglycerides can accumulate by congenital*

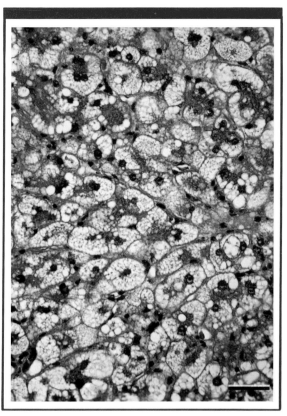

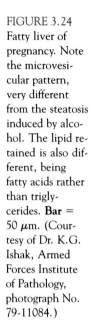

FIGURE 3.24 Fatty liver of pregnancy. Note the microvesicular pattern, very different from the steatosis induced by alcohol. The lipid retained is also different, being fatty acids rather than triglycerides. **Bar** = 50 μm. (Courtesy of Dr. K.G. Ishak, Armed Forces Institute of Pathology, photograph No. 79-11084.)

deficiency of acid lipase (*Wolman's disease of infants and an adult form called* **cholesteryl ester storage** *disease*) *(58). In this rare condition, both triglycerides and cholesterol esters accumulate in lysosomes, as occurs in other storage diseases due to enzyme deficiencies (p. 142). The deposits occur in most tissues, even in lymphocytes. A similar condition can be reproduced in only 4 hours by feeding egg yolk to rats (59).*

- *There is also a rare lipid-storage myopathy due to a defect in oxidative metabolism leading to* **carnitine deficiency** *(44). You will notice here an overlap with the effect of diphtheria toxin mentioned earlier.*
- *In the triglyceride-laden heart of diabetic mice a similar oxidation defect was found (57).*

Some conditions akin to steatosis are the following.
- **Triglyceride load as a normal condition.** *Strangely, the tubules in the renal cortex of the cat and other carnivores always contain lipid droplets. Since the kidney, like other tissues, oxidizes free fatty acids, the finding may be the result of lipoprotein uptake from the tubules (37).*
- **Phagocytosis leading to the accumulation of fat.** *In the convoluted tubules of the kidney, there is no doubt that true steatosis can develop as a result of metabolic disturbances (65, 73,*

89); however, in those diseases that imply leakage of plasma proteins through the glomerulus (lipoid nephrosis), the mechanism of lipid storage in the tubules is phagocytosis. The tubular epithelium reabsorbs lipoproteins from the lumen and accumulates droplets containing triglycerides, cholesterol, and phospholipids, as leftovers from digestion of the lipoproteins (37).
- **Lipid droplets in regenerating cells** *are common (38). There is no documented explanation; however, it is a fact that the respiratory metabolism of young cells and fetal cells depends more heavily on anaerobic glycolysis, which may make the cell less able to oxidize fatty acids.*
- **Lipid accumulation in cultured cells** *is another well-known phenomenon (80). True steatosis can result from anoxia, but most of the lipid is phospholipid from autophagocytosis (48, 49) and probably also from "overfeeding" with plasma loaded with lipoproteins.*
- **Renal cell carcinoma,** *which derives from the renal tubules, typically accumulates so much triglyceride that the tumor appears yellow. This is quite surprising because normal tubular cells of the human kidney contain few or no fat droplets.*

TO SUM UP: Droplets of triglycerides are mainly a symptom of cellular disease; they are rarely a cause of cellular disease. Oddly enough, a pathologist may diagnose alcoholic fatty livers every working day, yet never in a lifetime see an intracellular droplet actually filled with triglycerides. All a pathologist sees are empty vacuoles, *presumably* filled with triglycerides; histologic solvents have removed their content. This may explain why it took so long to discover that the droplets in the fatty liver of pregnancy contain something else, namely toxic fatty acids. Furthermore, lipids tend to dissolve into each other; perhaps not all the droplets glibly called "fat" are the same fat.

ACCUMULATION OF CHOLESTERYL ESTERS

Continuing our search for symptoms of cellular disease, we now turn to the hoarding of cholesteryl esters. *This particular form of excess storage is a true case of cellular indigestion.* All cells need cholesterol as a building block for their membranes, but when the supply exceeds the demand, the cells have no choice; they must store the excess ester in the form of droplets, mostly in lysosomes (Figure 3.25). The extreme but common example of this storage is offered by macrophages, whose uncontrolled appetite may lead them to swell enormously and to become bags of lipid droplets; in this bloated condition they are known internationally as **foam cells.** Bloated is an understatement: a foam cell may attain a diameter of 40–50 microns (112), which is 4–5 times above normal; the volume is therefore increased by a factor of 64–125.

> To identify droplets of cholesteryl esters, the method of choice is polarized light on sections of fresh tissue, as mentioned earlier; cholesteryl esters are birefringent (99). Normally such droplets are present in adrenal glands and in neural tissue prior to myelinization.

Because we are dealing with a case of cellular overload, it will help to review the sources of this overload. Mammalian cells obtain their cholesterol mainly from two sources: synthesis within the cell, which needs to be supplemented by uptake of low-density lipoproteins (LDL) via a receptor mechanism. The LDL particles (Figure 3.26) are assembled in the liver and can be considered as a door-to-door delivery system of cholesteryl ester. The cells then obtain cholesterol by hydrolyzing the ester. For phagocytic cells, there is a third source of cholesterol, namely phagocytosis. Macrophages are especially prone to obtain cholesterol by this mechanism because, as scavengers, they are often called upon to ingest cell debris, a rich

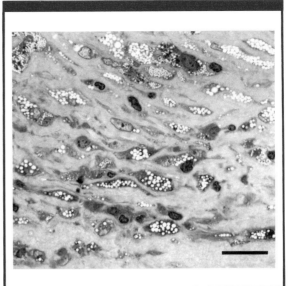

FIGURE 3.25 Foam cells in the intima of a human atherosclerotic artery. The cytoplasm appears foamy because it is packed with droplets of cholesterol esters. The larger foam cells are macrophage-derived; some of the smaller ones derive from smooth muscle cells. **Bar** = 25 μm.

source of membrane cholesterol. (Recall that in red cell membranes the cholesterol/phospholipid ratio is close to 1:1.)

THE CELL'S PROBLEMS IN DEALING WITH CHOLESTEROL

A cell overloaded with cholesterol faces a difficult challenge: cholesterol is one of the few molecules

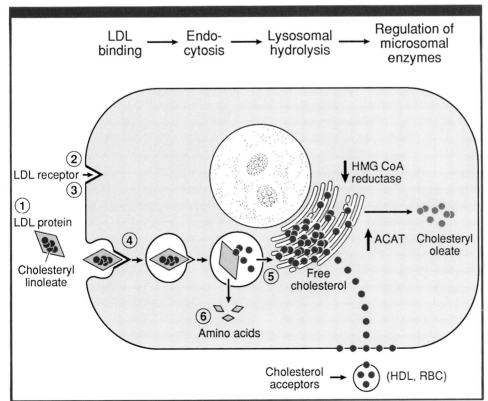

FIGURE 3.26 Steps in LDL uptake and breakdown by human macrophages and fibroblasts. Some of the cholesterol released is recycled to the cell membrane and then taken away by acceptors such as high-density lipoproteins (HDL) or red blood cells. (**HMG CoA reductase:** 3-hydroxy-3-methylglutaryl coenzyme A reductase. **ACAT:** acyl-coenzyme A: cholesterol acyl-transferase.) Sites at which mutations have been identified, leading to congenital defects, are (1) abetalipoproteinemia; (2) familial hypercholesterolemia (FH), receptor-negative; (3) FH, receptor-defective; (4) FH, internalization defect; (5) Wolman syndrome; and (6) cholesteryl ester storage disease. Modified from [100].)

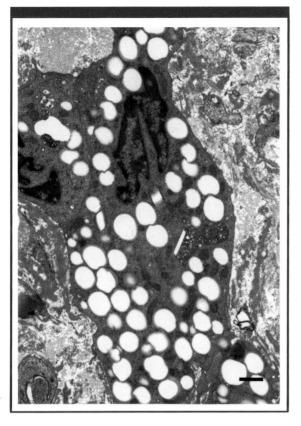

FIGURE 3.27
Foam cell in a
human athero-
sclerotic plaque.
There is a small
cholesterol crys-
tal in a lysosome.
Bar =1 μm.

This scenario is played out on the surface of arterial endothelium, which has direct access to plasma lipoproteins; but similar events occur on the other side of the endothelial barrier (105) because all classes of lipoproteins are present in the lymph (107). Since they are much too large to diffuse across the endothelial barrier, they must have been ferried across it by transcytosis (p. 596).

Foam cells are striking to behold but not fully understood. Why, for example, are all the droplets the same size? Why do they fail to fuse into one large droplet, as triglycerides do? Why do some droplets have membranes and others not? And why are they sometimes oval (Figure 3.27)? No expert could give us answers, except for speculating that the molecular arrangement of the esters within the droplet must impose a certain shape; the droplets are in fact liquid crystals, as shown by their birefringency.

*There is an alternative form of intracellular choles-
terol storage: rhomboid crystals of pure cholesterol,
occasionally found in living foam cells and in the
endothelium of hypercholesterolemic rats, presumably
as an indication of extreme cholesterol overload. The
cells containing such crystals appear to be in fine
shape despite the sharp object developing within them.*

CONDITIONS THAT FAVOR THE DEVELOPMENT OF FOAM CELLS

From what we have said, to find foam cells we will have to look for situations in which the supply of cholesterol is increased, either locally or generally. Here are some classic examples.

1) Death of Adipose Tissue This may occur, for example, after trauma. Dead fat cells release their content, and the surrounding macrophages digest the triglyceride and remain "stuck" with all the cholesterol dissolved within it. In the process they turn into foam cells (Figure 3.28) and may even fuse, as we will see shortly, giving rise to foamy giant cells called **Touton cells** (Figure 3.29) (92).

2) Atherosclerosis We will summarize this topic in Chapter 23, but here is the essence. In atherosclerosis, the first step appears to be that the endothelium "pumps" LDL lipoproteins into the arterial intima; monocytes then migrate from the blood into the intima, pick up the lipid, and become foam cells.

In view of these well-established facts, it came as an utter surprise to discover that *macrophages or monocytes incubated with particles of LDL refuse to*

that cannot be broken down in the body; it is also insoluble. It can be eliminated only through the liver, which incorporates it into micelles contain-ing bile acids and lecithin (106). These being the facts, any cell that takes up an excess of choles-terol (be it from LDL or from phagocytized debris) does not have the option of breaking it down; it can use a limited amount for its own membranes, but the rest must be esterified and stored in membrane-bound droplets. This mechanism is now well understood, thanks to the work of Michael Brown and Joseph Goldstein (93), who were awarded the Nobel Prize in 1985. A look at Figure 3.26 shows that the overloaded cell has, in fact, a safeguard. Some of the excess cholesterol can be carried to the cell surface and "offered" to any willing cholesterol acceptor that may be passing by. One such benefactor is known, namely high density lipoprotein (HDL) (94, 101). The details of this last and critical step, whereby a cell transfers its cholesterol to a passer-by, are not yet clear. For the time being, we may visualize an HDL particle bumping into the surface of the overloaded cell, picking up a few cholesterol molecules, incorporating them into its cholesterol-rich core, and floating away with them.

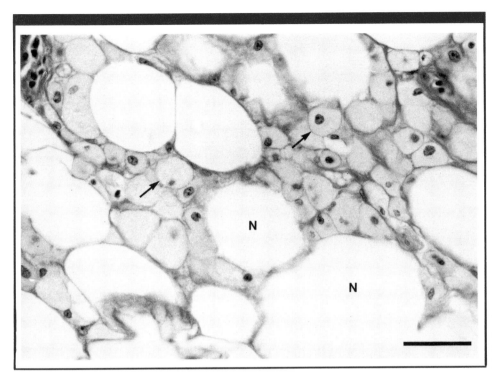

FIGURE 3.28
The lipid contained in necrotic fat cells (**N**) is taken up by macrophages, which become foam cells (**arrows**). **Bar** = 50 μm.

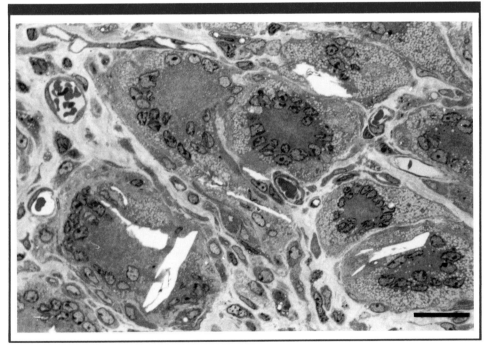

FIGURE 3.29
Touton cells, multinucleated giant cells that develop by fusion of foam cells. The nuclei are in the center, surrounded by cholesterol ester droplets. The intracellular crystals probably correspond to pure cholesterol. (These Touton cells were obtained experimentally by injecting a cholesteryl ester (N-nonanoate) in corn oil subcutaneously into the rat; the tissue was fixed two weeks later.) 1-μm section; toluidine blue stain. **Bar** = 25 μm.

phagocytize them. Later it was found that macrophages exposed to LDL down-regulate their surface receptors for LDL; they only take up LDL particles that have been "modified" (oxidized) by the endothelium, a process that may involve free radicals (108, 109). This is not an academic detail. It might make it possible to treat atherosclerosis with antioxidants, a hypothesis now being tested (111).

From atherosclerotic lesions, the foam cells can be isolated, studied, and even analyzed with the cell sorter (p. 15); this method helped to establish that some arterial "foam cells" (not quite as filled with lipid) derive from smooth muscle cells (97).

3) Housekeeping in the Lung The pulmonary alveoli and the small bronchi contain macrophages apparently adapted to live in the air. These cells work as scavengers: they keep the place clean, and for this deed they are rewarded by being coughed out or swallowed (p. 300). Their normal diet is mainly dust, but they are ready to take up also dead cells, surfactant, and lipoproteins that may have leaked into the alveoli. In so doing they turn into foam cells, whose presence in lower respiratory secretions can be considered a nonspecific marker of lung disease (95). When the bronchi are obstructed these free macrophages become numerous enough to produce a pattern called **lipid pneumonia** (110).

4) Xanthomas Xanthomas are yellow, tumorlike lumps of foam cells commonly found as a complication of hypercholesterolemia; the name xanthoma literally means "yellowma". The reader may ask why xanthomas develop locally, whereas hypercholesterolemia is a generalized condition. There is no good answer, except that many xanthomas develop in areas more exposed to trauma, such as the skin of the elbows. Some localizations remain mysterious: **xanthelasmas,** for example, are little yellow lumps that develop on the eyelid or at the nasal corner of the eye. Why should foam cells develop there (Figure 3.30)?

(5) Cholesterolosis of the Gall Bladder Occasionally, an excesss of cholesterol is deposited in the mucosa of the gall bladder (Figure 3.31).

Fibroblasts have LDL receptors, and, in fact, cultured fibroblasts were first used by Brown and Goldstein in their masterly studies. Thus, it is not too surprising to see long, thin, but foamy cells in inflamed tissues. This property of fibroblasts may also help understand the peculiar localization of xanthomas in tendons (104). A special variety of lipid-storing fibroblasts are the so-called Ito cells of the liver, which act as a reservoir of the fat-soluble vitamin A; their droplets contain cholesteryl esters and about 25 percent of triglycerides (98). Lipid-storing fibroblasts exist also in the lung (103).

TO SUM UP: The pathology of cholesteryl esters is largely the pathology of foam cells. Long a favorite of microscopists, these distinctive little monsters are a flag for certain local or general disturbances that lead to cholesteryl ester overload. However, we should remind the reader that cholesterol does more, in pathology, than creating storage problems; it is also involved in diseases of cell membranes (p. 128). Also, we said that cholesterol cannot be broken down. Then why is it that the world did not long ago become a vast, greasy dump of cholesterol crystals? Obviously there are bacteria that can deal with it (96, 102).

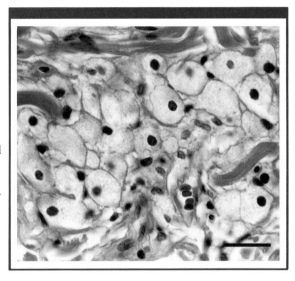

FIGURE 3.30 Macrophages loaded with lipid (foam cells). From a xanthelasma (a little yellow spot on an eyelid) that was removed for cosmetic reasons. **Bar** = 25 μm.

Accumulation of Glycogen and Related Materials

Glycogen is a readily available, water-soluble store of energy. As one would expect of fuel that must be at hand, most of it is free in the cytosol and is catabolized there; we made the same remark about triglyceride droplets.

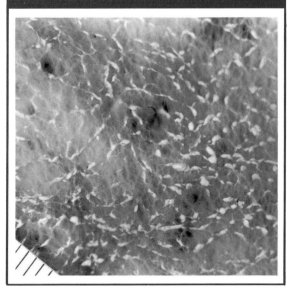

FIGURE 3.31 Mucosa of a gall bladder (close-up view). The white (actually yellowish) lumps and ridges represent submucosal accumulations of cholesterol-laden foam cells. This is the so-called cholesterolosis of the gall bladder. It is striking to the naked eye but apparently innocuous. Scale in mm.

An easy histochemical stain for glycogen is the PAS method (for periodic-acid–Schiff), based on the reactivity of aldehyde groups, which yields a red color. Other carbohydrate-containing macromolecules also give this reaction, but a simple test can help to identify them: glycogen can be removed by placing the unstained section in a dilute solution of "diastase" (in practice, saliva). By electron microscopy, glycogen appears in the form of aggregated alpha or isolated beta granules 150–300 Å in diameter, not always easy to distinguish from ribosomes; impregnation of glycogen with silver proteinate is helpful (p. 320). At very high powers, the beta particles appear to be composed of filaments 30 Å in diameter and up to 200 Å long, known as gamma particles. Occasionally, glycogen particles can be found in almost any organelle (113).

A persistent legend about glycogen is that it is dissolved by ordinary fixatives. Actually, no glycogen seems to be lost by the ordinary 3 percent glutaraldehyde solution used for electron microscopy. Some is lost, however, during the staining of histologic sections. This is why the cytoplasm of rat liver cells looks so ragged in histologic sections; the "empty" spaces correspond to glycogen deposits. This also explains a paradox: liver cells in sections of human liver taken postmortem look more compact and "nicer" than cells from liver biopsies (Figure 3.32). They are not nicer at all. They appear compact only because their glycogen stores were burned up during the agonal period.

Our knowledge of the cellular pathology of glycogen accumulation consists, so far, of a collection of interesting but isolated facts.

- *Young cells*, which lean more heavily on anaerobic glycolysis, *contain more glycogen than mature cells*; so do many tumor cells, which share many characteristics with young cells.
- *Anoxia is sometimes associated with excessive amounts of intracellular glycogen*, presumably because the cell is on the brink of death and can no longer metabolize its substrates. The mechanism probably underlies the appearance of glycogen and of triglycerides in cells around myocardial infarcts.
- *Diabetes can increase intracellular glycogen* (118). In untreated diabetes, tissues that depend on insulin for their glucose supply, such as liver and muscle, become glucose-starved and thus glycogen-depleted, whereas tissues insensitive to insulin become overloaded with glycogen; thus in rats with

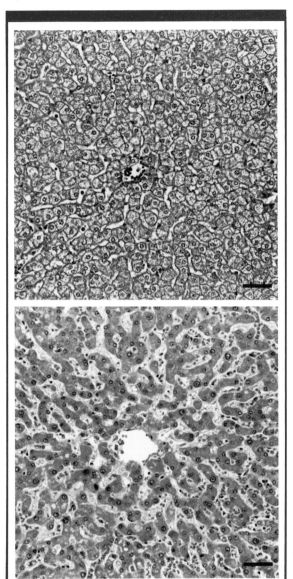

FIGURE 3.32 Different aspect of liver tissue obtained by biopsy (*top*) and by autopsy (*bottom*). The liver cells in the biopsy are filled with glycogen, which has virtually disappeared from the autopsy liver, presumably during the agonal period. **Bar** = 50 μm.

alloxan-induced diabetes, glycogen is reduced in the liver and increased in the brain. Large deposits of glycogen occur also in the kidney, in the straight portion of the proximal tubules, as can be demonstrated by microdissection (120); they are probably a consequence of glucose overload. Electron microscopy shows the glycogen both free and enclosed within large autophagocytic vacuoles called glycogenosomes (Figure 3.33) (117).

- *Glycogenic nuclei* are a cytologic puzzle. While studying diabetic tissues as long ago as 1883, Paul Ehrlich noticed glycogen in the nuclei of liver cells, a surprising observation because the nucleus rarely accumulates

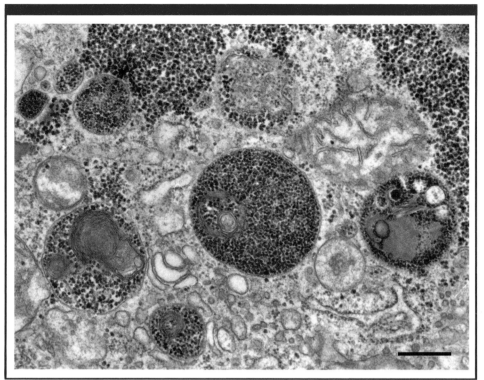

FIGURE 3.33
Accumulation of glycogen in a renal tubular cell of a rat made diabetic with streptozotocin (which kills pancreatic beta cells selectively). Many glycogen particles are free in the cytoplasm; others are contained in glycogenosomes as a result of autophagocytosis. **Bar** = 0.5 μm. (Reproduced with permission from [117].)

abnormal materials. However, this discovery turned out to be a disappointment because glycogenic nuclei are present also in normal livers (Figure 3.34), in the human myocardium, and in a variety of tumor cells (114). There is some evidence that nuclear glycogen is actually synthesized in the nucleus (115).

- *Lysosomal diseases offer the most striking pictures of intracellular glycogen storage,* due to the lack of a lysosomal enzyme (many glycogen-related enzymatic defects have been described). The buildup of glycogen in lysosomes is rather peculiar because cell biology tells us that glycogen should be degradable in the cytoplasm. The answer may be that, no matter how fast the cytoplasmic glycogen is degraded, whatever amount reaches the lysosomes is bound to remain undigested and to lead, over the years, to massive storage.

- *Corpora amylacea and Lafora bodies* are spherical bodies of neuropathologic interest; *both are glucose polymers* (polyglycosans) *and thus related to glycogen.* One may wonder why the central nervous system should develop such a wealth of glucose polymers; however, brain tissue is absolutely dependent on glucose as a source of energy and is also insulin-dependent. Perhaps the spherical bodies are the neuropathologic way to deal with an oversupply of glucose (118, 122).

The **corpora amylacea** have nothing to do with amyloid; the name means that they show concentric lines like starch granules (*amylon* is Greek for "starch") (Figure 3.35). They are extremely common and, it seems, totally harmless. In the grey matter, strangely enough, they arise in the

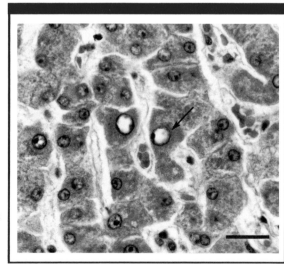

FIGURE 3.34
Glycogen-filled nuclei (**arrow**) in a normal human liver. **Bar** = 25 μm.

branches of fibrous astrocytes, causing them to swell enormously and to appear as extracellular. They can be found also in nerves. By electron microscopy they are fibrillar (119). Chemically they consist of a glycogenlike material (~80%) with phosphate and sulphate groups attached (123).

Lafora bodies are structurally similar but are pathologically far more significant. They were discovered in 1911 in the neurons in a case of myoclonic epilepsy and since then have been seen in other neurologic conditions. They may well represent a generalized metabolic disease because they are found in many tissues including the liver and skin. They can be degraded *in vitro* by amylase (118). Similar bodies can be seen to arise in the axons of diabetic rats (118).

> *Basophilic degeneration of the myocardium is a bizarre but not uncommon, age-dependent cellular change related to glycogen metabolism, in which a basophilic mass appears in many myocardial fibers. Chemical, enzymatic, and spectroscopic studies indicate that this material is related to glycogen (116, 121). By electron microscopy it is mostly fibrillar, like the corpora amylacea.*

Accumulation of Pigments

It may sound too simple to be scientific, but a change in color may be the first clue that something is wrong with a given tissue. The change may be obvious to the naked eye, or it may be apparent only through the microscope. Most of the coloring materials come from within, though some are environmental (156); they may be intracellular or extracellular. Chemically, they may be as different as soot and hemoglobin, but it is convenient to consider them as a group because they all convey the same general message: "Abnormal color—something may be wrong." Each pigment, of course, has its own particular significance.

> *We will never forget the case of a 52-year-old man with a round mass in his lung, discovered accidentally on an X-ray. A needle biopsy yielded some nondescript cells, plus one cell containing a few brown granules. We hoped they would represent an innocuous blood-derived pigment, but they gave the reactions of melanin. The presence of melanin in a mass within the lung makes it almost certain that a malignant melanoma has metastasized to the lung. This proved to be the case; a small melanoma of the back had escaped attention.*

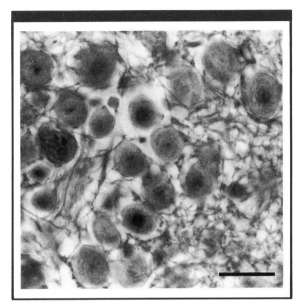

FIGURE 3.35 Cluster of corpora amylacea in the cortex of a human brain. These structures, which increase in number with age, are not associated with any known pathology. **Bar** = 50 μm. (Courtesy of Dr. T. W. Smith, University of Massachusetts Medical Center, Worcester, Mass.)

Coloring material is also a wonderful tool in experimental pathology, not only for staining sections but also for studies *in vivo*.

Although the term pigment is often used interchangeably with the term dye for any coloring material, we will follow tradition and use **dye** for colors (usually artificial) that form solutions and **pigment** for particulate, insoluble colors that form suspensions. Ordinary ink is a dye whereas India ink (a suspension of carbon black particles) and melanin are pigments. The distinction is important biologically because *exogenous dyes and pigments introduced into the body meet different fates.* We will return to this topic in the chapter on inflammation (p. 370).

EXOGENOUS PIGMENTS IN EVERYDAY LIFE: SOME EXAMPLES

The prototype of exogenous pigments is carbon black, a polite name for soot. This may sound like a homely topic, but it has taught us some major biologic lessons, due to two of its properties: it is virtually harmless, and it is so black that even minuscule grains are visible under the microscope. In other words, it is an ideal tracer.

OUR DAILY DOSE OF SOOT

City dwellers are condemned to breathe soot, which discolors the lungs for life. This blackening is called **anthracosis** (from Greek *ánthrax,* "charcoal"; in the lung, anthracosis is an example of **pneumoconiosis,** "lung-dust disease"). Any inhaled particles that measure less than 0.5 μm (128) can reach the alveolus, where they are engulfed by the resident alveolar macrophages. After this feat these macrophages acquire a new name, **dust cells** (Figure 3.36). Obviously the dust cells cannot remain in the alveolus or the air spaces would soon be clogged. Most of them escape along the bronchial tree, whence they are swept out by the cilia and then swallowed or coughed out. In the mouse, this cycle takes about 27 days (152).

> *Surprise! Some of the swallowed carbon black can be picked up again in the gut (151). Dust particles have been found in Peyer's patches, where they are probably picked up by the M cells, phagocytic epithelial cells specialized in taking up macro-molecules and even bacteria (p. 523). Another possible route from the lungs to the gut would be via the bloodstream, with leakage out of the venules in Peyer's patches (p. 300).*

How does the carbon pass from the alveolus to the connective tissue spaces of the lung? It obviously does get there because the interstitial spaces are loaded with blackened macrophages (Figure 3.37). Perhaps some alveolar macrophages crawl back into the tissue spaces. It is also possible that free carbon particles somehow cross the alveolar barrier and are phagocytized after they have trespassed into the tissue spaces. Most will remain inside the local macrophages for a lifetime. However, *a few carbon-laden dust cells find their way*

into the lymphatics, ending their journey in the nearest lymph node; the hilar nodes of city dwellers are often as black as coal. The lungs of coal miners are an unbelievable sight.

The dust cells that settle in a lymph node stay there until they die. How long that takes nobody knows; our guess is months or even years. At that point another macrophage will take up the pigment and again hold it until its death. So the cycle continues. A few loaded macrophages may escape into the thoracic duct and thence to the blood stream, but when they die their load of pigment will be picked up by "littoral phagocytes" (p. 299); soot is not an unusual sight in the human liver and spleen (138). This is a dead end for undigestible particles, which may seem inappropri-ate, but in the course of evolution there was little need to evolve a disposal route for the sinusoidal macrophages. Cities are a recent development, and soot, after all, is ugly but almost harmless.

TATTOOS

Tattooing is another cultural exposure to carbon black and more colorful pigments. After the particles are pricked into the skin, they are taken up by the local macrophages, aided by a few monocytes attracted out of the blood stream by the irritation; but *the macrophages of the skin remain where they are,* unlike those of the lung. Tattoo artists exploit this provincial attitude of skin macrophages, which, if undisturbed, tend to live out their long lives in the same place (Figure 3.38).

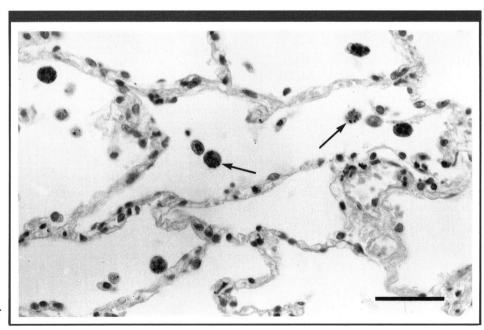

FIGURE 3.36
Alveolar macrophages turned into dust cells (**arrows**) in a human lung.
Bar = 50 μm.

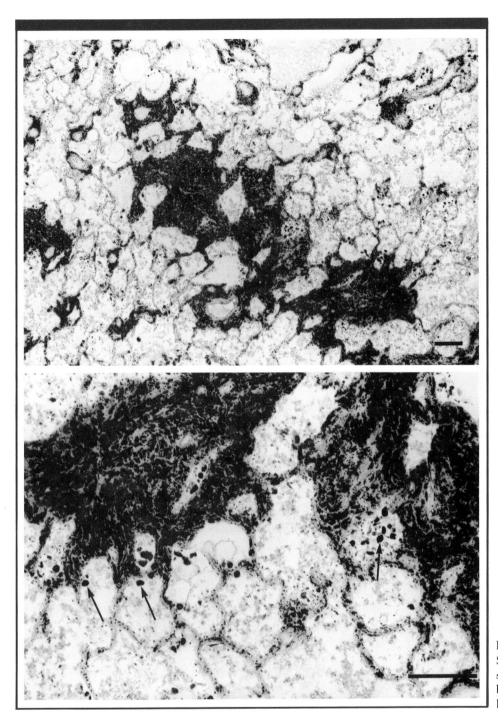

FIGURE 3.37
Sections of a miner's lung, lightly stained. Virtually all the black is carbon. **Arrows:** Single macrophages loaded with carbon. **Bar** = 200 μm.

At the time of the tattooing operation, however, the skin becomes inflamed and swollen. The lymphatics come into action and gradually pump away the fluid, including some particles of pigment. As soon as the particles reach a lymph node, they are trapped because lymph nodes act as filters. Perhaps, over the years, a few more particles—either free or in macrophages—will reach the node (tattoos do tend to fade with time), but the vast majority of pigment-laden macrophages will hold their position in the skin.

Should the tattooed area become inflamed once again, the macrophages will rise to the call, move around, multiply, and pick up bacteria or other extraneous matter. Thereafter, many will be drained away by the lymphatics, oblivious of their artistic role. The tattoo will be clouded or partially erased (Figure 3.39) (143).

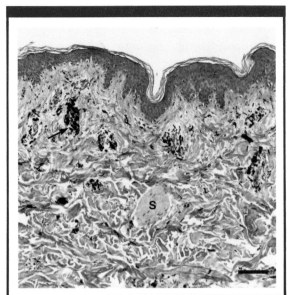

FIGURE 3.38 Tattooed human skin. The pigment is contained in clusters of macrophages (**arrow**). Note the lack of pigment in a bundle of smooth muscle cells (arrector pili, **S**). **Bar** = 100 μm.

Historically, the filtering function of the lymph nodes was discovered by Virchow through the autopsy of a soldier whose arm had been tattooed 50 years earlier. The red pigment of the tattoo, cinnabar, was also present in the nodes of the axilla (153) (Figure I.6). This mechanism is biologically very important because the lymph nodes are called to filter other unwanted particles, such as bacteria from foci of infection and metastatic cells from malignant tumors.

DRUG-INDUCED DISCOLORATIONS

Several drugs lead to abnormal colorations even though the drug itself is not necessarily colored. Tetracycline is well known for its property of becoming deposited in calcifying tissues, where it can be recognized by its yellow color and its golden fluorescence (126). The antibiotic is incorporated in the enamel as well as in the dentin (126). If tetracycline is administered to a pregnant woman, it becomes deposited in the growing teeth of the baby; the result is an unsightly discoloration of the deciduous teeth and the development of the enamel is inhibited (**enamel dysplasia**). We once saw the jaw of a slaughtered cow stained bright yellow by a mistake in the commercial feed, a huge overdose of tetracycline. Silver nitrate intake causes a generalized pigmentation (**argyria**), which is described on page 262.

ENDOGENOUS PIGMENTS

The gamut of colors available to mammalian tissues includes hues of yellow, brown, orange, red, and black; bile green is also available. Blue is

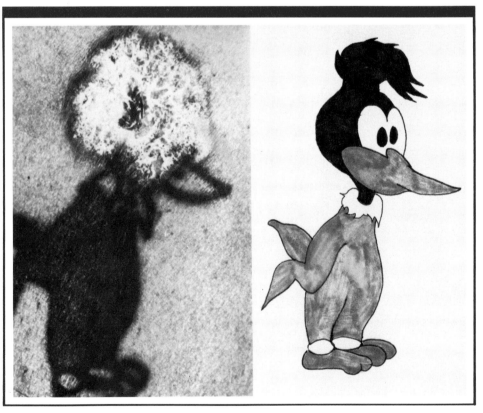

FIGURE 3.39
Macrophages become mobilized in inflammation. *Left:* Tattoo in the shape of Woody Woodpecker. At the top an accidental inflammatory reaction (dermatitis) has mobilized the macrophages, hence the drawing is scattered. *Right:* Control drawing for readers not familiar with Woody Woodpecker. (Reproduced with permission from Abel EA, Silberberg I, Queen D. Studies of chronic inflammation in a red tattoo by electron microscopy and histochemistry. Acta Dermatol (Stock) 1972;52:453–461.) (Drawing courtesy of William Silberberg.)

TABLE 3.1

Brown Pigments		
	NATURE	SIGNIFICANCE
Melanin	Polymer of hydroxyaromatics	In the skin: light protection ? Elsewhere: free-radical sink?
Lipofuscin	Polymer of oxidized lipids	Present in long-lived cells, index of aging, no "use" proven
Ferritin	Ferric oxyhydroxide (FeOOH) stored inside a protein hull	Principal storage form of iron
Hemosiderin	Denatured, partially digested ferritin	Present in lysosomes when ferritin is stored in excess

underrepresented because the blue plasma protein ceruloplasmin is always too dilute to show up. The blue color of the iris and the sexual skin of certain monkeys is due to interference phenomena, not to a sky-colored pigment. Monkey "blue skin" appears brown if transilluminated.

The three most common endogenous pigments are lipofuscin, melanin, and ferritin/hemosiderin. Being brown and intracellular, they look deceptively similar in histologic sections (Table 3.1).

LIPOFUSCIN

Lipofuscin, also known as age pigment or wear-and-tear pigment, is a very common, brown, granular, lipidic, intracellular material found in all animals, including worms and flies; even fungi have some. Because it increases in amount with age, it has fascinated biologists ever since it was discovered in 1842. It tells us something about the aging process (140, 144, 156).

Lipofuscin is a reminder that living matter is transient. Life depends on membranes and oxygen. Membrane lipids contain unsaturated fatty acids,

which are particularly susceptible to free radical damage, becoming peroxidized, cross-linked, and nonfunctional (p. 185). Of course there is a membrane-renewal system that depends in part on autophagocytosis and recycling of the molecular components; however, cross-linked lipids are more resistant to digestion. Therefore, every episode of autophagocytosis can lead, potentially, to a nondigestible residue: this is lipofuscin. The most common sources of lipofuscin are probably the mitochondria, which are particularly exposed to oxidation damage.

A good way to understand lipofuscin is to compare it with linoleum. Linoleum, as its name implies, is obtained from linseed oil. The British citizen who invented linoleum around 1860 discovered that if linseed oil is heated long enough in the presence of oxygen, it becomes darker and darker, less and less oily, and eventually turns into a solid. In more general terms, *if long-chain fatty acids are progressively oxidized, they gradually lose the typical properties of lipids. As their color slowly shifts from white to yellow to brown (Figure 3.40), they become less and less soluble in fat solvents, more and more cross-linked, and eventually turn into a solid mass.* The hardening of oil-based paints is based on the same process (131).

This process explains a peculiar property of lipofuscin. It can be stained with fat stains because it retains some of its lipid properties, but it can no longer be dissolved by the common fat solvents, which is why it is still present in sections of paraffin-embedded tissues. In fact, it is the only lipid that can be routinely stained with lipid stains in paraffin sections, although nobody ever tries to do so. The somewhat irregular stainability of

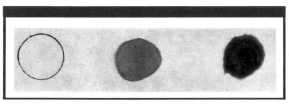

FIGURE 3.40
Progressive autooxidation of unsaturated fatty acids on filter paper. *Left circle:* Contains colorless fatty acids. *Center:* Same after 8 months incubation at 37°C in room air; the spot begins to turn brown. *Right:* After 18 months. (Reproduced with permission from [132].)

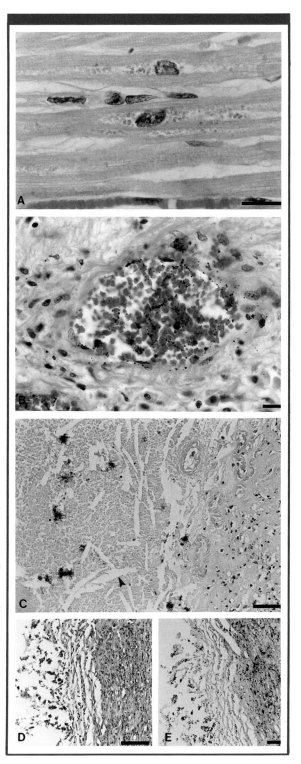

FIGURE 3.41
See color plate 3. Four common pigments seen in microscopic sections of animal tissues. *A-D:* hematoxylin and eosin stain. *A:* myocardial cells with lipofuscin granules (wear-and-tear pigment) collected in the space free of fibrils at either pole of the nucleus. **Bar** = 25 μm. *B:* black granules of hematin (formol pigment), a fixation artefact. The pigment has formed over red blood cells because it derives from their hemoglobin. **Bar** = 25 μm. *C:* clusters of bilirubin crystals in necrotic tissue, at the edge of the spleen infarct. *Arrowhead:* one of the several cholesterol crystals, as often seen in necrotic tissue. The nuclei at right belong mainly to macrophages surrounding the infarct. **Bar** = 100 μm. *D:* wall of an old hemorrhagic cyst (hematoma); the yellow-brown pigment in the lumen may be either hemosiderin/ferritin or bilirubin. **Bar** = 100 μm. *E:* similar area stained for iron (Perls Prussian blue reaction). The wall of the cyst contains much iron (hemosiderin, ferrritin) in macrophages; in the lumen, the pigment granules that do not stain for iron are bilirubin. **Bar** = 100 μm.

lipofuscin can be explained in terms of different stages of oxidation and polymerization.

By light microscopy, lipofuscin appears as yellow-brown grains somewhat larger than mitochondria, usually gathered in some part of the cytoplasm where other organelles leave space (Figure 3.41).

Histochemically, lipofuscin is basophilic and PAS positive; it can also be stained with acid fuchsin by the same acid-fast method used for Mycobacterium tuberculosis, *probably because its lipid behaves much like the lipid of that bacterium (131). Most important, it is autofluorescent: under UV light it emits a yellow-orange to green fluorescence, which* remains the best means of identification. If treated with H_2O_2 it becomes further oxidized and thus even more autofluorescent; this helps to distinguish it from melanin, another brown endogenous pigment, that is bleached by the same treatment. Lipofuscin can be extracted with a powerful lipid solvent, chloroform-methanol (144), and thus analyzed. It is not a definite compound but a random polymer of peroxidized lipids in which other molecules, especially proteins, can become copolymerized. Its composition varies depending on the organ and on the stage of oxidation; roughly half is lipid, the rest is mainly protein (129). It is sometimes mixed with melanin (p. 100).

By electron microscopy, the granules are seen to lie in the so-called **residual bodies,** which may become angular, reflecting the stiffness of the lipid polymer. The pigment itself appears as a dense, granular material that sometimes shows concentric "fingerprint" structures, presumably phospholipid remnants (Figure 3.42); other poorly digestible materials are often packed with lipofuscin, e.g., iron pigment, which may play a role in the further oxidation of the phospholipid.

Lipofuscin is abundant in neurons and myocardial cells, which can continue to accumulate oxidized lipids for as long as the individual survives. In the heart, the amount of lipofuscin increases progressively with age (Figure 3.43). Liver cells also contain a great deal of lipofuscin due to their long lives and high rate of autophagocytosis. A liver cell turns over all its organelles in less than a week (130). Labile cells such as those of the intestinal epithelium, with a life-span of about two days, do not have a chance to accumulate metabolic wastes. However, there is lipofuscin in fruit flies, which live only 40 days or so, and in dogs it develops 5.5 times faster than in man. This rate is proportional to the shorter life-span of the dog, suggesting that lipofuscin is a marker not only of age but of physiologic or "relative" age (144).

Besides age, another factor enhancing lipofuscin deposition is a high metabolic rate. This was shown in nerve cells (127) and even in houseflies, which were cleverly kept at various levels of activity (145, 157). The very busy eye muscles of mammals are also particularly rich in lipofuscin.

Dietary uptake of unsaturated fatty acids (a fashionable diet at the time of this writing) does not seem to affect lipofuscin deposition in man, but experiments on pigs fed large amounts of polyunsaturated fats have produced a "brown meat" with a rancid odor

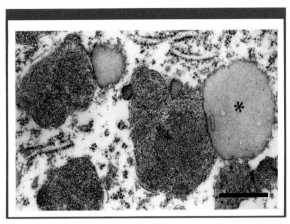

FIGURE 3.42
Granules of lipofuscin in a neuron of the human cortex, biopsied in the course of surgery for a brain tumor. The lipofuscin here appears filamentous; it is contained in residual bodies that also include droplets of lipid (*) **Bar** = 0.5 μm. (Courtesy of Dr. J.W. Boellaard, University of Tübingen, Germany.)

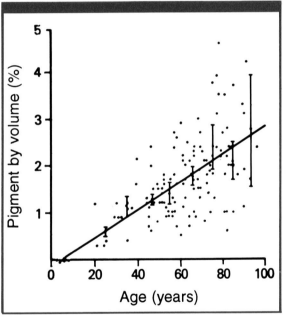

FIGURE 3.43
Progressive accumulation of lipofuscin in the human myocardium. (Reproduced with permission from [149].)

(125) characteristic of free radical damage. In the food industry, oxidation is a problem, hence the use of antioxidants. Malonaldehyde, a major by-product of free radical reactions, is used as an index of food oxidation; it is also the main cross-linking agent of lipofuscin (124). We may cautiously express the view that food additives may not necessarily be an evil in the specific case of antioxidants. Indeed, antioxidants have prolonged the life-span of creatures ranging from bacteria to fungi and laboratory rodents. There is even hope in an antioxidant therapy against atherosclerosis and against aging (141).

There is no proof that lipofuscin does any harm, although various theories of "lipofuscin damage" have been proposed (138). The general impression is that *lipofuscin increases with age but does not cause aging.* Perhaps a problem would arise if we lived much longer. Residual bodies stuffed with lipofuscin might become large enough to crowd out the other organelles, as happens in lysosomal diseases.

Can cells ever get rid of lipofuscin? Perhaps so, to a limited extent. Lysosomal enzyme inhibitors applied locally in the brain induce lipofuscin formation, suggesting a role for lytic enzymes (136). Although exocytosis of unwanted materials is hard to prove in mammalian cells, there is some evidence that neurons can transmit their lipofuscin to surrounding glial cells (127). Here also is a perplexing observation: it has been reported that drugs, such as centrophenoxine, that are effective against certain manifestations of senescence also dissolve lipofuscin (146, 147). Nobody is ready to believe that these drugs rejuvenate, but the findings do suggest that lipofuscin is not completely indigestible. The residual bodies in which it is lodged have been shown to contain several lysosomal enzymes (134). Perhaps lipofuscin is simply difficult to break down and is metabolized very slowly.

A few pathologic conditions involve lipofuscin. The brownish color of atrophic organs, especially heart and liver, is due to abundant lipofuscin, which increases both relatively (atrophic cells shrink) and absolutely (atrophy involves autophagocytosis, which produces more lipofuscin); hence the term **brown atrophy.** *Deficiency of vitamin E leads to excessive deposition of lipofuscin in several organs* (142, 144). This is understandable because lipofuscin is generated by oxidation, and nutritional lack of vitamin E means lack of an antioxidant. The pigment accumulates especially (for reasons unknown) in the smooth muscle cells of the uterus and of the gut. Here is one scenario that may occur in chronic pancreatic disease: pancreatic insufficiency → malabsorption of fat → lost fat carries with it the fat-soluble vitamin E → avitaminosis E with deposition of lipofuscin in the muscularis of the gut → "brown bowel syndrome" (157).

Melanosis coli has nothing to do with melanin. It is a visually striking but harmless condition in which the mucosa of the entire colon (or sometimes just a segment) is uniformly black, with a sharp limit toward the small intestine. The pigment—a variety of lipofuscin—is contained in macrophages in the mucosa; its presence is associated with the prolonged use of cathartics of the anthracene group (cascara

sagrada, senna, aloe, rhubarb) (148). An experimental study in guinea pigs suggests the following mechanism: intake of a given purgative → wave of cell death (apoptosis, p. 200) in the mucosal epithelium → phagocytosis of these dead cells by macrophages → loading of the macrophages with undigested lipid (154).

A rare group of inborn diseases of the nervous system, named **ceroid lipofuscinoses** *(155), are hereditary encephalopathies in which brain cells and many peripheral cells store abnormally large amounts of lipofuscin; some pigment can be found even in the urine.*

"Ceroid" versus lipofuscin Ceroid is a confusing term that has probably outlived its usefulness (131). The name was used in 1942 by Lillie to define a brown pigment seen in the liver of nutritionally deficient rats (129). Some experts then proposed that ceroid be applied to oxidized lipids of exogenous origin and lipofuscin to oxidized endogenous lipids (137). Microscopically the two are not distinguishable and so the distinction is rather academic. It is useful, however, to remember that exogenous lipids may also become oxidized and turn into brown residues as they do *in vitro.* Such is the brown pigment found in the sinusoidal phagocytes (p. 299) of patients fed intravenously with a fat emulsion (150). Unsaturated fatty acids injected into the skin of a rat can be found a whole year later in the local macrophages as brownish granules (133). At that time some of the lipid is still extracellular; it has also become oxidized as a brownish mass, proving that the oxidation also can take place outside cells.

Fats are easily oxidized in the presence of hemoglobin or hematin (156). This explains why, in areas of hemorrhage, fat cells often retain a yellow-brown content even in paraffin-embedded sections. The color represents oxidized fat, which has become insoluble (129, 135).

TO SUM UP: Lipofuscin is probably of no use to the cells that contain it, but it seems to be harmless. Its main fascination lies in its connection with wear and tear—that is, with age.

MELANINS

Brown granules inside a cell could belong to one of three main families: lipofuscin, melanin or iron pigments. There are several varieties of melanin; all are random polymers of hydroxyaromatics. They are very ancient molecules and extremely stable: melanin was found in the ink sacs of a fossilized squid that died 180 million years ago (166, 168). Although melanin comes from the Greek *mélas*, "black," not all melanins are black. In mammals the prevailing type is the dark brown **eumelanin** (roughly "melanin proper"); a subtype of eumelanin is neuromelanin, found in the nervous system. **Phaeomelanin** is yellow or red (*phaiós* is Greek for "grey"; the ancient Greeks had no word for "brown").

Eumelanin and Phaeomelanin Eumelanin is the brown-black pigment of the skin (163, 165, 166, 177, 178); for this reason the main impact of melanin on humankind has been, alas, in the form of social pathology. Eumelanin is present not only in the skin and hair but also in the pigmented epithelium of the eye, in the meninges (where melanomas occasionally arise), in a row of nuclei along the brain stem (the substantia nigra and the bluish-black locus coeruleus owe their color and their names to melanin), in the chromaffin system (adrenal medulla, sympathetic ganglia), and in a few other sites.

The reader may have enough recollection of embryology to remember that *the melanin-containing organs just listed are all of ectodermal origin, like the nervous system.* The pathophysiology of melanin includes many links between the nervous system, adrenals, and skin; just consider some of melanin's precursors: epinephrine, norepinephrine, and adrenochrome (Figure 3.44). We must also admit that these links are not self-evident; the skin, after all, could not be farther removed from the central nervous system. However, if there are still any skeptics who find it hard to believe that the melanocytes of the skin really have their ancestors in the central nervous system, Figure 3.45 provides final proof. This two-tone chick, which would normally be white, was born after an amazing feat of microsurgery by Nicole Le Douarin (169, 170). When it was still an embryo, a segment of its neural crest was replaced with a segment of neural crest from a quail. Following its inborn schedule, the graft sent out cells that migrated to the skin, where

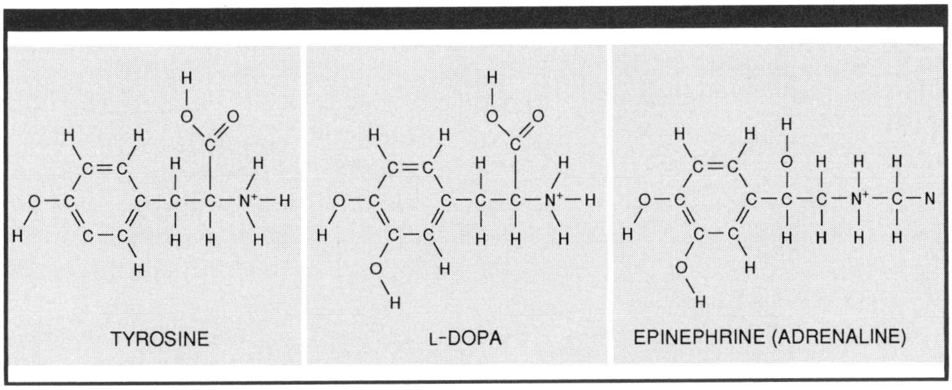

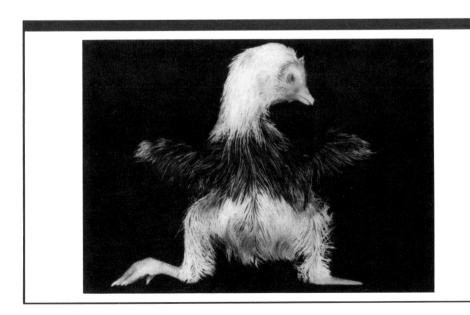

FIGURE 3.44
Melanin, as inert as it is, has some very dynamic predecessors, namely neurotransmitters derived from tyrosine (dopamine, norepinephrine, epinephrine). (Adapted from [79].)

TYROSINE   L-DOPA   EPINEPHRINE (ADRENALINE)

FIGURE 3.45
Proving the neural origin of melanocytes. When this white chick was an embryo, a segment of brown quail neural tube was grafted into its own neural tube, which resulted in a transverse stripe of brown quail color. (Reproduced with permission from [169].)

FIGURE 3.46
Distinctive appearance of heterochromatin in embryonic neuroblasts of two species of birds. *Top:* Quail. The heterochromatin forms a large centronuclear mass. *Bottom:* Chick. The heterochromatin is broken up in small scattered clumps. This difference makes it possible to follow the behavior and migrations of embryonic quail cells grafted into a chick. **Bar** = 10 μm. (Reproduced with permission from [169].)

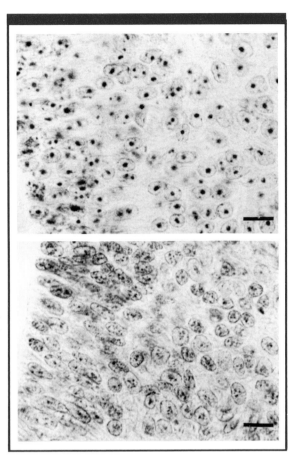

they became melanocytes. The migrating cells can actually be traced in microscopic sections because quail cell nuclei have distinctive nucleoli (Figure 3.46). The grafted chick hatched normally but with a transverse band of brown, quail-type feathers; this zone had been colonized by swarms of melanin-forming cells that wandered out from the segment of quail neural crest.

The pigment in skin is produced by the melanocytes and packed in granules (**melanosomes**) which, by electron microscopy, are membrane-bound and have a characteristic structure (Figure 3.47). These granules are transmitted to the surrounding epithelial cells (**keratinocytes**) in a manner that may be unique in biology: *each melanocyte actively implants its granules into the body of the cells close to it* (Figure 3.48) (160). Under pathologic conditions this activity can be disturbed, resulting in poor pigmentation (165).

Once in the keratinocyte, the melanosomes surround the nucleus, presumably to shield its DNA from radiation. In black skin the melanosomes—which are larger than those in white skin—remain free; in white skin they are taken up by autophagosomes and partially degraded. In other words, it is the number, size, and distribution of melanosomes, not of melanocytes, that determines skin color.

Chemically, eumelanin is an insoluble polymer of tyrosine, and phaeomelanin is an alkali-soluble polymer of tyrosine and cysteine. The latter is the typical pigment of red hair. There is evidence that all melanocytes produce a mixture of eumelanin and phaeomelanin. Eumelanin is easily synthesized *in vitro* but frustrating to study because it is insoluble, has little internal order, and has few characteristic spectroscopic bands. Its molecular weight is unknown because it has not yet been purified. Natural melanin includes 20–50 percent protein, as well as copper, iron, and zinc.

When studied by electron spin resonance, melanin gives a signal characteristic of organic free radicals. It has been proposed that the free radical nature of eumelanin is due to a quinone/hydroquinone/semiquinone equilibrium (163):

FIGURE 3.47
Four stages of melanosome development as seen by electron microscopy in cultured human melanocytes. The electron-dense material represents eumelanin. **Bar** = 0.1 μm. (Reproduced with permission from [161].)

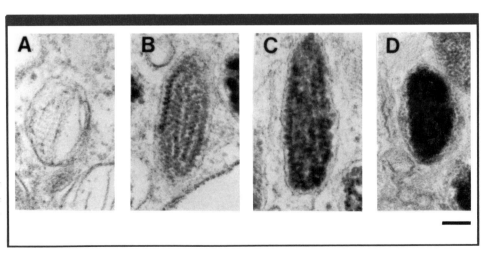

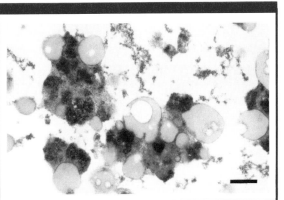

The redox properties of melanin have long been exploited in histochemistry. At pH 4, melanin granules reduce silver nitrate to metallic silver. This is the classic method for the histochemical detection of melanin (**Fontana reaction**), now being replaced by more specific but more expensive monoclonal antibodies.

Plant melanins are catechol melanins, unlike mammalian melanins, which are indole melanins (166). The blackening reaction of plants, as seen on a banana or a slice of apple, does not necessarily produce a polymer, but it does have links with melanin. Normally in plants, polyphenols and phenol oxidases are segregated in different compartments; when mixed as a result of damage, the oxidases turn the polyphenols into quinones, which are powerful oxidants and therefore antibacterial. As such, this reaction might be useful not only in plants (180) but possibly also in insects (181); nothing comparable is proven for mammals.

Neuromelanin, the melanin of the nervous system, is chemically a brown-black eumelanin like that of the skin. However, when studied by

electron microscopy, it has no specific ultrastructure. *It is not segregated in specific pigment cells such as melanocytes but resides in neurons* where it is contained in residual bodies (Figure 3.49) together with lipofuscin (158). It is present in a row of nuclei along the brainstem; the total amount of neuromelanin tends to decrease with age (144, 159) because the neuromelanin-containing neurons decrease in number. The distribution of neuromelanin- and catecholamine-containing neurons is very similar (172); it is tempting to conclude that neuromelanin has the purpose of detoxifying some molecule of the catecholamine

FIGURE 3.49
Residual bodies of human substantia nigra obtained at autopsy. The dark, electron-dense material is neuromelanin. **Bar** = 0.5 μm. (Courtesy of Dr. J.W. Boellaard, University of Tübingen, Germany.)

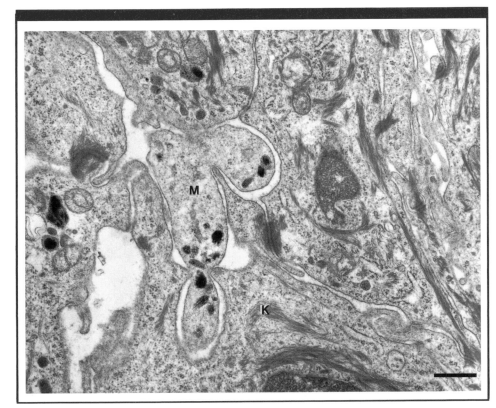

FIGURE 3.48
A natural autograft: a pseudopod of a melanocyte (**M**) containing melanosomes is being implanted into a keratinocyte. **K** = keratinocyte. In this particular case the grafting process is demonstrated in a basal cell carcinoma. **Bar** = 0.5 μm. (Reproduced with permission from [160].)

family. Catecholamines are derivatives of tyrosine, the basic monomer of skin melanin (Figure 3.44). Other interesting facts: albinos do have neuromelanin, although they have little or no melanin in the skin and in the eye (they have eyesight problems); carnivores, including man, have the largest amount of neuromelanin; rodents have none (159).

Melanin and lipofuscin can be associated. About 70 percent of the brown pigment in the myocardium is lipofuscin; 30 percent is melanin. The two pigments are associated also in the nerve cells (158), the liver, and possibly other organs (167, 173). What this correlation means is not clear, but there are similarities between the two pigments. Both are polymers resulting from the oxidative attack of certain substrates (amines and amino acids for melanin, unsaturated lipids for lipofuscin); the two processes might sometimes occur together and produce a mixed polymer (183).

The known functions of eumelanin are three:

- *Light absorption.* Eumelanin absorbs throughout the ultraviolet and visible regions of the spectrum; it converts light to heat and in the process becomes oxidized and darker (177). In essence, black skin proves to be a sunscreen rated at 13.4 (166). The sunscreen effect is beneficial because ultraviolet rays are carcinogenic. Dark-skinned people are much less susceptible to melanoma and to epidermal cancers than whites. Damage to the dermis is also reduced: solar elastosis (p. 260) is much more prevalent in the skin of blond and red-haired individuals.

Suntan and sunburn result from ultraviolet (UV) radiation. UV rays are classified as UV-A, the longest (400–315 nm), which cause suntanning and very weak inflammation; UV-B (315–280 nm), which also tan but cause sunburn; and UV-C (280–200 nm), which are germicidal but do not reach the earth's surface (166) (Figure 3.50). Suntanning occurs in two phases: (1) within minutes of exposure to UV rays there is an immediate darkening due to oxidation of melanin; (2) this fades in 6–8 hours and is followed by increased production and transfer of melanosomes from melanocytes to keratinocytes, evident after 2 days (164).

- *Free-radical sink.* A great deal of speculation has grown around this property of melanin. There is a free-radical theory of aging: does this imply that melanin could prolong life? The answer appears to be no, but it is certainly true that black skin ages better than white. Oddly enough, eumelanin produces potentially damaging free radicals when exposed to light (177).
- *Ion-exchange resin.* Melanin granules do behave as lumps of ion-exchange material but whether this amounts to a useful function is not clear. In practice, melanin, as an electron acceptor, binds many drugs, which act as electron donors. Among these are cocaine, epinephrine, the antidepressant phenothiasines (which block dopamine receptors) and especially chlorpromazine, an antidepressant used in the treatment of amphetamine poisoning. Patients treated with phenothiazines can develop an increased photosensitivity (165) and even a peculiar skin color ("purple people") (174).

Self-destruction of the melanocytes can be induced with certain drugs, which can therefore be applied locally to attenuate overpigmented areas. Among these is hydroxyanisole, a substituted phenol.

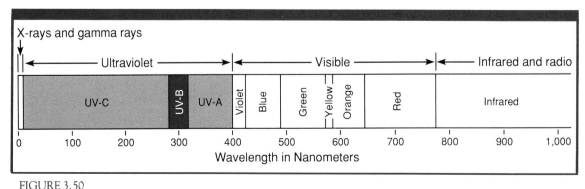

FIGURE 3.50
Electromagnetic spectrum, emphasizing the ultraviolet range. The wavelength band responsible for the most severe photobiologic effects is UV-B The UV-A band contributes to tanning, and the UV-C band is germicidal. (Adapted from [176].)

Apparently the melanosomes accept it as a substrate for melanogenesis, whereby tyrosinase converts it to damaging free radicals that kill the melanocyte (175).

Pathology of Melanin *The pathology of melanin is largely a matter of increased or decreased pigmentation* (165, 166). In either case, many chemical agents are involved; the defect may be a side effect of a drug (such as a chemotherapeutic agent against cancer) or the result of industrial exposure (171), and it may be permanent. Not all the mechanisms are known.

The best understood mechanism of depigmentation (161) is the autoimmune destruction of the melanocytes. Compared with other epidermal cells, such as keratinocytes, the melanocytes are unusually susceptible to immune damage. The white patches of depigmented skin known as **vitiligo** (an ancient Latin name of unknown origin) are thought to arise by such a mechanism (p. 575).

Albinism, due to a congenital partial or total absence of melanin, is found in man and many animals including rodents, birds, fish, and reptiles; it is basically due to lack of tyrosinase.

Patches of increased pigmentation appear when the adrenals are destroyed (Addison's disease). The pituitary responds to the drop in adrenal cortical hormones by increasing its adrenotropic output, which includes two melanizing hormones: ACTH, primarily a cortical stimulant (which also happens to stimulate melanocytes), and MSH, primarily a melanocyte stimulating hormone (which is also a weak adrenal stimulant).

Melanomas are tumors of melanocytes; typically they retain their ability to make melanosomes and thereappear as brown-black masses in man and other animals (Figure 3.51). At times, however, they contain so little melanin that they appear colorless and diagnosis is difficult unless special methods are used to detect a few telltale melanosomes (electron microscopy or histochemistry). If patches of vitiliginous skin are associated with melanoma, the prognosis of the melanoma is better (162).

TO SUM UP: Melanins are biologically very important but little understood. Their physicochemical properties are frustrating. Much remains to be learned.

FERRITIN AND HEMOSIDERIN

The rusty color of the two closely related intracellular pigments, ferritin and hemosiderin, reflects their vital function: iron storage. The cells in charge of the "iron bank" are largely the macrophages, but virtually any cell can be drafted to store iron in case of extreme overload.

In essence: **FERRITIN** *is a hollow protein loaded with iron. In a test tube it is brown, but when it is free in the cytoplasm it is invisible by light microscopy (except if stained histochemically for iron). The brown granules of iron-storing cells are autophagosomes loaded with semidigested ferritin mole-*

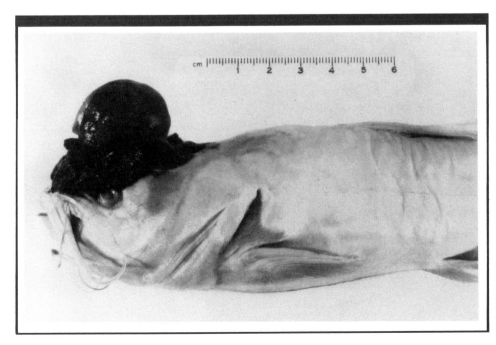

FIGURE 3.51
Brown bullhead with a primary melanoma of the head. (Courtesy of Dr. J.C. Harshbarger, Smithsonian Institution, Washington, D.C.)

cules, and this material is called **HEMOSIDERIN.** Ferritin and hemosiderin are normal products, but they may be present in excessive amounts.

Iron behaves, most appropriately, as a two-edged sword. On one hand, *iron is essential to life,* being the key to aerobic metabolism as well as to photosynthesis; in hemoglobin it is the key to oxygen transport. On the other hand, *iron is a highly toxic metal* (201, 225, 227) that mediates dangerous free-radical reactions (p. 184), and it favors the growth of bacteria and other parasites. Its pathophysiology reflects these conflicting roles. The precious but dangerous iron atoms are taken out of solution and tucked away as pigments, and their movements are tightly controlled.

Storage of Iron Because 70 percent of the body's iron is in hemoglobin, recovery from a large hemorrhage could be a long process if the iron had to be replaced by food intake (193, 197, 199). The

obvious solution is to have an easily accessible store of iron in nontoxic form (Figure 3.52). Nature's answer is ferritin, a beautiful molecule shaped like a hollow bead (called **apoferritin** when empty), in which iron atoms can be safely stockpiled in the nearly insoluble trivalent form (Figure 3.53).

The molecular weight of apoferritin is 441,000 daltons. The maximal loading capacity is about 4300 units of FeOOH (ferric oxyhydroxide), and the average ferritin molecule contains about 2000 of them. One or more crystals of FeOOH can be in the core; they also contain phosphate, perhaps as impurity. The protein subunits of apoferritin are of two kinds, H (for heart, or heavy) and L (for liver, or light); they are present in different proportions, which may explain the existence of several isoferritins (195). It takes about half a million ferritin molecules to provide the iron for one erythrocyte.

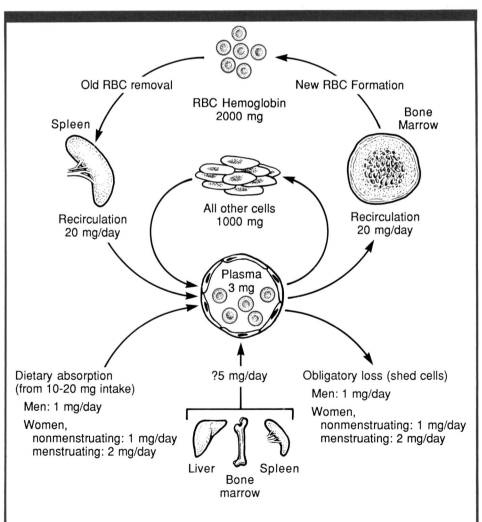

FIGURE 3.52
Economy of iron in the human adult. It involves balancing about 4000 mg in men and 3500 mg in women. Red blood cells carry 2000 mg and other cells about 1000 mg. The rest is stored in the liver, spleen, and bone marrow as ferritin and hemosiderin. Dietary absorption compensates for losses. It is assumed that there are exchanges between storage compartments and active compartments. (Adapted from [192].)

Old RBC removal   New RBC Formation

RBC Hemoglobin
2000 mg

Spleen   Bone
Marrow

Recirculation
20 mg/day   Recirculation
20 mg/day

All other cells
1000 mg

Plasma
3 mg

Dietary absorption
(from 10-20 mg intake)   ?5 mg/day   Obligatory loss (shed cells)

Men: 1 mg/day   Men: 1 mg/day

Women,
nonmenstruating: 1 mg/day
menstruating: 2 mg/day   Women,
nonmenstruating: 1 mg/day
menstruating: 2 mg/day

Liver   Spleen
Bone
marrow

In humans, 20–25 percent of total iron represents storage as ferritin and hemosiderin (192, 220) (Figure 3.52). Evolution invented this device a long time ago: ferritin exists in plants as **phytoferritin;** indeed it can be synthesized by virtually all animal and plant cells (191, 192, 198, 220).

The ferritin molecule recalls certain viruses. It consists of 24 very similar cylindrical subunits that are assembled to form a box 130 Å in diameter with rounded corners and an internal chamber of about 70 Å (see Figure 3.53). On each face there are four subunits and a pore about 10 Å in diameter. Ferrous ions diffuse through the pores into the hollow core where they assemble in crystals of ferric oxyhydroxide (FeOOH) (185, 200, 206). Ferrous ions, however, cannot fit into the crystal lattice; thus *the Fe^{2+} ions that diffuse into the pores are somehow oxidized to Fe^{3+} as they pass.* The reverse occurs when iron is extracted; this means that the reducing agents—whatever they may be—must diffuse into the pores and reach the surface of the crystal (Figure 3.53) (198). Iron can be mobilized from ferritin by superoxide from activated leukocytes (187).

By electron microscopy at very high powers, the protein shell of the ferritin molecules can be outlined by the procedure known as **negative staining** (Figure 3.54) (217). In ordinary transmission electron micrographs the shell is too transparent to create an image, but the iron core stands out as a tiny dot, which makes it one of the few molecules directly identifiable by electron microscopy. This property is exploited experimentally; when it is necessary to visualize macromolecules that are invisible by themselves, a standard trick is to bind them to ferritin molecules (Figure 3.55).

When a macrophage is challenged to store more iron (typically, by phagocytizing red blood cells), it immediately begins to synthesize more apoferritin molecules, which remain free in the cytosol and promptly pick up their load of iron atoms. Macrophages surrounding a mass of injected iron oxide show cytoplasmic ferritin particles within 4 hours (224); in tissue culture the delay shrinks to minutes (194). Soon the cytoplasm becomes crowded with ferritin molecules (Figure 3.56) (186). At some point, autophagocytosis sets in; that is, portions of the cytoplasm filled with ferritin molecules are rounded up and segregated into membrane-bound particles, which are typical autophagosomes but are also known as **siderosomes** (224). These are visible by light microscopy as brownish granules that stain positively for iron. Inside the siderosomes, the ferritin molecules are either loosely packed or crystallized (Figure 3.56), but in time they are digested by lysosomal enzymes. As the protein envelopes (apoferritin) are broken down, the iron cores become more and more crowded. The result is a dense mass in which the individual ferritin molecules are no longer visible. This material is **hemosiderin** (a name chosen by Virchow), which is now conceived as a mass of partially digested and denatured ferritin molecules mixed with loose iron cores of ferric oxyhydroxide, FeOOH (208, 224, 231). Histochemically, granules of hemosiderin react positively for iron, just like ferritin. There is no way to distinguish between ferritin and hemosiderin ex-

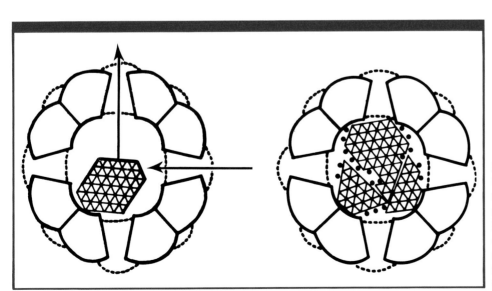

FIGURE 3.53
Cross section of two molecules of ferritin. *Left:* Molecule containing a single crystal of ferric oxyhydroxide. *Right:* Inner space nearly filled with crystals. Dots are phosphate and other ions bound to the crystal surface. (Reproduced with permission from [206].)

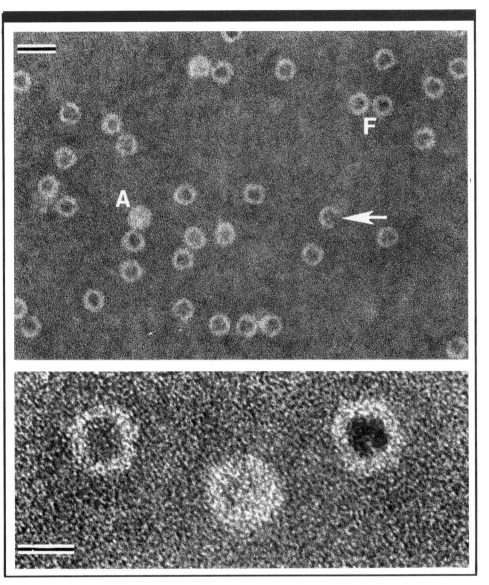

FIGURE 3.54
Ferritin molecules, negatively stained and seen by high-power electron microscopy. *Top:* The light rings represent the protein shell. **Arrow** points to a broken shell. **F:** Molecules loaded with iron. **A:** Molecule free of iron or not penetrated by the contrast medium. **Bar** = 200 Å. *Bottom:* The dense core at the left represents either a moderate iron load or penetration of the contrast medium. In the center is an apoferritin molecule without contrast. At the right, ferritin is heavily loaded with iron. **Bar** = 100 Å. (Reproduced with permission from [217].)

cept by electron microscopy or chemistry; however, in practice there is no need to make the distinction because *both pigments have the same significance: stored iron.* Hemosiderin develops when the cell is overloaded with ferritin.

Histochemical Reactions Both ferritin and hemosiderin react positively to the histochemical reaction for iron. With ferric ferrocyanide they yield the beautiful Prussian blue (Figure 3.57). Red blood cells, however, remain red because the iron of hemoglobin is tightly bound within the heme and is not available for the Prussian blue reaction.

There is no histochemical difference between ferritin and hemosiderin; however, by light microscopy, a diffuse blue stain of the cytoplasm suggests free ferritin, whereas hemosiderin is always present as granules, which correspond to phagosomes.

At autopsy, if the rusty color of an organ suggests the presence of excess iron pigment, it is easy to perform the Prussian blue test; a positive test can be quite spectacular (Figure 3.58). An even simpler but malodorous procedure is to wipe the surface of the tissue with ammonium sulfide: histochemically reactable iron instantly turns black due to the formation of iron sulfide. Both these color reactions date from the mid-1800s (221). Iron sulfide is also responsible for the black discoloration seen especially on the underside of the liver at autopsy. In this case H_2S is provided by colonic bacteria.

Travels of the Iron Atom How does the iron reach the cell or leave it? Not all the answers are available, but the itinerary of iron atoms inside the body is essentially as follows (197, 205, 213, 230) (Figure 3.52). Iron absorbed from the gut passes into the blood, where it is taken up by a carrier protein, **serum transferrin** (203, 209). Compared with tissue ferritin (which holds iron by "truck-loads"—up to 450,000 atoms), transferrin is rather like a bicycle; it can carry only two atoms. Cells that need iron bind transferrin to their membrane by means of specific receptors; the receptor complex is internalized, the iron is released, and the transferrin is returned to the surface for recycling. Incidentally, *there is no excretion of iron* (by the urine, bile, or other pathways), only a constant loss through the shedding of cells.

> *There is a serum ferritin (not transferrin!) that seems to be secreted by all body cells; it is slightly different from tissue ferritin and contains very little iron. Now here is another beautiful arrangement: the amount of this circulating ferritin is parallel to the amount of stored iron, wherever it may be (199). It would be nice to conclude that the serum ferritin level is what enables the intestinal mucosa to regulate the absorption exactly as required for replenishing the stores, but unfortunately the feedback mechanism remains a dilemma (192).*

Pathology of Iron Overload Both ferritin and hemosiderin are present in some phagocytes of the normal reticulo endothelial/mononuclear phago-

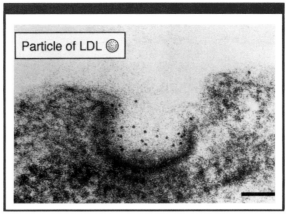

FIGURE 3.55
Ferritin as an electron microscopic label for invisible macromolecules. A pit in the membrane of a human fibroblast is picking up LDL particles, the size of which is indicated in the inset. The particles themselves are invisible, but the ferritin label indicates that they are present. **Bar** = 0.1 μm. (Reproduced with permission from [226].)

cyte system (RES/MPS; p. 297), but in cases of iron overload they can be present in excess or in cells that normally have no iron stores (**hemosiderosis**). Iron overload can be due to local or general causes. The most common local cause is hemorrhage into the tissues; the example traditionally used is that of the "black eye". A black eye is black and red from blood that infiltrates the tissues; later, as everybody knows, it acquires shades of purple, brown, green, and yellow. This display of colors is due to a variety of

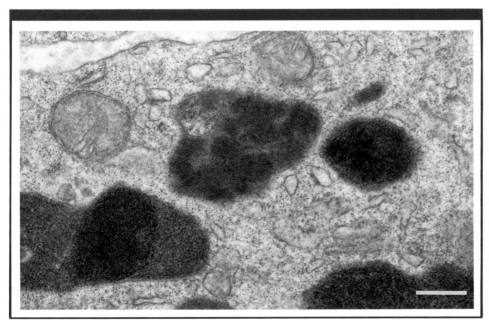

FIGURE 3.56
Part of a macrophage in the synovium of a knee joint subjected to constant bleeding. Several siderosomes are shown, one containing crystalline masses of ferritin. No ferritin is recognizable in the others; it was presumably transformed into hemosiderin. Many of the small dots in the cytosol correspond to free ferritin particles; they are more electron dense than the ribosomes. **Bar** = 0.3 μm. (Courtesy of Dr. J. Bhawan, Boston University School of Medicine, Boston, Mass.)

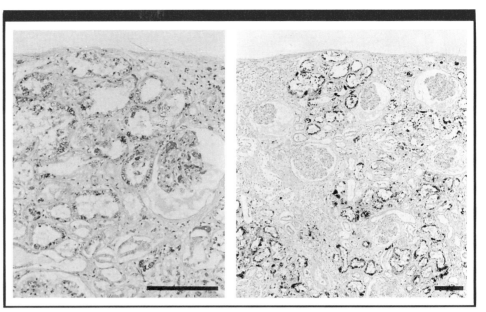

FIGURE 3.57
See color plate 4. Hemosiderosis in a human kidney, due to chronic low-grade hemolysis caused by a metallic prosthetic cardiac valve (St. Jude valve). *Left:* The dark (brown) deposits in the tubules represent hemosiderin derived from reabsorbed hemoglobin. Hematoxylin and eosin stain. *Right:* Same deposits stained for iron (Perls Prussian blue reaction). Bars = 200 μm.

pigments deriving from the extravasated red blood cells. The most colorful are actually iron-free.

The colorful "pathology of the black eye" due to hemoglobin breakdown makes one wonder whether the beautiful display of leaf colors in autumn may be due to a comparable chlorophyll breakdown. The answer is yes and no: the yellows and oranges are due mainly to carotenoids, normally present in the leaves but masked by the chlorophyll, and to phaeophytins consisting of chlorophyll that lost its magnesium. However, botanical experts tell us that not much is known on this topic.

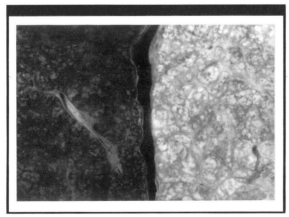

FIGURE 3.58
See color plate 5. Two slices of the same cirrhotic liver, from a case of hemochromatosis. *Right:* Fresh, untreated tissue. The rusty color betrays the presence of iron pigments (hemosiderin, ferritin). Lighter dots represent areas of regenerating liver. *Left:* Similar slice after a histochemical reaction for iron. The resulting Prussian blue shows that iron is everywhere, in the stroma as well as in the liver cells. Scale in mm.

When red blood cells are spilled into the tissue spaces they can survive for a short time, but eventually either they are phagocytized by macrophages or they hemolyze and their hemoglobin diffuses away (202, 216). The subsequent trials and tribulations of the hemoglobin molecules are many, but there is one common theme: *nature has devised many ways to recover the iron atoms.* It does so in two steps: the hemoglobin is retrieved, and its iron is extracted.

1. *Retrieval of hemoglobin.* Follow the diagram of Figure 3.59. If many red blood cells are lost by intravascular hemolysis, some of the hemoglobin dissolved in the plasma inevitably escapes through the glomeruli (remember that the glomerular filter is permeable to molecules smaller than ~60–70 kilodaltons, and hemoglobin is about 40 kilodaltons). However, on its way out along the kidney tubules, some of the hemoglobin is recovered by endocytosis (Figure 3.57). In the meantime, any hemoglobin that circulates free in the plasma is captured by a special protein, **haptoglobin** (*hápto* is Greek for "I bind"). The complex ends up in the liver, where it is recycled. If a great deal of free hemoglobin is present in the plasma, some of it is oxidized to **methemoglobin** (ferrihemoglobin), a chocolate-colored compound in which the four iron atoms are trivalent. Finally, some of the free hemoglobin will lose its hemes, but these too can be promptly captured by

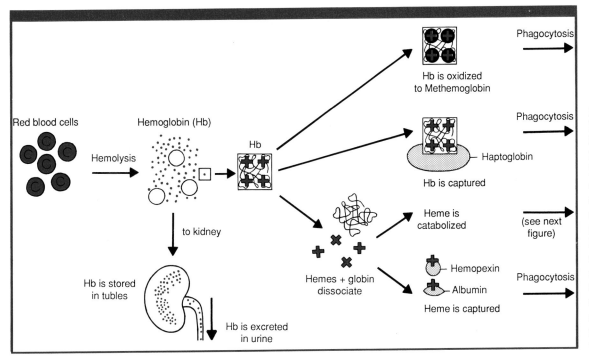

FIGURE 3.59 Possible fates of hemoglobin released by red blood cells. Any of the iron-containing molecules can be phagocytized. Phagocytosis (extreme right) is performed by the reticuloendothelial system (or mononuclear phagocyte system, p. 297).

albumin and by the protein **hemopexin,** and again the complexes are recovered by the liver.

Methemoglobin, when it is formed inside red blood cells, can be easily reduced to hemoglobin (210). When it develops in spilled blood it is presumably catabolized like hemoglobin. It is not recognizable microscopically. Lately it has become important in radiology due to its magnetic properties: recent brain hemorrhages are visible by nuclear magnetic resonance due to the contrast provided by their content of methemoglobin (188).

2. *Retrieval of iron.* Now let us see what happens to the hemes, the custodians of the iron (Figure 3.60). It so happens that the four hemes carried by each hemoglobin molecule can be detached fairly easily from the globin. Once they have left the globin, the hemes break open and the iron atom is freed. From then on, *the two parts of the original heme follow separate routes;* the broken ring gives rise to bilirubin (p. 113), and the iron finds its way into the surrounding cells, presumably by hitching a ride on transferrin molecules floating around.

How long does it take for ferritin or hemosiderin to appear? This question can be of medicolegal importance because the presence or absence of these pigments could help establish the date of an injury. Experimentally, after an injection of blood into the skin, a positive Prussian blue reaction was found at 24 hours in mice and rats (219) but not in rabbits (215). In humans, the first histochemically detectable traces of iron were found after 50–72 hours (227a), but—surprisingly—a definitive study is not available. At the biochemical level, as we have seen, the time required for ferritin synthesis is of the order of minutes.

A generalized iron overload occurs in **idiopathic hemochromatosis,** a hereditary disorder in which too much iron is absorbed or retained (192, 207, 223, 227), causing extensive iron deposits to develop in the skin, liver, pancreas, heart, and endocrine organs. The deposits are present both in phagocytic cells and in parenchymal cells and are often associated with scarring, especially of the liver and pancreas (Figure 3.58). It is not clear why the fibrous tissue increases, but the parenchymal cells are certainly injured. The symptoms are mainly those of liver damage, heart dysfunction, and multiple endocrine failures, especially pancreatic. (The disease was once called **bronze diabetes,** because of the brownish discoloration of the skin.) It was believed until recently that iatrogenic overload from repeated transfusions could not produce the full-blown disease because most of the iron was said to be stored in the reticuloendothelial system rather than in the parenchymal cells. Close scrutiny has shown,

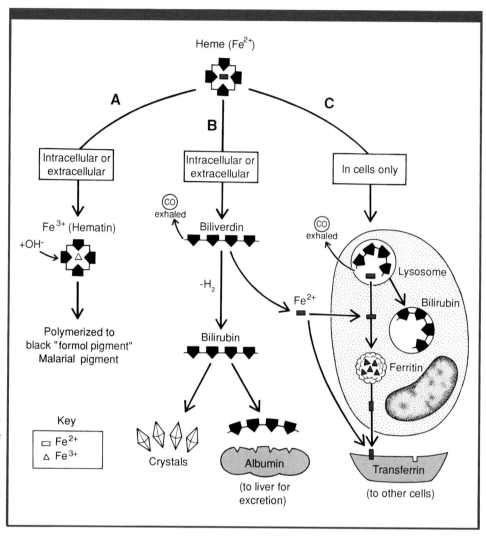

FIGURE 3.60
Three pathways contribute to the disposal of the heme molecule. **A**: The heme ring remains intact and polymerizes to black pigment. **B**: The heme ring is broken open and loses the iron; bilirubin is formed. **C**: The iron is incorporated into ferritin and recycled by transferrin.

however, that transfusion overload can also lead to organ damage (227). Thus, *hemochromatosis can be considered as a single clinical condition*, with many causes and various degrees of severity.

> The mechanism of cell damage in hemochromatosis is not fully understood. It seems that lysosomes stuffed with ferritin and hemosiderin are themselves damaged by the iron and become more fragile (184, 222). This could well be the result of free radical peroxidation: the Fe^{2+}/Fe^{3+} reaction entails a one-electron transfer, which means that it can catalyze many redox reactions in which injurious free radicals are formed, such as superoxide, hydrogen peroxide, and hydroxyl radical (p. 184) (223). Mitochondria can be damaged (201). Iron may also be involved in stimulating the fibrosis, but the evidence is meager (223). Perhaps the activated macrophages secrete cytokines that produce fibrosis.

Interestingly, it has been shown that large iron stores increase the risk of cancer (228) but also

that the hemochromatosis gene may have a protective value, perhaps by protecting against anemia (211).

Hemochromatosis is successfully treated by a method dear to Hippocrates: repeated bleeding.

Iron, Hemolysis, and Infection Let us summarize the astonishing cascade of molecular traps that are set for free iron and for iron-containing molecules (214):

- Free hemoglobin is bound by **haptoglobin** (1:1).
- Heme is captured by **hemopexin** (1:1).
- Excess heme is bound by **albumin** (2:1).
- Free iron in plasma is captured by **transferrin** (2:1).
- Free iron in secretions is captured by **lactoferrin** (2:1).
- Free iron is stored in **apoferritin** (about 4000:1).

What evolutionary pressures could have produced these trapping mechanisms? An obvious reason is the conservation of iron, but a strong case can be made also for the defense against infection (190).

Iron is so important for bacterial growth that it can be considered a virulence factor (189). When bacteria invade tissues, they find themselves in a world in which almost all the iron is hidden inside cells; there is some in the interstitial fluids, but it is almost entirely bound to transport proteins. What is left is far too little to support bacterial growth (204). Interestingly, transferrin was known as a bacteriostatic protein long before its role was understood. When it was added to bacterial cultures, it inhibited bacterial growth. Now we know that it did so by sequestering iron. To survive in such inhospitable juices, bacteria have elaborated complex iron-snatching mechanisms. Their main strategy is to secrete molecules called **siderophores** that have strong affinity for iron.

There is plenty of evidence that iron favors infection (229). In rats, a nonlethal dose of *Escherichia coli* injected into the peritoneum becomes lethal if accompanied by just 20 mg of hemoglobin (Figure 3.61) (196). *Extensive hemolysis is associated with infection,* especially in the peritoneum: a classic setting is the seepage of blood and bacteria into the peritoneal cavity from a strangulated loop of intestine (214). "Iron sepsis" can occur after an overdose of iron (218) and in infants even after therapeutic doses (196). A similar irony is that the well-meant refeeding of starved populations with low plasma transferrin levels may lead to saturation of transferrin and to increased attacks of malaria, suggesting that protozoan infections are also enhanced by iron (214). Hypoferremia may be an adaptation in parts of the world where infections are prevalent (212).

Once again, more is not necessarily better.

BILIRUBIN

If melanin influenced the course of history, bilirubin did so too, in a different way. As the name implies, bilirubin is the pigment of mammalian bile. Its bright yellow color (Fig. 3.41) struck the imagination of the Greeks and the Hindus so strongly that they considered "yellow bile" to be one of the four basic components of the human body. We still refer to this theory when we accuse someone of being bilious (243).

Bilirubin (240) is a stack of porphyrin rings that broke open and lost their iron (Figure 3.62). Once

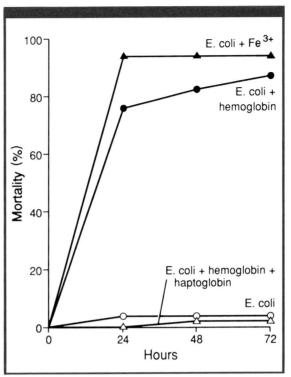

FIGURE 3.61
Iron favors infection. Mortality in rats inoculated intraperitoneally with 10^7 *Escherichia coli*, alone, with Fe^{3+} or with hemoglobin with or without, haptoglobin. It is obvious that hemoglobin and Fe^{3+} favor infection, whereas haptoglobin (which captures the hemoglobin) has a protective effect. (Adapted from [196].)

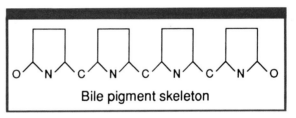

FIGURE 3.62
Skeleton of bile pigments. The porphyrin ring is broken open and the iron atom is lost. (Reproduced with permission from [241].)

broken, the beautiful porphyrin ring can never be mended and must be eliminated through the bile (Figure 3.60). When this exit is obstructed or overwhelmed, bilirubin levels in the blood rise and cause jaundice.

Genesis of Bilirubin Bilirubin can be formed anywhere in the body. It has been difficult to eradicate the erroneous belief that bile pigments are formed only in the liver—even Virchow knew better (247). The pathway from heme to bilirubin implies two major steps (235, 236, 238):

1. *Breaking open the heme ring,* an oxidative reaction. In the process, the iron atom drops off, and the resulting molecule is **biliverdin.** The broken methene bridge is

lost as carbon monoxide (CO). This CO is partly eliminated by the breath, so expired CO can be used as a measure of hemoglobin breakdown.

2. *Reducing biliverdin to bilirubin.*

Because all cells contain heme proteins as cytochromes, any cell type can form bilirubin during the catabolism of these particular proteins. Macrophages, however, produce bilirubin from heme on a much larger scale when they digest red blood cells; their phagosomes can accumulate enough bilirubin to appear as golden granules. This is why intracellular and extracellular bilirubin always appear—in due time—around hemorrhages. Virchow noticed its colorful crystals and reasoned that they were probably bilirubin; however, he was not absolutely sure, so he called it **hematoidin** (the name is now being dropped). He was quite carried away by its color (248):

> *"Hematoidin is one of the most beautiful crystals we are acquainted with. . . . When a young woman menstruates, and the cavity of the Graafian vesicle, from which the ovum has been extruded, becomes filled with coagulated blood, the haematine [hemoglobin] is gradually converted to haematoidine, and we afterwards find at the spot where the ovum had lain the beautiful deep-red colour of the haematoidine crystals, which remain as the last memorials of this episode."* [Note: bilirubin is orange-red when very concentrated: bilirubin stands for "bile red".]

> *A gold rim of extracellular bilirubin is commonly seen grossly in masses of necrotic tissue such as recent infarcts, 1–2 mm within the edge. This is not easily explained because heme breakdown is commonly described as an enzymatic intracellular process, and as such it should not occur in dead tissue. We propose to reconcile the facts as follows. The initial oxidative opening of the heme ring can be obtained also in vitro; it requires molecular oxygen and a reductant (so-called coupled oxidation) (245). The next, reducing step does require an enzyme, but enzymes might still be floating around in an area of cells that just died, and the proper combination of oxidation and reduction might well exist precisely at the periphery of an infarct.*

Light Microscopic Appearance The diagonsis of bilirubin is suggested by extracellular golden needles and rhomboids around a not-so-recent hemorrhage. Tiny, yellowish granules or crystals in macrophages can be distinguished from ferritin and hemosiderin if an iron reaction is negative; of course, bilirubin contains no iron (Figure 3.41). Still used is the Gmelin reaction with nitric acid

proposed in 1826 by the German chemist Gmelin, who also invented the terms ester and ketone.

> *There is a peculiar discrepancy in the behavior of bilirubin. Around a mass of spilled blood one would expect that the two heme-derived pigments, ferritin and bilirubin, would appear in roughly similar amounts and at the same time. They do not. In tissue sections, bilirubin appears late, in small amounts, and sometimes not at all. Perhaps it is easily carried away by albumin, or perhaps it does form (we do see a lot of yellow in a bruise) but being fat-soluble it is dissolved out of the tissue during the embedding procedure. Bilirubin can indeed be extracted from tissues with chloroform (247).*

Toxicity *Bilirubin is very toxic.* Oddly enough, its precursor biliverdin is harmless. Birds and reptiles wisely stop the heme breakdown at that point and simply eliminate the green pigment in the bile, but mammals take the trouble of actively converting the innocuous biliverdin into a toxic compound by adding two hydrogen atoms.

> *This oddity is perhaps explained by a problem introduced by the placenta. The fetus must get rid of its bile pigment by transferring it to the mother; the placenta, however, is impermeable to biliverdin but not to bilirubin (239).*

Being fat-soluble, bilirubin can cross cell membranes and kill cells, perhaps by a toxic effect on mitochondria (244). Fortunately, to reach any cell the bilirubin must float through extracellular water. Because its solubility in water is very low, toxic effects are usually avoided. Furthermore, what little does dissolve in water is promptly taken up by that all-purpose carrier molecule, albumin (p. 81). Only about 1 percent of bilirubin remains free. Albumin deposits its load of bilirubin in the liver, which conjugates it with glucuronic acid and excretes it in the bile. This mechanism protects us from bilirubin poisoning in all but the most severe cases of jaundice.

The toxicity of free bilirubin is well demonstrated in a strain of rats called Gunn rats, in which liver conjugation of bilirubin is deficient; bilirubin accumulates in the interstitium of the renal papillae, which becomes necrotic (233, 234) (Figure 3.63).

In the fetus and the newborn, however, liver conjugation of bilirubin is low because the necessary enzyme system (cytochrome P-450) is not yet fully developed. Danger can arise if the baby develops severe jaundice. This can happen either *in utero* by Rh or ABO incompatibility with the mother's blood or after birth when the newborn normally eliminates its excess of red blood cells, which are no longer needed because oxygen transport from the lungs is much more efficient than across the placenta. Whatever the cause of the jaundice in the newborn, the small amount of unconjugated bilirubin can cause damage in the central nervous system wherever the blood–brain barrier is not yet fully developed. Bilirubin seeps out of the capillaries and into cells of the gray matter, especially in basal nuclei, in amounts large enough to stain them yellow. Hence the German name **Kernicterus,** jaundice of nuclei. The condition is rare in our day; it results in death or brain damage (232, 246). One risk factor for kernicterus are drugs such as certain antibiotics that compete for albumin as a carrier (Figure 3.15).

The preventive treatment used in years past was a marvel of applied cell biology. Infants at risk for bilirubin toxicity were given phenobarbital in order to stimulate the formation in the liver of smooth endoplasmic reticulum and thus of P-450, which helps conjugate the bilirubin (p. 136). Today jaundiced neonates are exposed to bright light; this converts bilirubin to photoisomers (photobilirubin), which can be excreted in the bile even without conjugation (239, 242). Unfortunately, prolonged exposure to bright light **(phototherapy)** injured the tender retina of many newborns before this unexpected danger was discovered and the eyes were covered (237).

HEMATIN

Hematin, a black pigment derived from hemoglobin, is formed only under pathologic conditions (Figure 3.64). It is made of intact porphyrin rings that have been shed by the globin molecule (Figure 3.60); their iron is oxidized to trivalent, firmly bound, and histochemically not reactive. It does not give the Prussian blue reaction typical of hemosiderin and ferritin.

Hematin in pathology occurs largely as a nuisance, but it is interesting on several accounts.

*   *Hematin is a nuisance pigment.* Hematin, alas, develops artefactually in tissues that are being fixed in nonbuffered, acid formalin. The red blood cells shed their hemes and become peppered with black granules of hematin, to the dismay of aesthetically minded pathologists and to the confusion of medical students (Figure 3.41). This common artefact should not be misleading be-

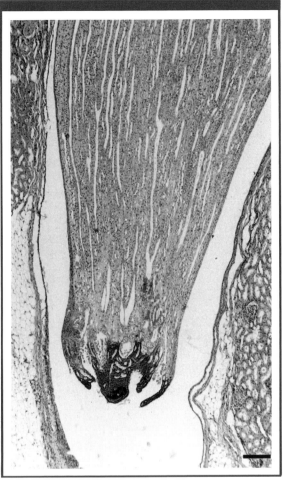

FIGURE 3.63 Longitudinal section of a renal papilla in a Gunn rat. These rats suffer from a congenital defect in the conjugation of bilirubin and become jaundiced; bilirubin is concentrated at the tip of the papilla. The papilla is necrotic and appears dark due to the heavy concentration of bilirubin. **Bar** = 100 μm. (Reproduced with permission from [233].)

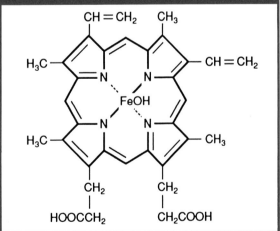

FIGURE 3.64 Hematin (also called ferriheme hydroxyl). The porphyrin ring is intact, and the oxidized iron is not available for histochemical reaction. (Reproduced with permission from [250].)

cause it would be unlikely for any black pigment to be riding piggyback on red blood cells; in malaria it would be *inside* the red blood cells, as we will see later. The lesson is that tissues should be fixed in buffered formalin at pH 6.9–7.5 (254).

- *Hematin develops in vivo in hematomas* (i.e., in blood spilled in the tissues). This is our own belief, based on microscopic experience; the literature is silent on the subject. The significance and fate of hematin in spilled blood are unknown.
- *Malarial pigment is a variety of hematin.* The malarial parasite *Plasmodium*, living inside a red blood cell, digests the hemoglobin and protects itself from the toxic heme products by polymerizing them into *hemozoin* (249, 251) (Figure 3.65). The antimalarial chloroquine works precisely by inhibiting this polymerization (255). When the parasitized red blood cells die, their black pigment ends up in the sinusoidal phagocytes (p. 299), hence the dusky color of the malarial liver and spleen. Once it is tucked away in the phagocytes, the pigment is harmless.

The only saving feature of hematin is that it can be used for the therapy of porphyrias, disorders of heme synthesis (252). Even there it is toxic.

TO SUM UP: The three main types of brown pigments (lipofuscin, melanin, blood-derived pigments) are biologically similar in that they are all part of normal life. However, *blood-derived pigments are unique in that they can be toxic*; iron itself is a dangerous atom, but hematin and heme-derived pigments are also toxic, and so is the iron-free bilirubin. Correspondingly, there are diseases caused by blood-related pigments (e.g. hemochromatosis, jaundice, porphyrias due to mistakes in heme biosynthesis) whereas there is no example of disease due to an effect of lipofuscin or melanin; indeed, melanin may be a detoxifying polymer.

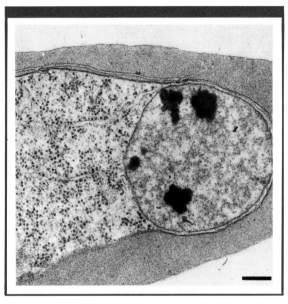

FIGURE 3.65 Malarial pigment (hemozoin, akin to hematin) in the food vacuole of the malarial parasite *Plasmodium gallinaceum* inside a red blood cell. **Bar** = 0.2 μm. (Reproduced with permission from [249].)

References

Vacuoles

1. Alberts B, Bray D, Lewis J, Raff M, Roberts K, Watson JD. Molecular biology of the cell, 2nd ed. New York: Garland Publishing, Inc., 1989.
2. Artigas J, Grosse G, Niedobitek F. Vacuolar myelopathy in AIDS. A morphological analysis. Pathol Res Pract 1990;86:228–237.
3. Biava CG, Dyrda I, Genest J, Bencosme SA. Kaliopenic nephropathy. A correlated light and electron microscopic study. Lab Invest 1963;12:443–453.
4. Buckley IK. Cellular injury in vitro: phase contrast studies on injured cytoplasm. J Cell Biol 1962;14:40–420.
5. Buckley IK. Phase contrast observations on the endoplasmic reticulum of living cells in culture. Protoplasma 1965;59:569–588.
6. Buckley IK. The lysosomes of cultured chick embryo cells. A correlated light and electron microscopic study. Lab Invest 1973;29:411–421.
7. Burg MB. Role of aldose reductase and sorbitol in maintaining the medullary intracellular milieu. Kidney Int 1988;33:35–641.
8. Burg MD, Kador PF. Sorbitol, osmoregulation, and the complications of diabetes. J Clin Invest 1988;81:635–640.
9. Buvat R. Origin and continuity of cell vacuoles. In: Reinert J, Ursprung H (eds). Origin and continuity of cell organelles. New York: Springer-Verlag, 1971, pp. 127–157.
10. Clegg JS, Seitz P, Seitz W, Hazlewood CF. Cellular responses to extreme water loss: the water-replacement hypothesis. Cryobiology 1982;19:306–316.
11. Clements RS Jr. The polyol pathway. A historical review. Drugs 1986;32(Suppl 2):3–5.
12. Cohn ZA, Benson B. The in vitro differentiation of mononuclear phagocytes. II. The influence of serum on granule formation, hydrolase production, and pinocytosis. J Exp Med 1965;121:835–848.
13. Cohn ZA, Ehrenreich BA. The uptake, storage and intracellular hydrolysis of carbohydrates by macrophages. J Exp Med 1969;129:30–225.
14. Dyck PJ. Resolvable problems in diabetic neuropathy. J NIH Res 1990;2:57–62.
15. Dyck PJ, Thomas PK, Asbury AK, Winegrade AI, Porte D Jr (eds). Diabetic neuropathy. Philadelphia: WB Saunders Company, 1987.
16. Glynn LE, Himsworth HP. The intralobular circulation in acute liver injury by carbon tetrachloride. Clin Sci 1948;6:235–245.
17. Greene DA, Lattimer SA. Altered myo-inositol metabolism in diabetic nerve. In: Dyck PJ, Thomas PK, Asbury AK, Winegrad AI, Porte D Jr (eds). Diabetic neuropathy. Philadelphia: WB Saunders Company, 1987, pp. 289–298.
18. Griffiths JB. Effect of hypertonic stress on mammalian cell lines and its relevance to freeze-thaw injury. Cryobiology 1978;15:517–529.

19. Joris I, Majno G. Cell-to-cell herniae in the arterial wall. Am J Pathol 1977;87:375–398.
20. Judzewitsch RG, Jaspan JB, Polonsky KS, Weinberg CR, Halter JB, Halar E, et al. Aldose reductase inhibition improves nerve conduction velocity in diabetic patients. N Engl J Med 1983;308:119–125.
21. Kirchain WR, Rendell MS. Aldose reductase inhibitors. Pharmacotherapy 1990;10:326–336.
22. Kohner EM, Porta M, Hyer SL. The pathogenesis of diabetic retinopathy and cataract. In: Pickup JC, Williams G (eds). Textbook of Diabetes, vol. 2. Oxford: Blackwell Scientific Publications, 1991, pp. 564–574.
23. Li MK, Kavanagh JP, Prendiville V, Buxton A, Moss DG, Blacklock NJ. Does sucrose damage kidneys? Br J Urol 1986;58:353–357.
23a. McManus ML, Churchwell KB, Strange K. Mechanisms of disease: regulation of cell volume in health and disease. N Engl J Med 1995;333:1260–1266.
24. Monserrat AJ, Chandler AE. Effects of repeated injections of sucrose on the kidney. Histologic, cytochemical and functional studies in an animal model. Virchows Arch [B] 1975;19:77–91.
25. Norris HT. Response of the small intestine to the application of a hypertonic solution. Am J Pathol 1973;73:747–764.
26. Riemenschneider T, Bohle A. Morphologic aspects of low-potassium and low-sodium nephropathy. Clin Nephrol 1983;19:271–279.
27. Rigdon RH, Cardwell ES. Renal lesions following the intravenous injection of a hypertonic solution of sucrose. A clinical and experimental study. Arch Intern Med 1942;69:670–690.
28. Robinson DG. Plant membranes. New York: John Wiley & Sons, 1985.
29. Rodgers GM, Taylor RN, Roberts JM. Preeclampsia is associated with a serum factor cytotoxic to human endothelial cells. Am J Obstet Gynecol 1988;159:908–914.
30. Shimamura T, Trojanowski S. Effects of repeated deprivation of drinking water on the structure of renal medulla of rats. Am J Pathol 1976;84:87–92.
31. Steinman RM, Brodie SE, Cohn ZA. Membrane flow during pinocytosis. A stereologic analysis. J Cell Biol 1976;68:665–687.
32. Stetz EM, Majno G, Joris I. Cellular pathology of the rat. Virchows Arch A Pathol Anat Histol 1979;383:135–148.
33. Trump BF, Janigan DT. The pathogenesis of cytologic vacuolization in sucrose nephrosis. An electron microscopic and histochemical study. Lab Invest 1962;11:395–411.
34. Zimmerman BR. Aldose reductase inhibitors. In: Dyck PJ, Thomas PK, Asbury AK, Winegrad AI, Porte D Jr (eds). Diabetic neuropathy. Philadelphia: WB Saunders Company, 1987, pp. 190–193.

Steatosis

35. Andersen T, Gluud C. Liver morphology in morbid obesity: a literature study. Int J Obesity 1984;8:97–106.
36. Bannister DW. Recent advances in avian biochemistry: The fatty liver and kidney syndrome. Int J Biochem 1979;10:193–199.
37. Bargmann W, Krisch B, Leonhardt H. Lipids in the proximal convoluted tubule of the cat kidney and the reabsorption of cholesterol. Cell Tissue Res 1977;177:523–538.
38. Bucher NLR, Malt RA. Regeneration of liver and kidney. Boston: Little, Brown and Company, 1971.
39. Cahill GF, Owen OE. Body fuels and starvation. Int Psychiatry Clin 1970;7:25–36.
40. Chien KR, Bellary A, Nicar M, Mukherjee A, Buja M. Induction of a reversible cardiac lipidosis by a dietary long-chain fatty acid (erucic acid). Am J Pathol 1983;112:68–77.
41. Combes B, Whalley PJ, Adams RH. Tetracycline and the liver. Prog Liver Dis 1972;4:589–596.
42. Dianzani MU. Reactions of the liver to injury: fatty liver. In: Farber E, Fisher MM (eds). Toxic injury of the liver, part A. New York: Marcel Dekker, Inc., 1979, pp. 281–331.
43. Eisele JW, Barker EA, Smuckler EA. Lipid content in the liver of fatty metamorphosis of pregnancy. Am J Pathol 1975;81:545–560.
44. Engel AG, Angelini C. Carnitine deficiency of human skeletal muscle with associated lipid storage myopathy: A new syndrome. Science 1973;179:899–901.
45. Fahimi HD, Kalmbach P, Stegmeier K, Stork H. Comparison between the effects of clofibrate and bezafibrate upon the ultrastructure of rat heart and liver. In: Greten H, Lang PD, Schettler G (eds). Lipoproteins and coronary heart disease. New York: Gerhard Witzstrock Publishing House, 1980, pp. 64–75.
46. Farber E, Fisher MM (eds). Toxic injury of the liver, pts. A and B. New York: Marcel Dekker, Inc., 1979.
47. Flatt JP. Body weight, fat storage, and alcohol metabolism. Nutr Rev 1992;50:267–270.
48. Gordon GB. Saturated free fatty acid toxicity. II. Lipid accumulation, ultrastructural alterations, and toxicity in mammalian cells in culture. Exp Mol Pathol 1977a;27:262–276.
49. Gordon GB. Lipid accumulation in the stationary phase of strain L cells in suspension culture. Lab Invest 1977b;36:114–121.
50. Gordon GB, Barcza MA, Bush ME. Lipid accumulation in hypoxic tissue culture cells. Am J Pathol 1977;88:663–678.
51. Hartroft WS. The sequence of pathologic events in the development of experimental fatty liver and cirrhosis. Ann NY Acad Sci 1954;57:633–645.
52. Hendrickse RG. Kwashiorkor: the hypothesis that incriminates aflatoxins. Pediatrics 1991;88:376–379.
53. Jelliffe DB, Jelliffe EFP. Causation of kwashiorkor: Toward a multifactorial consensus. Pediatrics 1992;90:110–113.
54. Kaplan MM. Acute fatty liver of pregnancy. N Engl J Med 1985;313:367–370.
55. Kern WH, Heger AH, Payne JH, DeWind LT. Fatty metamorphosis of the liver in morbid obesity. Arch Pathol 1973;96:342–346.
56. Korula J, Malatjalian DA, Badley BWD. Acute fatty liver of pregnancy. Can Med Assoc J 1982;127:575–578.
57. Kuo TH, Moore KH, Giacomelli F, Wiener J. Defective metabolism of heart mitochondria from genetically diabetic mice. Diabetes 1983;32:781–787.
58. Lake BD, Patrick AD. Wolman's disease: Deficiency of E600-resistant acid esterase activity with storage of lipids in lysosomes. J Pediatr 1970;76:262–266.
59. Lee M, Hatyashi H, Kato S, Sameshima Y, Hotta Y. Egg yolk-induced lipolysosome proliferation and fat infiltration of rat liver. Lab Invest 1982;47:194–197.
60. Leevy C. Fatty liver: A study of 270 patients with biopsy proven fatty liver and a review of the literature. Medicine 1962;41:249–276.
61. Lieber CS. Biochemical and molecular basis of alcohol-induced injury to liver and other tissues. N Engl J Med 1988;319:1639–1650.
62. Lombardi B. Considerations on the pathogenesis of fatty liver. Lab Invest 1966;15:1–20.

63. Luse SA, Wood WG. The brain in fatal carbon tetrachloride poisoning. Arch Neurol 1967;17:304–312.

64. MacMahon HE, Weiss S. Carbon tetrachloride poisoning with macroscopic fat in the pulmonary artery. Am J Pathol 1929;5:623–630.

65. Maunsbach AB, Wirsén C. Ultrastructural changes in kidney, myocardium and skeletal muscle of the dog during excessive mobilization of free fatty acids. J Ultrastruct Res 1966;16:35–54.

66. Nieth H, Schollmeyer P. Substrate-utilization of the human kidney. Nature 1966;209:1244–1245.

67. Novikoff AB, Novikoff PM. Microperoxisomes and peroxisomes in relation to lipid metabolism. Ann NY Acad Sci 1982;386:138–152.

68. Novikoff AB, Roheim PS, Quintana N. Changes in rat liver cells induced by orotic acid feeding. Lab Invest 1966;15:27–49.

69. Novikoff PM. Intracellular organelles and lipoprotein metabolism in normal and fatty livers. In: Arias I, Popper H, Schachter D, Shafritz DA (eds). The liver: biology and patholobiology. New York: Raven Press, 1982, pp. 143–167.

70. Novikoff PM, Roheim PS, Novikoff AB, Edelstein D. Production and prevention of fatty liver in rats fed clofibrate and orotic acid diets containing sucrose. Lab Invest 1974;30:732–750.

71. Ober WB, LeCompte PM. Acute fatty metamorphosis of the liver associated with pregnancy: a distinctive lesion. Am J Med 1955;19:743–758.

72. Palade GE. Functional changes in the structure of cell components. In: Hayashi T (ed). Subcellular particles. New York: The Ronald Press Company, 1959, pp. 64–83.

73. Perry MM, Siller WG. Incorporation of ³H-Oleic acid by the proximal convoluted tubule cells of the chick (gallus domesticus). Cell Tissue Res 1980;210:447–459.

74. Popper H, Thung SN, Gerber MA. Pathology of alcoholic liver diseases. Semin Liver Dis 1981;1:203–216.

75. Rappaport AM. Physioanatomical basis of toxic liver injury. In: Farber E, Fisher MM (eds). Toxic injury of the liver, part A. New York: Marcel Dekker, Inc., 1979, pp. 1–57.

76. Rarey KE, Davis JA, Deshmukh DR. Response of epithelial cells of the choroid plexus in the ferret model for Reye's syndrome. Lab Invest 1987;56:249–255.

77. Rhodin JAG. Histology. A text and atlas. New York: Oxford University Press, 1974.

78. Riely CA, Latham PS, Romero R, Duffy TP. Acute fatty liver of pregnancy. A reassessment based on observations in nine patients. Ann Intern Med 1987;106:703–706.

79. Rinaldi A, Tyndalo V. The complete book of mushrooms. New York: Crown Publishers, Inc., 1974.

80. Rothblat GH, Kritchevsky D. Lipid metabolism in tissue culture cells. Philadelphia: Wistar Institute Press, 1967.

81. Rubin E (ed). Alcohol and the cell. (Ann NY Acad Sci, vol. 492). New York: New York Academy of Sciences, 1987.

82. Rubin E, Lieber CS. Fatty liver, alcoholic hepatitis and cirrhosis produced by alcohol in primates. N Engl J Med 1974;290:128–135.

83. Schlunk FF, Lombardi B. Liver liposomes. I. Isolation and chemical characterization. Lab Invest 1967;17:30–38.

84. Slauson DO, Cooper BJ. Mechanisms of disease. Baltimore: Williams & Wilkins, 1982.

85. Suter PM, Schutz Y, Jequier E. The effect of ethanol on fat storage in healthy subjects. N Engl J Med 1992;326:983–987.

86. Trowell HC, Davies JNP, Dean RFA. Kwashiorkor. New York: Academic Press, 1982.

87. Waterlow JC (ed). Protein malnutrition. Cambridge: Cambridge University Press, 1955.

88. Waugh DA, Small DM. Identification and detection of in situ cellular and regional differences of lipid composition and class in lipid-rich tissue using hot stage polarizing light microscopy. Lab Invest 1984;51:702–714.

89. Wirthensohn G, Guder WG. Triacyglycerol metabolism in isolated rat kidney cortex tubules. Biochem J 1980;186:317–324.

90. Wittels B, Bressler R. Biochemical lesion of diphtheria toxin in the heart. J Clin Invest 1964a;43:630–637.

91. Wittels B, Bressler R. Lipid metabolism in the heart during fasting. Lab Invest 1964b;13:794–799.

Cholesterol

92. Aterman K, Remmele W, Smith M. Karl Touton and his "xanthelasmatic giant cell." A selective review of multinucleated giant cells. Am J Dermatopathol 1988; 10:257–269.

93. Brown MS, Goldstein JL. Lipoprotein metabolism in the macrophage: implications for cholesterol deposition in atherosclerosis. Annu Rev Biochem 1983;52:223–261.

94. Brown MS, Ho YK, Goldstein JL. The cholesteryl ester cycle in macrophage foam cells: continual hydrolysis and reesterification of cytoplasmic cholesteryl esters. J Biol Chem 1980;255:9344–9352.

95. Corwin RW, Irwin RS. The lipid-laden alveolar macrophage as a marker of aspiration in parenchymal lung disease. Am Rev Respir Dis 1985;132:576–581.

96. Druilhet RE, Traxler RW, Sobek JM. Bacterial utilization of cholesterol. Antonie van Leeuwenhoek 1968; 34:315–325.

97. Fowler S, Shio H, Haley NJ. Characterization of lipid-laden aortic cells from cholesterol-fed rabbits. IV. Investigation of macrophage-like properties of aortic cell populations. Lab Invest 1979;41:372–378.

98. French SW, Miyamoto K, Wong K, Jui L, Briere L. Role of the Ito cell in liver parenchymal fibrosis in rats fed alcohol and a high fat-low protein diet. Am J Pathol 1988;132:73–85.

99. Ginsburg GS, Atkinson D, Small DM. Physical properties of cholesteryl esters. Prog Lipid Res 1984;23:135–167.

100. Goldstein JL, Brown MS. Familiar hypercholesterolemia: pathogeneses of a receptor disease. Johns Hopkins Med J 1978;143:8–16.

101. Ho YK, Brown MS, Goldstein JL. Hydrolysis and excretion of cytoplasmic cholesteryl esters by macrophages: stimulation by high density lipoprotein and other agents. J Lipid Res 1980;21:391–398.

102. Imshenetskii AA, Nikitin LE, Nazarova TS, Efimochkina EF. Activities of cholesterol degrading microorganisms. Mikrobiologiya 1975;44:210–213.

103. Kaplan NB, Grant MM, Brody JS. The lipid interstitial cell of the pulmonary alveolus. Age and species differences. Am Rev Respir Dis 1985;132:1307–1312.

104. Kruth HS. Lipid deposition in human tendon xanthoma. Am J Pathol 1985;121:311–315.

105. Reichl D, Miller NE. The anatomy and physiology of reverse cholesterol transport. Clin Sci 1986;70:221–231.

106. Sedaghat A, Grundy SM. Cholesterol crystals and the formation of cholesterol gallstones. N Engl J Med 1980;302:1274–1277.

107. Sloop CH, Dory L, Roheim PS. Interstitial fluid lipoproteins. J Lipid Res 1987;28:225–237.

108. Steinberg D. Lipoproteins and atherosclerosis. A look back and a look ahead. Arteriosclerosis 1983;3:283–301.

109. Steinbrecher UP, Parthasarathy S, Leake DS, Witztum JL, Steinberg D. Modification of low density lipoprotein by endothelial cells involves lipid peroxidation and degradation of low density lipoprotein phospholipids. Proc Natl Acad Sci USA 1984;81:3883–3887.

110. Wright BA, Jeffrey PH. Lipoid pneumonia. Semin Respir Infect 1990;5:314–321.

111. Zimetbaum P, Eder H, Frishman W. Probucol: pharmacology and clinical application. J Clin Pharmacol 1990;30:3–9.

112. Zucker-Franklin D, Grusky G, Marcus A. Transformation of monocytes into "fat" cells. Lab Invest 1978;38:620–628.

Accumulation of Glycogen and Related Materials

113. Buja LM, Ferrans VJ, Levitsky S. Occurrence of intramitochondrial glycogen in canine myocardium after prolonged anoxic cardiac arrest. J Mol Cell Cardiol 1972;4:237–254.

114. Ghadially PN. Ultrastructural pathology of the cell and matrix, 2nd ed. London: Butterworths, 1982.

115. Karasaki S. Cytoplasmic and nuclear glycogen synthesis in Novikoff ascites hepatoma cells. J Ultrastruct Res 1971;35:181–196.

116. Kosek JC, Angell W. Fine structure of basophilic myocardial degeneration. Arch Pathol 1970;89:491–499.

117. Orci L, Stauffacher W. Glycogenosomes in renal tubular cells of diabetic animals. J Ultrastruct Res 1971;36:499–503.

118. Powell HC, Ward HW, Garrett RS, Orloff MJ, Lampert PW. Glycogen accumulation in the nerves and kidneys of chronically diabetic rats. A quantitative electron microscopic study. J Neuropathol Exp Neurol 1979;38:114–127.

119. Ramsey HJ. Ultrastructure of corpora amylacea. J Neuropathol Exp Neurol 1965;24:25–39.

120. Ritchie S, Waugh D. The pathology of Armanni-Ebstein diabetic nephropathy. Am J Pathol 1957;33:1035–1057.

121. Rosai J, Lascano EF. Basophilic (mucoid) degeneration of myocardium. A disorder of glycogen metabolism. Am J Pathol 1970;61:99–112.

122. Schwalbe H-P, Quadbeck G. Die Corpora amylacea immenschlichen Gihirn. Virchows Arch [A] 1975;366:305–311.

123. Stam FC, Roukema PA. Histochemical and biochemical aspects of corpora amylacea. Acta Neuropathol 1973;25:95–102.

Accumulation of Pigments—Lipofuscin

124. Balcavage WX, Alvager TKE. Reaction of malonaldehyde with mitochondrial membranes. Mech Ageing Dev 1982;19:159–170.

125. Barden H. The biology and chemistry of neuromelanin. In: Sohal RS (ed). Age pigments. Amsterdam: Elsevier/North-Holland Biomedical Press, 1981, pp. 155–180.

126. Bevelander G, Nakahara H. The effect of diverse amounts of tetracycline on fluorescence and coloration of teeth. J Pediatr 1966;68:114–120.

127. Brizzee KR, Ordy JM. Cellular features, regional accumulation, and prospects of modification of age pigments in mammals. In: Sohal RS (ed). Age pigments. Amsterdam: Elsevier/North-Holland Biomedical Press, 1981, pp. 101–154.

128. Cadle RD. Particle size. Theory and industrial applications. New York: Reinhold Publishing Corporation, 1965.

129. Casselman WGB. The in vitro preparation and histochemical properties of substances resembling ceroid. J Exp Med 1951;94:549–562.

130. de Duve C. A guided tour of the living cell, vol. 1. New York: Scientific American Books, Inc., 1984.

131. Elleder M. Chemical characterization of age pigments. In: Sohal RS (ed). Age pigments. Amsterdam: Elsevier/North-Holland Biomedical Press, 1981, pp. 203–241.

132. Gedigk P, Pioch W. Über die formale Genese lipogener Pigmente. Untersuchungen mit Estern hochungesättigter Fettsäuren. Virchows Arch [Pathol Anat] 1965;339:100–135.

133. Gedigk P, Totovic V. 4. Lysosomen und pigmente. Verh Dtsch Ges Pathol 1976;60:64–94.

134. Goldfischer S, Villaverde H, Forschirm R. The demonstration of acid hydrolase, thermostable reduced diphosphopyridine nucleotide tetrazolium reductase and peroxidase activities in human lipofuscin pigment granules. J Histochem Cytochem 1966;14:641–652.

135. Hartroft WS. The escape of lipid from fatty cysts in experimental dietary cirrhosis. In: Hoffbauer FW (ed). Conference on liver injury: Liver injury; transactions. New York: Josiah Macy, Jr Foundation, 1950, pp. 109–150.

136. Ivy GO, Schottler F, Wenzel J, Baudry M, Lynch G. Inhibitors of lysosomal enzymes: accumulation of lipofuscin-like dense bodies in the brain. Science 1984;226:985–987.

137. Kajihara H, Totovic V, Gedigk P. Zur Ultrastruktur und Morphogenese des Ceroidpigmentes. II. Spätveränderungen der Lysosomen in Kuppferschen Sternzellen der Rattenleber nach Phagocytose hochungesättigter Lipide. Virchows Arch B Cell Pathol 1975;19:239–254.

138. Koobs DH, Schultz RL, Jutzy RV. The origin of lipofuscin and possible consequences to the myocardium. Arch Pathol Lab Med 1978;102:66–68.

139. LeFevre ME, Green FHY, Joel DD, Laqueur W. Frequency of black pigment in livers and spleens of coal workers: correlation with pulmonary pathology and occupational information. Hum Pathol 1982;13:1121–1126.

140. Miquel J, Oro J, Bensch KG, Johnson JE Jr. Lipofuscin: fine-structural and biochemical studies. In: Pryor WA (ed). Free Radicals in Biology, vol. III. New York: Academic Press, 1977, pp. 133–182.

141. Munkres KD. Biochemical genetics of aging of Neurospora crassa and Podospora anserina: a review. In: Sohal RS (ed). Age pigments. Amsterdam: Elsevier/North-Holland Biomedical Press, 1981, pp. 83–100.

142. Raychaudhuri C, Desai ID. Ceroid pigment formation and irreversible sterility in vitamin E deficiency. Science 1971;173:1028–1029.

143. Silberberg I, Leider M. Studies on a red tattoo. Arch Dermatol 1970;101:299–304.

144. Sohal RS. Metabolic rate, aging, and lipofuscin accumulation. In: Sohal RS (ed). Age pigments. Amsterdam: Elsevier/North-Holland Biomedical Press, 1981, pp. 303–316.

145. Sohal RS, Donato H Jr. Effect of experimental prolongation of life span on lipofuscin content and lysosomal enzyme activity in the brain of the housefly, Musca domestica. J Gerontol 1979;34:489–496.

146. Spoerri PE, Glees P. The effects of dimethylaminoethyl p-chlorophenoxyacetate on spinal ganglia neurons and satellite cells in culture. Mitochondrial changes in the aging neurons. An electron microscopic study. Mech Ageing Dev 1974;3:131–155.

147. Spoerri PE, Glees P, El Ghazzawi E. Accumulation of lipofuscin in the myocardium of senile guinea pigs: dissolution and removal of lipofuscin following di-

methylaminoethyl p-chlorophenoxyacetate administration. An electron microscopic study. Mech Ageing Dev 1974;3:311–321.

148. Steer HW, Colin-Jones DG. Melanosis coli: studies of the toxic effects of irritant purgatives. J Pathol 1975;155:199–205.

149. Strehler BL, Mark DD, Mildvan AS, Gee MV. Rate and magnitude of age pigment accumulation in the human myocardium. J Gerontol 1959;14:430–439.

150. Thompson SW II. Lipogenic pigments related to treatment with exogenous lipid. In: Wolman M (ed). Pigments in pathology. New York: Academic Press, 1969, pp. 237–286.

151. Urbanski SJ, Arsenault AL, Green FHY, Haber G. Pigment resembling atmospheric dust in Peyer's patches. Mod Pathol 1989;2:222–226.

152. van Oud Alblas AB, van Furth R. Origin, kinetics, and characteristics of pulmonary macrophages in the normal steady state. J Exp Med 1979;149:1504–1518.

153. Virchow R. Cellular pathology as based upon physiological and pathological histology (translated from the second German edition by Britton Chance, 1859). New York: Dover Publications, 1971.

154. Walker NI, Bennett RE, Axelsen RA. Melanosis coli. A consequence of anthraquinone-induced apoptosis of colonic epithelial cells. Am J Pathol 1988;131:465–476.

155. Wolfe LS, Ng Ying Kin NMK, Baker RR. Batten disease and related disorders: new findings on the chemistry of the storage material. In: Callahan JW, Lowden JA (eds). Lysosomes and lysosomal storage diseases. New York: Raven Press, 1981, pp. 315–330.

156. Wolman M. Pigments in pathology. New York: Academic Press, 1969.

157. Wolman M. Factors affecting lipid pigment formation. In: Sohal RS (ed). Age pigments. Amsterdam: Elsevier/North-Holland Biomedical Press, 1981, pp. 265–281.

Melanin

158. Barden H. Further histochemical studies characterizing the lipofuscin component of human neuromelanin. J Neuropathol Exp Neurol 1978;37:437–451.

159. Barden H. The biology and chemistry of neuromelanin. In: Sohal RS (ed). Age pigments. Amsterdam: Elsevier/North-Holland Biomedical Press, 1981, pp. 155–180.

160. Bhawan J. Ultrastructure of melanocyte-keratinocyte interactions in pigmented basal cell carcinoma. Pigment Cell 1979;5:38–47.

161. Bolognia JL, Pawelek JM. Biology of hypopigmentation. J Am Acad Dermatol 1988;19:217–255.

162. Bystryn J-C, Pfeffer S. Vitiligo and antibodies to melanocytes. Prog Clin Biol Res 1988;256:195–206.

163. Chedekel MR. Photochemistry and photobiology of epidermal melanins. Photochem Photobiol 1982;35:881–885.

164. Edelstein LM. Melanin: a unique biopolymer. Pathobiol Annu 1971;1:309–324.

165. Fitzpatrick TB, Soter NA. Pathophysiology of skin. In: Smith LH, Thier SO (eds). Pathophysiology. The biological principles of disease. Philadelphia: WB Saunders, Co., 1981, p. 1745–1795.

166. Fitzpatrick TB, Szabó, Wick MM. Biochemistry and physiology of melanin pigmentation. In: Goldsmith LA (ed). Biochemistry and physiology of the skin. New York: Oxford University Press, 1983, pp. 687–712.

167. Gedigk P, Totovic V. Lysosomes and pigments. Verh Dtsch Ges Pathol 1976;60:64–94.

168. Goldsmith LA. Biochemistry and physiology of the skin. New York: Oxford University Press, 1983.

169. Le Douarin N. The neural crest. Cambridge: Cambridge University Press, 1982.

170. Le Douarin NM. Ontogeny of the peripheral nervous system from the neural crest and the placodes. A developmental model studied on the basis of the quail-chick chimaera system. Harvey Lect 1986;80:137–186.

171. Lerner EA, Sober AJ. Chemical and pharmacologic agents that cause hyperpigmentation or hypopigmentation of the skin. Dermatol Clin 1988;6:327–337.

172. Marsden CD. Brain melanin. In: Wolman M (ed). Pigments in pathology. New York: Academic Press, 1969, pp. 395–420.

173. Miquel J, Oro J, Bensch KG, Johnson JE Jr. Lipofuscin: fine-structural and biochemical studies. In: Pryor WA (ed). Free radicals in biology, Vol. III. New York: Academic Press, 1977, pp. 133–182.

174. Nahum LH. The purple-people syndrome. Conn Med 1965;29:332.

175. Riley PA. Mechanism of pigment-cell toxicity produced by hydroxyanisole. J Pathol 1970;101:163–169.

176. Scotto J, Fears TR, Fraumeni JF Jr. Solar radiation. In: Schottenfeld D, Fraumeni JF Jr (eds). Cancer epidemiology and prevention. Philadelphia: WB Saunders Company, 1982, pp. 254–276.

177. Sealy RC, Felix CC, Hyde JS, Swartz HM. Structure and reactivity of melanins: influence of free radicals and metal ions. In: Pryor WA (ed). Free radicals in biology, vol. IV. New York: Academic Press, 1980, pp. 209–259.

178. Smith LH Jr, Thier SO. Pathophysiology. The biological principles of disease. Philadelphia: WB Saunders Company, 1981.

179. Snyder SH. The molecular basis of communication between cells. Sci Am 1985;253:132–141.

180. Szent-Györgyi A. Bioelectronics. Science 1968;161:988–990.

181. Taylor RL. A suggested role for the polyphenol-phenoloxidase system in invertebrate immunity. J Invert Pathol 1969;14:427–428.

182. Wolman M (ed). Pigments in pathology. New York: Academic Press, 1969.

183. Wolman M. Factors affecting lipid pigment formation. In: Sohal RS (ed). Age pigments. Amsterdam: Elsevier/North-Holland Biomedical Press, 1981, pp. 265–281.

Ferritin and Hemosiderin

184. Abok K, Hirth T, Ericsson JLE, Brunk U. Effect of iron on the stability of macrophage lysosomes. Virchows Arch B Cell Pathol 1983;43:85–101.

185. Banyard SH, Stammers DK, Harrison PM. Electron density map of apoferritin at 2.8-A resolution. Nature 1978;271:282–284.

186. Bhawan J, Joris I, Cohen N, Majno G. Microcirculatory changes in posttraumatic pigmented villonodular synovitis. Arch Pathol Lab Med 1980;104:328–332.

187. Biemond P, van Eijk HG, Swaak AJG, Koster JF. Iron mobilization from ferritin by superoxide derived from stimulated polymorphonuclear leukocytes. Possible mechanism in inflammation diseases. J Clin Invest 1984;73:1576–1579.

188. Bradley WG Jr. MRI of hemorrhage and iron in the brain. In: Stark DD, Bradley WG Jr (eds). Magnetic resonance imaging. St. Louis: The CV Mosby Co., 1988, pp. 359–374.

189. Braun V. Iron supply as a virulence factor. In: Jackson GG, Thomas H (eds). The pathogenesis of bacterial infections. Berlin, Springer-Verlag, 1985, pp. 168–176.

190. Bullen JJ, Griffiths E (eds). Iron and infection. Chichester: John Wiley & Sons, 1987.

191. Crichton RR. Ferritin: structure, synthesis and function. N Engl J Med 1971;284:1413–1422.

192. Crosby WH. Hemochromatosis: current concepts and management. Hosp Pract 1987;22:173–192.

193. Deiss A. Iron metabolism in reticuloendothelial cells. Semin Hematol 1983;20:81–90.

194. Doolittle RL, Richter GW. Isoferritins in rat Kupffer cells, hepatocytes, and extrahepatic macrophages. Biosynthesis in cell suspensions and cultures in response to iron. Lab Invest 1981;45:567–574.

195. Drysdale JW. Ferritin phenotypes: structure and metabolism. Ciba Found Symp 1977;51:41–67.

196. Eaton JW, Brandt P, Mahoney JR, Lee JT Jr. Haptoglobin: a natural bacteriostat. Science 1982;215:691–693.

197. Emery T. Iron metabolism in humans and plants. Am Sci 1982;70:626–632.

198. Fairbanks VF, Klee GG. Ferritin. Prog Clin Pathol 1981;8:175–203.

199. Finch CA, Huebers H. Perspectives in iron metabolism. N Engl J Med 1982;306:1520–1528.

200. Ford GC, Harrison PM, Rice DW, et al. Ferritin: design and formation of an iron-storage molecule. Philos Trans R Soc Lond [Biol] 1984;304:551–565.

201. Ganote CE, Nahara G. Acute ferrous sulfate hepatotoxicity in rats. An electron microscopic and biochemical study. Lab Invest 1973;28:426–436.

202. Ghadially FN. Haemorrhage and hemosiderin. J Submicrosc Cytol 1979;11:271–291.

203. Gorinsky B. Transferrin: structure and function. In: Weatherall DJ, Fiorelli G, Gorini S (eds). Advances in red cell biology. New York: Raven Press, 1982, pp. 7–17.

204. Griffiths E. The iron-uptake systems of pathogenic bacteria. In: Bullen JJ, Griffiths E (eds). Iron and infection. Chichester: John Wiley & Sons, 1987, pp. 69–137.

205. Harding C, Heuser J, Stahl P. Receptor-mediated endocytosis of transferrin and recycling of the transferrin receptor in rat reticulocytes. J Cell Biol 1983;97:329–339.

206. Harrison PM, Banyard SH, Hoare RJ, Russell SM, Treffry A. The structure and function of ferritin. Ciba Found Symp 1977;51:19–40.

207. Hennigar GR, Greene WB, Walker EM, deSaussure C. Hemochromatosis caused by excessive vitamin iron intake. Am J Pathol 1979;96:611–624.

208. Hoy TG, Jacobs A. Ferritin polymers and the formation of haemosiderin. Br J Haematol 1981;49:593–602.

209. Huebers HA, Huebers E, Csiba E, Rummel W, Finch CA. The significance of transferrin for intestinal iron absorption. Blood 1983;61:283–290.

210. Jandl JH. Blood: Textbook of hematology. Boston: Little, Brown and Company, 1987.

211. Johnson RB. Advantageous hemochromatosis. N Engl J Med 1988;319:1155–1156.

212. Kent S, Weinberg E. Hypoferremia: adaptation to disease? N Engl J Med 1989;320:672.

213. Kimber RJ, Rudzki Z, Blunden RW. Clinching the diagnosis: 1. Iron deficiency and iron overload: serum ferritin and serum iron in clinical medicine. Pathology 1983;15:497–503.

214. Kluger MJ, Bullen JJ. Clinical and physiological aspects. In: Bullen JJ, Griffiths E (eds). Iron and infection. Chichester: John Wiley & Sons, 1987, pp. 243–282.

215. Lalonde J-MA, Ghadially FN. Ultrastructure of experimentally produced subcutaneous haematomas in the rabbit. Virchows Arch B Cell Pathol 1977;25:221–232.

216. Lalonde J-MA, Ghadially FN, Massey KL. Ultrastructure of intramuscular haematomas and electron-probe X-ray analysis of extracellular and intracellular iron deposits. J Pathol 1978;125:17–23.

217. Massover WH. The ultrastructure of ferritin macromolecules. III. Mineralized iron in ferritin is attached to the protein shell. J Mol Biol 1978;123:721–726.

218. Mofenson HC, Caraccio TR, Sharieff N. Iron sepsis: Versinia enterocolitica septicemia possibly caused by an overdose of iron. N Engl J Med 1987;316:1092–1093.

219. Muir R, Niven JSF. The local formation of blood pigments. J Pathol Bacteriol 1935;41:183–197.

220. Munro HN, Linder MC. Ferritin: structure, biosynthesis, and role in iron metabolism. Physiol Rev 1978;58:317–396.

221. Neumann E. Beiträge zur Kenntniss der pathologischen Pigmente. Virchows Arch Pathol Anat. Physiol Klin Med 1888;111:25–47.

222. O'Connell MJ, Ward RJ, Baum H, Peters TJ. Iron overload, lysosomes and free radicals. In: Reid E, Cook GMW, Luzio JP (eds). Cells, membranes, and disease, including renal. New York: Plenum Press, 1987, pp. 109–112.

223. Powell LW, Bassett ML, Halliday JW. Hemochromatosis: 1980 update. Gastroenterology 1980;78:374–381.

224. Richter GW. The cellular transformation of injected colloidal iron complexes into ferritin and hemosiderin in experimental animals. J Exp Med 1959;109:197–216.

225. Robotham JL, Lietman PS. Acute iron poisoning. A review. Am J Dis Child 1980;134:875–879.

226. Rubenstein E. Diseases caused by impaired communication among cells. Sci Am 1980;242:102–121.

227. Schafer AI, Cheron RG, Dluhy R, Cooper B, Gleason RE, Soeldner JS, Bunn HF. Clinical consequences of acquired transfusional iron overload in adults. N Engl J Med 1981;304:319–324.

227a. Sherman JM, Winnie G, Thomassen MJ, Abdul-Karim FW, Boat TF. Time course of hemosiderin production and clearance by human pulmonary macrophages. Chest 1984;86:409–411.

228. Stevens RG, Jones DY, Micozzi MS, Taylor PR. Body iron stores and the risk of cancer. N Engl J Med 1988;319:1047–1052.

229. Weinberg ED. The development of awareness of iron-withholding defense. Perspect Biol Med 1993;36:215–221.

230. Willingham MC, Hanover JA, Dickson RB, Pastan I. Morphologic characterization of the pathway of transferrin endocytosis and recycling in human KB cells. Proc Natl Acad Sci USA 1984;81:175–179.

231. Wixom RL, Prutkin L, Munro HN. Hemosiderin: nature, formation, and significance. Int Rev Exp Pathol 1980;22:193–225.

Bilirubin

232. Avery ME, Taeusch HW Jr (eds). Schaffer's diseases of the newborn, 5th ed. Philadelphia: WB Saunders Company, 1984.

233. Axelsen RA. Spontaneous renal papillary necrosis in the Gunn rat. Pathology 1973;5:43–50.

234. Axelsen RA, Burry AF. Bilirubin-associated renal papillary necrosis in the homozygous Gunn rat: light- and electron-microscopic observations. J Pathol 1976;120:165–175.

235. Berk PD, Berlin NI. Chemistry and physiology of bile pigments, Fogarty international center proceedings, No.

35. DHEW Publication No (NIH) 77-1100, U.S. Department of Health, Education, and Welfare. Public Health Service, National Institutes of Health, 1977.

236. Brown SB, Troxler RF. Heme degradation and bilirubin formation. In: Heirwegh KPM, Brown SB (eds). Bilirubin, vol. II. Boca Raton: CRC Press, 1982, pp. 1–38.

237. Glass P, Avery GB, Subramanian KNS, Keys MP, Sostek AM, Friendly DS. Effect of bright light in the hospital nursery on the incidence of retinopathy of prematurity. N Engl J Med 1985;313:401–404.

238. Gollan JL, Knapp AB. Bilirubin metabolism and congenital jaundice. Hosp Pract 1985;20:83–106.

239. Gollan JL, Schmid R. Bilirubin update: formation, transport, and metabolism. Prog Liver Dis 1982;8:261–283.

240. Heirwegh KPM, Brown SB (eds). Bilirubin, 2 vols. Boca Raton: CRC Press, Inc., 1982.

241. Lemberg R, Legge JW. Hematin compounds and bile pigments. New York: Interscience Publishers, 1949.

242. Lightner DA. Structure, photochemistry, and organic chemistry of bilirubin. In: Heirwegh KPM, Brown SB (eds). Bilirubin, volume I. Chemistry. Boca Raton: CRC Press, 1982, pp. 1–58.

243. Majno G. The healing hand. Man and wound in the ancient world. Cambridge: Harvard University Press, 1975.

244. Mustafa MG, King TE. Binding of bilirubin with lipid. A possible mechanism of its toxic reactions in mitochondria. J Biol Chem 1970;245:1084–1089.

245. O'Carra P, Colleran E. Nonenzymatic and quasi-enzymatic models for catabolic heme cleavage. In: Berk PD, Berlin NI (eds). International symposium on chemistry and physiology of bile pigments, Fogarty international center proceedings, No. 35. DHEW Publication No. (NIH) 77-1100. U.S. Department of Health, Education, and welfare. Bethesda: National Institutes of Health, 1977, p. 26.

246. Oski FA. Kernicterus. In: Avery ME, Taeusch HW Jr (eds). Schaffer's diseases of the newborn, 5th ed. Philadelphia: WB Saunders Company, 1984, pp. 633–635.

247. Rich AR, Bumstead JH. On the identity of haematoidin and bilirubin. Bull Johns Hopkins Hosp 1925;36:225–232.

248. Virchow R. Cellular pathology (translated from the 2nd German edition by B. Chance), 1859, Reproduced by Dover Publications, New York: 1971.

Hematin

249. Aikawa M, Huff CG, Sprinz H. Comparative feeding mechanisms of avian and primate malarial parasites. Milit Med 1966;131(suppl):969–983.

250. Budavari S, O'Neil MJ, Smith A, Heckelman PE (eds). The Merck index: An encyclopedia of chemicals, drugs, and biologicals, 11th ed. Rahway, NJ: Merck & Co., Inc., 1989, p. 732.

251. Fulton JD, Rimington C. The pigment of the malaria parasite Plasmodium berghei. J Gen Microbiol 1953;8:157–159.

252. Glueck R, Green D, Cohen I, Ts'ao C-h. Hematin: unique effects on hemostasis. Blood 1983;61:243–249.

253. Lemberg R, Legge JW. Hematin compounds and bile pigments. New York: Interscience Publishers, Inc., 1949.

254. Pizzolato P. Formalin pigment (acid hematin) and related pigments. Am J Med Technol 1976;42:446–439.

255. Wellems TE. How chloroquine works. Nature 1992;355:108–109.

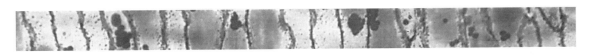

Symptoms of Cellular Disease: Pathology of the Organelles

CHAPTER 4

Pathology of the Plasma
Membrane

Pathology of the
Mitochondria

Pathology of the
Endoplasmic Reticulum
and Golgi Apparatus

Pathology of the
Lysosomes and
Peroxisomes

Pathology of the
Cytoskeleton

Pathology of the Nucleus

There are many ways to diagnose cellular disease. In Chapter 1 we used, as a guide to diagnosis, the presence of abnormal cellular contents. We will now see what we can learn by studying individual cellular organelles. Transposed to the clinical world, this approach would be the equivalent of studying changes of the liver, kidneys, skin, and so on. We will begin with the cell membrane, although its changes are very difficult or impossible to see.

Pathology of the Plasma Membrane

The skin of the cell—our elementary patient—is such a complex organ that we should briefly depict it before we come to grips with its woes.

In an evolutionary sense, the cell membrane is the oldest organelle: by enclosing a space it created a premise for life. Although it has a superficial analogy with the skin, it performs many more functions than the skin, being a physical boundary as well as an organ of contact, recognition, adhesion, communication, exchange, respiration, and even digestion. It should be visualized as a shifting, squirming carpet, made of an outer fluffy layer that coats a thinner sheet of soap-bubble texture, the bimolecular phospholipid leaflet. This sheet, actually a fluid (51), hangs together even though its molecules are not linked by covalent bonds. There are about 3 million molecules per square micrometer (μm) (1), constantly dancing about and rotating, stabilized by cholesterol molecules spaced between them. The cholesterol molecules themselves are so free that they can pop in and out of the sheet, changing places with cholesterol in the surroundings. Protein molecules float in this lipid layer; their deep end is sometimes anchored by ropelike elements of the cytoskeleton, conferring some stability to that part of the membrane. The fluffy overlay, the **glycocalyx** ("sweet cover"), is made of protein and carbohydrate molecules; it is actually more acid than sweet because enough H^+ ions can surround the cell to create an environment of pH 5 or lower (50). Chemically the glycocalyx may look relatively simple, but it is in fact extremely sophisticated. *The glycocalyx carries a code that is perhaps as important as the genetic code,* being in charge of the myriad recognition functions on which cell life depends (45).

The possibilities of diseases in such a system are almost infinite (2, 7, 8, 55, 60, 64, 65) (Figure 4.1). Some membrane defects are visible by high-power electron microscopy, especially when they consist of holes or protrusions; in fact, the larger protrusions (blebs) are easily seen even by light microscopy. However, most membrane changes are so subtle that only biochemical or immuno-chemical methods can detect them.

ACQUIRED DISORDERS OF THE CELL MEMBRANE

Most defects of the cell membrane are acquired by accident, through trauma, enzymes, toxins, and the like. Congenital diseases of the cell membrane are rare.

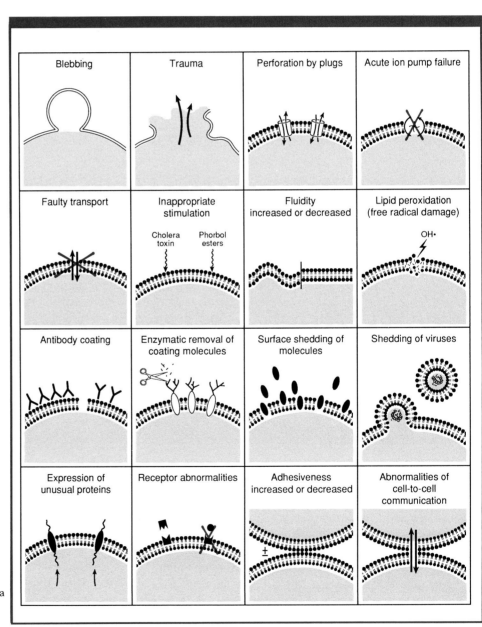

FIGURE 4.1
Disturbances of the cell membrane: a diagram of the 16 most common types.

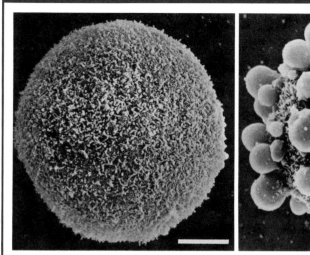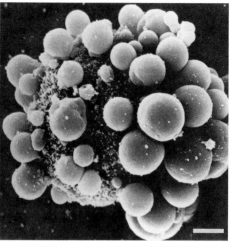

FIGURE 4.2
Left: Normal rat liver cell incubated in buffer. *Right:* Similar cell that is blebbing after 30 minutes incubation with two toxic agents (dicoumarol and menadione). The formation of blebs appears to reflect the inability of the cell to maintain normal links between cytoskeleton and surface membrane. Scanning electron microscopy. **Bars** = 3 μm. (Reproduced with permission from [25].)

BLEBBING

Blebbing is the most common symptom of acute cellular disease. Almost any type of insult will cause cells to develop protrusions, called **blebs,** that are shaped like blisters or balloons attached to the cell by a narrow neck (Figure 4.2). Blebs are very much like blisters; they contain fluid with few cytoplasmic organelles or none at all (61). Some blebs pinch off and float away, as has been observed *in vivo* (14); small ones can retract; some may ultimately explode. Blebbing occurs so quickly after cell damage, in seconds or minutes, that it has become (along with mitochondrial swelling) a very sensitive indicator of cellular suffering. However, if you see blebs on a published electron micrograph, beware; like swollen mitochondria, blebs can develop also as a result of poor fixation (26). It can be difficult to decide whether they are significant or artefactual. Specimens for ordinary histology are fixed with less rigorous standards than those required for electron microscopy, which means that paraffin sections are riddled with blebs. Fortunately, they are so tenuous that they are practically invisible; only the worried electron microscopist suspects them everywhere.

By light microscopy, a bleb can be clearly seen only when it is surrounded by a denser medium such as plasma, rather like an air bubble can be seen in water. The round holes so common in the plasma of blood vessels are nothing but blebs arising from endothelial cells or leukocytes (Figure 4.3). This simple fact has given rise to one of the most persistent errors of traditional histology: the colloid content of the thyroid follicles is described as having either a smooth or scalloped contour

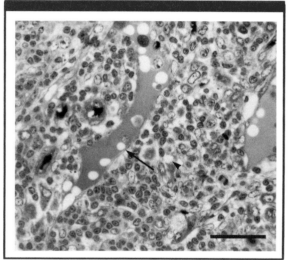

FIGURE 4.3
Blebs as a fixation artefact in a lymph node. Blebs arising from endothelial cells (**arrow**) are seen as punched-out holes in the plasma. Blebs arising in the interstitium (**arrowhead**) are not easily detected by light microscopy. **Bar** = 50 μm.

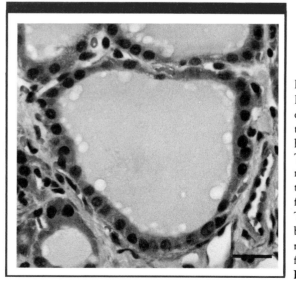

FIGURE 4.4
Blebbing of epithelial cells in the follicles of a human thyroid. The blebs are made visible by the colloid that fills the follicle. This example of blebbing is now recognized as a fixation artefact. **Bar** = 25 μm.

(Figure 4.4). The scalloping is supposed to indicate "digestion" by the thyroid cells (as if they had taken a bite out of the colloid), and it is still considered by many histologists as an indication of high thyroid activity. Then, in the late 1950s, electron microscopy appeared on the scene with its improved methods of fixation, and the scalloping disappeared—at least from electron microscopic material. The scalloping is caused by blebs protruding into the colloid and is an artefact of poorly fixed follicular epithelium!

Blebbing is not necessarily a threatening event for the cell. Controlled experiments (48) show that some blebs are reversible (p. 679). On the other hand, the bursting of a bleb in anoxic liver cells can be the final blow for a cell by causing a gash in the plasma membrane (23, 29).

Mechanism of Blebbing Electron micrographs suggest that, *in blebbing, the cell membrane is lifted away from the cytoplasm* as if it had become disconnected from the anchoring cytoskeleton. This interpretation is supported by much experimental evidence: phalloidin and cytochalasin B, which cause intense blebbing, are cytoskeletal poisons (19, 37).

> According to one view, the cytoskeletal disturbance that causes blebbing is related to an increase in cytosolic calcium (25, 39), which activates nonlysosomal proteolysis (37). It was therefore suggested that the target of this proteolytic activity is the cytoskeleton. This is probably true, but the increase of cytosolic calcium is not always found (29).

> A peculiar variant of blebbing occurs in the small intestine. If the mucosa is injured, for instance, by ischemia (62, 63) or ethanol (5), blebs develop from the basal surfaces of the epithelial cells rather than from their free surface. As a result, the cells become detached from the basement membrane: this explains the tendency of the intestinal epithelium to lift off leaving a wide subepithelial space. Why these cells bleb from their base is not clear; perhaps the free surface covered with microvilli is somehow not favorable to blebbing.
>
> In heart fibers, which are wrapped in sarcolemma, blebs caused by ischemia remain "squeezed" beneath the sarcolemma (44).

> Red blood cells rarely form blebs because their membranes are firmly anchored to their cytoskeletons, presumably a safety measure in view of their turbulent life. However, they do shed submicroscopic vesicles in vitro if they are depleted of ATP (52).

Ingenious cell biologists have turned blebbing into an experimentally useful tool. Chemically induced blebbing, followed by shedding of the blebs, has been used as a source of pure cell membranes (36). Ironically, the best method for obtaining such reproducible blebbing is to treat cells with formaldehyde, the standard fixative. It is no wonder that histologic sections are full of blebs.

FAILURE OF THE MEMBRANE PUMPS (ACUTE CELLULAR SWELLING)

Physiology teaches that most cells spend over 30 percent of their energy to keep their sodium pumps working (1, p. 137). If energy supplies suddenly fail (e.g., because the blood supply is cut off), the pumps will fail. Nobody can *see* a defective ion pump, but the result of its failure is dramatic and predictable—acute cellular swelling—a perfect example of Virchow's statement that pathology is physiology with obstacles. From these premises it should be obvious that *cellular swelling is common and can develop very rapidly and (up to a point) reversibly* (28). The internal organelles may or may not participate.

> Red blood cells do not visibly swell in ischemic tissues, although they do have sodium pumps. This is fortunate because red blood cells have to squeeze through capillaries; if they ever became bloated, they would block the passage altogether. (Perhaps they swell just a little. The hematocrit of venous blood is 1–2 percent higher than in arterial blood, which would amount to a 2.5–5 percent swelling.) It is likely that factors besides the sodium pump intervene in the pathogenesis of acute cellular swelling, such as the rigidity of internal structures.

Only extreme examples of swelling are easy to recognize in histologic sections: the affected cells appear larger and more transparent, as if an excess of water had diluted the cytoplasm; the obsolete term "hydropic degeneration" portrayed this aspect. Milder degrees of swelling are difficult to detect because a doubling of the volume implies only a 26 percent increase in diameter, which can easily escape notice (34).

What are the dangers of cellular swelling? First, *the distended membrane may become leaky.* This can be demonstrated by placing red blood cells in a hypotonic solution: they swell, eventually allowing the hemoglobin to escape. With the same experiment one can show that the holes in the membrane are reversible (49). Second, cellular swelling can be dangerous indirectly because it occupies space. Swollen cells can compress capillaries and inhibit blood flow, with catastrophic results, especially in the brain (p. 685); a similar complication can arise in the liver if the hepatocytes are bloated with water (Figure 3.5) or with fat (Figure 3.23).

Note: Cells can also swell, despite normal membrane function, by an increase in internal osmotic pressure (the sorbitol mechanism, p. 75). This type of swelling develops much more slowly.

INCREASED PERMEABILITY OF THE PLASMA MEMBRANE

Cells can tolerate small wounds (p. 180), but extensive leaks in the plasma membrane are lethal. Accordingly, killing cells by poking holes in their membranes is an ancient offensive strategy on this planet; it was discovered not only by snakes, fish, amphibians, insects, and plants but also by mammals. Our blood contains a special set of killer lymphocytes designed for destroying unwanted cells (such as virus-infected cells) plus an extraordinary set of proteins called complement, capable of assembling into a cell-killing machine; both these agents kill their target cells by perforating their plasma membranes. Fortunately for those cells that are wounded accidentally or perforated, *all cell membranes are fluid, and if perforated they self-seal very fast;* therefore, to be lethal, the holes have to be kept open, be numerous, or be very large. The offensive devices of "cellular warfare" meet all these criteria.

Phospholipases (Figure 4.5) are crude offensive

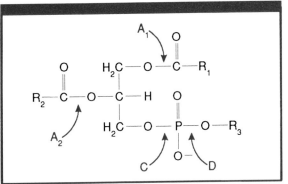

FIGURE 4.5 Stucture of a phospholipid molecule. **Arrows:** Bonds attacked by phospholipases A_1, A_2, C, or D. (Reproduced with permission from [54].)

devices found in almost all snake poisons (12, 13). These enzymes are dangerous in two ways: they can digest the cell membranes directly, and they can turn the phospholipid molecule into a detergent (i.e., into a membrane-destroying device) by snipping off one of its fatty acids. This works as follows. A phospholipid molecule such as lecithin is two-legged and roughly cylindrical; amputation of one leg makes it wedge-shaped. This wedge is **lysolecithin,** so called because it lyses red blood cells. It is easy to understand that lysolecithin molecules, due to their shape, will tend to assemble into rounded micelles (Figure 4.6); by this mechanism cell membranes are perforated or destroyed.

Small amounts of lysolecithin are normal metabolic products. Experimentally, lysolecithin fuses the membranes of adjacent cells (31).

Phospholipases are associated with plasma membranes and with lysosomes, probably in all cells. Large amounts are secreted in the pancreatic juice; this is why the spilling of this juice in acute pancreatitis is life-threatening.

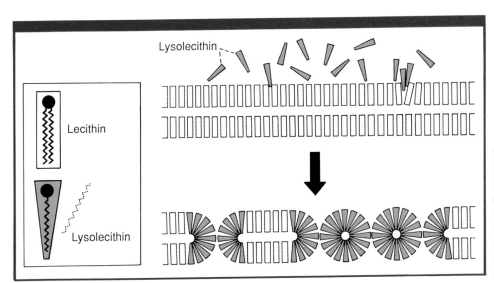

FIGURE 4.6 Disruption of cell membranes by lysolecithin. Lecithin is a normal component of cell membranes; when a phospholipase splits off one of its fatty-acid legs, it becomes lysolecithin, a wedge-shaped molecule that can break up lipid bilayers into micelles. (Modified from [31].)

FIGURE 4.7
Scanning electron micrographs of acanthocytes, spiny red blood cells deformed by an excess of cholesterol in their membranes. (Reproduced with permission from [6].)

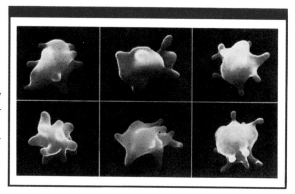

How can one find out if a cell membrane is leaky? The standard procedure is to expose the cell to a molecular marker that is normally excluded. In experimental animals, a standard method is to inject horseradish peroxidase *in vivo* and then find out if it has penetrated the cytoplasm (10). Another technique is to fix the tissue in the presence of colloidal lanthanum, which is visible by electron microscopy and which penetrates cells only if their membrane is leaky (24). In injured tissues, fibrinogen (a large globulin) can act as a natural tracer: if fibrin filaments appear inside a cell, this indicates that fibrinogen molecules have been allowed to penetrate (41).

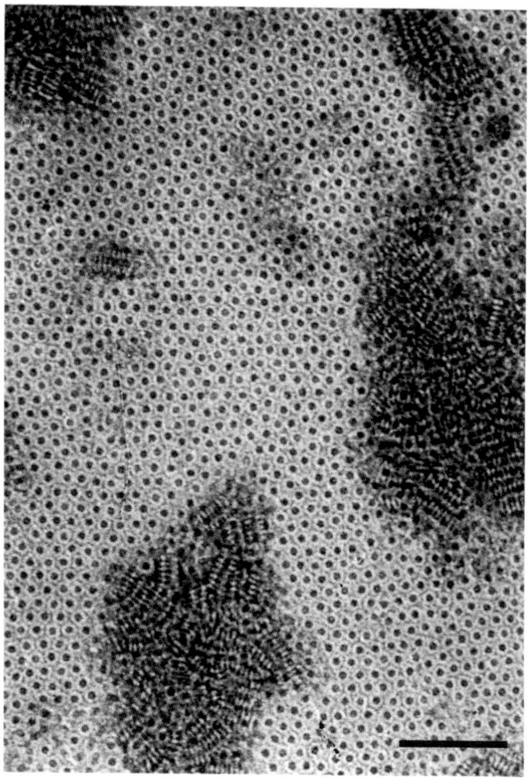

TOXIC INJURY OF THE CELL MEMBRANE

Under the microscope we cannot hope to see chemical defects in the cell membrane, but we can see their effects. Especially interesting are the chemical defects that lead to *changes in membrane fluidity.*

Excess Cholesterol Remember that cholesterol molecules are inserted into the cell membrane as stabilizers and that they can move in and out, exchanging with cholesterol in the surrounding fluid. In red blood cells their number is equal to that of the phospholipid molecules. If the plasma carries too much cholesterol, this excess equilibrates with the membranes of red blood cells, which become overloaded (25–65 percent) and stiffened (38). This causes the red blood cells to develop odd prickly shapes (Figure 4.7). These abnormal cells (acanthocytes, from *ácantha,* thorn) are removed by the spleen. This sequence can be produced experimentally, but it happens naturally in alcoholics with liver cirrhosis, who have an exces of cholesterol in their low-density lipoproteins (56).

> ***Saponins*** *are plant and echinoderm poisons that disrupt the cell membrane by combining with cholesterol; the principle is very effective (Figure 4.8) (4). Basically, these poisons act as detergents (saponin, soaplike). Primal people have known for millennia that saponins can be used not only as soap, but more imaginatively for catching fish; dissolved in water they destroy the function of the gills, and the fish turn belly up (58).*

FIGURE 4.8
Perforations produced by saponin in an artificial lipid membrane, a mixture of lecithin and cholesterol. Saponin binds with cholesterol and produces a disturbance in the cell membrane comparable to that produced by lysolecithin (Figure 4.6). **Bar** = 0.1 μm. (Courtesy of Dr. A.D. Bangham, Cambridge, England.)

Alcohol Alcohol is a mild anesthetic, and it acts on membranes much like other anesthetics. In acute alcoholic intoxication it has a "disordering" or "fluidifying" effect, which could explain the increased sensitivity to drugs of acutely intoxicated individuals (57). In chronic alcoholic intoxication the effect is opposite; an adaptive mechanism makes the membranes more rigid and less sensitive to drugs. This adaptation could well be linked with addiction (21).

Toxins Some toxins select protein targets on the cell membrane. One of the most potent of these is **tetrodotoxin,** the poison of the puffer fish (Figure 4.9). It blocks the sodium channels. When you order *fugu* in a Japanese restaurant, you depend on

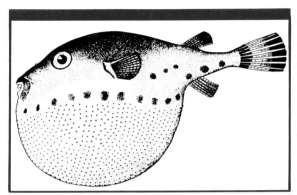

FIGURE 4.9
An enemy of sodium channels. Appropriately prepared, the puffer fish (*Spheroides spengleri*) is a delicacy of Japanese restaurants. The toxin produced by this fish (tetrodotoxin) is also present in the totally unrelated California newt. (Reproduced with permission from [20].)

the chef's ability to dissect out the toxic liver and ovaries (40). People of the Colombian forest poison their blowdarts with the secretion of a frog that is laced with **batrachotoxin,** which has the opposite effect: it kills cells by keeping sodium channels open (40). Countless other toxins affect the membranes of nerve endings.

DISORDERS OF MEMBRANE RECEPTORS

Woven into the cell membrane are myriads of receptors that can malfunction in many ways. The ills of these membrane receptors have also been called diseases of cell communication (42). A few examples follow.

Unmasking of a Hidden Receptor A receptor can be present but hidden by proteins. For example, endothelial cells exposed to leukocytic enzymes can reveal previously masked receptors for the Fc segment (the tail end) of immunoglobulin G (43). The unmasked receptors give endothelial cells the capacity to bind antigen–antibody complexes, which bristle with Fc segments. But complexes are dangerous. For the endothelial cell the ability to bind complexes is like catching a tiger by the tail (p. 530).

Overstimulation of a Receptor by a Toxin The classic example is overstimulation by cholera toxin. People infected with *Vibrio cholerae* have only one problem, phenomenal loss of fluid by the intestine, the so-called rice water diarrhea. This loss can amount to 20–30 liters in one day. And yet, intestinal biopsies show that the intestinal mucosa

is intact; there is no lesion or inflammatory reaction whatsoever. What happens is that the molecule of cholera toxin becomes attached to a specific glycolipid in the cell membrane, which acts as a receptor; the result—through a complex transduction mechanism mediated by a G protein (1)—is an irreversible stimulation of adenylate cyclase, leading to a steady secretion of sodium and water. The whole drama of cholera, therefore, boils down to excessive cell stimulation. The patient can be treated with the simple device of fluid intake, until the vibrio washes away. Other toxins, such as a coli toxin, act in a similar fashion (17).

Stimulation of a Receptor by an Antireceptor Antibody Antibodies can be developed against any protein, including receptors. When an antireceptor antibody binds to the receptor, in some cases the receptor "believes" that it is being stimulated by its legitimate ligand, and it responds accordingly. The hyperthyroidism of Graves' disease is due to the fact that the thyroid is being driven not only by the normal regulatory hormone, but also by an antibody. However, antireceptor antibodies may also have the opposite effect.

Blocking of a Receptor by an Antireceptor Antibody This is the mechanism of muscular weakness in *myasthenia gravis*. For reasons unknown, an antibody develops against the acetylcholine receptor. The antibody dutifully combines with the receptor, thereby preventing the acetylcholine from using it. Hence the lack of muscle stimulation (p. 575).

Attachment of Lectins to Membrane Components and the "Capping" Phenomenon Lectins are, to a large extent, laboratory tools (30). These molecules, derived mostly from plants (but also from bacteria and animals), were empirically found to have the property of combining specifically with carbohydrate components (ligands) of the cell surface (16, 22). Commercial catalogs of chemicals list them by the dozen, each with a different specificity; as such they are precious for experimental purposes, for example, as devices for identifying a given cell type *in vitro*. Some are potent cell-agglutinators (phytohemagglutinins); others are used as mitogens, and that may be one of their functions in plants (22).

A widely used lectin is Concanavalin A (Con A), extracted from the jack bean, which combines

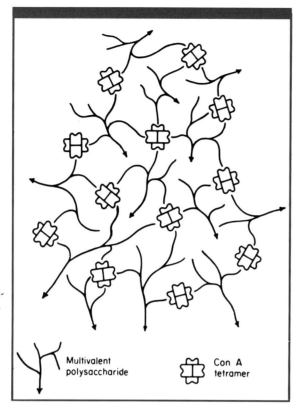

FIGURE 4.10
The chain-end mechanism, whereby tetravalent concanavalin A is thought to aggregate and precipitate polysaccharides or glycoproteins. (Reproduced with permission from [22].)

Multivalent polysaccharide   Con A tetramer

with specific carbohydrate groupings on chain ends (Figure 4.10). When lymphocytes are exposed to this lectin, at first a diffuse bonding of Con A molecules occurs all over the cell surface. Then, as the cell moves about, it gathers all the binding sites to one spot, or **cap,** corresponding to its tail end (uropige). Ultimately, it internalizes the cap into a phagosome (Figure 4.11). The capping sequence has been studied extensively in relation to antibody binding (47).

CONGENITAL DISORDERS OF THE CELL MEMBRANE

No known disease affects *all* cell membranes, perhaps because it would be incompatible with

life. Diseases linked to defects in the cell membrane are many but are poorly understood at the molecular level. One of these, lactase deficiency, is extremely common; the others are rather rare. Fortunately, even the most severe are not in themselves lethal.

Lack of a Receptor An example: The cell membranes of patients with familial hypercholesterolemia have virtually no low-density lipoprotein (LDL) receptors. Thus, cholesterol-bearing particles are forced to accumulate in the blood (11).

Inadequate Number of Receptors A reduced number of insulin receptors is found in the most common variety of diabetes, which develops in adults and is characterized by insulin resistance (diabetes type II).

BRUSH BORDER DISEASES

A large group of membrane disorders affect the epithelium of the gut and of the proximal convoluted tubules of the kidney—mesodermal derivatives that are structurally and functionally very similar: both have microvilli and are specialized for absorption. Congenital defects arise through deficiency or lack of a protein component in the membrane (15). (Note: There is evidence that the brush borders can be affected also secondarily, that is, during the regeneration of intestinal cells.)

Deficiency of Lactase in the Gut This deficiency leads to lactose intolerance, that is, to gastrointestinal disturbances after ingestion of milk and its products (except butter). Because northern Europeans and their North American descendants are generally spared, medical textbooks written in these regions have nearly ignored this condition. Actually, lactase deficiency is so common that it raises a philosophical problem: because it affects most of humanity, perhaps it should not be considered a disease at all. It is the biologically

FIGURE 4.11

Capping phenomenon demonstrated in mouse lymphocytes. *Left:* Mouse lymphocyte incubated with the ligand Con A and photographed by immunofluorescence. The ligand is bound over most of the surface. *Center:* After further incubation, the ligand–receptor complex is aggregated into patches. *Right:* Later, a single cap is formed. (Reproduced with permission from [9].)

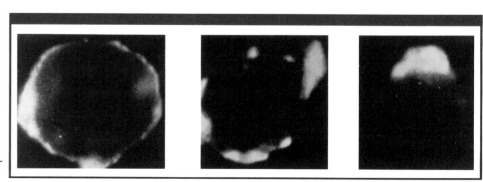

sensible condition whereby the enzyme for digesting lactose disappears after the infant is weaned and milk ceases to be a natural food. In human history milk products are a recent acquisition, not shared by large parts of Asia and Africa. Evolution has not yet had the time to fully acknowledge the use of milk by adults. It could be argued that lactase persistence is the disease (27).

Cystinuria Cystinuria is a rare defect in intestinal and renal reabsorption of dibasic amino acids and cystine. As in the other conditions of this group, the brush border appears normal by electron microscopy. Clinically, the intestinal defect itself is of no consequence, but cystine is poorly soluble, and because the kidney tubules fail to reabsorb it, it precipitates as stones in the urinary pathways, causing all the complications of urolithiasis: infections and even renal failure and death.

Hypophosphatemia In this rare condition the absorption of phosphate is defective. Again, both kidney and gut are affected; the loss of phosphate, a building block of bone mineral, results in poorly calcified bones. The resulting disease recalls rickets due to the deficiency of vitamin D, but it is, predictably, vitamin D resistant.

MUSCULAR DYSTROPHY

A condition that represents a widespread membrane defect is muscular dystrophy, in which the dominating clinical defect concerns striated muscles, but membrane defects have been described in blood cells and other tissues (46). It has been reported that about 5 percent of a patient's muscle fibers show missing patches of plasma membrane, which could account for a clinical sign: high blood levels of creatine phosphokinase, a muscular enzyme (35). However, this structural membrane defect may be secondary to muscular breakdown. Muscular dystrophy was shown to reflect the absence of a protein, dystrophin, that may strengthen the plasmalemma by anchoring elements of the cytoskeleton to the surface membrane (3, 18, 66).

TO SUM UP: The cell membrane is involved in a tremendous variety of pathologic conditions, ranging from the ubiquitous cell blebbing to rare congenital defects. We have chosen the most striking examples, but one could make the point that *practically all diseases involve the cell membrane.* Inflammation includes many membrane phenomena, including leukocyte adhesion to the endothelium, leukocyte aggregation, and cell fusion. Immunology is to a large extent centered on cell membrane effects because the cell surface of each species defines what is "self." Infection by bacteria (17) and viruses depends a great deal on specific surface interactions: this is how gonococci, for example, and vaccinia virus select their targets. Much of tumor biology is also a matter of altered cell surfaces. A pathology of intercellular communication via intercellular junctions is just beginning to develop.

Finally, remember that myelin is made of Schwann cell membranes wrapped many times around an axon: this means that the so-called demyelinating diseases of the nervous system, such as multiple sclerosis, are really diseases of the cell membrane. Indeed, in the 1950s, when the nature of myelin was discovered by electron microscopy, biochemists who had thought of themselves as myelin experts suddenly found themselves catapulted into the position of cell membrane experts.

Pathology of the Mitochondria

A great deal has been learned about normal mitochondria since they were first isolated in the late 1940s and identified as the cell's power plant (76). Regarding mitochondrial pathology, the correlation between structural and functional abnormalities is still sketchy. However, there are some exciting developments. The most startling of all has been the concept that *mitochondria may be the descendants of archaic bacteria,* the remnants of infection of a primal cell (83, 94). Evidence for this possibility is that they have their own DNA and their own mechanisms of transcription and translation. Because mitochondria do have their own DNA, it should also be possible to inherit certain diseases by a mitochondrial, nonmendelian inheritance. When the ovum is fertilized, most of the mitochondria are contributed by the mother (there is very little space for mitochondria in a spermatozoon's head). Diseases inherited in this manner should affect both sexes but be transmitted by maternal inheritance only (in contrast to X-linked recessive transmission) (94). Indeed many such mitochondrial diseases have been identified; they have a wide variety of systemic effects, but mainly neurologic and muscular (86, 75a).

FUNCTIONAL ANOMALIES

Mitochondrial Myopathies Mitochondrial myopathies are diverse and rare, but biologically very interesting (69). Clinically they affect both muscle and brain in varying measures, hence the alternative name mitochondrial encephalomyopathies. The biochemical defect can be in the utilization of substrate, in the coupling of oxidation and phosphorylation, or in the respiratory chain. Diagnosis is difficult because biochemical studies require a large sample of tissue. Electron microscopy shows a variety of changes that are suggestive but hard to interpret, such as the bizarre "parking lot mitochondria" shown in Figure 4.12.

"Mitochondrial Fever" What thoughts would go through your mind if you had to work out the condition of a young woman, who has been fatigued since childhood, thin, feverish, intolerant of heat, sweating profusely, and showing a twice normal metabolic rate? Perhaps hyperthyroidism, but what if the laboratory data indicate a normal thyroid? Such was the case worked out by R. Luft and colleagues in Sweden in 1962 (79). The woman suffered from uncoupling of oxidation and phosphorylation in the mitochondria, which therefore produced heat rather than energy! "Luft's disease" was the first recognized disease of the mitochondria. It should not be confused with malignant hyperthermia, a disorder of muscle metabolism (p. 490).

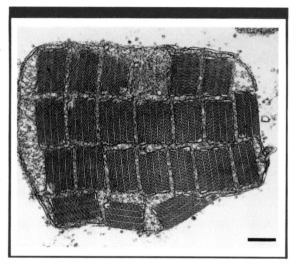

FIGURE 4.12
The astonishing "parking lot mitochondrion." These paracrystalline inclusions are one of many mitochondrial changes found in congenital myopathies. Their significance is unknown. (Reproduced with permission fom [80].)

STRUCTURAL ANOMALIES

Mitochondriomas Mitochondria replicate within the cell much like bacteria; sometimes they do so in excess, filling up the cell and crowding the other organelles. For reasons unknown, this happens characteristically in two tumors of the salivary glands, called Warthin's tumor and oncocytoma (88, 90, 91) and occasionally in other cells, such as in the liver (Figure 4.13) (81). In every case, histologically, the cell body stains strongly with eosin; only the electron microscope can show the real reason for this unusual feature: the cytoplasm is largely replaced by a compact mass of mitochondria. It has been proposed that this phenomenon should be interpreted as a benign tumor of the mitochondria, or mitochondrioma. Real bacteria, incidentally, are not known to form "tumors" (p. 716).

Electron Microscopic Changes of Mitochondria There are enough of these changes to fill a monograph (68) (Figure 4.14). Most common, almost ubiquitous, is mitochondrial swelling mentioned in reference to vacuoles (p. 72); it requires active respiration, but the respiration becomes uncoupled from phosphorylation (77, 78), which means that the mitochondria are producing heat rather than energy as ATP. Bizarre shapes of mitochondria can be induced by many toxic agents, including ethyl alcohol, as shown in

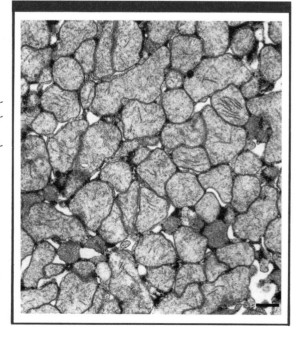

FIGURE 4.13
Abnormal crowding of mitochondria in a liver cell, possibly representing a "benign tumor" of mitochondria. This example was an accidental finding in a case of biliary cirrhosis. **Bar** = 0.5 μm. (Reproduced with permission from [81].)

human volunteers (84). Giant mitochondria are found in many organs, especially heart and muscle (68).

> *The agents that induce giant mitochondria are many but their mechanism of action is not known (68, 85, 93). The most spectacular effects are obtained with a copper chelating agent, cuprizone (89). Other reported causes include alcohol, reserpine, hypophysectomy, jaundice, viral hepatitis, and nutritional deficiencies.*

Calcium Deposits Calcium hoarding by the mitochondria could be a defensive mechanism, as an extension of normal functions (p. 231). The mitochondria (and the endoplasmic reticulum) normally behave as calcium sinks for the cytoplasm, where the calcium ion concentration is kept extremely low (less than 10^{-7} M). As excess calcium is pumped into the mitochondria, part of it is thought to precipitate as phosphate in the mitochondrial matrix; this removes the calcium from solution and makes the work of the pump easier. In osteoblasts, for which calcium metabolism is a primary function, large masses of calcium salts are found in the mitochondria. In other cells, amorphous or crystalline masses of calcium salts develop under pathologic conditions (70, 72, 92). These masses are not necessarily tombstones; they can just represent calcium overload. We will return to this topic in discussing calcification (Chapter 6).

> *Different configurations of the mitochondria were emphasized in the late 1960s as expressions of different functional conditions (67, 74, 75). Remember that mitochondria have an outer and an inner membrane, and therefore an outer space (between the membranes) and an inner space (filled with matrix). The supposed orthodox configuration is that usually seen on electron micrographs: the cristae appear as darker structures against a light matrix. In the condensed configuration the matrix becomes denser, thus the cristae appear as lighter, broader, and irregular streaks against a dark background (Figure 4.15) (87). The two configurations still exist, but they have faded out of the literature; their meaning is unclear except that they probably represent osmotic changes.*
>
> *Glycogen inclusions are sometimes found in the mitochondria. The granules of glycogen are too large to traverse the mitochondrial membrane, and even if the glycogen developed from excess glucose, cytosolic enzymes would be required for polymerizing glucose to glycogen; it is therefore assumed that this change may reflect an abnormality in the permeability of the mitochondrial membrane (71).*

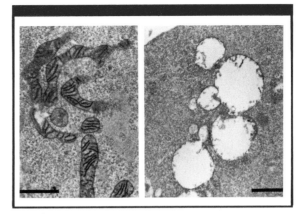

FIGURE 4.14
Example of toxic mitochondrial damage. *Left:* Normal mitochondria of Sertoli cell. *Right:* Mitochondrial swelling induced by gossypol, a disesquiterpene found in cottonseed, which has been used as a male contraceptive in China. **Bars** = 1 μm. (Reproduced with permission from [82].)

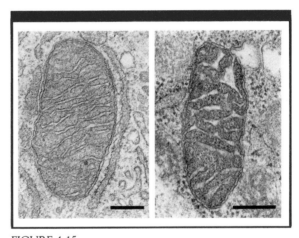

FIGURE 4.15
Two possible configurations of mitochondria. *Left:* "Orthodox" configuration, from a normal human myelocyte. *Right:* "Condensed" configuration, from a myelocyte of a patient who had been treated for 5 days with chloramphenicol, an antibiotic that is also an inhibitor of mitochondrial protein synthesis. **Bars** = 0.2 μm. (Reproduced with permission from [87].)

Pathology of the Endoplasmic Reticulum and Golgi Apparatus

Like other sections on subcellular pathology, this one could not have been written before 1950. That was about the time when two of the founding fathers of cell biology discovered the membranous part of the endoplasmic reticulum

(ER) (120, 121) and its accompanying ribosomes (117).

Before then, some "ER" pathology had been seen, but its meaning, of course, could not be understood. For example, pathologists had learned to associate cytoplasmic basophilia with "busy cells," cells actively producing protein either for secretion or for their own growth, but they could not possibly guess that the basophilia is due to the nucleic acids of the protein-building machines, the ribosomes. Similarly, there was no way to guess that some vacuoles and some "protein granules" represent the retention of fluid or proteins in expansions of ER cisternae, or that cells supposedly killed by toxic agents were really the victims of free radicals produced by their own ER.

PATHOLOGY OF THE RIBOSOMES

When seen by electron microscopy, the basophilic component of the ER may show some interesting anomalies. Some toxic agents cause polysomes to disperse as free ribosomes (Figure 4.16) (112) or cause the ribosomes to become detached from the cisternae (p. 188). The ribosomes can also aggregate into orderly crystals; this has been shown

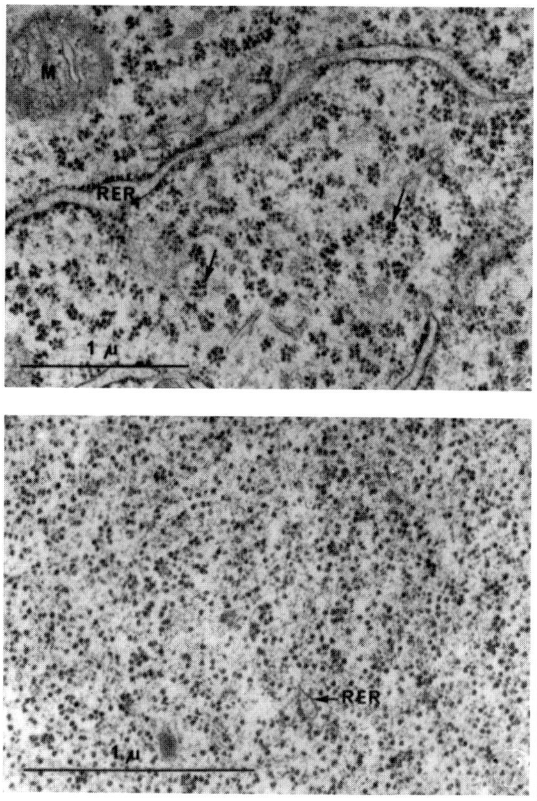

FIGURE 4.16 A subtle symptom of cellular disease: the dispersal of polysomes (*top*), which become free ribosomes (*bottom*). Mouse embryo cells 2 hours after treatment with an inhibitor of DNA synthesis, fluoro-deoxyuridine (FUdR). The other organelles remained normal. **Bars** = 1 μm. (Reproduced with permission from [112].)

under conditions that imply a shutdown of protein synthesis, such as may occur with cooling or in the course of programmed cell death (p. 205).

RETENTION OF FLUID OR PROTEINS: ER STORAGE DISEASES

It is still unclear why the ER should retain fluid and swell into vacuoles, but it often does so (p. 74) (98). For reasons unknown, the perinuclear cisterna in dying cells is especially prone to swell and to create a clear halo hugging the nucleus (Figure 4.17) (96).

The retention of proteins in the ER is better understood. Recent studies have shown that the ER exerts a *quality control* over protein secretion, by retaining and destroying misfolded or unassembled molecules, sometimes complexed with heat shock proteins (108, 110). Congenitally defective proteins are retained presumably because they are mismatched with the ER machinery (108); they tend to form aggregates, perhaps because of poor solubility (why they escape destruction is not clear) and develop into masses that distend the cisternae and are visible even by light microscopy. This phenomenon has been called "cellular constipation," an inelegant term, but the cell—our elementary patient—has many human attributes.

Some examples: plasma cells occasionally contain rounded, eosinophilic "granules" of protein known as **Russell bodies** (incidentally; we checked Dr. W. Russell's paper; whatever he saw in 1890 (125) had nothing to do with what we now call Russell bodies). Remember that plasma cells are busily producing antibody proteins (immunoglobulins), which is why they are filled with basophilic ER. So it did not come as a great surprise when it turned out that the Russell bodies are globs of immunoglobulin; the electron microscope showed that they lie within expansions of the ER (124, 126, 134). The precise mechanism is not known, but it may be related to overstimulation of the plasma cells (126).

In the case of the Russell bodies, the constipation seems to be accidental. In other situations it is congenital; the ER is completely or partially unable to export its product due to some molecular defect. This mechanism is shared by a few conditions known as endoplasmic reticulum storage diseases, a relatively new category (99) (Figure 4.18).

ALPHA-1-ANTITRYPSIN DEFICIENCY

The best-known example of ER storage diseases is alpha-1-antitrypsin deficiency. This very technical name covers a fascinating story (105). The liver normally synthesizes and secretes into the plasma a protein that has the property of inhibiting trypsinlike enzymes, hence its name: alpha-1-antitrypsin. Why is it made? Normally many granulocytes end their short lives by breaking up in the narrow capillaries of the lungs. In so doing they spill dangerous enzymes that must be neutralized immediately. Especially dangerous is elastase, a direct threat to the elastic framework of the lung. Now, *alpha-1-antitrypsin is also a potent elastase inhibitor,* and individuals with low plasma levels of this enzyme develop emphysema, a breakdown of the pulmonary alveolar structure.

The liver cells of some affected individuals do manufacture the inhibitor protein but cannot secrete it because it is defective by a single amino-acid substitution (97). As a result, the protein becomes compacted in the ER, especially in the liver cells, where the little lumps can easily be seen histologically (Figure 4.19). Although the connection is easy to see now, we are impressed with the insight of those who originally connected tiny granules in liver cells with a problem in the lungs, (104).

> *Similar granules have been found in many other tissues by using alpha-1-antitrypsin antibodies (101). The prognosis of emphysema in alpha-1-antitrypsin deficiency is far worse for smokers, another good reason for not smoking (105).*

Many students are confused by the paradox of excess storage associated with deficiency, but the paradox is only apparent: the *amount of circulating protein is too low precisely because much of the product is being hoarded.*

> *Alpha-1-antitrypsin deficiency, a Swedish discovery (104), is common and has many variants of different severity; the homozygous state is found in 1:1750 individuals, the heterozygous in 1:20 (113). It can be reproduced experimentally in rats by treatment with galactosamine (97), as well as in transgenic mice who have received the defective human gene (100) (Figure 4.20).*
>
> *Few other ER storage diseases are known as yet. In one the hoarded molecule is alpha-1-chymotrypsin, in another it is fibrinogen (Figure 4.21) (118).*
>
> *Nature played a peculiar trick on turkeys: they too can be afflicted by an alpha-1-antitrypsin deficiency, but as a lysosomal storage disease: presumably the enzyme is sent to the wrong address (99).*

DISORDERS OF THE ENDOPLASMIC RETICULUM RELATED TO DETOXIFICATION

This is a strange phenomenon. The endoplasmic reticulum is equipped with an oxidase called

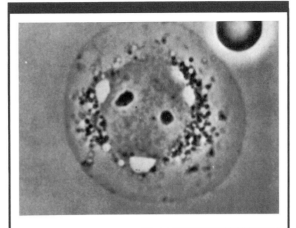

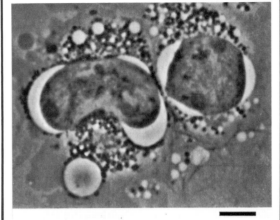

FIGURE 4.17 Vacuoles arising in the perinuclear cisterna. This common expression of cellular suffering is shown here in dying leukocytes. *Top:* Early stage. *Bottom:* advanced stage. **Bar** = 5 μm. (Reproduced with permission from [6].)

cytochrome **P-450,** which has the role of metabolizing and inactivating certain toxic substrates. Sometimes, instead of producing inactive molecules, the P-450 oxidase produces free radicals, which can injure and even kill the cell.

> *The liver is the principal site of detoxification and therefore the richest store of cytochrome P-450. Most toxic agents are taken in by mouth, and the gut is a very poor protective barrier against them (123).* Thus, toxic agents are massively absorbed and transported directly to the liver. However, most, if not all, cell types contain some P-450, which explains how endothelial damage by the ER "detoxyfying" mechanism can occur also in the lung (103).

Cytochrome P-450 (so named after its maximum spectrophotometric absorption, which is close to 450 nm) is built into the membrane of the smooth and rough ER in most (probably all) organs (128, 133). Slightly different varieties are found in mitochondria and, not surprisingly, in bacteria (116). There are many isozymes of P-450 (115), but not all are "dangerous": in some organs they are involved in the metabolism of *endogenous*

FIGURE 4.18
Left: Diagram of the endoplasmic reticulum storage diseases. Condensation (aggregation) of protein in the cisternae of the endoplasmic reticulum impairs their exportation toward the Golgi apparatus. (Adapted from [127].) *Right:* Example of endoplasmic reticulum disease. Detail from a human liver cell in a case of alpha-1-antitrypsin deficiency. The granular masses of defective alpha-1-antitrypsin are clearly within cisternae of the ER (•). **Bar** = 0.5 μm. (Reproduced with permission from [119].)

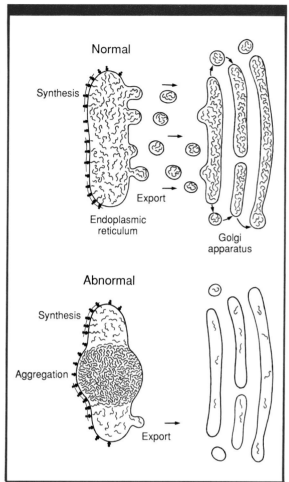

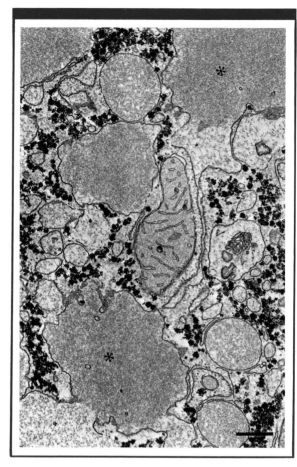

substrates (111), such as steroid hormones, which are not known to create toxic products. However, in the liver, P-450 enzymes are specialized for metabolizing *exogenous* lipid-soluble substrates ("xenobiotics"), which happen to include a number of drugs and pollutants. This particular set of enzymes is **inducible,** that is, it is synthesized in response to toxic substrates.

This potentially suicidal mechanism was discovered around 1960 as a result of efforts to understand the fatty liver caused by carbon tetrachloride, an industrial lipid solvent (122, 123) (p. 187). R.O. Recknagel, a biochemist and toxicologist, proposed that the CCl_4 molecule gave rise to highly toxic free radicals while being "detoxified" in the liver. This concept fit very well with electron microscopic studies of the liver after CCl_4 poisoning: they showed clear-cut damage to the ER evidenced by detachment of the ribosomes and "collapse" (flattening) of the cisternae (106, 129). These events are more fully analyzed in the section on free radical pathology (p. 182).

Today it is clear that, when challenged with fat-soluble drugs or toxic agents, the ER responds in two ways: hyperplasia and self-destruction, as just noted. The hyperplasia can be demonstrated in rats with therapeutic doses of barbiturates: the smooth ER expands greatly in a matter of days. Similar abnormalities are found in human liver (Figure 4.22). When examined by cell fractionation, the hypertrophic ER is found to contain large amounts of cytochrome P-450. This means that the enzyme has been induced: in some cases the normal P-450 enzyme is being synthesized more actively, and in other cases a new variety of P-450 is generated.

Now, supposing that a liver contains a great deal of hyperplastic ER produced in response to a given xenobiotic agent, will it be protected if it is exposed to a second agent? The answer is "It depends."

- *One poison followed by another may make the second more—or less—dangerous depending on the interplay between them at the level of the P-450, as shown in the following examples.*

- *Heavy smokers require higher doses of certain drugs* because their liver ER, having become hyperplastic by detoxifying nicotine, destroys them at a faster rate. The drugs include caffeine (109) (heavy smokers need more coffee for the same effect), beta blockers, and theophylline (114). In other words, if the effects of ER hyperplasia are not taken into account, heavy smokers who fall ill run the risk of inadequate therapy.

- *Insomniacs become distressingly tolerant to barbiturates:* they have developed so much smooth ER that the barbiturate is destroyed before it can induce sleep.

- *A small dose of CCl₄ protects a rat against a second lethal dose (for about 3 days)* (131). The reason: much of the liver ER is destroyed, which removes the source of the cytochrome P-450. By the same token, CCl₄ protects against a lethal dose of the mushroom poison phalloidin (107).

- *Removing two-thirds of the liver 4 days before a dose of CCl₄ protects rats from its lethal effect* (130): regenerating liver cells have an inefficient or immature P-450.

- *Newborn rats are insensitive to CCl₄* (102). The reason: much like regenerating liver, the liver of baby rats does not yet have enough P-450.

Why has the endoplasmic reticulum developed this dangerous set of enzymes? The answer is that *the mechanism evolved for processing internal or natural molecules;* the enormous output of synthetic chemicals by our society was not anticipated by evolution.

Another important practical aspect of P-450 biology is that *the response of any single patient to certain drugs and even to certain carcinogens depends on his or her enzymatic make-up,* which is genetically determined: hence the new field of pharmacogenetics (132).

TO SUM UP: The pathology of the endoplasmic reticulum reflects the two main functions of this organelle. First, *detoxification.* Thanks to an industrial poison, CCl₄, it was discovered that this process sometimes goes awry: the ER can create dangerous free radicals, poisons, or carcinogens out of previously harmless molecules. A side product of these studies was the opening of a new field, free radical pathology. Because the ER is not identical in all of us, what happens to each one of us in life depends in part on the ER that we inherit. Second, *synthesis.* Pathologic storage can occur in the ER as it does in

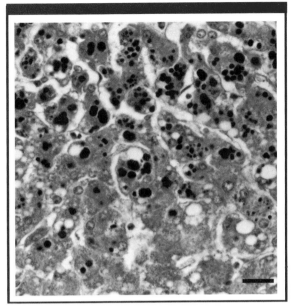

FIGURE 4.19
Liver of a patient suffering from alpha-1-antitrypsin deficiency. Periodic acid–Schiff stain, whereby glycoproteins are stained a deep red. The dark granules in many hepatocytes correspond to masses of alpha-1-antitrypsin retained in the ER. The liver cells in the lower part of the field contain fat droplets. This abnormality may not be a part of the disease because this patient became depressed and resorted to alcohol abuse. **Bar** = 25 μm.

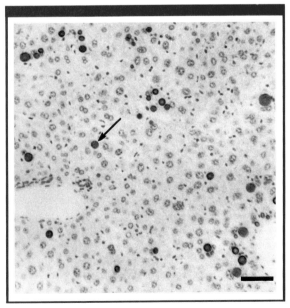

FIGURE 4.20
Globules of human alpha-1-antitrypsin in the liver of a transgenic mouse carrying a human gene for defective alpha-1-antitrypsin. The globules (**arrow**) are stained brown with an antibody against alpha-1-antitrypsin conjugated to peroxidase. **Bar** = 50 μm. (Courtesy of Dr. M.J. Finegold, Texas Children's Hospital.)

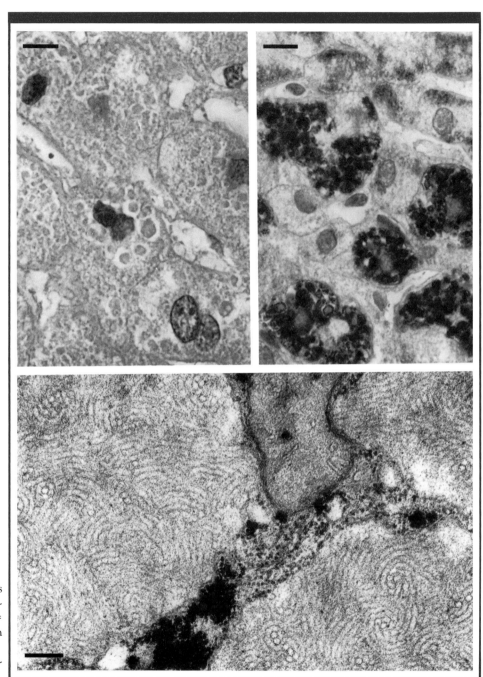

FIGURE 4.21
Fibrinogen storage disease, a newly discovered ER storage disease. *Top left:* Histological aspect of liver cells (note the large granules). **Bar** = 10 μm. *Top right:* Dark stain corresponds to specific antibody staining, identifying the material as fibrinogen. **Bar** = 10 μm. *Bottom:* Electron micrograph of the granule content. **Bar** = 0.2 μm. (Courtesy of Dr. U. Pfeifer, University of Würzburg, Germany.)

lysosomes. So far there is only one major ER storage disease, but it is very common.

In closing, the reader might be interested to know how the ER received its name, because the ER as we now see it is not obviously endoplasmic or reticular.

In 1944 the electron microscope existed but could not be used for the study of cells and tissues: there was no method for cutting tissue sections thin enough to be traversed by the electron beam. Then, Dr. Keith R.

Porter, later the inventor of the Porter–Blum ultramicrotome, came upon the idea of preparing cultures of fibroblasts on cellophane. When grown in this manner, fibroblasts spread out and develop extremely thin, veil-like expansions. There was reason to hope that these expansions might be thin enough to allow the passage of electrons. So they were; their outer, thinner parts were empty, but a little closer to the cell center they contained a peculiar network of interconnected cords. Today we know that this surprising arrangement was due to the very special condition of the cells. The ER as seen in modern ultrathin sections appears as a stack of interconnected pancakes. Somehow, as it was squeezed in the expansions of Porter's very flat cells, the ER assumed the aspect of a network—such as no contemporary electron microscopist has ever seen. In any event, the network that Porter saw occupied the inner portion of the cytoplasm without reaching the edge of the cell: so it was a reticulum and it was endo-plasmic (120, 121) (Figure 4.23).

PATHOLOGY OF THE GOLGI APPARATUS

To the relief of many a student, the Golgi apparatus contributes little to pathology at least in comparison with other organelles (138a). It is practically invisible by light microscopy except in plasma cells: the typical half-moon of clear cytoplasm separating the nuclei of plasma cells from the basophilic cytoplasm is nothing but the negative image of the Golgi apparatus, enlarged in relation to the amount of globulin synthesis. Little was learned from electron microscopy (138, 139) except that the Golgi cisternae sometimes swell (136).

However, where there is function, there is malfunction. The basic task of the Golgi apparatus is to sort the proteins supplied by the endoplasmic reticulum and target them to various addresses: lysosomes, secretory granules, or the cell surface. In rare cases this function is flawed: *the lysosomal enzymes are secreted but deprived of their proper address, and their undigested substrates accumulate in large cellular inclusions;* hence the name **I-cell disease** (Figure 4.24) (135). We will return to this disease in relation to lysosomes.

The Golgi apparatus attaches "address labels" to proteins and lipids by means of specific glycosylation reactions. It so happens that all the lysosomal enzymes are provided with the same label or "recognition marker" (mannose-6-phosphate) (137), which means that a defect in the "addressing" enzymes can affect all the lysosomal hydrolases. In I-cell disease most hydrolytic enzymes are missing in the lysosomes themselves, but they are present in the extracellular fluid: this indicates a defect in the addressing system. For reasons unknown, not all cell types are affected.

Pathology of the Lysosomes and Peroxisomes

As the cell's principal digestive organs, the lysosomes are involved in most diseases, but in addition, they have over 50 diseases of their own; the literature is mountainous (154, 155, 157, 158,

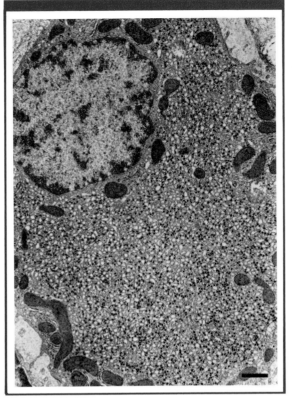

FIGURE 4.22 Hyperplasia of the smooth ER in a hepatocyte. All other organelles are displaced toward the periphery. By light microscopy the cytoplasm of such cells has an eosinophilic "ground glass" appearance. From a 53-year-old man on long-term prednisone treatment for chronic active hepatitis. **Bar** = 1.0 μm. (Reproduced with permission from [119].)

168, 189). After lysosomes were formally identified and described in 1955, it turned out (as is usual in such discoveries) that they had been seen before (144). But their rediscovery is unique in one respect: like the planet Neptune, they were predicted before they were seen.

About 1955, DeDuve and collaborators were studying the distribution of enzymes in various fractions of liver-cell homogenates that had been separated by ultracentrifugation. From this analysis they predicted that acid phosphatase would be found to be contained in special granules, distinct from all other known organelles. A histochemical method for acid phosphatase then enabled Novikoff to see the granules: almost overnight the lysosomes ceased to be a "concept" and became established as real organelles. Soon thereafter it was realized, to everyone's delight, that the unexplained granules of the blood-borne granulocytes were nothing but special varieties of lysosomes (152). Comparable organelles were later found in plants.

Today we know that some catabolic functions are performed in the cytosol (p. 43), but the bulk of intracellular digestion is performed in the lysosomes by enzymes, of which at least 60 have been identified. Presumably not all of these enzymes are present in all cells, but acid phosphatase is always present. It has therefore

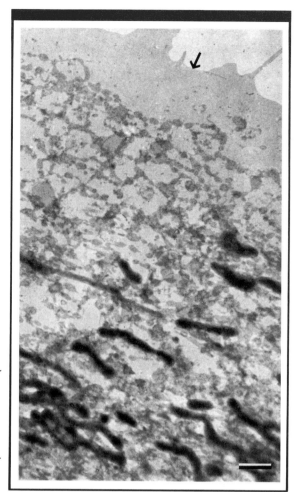

FIGURE 4.23 How the endoplasmic reticulum got its name. In the thin expansions of cultured cells, viewed by electron microscopy, it appears like a "reticulum" limited to the "endoplasm." **Arrow:** Ectoplasm. **Bar** = 1 μm. (Courtesy of Dr. K.R. Porter, University of Pennsylvania, Philadelphia, PA.)

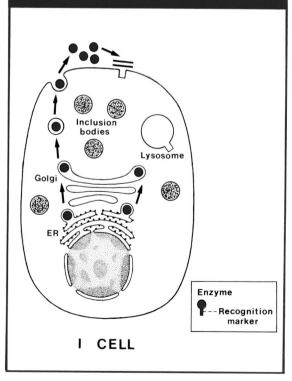

I CELL

FIGURE 4.24 Cellular disturbance in I-cell disease (compare with Figure 4.33). In I-cell disease the cells are unable to produce the enzyme recognition marker, which is essential for the intracellular transport of enzymes to the lysosomes as well as for the extracellular pathway. As a result, the hydrolytic enzymes cannot complete either pathway. (Adapted from [1].)

retained its key function as a marker enzyme: *the standard procedure for proving, by light or electron microscopy, that an unknown organelle is a lysosome is to react it for acid phosphatase* (Figure 4.25).

The lysosome family is an untidy-looking group under the electron microscope. Unlike the highly stylized mitochondria, lysosomes vary in shape, size, and content because of their diversified and adventurous life cycle. Born as small **primary lysosomes** that bud off the Golgi apparatus, they sooner or later fuse with other vesicles, into which they pour their enzyme-rich contents. These other vesicles may have arisen from phagocytosis (phagosomes), pinocytosis (pinosomes), or autophagocytosis (p. 42). The result of any of these fusions is a **secondary lysosome.**

Micropinocytic vesicles, which are much smaller than primary lysosomes, also find their way into the primary lysosomes, where their membranes are recycled. This amounts to saying that lysosomes are a major site of phospholipid recycling: a property that lies at the root of many lysosomal diseases.

Whatever the lysosomes are unable to digest they simply retain; these leftovers may be foreign particles, heavily oxidized lipids from the cells' own catabolism (lipofuscin, p. 97), or chemicals that are undegradable by available enzymes. Lysosomes stuffed with such residues have been called **residual bodies** or *tertiary lysosomes* (189),

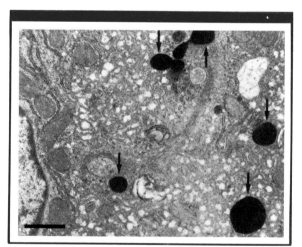

FIGURE 4.25
Demonstration of acid phosphatase in the lysosomes (**arrows**) of a liver cell in the guinea pig. The histochemical reaction is based on capturing, by means of cerium ions, the inorganic phosphate released during the enzymatic hydrolysis of phosphate-containing substrates. **Bar** = 1 μm. (Reproduced with permission from [193].)

but some electron microscopists refer to them irreverently as the garbage cans of the cell. As the stuffing continues, lysosomes may swell, up to several micrometers under extreme conditions (168). Incidentally, how the lysosomes manage not to digest themselves is not yet clear.

Garbage disposal, for metazoan cells, is a problem. The option of simply hoarding the wastes is only a short-term solution. Protozoans are much more effective: they get rid of bulky residues by a process referred to as defecation (biologists push anthropomorphism to the point of placing a little bottom [or cytopige] at the "rear end" of proto-zoans) (181). The trouble with our own metazoan cells is that they live on such refined foods and fuels (amino acids, glucose) that they are rarely faced with the need to evacuate solid residues; as a result, they have developed almost no ability to do so. It can also be that evolution downplayed evacuation of residues in metazoans because dumping the lysosomal enzymes into the tissue spaces would be dangerous to the surrounding cells (155). Whether mammalian cells ever "defecate" has been much debated (189). However, movies have documented beyond doubt that human leukocytes eject phago-cytized bacteria. Exocytosis, of course, is routinely performed by mammalian cells as secretion.

In plants the problem of getting rid of cellular leftovers is especially complex, because plants have no guts and no kidneys. Therefore, the cells dump some of their catabolites in the extracellular space, where they are polymerized and stored as resin.

Much of what we know about the pathology of lysosomes has been gleaned from studies of granulo-cytes, simply because they are such a convenient source of "granules." We have learned that lyso-somes contribute to cellular pathology in several ways:

- massive release of enzymes into the cell itself
- massive release of enzymes to the extra-cellular spaces
- failure of the lysosomes to fuse with phagosomes
- failure of the lysosomes to digest.

MASSIVE RELEASE OF LYSOSOMAL ENZYMES INTO THE CELL

It does not take much imagination to realize that a collection of little enzyme bombs sitting in the cytoplasm could represent a serious hazard for the cell. At the whole-body scale, we are reminded of the pancreas, another time bomb full of enzymes that poses a threat to the individual (p. 213). Indeed, soon after lysosomes were discovered, a colorful theory was proposed: lysosomes might act as "suicide bags" in giving a dying cell the *coup de grâce* (189). Studies on cell death showed that this event is the exception, not the rule (p. 196). Though it turns out to be true that cells *can* commit suicide, they do so without firing off their lysosomes; instead something happens to their DNA (p. 200).

On the other hand, we must briefly dwell on the exception: the lysosomes may become a hazard to the cell if they are broken open from inside. Imagine a situation in which a phagocytic cell takes in a microscopic crystal. The result may be as dangerous to the cell as swallowing a razor blade: the phagosome breaks open. The razor blade analogy is not quite exact, because breaking open the phagosome may occur not by a simple puncture but by a physicochemical interaction between the surface of the crystal and the phagosomal membrane (197). Because phago-somes are full of lysosomal enzymes, the cell can die of this accident. The victim is usually a phagocyte; the crystals can be of several sorts (151). The so-called **crystal-induced diseases** include gout (197), silicosis (141, 175), and pseudogout, a form of arthritis caused by micro-scopic crystals of calcium pyrophosphate (p. 243) (185). In this group of diseases the lysosomes are not giving the *coup de grâce* to dying cells; they are killing healthy ones outright.

MASSIVE RELEASE OF LYSOSOMAL ENZYMES TO THE EXTERIOR

Spillage of enzymes into extracellular space occurs in two very different circumstances. In *inflamma-tion*, leukocytes spill enzymes while they phago-cytize and when they die; the result may or may not be an advantage (p. 322). In *shock*, virtually all tissues in the body are poorly perfused with blood. This causes generalized cell damage, whereby lysosomal enzymes are thought to spill out of the cells; hence the therapy with corticoids, which stabilize the lysosomal membranes.

FAILURE OF LYSOSOMES TO FUSE WITH PHAGOSOMES

Failure to fuse is really not a disease but the result of a cunning survival strategy devised by certain parasites (143, 164, 165, 173). Imagine that a

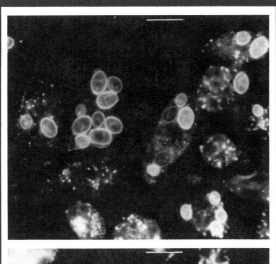

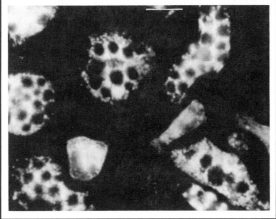

FIGURE 4.26

Prevention of fusion between phagosome and lysosome in cultured macrophages by sulfatides of *Mycobacterium tuberculosis*. *Top:* Live macrophages after 45 minutes incubation with live yeasts; staining of lysosomes with acridine orange and examination in fluorescent light. Phagocytized yeasts are fluorescent because the marker dye of the lysosomes has emptied itself into the phagosomes. This is the normal response. *Bottom:* These macrophages were pretreated with sulfatide for 18 hours, then stained with acridine and incubated with live yeasts for 2 hours. The macrophages are filled with packed lysosomes surrounding dark spaces, which represent unstained yeasts inside nonfused phagosomes. **Bars** = 10 μm. (Reproduced with permission from [163].)

macrophage ingests a *Mycobacterium tuberculosis* (which it habitually does as part of the body's defense against tuberculosis). The bacillus, now trapped in the phagosome, somehow prevents surrounding lysosomes from fusing with phagosomes. The result is that the bacillus survives. This has a major impact: *the macrophage becomes a haven for the very bacteria it is supposed to destroy.* The bacillus, safe inside the macrophage, may actually be transported to a distant site—rather like Jonah,

who was vomited up on dry ground by the whale, three days after ingestion. Fortunately, most macrophages tend to stay put, but alveolar macrophages could certainly be coughed out into the air with their virulent load.

This bacterial strategy sounds admirable, but how does it work? How do bacteria prevent lysosomes from fusing with the phagosomes? After several years of debates, the safest conclusion is that different mechanisms exist (197). For *M. tuberculosis* a mechanism was worked out starting from a clue provided by the bacillus itself. It was noticed that the virulence and infectivity of this bacillus correlated with the production of sulfatides, strongly acidic glycolipids. This suggested that these "virulence factors" might act by preventing phagosome–lysosome fusion. Indeed, when the sulfatides were administered to cells in tissue culture, the lysosomes were inhibited just as in the natural tuberculosis infection (Figure 4.26) (163, 165). A different trick is used by a protozoan, *Toxoplasma* (173, 174). While it is being phagocytized, it manages to "choose" the patch of membrane that will imprison it: that particular patch of membrane will lack the signals needed for fusion with lysosomes, and so the *Toxoplasma* will live happily ever after (Figure 4.27) (172).

FAILURE OF LYSOSOMES TO DIGEST

For digestive organelles, lack of digestion is the ultimate failure. It can occur in several settings: (a) *the lysosomes are normal* but they are presented with an object or bacterium that they cannot digest; (b) *the lysosomes are congenitally abnormal,* lacking one particular enzyme; (c) *the lysosomes have become abnormal* by taking up a drug or other molecule that makes digestion impossible.

NORMAL LYSOSOMES PRESENTED WITH UNDIGESTIBLE MATERIAL

As we just discussed, the indigestible material remains stored in residual bodies. Perhaps some of it, at some later date, can be extruded—but not much is known about this.

CONGENITALLY ABNORMAL LYSOSOMES (LYSOSOMAL STORAGE DISEASES)

There is a group of about 40 diseases—individually rare but collectively fairly common—characterized by the lack or malfunction of a lysosomal enzyme. They are inherited in a mendelian autosomal recessive pattern and are often fatal, whether they occur in humans, cats, dogs, or

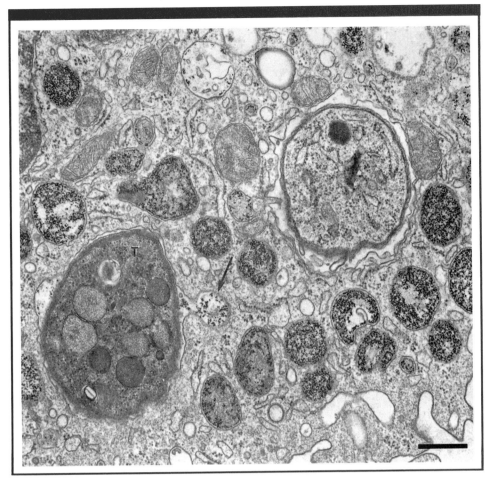

FIGURE 4.27
Inhibition of phagosome–lysosome fusion in a macrophage that phagocytized live Toxoplasma, as well as dead, glutaraldehyde-fixed Toxoplasma as control. The lysosomes of this macrophage were previously labeled with particles of thorotrast (**black dots**); then the macrophage was exposed to Toxoplasma and fixed 1 hour later. At lower left, a dead *Toxoplasma* (**T**), recognizable by its increased electron density, lies tightly wrapped in a phagosomal membrane that contains thorotrast particles; a lysosome loaded with thorotrast particles is just fusing with it (**arrow**). At top right, a living *Toxoplasma* is also wrapped in a phagosomal membrane, but there are no thorotrast particles in the phagosome and no lysosomes are fusing with it. **Bar** = 0.5 μm. (Reproduced with permission from [173].)

other animals (161, 178, 179, 195). The enzymatic defect leads primarily to stuffing of the lysosomes with the substrate of the affected enzyme, in some cell types more than in others, depending on the disease; the cells become bloated with huge lysosomes and eventually may even die.

> Most commonly the enzymatic deficiency is due to the fact that a lysosomal enzyme is missing, but at least five other genetic mechanisms can lead to the same result (142): the enzyme may be present but inactive; it may be synthesized but fail to reach the lysosomes; it may be unstable at the acid lysosomal pH; an activator protein can be missing; or there may be a defect in the transport of the degradation product. An acquired mechanism is also known: the enzyme may be blocked by an inhibitor, such as a drug. It follows that the same disease may be produced by several mechanisms.

The lysosomal storage diseases are usually classified on the basis of the substrate that accumulates, the main groups being glycogen and glycoproteins, mucopolysaccharides, sphingolipids, lipids (triglycerides and cholesteryl esters), and mucolipids (Table 4.1). Being experiments of nature, these diseases have shown us new vistas on lysosomal function. Without attempting to review them, we will answer some of the questions that concern the group as a whole.

How do Storage Diseases Reveal Themselves?

Pediatricians see most cases, for obvious reasons. Typically, the child is normal at birth but fails to thrive. Neurological symptoms and/or a large liver and spleen may be present. A liver biopsy may suggest the diagnosis (Figure 4.28) (192). Occasionally, the child has a particular facies; hence, for example, the alternative name *gargoylism* for Hurler's disease, a mucopolysaccharidosis (Figure 4.29). (Gargoyles are the grotesque figures used as water spouts on Gothic cathedrals; see Figure 4.30). Other physical signs vary, but a few themes predominate: stunted growth, mental retardation, blindness, deafness, heart and muscle dysfunction,

TABLE 4.1

Summary of Lysosomal Storage Diseases

Disorder	Enzyme Deficiency	Stored Material	Unique Manifestations
Tay-Sachs and var., G_{M2} gangliosidosis	Hexosaminidase A	G_{M2} ganglioside	Macrocephaly, hyperacusis in infantile form; increased in Ashkenazi Jews
Krabbe, galactosylceramide lipidosis	Galactosylceramide β-galactosidase	↑ Galactocerebroside/ sulfatide ratio	Extreme irritability, ↑ CSF protein, fever, globoid cell neuropathology
Metachromatic leukodystrophy, sulfatide lipidosis	Arylsulfatase A (cerebroside sulfatase)	Galactosyl sulfatides	↑ CSF protein and early gait abnormalities in late infantile form; peripheral neuropathy
Niemann-Pick, sphingomyelin lipidosis	Sphingomyelinase in types A and B but not type C	Sphingomyelin, cholesterol	Pulmonary infiltrates, brownish skin, infantile neuronopathic form increased in Ashkenazi Jews, sea-blue histiocytes
Gaucher, glucosylceramide lipidosis	β-Glucocerebrosidase	Glucosylceramide	Adult form includes ↑ acid phosphatase, pathologic fractures; Ashkenazi Jewish predilection
Fabry, trihexosyl ceramidosis	α-Galactosidase A	Trihexosylceramide	Cutaneous angiokeratoma, vascular thromboses, hypohydrosis
Pompe, glycogen storage type II	Acid maltase (α-1,4- and 1,6-glucosidase)	Glycogen	Lethal skeletal and cardiac myopathy in infantile form; primarily skeletal myopathy in adults
Morquio, mucopolysaccharidosis IV	N-Acetylgalactosamine-6-sulfate sulfatase	Keratan sulfate	Severe deformity, odontoid hypoplasia, aortic regurgitation
Mucolipidosis II, I-cell disease	UDP-N-acetylglucosamine (GlcNAc):glycoprotein GlcNAc-1-phosphotransferase	Glycoproteins, glycolipids	Coarse facies, inclusions in cultured fibroblasts, normal mucopolysacchariduria
Neuronal ceroid lipofuscinoses	Unknown	"Ceroid" lipofuscin	Electron microscopy helpful, degree of genetic heterogeneity unknown

Adapted from Beaudet, AL Lysosomal storage diseases. In: Wilson, JD, Braunwald E, Isselbacher KJ, Petersdorf RG, Martin JB, Fauci AS, and Root RK, Harrison's principles of internal medicine. 12th ed. New York: McGraw-Hill, Inc., 1991: 1845–1854.

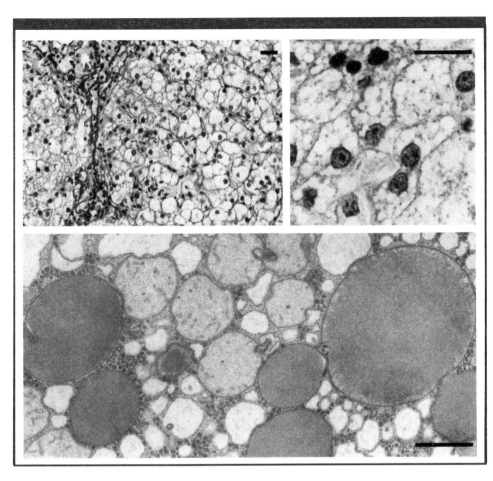

FIGURE 4.28

Cholesteryl ester storage disease. *Top left:* Histologic aspect of the liver. **Bar** = 25 μm. *Top right:* Detail, showing foamy aspect of liver cells. **Bar** = 25 μm. *Bottom:* Electron microscopy shows membrane-bound granules filled with lipid material. **Bar** = 1 μm. (Courtesy of Dr. U. Pfeifer, University of Würzburg, Germany.)

a clouded cornea due to large, light-diffracting lysosomes in corneal cells. Yet some lysosomal disorders can appear in adult life; this is possible because the enzyme activity is not necessarily missing; it may be simply reduced.

What Organs or Tissues are Affected? In principle the enzymatic defect should occur in all cells, and at the level of the microscope some pathologic storage tends to occur everywhere; but *extreme overloading with substrate occurs where the metabolism of that substrate is most active.* For instance, absence of glucose-6-phosphatase (von Gierke's disease) leads to hepatomegaly by glycogen overloading of the liver cells; sphingomyelin (Niemann-Pick's disease) can show a predilection for the brain. However, the preferences are not always explainable and may depend on the age of onset. It is important to remember that hepatomegaly sometimes has an entirely different mechanism: the overloaded cells are not the liver cells but the Kupffer cells and the entire system of sinusoidal (littoral) macrophages (p. 299). This happens, for example, in Gaucher's disease. The substrate is a

lipid from the membranes of dying blood cells and is therefore poured in large amounts directly into the bloodstream, where it follows the fate of any abnormal material: phagocytosis by the sinusoidal macrophages (mainly in the liver and spleen), except that the macrophages too are unable to digest it.

What Happens to the Overloaded Cells? Signs of cell dysfunction are obvious in the central nervous system: the abnormal storage occurs in the cell body of the neurons—in the grey matter—but myelin development is impaired in the axons, in the white matter (176). The space-occupying aspect of storage should disturb some cells, and overloaded liver macrophages eventually do cause pressure atrophy of liver cells and other parenchymal cells. However, purely mechanical explanations are often suspect. In fact, some of the tissue changes, such as liver cirrhosis, have been ascribed to damage by enzymes spilled by the macrophages during phagocytosis (150), a phenomenon known as regurgitation (p. 404). Oddly enough, there can also be signs of general

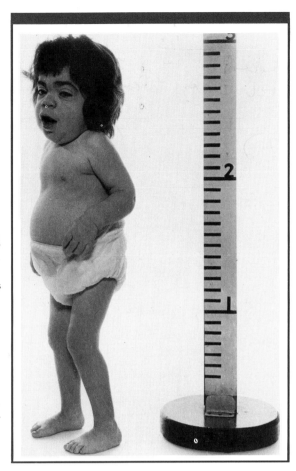

FIGURE 4.29 Five-year-old girl with a lysosomal disease, muco-polysaccharidosis type I (also called Hurler's disease or gargoylism). Scale in feet shows stunted growth (height appropriate for a 3-year-old). (Reproduced with permission from [149].)

enzymatic activity is present in the nervous system). The clinical severity varies; some patients are devastated in their twenties whereas others, who may have up to 40 percent of the normal level of the critical enzyme, β-glucocerebrosidase, live fairly symptom-free into their seventies.

Regarding the pathogenesis, **obsolete leukocytes** *are the most important source of glucocerebroside quantitatively followed by red cells and neural tissue. Knowing this, the result can be predicted. Leukocytes and red cells are normally broken down and their products recycled by the phagocytic cells of the liver, spleen, and bone marrow, the three main locations of sinusoidal macrophages. Thus, in the adult disease the cells condemned to become most overloaded with glucocerebroside are the macrophages exposed to the blood stream. As more of them become filled up, some die and some divide; the new cells pick up and inherit the content of the old ones, and so the cycle continues. Liver, spleen, and bone marrow become massively filled with stuffed phagocytes, also called Gaucher cells (Figure 4.32). Secondary problems then arise. The blood-forming bone marrow is crowded out by Gaucher cells, leading to anemia and thrombocytopenia. The bone itself, compressed from inside, becomes thinner and may fracture (Miss Wheelchair America for 1987 was a Gaucher patient); the liver cells are also compressed but usually without major consequence because mammals can get by on a fraction of their liver mass. The spleen enlarges, leading to a syndrome of excessive splenic function (p. 603) (spleens of 12 kg have been recorded, and splenectomy can be of some relief).*

The infantile form (Type II) is deservedly called acute neuropathic or malignant. Typically, the baby looks normal at delivery. The problems begin at about 3 months, due to Gaucher cells infiltrating the central nervous system or the peripheral tissues: failure to thrive, difficult feeding, neuromuscular symptoms, large liver and spleen, spasticity, strabismus, and persistent retroflexion of the head. Death occurs within 2 years, often as a result of infection superimposed onto lungs filled with Gaucher cells.

lysosomal overactivity (183), perhaps reflecting increased compensatory manufacture of new but ineffective lysosomes. Also, the overstuffed lysosomes may be unable to fulfill other functions and show signs of secondary disturbances (156, 190) (Figure 4.31). Finally, in one group of lysosomal storage diseases, the sphingolipidoses, it was found that protein kinase C was inhibited, an event that could lead to general impairment of signal transduction within the cell (166).

An Example: Gaucher's Disease To better understand the sequence and the localizations of lysosomal storage diseases it will help to follow them in Gaucher's disease (148), where the stored metabolite is a glucocerebroside, normally an intermediary in lipid metabolism of cell membranes (191).

The adult form (Type I) of Gaucher's disease is more common and much less severe than the infantile form and is characterized by splenomegaly, hepatomegaly, anemia, thrombocytopenia, and erosion of the inner cortex of the long bones. Typically, there are no neuropathic symptoms (perhaps because enough

A Lesson from Lysosomal Storage Diseases: Lysosomal Enzymes are Normally Secreted and then Recaptured This bizarre but important fact of normal cell biology was learned by culturing cells from patients with lysosomal storage diseases. These cultured cells, by the way, continue to manifest the abnormality and develop "granules" (stuffed lysosomes). Using fibroblasts cultured from various patients, Elizabeth Neufeld and her group at the National Institutes of Health made a surprising observation (187, 188). If cells from a storage disease are cultured together with normal fibroblasts, the diseased cells are cured and the storage granules reabsorbed. It was therefore assumed, at first, that the normal cells secreted some unknown "corrective factor": later it turned out that the factor was simply the missing enzyme, supplied by the normal cells present in the culture. This made it possible to understand an even more surprising result: cells with two different storage diseases cured each other! Clearly this happened because each cell type lacked an enzyme that was present in the other cell type. This result offered hope for therapy at the whole-body level, but it also meant that a certain amount of lysosomal enzymes must normally be secreted by the cells. Following this lead, a new facet of normal lysosomal physiology was discovered. *The cells supply their lysosomes with enzymes by two pathways: one runs from the Golgi apparatus to the lysosome, the other leads to the cell surface. Thus, the enzyme is secreted and then recaptured, with some loss, and carried back to the lysosome* (Figure 4.33). Now we understand, at long last, why small amounts of lysosomal enzymes from many organs are present in the blood.

At this point we can return to the I-cell disease mentioned in relation to the Golgi apparatus. In this disease all the enzymes synthesized for the lysosomes are defective because they all lack the label addressing them to the lysosomes (Figure 4.24). The same label is required for recapture after secretion; therefore, if I-cells are cultured with cells of any lysosomal disease, the I-cells are unable to perform a cure because no I-cell enzyme can be recaptured.

Diagnosis and Therapy of Lysosomal Storage Diseases The disease is first suspected clinically, then confirmed by biopsy. In a pregnant woman, the diagnosis of fetal disease can be made by amniocentesis between the second and third month of pregnancy; specialized laboratories can then test the fluid for the expected defect (reduced enzyme, excess substrate) or provide cells that can be cultured and tested in similar fashion. A recent development is first-trimester biopsy of the chorionic villi by passing an ultrasound-directed catheter through the cervix. This method can yield enough cells for chromosomal, biochemical, and DNA studies and has the advantage of speed. Because it avoids the 2–4 weeks needed for the cells to grow, the pregnancy can be interrupted earlier (153, 170, 177).

Therapy entered a new era in 1991 with the intravenous administration of the missing enzyme,

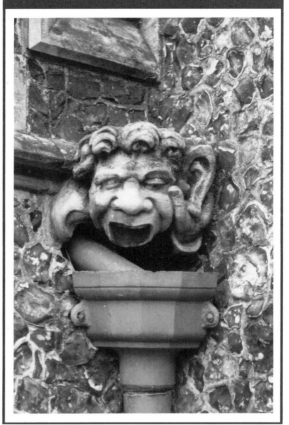

FIGURE 4.30
Gargoyle on the Parish Church of St. Peter and St. Paul, Tring, Hertfordshire, England. The depressed nasal bridge, wide nostrils, thick lips, and irregular teeth recall the features of children with Hurler's disease (gargoylism). (Courtesy of Professor D. Robinson, Queen Elizabeth College, University of London. Reproduced with permission from [146].)

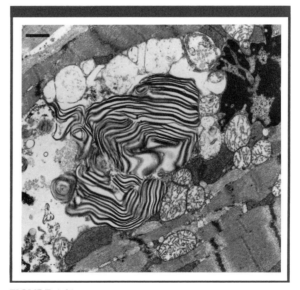

FIGURE 4.31
Zebra bodies: A manifestation of cellular disease in gargoylism, a lysosomal disorder characterized by the generalized accumulation of glycosaminoglycans. The zebra bodies represent the accumulation of phospholipids, which may be the consequence of a secondary lysosomal disturbance and may contribute to cardiac failure in these patients. (Myocardium of a 23-year-old man; tissue obtained at autopsy.) **Bar** = 1 μm. (Reproduced with permission from [190].)

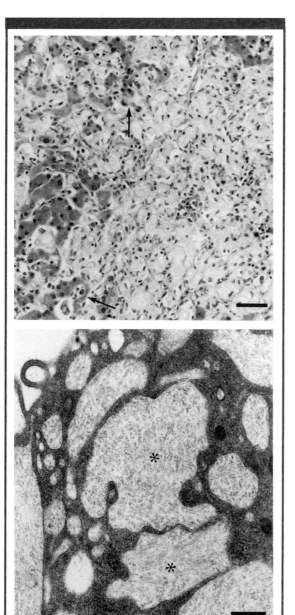

FIGURE 4.32 Liver in Gaucher's disease. *Top:* The cords of liver cells are atrophic (**arrows**) and largely replaced by masses of large clear cells: macrophages loaded with undigested phospholipid. **Bar** = 100 μm. *Bottom:* An electron microscopic view: Part of a Gaucher cell from the bone marrow. Retained phospholipid (·) appears as a tangle of thin-walled, twisted tubules 300–600 Å in diameter. **Bar** = 0.5 μm. (Reproduced with permission from Iancu TC. The ultrastructural spectrum of lysosomal storage diseases. Ultrastruct Pathol 1992;16:231–244.)

which is extracted from human tissues and targeted to macrophages, the cells that need it most (145, 148). The results are extremely encouraging and hopefully the cost will decrease (for a single patient it has "dropped" to $100,000 per year) (160). Another breakthrough came from liver transplantation for Type IV glycogen storage disease and Gaucher's disease: liver function improved, as expected; in addition, *the abnormal deposits throughout the body regressed,* whereas the team that carried out this study had assumed that the disease would continue its relentless course (196). How would our readers explain this happy turn of events?

Remember the "correction phenomenon" observed in vitro: This is the in vivo counterpart. The cells of the implanted liver secrete lysosomal enzymes that circulate in the blood stream and are picked up by the defective cells. Furthermore, in this study it was found that Kupffer cells emigrated from the implanted liver, settled elsewhere in the body, and presumably continued to produce their normal enzymes (10–15 percent of liver cells are Kupffer cells).

DRUG-INDUCED (IATROGENIC) LYSOSOMAL DISEASES

Strange but true: lysosomes can be disturbed by therapeutic agents, in fact by a number of lysosomotropic molecules, some of which are otherwise harmless dyes.

Biologists have long known that the so-called neutral red given in vivo will stain the macrophages, especially if they are very busy phagocytizing (Figure 5.38). This can now be explained: the red dye accumulates in the lysosomes. Another cationic dye, acridine orange (which has a beautiful fluorescence), gives striking pictures of primary and secondary lysosomes (Figure 4.26).

There are many lysosomotropic drugs, which diffuse through the plasma membrane and into the lysosome. Like the dyes, they are cationic as well as amphipathic; that is, their polar end makes them water soluble, and their nonpolar end enables them to penetrate cell membranes. Once a drug is inside the lysosome, the acid environment modifies it in such a way that it is trapped (183). A classic drug of this type is **chloroquine,** which happens to be an antimalarial drug; it also has the property of raising the internal pH of the lysosome, thus inactivating its enzymes. For this reason it has become a standard tool in lysosome research. Now we can explain the demise of the malarial parasite. Its aggressive strategy is based on invading the red blood cell, which is devoid of lysosomes and therefore defenseless. When the chloroquine comes along, it stops digestion within the lysosomes of the parasite, and the creature starves to death (180).

Obviously, lysosomotropic drugs can be useful, but there is the other side of the coin: they can create iatrogenic lysosomal diseases. Once inside the lysosomes the drugs can combine with molecules that are to be processed, usually phospholipids, and make them resistant to breakdown. The result, seen under the electron microscope, is a typical storage disease (Figure 4.34) (169, 171). Clinical symptoms include muscular weakness, tremor, and mild clouding of the cornea, as seen in

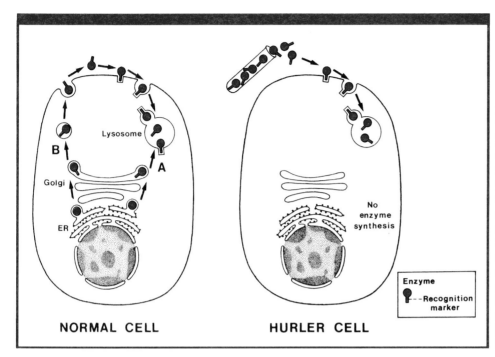

FIGURE 4.33
The roundabout ways of normal lysosomal enzymes. *Left:* the normal condition. As soon as the molecules are synthesized, some migrate directly to the lysosomes (**A**) and some leave the cell and are recaptured (**B**). This odd mechanism was discovered by studying lysosomal disease. *Right:* Cells from a case of Hurler's disease are incapable of synthesizing one enzyme (alpha-L-iduronidase) but can still pick it up and store it in their lysosomes if it is supplied from the outside. *This is a general rule for lysosomal storage diseases.* (Adapted from [1].)

congenital lysosomal diseases (167). Fortunately, these changes, which are seen after months of drug use, are reversible. Chloroquine myopathy is a fine example (184) (Figure 4.35).

> *Drugs that cause lysosomal storage diseases include antidepressants, inhibitors of cholesterol biosynthesis, vasodilators, antihistamines, anticancer agents, antibiotics (183), and the antiarrhythmic drug amiodarone. Cells affected, besides the cornea, include spleen phagocytes, which normally degrade blood cells; Sertoli cells, which normally degrade residues shed by spermatids; alveolar macrophages, which normally degrade surfactant; and retinal pigment epithelium, which normally renews visual cell membranes. In the retinal pigment epithelium cells, the outer segment of each rod contains a large stack of membranes which, in the rat, is totally renewed every 9 days. For the drug-induced storage effects to occur, chronic administration is required. Note the difference from congenital lysosomal disorders: in the drug-induced conditions just listed the lysosomes are only frustrated by adulteration of their substrate; there is no depletion or inhibition of their enzymes. An experimental model closer to the congenital condition would require a drug that reduces or inhibits a specific lysosomal enzyme. This has been achieved for Niemann-Pick's disease (194).*

TO SUM UP: Lysosomes suffer from many congenital and acquired diseases. As unplanned experiments—natural or man-made—they have taught us some basic lessons in cell biology.

PATHOLOGY OF THE PEROXISOMES

In our cholesterol-conscious culture, the peroxisomes attracted considerable interest when it was found that various hypolipidemic drugs, as well as aspirin, caused the number of these organelles to increase in the liver (Figures 4.36, 4.37) (199, 200, 201). This is still a puzzle, and so is the

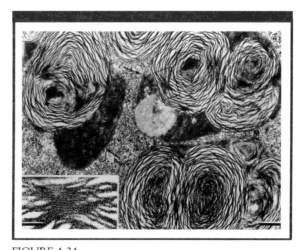

FIGURE 4.34
Drug-induced lysosomal disease: lamellated inclusion bodies in the liver cell of a guinea pig treated with chlorphentermine, an appetite suppressant, for 2 weeks. **Arrows**: membrane belonging to the remnants of a lysosome. **Bar** = 0.3 μm. *Inset:* Periodicity of the lamellar material (40–50 Å). **Bar** = 0.1 μm. (Reproduced with permission from [182].)

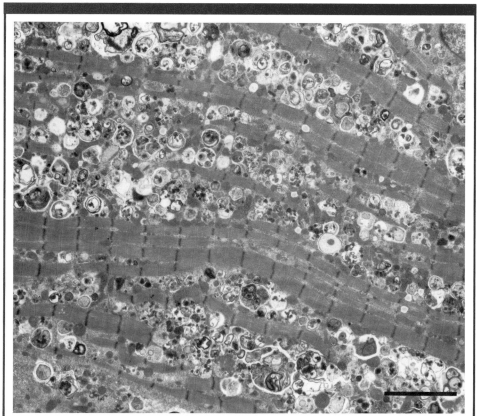

FIGURE 4.35
A drug-induced lysosomal disease: chloroquine myopathy. The patient, a 79-year-old lady with rheumatoid arthritis, had taken hydroxychloroquine for 6 years. During the last 3 months she developed weakness and fatigue. This muscle biopsy shows part of a striated muscle cell in which the bundles of fibrils are dissociated by myriads of myelin figures (phospholipids) some of which are clearly inside lysosomes. **Bar** = 5 μm. (Courtesy of Dr. U. De Girolami, Brigham and Women's Hospital, Boston, MA.)

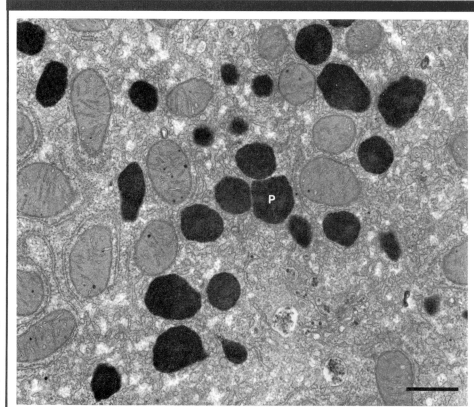

FIGURE 4.36
Increased number of peroxisomes in rat liver cells after administration of a hypocholesterolemic agent. Normally, the number of peroxisomes is about half the number of mitochondria; here they are more numerous. **Bar** = 0.5 μm. (Reproduced with permission from [199].)

observation that these disparate peroxisome proliferators are also carcinogenic for the liver (203).

Peroxisomes are ubiquitous organelles that are also present in protozoa and plants; they are small (0.5 μm or less) and numerous, about 1000 per liver cell (compared with 2000 mitochondria), and account for about one-fifth of the oxygen uptake of the liver (204). Their 15 (or so) enzymes include oxidases producing H_2O_2 and catalases destroying it. They are specialized in the beta-oxidation of long-chain fatty acids (C24–26) in contrast with the mitochondria, whose appetite is directed to shorter chains. They also synthesize plasmalogens, a unique category of phospholipids present in myelin and in platelet activating factor (p. 347) (202). Other possible roles include protecting the cell against buildup of H_2O_2, degrading bacterial walls, and providing an accessory pathway for the oxidation of lipids.

Rare congenital diseases are known in which peroxisomes are almost absent, diminished, or lacking an enzyme (202). The first category is represented by the Zellweger syndrome (205, 206), in which severe demyelination probably reflects the lack of plasmalogens in the myelin. In this syndrome the enzymes of the peroxisomes seem to be normal; the defect lies in the protein that translocates the enzymes into the peroxisomes (205, 206). This may be the first reasonably documented case of "translocation pathology" (203).

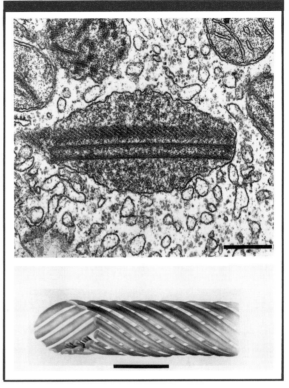

FIGURE 4.37 Effect of aspirin on peroxisomes in rat liver. *Top:* The treatment induces the appearance of rigid tubules, which are probably crystals of enzyme molecules. **Bar** = 0.4 μm. *Bottom:* Reconstructed model of the crystal. **Bar** = 110 nm. (Reproduced with permission from [201]).

Pathology of the Cytoskeleton

The term skeleton is not quite appropriate for the cell's three major sets of fibrils (or filaments) because some of their functions are more like those of muscle. For this reason, the pathology of the cytoskeleton is a mixed bag. We will be describing abnormal lumps of truly cytoskeletal fibrils as well as dynamic events, such as cilia that fail to whip as they should. Interestingly, *a number of natural poisons are targeted against components of the cytoskeleton.*

The cytoskeleton as it is known today includes three kinds of filamentous structures:

- **Thin filaments** (~60 Å), made of actin, a component of the contractile system.
- **Intermediate filaments** (80–100 Å), which come in five varieties and may in fact be motionless.
- **Microtubules** (240 Å), hollow rods long held to function only as cellular bones,

but now recognized as being highly mobile.

PATHOLOGY OF THE THIN FILAMENTS

The thin filaments (actin) are maximally developed in muscle cells and as such have a pathology specific to those cells. Here we will deal only with abnormalities of more general interest.

Rigor Mortis *Rigor, that archetypal expression of death, occurs when myosin heads become locked to the actin filaments* (Figure 4.38). This tight bond is due to the lack of ATP and can be released by ATP unless rigor is advanced (212). Despite its name, rigor "mortis" can develop also in the living body, for example in a recent myocardial infarct (226) or in a limb suddenly deprived of its blood supply. It may come as a shock to learn that rigor mortis has been studied extensively by the meat industry, the reason being that nobody would choose to buy a steak in rigor.

The essentials of the onset of rigor are as follows. If muscles are rich in glycogen, like those of well-fed nonexercised animals, glycolysis after death causes a sharp drop in pH to ~5.6. This is the setting of acid rigor, in which the contracture appears late (e.g., 11 hours at 17°C) and resolves by itself relatively fast,

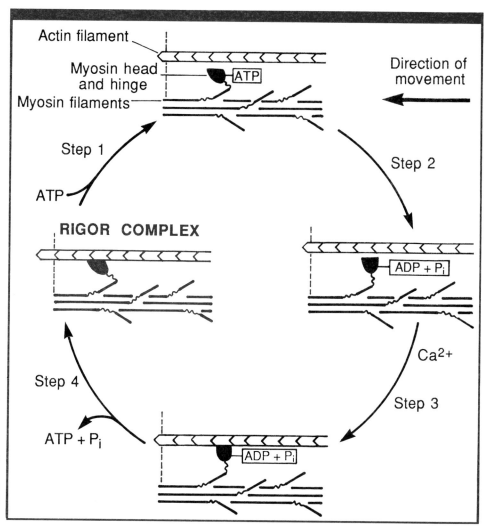

FIGURE 4.38
Genesis of rigor mortis: myosin-ATPase cycle during muscle contraction. If the supply of ATP runs out, the myosin head remains locked to the thin filament, in the so-called rigor complex (Step 4). Normally this lock is released by the binding of ATP to the myosin head, as shown in the next step of the cycle. (Adapted from [218].)

perhaps because the attached myosin heads are denatured and lose their grip. If muscles have little glycogen, like those of an animal that has been hunted down or a steer that struggled before death, the pH remains around 7.1–7.2; rigor sets in very rapidly, often with some shortening of the muscle, and may never resolve until putrefaction sets in. This is alkaline rigor. The alkaline pH gives the flesh its dark red color (212).

Drug-Induced Abnormalities Beyond this macabre involvement with rigor mortis, *actin filaments are the target of several drugs and potent toxins* (217). Phalloidin, a toxin of the deadly mushroom *Amanita phalloides* (Figure 3.21), binds specifically to actin filaments (244); this gives it a practical use: it can be chemically bound to fluorescent dyes and used very effectively for the microscopic demonstration of actin by UV light (Figure 4.39). *Cytochalasin B* (extracted from Kodo millet, a grain crop) prevents the polymerization of actin filaments (Figure 4.39);

it is so poisonous that in ancient India it was used to kill tigers (242). It also has the amazing properties of causing cells to extrude their nuclei (237) and of preventing cellular cleavage without preventing mitosis (215). *Cytochalasins*, incidentally, are a group of compounds that relax cells (from *chàlasis*, slackening).

Jaundice can be the result of a cytoskeletal disturbance in the liver. The finest roots of the bile ducts are encircled by a coat of fibrils including actin. Drugs that interfere with actin, such as phalloidin and cytochalasin B, produce structural and functional changes in the canaliculi, as well as jaundice (230, 231).

PATHOLOGY OF INTERMEDIATE FILAMENTS

The intermediate filaments are divided into five classes, each typical (within limits) of a particular type of cell:

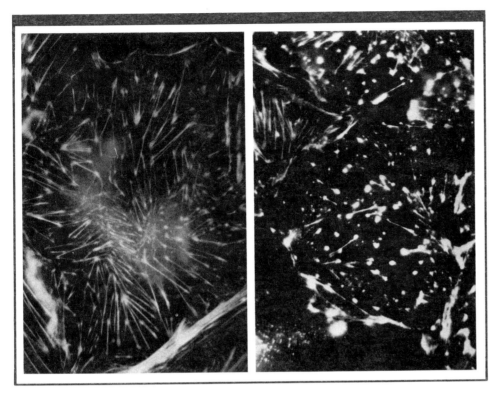

FIGURE 4.39
Disruption of actin-containing fibers (stress fibers) by cytochalasin D in cultured cells. The stress fibers are demonstrated by fluorescence microscopy, utilizing a fluorescent molecule (rhodamine) linked to phalloidin, which has a high affinity for actin. *Left:* Normal cell. *Right:* Cell after 10 minutes of exposure to cytochalasin D; most of the stress fibers have disappeared. (Courtesy of M. Schliwa, University of California, Berkeley, CA.)

- **Cytokeratin filaments,** typical of epithelial cells
- **Desmin filaments,** muscle cells
- **Vimentin filaments,** connective tissue cells
- **Neurofilaments,** neurons
- **Glial filaments,** astrocytes

This list is a challenge to the newcomer's memory, but in the practice of medicine it is an advantage because it helps trace the ancestry of bizarre tumor cells when all other criteria fail (p. 933). Only the cytokeratin filaments and the neurofilaments are known to have a significant pathology, and will be discussed below.

CYTOKERATIN FILAMENTS

Hyaline masses of cytokeratin filaments are common in the liver cells of alcoholics (Figure 4.40). (The term *hyaline* means "glassy, structureless.") In 1911, when Frank B. Mallory first described these inclusions in the liver of alcoholics at Boston City Hospital, he had good reasons to call them alcoholic hyalin. Today, however, it is best to call them **Mallory bodies** because they have turned up in many other conditions besides alcoholism. In ordinary sections they appear as eosinophilic clumps; their fibrillar nature is seen by electron microscopy (Figure 4.41) in patterns suggesting three variants (219) (Figure 4.42). Tests with various types of anticytokeratin antibodies (there are at least 20 human cytokeratins) show that the fibrils of Mallory bodies are similar to liver and to epidermal keratin (223), perhaps slightly abnormal (224). Why Mallory bodies form is unclear (225).

Inclusions similar to Mallory bodies but unrelated to alcohol abuse have been found (a) in the liver (in obesity, especially after repeated fasting; after jejunal bypass as a surgical treatment; and in jaundice and other biliary disorders); (b) in the pulmonary epithelium in asbestosis; and (c) in some tumors of the liver and lung (223). They can be produced experimentally in mice, oddly enough, by injecting anti*tubulin* drugs (221); if the drug is withdrawn, they disappear.

Crooke's hyalin, another type of intracellular hyalin, develops in the pituitary basophil cells (which secrete the adrenal cortical stimulant ACTH) as a response to excessive plasma levels of ACTH or glucocorticoids. Like the Mallory bodies, Crooke's hyalin consists of cytokeratin filaments. Apparently, the basophil cells, inhibited from secreting ACTH, produce excess cytokeratin. The hormonal imbalance may be due, for example, to an adrenal tumor or adrenal hyperplasia (Cushing's syndrome), or even to therapeutic doses of ACTH or corticoids (227).

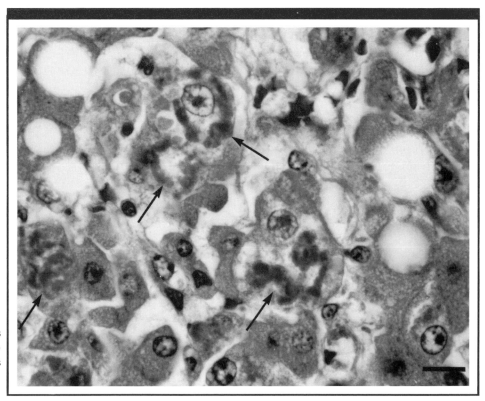

FIGURE 4.40
Mallory bodies (**arrows**) in liver cells of an alcoholic. **Bar** = 25 μm. (Courtesy of Dr. K.G. Ishak, Armed Forces Institute of Pathology, Washington, D.C.)

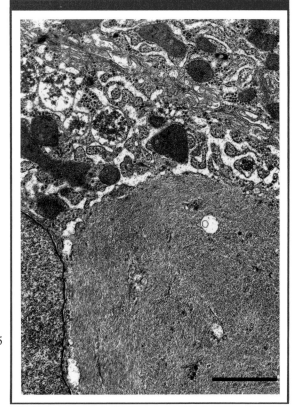

FIGURE 4.41
Typical Mallory body (type I) in alcoholic liver disease. **Bar** = 5 μm. (Reproduced with permission from [231].)

Neurofilaments In the nervous system, neurofilaments are present in the axon and in parts of the perikaryon; they are thought to provide mainly structural support. Several drugs and toxic agents, including (rather paradoxically) anti*tubular* agents, cause abnormal accumulations of neurofilaments in the neurons or in the axons; swellings of the axons overfilled with neurofilaments become clinically apparent as neuropathies. One such drug is antabuse for the treatment of alcoholism (213). Aluminum intoxication produces similar lesions (241).

PATHOLOGY OF THE MICROTUBULES

Microtubules were discovered by electron microscopy in the 1960s; before then, electron microscopists, who always worry about artefacts, fixed their specimens with osmium tetroxide and in the cold—which just happens to create an artefact of its own by disassembling the microtubules. Eventually, fixation at room temperature—and with glutaraldehyde—in Keith Porter's laboratory opened the door to a new cellular structure.

Microtubules are naturally unstable structures made from tubulin units free in the cytoplasm. They are constantly disassembled and reassembled, and may

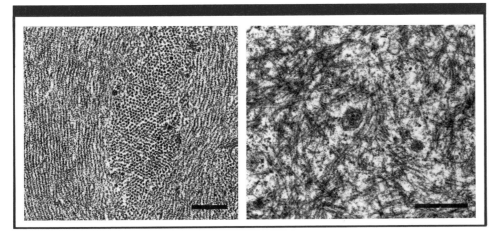

FIGURE 4.42
Fine structure of Mallory bodies. Type I (*left*) and type II (*right*) in alcoholic liver disease. Type III Mallory bodies are extremely electron dense and structureless. **Bars**: left = 1 μm, right = 0.5 μm. (Reproduced with permission from [231].)

grow at one end while dissolving at the other. They provide rigidity and polarity to the cell, but also exert a more sophisticated function by means of proteins that come to settle on their surface and act as molecular cilia. Thanks to this arrangement, microtubules placed on a glass surface propel themselves in a straight line as if driven by an invisible force (211). By the same mechanism, microtubules inside a living cell act as engines that propel microvesicles, secretory granules, and other organelles from one part of the cell to another. Microtubules are essential during mitosis and also represent the skeleton of cilia and of eukaryotic flagella. Therefore, interfering with the structure and function of the microtubules can be disastrous to the cell and to the whole organism.

Antitubular Drugs Microtubules are the targets of many drugs, which have in common the property of binding to molecules of **tubulin,** the building blocks of microtubules, thereby preventing their assembly. *Because a spindle of tubules is essential for the cellular ritual of mitosis, these drugs can behave as antimitotic poisons, and therefore as antitumor agents.*

The prototype of the group is colchicine, obtained from the meadow saffron (Figure 4.43), one of the oldest specific drugs, which was used for the treatment of gout as early as the sixth century (218). Unfortunately, colchicine is very toxic. Given orally it causes diarrhea because, being an antimitotic, it stops mitoses in metaphase in the rapidly regenerating intestinal epithelium, just as X-rays do.

An acute attack of gout occurs when a wave of neutrophils massively phagocytizes crystals of urate in a joint (p. 243). This extremely painful episode can be dramatically interrupted by colchicine taken by mouth. The effect of colchicine is probably antileukocytic; that is, the disassembly of mi-

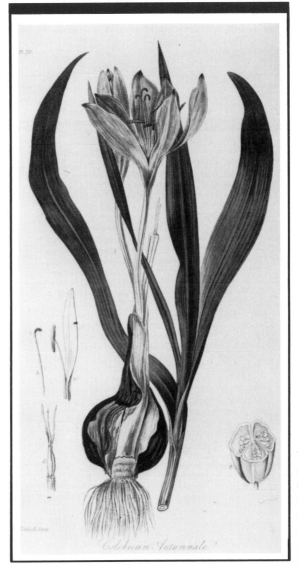

FIGURE 4.43
The source of colchicine, *Colchicum autumnale*, the meadow saffron. (Reproduced with permission from [232].)

crotubules prevents the leukocytes from running to the scene and phagocytizing the crystals of urate. Other antitubule agents share this antigout effect. Intravenous colchicine is still used for gout, but it has a very low benefit-to-toxicity ratio (238).

In the 1800s, frequent cases of colchicine poisoning (some occurred during the treatment of gout) led to the study of its effects in experimental animals and to the discovery that colchicine arrested mitoses (Figure 4.44). In 1937 it was found that colchicine increases the number of chromosomes in plants; since then it has been a major botanical tool for producing experimental polyploids (221). Until 1956, the exact number of chromosomes in humans was unclear; it was set at 46 thanks to colchicine. Eventually, colchicine also led to the discovery of tubulin, to which it binds stoichiometrically (221).

The antitubulin poisons include the **vinca alkaloids,** derived from the Madagascar periwinkle, which today are an essential weapon against cancer; **podophyllotoxin,** obtained from the root of the May apple (*Podophyllum*), once used by the Penobscot tribe to treat warts (243); and **griseofulvin,** isolated from *Penicillium griseofulvum,* a

fungistatic (245) (Figure 4.45). Colchicine, incidentally, is too toxic for use as an antitumor agent.

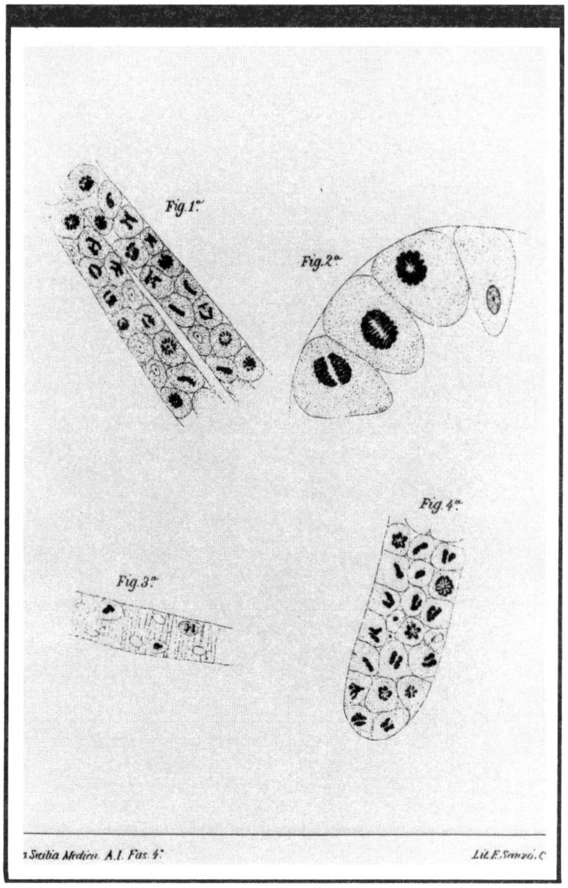

The cellular effect of these drugs, as observed on isolated cells, is no less than spectacular: the microtubules break up or disappear entirely (Figure 4.45). Most of the therapeutic effects can be explained by this mechanism. However, the blockage of mitoses does not tell the whole story. Colchicine, for instance, is 1000 times more toxic to the lymphocytes of lymphatic leukemia than to normal lymphocytes, a property that was proposed as a diagnostic test (240).

PATHOLOGY OF THE CILIA

Cilia are highly specialized assemblies of microtubules and other proteins. Sperm tails are essentially the same as cilia, only longer (Figure 4.46). Cilia can be damaged by infection and, in the upper airways, by smoke, hay fever, or the common cold (207); they can fall off or disappear by several different mechanisms (Figure 2.40) (214). *The best-known ciliary defects are congenital.*

Immotile Cilia Syndrome The first report of genetically abnormal cilia came some 30 years ago with the discovery of a unicellular alga that could not swim because its flagella were motionless (210). Then in 1975 a paper appeared describing the condition of a man whose spermatozoa were motionless (228). A Swedish cell biologist and expert on cilia, Björn Afzelius, confirmed the existence of this disease in a fertility clinic in Stockholm—but he went one step further: cilia are cilia, he thought, wherever they may be; perhaps the patients with immotile spermatozoa also suffered from immotile cilia in the bronchi? A quick look at some patients' files proved him right: immotile spermatozoa went along with chronic bronchitis and sinusitis (210). Thus was born the immotile cilia syndrome.

Afzelius was well qualified to discover this syndrome. Back in 1959, on a sunny day, while studying his electron micrographs on the beach, he had discovered the dynein arms, the engine that drives the cilia. It is missing in some cases of immotile cilia syndrome (Figure 4.47) (210).

After the immotile cilia syndrome was recognized, it turned out that some of the patients suffered from a triad of conditions long known as the utterly mysterious Kartagener syndrome: **bronchiectasis** (bronchial dilatations), **chronic sinusitis,** and **situs inversus viscerum** (heart on

FIGURE 4.44 Effect of colchicine poisoning on the epithelial lining of the stomach and intestines, as seen by B. Pernice in 1889, in dogs that 24–48 hours previously were given a dose of tincture of colchicine by mouth. Pernice's conclusion was not that mitoses were arrested but that the cells were "stimulated and excited" by the colchicine. (Reproduced with permission from [229].)

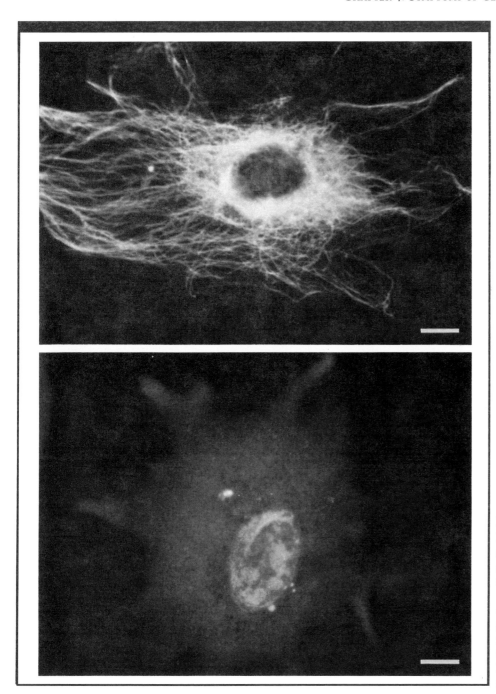

FIGURE 4.45
Disruption of microtubules by griseofulvin, a mold metabolite of the genus *Penicillium*, used as a fungistatic. *Top:* Normal cultured cell (mouse 3T3 cell). *Bottom:* Similar cell after 18 hours of exposure to griseofulvin. Comparable effects are induced by colchicine and by vinblastine, which also bind to tubulin. **Bars** = 5 μm. (Reproduced with permission from [245].)

the right, liver on the left, etc.). Now the first two components of the triad are easy to understand. As for the situs inversus, it could be due to a ciliary problem in very early embryologic development (207). Female infertility also may occur (there are cilia in the Fallopian tubes) but not in all cases. Today, 20 types of abnormal cilia are known; the incidence of such defects is about 1 per 15,000 births. Dogs and mice are also affected.

The most amazing part of this story is that several major and apparently unrelated problems, such as male and female infertility, a chronic cough, and even a right-sided heart, could be due to one molecular defect.

TO SUM UP: A striking feature of cytoskeletal pathology is its close correlation with poisons. Some powerful plant toxins, phalloidin and the cytochalasins, are targeted to actin; alcohol and antabuse (an intriguing association) target inter-

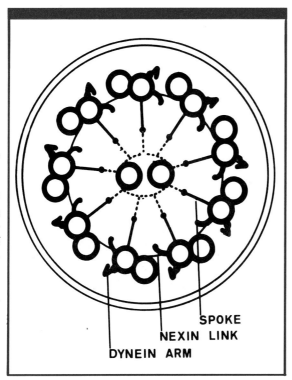

FIGURE 4.46 Diagram of the cross-section of a cilium or of the central portion of a spermatozoon's tail. The 9 + 2 microtubules are held together by three kinds of connections as indicated; the dynein arms are believed to be responsible for the motility. (Reproduced with permission from [221].)

SPOKE
NEXIN LINK
DYNEIN ARM

mediate filaments; many plant poisons disrupt the microtubules. We are tempted to suggest that plants, in their competition with mammals, discovered that breaking up the cytoskeleton is an efficient way to kill mammalian cells. Pharmacologists have followed this lead in using some of these plant poisons to kill cancer cells.

In closing this review of cytoskeletal pathology we should recall that 20 percent of the cell's bulk consists of the *microtrabecular lattice,* the ultimate cytoskeleton. It is an extremely fine, three-dimensional network of fibrils, described by the same Keith Porter who discovered the endoplasmic reticulum and the microtubules (234–236) (Figure 4.48). Practically nothing is known about its role in disease.

Pathology of the Nucleus

Unlike any other organelle, the nucleus can be studied in several totally different ways; correspondingly, there are different types of nuclear pathology. Basically, the nucleus is the custodian of an enormous treasure, the genome: It has been calculated that the DNA of a single human sperm or ovum contains 3×10^9 base pairs, more than 100 times the number of letters and punctuation marks in a set of the *Encyclopaedia Britannica.* This mind-boggling system is under constant repair by a maintenance crew of at least 30 specialized enzymes, without which we would die much sooner from DNA damage (250). This crew, of course, has its own set of disturbances, some of which predispose to cancer, and will be dealt with in Chapter 29. We might conclude that just *looking* at the nucleus is rather like staring at a textbook of genetics, closed. Indeed, if we only study the nucleus under the microscope, and

FIGURE 4.47 A classic cytoskeletal disease, the immotile cilia syndrome. *Left:* Cross section of the tail of a normal human spermatozoon; it is essentially a cilium. **Arrowheads:** Dynein arms. *Right:* Cross section through the tail of a spermatozoon from a patient with the immotile cilia syndrome. The dynein arms are missing. Lacking the dynein molecule, the spermatozoa are motionless; hence these individuals are sterile. **Bars** = 0.1 μm. (Courtesy of Dr. B.A. Afzelius, University of Stockholm, Stockholm, Sweden.)

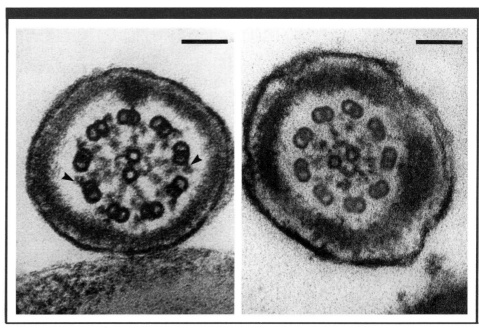

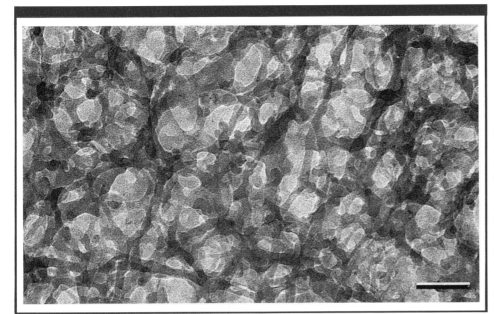

FIGURE 4.48
A high-voltage electron micrograph showing the ultimate structure of the cell, described by K.R. Porter et al. as "microtrabecular lattice" (235). It has been suggested that each trabecula may contain a central filament of F-actin (215). The three-dimensional effect is due to the depth of focus of the million-volt electron microscope. **Bar** = 0.1 μm. (Courtesy of Dr. K.R. Porter, University of Pennsylvania, Philadelphia, PA.)

follow its visible changes in disease, we will gather very little information. The nucleus by its very nature must be extremely stable; it cannot afford great variations in structure. Thus, before the DNA revolution, the nucleus held the reputation of being microscopically a rather dull structure.

Things began to change in 1949 when it was discovered, quite accidentally, that "just by *looking*" at a nucleus one could tell the sex of its owner (246). The scientific community was shocked; we recall an eminent anatomist muttering "I can't face it." Yet today sex chromatin belongs to basic biology. Then came the microscopic study of chromosomes, which grew into science of its own, cytogenetics. In the 1980s molecular biology appeared on the scene. Suddenly it became possible to isolate genes, to insert them into bacteria, and to create transgenic animals by the methodology of recombinant DNA. An offshoot of this science is *molecular pathology* which aims at correlating DNA and disease. Parallel to these developments, the traditional morphology of the nucleus has progressed, in quality as well as in range, by the use of the fluorescence-activated cell-sorter, or FACS (p. 15).

Genetics used to be the only tool for exploring the genome. Today, the nucleus and its DNA can be studied in many other ways, requiring various specializations:
- biochemistry
- morphology of the intact nucleus (including the FACS)
- morphology of the chromosomes (cytogenetics)
- molecular biology (including transgenic animals)
- molecular pathology
- biology of DNA repair

We can only review the essentials of nuclear morphology, and provide a bird's eye view of other approaches.

MICROSCOPY OF THE NUCLEUS

In searching for signs of cellular disease, we can learn a lot by using the microscope simply to examine the size, shape, and structure of the nucleus. Tumor diagnosis hinges very much on such considerations.

Nuclear size can increase tremendously when quiescent cells are suddenly activated to a high level of protein synthesis, as best demonstrated by fibroblasts around a focus of injury (Figure 4.49). At the same time the heterochromatin becomes dispersed, and the nucleolus enlarges. A large nucleolus is the hallmark of heightened protein synthesis.

In most cells about 90 percent of the chromatin is thought to be transcriptionally inactive (247) and appears as dense masses of heterochromatin. A small fraction of the heterochromatin is permanently "turned off"; that is, it is never transcribed (constitutive heterochromatin). The rest is facultative heterochromatin, which probably reflects the level of

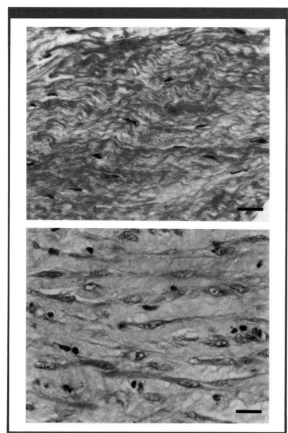

FIGURE 4.49
Effect of cellular
activation on the
nucleus. *Top:*
Quiescent fibro-
blasts in the scar
of an old myocar-
dial infarct. *Bot-
tom:* Activated
fibroblasts in the
wall of an ab-
scess. Note the
enlarged, clear
nuclei. **Bars =
25 μm.**

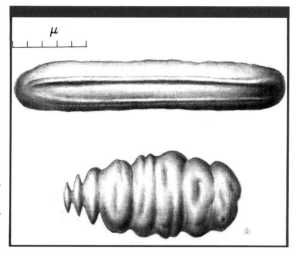

FIGURE 4.50
Deformation of
myocardial nu-
clei by myocar-
dial contraction:
an artist's view.
Top: relaxed con-
dition. *Bottom:*
contracted condi-
tion. (Adapted
from [249].)

*transcriptional activity in various cell types: embry-
onic cells have very little of it, highly specialized cells
such as lymphocytes have a great deal.*

Nuclear size can also reflect nuclear ploidy, which
represents another vital concern in tumor diagnosis. In practice, (a) a large, pale nucleus suggests
an active transcriptional state; (b) a large and very
basophilic nucleus suggests excessive DNA con-

tent; (c) a small and very basophilic nucleus
suggests a low level of activity (transcription
turned off).

In contractile cells, *the oblong nucleus becomes
wrinkled like an accordion when the cell contracts*
(Figure 4.50). This phenomenon gave the first
hint that endothelial cells are contractile; it also
helped identify the contractile modulation of
fibroblasts (p. 472). *Grotesque nuclear shapes are
typical of malignant tumors.*

The rock bottom of nuclear pathology is that *if
the nucleus has disappeared, the cell must have been
dead for a long time.* This notion, however
rudimentary, is very practical in histopathology:
an area without nuclei is (usually) a cemetery of
cells. The nucleus can break down in three ways: it
can slowly lose its affinity for basic dyes and fade
away (**karyolysis,** typical of ischemic cell death);
conversely, it can shrivel into a dense, highly
basophilic mass (**pyknosis,** from *pyknós,* dense);
or it can become pyknotic and then break up into
small pieces (**karyorhexis**) (Figure 4.51). Pyknosis
and karyorhexis are important because they suggest that the cell may have committed suicide
(apoptosis, p. 200).

> *The nucleus is the only cellular organelle to suffer the
> indignity of being expelled from the cytoplasm, such
> as during the maturation of erythrocytes (261). With
> cytochalasin it is possible to produce this phenomenon
> at will in other cells. An enucleated cell is called a
> **cytoplast.***

The electron microscopy of the nucleus has
been somewhat disappointing, because chromosomes are simply not visible on routine ultrathin
sections. However, *the nucleolus shows characteristic
ultrastructural changes under the influence of inhibitors
of protein synthesis,* such as actinomycin or
ethionine; that is, its components become segregated into two or three discrete masses (Figure
4.52) (251, 266).

Nuclear inclusions listed to date are so many that
only an atlas can do them justice (254): they
include cellular organelles that were perhaps
trapped during mitosis, droplets of lipid, glycogen,
or protein, membrane infoldings, viruses, fibrils,
crystals, and tubules; most are unexplained and
visible only by electron microscopy. Easily seen by
light and electron microscopy are the *lead inclusion
bodies* found in epithelial cells of the renal
convoluted tubules and in liver cells as a result of
chronic lead intoxication (Figure 4.53) (256, 262,

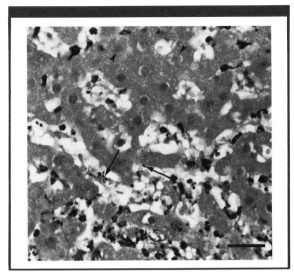

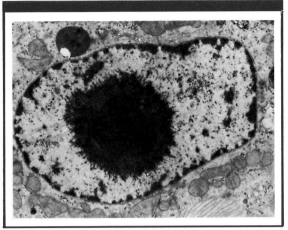

FIGURE 4.53
Lead inclusion body (dense mass) in a nucleus. From the proximal convoluted tubule of a man professionally exposed to lead. (Reproduced with permission from [255].)

FIGURE 4.51
Two ways of nuclear demise: karyolysis (**arrowheads**) and karyorhexis (**arrows**). The moon-shaped vacuoles around the karyolytic nuclei represent swelling of the perinuclear cisterna of the endoplasmic reticulum. From a fragment of rat liver implanted into the peritoneum. Stage = 24 hours. **Bar** = 25 μm.

possibly because the toxic lead is safely sequestered in the mass. Lead inclusion bodies have turned up in plants growing by the roadside, another sign of environmental pollution (267).

THE STUDY OF CHROMOSOMES: CYTOGENETICS

A great deal can be learned from the direct microscopic study of chromosomes, which can be visualized only in dividing cells. The basic principle is to start with a cell culture (e.g., white blood cells) and to treat it with colchicine, which arrests the mitoses in metaphase (p. 155). At this stage, using a nuclear stain, the chromosomes are

268). The fact that lead would choose to precipitate in the nuclei of just those two tissues is another example of the myriad of unexplained specificities of drugs and toxic agents. Cells with lead inclusion bodies look remarkably unaffected,

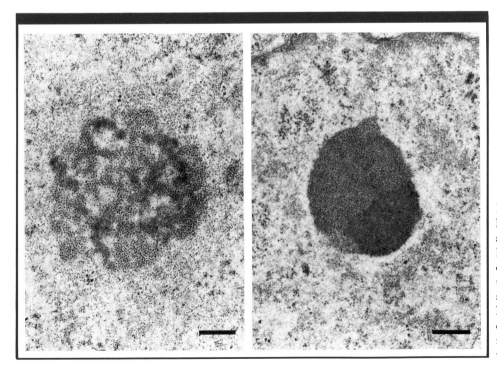

FIGURE 4.52
Effect of a protein synthesis inhibitor, actinomycin D, on the nucleolus of liver cells (rat). *Left:* Normal liver nucleolus, showing the typical lacy structure. *Right:* Nucleolus 2 hours after actinomycin (1 μg/g body weight). Nucleolar components have separated out into two and possibly three masses. **Bars** = 0.5 μm. (Reproduced with permission from [250].)

visible—but clustered and not individually recognizable. By a fortunate accident it was discovered that distilled water swells the mitotic cells; using this trick it is possible to obtain "spreads" of the metaphase chromosomes. With some luck, one or more of the spreads will be perfect, with all the chromosomes separated. The best mitoses are then photographed and suitable enlargements are printed. The next step is very empirical but it works: from one such enlargement, all the images of chromosomes are cut out with scissors, identified by size and shape, paired, and pasted on a sheet in a standard order. This display is called a **karyotype** (Figure 4.54): in humans it consists of 22 pairs of autosomes, plus two sex chromosomes, XX in females and XY in males. Some applications of this technique are discussed in Chapter 29.

MOLECULAR BIOLOGY: TRANSGENIC ANIMALS

Transgenic mice appeared on the scene in 1980. The term transgenic, as our readers surely know, means that these creatures carry sequences in their genome that have been inserted by laboratory techniques (260, 265, 269). The most common way to produce a transgenic animal is to microinject the DNA sequence of interest into the nucleus of a one-cell embryo; this sequence will then integrate into the genome (randomly, at least by the current techniques), and the altered genome is then transmitted to the offspring in mendelian fashion. This revolutionary development is now taken for granted, for the study of normal as well as of defective genes, including the tumor-related oncogenes.

MOLECULAR GENETICS: METHODS OF MOLECULAR PATHOLOGY

Although the topic of molecular genetics is beyond the scope of our book, the reader should be aware of recent techniques that have had an enormous impact on medical science (252, 253, 258, 260, 261a). When applied to problems of pathology these methods are currently known as molecular pathology. This term is here to stay, but it is an obvious misnomer. It seems to imply the study of pathology at the level of all molecules, whereas it is focused on the pathology of DNA, RNA and their products.

The techniques that we will sketch here are derived from the same DNA wizardry that led to

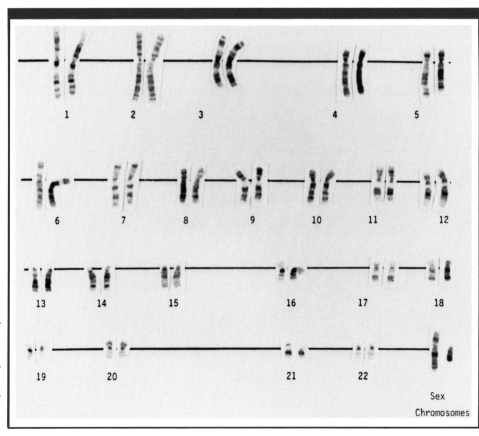

FIGURE 4.54
Normal human karyotype (male), displayed in the standard manner. The bands on the chromosomes were obtained by treatment with trypsin followed by Giemsa stain. (Courtesy of Dr. P.L. Townes, University of Massachusetts Medical Center, Worcester, MA.)

transgenic animals, but all are *in vitro* methods. They all rely on the same basic principle: the DNA molecule is made of two parallel and complementary strands held together by hydrogen bonds. If the DNA molecule is gently heated (i.e., heat denatured), the two strands come apart; then if they are brought into proximity, they show the uncanny ability to reanneal exactly in the same position (Figure 4.55). This means that a short piece of artificially prepared single-stranded DNA, mixed with single-stranded DNA, will anneal or **hybridize** with the complementary segment of DNA—if any such segment is present. These short pieces of artificially prepared DNA, called **probes,** will hybridize whether the complementary DNA is in solution or in the nuclei of histologic sections.

The same principles apply to RNA. Thus, hybridization may occur as DNA/DNA, RNA/RNA, or DNA/RNA.

Hybridization is not to be confused with recombination, which refers to the end-to-end attachment of double-stranded DNA fragments, which have "sticky ends."

The scientific applications of hybridization are limitless as long as the necessary DNA and RNA probes are at hand. These probes are obtained commercially, and producing them is part of this new science (they are prepared by cloning genes or cDNA fragments in bacterial cells; they can also be produced by amplification using the polymerase chain reaction, PCR) (258).

The **polymerase chain reaction** is a magnificent trick for multiplying enzymatically the amount of DNA in very small samples; within a matter of hours a tiny sample can be amplified a million times. So important is this method that polymerase was nominated as Molecule of the Year—the first—in 1989 (259).

This methodology can be applied to tissue sections or to tissue extracts; each has its advantages. *In* **histologic sections,** *DNA or RNA probes can be made visible by any one of the methods shown in Figure 4.56.* The beauty of this microscopic method is its sensitivity; even a single cell shows up if it contains the specific DNA (Figure 4.57), whereas the *in vitro* method to be described later, the Southern blot, requires about one million cells (252). The DNA molecule is so resistant to change that the probes can be used on tissues that have been long since fixed and embedded in paraffin, and even on tissues of ancient mummies (263).

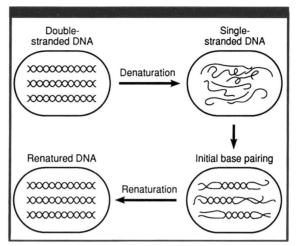

FIGURE 4.55

A basic procedure of molecular biology: denaturation (melting) and renaturation (reannealing) of DNA. Gentle heating causes the double-stranded DNA to unwind into two single strands; upon cooling, the single strands "find" each other and reanneal in the same sequence as in the original DNA. (Adapted from [251].)

Here are two of the questions that can be answered by using probes on histologic sections. Is viral genome present in the cells? Is a given gene activated? The latter very subtle question can be answered by searching for the appropriate mRNA; it can also be answered by looking for the gene product, if the specific antibody is available.

The standard method for examining the DNA in **tissue extracts** *is the so-called Southern blot,* named after Dr. Edward M. Southern of Dallas, Texas. This and related methods are mentioned so often in the literature that it may be helpful to outline them here.

The basic principle of the **Southern blot** is shown in Figure 4.58. The DNA, obtained from a cell lysate, is digested into segments using an appropriate restriction endonuclease (an enzyme that recognizes a particular base sequence and cuts the DNA molecule only at the sites where that sequence occurs). The digest is then drawn electrophoretically along a plate of agarose gel; the shorter segments migrate farther, and to assess their molecular weight, standard molecules of known molecular weight are run alongside. Then the agarose gel is soaked in alkali to denature the DNA. Next, the whole mass of electrophoresed fragments is transferred to another gel (usually a sheet of nitrocellulose) that is more suitable for the following step of the procedure. To accomplish the transfer the sheet of nitrocellulose is placed over the agarose and

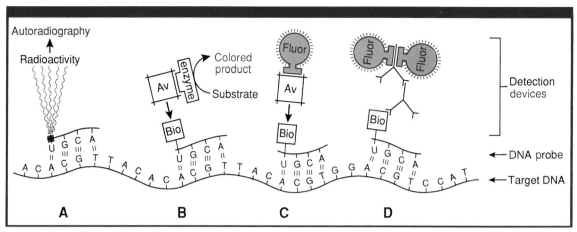

FIGURE 4.56

Basic principle of *in situ* hybridization, aimed at identifying specific sequences in nuclear DNA (target DNA). The key is to have a specific DNA probe (here labeled UGCA) that hybridizes with the DNA sequence that is to be identified. Once hybridized, the probe is made visible—in tissue sections—by one of four methods. **A**: With a radioactive label, to be detected by autoradiography. **B**: By enzyme histochemistry; the probe is labeled with biotin, and then the biotin is bound to avidin, a protein, which in turn carries an enzyme capable of producing a colored product. **C**: A variant of **B** in which the avidin carrier is bound to a fluorescent molecule. **D**: Double-antibody method, also based on fluorescence. (Adapted from [257].)

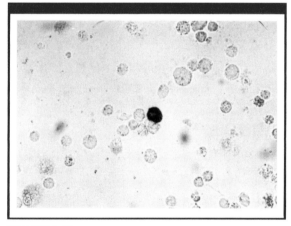

FIGURE 4.57

Detection of HIV-1-infected lymphocytes by means of *in situ* hybridization, in the peripheral blood of a hemophilic patient infected with HIV-1 by treatment with contaminated Factor VIII. During the early symptom-free interval, lymphocytes were obtained by centrifugation and placed on a slide. A biotinated HIV genomic probe was hybridized to the cells and detected by alkaline phosphatase linked to streptavidin. The histochemical reaction for alkaline phosphatase produced a dark brown deposit (black cell in center). This positive reaction indicates the presence of viral RNA. Note that only one of many lymphocytes expresses HIV RNA. This is typical for this phase of the disease: 1/1000–1/10,000 of the blood lymphocytes are usually positive. (Courtesy of Dr. R. H. Singer, University of Massachusetts Medical School, Worcester, MA.)

covered with a stack of absorbent paper, which acts as a wick, drawing water and DNA from one gel into the other. In the end, the DNA fragments are distributed in the same way in the nitrocellulose gel as they were in the agarose. The nitrocellulose sheet is then immersed in a solution containing a radioactive probe, selected according to the purpose of the test. The probe hybridizes with the complementary DNA, and its location is determined by autoradiography. The final product is an autoradiograph.

Northern blots (a pun on the name of Dr. Southern) are the RNA equivalent of Southern blots. The joke has been extended to **Western blots,** used for sizing polypeptides by gel electrophoresis. The **Dot-blot** is a simpler and faster variety of hybridization in which a known amount of DNA or RNA is dripped onto a membrane as a 4-mm dot and is then denatured and hybridized; the intensity of the radioactive dot is compared with that of dots prepared with known standards.

Restriction fragment length polymorphisms or RFLP (we agree that the name is repulsive) are harmless but useful oddities of the DNA molecule that can be brought out by Southern blots. Let us first clarify the name. An RFLP is a change in the length of the DNA fragments that are produced by restriction enzymes. DNA polymorphisms represent variations in genetic material between individuals; they occur every 200–500 base pairs (252). Some polymorphisms occur in or near

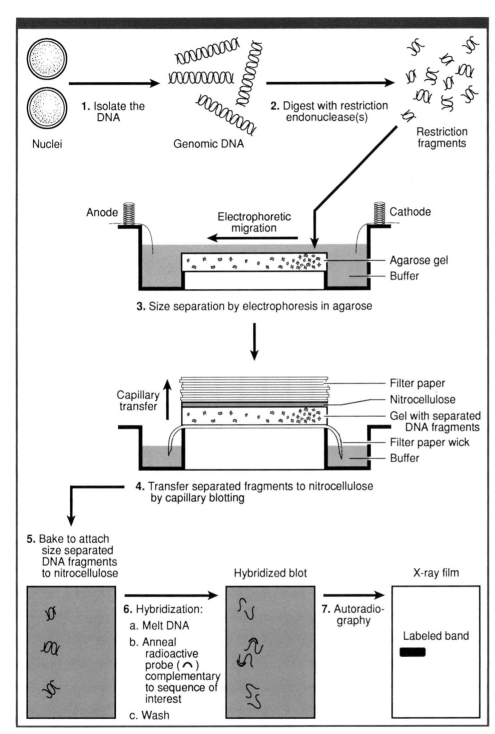

FIGURE 4.58
Southern blot hybridization: a method used for characterizing the organization of DNA that surrounds a specific nucleic acid sequence, e.g., a particular gene. (Adapted from Abbas AK, Lichtman AH, Prober JS. Cellular and molecular immunology. Philadelphia: W.B. Saunders Company, 1991, p. 73.)

genes and may be associated with phenotypic changes and disease. Others occur in noncoding DNA and may have no obvious effect on the phenotype; however, they are of interest for two reasons: (1) they represent an individual (innocuous) trait that can be used for "molecular fingerprinting," which is of great value in forensic medicine; (2) for reasons unknown, polymorph-

isms may be linked with a specific abnormal trait; if the trait is recessive, an RFLP may be present to indicate that the individual carries the gene. Carriers of the gene can therefore be identified.

Polymorphisms can be detected on Southern blots. After digestion of the DNA with a particular restriction enzyme, the pattern of bands on a Southern blot depends on the size of the frag-

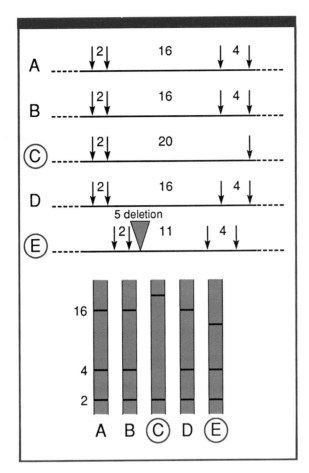

FIGURE 4.59

Hypothetical restriction map of part of the X chromosome from five males. *Top:* Horizontal lines represent DNA molecules cut by a restriction enzyme at certain points (**arrows**). Numbers represent lengths of restriction fragments in kilobases. Individuals **A**, **B**, and **D** have identical restriction maps with this enzyme. **C** and **E** illustrate restriction fragment length polymorphisms: **C** due to a point mutation that abolishes one of the restriction sites and **E** due to a deletion in the largest fragment between two adjacent restriction sites. *Bottom:* Agarose gel and electrophoresis of restriction fragments illustrated above. The polymorphism between individuals is obvious. (Reproduced with permission from [254].)

ments. Suppose that a deletion in an intron has deleted precisely a base sequence recognized by the restriction enzyme: no cut will be made at that spot, and the result will be a larger and slower-moving DNA fragment (Figure 4.59).

A closing thought. Today molecular genetics is everywhere, but how did it all start? Our readers should know of the forgotten hero of this saga, Frederick Griffith, a little-known British medical officer so dedicated to his work that he was killed

FIGURE 4.60

The classic transformation experiment by Avery et al. in 1944. At left, small colonies of pneumococcus Type II, "rough" variant, are growing on agar. At right, colonies of the *same* pneumococcus grown in the presence of "transforming principle" (DNA) obtained from Type III pneumococci. The smooth, glistening, mucoid colonies are typical of pneumococcus Type III. The conclusion is that exogenous DNA has been able to transform pneumococci Type II into Type III. (Reproduced with permission from [247].)

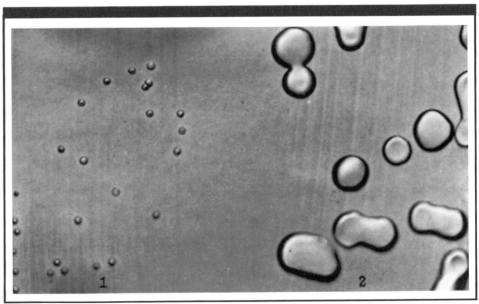

in his laboratory during an air raid over London in 1941 (257, 264). In 1928 he made a critical observation. Having noticed some unexplained shifts in the types of pneumococci in the population of his district, he tried to find out whether one type of pneumococcus could be turned into another. He did so *in vivo* by injecting mice with live pneumococci of a nonvirulent strain, together with dead pneumococci from a virulent strain: the mice died of infection with the virulent strain. Griffith concluded that something coming from the dead virulent bacteria had transformed the nonvirulent bacteria; in 1944 that "something" was identified as DNA by Avery, MacLeod, and McCarty at the Rockefeller Institute (Figure 4.60) (247).

References

Pathology of the Cell Membrane

1. Alberts B, Bray D, Lewis J, Raff M, Roberts K, Watson JD. Molecular biology of the cell. New York: Garland Publishing, Inc., 1989.
2. Andreoli TE, Hoffman JF, Fanestil DD (eds). Physiology of membrane disorders. New York and London: Plenum Medical Book Co., 1978.
3. Arahata K, Ishiura S, Ishiguro T, et al. Immunostaining of skeletal and cardiac muscle surface membrane with antibody against Duchenne muscular dystrophy peptide. Nature 1988;333:861–863.
4. Bangham AD, Horne RW. Negative staining of phospholipids and their structural modification by surface-active agents as observed in the electron microscope. J Mol Biol 1964;8:660–668.
5. Beck IT, Dinda PK. Acute exposure of small intestine to ethanol: effects on morphology and function. Dig Dis Sci 1981;26:817–838.
6. Bessis M. Living blood cells and their ultrastructure. Berlin: Springer-Verlag, 1973.
7. Bianchi G, Carafoli E, Scarpa A (eds). Membrane pathology. (Ann NY Acad Sci, Vol 488). New York: The New York Academy of Sciences, 1986.
8. Bolis L, Hoffman JF, Leaf A (eds). Membranes and disease. New York: Raven Press, 1976.
9. Bourguignon LYW, Bourguignon GJ. Capping and the cytoskeleton. Int Rev Cytol 1984;47:195–224.
10. Boutet M, Hüttner I, Rona G. Permeability alteration of sarcolemmal membrane in catecholamine-induced cardiac muscle cell injury. Lab Invest 1976;34:482–488.
11. Brown MS, Goldstein JL. Familial hypercholesterolemia: defective binding of lipoproteins to cultured fibroblast associated with impaired regulation of 3-hydroxy-3-methylglutaryl coenzyme A reductase activity. Proc Natl Acad Sci USA 1974;71:788–792.
12. Bücherl W, Buckley E (eds). Venomous animals and their venoms. Volume II. Venomous vertebrates. New York: Academic Press, 1971.
13. Bücherl W, Buckley EE, Deulofeu V (eds). Venomous animals and their venoms. Volume I. Venomous vertebrates. New York: Academic Press, 1968.
14. Buckley IK. Tissue injury by high frequency electric current: observations with the Sandison-Clark ear chamber. Aust J Exp Biol Med Sci 1960;38:211–226.
15. Crane RK, Menard D, Preiser H, Cerda J. The molecular basis of brush-border membrane disease. In: Bolis L, Hoffman JF, Leaf A (eds). Membranes and disease. New York: Raven Press, 1976, pp. 229–241.
16. Damjanov I. Lectin cytochemistry and histochemistry. Lab Invest 1987;57:5–20.
17. Eidels L, Proia RL, Hart DA. Membrane receptors for bacterial toxins. Microbiol Rev 1983;47:596–620.
18. England SB, Nicholson LVB, Johnson MA, et al. Very mild muscular dystrophy associated with the deletion of 46% of dystrophin. Nature 1990;343:180–182.
19. Frimmer M, Petzinger E. Mechanism of phalloidin intoxication I: cell membrane alterations. In: Popper H, Bianchi L, Reutter W (eds). Membrane alterations as basis of liver injury. Falk Symposium 22. Baltimore: University Park Press, 1977, pp. 293–299.
20. Fuhrman FA. Tetrodotoxin. Sci Am 1967;217:60–71.
21. Goldstein DB. The effects of drugs on membrane fluidity. Annu Rev Pharmacol Toxicol 1984;24:43–64.
22. Goldstein IJ, Poretz RD. Isolation, physicochemical characterization, and carbohydrate-binding specificity of lectins. In: Liener IE, Sharon N, Goldstein IJ (eds). The lectins: properties, functions, and applications in biology and medicine. Orlando: Academic Press, Inc., 1986, pp. 33–247.
23. Herman B, Nieminen AL, Gores GJ, Lemasters JJ. Irreversible injury in anoxic hepatocytes precipitated by an abrupt increase in plasma membrane permeability. FASEB J 1988;2:146–151.
24. Hoffstein S, Gennaro DE, Fox AC, Hirsch J, Streuli F, Weissmann G. Colloidal lanthanum as a marker for impaired plasma membrane permeability in ischemic dog myocardium. Am J Pathol 1975;79:207–218.
25. Jewell SA, Bellomo G, Thor H, Orrenius S, Smith MT. Bleb formation in hepatocytes during drug metabolism is caused by disturbances in thiol and calcium ion homeostasis. Science 1982;217:1257–1259.
26. Johnston WH, Latta H, Osvaldo L. Variations in glomerular ultrastructure in rat kidneys fixed by perfusion. J Ultrastruct Res 1973;45:149–167.
27. Kretchmer N. Memorial Lecture: lactose and lactase—a historical perspective. Gastroenterology 1971;61:805–813.
28. Leaf A, Macknight ADC. Ischemia and disturbances in cell volume regulation. In: Andreoli TE, Hoffman JF, Fanestil DD (eds). Physiology of membrane disorders. New York: Plenum Medical Book Company, 1978, pp. 1093–1100.
29. Lemasters JJ, DiGuiseppi J, Nieminen A-L, Herman B. Blebbing, free Ca²⁺ and mitochondrial membrane potential preceding cell death in hepatocytes. Nature 1987;325:78–81.
30. Liener IE, Sharon N, Goldstein IJ (eds). The lectins: properties, functions, and applications in biology and medicine. Orlando: Academic Press, Inc., 1986.
31. Lucy JA. The fusion of cell membranes. In: Weissmann G, Claiborne R (eds). Cell membranes: biochemistry, cell biology & pathology. New York: HP Publishing Co., Inc., 1975, pp. 75–83.
32. Lucy JA. Is there a membrane defect in muscle and other cells? Br Med Bull 1980;36:187–192.

33. Lucy JA, Glauert AM. Structure and assembly of macromolecular lipid complexes composed of globular micelles. J Mol Biol 1964;8:727–748.

34. Majno G, La Gattuta M, Thompson TE. Cellular death and necrosis: chemical, physical and morphologic changes in rat liver. Virchows Arch Pathol Anat 1960;333:421–465.

35. Mokri B, Engel AG. Duchenne dystrophy: electron microscopic findings pointing to a basic or early abnormality in the plasma membrane of the muscle fiber. Neurology 1975;25:1111–1120.

36. Moldovan NI, Radu AN, Simionescu N. Endothelial cell plasma membrane obtained by chemically induced vesiculation. Exp Cell Res 1987;170:499–510.

37. Nicotera P, Hartzell P, Davis G, Orrenius S. The formation of plasma membrane blebs in hepatocytes exposed to agents that increase cytosolic Ca^{2+} is mediated by the activation of a nonlysosomal proteolytic system. FEBS Lett 1986;209:139–144.

38. Ostwald R. Cholesterol and membranes. In: Dupont J (ed). Cholesterol systems in insects and animals. Boca Raton: CRC Press, Inc., 1982, pp. 51–75.

39. Phelps PC, Smith MW, Trump BF. Cytosolic ionized calcium and bleb formation after acute cell injury of cultured rabbit renal tubule cells. Lab Invest 1989; 60:630–642.

40. Putney JW, Jr, Askari A. Modification of membrane function by drugs. In: Andreoli TE, Hoffman JF, Fanestil DD (eds). Physiology of membrane disorders. New York: Plenum Medical Book Company, 1978, pp. 417–445.

41. Rona G, Hüttner I, More RH. Fibrin as a natural tracer in cardiac muscle cell injury. Thromb Diath Haemm Suppl 1973;56:21–33.

42. Rubenstein E. Diseases caused by impaired communication among cells. Sci Am 1980;242:102–116, 120–121.

43. Ryan US, Schultz DR, Ryan JW. Fc and C3b receptors on pulmonary endothelial cells: induction by injury. Science 1981;214:557–558.

44. Sage MD, Jennings RB. Cytoskeletal injury and subsarcolemmal bleb formation in dog heart during in vitro total ischemia. Am J Pathol 1988;133:327–337.

45. Schnaar RL. The membrane is the message. The Sciences 1986;May/June:34–40.

46. Schotland DL, Bonilla E, van Meter M. Duchenne dystrophy: alteration in muscle plasma membrane structure. Science 1977;196:1005–1007.

47. Schreiner GF, Unanue ER. Membrane and cytoplasmic changes in B lymphocytes induced by ligand-surface immunoglobulin interaction. Adv Immunol 1976;24:37–165.

48. Schwartz P, Piper HM, Spahr R, Spieckermann PG. Ultrastructure of cultured adult myocardial cells during anoxia and reoxygenation. Am J Pathol 1984;115:349–361.

49. Seeman P. Transient holes in the erythrocyte membrane during hypotonic hemolysis and stable holes in the membrane after lysis by saponin and lysolecithin. J Cell Biol 1967;32:55–70.

50. Silver IA, Murrills RJ, Etherington DJ. Microelectrode studies on the acid microenvironment beneath adherent macrophages and osteoclasts. Exp Cell Res 1988;175: 266–276.

51. Singer SJ, Nicolson GL. The fluid mosaic model of the structure of cell membranes. Science 1972;175:720–731.

52. Snyder LM, Fairbanks G, Trainor JP, Fortier NL, Jacobs JB, Leb L. Properties and characterization of vesicles released by young and old human red cells. Br J Haematol 1985;59:513–522.

53. Snyder LM, Lutz HU, Sauberman N, Jacobs J, Fortier NL. Fragmentation and myelin formation in hereditary xerocytosis and other hemolytic anemias. Blood 1978;52: 750–761.

54. Stryer L. Biochemistry, 3rd ed. New York: WH Freeman and Company, 1988.

55. Tao M (ed). Membrane abnormalities and disease. Volumes I and II. Boca Raton, CRC Press, Inc., 1982.

56. Tao M, Conway RG. Biochemical aspects of normal and abnormal erythrocyte membranes. In: Tao M (ed). Membrane abnormalities and disease, volume I. Boca Raton, CRC Press, Inc., 1982, pp. 43–90.

57. Taraschi TF, Rubin E. Biology of disease: effects of ethanol on the chemical and structural properties of biologic membranes. Lab Invest 1985;52:120–131.

58. Teixeira JRM, Lapa AJ, Souccar C, Valle JR. Timbós. Ichthyotoxic plants used by Brazilian indians. J Ethnopharmacol 1984;10:311–318.

59. Trump BF, Berezesky IK, Phelps PC, Jones RT. An overview of the role of membranes in human disease. In: Trump BF, Laufer A, Jones RT (eds). Cellular pathobiology of human disease. New York: Gustav Fischer, 1983, pp. 3–48.

60. Trump BF, Laufer A, Jones RT (eds.) Cellular pathobiology of human disease. New York: Gustav Fischer, 1983.

61. Trump BF, Penttila A, Berezesky IK. Studies on cell surface conformation following injury. Virchows Arch. B Cell Pathol 1979;29:281–296.

62. Wagner R, Gabbert H, Höhn P. The mechanism of epithelial shedding after ischemic damage to the small intestinal mucosa. A light and electron microscopic investigation. Virchows Arch B Cell Pathol 1979;30:25–31.

63. Wagner R, Gabbert H, Höhn P. Ischemia and postischemic regeneration of the small intestinal mucosa. A light microscopic and autoradiographic study. Virchows Arch B Cell Pathol 1979;31:259–276.

64. Wallach DFH (ed). Plasma membranes and disease. London: Academic Press, 1979.

65. Weissmann G, Claiborne, R (eds). Cell membranes: biochemistry, cell biology & pathology. New York: HP Publishing Company, Inc., 1975.

66. Zubrzycka-Gaarn EE, Bulman DE, Karpati G, et al. The Duchenne muscular dystrophy gene product is localized in sarcolemma of human skeletal muscle. Nature 1988;333: 466–469.

Pathology of the Mitochondria

67. Bereiter-Hahn J, Vöth M. Metabolic control of shape and structure of mitochondria in situ. Biol Cell 1983;47:309–322.

68. Carafoli E, Roman I. Mitochondria and disease. Mol Aspects Med 1980;3:295–429.

69. DiMauro S, Bonilla E, Zeyiani M, Nakagawa M, DeVivo DC. Mitochondrial myopathies. Ann Neurol 1985;17: 521–538.

70. DeRobertis EDP, DeRobertis EMF. Cell and molecular biology. Philadelphia, Saunders College, 1980.

71. Ferrans VJ. Cardiac hypertrophy: morphological aspects. In: Zak R (ed). Growth of the heart in health and disease. New York: Raven Press, 1984, pp. 187–239.

72. Greenawalt JW, Rossi CS, Lehninger AL. Effect of active accumulation of calcium and phosphate ions on the structure of rat liver mitochondria. J Cell Biol 1964;23:21–38.

73. Hackenbrock CR. Ultrastructural bases for metabolically linked mechanical activity in mitochondria. I. Reversible ultrastructural changes with change in metabolic steady

state in isolated liver mitochondria. J Cell Biol 1966;30: 269–297.

74. Hackenbrock CR. Ultrastructural bases for metabolically linked mechanical activity in mitochondria. II. Electron transport-linked ultrastructural transformations in mitochondria. J Cell Biol 1968; 37:345–369.

75. Harris RA, Williams CH, Caldwell M, Green DE, Valdivia E. Energized configurations of heart mitochondria in situ. Science 1969;165:700–702.

75a. Johns DR. Mitochondrial DNA and disease. N. Engl J Med 1995;333:638–644.

76. Lane MD, Pedersen PL, Mildvan AS. The mitochondrion updated. Science 1986;234:526–527.

77. Lehninger AL. Respiration-linked mechanochemical changes in mitochondria. In: Kasha M, Pullman B (eds). Horizons in biochemistry. New York: London, Academic Press, 1962, pp. 421–435.

78. Lehninger AL. Water uptake and extrusion by mitochondria in relation to oxidative phosphorylation. Physiol Rev 1962;42:467–517.

79. Luft R, Ikkos D, Palmieri G, Ernster L, Afzelius B. A case of severe hypermetabolism of nonthyroid origin with a defect in the maintenance of mitochondrial respiratory control: a correlated clinical, biochemical, and morphological study. J Clin Invest 1962;41:1776–1804.

80. Morgan-Hughes JA. Mitochondrial myopathies. In: Mastaglia FL, Walton J (eds). Skeletal muscle pathology. Edinburgh: Churchill Livingstone, 1982, pp. 309–339.

81. Pfeifer U. Ultrastructural pathology of the human liver. In: Csomós G, Thaler H (eds). Clinical hepatology. Berlin: Springer-Verlag, 1983, pp. 159–194.

82. Robinson JM, Tanphaichitr N, Bellvé AR. Gossypol-induced damage to mitochondria of transformed Sertoli cells. Am J Pathol 1986;125:484–492.

83. Roodyn DB, Wilkie D. The biogenesis of mitochondria. London: Methuen & Co., Ltd., 1968.

84. Rubin E, Beattie DS, Toth A, Lieber CS. Structural and functional effects of ethanol on hepatic mitochondria. Fed Proc 1972;31:131–175.

85. Schaffino S, Severin E, Hanzlíková V. Intermembrane inclusions induced by anoxia in heart and skeletal muscle mitochondria. Virchows Arch B Cell Pathol 1979;31: 169–179.

86. Sherman J, Angulo M, Boxer RA, Gluck R. Possible mitochondrial inheritance of congenital cardiac septal defects. N Engl J Med 1985;313:186–187.

87. Smith U, Smith DS, Yunis AA. Chloramphenicol-related changes in mitochondrial ultrastructure. J Cell Sci 1970;7:501–521.

88. Sun CN, White HJ, Thompson BW. Oncocytoma (mitochondrioma) of the parotid gland. Arch Pathol 1975;99:208–214.

89. Suzuki K. Giant hepatic mitochondria: production in mice fed with cuprizone. Science 1969;163:81–82.

90. Tandler B, Hutter RVP, Erlandson RA. Ultrastructure of oncocytoma of the parotid gland. Lab Invest 1970;23: 567–580.

91. Tandler B, Shipkey FH. Ultrastructure of warthin's tumor. I. Mitochondria. J Ultrastruct Res 1964;11:292–305.

92. Thomas RS, Greenawalt JW. Microincineration, electron microscopy, and electron diffraction of calcium phosphate-loaded mitochondria. J Cell Biol 1968;39:55–76.

93. Wakabayashi T, Asano M, Kawamoto S. Induction of megamitochondria in the mouse liver by isonicotinic acid derivatives. Exp Mol Pathol 1979;31:387–399.

94. Wallace DC. Mitochondrial genes and disease. Hosp Pract 1986;21:77–92.

Pathology of the Endoplasmic Reticulum

95. Berg NO, Eriksson S. Liver disease in adults with alpha-1-antitrypsin deficiency. N Engl J Med 1972;287:1264–1267.

96. Bessis M. Cell death. Triangle 1970;9:191–199.

97. Bolmer S, Kleinerman J. Isolation and characterization of α_1-antitrypsin in PAS-positive hepatic granules from rats with experimental α_1-antitrypsin deficiency. Am J Pathol 1986;123:377–389.

98. Buckley IK. Phase contrast observations on the endoplasmic reticulum of living cells in culture. Protoplasma 1964;59:569–588.

99. Callea F, Brisigotti M, Fabbretti G. Bonino F, Desmet VJ. Hepatic endoplasmic reticulum storage diseases. Liver 1992;12:357–62.

100. Carlson JA, Rogers BB, Sifers RN, et al. Accumulation of PiZ α_1-antitrypsin causes liver damage in transgenic mice. J Clin Invest 1989;83:1183–1190.

101. Carlson JA, Rogers BB, Sifers RN, Hawkins HK, Finegold MJ, Woo SLC. Multiple tissues express alpha_1-antitrypsin in transgenic mice and man. J Clin Invest 1988;82:26–36.

102. Dawkins MJR. Carbon tetrachloride poisoning in the liver of the new-born rat. J Pathol Bacteriol 1963;85: 189–196.

103. Durham SK, Boyd MR, Castleman WL. Pulmonary endothelial and bronchiolar epithelial lesions induced by 4-ipomeanol in mice. Am J Pathol 1985;118:66–75.

104. Eriksson S. Discovery of α_1-antitrypsin deficiency. Lung 1990;Suppl:523–529.

105. Eriksson S. Alpha_1-antitrypsin deficiency: lessons learned from the bedside to the gene and back again. Historic perspectives. Chest 1989;95:181–189.

106. Farber E, Liang H, Shinozuka H. Dissociation of effects on protein synthesis and ribosomes from membrane changes induced by carbon tetrachloride. Am J Pathol 1971;64:601–617.

107. Floersheim GL. Schutzwirkung hepatotoxischer Stoffe gegen letale Dosen eines Toxins aus Amanita phalloides (phalloidin). Biochem Pharmacol 1966;15:1589–1593.

108. Hurtley SM, Helenius A. Protein oligomerization in the endoplasmic reticulum. Annu Rev Cell Biol 1989;5: 277–307.

109. Jusko WJ. Smoking effects in pharmacokinetics. In: Benet LZ, Massoud N, Gambertoglio JG (eds). Pharmacokinetic basis for drug treatment. New York: Raven Press, 1984, pp. 311–320.

110. Klausner RD, Lippincott-Schwartz J, Bonifacino JS. The T cell antigen receptor: Insights into organelle biology. Annu Rev Cell Biol 1990;6:403–431.

111. Kupfer D. Endogenous substrates of monooxygenases: fatty acids and prostaglandins. Pharmacol Ther 1980;11: 469–496.

112. Langman J, Cardell L. Ultrastructural observations on FUdR-induced cell death and subsequent elimination of cell debris. Teratology 1978;17:229–270.

113. Lieberman J, Mittman C, Schneider AS. Screening for homozygous and heterozygous α_1-antitrypsin deficiency. Protein electrophoresis on cellulose acetate membranes. JAMA 1969;210:2055–2060.

114. Luczynska C, Wilson K. The clinical significance of the effects of cigarette smoking on drug disposition. Methods Find Exp Clin Pharmacol 1983;5:479–487.

115. Nelson DR, Kamataki T, Waxman DJ, et al. The P450 superfamily: update on new sequences, gene mapping, accession numbers, early trivial names of enzymes, and nomenclature. DNA Cell Biol 1993;12:1–51.

116. Ortiz de Montellano PR. Cytochrome P-450. New York: Plenum Press, 1986.
117. Palade G.E. A small particulate component of the cytoplasm. J Appl Phys 1953;24:1419.
118. Pfeifer U, Ormanns W, Klinge O. Hepatocellular fibrinogen storage in familial hypofibrinogenemia. Virchows Arch Cell Pathol 1981;36:247–255.
119. Phillips MJ, Poucell S, Patterson J, Valencia P. The liver: an atlas and text of ultrastructural pathology. New York: Raven Press, 1987.
120. Porter KR. Electron microscopy of basophilic components of cytoplasm. J Histochem Cytochem 1954;2:346–373.
121. Porter KR, Claude A, Fullam EF. A study of tissue culture cells by electron microscopy. Methods and preliminary observations. J Exp Med 1945;81:233–246.
122. Recknagel RO, Ghoshal AK. Lipoperoxidation as a vector in carbon tetrachloride hepatotoxicity. Lab Invest 1966;15:132–146.
123. Recknagel RO, Glende EA, Jr, Hruszkewycz AM. Chemical mechanisms in carbon tetrachloride toxicity. In: Pryor WA (ed). Free radicals in biology. Vol. III. New York: Academic Press, 1977, pp. 97–132.
124. Rifkind RA, Osserman EF, Hsu KC, Morgan C. The intracellular distribution of gamma globulin in a mouse plasma cell tumor (X5563) as revealed by fluorescence and electron microscopy. J Exp Med 1962;116:423–432.
125. Russell W. An address on a characteristic organism of cancer. Br Med J 1890;2:1356–1360.
126. Shultz LD, Coman DR, Lyons BL, Sidman CL, Taylor S. Development of plasmacytoid cells with Russell bodies in autoimmune "viable motheaten" mice. Am J Pathol 1987;127:38–50.
127. Sifers RN, Finegold MJ, Woo SLC. Alpha-1-antitrypsin deficiency: accumulation or degradation of mutant variants within the hepatic endoplasmic reticulum. Am J Respir Cell Mol Biol 1989;1:341–345.
128. Singer HA, Saye JA, Peach MJ. Effects of cytochrome P-450 inhibitors on endothelium-dependent relaxation in rabbit aorta. Blood Vessels 1984;21:223–230.
129. Smuckler EA, Iseri OA, Benditt EP. An intracellular defect in protein synthesis induced by carbon tetrachloride. J Exp Med 1962;116:55–72.
130. Ugazio G, Danni O, Mililo P, Burdino E, Congiu AM. Mechanism of protection against carbon tetrachloride toxicity. I. Prevention of lethal effects by partial surgical hepatectomy. Drug Chem Toxicol 1982;5:115–124.
131. Ugazio G, Koch RR, Recknagel RO. Mechanism of protection against carbon tetrachloride by prior carbon tetrachloride administration. Exp Mol Pathol 1972;16:281–285.
132. Vesell ES. Pharmacogenetic perspectives: genes, drugs and disease. Hepatology 1984;4:959–965.
133. Waterman MR, John ME, Simpson ER. Regulation of synthesis and activity of cytochrome P-450 enzymes in physiological pathways. In: Ortiz de Montellano PR (ed). Cytochrome P-450. New York: Plenum Press, 1986, pp. 345–386.
134. Weinstein T, Mittelman M, Djaldetti M. Electron microscopy study of Mott and Russell bodies in myeloma cells. J Submicrosc Cytol 1987;19:155–159.

Pathology of the Golgi Apparatus

135. Alberts B, Bray D, Lewis J, Raff M, Roberts K, Watson JD. Molecular biology of the cell. New York: Garland Publishing, Inc., 1983.
136. Bainton DF, Takemura R, Stenberg PE, Werb Z. Rapid fragmentation and reorganization of golgi membranes during frustrated phagocytosis of immobile immune complexes by macrophages. Am J Pathol 1989;134:15–26.
137. Farquhar MG, Bergeron JJM, Palade GE. Cytochemistry of Golgi fractions prepared from rat liver. J Cell Biol 1974;60:8–25.
138. Ghadially PN. Ultrastructural pathology of the cell and matrix, 2nd ed. London: Butterworths, 1982.
138a. Gonatas NK. Rous-Whipple Award Lecture. Contributions to the physiology and pathology of the Golgi apparatus. Am J Pathol 1994; 145: 751–761.
139. Tartakoff AM. The Golgi complex: crossroads for vesicular traffic. Int Rev Exp Pathol 1980;22:227–251.

Pathology of the Lysosomes

140. Alberts B, Bray D, Lewis J, Raff M, Roberts K, Watson JD. Molecular biology of the cell, 2nd ed. New York: Garland Publishing, Inc., 1983.
141. Allison AC, Morgan DML. Effects of silica, asbestos, and other particles on macrophage and neutrophil lysosomes. In: Dingle JT, Jacques PJ, Shaw IH (eds). Lysosomes in applied biology and therapeutics, vol. 6. Amsterdam: North-Holland Publishing Co., 1979, pp. 149–159.
142. Alroy J, Warren CD, Raghavan SS, Kolodny EH. Animal models for lysosomal storage diseases: their past and future contribution. Hum Pathol 1989;20:823–826.
143. Armstrong JA, D'Arcy Hart P. Response of cultured macrophages to Mycobacterium tuberculosis, with observations on fusion of lysosomes with phagosomes. J Exp Med 1971;134:713–740.
144. Aterman K. The development of the concept of lysosomes. A historical survey, with particular reference to the liver. Histochem J 1979;11:503–541.
145. Barton NW, Brady RO, Dambrosia JM, et al. Replacement therapy for inherited enzyme deficiency-macrophage-targeted glucocerebrosidase for Gaucher's disease. N Engl J Med 1991;324:1464–1470.
146. Baum H, Gergely J. Molecular aspects of medicine, vol. 2. Oxford: Pergamon Press, 1980.
147. Beaudet AL. Lysosomal storage disease. In: Wilson JD, Braunwald E, Isselbacher KJ, et al. (eds). Harrison's principles of internal medicine, 12th ed. New York: McGraw-Hill, Inc., 1991.
148. Beutler E. Gaucher's disease. N Engl J Med 1991;325:1354–1360.
149. Benson PF, Fensom AH. Genetic biochemical disorders. Oxford: Oxford University Press, 1985.
150. Brady RO, Barranger JA. Glucosylceramide lipidosis: Gaucher's disease. In: Stanbury JB, Wyngaarden JB, Frederickson DS, Goldstein JL, Brown MS (eds). The metabolic basis of inherited disease. 5th ed. New York: McGraw-Hill Book Company, 1983, pp. 842–856.
151. Cherian PV, Schumacher HR Jr. Immunochemical and ultrastructural characterization of serum proteins associated with monosodium urate crystals (MS) in synovial fluid cells from patients with gout. Ultrastruct Pathol 1986;10:209–219.
152. Cohn ZA, Hirsch JG. The isolation and properties of the specific cytoplasmic granules of rabbit polymorphonuclear leucocytes. J Exp Med 1960;112:983–1004.
153. D'Alton ME, DeCherney AH. Prenatal diagnosis. N Engl J Med 1993;328:114–120.
154. de Duve C. The lysosome. Sci Am 1963;208:64–72.
155. de Duve C. A guided tour of the living cell. Vol I. New York: Scientific American Books, 1984.
156. DeGasperi R, Alroy J, Richard R, et al. Glycoprotein

storage in Gaucher disease: lectin histochemistry and biochemical studies. Lab Invest 1990;63:385–393.

157. Dingle JT. Lysosomes in biology and pathology. Vol 3. New York: Elsevier-North Holland Publishing Co., 1973.

158. Dingle JT, Dean RT. Lysosomes in biology and pathology, vol 5. Amsterdam: North-Holland Publishing Company, 1976.

159. Dingle JT, Jacques PJ, Shaw IH. Lysosomes in applied biology and therapeutics. Volume 6. Amsterdam: North-Holland Publishing Company, 1979.

160. Figueroa ML, Rosenbloom BE, Kay AC, Garver P, Thurston DW, Koziol JA, Gelbart T, Beutler E. A less costly regimen of alglucerase to treat Gaucher's disease. N Engl J Med 1992;327:1632–1636.

161. Glew RH, Basu A, Prence EM, Remaley AT. Lysosomal storage disease. Lab Invest 1985;53:250–269.

162. Goldman R. Ion distribution and membrane permeability in lysosomal suspensions. In: Dingle JT, Dean RT (eds). Lysosomes in biology and pathology. Volume 5. Amsterdam: North-Holland Publishing Company, 1976, pp. 309–336.

163. Goren MB, Hart PD, Young MR, Armstrong JA. Prevention of phagosome-lysosome fusion in cultured macrophages by sulfatides of Mycobacterium tuberculosis. Proc Natl Acad Sci USA 1976;73:2510–2514.

164. Goren MB, Swendsen CL, Fiscus J, Miranti C. Fluorescent markers for studying phagosome-lysosome function. J Leukocyte Biol 1984;36:273–292.

165. Goren MB, Vatter AE, Fiscus J. Polyanionic agents do not inhibit phagosome-lysosome fusion in cultured macrophages. J Leukocyte Biol 1987;41:122–129.

166. Hannun UA, Bell RM. Lysosphingolipids inhibit protein kinase C: implications for the sphingolipidoses. Science 1987;235:670–674.

167. Harris L, McKenna WJ, Rowland E, Krikler DM. Side effects and possible contraindications of amiodarone use. Am Heart J 1983;106:916–923.

168. Holtzman E. Lysosomes: a survey. New York: Springer-Verlag, 1976.

169. Hortsmann G, Lüllmann-Rauch R. Mucopolysaccharidosis-like alterations in cardiac valves of rats treated with tilorone. Virchows Arch (Cell Pathol) 1985; 48:33–45.

170. Jackson LG. First-trimester diagnosis of fetal genetic disorders. Hosp Pract 1985;20:39–48.

171. Jägel M, Lüllmann-Rauch R. Lipidosis-like laterations in cultured macrophages exposed to local anesthetics. Arch Toxicol 1984;55:229–232.

172. Joiner KA, Fuhrman SA, Miettinen HM, Kasper LH, Mellman I. Toxoplasma gondii: fusion competence of parasitophorous vacuoles in Fc receptor-transfected fibroblasts. Science 1990;249:641–646.

173. Jones TC, Hirsch JG. The interaction between Toxoplasma gondii and mammalian cells. II. The absence of lysosomal fusion with phagocytic vacuoles containing living parasites. J Exp Med 1972;136:1173–1194.

174. Jones TC, Yeh S, Hirsch JG. The interaction between Toxoplasma gondii and mammalian cells. I. Mechanism of entry and intracellular fate of the parasite. J Exp Med 1972;136:1157–1172.

175. Kane AB, Stanton RP, Raymond EG, Dobson ME, Knafelc ME, Farber JL. Dissociation of intracellular lysosomal rupture from the cell death caused by silica. J Cell Biol 1980;87:643–651.

176. Kaye EM, Alroy J, Raghavan SS, et al. Dysmyelinogenesis in animal model of GM₁ gangliosidosis. Pediatr Neurol 1992;8:255–261.

177. Kleijer WJ, Janse HC, Vosters RPL, Niermeijer MF, van de Kamp JJP. First-trimester diagnosis of mucopolysaccharidosis IIIA (Sanfilippo A disease). N Engl J Med 1986;314:185–186.

178. Kolodny EH, Cable WJL. Inborn errors of metabolism. Ann Neurol 1982;11:221–232.

179. Kornfeld S, Sly WS. Lysosomal storage defects. Hosp Pract 1985;20:71–82.

180. Krogstad DJ, Schlesinger PH, Gluzman IY. Antimalarials increase vesicle pH in Plasmodium falciparum. J Cell Biol 1985;101:2302–2309.

181. Kudo, RR. Protozozoology. Springfield: Charles C Thomas, 1966.

182. Lüllmann-Rauch R, Reil GH. Chlorphentermine-induced ultrastructural changes in liver tissues of four animal species. Virchows Arch [B] 1975;13:307–320.

183. Lüllmann-Rauch R. Drug-induced lysosomal storage disorders. In: Dingle JT, Jacques PJ, Shaw IH (eds). Lysosomes in applied biology and therapeutics Vol 6. Amsterdam: North-Holland Publishing Company, 1979, pp. 49–130.

184. MacDonald RD, Engel AG. Experimental chloroquine myopathy. J Neuropathol Exp Neurol 1970;29:479–499.

185. McCarty DJ. Crystal deposition joint disease. Annu Rev Med 1974;25:279–288.

186. Neufeld EF. Lysosomal storage diseases. Annu Rev Biochem 1991;60:257–280.

187. Neufeld EF, Cantz MJ. Corrective factors for inborn errors of mucopolysaccharide metabolism. Ann NY Acad Sci 1971;179:580–587.

188. Neufeld EF, Lim TW, Shapiro LJ. Inherited disorders of lysosomal metabolism. Annu Rev Biochem 1975;44:357–376.

189. Novikoff AB. Lysosomes: a personal account. In: Hers G, Van Hoof F (eds). Lysosomes and storage disease. New York: Academic Press, 1973, pp. 1–41.

190. Perkins DG, Haust MD. Ultrastructure of myocardium in the Hurler syndrome. Possible relation to cardiac function. Virchows Arch (Pathol Anat) 1982;394:195–205.

191. Peters SP, Lee RE, Glew RH. Gaucher's disease, a review. Medicine 1977;56:425–442.

192. Pfeifer U, Jeschke R. Cholesterylester-Speicherkrankheit. Virchows Arch B Cell Pathol 1980;33:17–34.

193. Robinson JM, Karnovsky MJ. Ultrastructural localization of several phosphatases with Cerium. J Histochem Cytochem 1983;31:1197–1208.

194. Sakuragawa N, Sakuragawa M, Kuwabara T, Pentchev PG, Barranger JA, Brady RO. Niemann-Pick disease experimental model: sphingomyelinase reduction induced by AY-9944. Science 1977;196:317–319.

195. Stanbury JD, Wyngaarden JB, Frederickson DS, Goldstein JL, Brown MS. The metabolic basis of inherited disease. 5th ed. New York: McGraw-Hill, 1983.

196. Starzl TE, Demetris AJ, Trucco M, et al. Chimerism after liver transplantation for type IV glycogen storage disease and type 1 Gaucher's disease. N Engl J Med 1993;328:745–749.

196a. Sturgill-Koszycki S, Schlesinger PH, Chakraborty P, Haddix PL, Collins HL, Fok AK, Allen RD, Gluck SL, Heuser J, Russell DG. Lack of acidification in mycobacterium phagosomes produced by exclusion of the vesicular proton-atpase. Science 1994; 263: 678–683.

197. Weissmann G. The molecular basis of acute gout. In: Weissmann G, Claiborne R (eds). Cell membranes: biochemistry, cell biology and pathology. New York: HP Publishing, 1975: 257–266.

198. Weissmann G, Claiborne R (eds). Cell membranes: biochemistry, cell biology and pathology. New York: HP Publishing. 1975.

Pathology of the Peroxisomes

199. Baumgart E, Stegmeier K, Schmidt, FH, Fahimi HD. Proliferation of peroxisomes in pericentral hepatocytes of rat liver after administration of a new hypocholesterolemic agent (BM 15766). Sex-dependent ultrastructural differences. Lab Invest 1987;56:554–564.

200. Fahimi HD, Kalmbach P, Stegmeier K, Stork H. Comparison between the effects of clofibrate and bezafibrate upon the ultrastructure of rat heart and liver. In: Greten H, Lang PD, Schettler G (eds). Lipoproteins and coronary heart disease. New York: Gerhard Witzstrock Publishing House, 1980, pp. 64–75.

201. Hruban Z, Gotoh M, Slesers A, Chou S-F. Structure of hepatic microbodies in rats treated with acetylsalicylic acid, clofibrate, dimethrin. Lab Invest 1974;30:64–75.

202. Moser HW, Goldfischer SL. The peroxisomal disorders. Hosp Pract 1985;20:61–70.

203. Rao MS, Reddy JK. Peroxisome proliferation and hepatocarcinogenesis. Carcinogenesis 1987;8:631–636.

204. Riede UN, Fringes B, Moore GW. Peroxisomes in cellular injury and disease. In: Trump BF, Laufer A, Jones RT (eds). Cellular pathobiology of human disease. New York: Gustav Fischer, 1983, pp. 139–174.

205. Santos MJ, Imanaka T, Shio H, Small GM, Lazarow PB. Peroxisomal membrane ghosts in Zellweger syndrome—aberrant organelle assembly. Science 1988;239:1536–1538.

206. Shimozawa N, Tsukamoto T, Suzuki Y, et al. A human gene responsible for Zellweger syndrome that affects peroxisome assembly. Science 1992;255:1132–1134.

Pathology of the Cytoskeleton

207. Afzelius BA. The immotile-cilia syndrome and other ciliary diseases. Int Rev Exp Pathol 1979;19:1–43.

208. Afzelius BA. "Immotile-cilia" syndrome and ciliary abnormalities induced by infection and injury. Am Rev Resp Dis 1981;124:107–109.

209. Afzelius BA. Disorders of ciliary motility. Hosp Pract 1986;21:73–80.

210. Afzelius BA, Eliasson R, Johnsen O, Lindholmer C. Lack of dynein arms in immotile human spermatozoa. J Cell Biol 1975;66:225–232.

211. Allen RD. The microtubule as an intracellular engine. Sci Am 1987;256:42–49.

212. Bendall JR. Postmortem changes in muscle. In: Bourne GH (ed). The structure and function of muscle. 2nd ed. Vol II. New York: Academic Press, 1973, pp. 243–309.

213. Bilbao JM, Briggs SJ, Gray TA. Filamentous axonopathy in disulfiram neuropathy. Ultrastruct Pathol 1984;7:295–300.

214. Bloodgood RA. Resorption of organelles containing microtubules. Cytobios 1974;9:143–161.

215. Carter SB. Effects of cytochalasins on mammalian cells. Nature 1967;213:261–264.

216. Clegg JS. Interrelationships between water and cellular metabolism in Artemia cysts. XI. Density measurements. Cell Biophys 1984;6:153–169.

217. Cooper JA. Effects of cytochalasin and phalloidin on actin. J Cell Biol 1987;105:1473–1478.

218. Copeman WSC. A short history of the gout and the rheumatic diseases. Berkeley: University of California Press, 1964.

219. Darnell J, Lodish H, Baltimore D. Molecular cell biology. New York: Scientific American Books, 1986.

220. Denk H, Franke WW, Kerjaschki D, Eckerstorfer R. Mallory bodies in experimental animals and man. Int Rev Exp Pathol 1979;20:77–121.

221. Dustin P. Microtubules. 2nd ed. Berlin: Springer-Verlag, 1984.

222. Eliasson R, Mossberg B, Camner P, Afzelius BA. The immotile-cilia syndrome. N Engl J Med 1977;297:1–6.

223. French SW. Present understanding of the development of Mallory's body. Arch Pathol Lab Med 1983;107:445–450.

224. Hazan R, Denk H, Franke WW, Lackinger E, Schiller DL. Change of cytokeratin organization during development of Mallory bodies as revealed by a monoclonal antibody. Lab Invest 1986;54:543–553.

225. Irie T, Benson NC, French SW. Electron microscopic study of the in vitro calcium-dependent degradation of Mallory bodies and intermediate filaments in hepatocytes. Lab Invest 1984;50:303–312.

226. Lowe JE, Jennings RB, Reimer KA. Cardiac rigor mortis in dogs. J Mol Cell Cardiol 1979;11:1017–1031.

227. Neumann PE, Horoupian DS, Goldman JE, Hess MA. Cytoplasmic filaments of Crooke's hyaline change belong to the cytokeratin class. Am J Pathol 1984;116:214–222.

228. Pedersen H, Rebbe H. Absence of arms in the axoneme of immobile human spermatozoa. Biol Reprod 1975;12:541–544.

229. Pernice B. Sulla cariocinesi delle cellule epiteliali e dell'endotelio dei vasi della mucosa dello stomaco e dell'intestino, nello studio della gastroenterite sperimentale (nell'avvelenamento per colchico). Sicilia Med 1889;1:265, 279.

230. Phillips MJ, Oda M, Funatsu K. Ece for microfilament involvement in norethandrolone-induced intrahepatic cholestasis. Am J Pathol 1978;93:729–744.

231. Phillips MJ, Poucell S, Oda M. Mechanisms of cholestasis. Lab Invest 1986;54:593–608.

232. Phillips MJ, Poucell S, Patterson J, Valencia P. Alcoholic liver disease and cirrhosis. In: Phillips MJ, Poucell S, Patterson J, Valencia P (eds). The liver. An atlas and text of ultrastructural pathology. New York: Raven Press, 1987, pp. 393–446.

233. Plenck JG. Icones Plantarum Album, Centuria II/125, 1789.

234. Porter KR. The cytomatrix: a short history of its study. J Cell Biol 1984;99 (Pt. 2):3s–12s.

235. Porter KR, Anderson KL. The structure of the cytoplasmic matrix preserved by freeze-drying and freeze-substitution. Eur J Cell Biol 1982;29:83–96.

236. Porter KR, Beckerle M, McNiven M. The cytoplasmic matrix. Mod Cell Biol 1983;2:259–302.

237. Poste G, Lyon NC. Enucleation of cultured animal cells by cytochalasin B. In: Tanenbaum SW (ed). Cytochalasins—biochemical and cell biological aspects. Amsterdam: North-Holland Publishing Company, 1978, pp. 161–189.

238. Roberts WN, Liang MH, Stern SH. Colchicine in acute gout. JAMA 1987;257:1920–1922.

239. Rungger-Brandle E, Gabbiani G. The role of cytoskeletal and cytocontractile elements in pathologic processes. Am J Pathol 1983;110:361–392.

240. Schrek R, Stefani SS. Toxicity of microtubular drugs to leukemic lymphocytes. Exp Mol Pathol 1981;34:369–378.

241. Selkoe DJ, Magner AM, Shelanski ML. Pathology and biochemistry of the neurofilament in experimental and human neurofibrillary degeneration. Aging 1979;8:121–139.

242. Tanenbaum SW. Microbiological, preparative and analytical aspects of cytochalasin production. In: Tanenbaum SW (ed). Cytochalasins—biochemical and cell

biological aspects. Amsterdam: North-Holland Publishing Company, 1978, pp. 1–14.

243. Vogel VJ. American indian medicine. Norman: University of Oklahoma Press, 1970.

244. Watanabe S, Phillips MJ. Acute phalloidin toxicity in living hepatocytes. Evidence for a possible disturbance in membrane flow and for multiple functions for actin in the liver cell. Am J Pathol 1986;122:101–111.

245. Weber K, Wehland J, Herzog W. Griseofulvin interacts with microtubules both in vivo and in vitro. J Mol Biol 1976;102:817–829.

Pathology of the Nucleus

246. Alberts B, Bray D, Lewis J, Raff M, Roberts K, Watson JD. Molecular biology of the cell. New York: Garland Publishing Co., 1983.

247. Avery OT, MacLeod CM, McCarty M. Studies on the chemical nature of the substance inducing transformation of pneumococcal types. Induction of transformation by a deoxyribonucleic acid fraction isolated from Pneumococcus Type III. J Exp Med 1944;79:137–158.

248. Barr ML, Bertram EG. A morphological distinction between neurones of the male and female, the behaviour of the nucleolar satellite during accelerated nucleoprotein synthesis. Nature 1949;163:676–677.

249. Bloom S, Cancilla PA. Conformational changes in myocardial nuclei of rats. Circ Res 1969;24:189–196.

250. Bohr VA, Evans MK, Fornace AJ Jr. DNA repair and its pathogenetic implications. Lab Invest 1989;61:143–161.

251. Farber E. Biochemical pathology. Annu Rev Pharmacol 1971;11:71–96.

252. Fenoglio-Preiser C (ed). Advances in pathology, vol 2. Chicago: Year Book Medical Publishers, Inc, 1989.

253. Fox JE. Molecular genetics—an overview for the clinician. Child Hosp Q 1989;1:43–47.

254. Ghadially FN. Ultrastructural pathology of the cell and matrix. 2nd ed. London: Butterworths, 1982.

255. Goudie RB. DNA technology in histopathology. In: Anthony PP, MacSween RNM (eds). Recent advances in histopathology, No. 14. Edinburgh: Churchill Livingstone, 1989, pp. 1–21.

256. Goyer RA, Cherian MG. Tissue and cellular toxicology of metals. In: Brown SS (ed). Clinical chemistry and chemical toxicology of metals. Amsterdam: Elsevier Biomedical Press, 1977, pp. 89–103.

257. Griffith F. The significance of pneumococcal types. J Hyg 1928;27:113–159.

258. Grody WW, Gatti RA, Naeim F. Diagnostic molecular pathology. Mod Pathol 1989;2:553–568.

259. Guyer RL, Koshland DE Jr. The molecule of the year. Science 1989;246:1543–1546.

260. Jaenisch R. Transgenic animals. Science 1988;240:1468–1474.

261. Kerkhoven P, Marti HR, Hug G. Electronmicroscopic and biochemical observations on erythroid cells in congenital dyserythropoietic anemia type II. Virchows Arch A Pathol Anat Histol 1974;363:1–15.

261a. Korf B. Molecular medicine: Molecular diagnosis (Part one). N Engl J Med 1995; 332:1218–1220.

262. McLachlin JR, Goyer RA, Cherian MG. Formation of lead-induced inclusion bodies in primary rat kidney epithelial cell cultures: effect of actinomycin D and cycloheximide. Toxicol Appl Pharmacol 1980;56:418–431.

263. Pääbo S. Ancient DNA: extraction, characterization, molecular cloning, and enzymatic amplification. Proc Natl Acad Sci USA 1989;86:1939–1943.

264. Portugal FH, Cohen JS. A century of DNA. Cambridge: The MIT Press, 1977.

265. Scarpelli DG, Migaki G, Pletcher JM (eds). Transgenic animal models in biomedical research. Washington DC: Armed Forces Institute of Pathology, 1991.

266. Schoefl GI. The effect of actinomycin D on the fine structure of the nucleolus. J Ultrastruct Res 1964;10:224–243.

267. Skaar H, Ophus E, Gullvag BM. Lead accumulation within nuclei of moss leaf cells. Nature 1973;241:215–216.

268. Walton J, Buckley IK. The lead-poisoned cell: a fine structural study using cultured kidney cells. Exp Mol Pathol 1977;27:167–182.

269. Westphal H. Transgenic mammals and biotechnology. FASEB J 1989;3:117–120.

Cell Injury and Cell Death

CHAPTER 5

> Cell Injury and
> Response
> Cell Death
> Necrosis

In Chapter 4 we dealt with the pathology of individual organelles; we will now consider the effects of injury on the cell as a whole.

As to the meaning of **injury,** dictionaries equate it with damage, which is good enough. The damage may be structural and/or functional. The main point is that the term injury does not include the response. Think of the term *wound,* which refers only to the damage; inflammation and repair are the responses.

Depending on the nature and intensity of the injury, cells may respond with an increased or decreased level of activity (Figure 5.1).

The notion of increased activity as a result of injury might lead us into an argument about what is injury and what is stimulation. In fact, a new word has crept into the recent literature, **cellular perturbation** (167, 213), which implies an intermediate situation: a stimulus induces pathology by eliciting an inappropriate response (e.g., an endothelial cell is led to express a blood-clotting protein).

Cell Injury and Response

Cells can be hurt by myriads of agents, physical (such as trauma or heat), chemical (toxins), or biological (bacteria, viruses). The catalog of cellular responses is much shorter, because cells have a limited number of ways to react. A number of cellular responses were described in Chapters 3 and 4; we now present one that is triggered by any form of injury: the so-called heat shock or cellular stress response. This basic phenomenon came into the limelight in the late 1980s.

THE HEAT-SHOCK OR CELLULAR STRESS RESPONSE

What follows is one of the broadest known generalizations regarding disease. *All the cells that have been tested—cells from animals, plants, and yeasts down to the simplest prokaryotes—when submitted to a stress such as a mild increase in temperature, temporarily turn down their usual protein synthesis and turn up the synthesis of certain selected proteins that have been called **heat-shock proteins*** (HSPs) (243). Because the response can be induced by virtually any type of stressing agent, the term **stress proteins** is also used. The response develops within minutes (243) and lasts only a day or so. This time limit is probably a matter of survival: the cell cannot afford to turn off its regular protein synthesis indefinitely. In humans the stress response is triggered, for example, by ischemia, inflammation, fever, alcohol, and tissue damage in general (160).

THE HEAT-SHOCK PROTEINS

The discovery of heat-shock proteins was slow in coming because it depended heavily on modern methods of protein electrophoresis on gels. It was

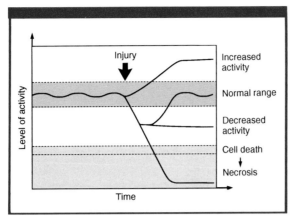

FIGURE 5.1

Responses of cells to injury. The activity of normal cells oscillates around a steady state, the physiologic range. After injury (**arrow**) cells may respond by increased activity (such as by the heat-shock response), by reversibly or irreversibly decreased activity, and eventually by cell death and necrosis. Enzymatic activity can persist for some time also in necrotic cells. (Adapted from [157].)

made in 1962 through an odd experiment on fruit flies, an experiment so odd that it might have qualified for the Golden Fleece Award distributed in recent times by a U.S. senator to the government-funded perpetrators of "irrelevant" scientific experiments.

Working in a genetics laboratory in Naples, Dr. Ferruccio Ritossa chose to study the effect of slight warming on the salivary gland chromosomes of fruit fly larvae. After 30 minutes at 30°C (25°C being normal for the flies) he noticed that "puffs" appeared at certain sites—and always the same sites—on two chromosomes (Figure 5.2). The effect was reversible and could be elicited also with toxic chemicals (dinitrophenol, salicylate). It was known at that time that the puffs corresponded to sites of DNA uncoiling, a sign of enhanced transcription (RNA synthesis). In other words, the puffs represented activated genes. Twelve years later, in Geneva, A. Tissières and coworkers (226) showed by gel electrophoresis that protein synthesis was in fact enhanced: heat shock induced the appearance or increase of six proteins, accounting for about 30 percent of the total protein synthesis; the production of most other proteins was decreased. It seemed that the cell's protein-building machinery was being preempted for the manufacture of a small group of proteins. Within a few years similar results were obtained with all kinds of cells, from E. coli to slime molds and human tumors (198), and with all kinds of stressors.

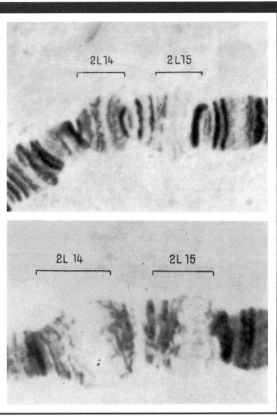

FIGURE 5.2

The original "puffing chromosomes" of Ritossa, which led to the discovery of heat-shock proteins. *Top:* brackets indicate two normal regions in salivary gland chromosomes of a larva of *Drosophila* reared at 25°C. *Bottom:* the same regions after receiving a thermal shock, administered by warming the larva for 30 minutes at 30°C. The key point is that the puffing occurred only in these regions, suggesting a specific phenomenon induced by heat. (Reproduced with permission from [191].)

The heat-shock response is about as ancient as it could be: the genes that code for its proteins have changed little in 3 billion years (248, 259). For example, if the amino acid sequences of equivalent heat-shock proteins from prokaryotes and eukaryotes are compared, they are about 50 percent homologous, and many of the other residues are similar (259). Clearly the heat-shock response must play a key role for survival, and whatever that role may be, it must be intracellular because *the HSPs are not secreted.* The stressed cell keeps them for itself. Other facts have emerged: *most of the HSPs are constitutive,* that is, they are always present in normal cells at low levels, as is well demonstrated by gel electrophoresis (Figure 5.3), and *all are key players in the cell's metabolism* (17).

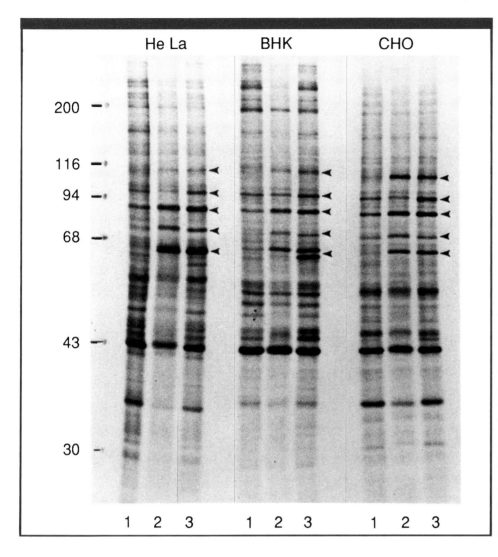

FIGURE 5.3
Gels of various mammalian cell lines showing heat-shock proteins after labeling with ^{35}S-methionine. **HeLa**: HeLa cells. **BHK**: Baby hamster kidney cells. **CHO**: Chinese hamster ovary cells. For each cell line, *lane 1* shows normal growth conditions, *lane 2* the effect of heat shock, and *lane 3* the effect of exposure to an amino acid analog of proline. **Arrowheads** point to heat-shock proteins. Note that the latter also exist in the normal control, although in lesser amounts. Figures at left indicate molecular mass in kilodaltons. (Reproduced with permission from [245].)

The heat-shock or stress proteins are presently designated by HSP followed by the molecular mass in kilodaltons. The ranges of HSP molecular weights fall into groups: nearly all species express "universal" HSPs in the ranges of 90, 70, and 20–30 kD. A fourth HSP is much smaller (76 residues) and has its own name: **ubiquitin.** It was discovered accidentally during a search for thymic hormones and found to be truly ubiquitous years before it was recognized as an HSP (24).

Functions of Heat-Shock Proteins The colorful names of **unfoldases** or **chaperonins** for the members of the HSP 70 family indicate that under normal conditions *these molecules bind to other proteins, recognize those that are incorrectly folded or glycosylated, repair them, and accompany them to their proper destination within the cell* (17,

254) (Figure 5.4). Some assist in the translocation of proteins across membranes or take part in disassembling clathrin-coated vesicles, perhaps as a device for shutting down nonessential activity (17). These normal functions help us understand what the heat-shock proteins accomplish under pathologic conditions. It has been suggested that the proteins of the HSP 70 family intervene to "save" as many protein molecules as they can, whereas those beyond salvage are degraded with the help of ubiquitin (254). Ubiquitin, as we have seen, becomes covalently bound to denatured proteins and targets them for destruction (p. 43). This role of denatured proteins may explain why heat shock remains the most effective type of stress for studying the cellular stress response: heat is the most effective agent for denaturing proteins.

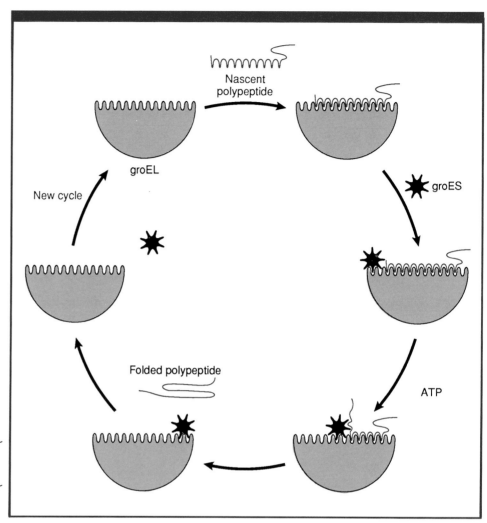

FIGURE 5.4
Hypothetical scheme showing how two heat-shock proteins (groEL and groES) may collaborate in folding nascent polypeptides into the proper shapes. A similar model can be proposed for correcting the shapes of denatured proteins. (Adapted from [160].)

Role of Heat-Shock Proteins in Cell Survival
Many experiments—both *in vivo* and *in vitro*—show that *cells challenged with mild heat become* **thermotolerant,** *that is, they can survive later exposure to a lethal temperature* (12, 254). Cultured fibroblasts grown at 37°C will survive a 30-minute thermal shock at 45°C, but if they are microinjected with an antibody against HSP 70, they die (Figure 5.5) (189). Various injurious agents bestow protection against other injurious agents (this is called **cross-protection**). For example, recovery from anoxia increases cellular thermotolerance as well as HSP synthesis; exposure to heat increases a cell's tolerance to adriamycin (48, 131). This works also *in vivo:* in rats maintained for 15 minutes at a body temperature of 41°C (reached by breathing air at 41–42°C), the retina is less sensitive to damage by bright light (12).

Morphology of the Heat-Shock Response Early in the heat-shock response, HSP 72 has been found to localize in the nucleolus; later, during recovery, it diffuses into the cytoplasm to areas rich in ribosomes (248). This distribution suggests that *HSP 72 may be involved in "rescuing" the complex molecular machinery involved in transcription and translation* (248).

The structural changes that occur during heat shock are mild and not necessarily related to the HSPs: condensation of the chromatin, appearance of bundles of filaments in the nucleus (178, 247), and breakup of the Golgi apparatus. The intermediate filament network tends to collect around the nucleus (243) as if it were providing it with a protective wrapping; however, HSPs tend to oppose this effect (246).

Functional changes during heat shock include a shift to anaerobic metabolism, with subtle changes in mitochondrial morphology. Also during the stress response, the cells abruptly stop growing (243), which fits with the survival plan: in an emergency, growth is a low priority.

How does the cell perceive the stress and transduce the information to the heat-shock genes? Studies on HSP 70 have shown that cells contain a protein, HSF (for heat-shock-transcription factor) which is normally inactive; heat causes it to undergo a conformational change whereby it binds to heat-shock genes and activates them. This happens in minutes (159a). For mammalian cells the critical temperature is about 42°C; interestingly, the cells of the mouse testis—which are accustomed to live at 30°C—are triggered at 36–38°C (193a).

For agents other than heat the transduction system is not so clear. For example, the injection of denatured proteins into the cytoplasm triggers the stress response (249). It has been suggested that the heat-shock genes could be turned on by the exhaustion of the normal ubiquitin stores (164).

Bacterial Stress Proteins: A Two-Edged Sword?
It may have occurred to the reader that the near-identity between bacterial and mammalian heat-shock proteins may create a problem. Suppose that virulent bacteria, attacked by their host, generate their own heat-shock proteins, and die; further suppose that the host produces an immune response against these proteins. Could this lead to a two-pronged attack against the bacterial *and* the similar self-proteins? This and other scenarios are possible:

- Could it be that contact with bacterial HSPs since infancy might lead to immunity toward those bacteria in the adult?
- Conversely, could it be that HSPs produced by bacteria might fail to trigger an immune response because they are not recognized as foreign?
- Would it be possible to use bacterial HSPs as polyvalent vaccines?

The answers are just beginning to come in. For example, bacterial HSPs do induce antibodies in patients suffering from tuberculosis and leprosy (258). Also, there is strong evidence linking stress proteins with rheumatic disease, that is, with some forms of arthritis (254, 258). We expect interesting developments in this area. In the meantime, the heat-shock response is being drafted for useful purposes: using recombinant DNA technology, experts have engineered "stress reporter" fruit flies that turn blue when exposed to teratogens (agents that disturb fetal development) and worms that turn blue when exposed to toxic agents (244).

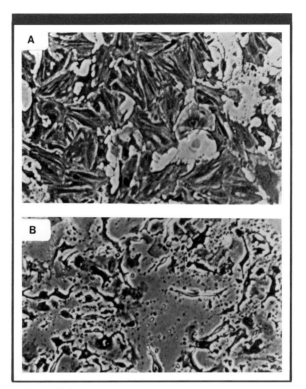

FIGURE 5.5
Cells individually microinjected with antibodies against heat-shock proteins are unable to survive a heat-shock challenge. The two panels show rat fibroblasts that have been submitted to heat shock at 43°C for 2 hours. *Top*: cells microinjected with a "control" antibody have survived. *Bottom*: cells microinjected with antibody against 72/73-kD stress proteins have not survived the heat shock. (Reproduced with permission from [189].)

A final thought on heat-shock proteins: we find especially attractive the concept that they are involved in the general repair of cell proteins. We had always found it somewhat unfair that the DNA alone should be endowed with repair enzymes, even though DNA repair must be a high priority; it seems that this "unfairness" simply reflected our ignorance.

The stress response of the liver. *In closing this discussion of cellular stress response, we should point to another analogy between the cell—the elementary patient—and the body as a whole. Severe, acute disease—such as trauma or infection—causes the liver to alter its pattern of protein synthesis, a phenomenon known as the* **acute phase response** *(p. 491). It is not a heat-shock response: we are dealing with proteins that are secreted into the plasma rather than retained in the cell like HSPs; also, this reaction is slower and more prolonged than the heat-shock response. However, the purpose is the same:*

survival of the cell for the heat-shock proteins and survival of the body for the acute phase proteins.

CELL WOUNDS

Having examined the overall response of cells to stress, we will now see how they respond to the challenge of a wound.

Cells are sturdy; consider that we walk on them at every step. They can stand microsurgery with the laser, which can destroy minuscule targets such as one arm of a single chromosome (19). They have been seen to survive and even to divide(!) after surgical removal of the nucleus (137). Muscle fibers can be impaled many times with 0.5-μm microelectrodes and still maintain their resting potential (56), thus enabling electrophysiologists to make a living. And think of the enormous trauma endured by glial cells when they are isolated from a brain mash; yet they can be cultured (44).

Wounds in Individual Cells The healing of tiny cellular wounds is difficult to study, but experiments with large cells such as amebae and the eggs of marine animals have begun to answer some questions. In a little known book that appeared just before the era of cell biology, the eminent physiologist L. V. Heilbrunn summarized his studies on wounded muscle cells and marine eggs (103). If the egg of a starfish kept in seawater is punctured, a blob of protoplasm begins to flow out of the opening, but it soon appears to coagulate, and the outflow stops. Heilbrunn called this the **surface precipitation reaction** (SPR). If calcium was removed from the seawater, the SPR did not occur, and the cell seemed to bleed itself to death (Figure 5.6). These beautiful studies have never been duplicated. More recent data suggest that several processes are at work in the healing of cell wounds. Tiny wounds (~0.5 μm or less) probably heal by physical forces, just like punctures in artificial lipid membranes (56, 171). Larger cell wounds appear to heal by a combination of three mechanisms:

- *Purse-string contraction of the cell cortex*, which results from the actin–myosin system that lines the deep surface of the plasma membrane in most cells. This system should be ideally suited to contract around a wound. It seems to do so in wounds in the cortex of frog eggs (Figure 5.7) (23). When the enormous cells of certain marine algae are wounded, cellular contraction occurs, and calcium is required (123).
- *New membrane formation*, which has been elegantly shown by spearing a single ameba with the tip of an eyelash (216, 217).
- *Calcium-dependent coagulation of the cytoplasm.* This effect, postulated by Heilbrunn, has been confirmed in a few other cell types (171), although the molecular significance of this coagulation is not yet clear (56). We could be dealing with a process similar to blood clotting (as Heilbrunn suggested) or with a change akin to the protein denaturation of coagulative necrosis. The "clots" that develop on the stumps of severed muscle cells should be seen in this light (Figure 2.17).

These three mechanisms of cellular wound healing recall those at work in bodily wound healing: the clotting of the cytoplasm recalls the clotting of the blood, and it is also calcium-dependent; *the formation of new cell membrane recalls the gliding of epithelial cells* over small wounds (e.g., in the cornea); and *the contraction of cell fibrils recalls the contractile activity of the fibroblasts* (p. 472). In the last case, even the molecular mechanism is the same as in the purse-string contraction of cell wounds: a beautiful example of natural economy.

Wounds in a Sheet of Communicating Cells In many cellular systems there is cell-to-cell commu-

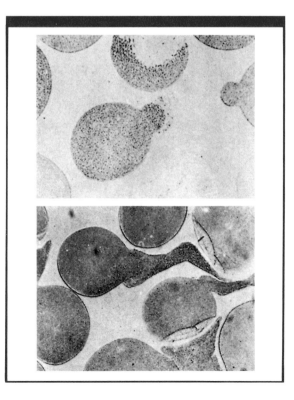

FIGURE 5.6 Effect of mechanical damage on starfish eggs. *Top:* Egg punctured in seawater. The small amount of escaping cytoplasm has coagulated and temporarily healed the injury. *Bottom:* In calcium-free seawater the cytoplasm fails to coagulate, and the cytoplasm bleeds out into the medium. (Reproduced with permission from [103].)

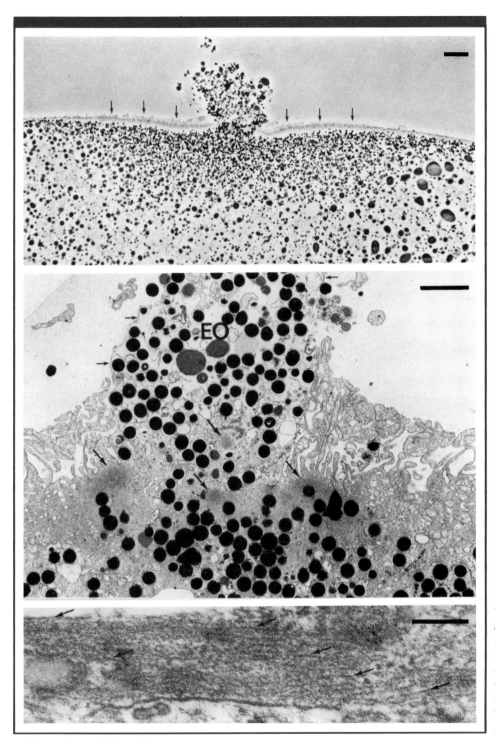

FIGURE 5.7

Top: A punctured frog egg spills some of its yolk granules. **Bar** = 2μm. *Center:* detail of the punctured site. (EO = exovate. **Bar** = 2μm. *Bottom:* The puncture wound heals in purse-string fashion by the contraction of filaments (**arrows**) arranged in bundles. **Bar** = 0.2 μm. (Reproduced with permission from [23].)

nication via "gap junctions," channels permeable to small molecules (up to 900 kD). If a cell is wounded, do its neighbors "know" about it? This question has been studied in several *in vitro* systems by injecting dyes into single cells. If a sheet of epithelial cells is wounded, the cells on the margin of the wound are torn open and exchange freely with the exterior medium. However, within minutes, the junctions with their neighbors are sealed off; to this effect, calcium or other divalent cations are required (136, 171). In endothelial sheets, communication was markedly reduced in 30 minutes; then it returned to normal and actually increased for some time (179).

Cell-to-cell communication is important in heart pathology. Heart cells are all functionally interconnected. Around a myocardial infarct, millions of dead cells are connected with surrounding live cells. This means that intracellular ions could leak out of the live, injured cells and initiate a lethal wave of depolarization. Fortunately, within 2–6 minutes a "healing-over" reaction occurs, indicating that a new ionic barrier is built up near the traumatized ends of the live cells and maintains the gradient of ionic concentration (54). Calcium is essential for this highly focal coagulation (57). Thanks to this ionic barrier a myocardial infarct can be sealed off and prevented from disrupting the function of the entire heart. The precise nature of the seal is not clear; it may be similar to the cytoplasmic coagulation discussed earlier.

Electrical effects of cell wounds are exploited in cardiology; recent myocardial infarcts, for example, affect the electrocardiogram because the live but injured part of the myocardium is negative with respect to the normal heart (98). Injury currents are mild and generally neglected in pathology; they were once thought to be involved in generating thrombi, but this was not confirmed. Biologists now believe that they can affect regeneration (p. 34) and be strong enough, in theory, to affect the orientation of surrounding cells (p. 355).

TOXIC CELL INJURY AND FREE RADICAL PATHOLOGY

Toxic cell injury used to be a depressing topic and quite hopeless, because each toxic agent seemed to act by a different mechanism. Some agents are respiratory poisons; others, as we have seen, block membrane pumps; others yet interfere with the cytoskeleton, inhibit protein synthesis, stuff the lysosomes, or damage the endoplasmic reticulum. A large number of poisons such as alcohol have multiple effects, while others are extraordinarily specific for a single minuscule target, such as gossypol, which destroys only the mitochondria of the Sertoli cells (Figure 4.14).

And then, quite suddenly, some unity was discovered in all this variety: *many toxic agents in their natural state are actually innocuous molecules, but they generate highly toxic **free radicals** as they are processed by enzymes in the endoplasmic reticulum.* This generalization has been extremely helpful; the variety of toxic activities still exists, but it becomes more manageable.

This discovery came in the 1960s from the study of liver damage by carbon tetrachloride, mentioned in Chapter 4 as causing cellular swelling and steatosis (p. 136). Later it turned out that *free radicals are involved in many pathologic and physiologic events,* far beyond the field of toxic agents; in fact they are turning up in all branches of pathology (7, 100, 218).

Although free radicals made their debut in pathology quite recently, they had been waiting for a long time (7, 100, 218). Two billion years ago, after the anaerobic blue-green algae had produced enough oxygen by photosynthesis, new types of cells evolved to exploit it for a life based on respiration. But these new cells were caught in a bind, as we are to this day: *oxygen is life-giving but toxic; no breathing animal can survive in pure oxygen.* Survival in our atmosphere is based on a precarious system of chemical mechanisms that minimize the production of oxygen-derived free radicals and inactivate (scavenge) those that are inevitable.

The reality of oxygen toxicity dawned on the medical profession quite late. Before 1967, when a critically ill patient was kept for many days on a respirator delivering pure oxygen and then died of a peculiar lung disease, suspicions centered on a virus or on the machine itself (166). Today, with the perfect clarity of hindsight (80), it is obvious that the toxicity of oxygen should have been predicted from its electronic structure, because its reduction to water can proceed through a series of steps that generates highly reactive free radicals (73, 79). This is why this field is so closely linked with the metabolism of oxygen. However, let it be clear that *many free radicals have nothing to do with oxygen,* at least initially.

The existence of free radicals in the world of chemistry was established by the turn of the century but remained shrouded in controversy, not all of which has disappeared. The food industry was the first to realize the importance of free-radical chemistry: by the 1940s it was clear that free radicals could explain the rancidity of foods. The great leap from cans of rancid peanuts to live people came about twenty years later, when it was realized that free radicals play a role in normal physiology, in disease, and even in aging (50) (are we slowly turning rancid?). The discovery, as mentioned earlier, was made not directly through the toxicity of oxygen but through studies of carbon tetrachloride poisoning.

HOW DO FREE RADICALS RELATE TO DISEASE?

Let it be clear that we could not live without free radicals; however, they often cause damage. It should be helpful to begin with a bird's-eye view of the situations in which free-radical reactions are relevant to pathology. Here are a few.

- *Leukocytes use oxygen-derived free radicals for killing bacteria.* The price paid for this marvelous adaptation is that the same free radicals can turn against the leukocytes themselves or against any nearby tissue.
- *Because leukocytes produce free radicals even in the absence of bacterial stimulation,* many inflammatory diseases involve free-radical-induced damage, especially in the joints and lungs.
- *Injury spills blood, which releases iron;* iron catalyzes free-radical reactions that increase the damage, especially in the central nervous system.
- *Injury releases arachidonic acid from cell membranes;* the subsequent metabolism of arachidonic acid involves lipid peroxidation with release of free radicals (37).
- *Ischemia,* in theory, should be relieved by reperfusion; but when oxygen-rich blood is returned to the ischemic tissue, it raises havoc by a mechanism based on oxygen-derived free radicals (p. 687).
- *Organ preservation for transplants* is jeopardized by similar reperfusion problems.
- *Sunlight* damages the skin by singlet oxygen and free-radical mechanisms.
- *X-rays* kill tumors and cause tissue damage, in part by producing free radicals.
- *Tumors* are caused by many mechanisms; one is thought to be DNA damage by free radicals.
- *Many drugs, toxic agents, and pollutants* cause damage because they are metabolized in such a way as to produce injurious free radicals; the long list includes, besides CCl_4, cigarette smoke, antibiotics, anticancer agents, and the ill-famed paraquat (221).
- *Atherosclerosis,* the great killer in Western cultures, involves the peroxidation of low-density lipoprotein (LDL), so much so that an antioxidant therapy is now being tested (p. 658).
- *Aging;* yes, there is also a free-radical theory of aging (50, 186).

We will spare you allergy, frostbite, and much more. This partial list should suffice to prove that this chapter—perhaps rather dry for some tastes—is justified.

WHAT ARE FREE RADICALS?

Free radicals are atoms or molecules with an unpaired electron in the outermost orbital. As such they are unstable and therefore highly reactive. Some last just milliseconds, and their existence can be established only indirectly: much of the controversy that still surrounds free radicals stems from this fact. They also tend to form chain reactions, which could be very destructive if the cells were not prepared to stop them by a number of defensive mechanisms. The brief existence of free radicals, reminiscent of a flare, has three phases: *initiation, propagation,* and *termination.* Because they are so reactive and easily trapped, free radicals can travel only very short distances within a cell, probably fractions of a micrometer. If this were not so, the DNA in the nucleus would be at the constant mercy of metabolic events in the endoplasmic reticulum and the mitochondria.

How, in a living tissue, can any atom or molecule find itself limited to a single electron in an outer orbit? This accident can occur in several ways.

- *Energy supplied by the environment can split the covalent bond between two atoms* in such a way that one electron remains attached to either side (homolytic fission). This is what happens when tissues are irradiated: water molecules are split into free radicals (**radiolysis**) which account for much of the tissue damage. The energy of sunlight does something similar to the skin (**photolysis**).
- Even without the application of external energy, *susceptible atoms can capture an electron,* for instance, an electron that strays off the electron transport chain in a mitochondrion. Normally, the electron-transfer reactions are carried out by enzymes that are firmly embedded and properly ordered in lipid membranes, so that the production of free radicals is minimized; but this order can be broken.

Under normal conditions, about 1 percent of the electrons that pass along the transport chain stray away and react with molecular oxygen; fortunately, the resulting free radical is captured by defensive free-radical scavengers (to be discussed shortly) and damage is avoided (95). The rate of this electron escape is directly proportional to the partial pressure of oxygen. In a person breathing 100 percent O_2 the mitochondria of the pulmonary alveolar cells may produce five times the usual amount of free radicals, too much for the scavenger mechanisms to absorb.

- *Several oxidative enzymes can produce free radicals* (Figure 5.8) (79), in some cases because the substrate diffuses away from the enzyme surface before it is wholly oxidized or reduced to an even electron number (185).

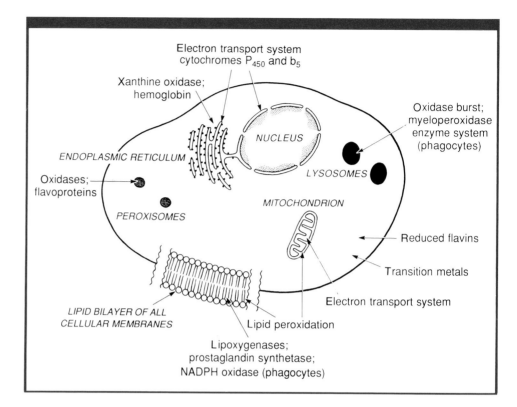

FIGURE 5.8
Cellular sources of free radicals.
(Adapted from [141].)

The enzymes involved in redox reactions contain heavy metals such as Fe, Cu, and Zn (hence their color and their name: cytochromes). This is a key point: the so-called transitional metals, which can change valence, take part in electron transfers as acceptors or donors; when they are loose in the tissues they continue in these roles and generate free radicals in an uncontrolled fashion. Iron is the chief offender (6, 101, 159, 222).

THE ABC OF FREE-RADICAL REACTIONS IN BIOLOGICAL SYSTEMS

Let us begin by explaining the chain of events leading to the destruction of alveolar cells in the

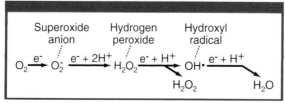

FIGURE 5.9
The univalent pathway for the reduction of molecular oxygen to water. During this stepwise addition of electrons, toxic free-radical by-products appear. This does not occur when oxygen is reduced quadrivalently by the mitochondrial cytochrome oxidase system. (Reproduced with permission from [55].)

lungs of an animal exposed to 100 percent oxygen (p. 182). We know that cells derive most of their ATP from the stepwise reduction of oxygen to water by the mitochondrial transport system; each electron is conveyed along an orderly chain of enzyme molecules woven into the mitochondrial membrane. Although four electrons are needed for reducing each atom of oxygen, an oxygen atom can accept fewer than four; and in so doing it turns into one of several toxic free radicals, as summarized in Figure 5.9.

If oxygen accepts *one* electron, it becomes **superoxide anion radical:**

$$O_2 + 2e^- \longrightarrow O_2^- \text{ (superoxide anion radical)}$$

Superoxide itself is not a very powerful oxidant; however, it can easily donate its electron to any nearby atom of Fe^{3+}, thereby reducing it to **divalent Fe:**

$$O_2^- + Fe^{3+} \longrightarrow O_2 + Fe^{2+}$$

If O_2 accepts *two* electrons, it produces the old-time antiseptic, **hydrogen peroxide:**

$$O_2 + 2e^- + 2H^+ \longrightarrow H_2O_2 \text{ (hydrogen peroxide)}$$

Now, in the presence of divalent Fe, hydrogen peroxide produces OH·, the **hydroxyl radical,** which is the most reactive of all biological free radicals and the most potent biological oxidizing agent known:

$$H_2O_2 + Fe^{2+} \longrightarrow HO\cdot + OH^- + Fe^{3+}$$

Hydroxyl radical, HO· (also written OH·), is the real villain of most free-radical reactions in biology; it can react with almost any organic molecule. In fact, a classic method for hydroxylating organic molecules is Fenton's reagent, a mixture of H_2O_2 and iron salts, which produces the reaction we have just outlined (95).

The last two reactions occur in the presence of iron, which acts as a catalyst; they can be summed up as follows, leaving out the Fe:

$$O_2^- + H_2O_2 \xrightarrow{\text{Fe}} OH\cdot + OH^- + O_2$$

This fundamental reaction has been called the iron-catalyzed Haber–Weiss reaction or the superoxide-driven Fenton reaction. Iron atoms for these reactions, inside and outside the cell, can be supplied by ferritin, transferrin, hemoglobin, and other heme-containing molecules. Here is an example: in blunt injuries to the central nervous system, blood escapes into the white or grey matter; part of the ensuing cellular damage is attributed not to trauma *per se* but to free radicals generated by the hemoglobin of spilled red blood cells (59) and by the iron transported by the plasma (250) (p. 214). We chose the central nervous system as an example, because this tissue is especially sensitive to free-radical damage on account of its high phospholipid content.

HOW FREE RADICALS CAUSE DAMAGE

When a potent oxidizer such as OH· is set loose inside or near a cell, it can initiate a series of reactions that have irreparable effects on macromolecules. *Lipid, protein, carbohydrate, and even DNA molecules can be bent out of shape, broken, or cross-linked* (Figure 5.10). It is worth noting that commercial polymers such as Teflon, vinyl plastics, and even rubber are solidified (i.e., cross-linked) with the help of free radicals. Something similar happens normally *in vivo*: age pigment, lipofuscin, is made of cross-linked lipid (p. 97). On the other hand, in arthritis, the breakdown of hyaluronic acid, the essential macromolecular lubricant of all joints, is also attributed to free radicals.

Lipids are prime molecular targets for free radicals, which means that cell membranes are especially at

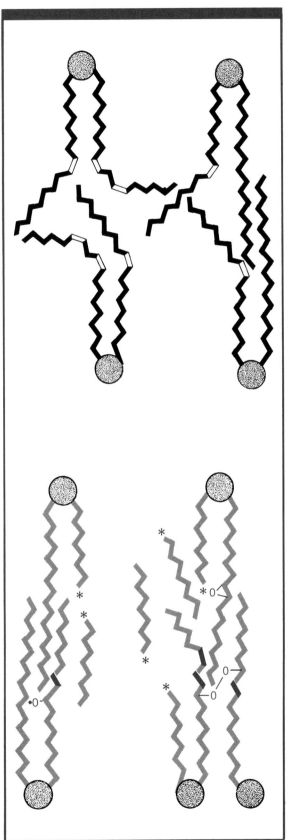

FIGURE 5.10
Types of damage that free radicals can produce in phospholipid molecules. *Top:* Four normal phospholipid molecules forming the skeleton of the plasma membrane. The circles are glycerophosphate head groups. In the fatty acid tails, unsaturated bonds create a bend with an angle of 123°. *Bottom:* As a result of free-radical attack, the fatty acid chains can be bent out of shape, broken, or cross-linked. •: Negative charge of carboxylic groups. -O·: Oxygen atoms. (Adapted from [58].)

risk. We will use them to illustrate the basic reactions.

Initiation Consider the basic structure of the bimolecular leaflets, with the water-soluble, polar ends of the phospholipid molecules on the outer surfaces and the nonpolar ends pointing inward. Oxygen is 7 or 8 times more soluble in nonpolar solvents than in water, which means that it is more available in this midzone of the cell membrane (33). Here lie precisely those parts of the phospholipid molecules—the polyunsaturated fatty acids—that are most susceptible to free-radical damage. Polyunsaturated fatty acids (PUFA) have an Achilles heal: the hydrogens on carbons between two double bonds are easily abstracted. A free radical comes along and abstracts the hydrogen, whereupon the double bonds rearrange themselves. This rearrangement causes the molecule to change shape because the normal *cis* form bends the chain to 123 degrees, whereas the *trans* form is straight (Figure 5.10).

Propagation Now comes the phase of propagation. For instance,

$$PUFA\cdot + O_2 \rightarrow PUFA-OO\cdot$$
$$PUFA-OO\cdot + PUFA$$
$$\rightarrow PUFA-OOH + PUFA\cdot$$

Another set of reactions causes the fatty-acid chains to break up and yield **malonaldehyde** (60).

The smell of rancid foods is due to such aldehydes and to other lipid oxidation products (49, 74), but it has a useful counterpart: malonaldehyde can be used for quantitating free-radical reactions.

Termination Eventually, before the whole cell and its neighbors are involved, *terminating reactions* set in. Note that in all the following examples, *the final result is that the fatty acids have been polymerized;* in other words, the net effect of the free-radical assault is a molecular lesion:

$$PUFA\cdot + PUFA\cdot \rightarrow PUFA-PUFA$$
$$PUFA-OO\cdot + PUFA-OO\cdot \rightarrow$$
$$O_2 + PUFA-OO- PUFA$$
$$PUFA-OO\cdot + PUFA \rightarrow PUFA-OO-PUFA$$

Other and more favorable terminating options occur when the roving free radical bumps into a scavenger enzyme, or a scavenger phenolic compound such as vitamin E, embedded in the cell membrane. Such large molecules take part in free-radical reactions without propagating them: even though they acquire the change of a free radical, they can be considered "frozen," immobilized free radicals (95):

$$PUFA\cdot + (vit. E)OH \rightarrow PUFA-H + (vit. E)\cdot$$

The (vit. E)OH can then be regenerated by reacting with reduced glutathione (GSH) to yield

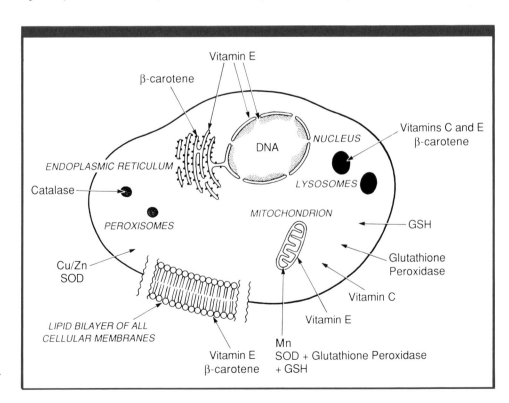

FIGURE 5.11
Cellular scavengers of free radicals. (Adapted from [141].)

GSSG, which in turn is reduced by glutathione reductase:

$$(\text{vit. E})O\cdot + GSH \rightarrow (\text{vit. E})OH + GS\cdot$$
$$GS\cdot + GS\cdot \rightarrow GSSG$$
$$GSSG + NADPH + H^+ \rightarrow 2GSH + NADP^+$$

DEFENSES AGAINST FREE RADICALS

Cells appear to have at least two neatly coordinated lines of defense: scavenger enzymes and antioxidants (Figure 5.11).

The first line of defense is a twin set of enzymes that eliminates the two principal reactants, superoxide radical (O_2^-) and hydrogen peroxide (H_2O_2), so that they cannot interact by the Haber–Weiss reaction and produce the dangerous hydroxyl radical OH·. Each of the two free radicals is counteracted by a specific type of enzyme:

Superoxide Dismutase This enzyme (called SOD) eliminates O_2^-:

$$O_2^- + O_2 + 2H \xrightarrow{\text{SOD}} H_2O_2 + O_2$$

SOD, an inducible enzyme, is present in several isoenzyme forms: some are free in the cytosol, poised to catch superoxide radicals wherever they may appear, and some are in the mitochondria, where most of the oxidative metabolism occurs. On the other hand, SOD is present only in trace amounts in plasma and extracellular fluids, which means that free-radical reactions outside cells are not readily held in check (80). True to its important function, SOD is very stable and one of the most active enzymes known.

SOD was discovered in 1938 in ox blood as a blue-green, copper-containing protein of unknown function and was called hemocuprein. Then cupreins were found in several tissues. In 1969 it was shown that they all represented SOD and contained zinc as well as copper (79). The metal atoms act as electron exchangers.

An intellectually satisfying detail: aerobic bacteria also contain SOD, in which the copper is replaced by iron or manganese. Bacterial SOD belongs to a totally different evolutionary development, as shown by its amino acid sequence. Guess which SOD is present in mitochondria? The bacterial type—one more bit of evidence that bacteria and mitochondria are close relatives (79).

Catalases and Peroxidases These enzymes eliminate H_2O_2, the other potentially dangerous substrate; both have hematin as a prosthetic group. Catalases act directly on H_2O_2, whereas peroxi-dases require a cosubstrate (reductant) other than H_2O_2 as electron donors (79).

$$H_2O_2 + H_2O_2 \rightarrow 2H_2O + O_2 \quad \text{(catalases)}$$
$$H_2O_2 + RH_2 \rightarrow 2H_2O + R \quad \text{(peroxidases)}$$

Antioxidants The second line of defense is a group of water- and lipid-soluble antioxidants. While SODs and catalases/peroxidases hold to a minimum the two precursors of OH·, the small amount of OH· and other radicals that may yet form are being neutralized by antioxidants strategically distributed in the membranes and the cytosol:

Vitamin E
  (alpha-tocopherol)
beta-carotene   *in the lipid phase*
  (precursor of
  vitamin A)
ascorbic acid   *in the watery phase*
glutathione

In the extracellular spaces there is little or no superoxide dismutase; however, the plasma contains powerful scavengers, notably **ceruloplasmin.**

EXAMPLES OF FREE-RADICAL DISEASE

As we mentioned earlier, the trailblazer of this research was carbon tetrachloride poisoning—or rather Dr. R.O. Recknagel (p. 136). Only 2 hours after administration of the poison, electron microscopy of the liver already shows quite clearly that something is happening to the endoplasmic reticulum; the cisternae seen in profile become very thin and collapsed, as if they had lost their content (Figure 5.12) (65). Today the molecular events are largely understood. The P-450 enzyme system, embedded in the membrane of the endoplasmic reticulum, adds an electron to the CCl_4 and splits it into a Cl^- ion and the highly reactive free radical CCl_3^-, which attacks the membranes of the ER (Figure 5.13). This mechanism explains the toxic effects on the liver of many drugs (165), of environmental agents, and even of carcinogens (230).

Another classic example of free-radical injury (77, 146) is lung damage from exposure to pure oxygen. Adult rats breathing O_2 at one atmosphere die of pulmonary edema in less than 60 hours (73); histology shows destruction of the alveolar epithelium and of the underlying capillary endothelium (147). Chronic lung damage is caused by environmental pollutants, including ozone, NO, NO_2, and cigarette smoke, which initiate free-radical reactions.

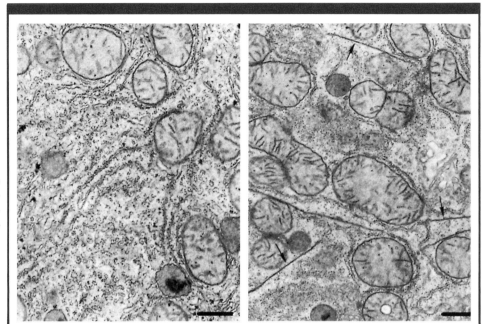

FIGURE 5.12
Effect of CCl₄ on rat liver. *Left:* Control (part of a liver cell). Note abundant endoplasmic reticulum and polyribosomes. *Right:* Two hours after intragastric administration of CCl₄. The rough ER cisternae have collapsed into thin, rigid plates; ribosomes have become detached; polyribosomes have broken up. **Bars** = 0.5 μm. (Reproduced with permission from [65].)

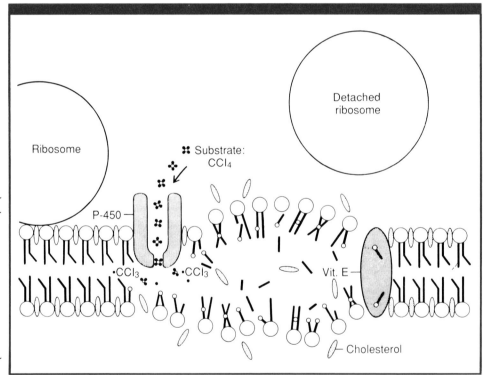

FIGURE 5.13
Artist's view of the catastrophic events in the membrane of the endoplasmic reticulum when the P-450 enzyme system metabolizes CCl₄. The CCl₄ breaks down into free radicals, which attack the surrounding phospholipid molecules (particularly their fatty acid tails), causing them to be deformed, cross-linked, or split; the chain reaction is then stopped by a molecule of vitamin E, which scavenges lipid peroxyl radicals. As a result of the membrane damage, the ribosomes become detached.

Besides X-ray radiation, sunlight can be toxic (62, 71). Sunbathers protect themselves with sunscreen creams, and some aerobic bacteria protect themselves with SOD, but to strict anaerobes sunlight is lethal. The aerobe *Sarcina lutea* is yellow (lutea) because it contains the orange-yellow antioxidant beta-carotene in its membrane; the coating works like a suntan and makes the bacterium photoresistant. Indeed, the carotene-free mutant dies when exposed to light, becoming the victim of light-generated singlet oxygen and free radicals (Figure 5.14). This may sound like trivial information, but in 1970 it led Micheline Mathews-Roth and her collaborators to discover that previously incurable photosensitive patients could be treated with an antioxidant, β-carotene, a precursor of vitamin A. The inspiring thought: what is good for bacteria might also be good for people (149).

> These photosensitive patients suffered from erythropoietic protoporphyria, a congenital anomaly in the metabolism of blood porphyrins (the ring-shaped, tetrapyrrolic, iron-free precursors of the heme in hemoglobin). Porphyrins have long been known as photosensitizers. Due to the lack of an enzyme, an excess of protoporphyrin accumulates in the blood and tissues. The precise chain of events is not clear, but it is believed that when protoporphyrin is struck by light, it generates free-radical reactions and singlet oxygen; therefore, exposing the skin to sunlight causes itching, burning, blisters, and even ulcerations and scarring. For some of these patients, condemned to lead a nocturnal life, treatment with beta-carotene makes it possible to reappear and work in broad daylight (149) (Figure 5.15).

How does one know that a disease is caused by free radicals? Ultimate proof is perhaps impossible. Many biochemical and biophysical methods are available for detecting and measuring free radicals (219). There are also some revealing experiments of nature: patients who lack glutathione peroxidase in their red blood cells suffer from hemolytic anemia because the red cell membranes are open to attack by H_2O_2. A similar defect is known for platelets in Glanzmann's thrombocytopenia (79). However, *the most compelling proof that a disease is caused by free radicals is the effect of prevention or treatment with antioxidants and/or with free-radical scavengers.*

Experimentally, many reports indicate that treatment with superoxide dismutase (SOD), for instance, reduces X-ray damage or prolongs the life of rats exposed to pure oxygen (7, 218, 231). Cloned human SOD is now available and its clinical uses are being explored (7, 31); however, any therapy aimed at suppressing free radicals will not be without hazard because, after all, leukocytes need to retain their oxygen-radical generating mechanisms if they are to protect us from bacteria (16).

> There are other problems. SOD injected intravenously is removed so fast by the littoral phagocytes (p. 299) that its half-life is of the order of minutes. The same is true for catalase. Furthermore, these enzymes are needed also, and perhaps, especially inside the cells where many free-radical reactions are initiated. Yet only a tiny fraction of the circulating

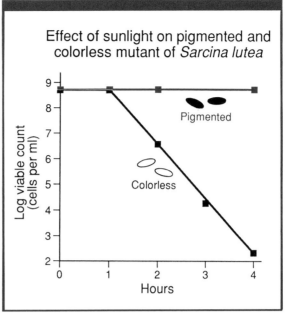

Effect of sunlight on pigmented and colorless mutant of *Sarcina lutea*

FIGURE 5.14 The bacterium *Sarcina lutea* is protected from the lethal effect of sunlight by its natural carotenoid pigment. (Adapted from [150]).

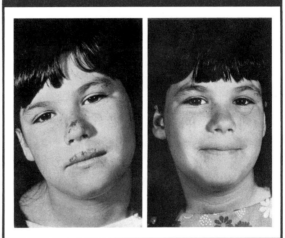

FIGURE 5.15 *Left:* Child with skin lesions typical of protoporphyria, an oversensitivity to light. *Right:* Same child after treatment with β-carotene, a precursor of vitamin A. (Courtesy of Dr. M. Mathews-Roth, Channing Laboratory, Harvard University, Boston, MA.)

> enzyme is picked up by the endothelium, and even less is transcytosed into the tissues. Several tricks have been devised to evade the littoral phagocytes, with some success: packing the enzymes in liposomes (p. 212), in the hope that these will fuse with the endothelium of various organs and not just with phagocytes; and linking the enzyme with polyethylene glycol, which facilitates nonspecific cellular uptake and also makes the enzyme nonimmunogenic (16).

TO SUM UP: The study of free radicals has opened a window on some new mechanisms of disease, and therapeutic developments are bound to follow. A hot area of research is free-radical injury to the central nervous system. Myelin is made of cell membranes, which makes it a preferential target for free radicals; and injury spills red blood cells, which supply iron, a catalyst of free-radical reactions. Other major areas of interest are inflammation (free radicals are now listed among the chemical mediators of inflammation) and ischemia, a topic closely related to oxygen supply (p. 687). Free-radical research has come a long way since the cans of rancid peanuts.

Cell Death

The ultimate effect of cell injury is cell death. This topic, once considered the dullest in pathology, has become extremely fashionable since it was realized that many of us die, after all, of cell death

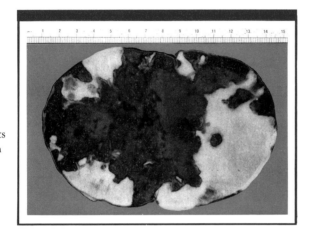

FIGURE 5.16 Multiple infarcts (white areas) in the enlarged spleen of a woman with a long history of heart disease.

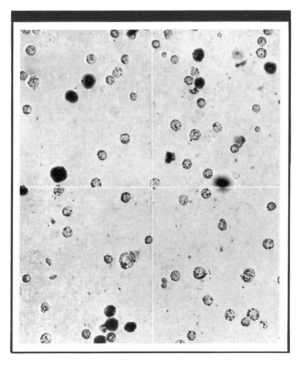

FIGURE 5.17 Dye exclusion test for identifying dead cells in a suspension of Ehrlich ascites carcinoma. The cells that have been permeated by the black dye (nigrosin) are dead. (Reproduced with permission from [111].)

in the form of infarcts. Another incentive for studying cell death has been the rise of organ banks to support organ grafts: suddenly it became urgent to find out how and why cells die. Whole books on cell death are now commonplace (29, 30, 53, 156, 184, 227, 227a).

Cell death occurs in a variety of settings somewhat reminiscent of the human condition:
- by *accident*, such as failure of the blood supply;
- by *suicide*: virtually every cell type is ready to perform this ultimate sacrifice. If it receives the appropriate signal, it blindly complies, and switches on an active mechanism that leads to self-destruction;
- by *killer cells* that are specialized for this aggressive duty.

Such are, so to say, the social settings of cell death; as regards the microscopic, biochemical and functional changes of dying cells, we can expect a great deal of variability: cells killed **accidentally** by trauma, heat, dehydration, poisons, histologic fixatives, or lack of oxygen will presumably die different deaths, and dying neurons will presumably develop changes different from those of dying lymphocytes. However, in practice, only one form of accidental cell death is well understood, because it is very common, easy to produce experimentally on a massive scale, and therefore easy to sample: *ischemic cell death*. Typically, ischemic cell death is accompanied by cellular swelling; we therefore proposed that it be called *oncosis* (from the Greek *ónkos*, swelling), a name coined almost a century ago by von Recklinghausen (142a). As regards **cell death by suicide**, it often occurs by a modality called *apoptosis*, which involves cell shrinkage (it was originally called "shrinkage necrosis"). Oddly enough, apoptosis—so typical of cell suicide—usually occurs in cells assassinated by killer cells.

When is a cell dead? The reader may recall that we had a hard time defining clinical death (p. 3); it is no easier to define cell death. There is no certain way to find out exactly when a cell dies. On the other hand, after a cell has been dead for some time, say 12–24 hours, it undergoes secondary morphologic changes, such as the breakdown of the nucleus, that are summed up by the term **necrosis** (which we will discuss later). Necrosis is easily recognized, but experts are still seeking techniques for identifying cells that died within minutes or hours. One of the difficulties is distinguishing reversible injury from recent death;

increased membrane permeability, for example, may occur in both situations.

The diagnosis of cell death, if such a diagnosis is possible, should probably rely on functional rather than morphologic criteria. The most used criterion is increased permeability of the cell membrane, which is easily tested on isolated cells either in suspension or in tissue culture. A suitable dye is placed in the medium; if the cells exclude it, they are alive; if they soak it up, they are presumed dead (dye exclusion test). Nigrosin (a black dye) and trypan blue are often used in this manner (Figure 5.17). Another method applicable to cell suspensions or cultures is to label all the cells with radioactive chromium while they are still alive. Exactly how and where the chromium is bound in the cell is not clear, but in practice it is released when the cell dies. Thus, the amount of chromium released into the medium is an indication of cell death (27, 193, 253). A complicating factor is that some release occurs before death as a result of injury (41). On tissue sections there is no foolproof method for identifying cells that are dying or just died, with one major exception: the modality of cell death called apoptosis can be identified by its distinctive nuclear changes as well as by a histochemical method based on molecular pathology, as we will explain further.

CELL DEATH WITH SWELLING: ONCOSIS

This form of cell death is typically the result of ischemia. The swelling, as will be discussed below, is due to the failure of ionic pumps in the cell membrane, through lack of energy supply; we can therefore expect that oncosis will also be induced by poisons that interfere with the cell's energy metabolism, or with the integrity of the cell membrane. Ischemia kills cells within a time span that varies between minutes (for neurons) and hours (for fibroblasts).

It follows that one of Nature's best models of oncosis should be the infarcts, so commonly seen in human hearts, brains, kidneys, and other organs. Infarcts, in a real sense, multiply and enlarge the cellular features of oncosis and of the necrosis that follows. Overall, the study of human or experimental infarcts teaches us some important lessons. First of all, as the cells swell and die, little can be seen by the naked eye and even with the microscope; however, *after* the cells have died, striking changes occur that anatomists have observed for centuries: in most solid organs the infarcts become firm and white in a matter of days; by contrast, some necrotic tissues appear to disintegrate and liquefy. These two opposite trends represent the multiplied effects of cellular changes: *while the cells are dying, their*

proteins are caught between two possible fates: denaturation (i.e., coagulation) and autolysis (dissolution by their own enzymes). This is one of the basic rules of cell death. Both mechanisms of protein demise are at work even after cell death; this dualism is reflected, as we will see, in the ancient terms *liquefaction necrosis* and *coagulation necrosis*.

The two mechanisms are best observed in action in second-rate fish markets: fish fillets should be soft and semitransparent, but after they have been displayed for a day or two they look stiff, opaque, and whitish as if they had been partly cooked; this appearance— long known in pathology as parboiled (partially boiled)—is due to protein denaturation. On the other hand, outdated shellfish become flabby and seem to liquefy: this is autolysis.

The terms *coagulation* and *denaturation* in the context of cell death are used interchangeably, because denatured proteins tend to coagulate. Overall, in dying and dead tissues, the balance between the two processes depends on the enzyme content of the cells. *In the end, coagulation usually prevails.*

Oncosis: A Simple Experiment To study the features of oncosis (such as the changes in cell volume, or the time course of protein denaturation and autolysis), we must turn to experimental infarcts (143). Note that the liver has been used for most experimental studies of cell death: we should keep in mind that the data are *probably* applicable to other tissues, but with some changes.

Let us prepare little cubes of fresh, sterile, rat liver, 1 cm on edge, and introduce them into the peritoneal cavities of other rats. We recover and examine these implants after various periods of time. Under these circumstances we can assume that the implanted liver cells are dying of blood deprivation; immunologic phenomena are not involved, at least up to 24 hours. The basic changes are summarized in Figures 5.18 and 5.19.

- *Immediately the implants begin to swell,* as shown by an increase in weight
- Their internal pH drops precipitously
- The amount of extractable protein and of protein breakdown products rises, then falls
- in the meantime the implants become paler and paler to the naked eye

Translating these changes into cellular terms, we have:

- *The swelling (weight gain) of an implant means that the liver cells are starved of oxygen;* thus, the membrane ion pumps run down,

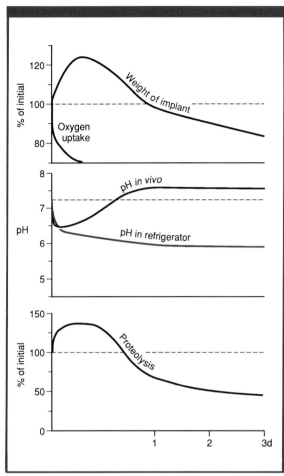

FIGURE 5.18

Changes occurring over 5 days in a mass of dying and dead tissue (oncosis → necrosis). **Black curves:** Fragments of rat liver implanted in the peritoneum. **Red curve:** rat liver stored in a refrigerator. *Top:* The implants swell, then shrink as the cells burst; the ability to take up oxygen (tested *in vitro*) reflects the condition of the mitochondria. *Center:* Tissue pH drops precipitously *in vivo*, then rises if the acid can diffuse away (which does not occur *in vitro*). *Bottom:* The amount of extractable protein rises (autolysis) then falls as protein denaturation prevails. See Figure 5.19. (Adapted from [143].)

and the cells swell as fluid is absorbed (in this setting) from the peritoneal cavity.

- *The drop in pH occurs because the cells must turn to their glycogen supplies* and limp along for some time by glycolysis, producing lactic acid, which cannot be removed because the tissue has no circulation. In the meantime, some enzymes leak out of the lysosomes, and finding themselves in an acid pH (optimal for lysosomal hydrolases), they attack all the cytoplasmic components. Eventually

the pH returns to normal because the cell membranes are broken down, enabling the acids to diffuse away and be removed by the blood stream of the surrounding live tissues.

- *The percentage of extractable protein and peptides rises as the cells begin to digest themselves, then falls as denaturation prevails.* Denaturation is what makes dead tissue turn white (Figure 5.20), as we will explain shortly.

Microscopic Aspect of Dying and Dead Tissues

The changes along this deadly path are comparatively slow and hard to see by light microscopy (Figure 5.20). The early swelling is not obvious (a doubling in volume implies only a 26 percent increase in diameter); the mitochondria and ER may swell, but this is best seen by electron microscopy; the cytoplasmic basophilia fades away slowly because the ribosomes are partly denatured and partly digested by lysosomal ribonucleases; the nucleus eventually breaks down and disappears (p. 160); by 24 hours or so the cell is an *eosinophilic mass* with little or no structural detail. *Some time during this sequence the cell must have died.* But when?

The point of no return, beyond which the liver cell is no longer retrievable, can be determined—*in vivo*—by another simple experiment: all we need to do—in a series of rats—is to clamp the circulation to a liver lobe for increasing times and then allow the circulation to return. One day later, if the lobe looks grossly normal, the cells have survived; *if the lobe has become white and firm, the cells have died.* This approach sets the point of no return in this system at 2–2.5 hours (18, 76). Now, returning to liver implants, if we examine the cells by light microscopy after 2–3 hours, we will see nothing to tell us that they differ significantly from those of normal controls (Figure 5.20): as expected, histologic sections do not give us the time of cell death.

Why does the dead tissue become firmer and white? Common sense suggests protein denaturation, but proving it is not simple, because there is no histochemical method specific for denatured protein. In ordinary histologic sections *coagulated cells are eosinophilic* (which explains why neuropathologists sometimes speak of *red neurons* in injured brain tissue), but this is of course very nonspecific. The best way to demonstrate denatured proteins in a tissue is to examine thin slices of fresh, unfixed frozen sections using three types of illumination:

- By **transmitted light,** the implants become

more and more opaque, as would be expected from the precipitation (coagulation) of denatured proteins.

- By **dark-field illumination,** the earliest signs of protein precipitation lie far beneath the limits of visibility by ordinary light microscopy, yet they can be beautifully visualized by means of the **Tyndall effect:** the optical phenomenon whereby, to an observer in a dark room, a ray of sunlight renders visible particles of dust that would be invisible in diffuse light. Each particle shines like a bright star. Under the microscope, this effect is obtained by illuminating the object from the side (dark-field microscopy) rather than from beneath. In this way one can visualize particles of ultramicroscopic size. Indeed, slices from a series of implants at different stages show a progressive increase in brightness (Figure 5.21).
- By **ultraviolet microscopy,** denatured proteins become autofluorescent, and slices of the implants show a progressive increase in autofluorescence (Figure 5.22).

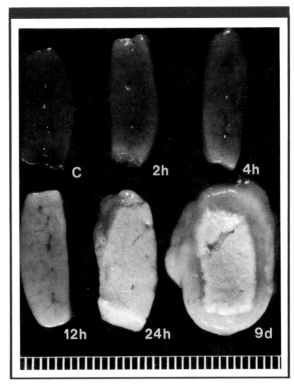

FIGURE 5.19 Gross aspect of rat liver, normal (**C**) and after it was implanted in the peritoneal cavity for 2, 4, 12, and 24 hours, and for 9 days. Increasing whiteness is due to protein denaturation. After 9 days the implant is wrapped in omentum. Scale in mm. (Reproduced with permission from [143].)

Protein Denaturation These results tell us, in essence, that infarcts become white, opaque, and firm for the same reason that transparent egg white becomes white, opaque, and firm when boiled; the whiteness of snow, compared with the transparency of water, is based on the same Tyndall effect. As to the "dryness" of coagulated tissue, it is so only in appearance: a hard-boiled egg also appears

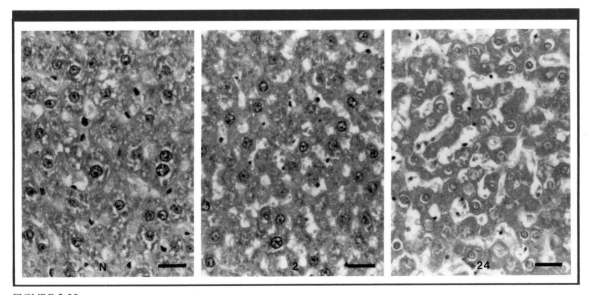

FIGURE 5.20
The difficulty of recognizing cell death by light microscopy. *Left:* Normal rat liver (**N**). *Center:* Section from a fragment of liver that has been implanted into the peritoneal cavity of another rat for 2 hours. Most of these cells are dead, but cannot be recognized as such on this routine microscopic section. *Right:* Section from a 24-hour liver implant. The cells are now clearly necrotic. The white halos around the nuclei are due to swelling of the perinuclear cisternae. **Bars** = 25 μm.

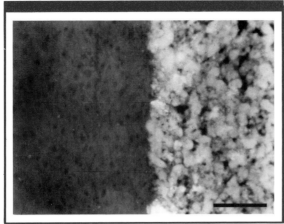

FIGURE 5.21

Precipitation of proteins in coagulation necrosis, as seen in fresh, unfixed sections of rat liver examined by dark field microscopy. *Left:* normal liver. *Right:* liver implant after 24 hours. The brightness is due to light diffraction by clumps of coagulated proteins. The earliest change is already visible, after only 30 minutes of anoxia. **Bar** = 100 μm. (Reproduced with permission from [143].)

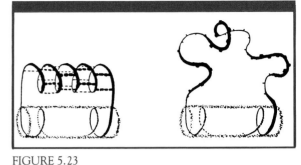

FIGURE 5.23

Denaturation of a protein molecule, artist's view. *Left:* Normal coiled structure; the coils are held together by bonds of various kinds. *Right:* The molecule becomes uncoiled. Side chains are exposed and available for binding with other compounds. This explains the greater reactivity of denatured proteins. (Modified from [113].)

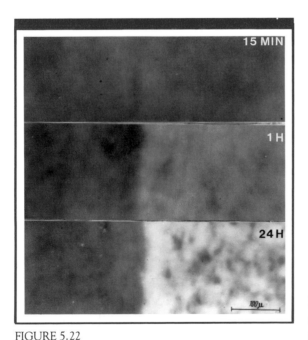

FIGURE 5.22

Sections of unfixed rat liver (*left*, normal, *right*, implanted) viewed by ultraviolet light. The implants had been left in the peritoneal cavity for the time intervals indicated. Autofluorescence indicates protein denaturation. Note that protein denaturation begins while the cells are still alive, because it is already obvious at 1 hour, whereas it takes $2-2\frac{1}{2}$ hours of ischemia to kill liver cells. (Reproduced with permission from [143].)

dry but in fact contains the same amount of trapped water as a fresh egg (143).

A look at the time sequence of the various changes in dying tissue reveals an important fact: *protein lysis and coagulation are both occurring while the cell is still alive.*

> *Protein denaturation implies an uncoiling of the tertiary molecular structure (Figure 5.23) (113); this exposes "buried" side chains, with several physicochemical results: denatured proteins become more reactive; they tend to aggregate; and some of the exposed radicals, if irradiated with ultraviolet light, emit visible light (i.e., become autofluorescent) (2, 25, 220).*

> *Why is the sky blue? We are referring again to the Tyndall effect. Using gold colloids the smallest particles visible by dark-field microscopy are of the order of 50 Å (151). Theoretically, however, there is no limit to the size of an object that can be visualized by light diffraction as long as sufficient illumination is provided (144). After all, the sky is blue because of the light scattered by individual gas molecules in the atmosphere (208).*

Protein denaturation is perhaps the most prevalent and the least studied of all pathologic cellular changes; until recently it was of interest (behold) only to the food industry (126). Yet it was recognized as early as 1886 by Weigert, one of Virchow's disciples, as *Koagulationsnekrose* (coagulation necrosis) (143). In one respect this term is ambiguous: it leaves open the question whether cell death is caused by or followed by coagulation. From what we have just said, however, the ambiguity is appropriate: *protein denaturation begins*

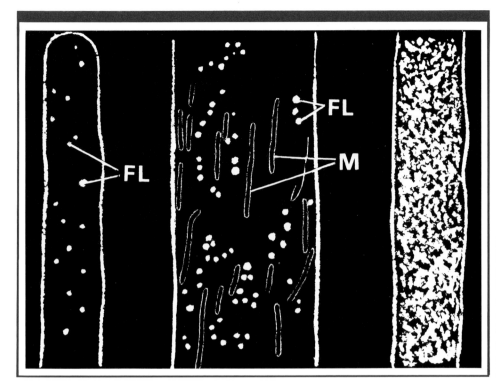

FIGURE 5.24
Denatured proteins in dead cells of plants. Three filaments of the fungus *Saprolegnia* seen by dark-field microscopy. *Left* and *center:* Two normal filaments. **FL**: Free lipid droplets. **M**: Mitochondria. *Right:* A dead filament; its cytoplasm is filled with precipitated proteins that diffract the light. (Slightly retouched from [97].)

in the live cell, takes part in the killing, and then continues in the dead cell. A major function of the heat-shock proteins is precisely to oppose denaturation *in vivo*. We can venture to guess that a dying cell must be a busy place for ubiquitin, the monitor of denatured proteins (p. 43).

Protein denaturation has been observed also in plants (Figure 5.24) (97) and must be a general phenomenon. It has one striking clinical manifestation: the cataract (Figure 5.25). The progressive changes in a cataractous lens, although very slow (months and years), are in many ways parallel to those in the liver implants (143). As the cells of the crystalline lens die, water content and diffusible protein rise and then drop; the pH drops and then returns to normal; opacity and calcium content rise progressively.

By electron microscopy the aggregates of denatured protein, if large enough, become recognizable as fluffy masses. During autolysis in vitro, within 1 hour the mitochondria swell and acquire small smudgy masses of osmiophilic material (109, 228). These masses are not lipid soluble, not rich in calcium, but digestible by proteases (108); they probably represent aggregates of denatured protein. All those who use fluorescence microscopy are familiar with the fact that dead cells are autofluorescent, but the phenomenon is known only as a nuisance. For obvious reasons, there are some

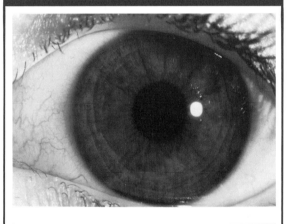

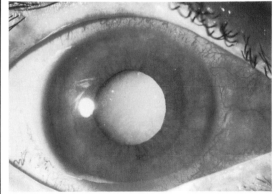

FIGURE 5.25
See color plate 6. *Top:* Normal human eye. *Bottom:* Eye with a cataractous lens. The whiteness, due to protein denaturation, is common to most necrotic tissues. (Courtesy of Dr. J. Babel, Geneva, Switzerland.)

studies on protein fluorescence in the crystalline lens (25).

The mechanism of protein denaturation in cells is not known. The initial drop in pH may be relevant initially, but the process continues even after the pH has returned to normal. Calcium may be involved (67, 68); indeed, denaturation occurs faster *in vivo* than in isolated tissues incubated at 37°C (143), suggesting that calcium supplies from the living tissues facilitate the process.

What is the biological significance of protein denaturation? We see it as a *protective device* on two counts. First, the dying cells are loaded with lysosomal proteolytic enzymes, ready to initiate self-digestion (autolysis). The products of protein digestion (peptides) are powerful irritants and set off an acute inflammatory reaction. *Denaturation puts a stop to autolysis (and to the acute inflammatory response) by inactivating the enzymes and removing their substrates.* Second, proteins released by dying cells can diffuse into the blood stream and become antigens, because intracellular proteins can be recognized by the immune system as nonself. *Denaturation interrupts this sequence by making the proteins insoluble and nonantigenic.*

Support for the latter suggestion comes from the cataract: if a crystalline lens is injured by trauma and not removed, its spilled proteins can give rise to antibodies that attack the lens in the other eye (**phacoanaphylactic ophthalmitis** [72]).

These concepts will be essential for understanding the evolution of an inflammatory reaction around infarcts (p. 439).

> *Mild denaturation of soluble proteins is thought to increase their antigenicity, but in coagulation necrosis we are dealing with profound denaturation with loss of solubility; the aggregated proteins are no longer able to diffuse into the bloodstream, and histology shows that no immune response develops locally against the coagulated mass.*

> *Because the exposed groups of the uncoiled proteins make them more sticky, it has been postulated that denaturation is the mechanism whereby obsolete plasma protein molecules are recognized by phagocytic cells and are picked up and destroyed (224, 238, 239).*

THEORIES OF CELL DEATH: WHAT IS THE FINAL BLOW TO THE ONCOTIC CELL?

We have insisted on **protein denaturation** because, as the term **coagulation necrosis** implies, it is a key feature of accidental cell death. While this change progresses, the cell's metabolism is disrupted and much else is going on. This is a hot area of research. If we knew exactly why a cell becomes irreversibly injured, we might be able to improve the therapy of infarcts; we might even be able to preserve organs better in organ banks, a field that has made little progress in recent years. The hope is to identify some critical cellular malfunction as obvious as "heart failure" and "respiratory failure" are for the body as a whole.

Of course, to hope that any one change can be singled out as *the* critical event may be unrealistic because there are many cell types and many causes of cell death. However, some interesting facts have emerged. The overall approach has been to choose a tissue, injure the cells in some way (*in vivo* or *in vitro*), and then test which cellular organelle or which function might be closing the door to survival. Some theories died, but even those contained some truth. Here are the milestones along this path. The first three mechanisms were tested on ischemic tissues.

- (1) The **lysosomal theory** remains just a theory. It was an outgrowth of the enthusiasm that surrounded the discovery of these organelles. Ischemic cells were supposedly killed from inside by release of lysosomal enzymes: this rather sensational "suicide bag" concept did not fit the facts (66). When cells do commit suicide, as we have seen, they do not use lysosomes (crystal-induced cell suicide seems to be the only exception, p. 141).

- (2) The **mitochondrial theory** has much more to it. Progressive mitochondrial damage is biochemically obvious (157). At the electron microscopic level this damage has been classified into half a dozen grades (157); the most significant of these is the appearance of proteinaceous flocculent densities that appear to be the most reliable ultrastructural sign of irreversible damage.

- (3) The **protein denaturation theory** has already been discussed; today we can add that cells dying by ischemia try to rescue their proteins from denaturation by turning on the heat-shock response. However, if the ischemia persists, the response is bound to fail. It is not known whether protein denaturation might be the final blow; it certainly continues long after cell death (143).

Another set of theories was tested on models of toxic rather than ischemic injury. The new line of thought was that specific metabolic poisons would more precisely dissect the mechanisms of cell death, in contrast with the indiscriminate massacre of ischemic injury. The main target was the liver, which bears the brunt of many toxic insults; especially useful was intoxication with **ethionine,** the ethyl analog of methionine and an inhibitor of protein synthesis. Ethionine induces many specific biochemical and morphologic changes, but not cell death; in other words, *ethionine offers the possibility of finding out what can be done to a cell without killing it.* As a result, three more theories died.

- (4) **Drop in ATP**
- (5) **Inhibition of protein synthesis**
- (6) **Loss of potassium and increase in sodium**

None of these chemical changes can be responsible for cell death because ethionine produces all three, and they can be sustained for 24–48 hours without killing the cells (66):

- (7) While all these theories were being tested, 40 years of studies on carbon tetrachloride poisoning of the liver ended with the discovery of free-radical damage and another theory of cell death: **lipid peroxidation** became a new candidate for ultimate cell killer. However, the role of free radicals in autolysis and in ischemic cell death remained unclear (157), and so the search continued.

- (8) **Increased permeability of the plasma membrane** was long recognized as a possible component of cell injury and death, as proven by the very existence of the dye-exclusion tests. But how would it kill the cell? The first and simplest thought was an escape of potassium and an influx of sodium; disappointingly, it turned out that major fluxes of these ions did not necessarily cause cell death (110). Therefore this eighth mechanism lay dormant until 1979 when it was proposed that the critical ion shift resulting from increased permeability concerned neither potassium nor sodium but calcium, and that an influx of calcium was the final common pathway. Then came a combined theory:

- (9) **Increase in membrane permeability followed by influx of calcium** (38, 67, 68, 210). Calcium ions are biologically very active and liable to disrupt the myriad of interrelated metabolic reactions inside the cell. J.L. Farber proposed that a phospholipase, present in many cell mem-

branes including the mitochondria, is activated by calcium, leading to membrane disruption. *This theory is currently the most popular.* Some of the calcium may come from the ER and especially from the mitochondria: remember that the calcium content of the mitochondria is 1000 to 10,000 times greater than in the cytoplasm (10^{-3} vs. 10^{-6}–10^{-8}M). Whatever its source, the excess of free calcium can activate other enzymes besides phospholipases: *an ATPase* (38), which destroys what little ATP is generated; *proteases* (212), which may explain both the cytoskeletal damage (83, 211) and the surface blebbing; *endonucleases,* which may explain some of the nuclear changes.

The membrane damage caused by phospholipases is at least threefold: phospholipids are lost, and their breakdown products are membrane-toxic. By snipping a fatty acid from the phospholipid molecules, the phospholipase creates "one-legged" lysophospholipids. The wedge shape of these molecules causes them to break up the lipid bilayer into micelles (Figure 4.6); in the meantime the fatty acids, being fat soluble, also insert themselves into the membranes, contributing to the molecular disorder (Table 5.1) (46, 52).

Why should the cell membranes contain such dangerous enzymes as phospholipases? We are dealing

---

TABLE 5.1

Possible Mechanisms of Plasma Membrane Damage during Ischemic Cell Death (Oncosis)

Stretching, secondary to cellular swelling
Loss of phospholipids*
Increased disorder due to insertion of fatty acids*
Increased disorder due to insertion of lysophospholipids*
Loss of connection with cytoskeleton, resulting in blebbing
Bursting of blebs

*Due to phospholipases; may affect internal membranes as well

with one of nature's many two-edged swords. Phospholipases have many essential functions, including phospholipid turnover and protein kinase activation (202). In the plasma membrane they are the key to eicosanoid metabolism. By cleaving arachidonic acid from phospholipid molecules, they initiate the cascade that leads to the production of prostaglandins and leukotrienes, important mediators of inflammation (p. 345).

So how can we envision the drama of accidental cell death? The drama may vary from one tissue to another and with the type of injury, but for ischemic cell death of liver cells we can suggest the following plot, drawn from many sources. The reader should try to see it as a movie:

1. Mitochondrial ATP production stops.
2. The ATP-driven membrane ionic pumps run down.
3. Sodium and water seep into the cell.
4. The cell swells, and the plasma membrane is stretched.
5. Glycolysis enables the cell to limp on for a while.
6. The cell initiates a heat-shock (stress) response, which will probably not help if the ischemia persists.
7. The pH drops.
8. Calcium enters the cell.
9. Calcium activates phospholipases, causing the cell membranes to lose phospholipid and producing lysophosphatides and fatty acids, both of which cause more membrane damage, initiating a vicious circle.
   - Calcium activates proteases, damaging cytoskeletal structures, attacking membrane proteins, which is followed by **blebbing.**
   - Calcium activates ATPase, causing more loss of ATP.
   - Calcium activates endonucleases, causing the nuclear chromatin to clump.
10. Protein denaturation starts (calcium may be involved).
11. All cell membranes are damaged.
12. The ER and other organelles swell.
13. At some point the cell dies, possibly killed by the burst of a bleb.

Some of these concepts have been tested for therapeutic application. Calcium channel blockers do retard cell death experimentally (39); and calcium ionophores, which allow a flow of calcium into the cell, induce it (67, 68). Calcium channel blockers are indeed used in cardiac therapy, but their mechanism of action is difficult to assess because they have several effects, such as vasodilatation; whether they can reduce the size of infarcts is not clear (38).

Note: *Fast or slow cell death may produce different sequences of events.* This is best seen in myocardial infarcts, where the myocardial fibers die suddenly or slowly depending on the distance from the nearest blood supply. As shown in Figure 5.26, in the center of the infarct, where the lack of oxygen and nutrients is total, the cells just coagulate (if there is an initial phase of swelling, it is soon reversed). By contrast, cells that lie close to the inner surface of the ventricle can survive for some time on oxygen and nutrients diffusing from the blood in the ventricular cavity; they swell and slowly "melt away" by a process akin to autolysis, leaving an empty tube of basement membrane; there is no hint of coagulation. This process is called *myocytolysis.*

Massive cell death within the live body is modified by its live surroundings; we can therefore expect it to be different from massive cell death in organs separated from the body. For example, in liver tissue displayed in a butcher's shop the cells die of ischemia, but all the changes in the dying and dead cells are produced by the cell's own

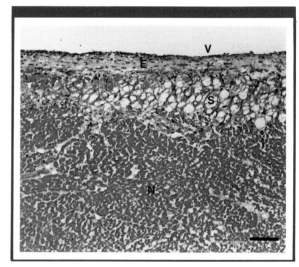

FIGURE 5.26
Myocardial infarct showing two varieties of ischemic cell death, depending on the distance from the nearest blood supply. **E:** endocardium. **S:** empty-looking myocardial fibers that swelled and died a slow death (myocytolysis), being partly nourished by blood flowing in the ventricle (**V**). **N:** necrotic, shrunken myocardial fibers that underwent coagulation necrosis. **Bar** = 100 μm.

content; nothing is added to the tissue's internal milieu, and nothing is removed. This is *autolysis*.

AUTOLYSIS

When cells die in tissues that have been separated from the body and in the whole body after death, some of the lysosomal hydrolytic enzymes are spilled out; they find an acid pH favorable to their activity, and some degree of self-digestion ("autolysis") takes place. However, the term *postmortem autolysis* is misleading because protein denaturation does occur at the same time, although much more slowly than in an infarct; in a refrigerator it takes months rather than hours (143).

Fortunately for those who study disease, the process of postmortem autolysis is fairly slow. The breakdown is most severe in organs that are loaded with digestive enzymes, mainly the pancreas, which literally self-destructs in a few hours. For obscure reasons, the adrenal medulla also tends to liquefy: this is why early anatomists thought that the adrenals were empty bags (hence the name **adrenal capsules** in the older literature). Histologically, the destructive effects of lysis and denaturation vary from tissue to tissue; eventually the nuclei can no longer be stained (**karyolysis**). In the kidney, for instance, the glomeruli are relatively resistant, whereas the convoluted tubules autolyze very fast, perhaps because they contain more lysosomes. To the inexperienced eye, tubular autolysis can be mistaken for tubular necrosis due to circulatory failure or toxic agents (Figure 5.27). This "disappearance" of the nuclei may be only apparent; chemical analysis has shown that 50 percent of the DNA is still present in tissue autolyzing *in vitro* at 37°C when the nucleus in histologic sections appears only as a ghost (229).

Obviously, it is best to perform autopsies as early as feasible. After 12 hours many structures are already marred by artefacts. Changes that occur within 3–5 hours can still be reversed if small samples are incubated in an oxygenated medium (14, 69, 209).

Does autolysis occur *in vivo*? It certainly does. As we mentioned earlier, whenever a cell dies, its proteins are caught between two fates: lysis, mainly by the cell's own enzymes, and denaturation, somehow favored by the surrounding live tissues, perhaps because they supply calcium. It follows that in the centers of very large infarcts autolysis prevails.

Autolysis raises an interesting question: when the whole body has been dead for 24 hours, why

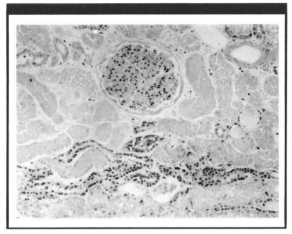

FIGURE 5.27
Postmortem autolysis in a human kidney, as often seen when the autopsy is performed as late as 18–24 hours after death. The nuclei in most of the tubules are no longer stainable. There is no doubt that this change occurred *post mortem* because necrosis of the tubules in a living kidney would have elicited a lively inflammatory reaction, and no such response is seen.

does it not appear like a massively coagulated infarct of the same age? The answer is that *postmortem autolysis and necrosis in vivo are very different phenomena*. Around a focus of necrosis, the circulation removes the breakdown products (thereby accelerating the breakdown reactions); it also removes pigments that are diffusing out, such as hemoglobin and its breakdown products, thus enhancing the whiteness of the necrosis; it supplies calcium (probably the main accelerator of denaturation) and other materials, including cells and enzymes that digest the tissues from outside (**heterolysis**). Therefore, paradoxically, the net effect of the surrounding blood flow is to accelerate the destruction. For example, a segment of kidney deprived of its blood supply dies, and after 2 or 3 days it will appear as a firm, white mass of necrotic tissue (white infarct); by contrast, if the kidneys are left in place after death, they will change aspect, but no matter how long we may wait, they will never look like a white infarct.

Some useful lessons have been learned from the study of tissue samples autolyzing in vitro (109, 143, 168, 228, 229), including contributions from food technology (126). (a) Refrigeration, of course, slows down the process. (b) Lysosomes in autolyzing tissues remain fairly well preserved (228, 229) and contain histochemically demonstrable acid phosphatase even after 4 hours of incubation at 37°C

(90) (another blow to the suicide bag hypothesis). (c) Mitochondria lose their small dense granules (probably loaded with divalent cations) within 15 minutes; this can probably be taken as an index of ischemia in vivo.

On a more tasteful note, the sweetening that occurs as fruit ripens is partly an autolytic process; tasteless starch breaks down to tempting sucrose, glucose, and fructose. The chemical breakdown, however, occurs within the living cell (93, 94).

Autolysis in Bacteria In bacteria, autolysis is part of life. Enzymes called *autolysins* break down the bacterial wall, especially during cell division; antibiotics of the beta-lactam group (including penicillin) favor the action of autolysins in dividing bacteria, so that the wall becomes thinner, expands, and may eventually burst (225). If the wall contains endotoxins—as is the case for gram-negative bacteria—a dying bacterium that undergoes autolysis, releasing endotoxin and other irritating fragments of its wall, can be more irritating than a live bacterium (32a).

CELL DEATH WITH SHRINKAGE: APOPTOSIS

Apoptosis is a distinctive form of cell death, or more precisely a form of cell suicide. It occurs in so many normal and abnormal processes—embryogenesis, growth, atrophy, toxic injury,

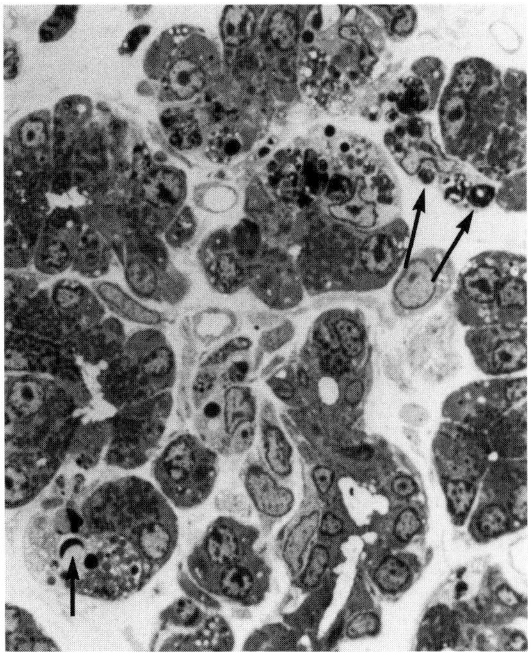

FIGURE 5.28 Parotid gland 24 hours after obstruction of the duct. Note the marginated, sharply defined, condensed chromatin in apoptotic nuclear fragments (**short arrow**) and partly degraded apoptotic bodies within macrophages (**long arrows**). (Reproduced with permission from [236].)

virus infections, immune responses, tumors—that it is now viewed as an essential component of life, *an equal and opposite force to mitosis* (28).

The concept of apoptosis was born in Australia about 1971 (114, 118). It was meant to describe, at first, a novel form of cell death seen during atrophy. The first inkling came from the histology of rat livers after ligation of a major branch of the portal vein, a procedure that causes rapid atrophy of the corresponding liver lobes (114). Some cells appeared to shrink and die without a phase of swelling, hence the earlier name "shrinkage necrosis." The nucleus became pycnotic in a distinctive manner: the condensed chromatin became plastered against the nuclear membrane in the shape of half-moons (Figure 5.28). Furthermore, the dying cells were scattered here and there among normal cells, quite unlike what happens in an infarct. This type of cell death was recognized as an entity and called *apoptosis*, a Greek term for "falling off" (e.g., of leaves from a tree or petals from a flower) (118), which aptly describes the dropping out of scattered cells.

These early observations have been confirmed many times in tissues undergoing rapid atrophy (115, 237): in the premenstrual human endometrium (106), in kidney tubules after ligature of the ureter (Figure 2.44) (89), in capillary endothelial cells during the involution of the corpus luteum (8), in the rat prostate after castration (117), and in many other systems.

At first apoptosis was defined by purely morphologic criteria, and especially by the changes of the nucleus; later it was discovered that the nuclear changes typical of apoptosis are associated with a definite type of DNA breakdown recognizable by gel electrophoresis. Today we can therefore define apoptosis as *a special variety of cell death characteristic by its morphology and by the type of DNA breakdown*. Its typical features can be summarized as follows (Figures 2.35, 5.29):

- The cell shrinks and its cytoplasm becomes dense.
- The chromatin aggregates into sharply defined, dense masses against the nuclear membrane.
- The nucleus may eventually break up into rounded fragments (**karyorhexis**).
- The cell emits (**budding**) protrusions that tend to break off as small, rounded eosino eosinophilic bodies (apoptotic bodies) that may contain nuclear fragments.

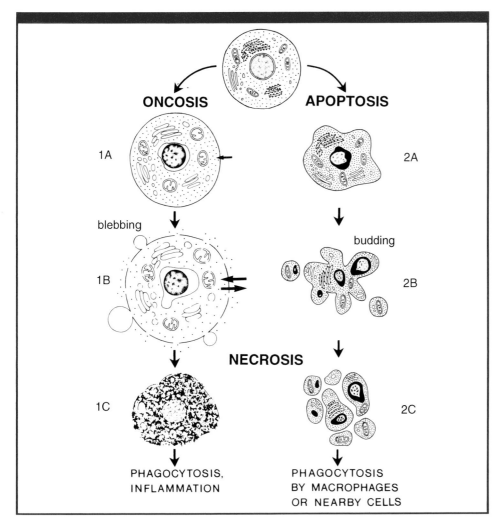

FIGURE 5.29
Two modes of cell death, which may occur in the same cell type. *Left: oncosis.* **1A:** the cell and some of it organelles swell. **1B:** permeability is increased, blebbling occurs. **1C:** the cell undergoes coagulation necrosis (the less common liquefaction necrosis is not indicated). Cells that die in this manner attract mainly neutrophils. *Right: apoptosis.* **2A:** the cell shrinks and becomes more dense, the chromatin undergoes condensation and margination. **2B:** the cell undergoes *budding* (not blebbling); some buds break off and become free apoptotic bodies, with or without nuclear inclusions. **1C:** the remains of the apoptotic cell that remain free undergo necrosis; others are phagocytized by macrophages and by neighboring cells. *Note that necrosis (secondary changes in dead cells) can follow oncosis as well as apoptosis.* Nuclear breakdown occurs by karyolysis (in oncosis), and by pyknosis and karyorhexis (in apoptosis). (Reproduced with permission from [142a]).

- Macrophages or neighboring cells phagocytize the debris.
- Biochemical feature: a characteristic, nonrandom, internucleosomal cleavage of the DNA (see further).

Figure 5.29 illustrates the main differences between apoptotic and oncotic cell death: in the latter the doomed cell tends to swell, the chromatin breaks up and eventually undergoes **karyolysis,** and the debris of the dead cell attract neutrophils.

In real life the sequence of apoptosis is quite abrupt (161): the shrinkage and budding are over in minutes, and the apoptotic bodies are digested in a few hours (237). A rapidly shrinking tissue may show only a scattering of nuclear remains, easily overlooked (which explains why apoptosis was discovered so late). In fact, the apoptotic drama is lost in histologic sections.

However, by a stroke of good fortune, the entire sequence of apoptosis was captured cinematographically by a pioneering French hematologist, Marcel Bessis, 16 years before apoptosis was discovered (20): a leukocyte dying under the objective threw out bulky pseudopodia (the "budding" seen in fixed sections), then suddenly broke up into a cluster of separate bodies (Figure 5.30). The electron micrograph of an apoptotic cell shown in Figure 5.31 illustrates this same, almost explosive breakup.

Zeiosis *(from the greek zeio, "I boil") is sometimes used to describe the "budding" of a cell dying by apoptosis. The term should be avoided because it was created to mean something quite different. In 1951, Costero and Pomerat (47) were studying cultures of human brain cortex maintained in vitro; among the various regressive phenomena, they noticed that some dendrites, seen in accelerated motion pictures, showed multiple blebs that appeared as "vesicles which are filled and blow out without interruption*

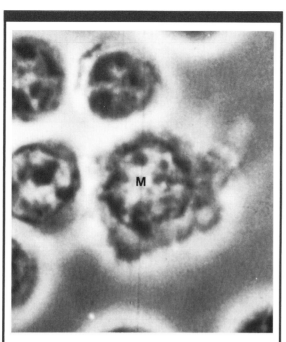

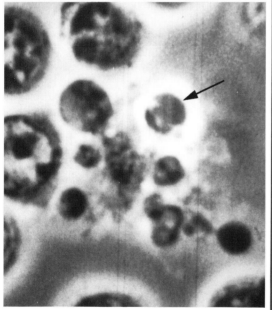

FIGURE 5.30 Apoptosis recorded on film before it had a name. Two frames of a movie taken by M. Bessis in 1955, showing the death of a white blood cell (probably a monocyte, M) maintained *in vitro* at 37 C. *Top:* the cell just before it began to die; in later frames it began to throw out pseudopodia (the "budding" process) and at 33 minutes (*bottom*) it suddenly broke apart into what we now call apoptotic bodies. **Arrow:** this fragment appears to contain "half-moons" of condensed chromatin typical of apoptosis.

resembling the behavior of a very dense fluid under intense boiling," hence the name.

The apoptotic bodies, with or without condensed nuclear remnants, are disposed of in several ways. Those arising from epithelial surfaces may be extruded into the lumen; otherwise, they are taken up by macrophages that may be lying nearby or, more surprisingly, by the adjacent cells (Figure 2.35). What causes these former neighbors, ordinarily not phagocytic, to devour the corpse of one

of their kind is not known. As to the macrophages, they must somehow be alerted to the presence of an obsolete cell and then recognize it as legitimate prey. It was recently shown that obsolete neutrophils and lymphocytes are recognized by macrophages via their vitronectin receptor, which happens to be involved also in cell anchorage (197). The cell membrane was also shown to lose its characteristic asymmetry, and thus to expose more negatively charged phospholipids (122a).

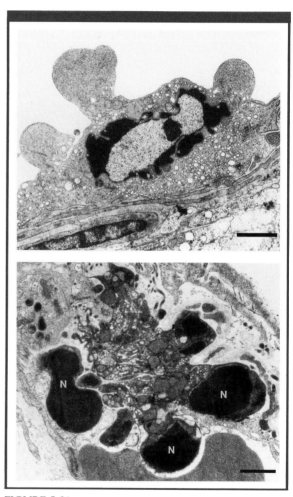

FIGURE 5.31
Typical nuclear changes of apoptosis, as seen in the course of atrophy (cell deletion). Tissue is from breasts of mice and rats during involution after lactation. *Top:* Rat mammary gland, 4 days after weaning; apoptosis of an endothelial cell. Note the peculiar clustering of the chromatin against the nuclear membrane and the deformation of the latter. **Bar** = 2 μm. *Bottom:* Mouse mammary gland 2 days after weaning. Note the budding of the endothelial cell; each bud contains a fragment of the nucleus (**N**). **Bar** = 1 μm. (Reproduced with permission from [235].)

Biochemical Mechanisms of Apoptosis At this time, the distinctive biochemical feature of apoptosis is the cleavage of the nuclear DNA (4, 35, 45, 116, 237, 257, 122a). Because the cuts fall between nucleosomes, the resulting DNA fragments represent multiples of approximately 185 base pairs; hence the characteristic **ladder pattern** seen by gel electrophoresis (Figure 5.32). By contrast, in accidental cell death, electrophoresis of the DNA produces a long smudge, meaning that the DNA has been chopped indiscriminately into pieces of random length. In apoptosis the cutting is probably due to an endonuclease activated by calcium (154). Why the dying cell should turn against its DNA is not clear. Perhaps it is "destroying its files" to prevent the accidental transfer of genetic information, as might conceivably happen when the apoptotic bodies are phagocytized (116). This line of reasoning has been carried one step further. Perhaps all cells contain a triage mechanism that recognizes whether the DNA has been damaged severely enough to increase the risk of heritable changes, and if the answer is yes, it condemns the cell to suicide. Viewed in this light, apoptosis would be a guardian of genetic fidelity; its philosophic significance would not be suicide, but survival (227).

Whatever may be the biological advantage of internucleosomal cleavage of the DNA, a technical advantage became obvious to the molecular biologists: they were able to find a color reaction for detecting nicks in the DNA, whereby we now have a beautiful histochemical method for detecting apoptosis in tissue sections (86).

The self-destruction of the chromatin certainly fits with the notion of cell suicide, but there is even more compelling evidence: *in some cases apoptosis can be prevented by inhibitors of protein synthesis (145, 256, 257).* This suggests that the cell may need to manufacture some tool necessary for killing itself (135). Recent studies on metamorphosis in moths have suggested that killer proteins may be produced (13).

Exactly what the cell is synthesizing at the last minute is not clear. It should not be endonuclease because it is already there (107). The need for protein synthesis in cells pushed to commit suicide may remind the reader of heat-shock proteins, which are also synthesized in times of stress. Could there be a link between stress proteins and cell suicide (135, 237)? The answer is bound to come shortly.

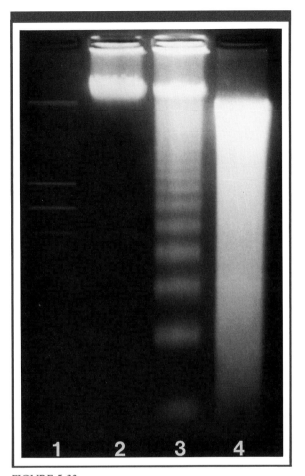

FIGURE 5.32

Comparing the DNA breakdown in apoptosis and accidental cell death. Agarose gel electrophoresis of DNA extracted from cultures of mouse cells, stained with ethidium bromide and photographed under ultraviolet light. *Lane 1:* Molecular weight markers. *Lane 2:* Control culture. *Lane 3:* Culture heated for 30 minutes to 44°C, extracted 8 hours later, when it showed typical, extensive apoptosis. *Lane 4:* Culture submitted to repeated freezing and thawing, and extracted 72 hours later, when it showed massive "necrosis" (accidental cell death). (Reproduced with permission from [116].)

A process as fundamental as apoptosis should be under genetic control, and indeed it is. In some models the oncogene c-*myc* induces apoptosis, whereas the oncogene *bcl-2* suppresses it (34). These initial studies raise the hope that the up- or down-regulation of certain genes may some day be used in fighting cancer cells.

When and Where does Apoptosis Occur?
Apoptosis was discovered in tissues undergoing *atrophy*; under those conditions it corresponded to

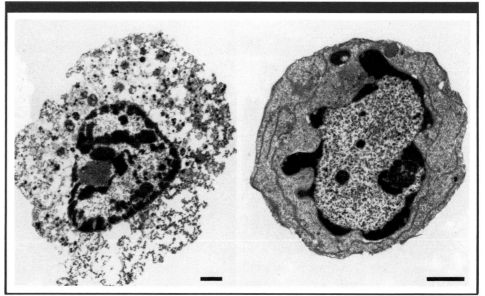

FIGURE 5.33
The two principal modes of cell death in cultured cells of the same line (a mastocytoma). *Left:* Swollen, necrotic cell that died of anoxia (presumably by oncosis) after incubation for 30 hours in 95% N_2 + 5% CO_2. *Right:* Apoptosis 4 hours after a heat shock (30 minutes at 43°C). Apparently the "suicide program" of this cell was turned on by the heat. **Bars** = 0.2 μm. (Courtesy of Dr. B.V. Harmon, Medical School, Herston, Queensland, Australia.)

the form of cell suicide required for deleting a percentage of the cell population (p. 41). Then the features of apoptosis were recognized in *cell death by killer cells* (p. 332, 510) and in *programmed cell death*, as it occurs in the embryo and in many mature tissues in which cell renewal is constant, such as the epidermis (86). If the list ended here we might conclude that apoptosis is a ritual whereby the body removes its unwanted cells, but the story is more complicated: apoptosis is sometimes seen also in cells killed by a variety of agents such as ischemia, toxic agents, and anticancer drugs (34). This means that *probably any cell can undergo apoptosis* if the conditions are right. For example, Figure 5.33 shows two cells of the same tumor, killed *in vitro*; one has developed apoptosis, the other accidental cell death. Some drugs can induce either form of cell death (127). Apoptosis can also be induced by *viruses*; the rounded, eosinophilic bodies seen in the liver in cases of viral hepatitis are thought to arise in this manner (237) (Figure 5.34). Finally, those utterly fashionable molecules, the *cytokines* (p. 349) have found their way also into this chapter: for example, tumor necrosis factor (TNF) induces apoptosis in cultured endothelial cells (192). This may explain the hemorrhagic necrosis caused by TNF in living tumors (p. 351).

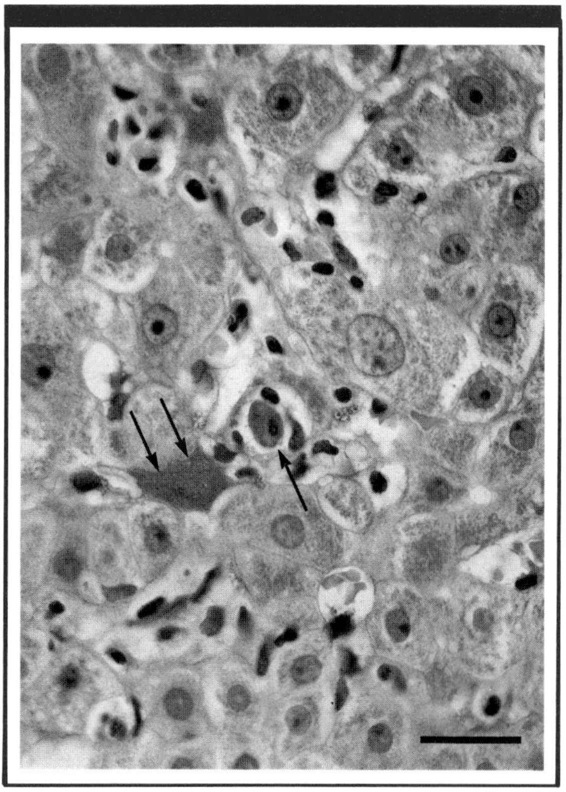

FIGURE 5.34
Liver in a case of hepatitis, showing the death of two isolated cells (**arrows**), which turn into eosinophilic bodies. **Bar** = 25 μm. (Courtesy of Dr. K.G. Ishak, Armed Forces Institute of Pathology, Washington, DC.)

Lysosomal enzymes are not involved in the suicide of self-deleting cells (9); when lysosomes do intervene, as during insect metamorphosis, they attack only mitochondria and ribosomes and spare the nuclei, which seems most appropriate (133).

Apoptosis: loose ends. Although the basic facts of apoptosis are clear, a number of questions need to be answered. For example: (a) Apoptosis usually hits single cells scattered within a population. How are these cells selected? (b) In myocardial infarcts—a classic setting for oncosis—histochemistry for apoptosis shows many positively stained cells, and gel electrophoresis of DNA extracts show the ladder pattern typical of apoptosis (108a): what is going on here? Perhaps some myocardial cells, sensing the impending catastrophe, prefer to kill themselves? (c) It is said that the permeability of the cell membrane, as demonstrated by dye exclusion, is intact in extruded apoptotic bodies (237), but this requires further study. (d) Does protein denaturation occur in apoptosis, as the dense cytoplasm suggests? There is no answer yet. (e) Some inhibitors of protein synthesis prevent aoptosis, but others, such as diphtheria toxin and ricin, cause it (237). (f) An influx of calcium is said to activate the endonucleases and trigger apoptosis, but an influx of calcium occurs also in accidental cell death, yet the nuclear changes are different. (g) Because there are many examples of cell death intermediate between apoptosis and accidental cell death, it is best to consider these two modes as the extremes of a spectrum (257). (h) Cell suicide is prevalent in plants, but it does not take the form of apoptosis (82).

Finally, we must warn our readers that the literature on cell death is profoundly confusing, mainly because most authors fail to distinguish between cell death (defined by the "point of no return") and necrosis (changes that occur after cell death). Worse yet, accidental cell death is generally referred to as "necrosis." To say that a cell dies by necrosis is just like saying that clinical death occurs by post-mortem autolysis. We have attempted to bring the ship back on course by re-introducing the ancient term oncosis for "cell death with swelling" (the main form of accidental cell death) as opposed to apoptosis, "cell death with shrinkage" (143a).

The biology of apoptosis is advancing by leaps and bounds. Recent advances include a role for the mitochondria and for cytoplasmic components (108a).

PROGRAMMED CELL DEATH

Just as leaves can be programmed to shrivel up and die at a certain time of the year, many cells are programmed to die at a fixed time, as a normal part of tissue function (30, 53, 133, 156, 227). Human granulocytes die and are replaced at the rate of 1.3 million per second (204). The basal cells of the skin continue to produce new cells, which work their way toward outer layers, die, and flake off; the cycle takes 3–4 weeks, which means that we shed our skins much more often than snakes. *These normal cycles of cell life and death cannot be interrupted without threatening the survival of the individual.* In other words, the basic rule of life on this planet applies also to the world of cells: life and death are two sides of a coin. There is no better illustration of this concept than the famous

stone puma created by a pre-Columbian Aztec sculptor. Seen from the front the puma is alive; seen from the back it is a skeleton (Figure 5.35).

Cells programmed for deletion usually (but not always) die by apoptosis; therefore, programmed cell death in some models can be prevented by inhibitors of protein synthesis (63). Interestingly, in some forms of programmed cell death the ribosomes aggregate into crystals, a neat way to be put out of commission (Figure 5.36) (162, 170, 182).

Programmed cell death starts in the embryo, where it plays a major role: whole groups of cells die on schedule (88) as if they were deleted from the local development program (27). *Sometimes the deletion occurs because an organ has become obsolete;* such is the case of the pronephros. Cataclysmic examples of this kind occur during insect metamorphosis (134). *Nature also uses cell death to impart shape* (194, 195, 241), much as a sculptor hammers chips off a block of marble; this is how five digits are carved out of the rudimentary hand or foot, which initially looks like a solid paddle (9) (Figure 5.37). In the chick embryo, about the fourth day, a mass of cells dies in order to outline the rudimentary shape of the wing (Figure 5.38); if these cells are cut out and grafted to another part of the embryo, where their self-sacrifice would not seem to be called for, they die anyway according to the original schedule (196).

Another fetal event dependent on cell death is the fusion of the two palatal shelves to produce a complete palate. For the two shelves to fuse, the covering epithelium must disappear, and it does so by apoptosis. There is some evidence that cortisone can prevent the fusion, suggesting a mechanism for certain malformations such as cleft palate (91).

Even tumors show programmed cell death (29). Those that arise from cells with an inborn deletion program, such as the epidermis, continue to express it: the malignant stem cells continue to multiply, producing cells that differentiate and progress to their death (p. 749) (27).

In plants, cell death explains the development of bark, thorns, and vessels, all of which are formed by the programmed death of long rows of cells (82).

In essence, *programmed cell death occurs by cell suicide in response to a signal.* Where does the signal come from? Cells that differentiate toward their own death, such as the keratinocytes of the epidermis, must have their own built-in suicide

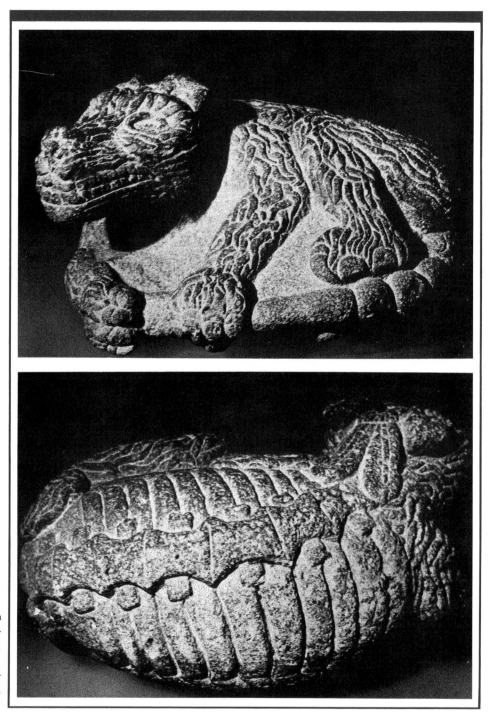

FIGURE 5.35
Life and death are inseparable. This concept is beautifully illustrated by this Aztec sculpture of a puma, from the Museum of Anthropology in Mexico City. *Top:* Viewed from the front, the puma is alive. *Bottom:* Viewed from the back, it is a skeleton. (Courtesy of the Museum of Anthropology, Mexico City, Mexico.)

program. *In some cases the signal for suicide is delivered by hormones or similar messengers* (Table 5.2). For instance, during metamorphosis of the silk moth, the normal breakdown of the intersegmental muscles can be inhibited by parasympathicomimetic drugs (e.g., physostigmine); this suggests that the signal for cellular breakdown, in that system, is the lack of motor-nerve impulses (134). Also, it is long known that stress causes the thymus to shrink; this can now be explained: lymphocytes, even malignant ones, undergo apoptosis in response to glucocorticoids (251). *In other situations the trigger is lack of a growth factor,* and correspondingly, an extra supply of the factor suppresses or reduces the programmed cell deletion (13). For example, nerve growth factor reduces cell death in the embryonic nervous system (130, 172), and erythropoietin controls red cell produc-

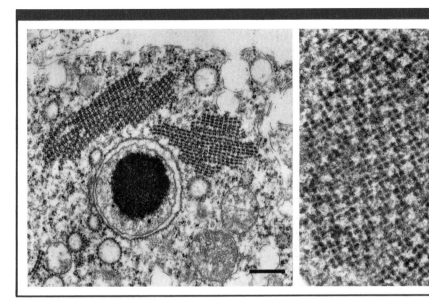

FIGURE 5.36
Crystallization of ribosomes during programmed cell death in a chick embryo. *Left:* In the limb bud ("posterior necrotic zone"). **Bar** = 0.5 μm. (Courtesy of N. Karle Mottet, M.D., Professor of Pathology, University of Washington School of Medicine, Seattle.) *Right:* In the spinal cord. **Bar** = 0.1 μm. (Reproduced with permission from [170].)

tion by preventing programmed cell death in red cell progenitors (121).

REPRODUCTIVE AND OTHER TYPES OF CELL DEATH

Radiation can kill cells directly, but in low doses it only stops them from multiplying. The same effect is produced by many cytotoxic chemicals, also called radiomimetic for this very reason. The mechanism is damage to the DNA, best recognized microscopically as chromosomal abnormalities (p. 832). Some irradiated cells become gigantic (Figure 5.39). Many factors affect the extent of the damage: type and dosage of radiation, temperature, presence of protecting and sensitizing agents (especially oxygen), and stage of the mitotic cycle (104). Most affected are those tissues in which mature cells are produced by a relatively small number of rapidly dividing precursor cells, such as the bone marrow, the epidermis, the lining of the gut, and the testicular tubules. Cells thus deprived of their reproductive capacity may appear microscopically normal; their defect can be brought to light experimentally by testing their ability to form colonies. This "hidden injury" is one of the long-term effects of radiation and cytotoxic therapy.

Could there be other types of cell death? The answer is definitely yes. Apoptosis was unknown until the 1970s. Other ways of cell death are bound to come up. For example: the embryonic

TABLE 5.2

Signals for Cell Suicide in Programmed Cell Death

CELL SYSTEM	SIGNAL
Tadpole tail	Thyroxine
Mullerian ducts	Androgen
Thymocytes	Glucocorticoids
Insect labial gland	Ecdysterone
Insect intersegmental muscle	Lack of neurotransmitter
Neurons	Lack of nerve growth factors
Mammary gland	Lack of prolactin
Rat prostate	Castration

Modified from Lockshin R A, and Zakeri-Milovanovic Z. Nucleic acids in cell death. In: Davies I, and Sigee D C (eds.), Cell Ageing and Cell Death. Cambridge: Cambridge University Press, 1984, pp. 243–268.

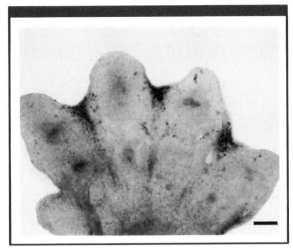

FIGURE 5.37
Section through the hind foot of a rat fetus at day 17,
stained for acid phosphatase. The strong reaction in the
interdigital tissues corresponds to areas where macrophages
are busily removing the debris of dead tissue. The
histochemical reaction is actually revealing the lysosomes
and phagosomes of the macrophages. **Bar** = 200 μm.
(Reproduced with permission from [9].)

central nervous system contains about twice as
many cells as will be needed (144a); the excess is
pruned away by programmed cell death, according
to *three* morphologically distinct mechanisms.
Only one of these corresponds to apoptosis

(199a). Some bizarre manifestations of cell death,
still unclassified, were made by Marcel Bessis in
the cinematographic recordings mentioned earlier
(20). The protagonists were leukocytes allowed to
die in a thin layer of fluid between glass slide and
coverslip. Here are two of their performances:

- In one neutrophil, the three lobes of the
  nucleus merged into one—perhaps a special
  case of pyknosis; this means that some of
  the mononuclear cells observed in inflammatory exudates could be obsolete neutrophils.
- Another granulocyte expelled the content
  of its nucleus, recalling the nuclear extrusion known to occur during the maturation
  of red blood cells and under the effect of
  cytochalasin (p. 152).

Nobody could ever guess that such events take
place by looking at fixed cells, let alone homogenized cells in test tubes.

A final teaser: there is no name for cell death by
histologic fixatives, which, under ideal conditions,
leaves no morphologic trace. Instant mummifica-
tion?

*Can cells be protected against injury and death?
Corticoids are thought to toughen cell membranes, as
reflected in some of their clinical applications, but
little is known of the molecular mechanism (199,
207). Some "cardioprotection" against ischemic
damage has been obtained with transforming growth*

FIGURE 5.38
Programmed cell
death. *Left:*
Wing bud of a 4-
day chick em-
bryo stained with
neutral red and
cleared (whole
mount). **Arrow**
points to a popu-
lation of macro-
phages stained
with neutral red
and loaded with
the debris of
dead cells. *Right:*
Squash prepa-
rations to show
the living macro-
phages (**arrow**)
filled with large
phagosomes. (Re-
produced with
permission from
[194].)

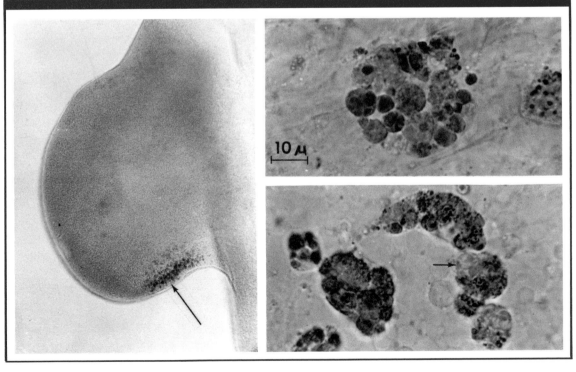

factor-beta (TGF-beta) (128), but the mechanism is at least in part antiinflammatory rather than cell preserving. The rather misleading term cytoprotection is used for drugs (prostaglandins) said to protect the gastric mucosa against injurious agents such as alcohol (124); the effect may be due to increased blood flow rather than to a real cellular protection. The search for cell protectors continues; even ginseng has been tested (81). Glycine and alanine are hopeful leads; in vitro they protect a variety of cells from hypoxic death, by a mechanism apparently unrelated to amino acid metabolism (233).

TO SUM UP: newcomers tend to confuse the *different morphologic expressions* of cell death (accidental cell death, apoptosis, reproductive cell death) with the *different settings* of cell death (such as ischemia, programmed cell death, cell killing). In somewhat oversimplified terms, it helps to remember the following:

- Morphologically, most cells die in one of two ways: they either swell while their nucleus fades away by karyolysis, or shrink while the nucleus becomes very dense and breaks up by karyorhexis, a modality called apoptosis.
- The swelling modality is usually seen in accidental cell death, especially by ischemia. We called it *oncosis* (some call it *necrosis*, an inappropriate and confusing term).
- Apoptosis can occur as a *spontaneous* phenomenon in cells that commit suicide because their time has run out; a classic example is programmed cell death in the embryo. The suicide appears to be due to an automatic, genetically planned suicide program.
- Apoptosis can also be *induced* in virtually any cell type. This self-destruction can be triggered by killer cells, as well as by a wide variety of stimuli. In these cases the cells appear to switch on a genetic suicide program available, but not bound to be expressed.

Necrosis

After cells have died, they slowly proceed to lose all remnants of organized structure: this is necrosis, a varied and interesting process despite its morbid name. If extensive enough, it has effects on the

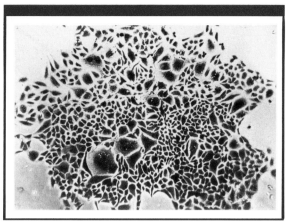

FIGURE 5.39 Changes induced by irradiation in a colony of cultured HeLa human cancer cells. The large "monster" cells have lost their reproductive capacity but still carry on metabolic functions. (Reproduced with permission from [187].)

body locally and generally, and within a few hours or days the necrotic mass itself undergoes three dynamic changes:

- *Calcium salts* accumulate.
- *Membrane cholesterol* becomes free and crystallizes.
- *Membrane phospholipids* form beautiful but pointless myelin figures.

Besides these relatively peaceful biochemical changes, a necrotic mass may be drastically modified by environmental effects and turn into *gangrene:* an ancient and convenient clinical term that refers to necrosis modified either by exposure to air resulting in drying (dry gangrene), or by infection that turns it into a mixed bacterial culture (wet gangrene). Because both forms of gangrene are especially unsightly in animals, we will illustrate them in fruit (Figure 5.40).

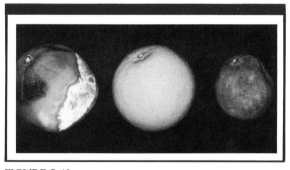

FIGURE 5.40
See color plate 7 .   The notion of dry and moist gangrene illustrated with oranges. *Center:* normal orange. *Left:* an orange that became dehydrated over several weeks at room temperature; it sustained no fungal or bacterial growth. A similar sequence applies to the umbilical cord. *Right:* moist gangrene. This orange became infected before it had the time to dry, and is now being overgrown with fungi and bacteria.

FIGURE 5.41 A "stone baby" (lithopedion) illustrated by Cruveilhier around 1842. A Parisian woman of 35, with one child, became pregnant. Toward the fourth or fifth month she suffered a prolonged episode of abdominal pain; then her abdomen shrank back to normal, the pain abated, and her periods reappeared. She had two more children, although she always felt that she had some kind of "foreign body" in her belly. In 1823, at age 77, she developed a strangulated hernia, was operated on, and died. At autopsy, this mummified, calcified fetus was discovered in the abdomen (51).

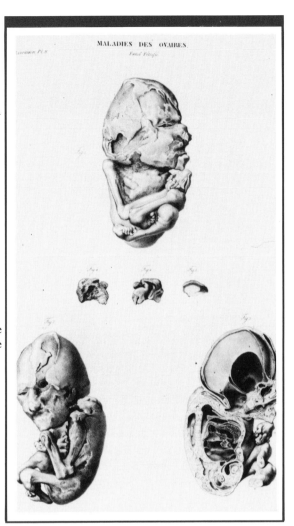

MALADIES DES OVAIRES

CALCIUM DEPOSITION

Calcium begins to accumulate immediately, even before the cell dies (142). At first the deposits are not microscopically visible, but soon (hours, days) they appear as basophilic granules, usually smaller than nuclei. Occasionally the necrotic mass undergoes massive calcification. Because we are accustomed to think of cells as people, we visualize the macrophages nibbling at the necrotic mass as having a gritty meal. The complex process of calcification will be discussed later (Chapter 6). To underscore its importance, we will mention here only the most spectacular example, rarely seen in our days: the so-called lithopedion, or stone baby (Figure 5.41), in which the calcification actually makes the fetus stonelike.

Today, the symptoms of tubal pregnancy call for immediate surgery. However, if a tubal pregnancy remains undiagnosed, it leads to rupture of the tube; thereby the embryo (or fetus) finds itself loose in the peritoneal cavity and dies. During past centuries, it was common for the "lost baby," incubated in the aseptic environment of the peritoneum, to undergo coagulative necrosis and then to calcify into a permanent lithopedion (261). This still happens occasionally (158).

There is a great deal of cholesterol in the plasma membranes: roughly half of the total lipid. When the cells die, the cholesterol slips out of the membranes, in which it was floating almost freely, as you recall, not being held by covalent bonds. Because cholesterol is insoluble in water, it crystallizes into thin, flat rhomboid plates that have long attracted the curiosity of microscopists (Figure 5.42). In frozen sections they are birefringent; in paraffin sections they have been dissolved out, leaving the familiar cigar-shaped **cholesterol clefts,** which are cross sections of plates (Figure 5.43). The typical cigar shape, however, is an artefact due to tissue shrinkage; in tissues fixed for electron microscopy the clefts are always rectangular (Figure 5.44).

What happens next to the cholesterol crystals? Being insoluble in water they would persist indefinitely were it not for the macrophages, which are able to esterify cholesterol and then get rid of any excess via the HDL-lipoprotein pathway. From then on, there are only two ways for the body to rid itself of cholesterol: it can either excrete it through the bile (as the name implies:

The drying up, however ugly, is a favorable development relative to wet gangrene because bacteria cannot grow in dry tissue. An example of dry gangrene in mammals is the stump of the normal umbilical cord. The cord dies, dries up, and its connection with the live tissues is eventually severed; neutrophil enzymes do the actual surgery. Toes deprived of blood flow (e.g., by atherosclerotic arteries) share the same fate, and so do dead autumn leaves.

Wet gangrene is an ominous event. Bacteria swarming in the necrotic mass can easily diffuse into live tissue and into the bloodstream. *Gas gangrene* earns its name from anaerobic bacteria that produce visible and palpable bubbles of gas within the tissues. A typical setting: in a limb crushed in a motorcycle accident, the injured tissues lose most or all of their blood supply and become a pasture for anaerobic bacteria picked up from the soil.

chole-sterol means "bile sterol") or shed whole cells, cholesterol and all (p. 87).

MYELIN FIGURES

Myelin figures are stacks of phospholipid bilayers in the shape of spheres, cylinders, and spirals that develop wherever cells are destroyed. They are liquid crystals (206) and reflect the natural tendency of phospholipids to form bilayers. Because of their ordered molecular arrangement they can be birefringent, but in ordinary histologic sections they are usually invisible because they stain poorly. Presumably, when the cell dies, proteolysis severs all links between cell membranes and cytoskeleton, and the phospholipids become free to follow the laws of physical chemistry. Phospholipids with a negative charge, such as phosphatidyl serine, swell the most (205).

Myelin figures grow like ghosts out of dead cells and are best seen if a fragment of tissue is allowed to die in water (32) (Figure 5.45). By electron microscopy, myelin figures can also be seen inside cells (Figure 4.31). In general, to the electron microscopist, *myelin figures (especially those free in tissue spaces) indicate that cell damage has occurred.*

The discovery of myelin figures by Virchow is a beautiful example of intuition and synthesis based on an extremely simple experiment. In his Cellular Pathology (1858) he explains that if bits of nerves are teased in water, their myelin sheaths expand into peculiar figures (Figure 5.46) (234). Anyone else would have dismissed these figures as unimpressive artefacts; but Virchow used them to argue, quite prophetically, that they represent a basic material present in all cells. What he really saw was phospholipid. In reading his words, remember that he had described and named myelin but still knew nothing of phospholipids or cell membranes:

"Now it is very remarkable that this same substance [myelin] is one which most extensively prevails in the animal body. I had, curiously enough, in the first instance in the examination of lungs come across forms which presented very similar qualities to those we observe in the medulla of the nerves. Although this was very surprising, yet I did not really think there was an actual correspondence until I was gradually led [] to examine a number of tissues chemically. The result showed, that there scarcely exists a tissue rich in cells in which this substance does not occur in large quantity [] It is the same substance which forms the principal constituent of the yellow mass of yolk in the hen's egg [perfectly true], whence its taste and peculiarities, especially its peculiar tenacity and viscidity which are employed for the higher technical purposes of the kitchen, are familiar to everyone" (234).

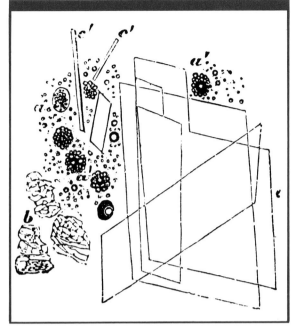

FIGURE 5.42 Microscopic crystals of cholesterol obtained from the necrotic center of an atheromatous plaque in an artery. Their typical shape is rhomboid, as shown in this drawing from 1873. (Reproduced with permission from [190].)

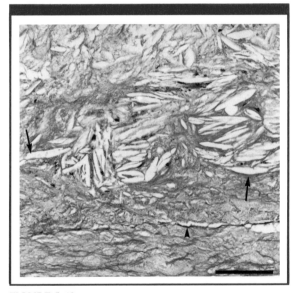

FIGURE 5.43
Empty, cigar-shaped clefts (**arrows**) left by dissolved cholesterol crystals in the necrotic core of an atherosclerotic plaque. Histologic section. **Arrowhead**: Internal elastic lamina (separating intima from media). Cholesterol crystals are common in any necrotic mass; here they are especially prominent because the dead cells (foam cells) were loaded with cholesteryl ester. **Bar** = 100 μm.

If we replace Virchow's myelin with phospholipids, we can readily understand why this key substance seemed to be present "in large quantities" in all cells. Virchow would have been delighted but not surprised to know that myelin and myelin figures, under the electron microscope, are very much alike (215).

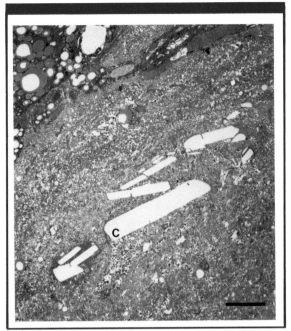

FIGURE 5.44 Crystals of cholesterol (**C**) in the necrotic core of a human atherosclerotic plaque as seen by electron microscopy. Part of a foam cell appears in the upper left corner. **Bar** = 5 μm.

Note also in passing that he found phospholipid in the lung; he may well have discovered surfactant, the phospholipid that plays a key role in lung physiology, but it was not described until the 1950s (43, 141a).

From myelin figures to liposomes Once an interesting artefact, myelin figures have now leaped into prominence and even into commerce as **liposomes,** suspensions of standardized, spherical, microscopic myelin figures (152, 173–175) (Figure 5.47). They were born in the 1960s from studies of phospholipid emulsions (10). It had been clear for some time that phospholipid bilayers resembled cell membranes and could even be perforated by saponins just like them (11, 139); then Sessa and Weissmann (200, 201) proposed that spheres of such membranes, liposomes, could be made to represent actual models of cells by trapping in their cavity or incorporating into their membranes enzymes and a variety of water-soluble and lipid-soluble molecules. Because liposomes can be fused with real cells, they are used *in vitro* for transfection. Drug delivery by liposomes *in vivo* is another development (Figure 5.48) (92). The ultimate hope is that some day they may be injected intravenously and targeted to deliver their load in any selected organ, but at the present state of the art, when injected intravenously they are largely phagocytized by the sinusoidal phagocytes of the liver, spleen, and bone marrow (p. 299). This is a nuisance, except for those cases in which

the sinusoidal phagocytes happen to contain the target: a parasite.

Imagine this scenario. Certain fungal and parasitic agents hide and survive within phagosomes of the sinusoidal phagocytes. The phagocytic cells take up the parasites and cannot get rid of them. In essence, they nurture them. A classic case is Kala-azar (a tropical disease caused by the protozoan Leishmania donovani), which can be treated with antimonials, except that these compounds are very toxic if given intravenously (183). But if the antimonials are packaged in liposomes, they can be delivered into the blood quite safely; the liposomes are taken up by the sinusoidal phagocytes and then fused with the secondary phagosomes containing the parasites. It would be difficult to conceive a more advantageous delivery of the drug: the therapeutic index is multiplied by several hundred times (242).

Thus, myelin figures, that homely product of necrosis, are on the way to becoming a therapeutic weapon. Part of their fascination is that they bring biologists closer to an ancient dream: the artificial cell. The first cell, after all, must have been a globule about as simple as a liposome; and all living organisms, as George Palade once said, must represent a direct expansion of that original globule (176).

CELL DEATH AND NECROSIS IN SPECIAL TISSUES

The basic rules of cell death and necrosis do not change from tissue to tissue, but cells differ; thus, special problems arise in each type of tissue. The main examples follow.

DEATH OF ADIPOSE TISSUE

Focal death of adipose tissue (also called fat necrosis or steatonecrosis) is not uncommon, especially after trauma or (in the abdomen) by spilling of pancreatic enzymes (Figure 5.49). *The distinctive biological feature of adipose tissue necrosis is that the fat released by the cells becomes an irritant.* First the macrophages feast on it and turn into foam cells or even into multinucleated Touton cells (Figure 5.50). Then the fibroblasts take part in the action and lay down an abundance of collagen (Figure 5.51), which feels—if it can be palpated through the skin—like a firm mass. Now imagine a trauma to the female breast (e.g., by a car accident); a firm lump of fat necrosis can lead to a difficult differential diagnosis with a tumor, benign or malignant.

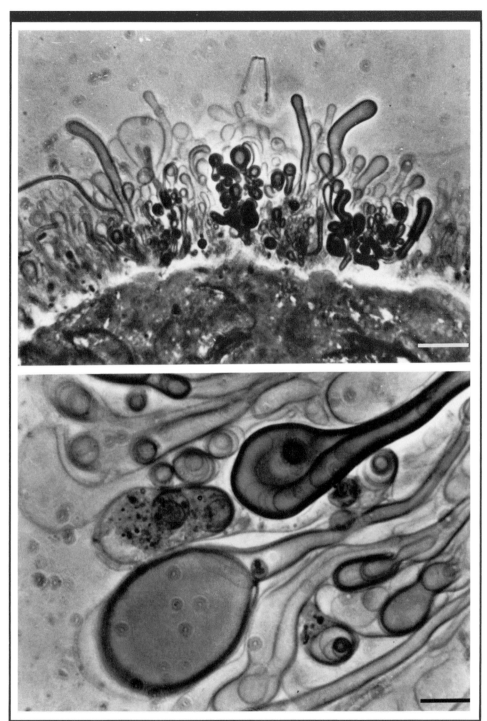

FIGURE 5.45
Myelin figures emerging from the edge of a piece of tissue (placenta) that was allowed to die in saline beneath a coverslip. *Top:* The phospholipid structures are enhanced by staining with Sudan black. *Bottom:* Multiple layers are visible in several of the myelin figures. Phase contrast microscopy. **Bars** = 10 μm. (Reproduced with permission from [32].)

The lively tissue reaction occurs because the triglycerides break down giving rise to fatty acids, which are irritants. Some are probably inactivated by binding with the ever-present carrier, albumin. Another fraction of free fatty acids combines with calcium and becomes soap. Calcium soaps are recognizable in frozen sections as bundles of needles.

Fat necrosis in the abdominal cavity due to the spilling of pancreatic enzymes is a catastrophic event that occurs when the digestive enzymes are activated in the living pancreas. The cause of this explosive activation is not always clear; trauma, ischemia, infection, a huge meal, or alcoholic debauch are sometimes involved. What-

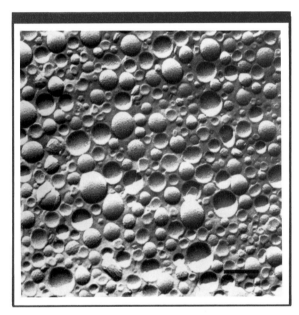

cells in which this substance quantity; still it is only in tl serve substa in all contai in the only sc

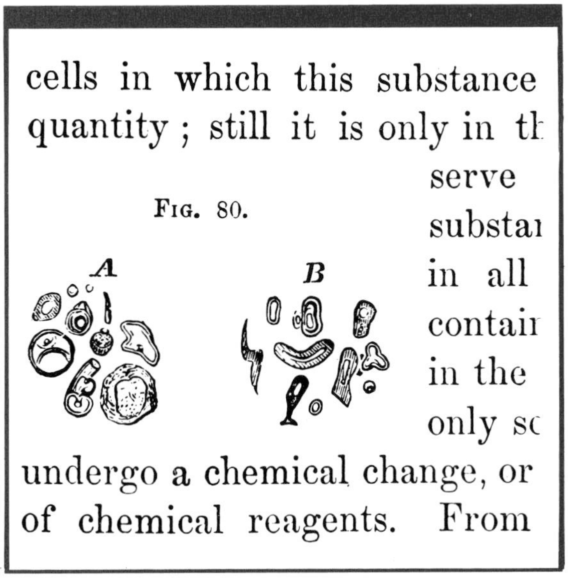

FIG. 80.

A   B

undergo a chemical change, or of chemical reagents. From

FIGURE 5.46 Myelin figures as drawn in 1858 by Virchow, who obtained them from nerves macerated in water.

FIGURE 5.47 Liposomes, in a freeze-fracture electron micrograph of vesicles prepared from egg phospholipid. **Bar** = 0.2 μm. (Reproduced with permission from [152].)

drops). Histologically these candle drops consist of necrotic fat cells surrounded by a halo of inflammation. *When fat necrosis is very extensive, the mass of dead cells and fatty acids can drain enough calcium from the plasma (forming calcium soaps) to induce hypocalcemic tetany.*

Fat cells can sometimes be killed from inside by a crystallization of their own fat droplet. This can happen if the temperature drops beneath the melting point of the triglycerides, as in hypothermia, or because the triglycerides have an abnormally high melting point. This occurs physiologically in the newborn (78).

DEATH OF CENTRAL NERVOUS TISSUE

Nervous tissue is special in many ways. Not surprisingly, the pathology of cell injury and cell death is also special (85). We will mention just three unusual features:

(a) *Liquefaction.* When a mass of brain tissue dies as a result of ischemia, many neuron cell bodies undergo coagulation necrosis (and turn into "red neurons" [84]) but the white matter and the tangle of cell processes in the grey matter (called "neuropil") break down into a milky fluid, a change that requires 5–10 days. Brain tissue does not contain more hydrolases than other organs, but the dead fibers and fibrils tend to break up into droplets, whereby the tissue disintegrates, producing the familiar "brain softening" (Figure 5.53). The resulting emulsion contains, besides myelin figures, large numbers of foam cells derived from blood monocytes and from the local population of macrophages (the **microglia**).

(b) *Excitotoxicity.* This recently described phenomenon could occur only in the brain. Dying neurons release their large stores of neurotransmitters, especially *glutamate. Excessive binding of glutamate to neuron receptors causes an influx of calcium, which initiates the demise of the cells* (40, 262). This mechanism, known as excitotoxicity, has important implications for the pathogenesis of nervous tissue damage by ischemia and other causes (132a, 249); it has also opened the possibility of therapy with receptor antagonists (15).

(c) *Free radical damage.* Almost any type of injury to the brain or cord will cause some red blood cells to spill into the tissue. In other organs these stray red blood cells would be quickly picked up by macrophages; in central nervous tissue this process is slower, and the iron of hemoglobin has the time to mediate free radical reactions, to which this tissue is especially sensitive.

ever the initial cause may be, masses of adipose tissue are damaged by the enzymes not only in the peritoneal cavity but even as far as the thoracic cavity or in the bone marrow. The lethal blow to the fat cells is probably given by pancreatic phospholipases that attack their membranes. Strangely enough, although the enzymes are spilled all over the peritoneal cavity, the resulting fat necrosis is typically focal; it presents as whitish, pea-sized, superficial spots on the omentum and wherever adipose tissue is present. These spots look very much like wax dropped from a candle (Figure 5.52), hence their very descriptive French name, *taches de bougie* (candle

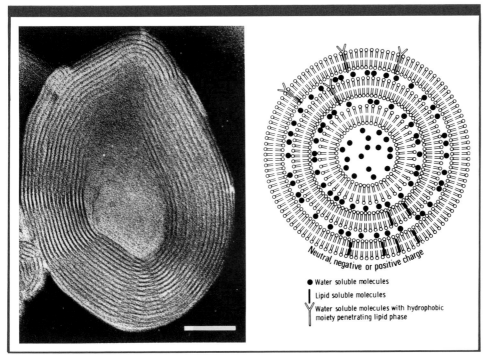

FIGURE 5.48
Left: A multilayered liposome as seen by electron microscopy in cross section. *Right:* Diagram of such a liposome, showing three bilayers of polar phospholipids alternating with aqueous compartments. Both water-soluble and lipid-soluble molecules can be inserted in such a structure, as indicated. **Bar** = 0.1 μm. (Reproduced with permission from [92].)

DEATH OF BONE TISSUE

Bone necrosis always occurs in fractures and sometimes after X-irradiation. The behavior of dead bone is unique in several respects. Bone is inhabited by *osteocytes,* cells imprisoned within the calcified matrix and communicating with each other and with bone surfaces by a network of microscopic canals. Whenever a group of osteocytes dies, the bone itself remains for a time outwardly and chemically unchanged; it does not become decalcified but simply loses its microscopic tenants (Figure 5.54). However, over days, weeks, and months, *the osteoblasts on the bone surfaces somehow receive the message that the bone tissue beneath them is dead; osteoblasts appear and slowly erode all the dead tissue while osteoblasts replace it with new bone.* After a fracture this process requires several months.

However, if the necrotic bone becomes infected, the sequence of events is entirely different. This can happen, for example, in an open fracture, or in the jaw after irradiation for a tumor in the mouth, which is a great source of bacteria. Once the necrotic bone is permeated with bacteria, the bone-resorbing cells no longer attack it; instead, they carve their way around it and isolate it. From this point on, the dead infected bone becomes an infected foreign body (a **sequestrum**), which can persist for years and continue to maintain the infection unless it is removed surgically. *Foreign bodies in general have the peculiar property of sustaining infection* (p. 478).

DEATH OF MYOCARDIAL TISSUE

Heart fibers are unique in that they beat. When they suddenly die, in an infarct, they cease to beat within one minute. We now have the situation of live, pulsating fibers rhythmically tugging at the ends of paralyzed but still live fibers. The result is that the paralyzed fibers are progressively drawn out and become long, thin, and wavy (26). Exactly how fast this occurs has not yet been determined, but the delay is certainly less than 3 hours and perhaps as short as 30 minutes. The wavy fibers, initially, probably represent a reversible injury. *Thus, the heart offers a unique exception to the rule that cell death cannot be recognized before 6–8 hours* (p. 192).

NECROSIS OF HOLLOW ORGANS

So far we have discussed necrosis in solid organs, such as the brain or liver. Special problems arise when necrosis occurs in the wall of hollow organs such as the gut or the gall bladder. An example: if a segment of the intestine dies (e.g., by ischemia), the necrotic mucosa can no longer function as a barrier to the bacteria contained in the lumen; the muscular layer is paralyzed, peristaltic movements cease, and thus the necrotic segment of gut acts as an obstruction; the bacteria in the lumen produce

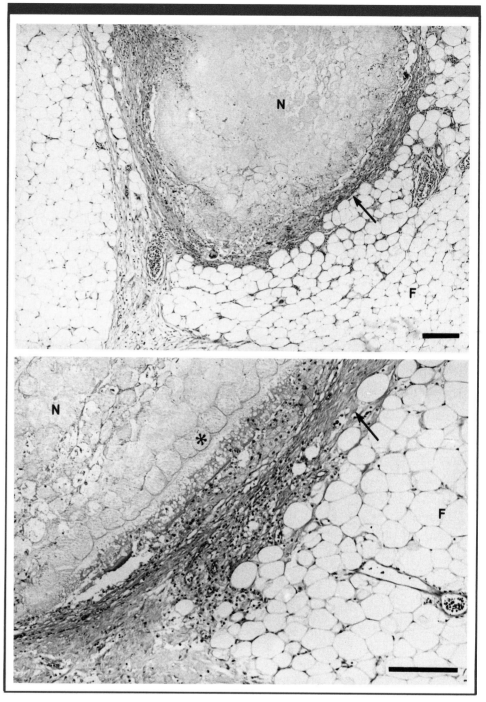

FIGURE 5.49
Necrosis of fat tissue (**N**) in a case of acute pancreatitis. *Top:* topographic view. *Bottom:* detail. The outlines of some dead fat cells (·) are still recognizable. **F**: Normal fat tissue. **Arrow:** Fibrous layer, indicating that the necrosis occurred several days previously. **Bars** = 200 μm.

gas, which stretches the weakened wall and may cause it to burst.

> *Epithelial cells that slough off from the mucosa of an injured hollow organ, such as an ischemic intestine, are generally thought to be dead; this may be wrong. In renal ischemia, renal tubules shed many of their epithelial cells into the urine and eventually produce the histologic picture of "acute tubular necrosis." However, when cultured, 25–30 percent of the cells*

> *shed in the urine are found to be still alive. Shedding therefore precedes cell death (187a).*

MOLECULES RELEASED BY INJURED, DYING, AND DEAD CELLS

Injured cells begin to spill their soluble contents even when the damage is reversible (1); when they die they release what is left. The material leaching out of dying and dead tissue is relevant to pathology for several reasons:

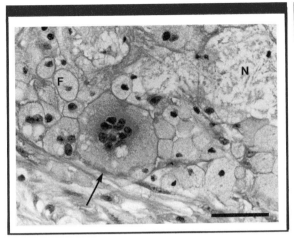

FIGURE 5.50
Cellular responses to necrotic fat cells (**N**). **F**: foam cells (macrophages loaded with cholesteryl esters). The cholesteryl esters were dissolved in the triglycerides released by the necrotic fat cells. **Arrow**: typical Touton cell, derived by fusion of foam cells. **Bar** = 50 μm.

- It is irritating to the surrounding normal tissues and sets up a local inflammatory response (p. 437).
- It may also have general effects, either toxic or injurious in some other way.
- It may attain blood levels high enough to be measured and thus become useful for diagnostic purposes.

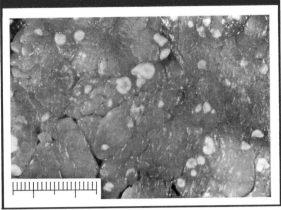

FIGURE 5.52
Small foci of fat necrosis ("candle drops") on retro-peritoneal fat in a case of acute hemorrhagic pancreatitis. Scale in mm. (Courtesy of Dr. E. Soto, St. Vincent Hospital, Worcester, MA.)

The spilling is exploited *in vitro* and *in vivo* to measure the extent of cell damage and death; *in vivo*, the spilling raises the further issue of possible effects on surrounding tissues (inflammation) or even at a distance when the release is massive. Classic experimental and clinical settings in which this massive release can occur are infarction, especially of the heart (Figure 5.55), and the release of a tourniquet left too long in place.

The principal molecules released by dying and dead cells (besides excitotoxins, p. 214) are potassium, enzymes, uric acid, myoglobin, and other proteins.

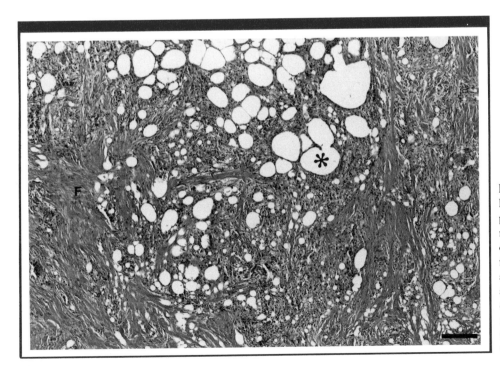

FIGURE 5.51
Long-term result of trauma on adipose tissue: intense fibrosis (**F**) as a reaction to shattered fat cells. The clear spaces (∗) are droplets of free fat, which produced a macrophage response as well as a fibroblast response. When this sequence of events occurs in the female breast, the firm fibrotic lump may suggest the clinical diagnosis of tumor. **Bar** = 200 μm.

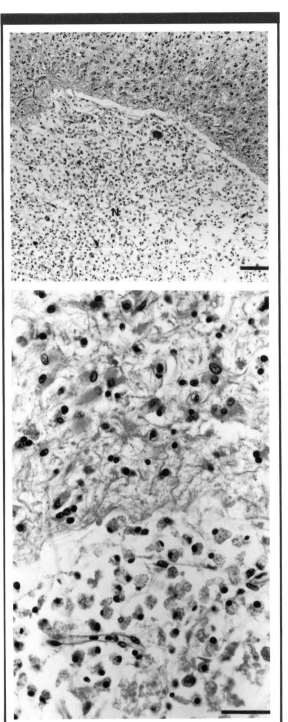

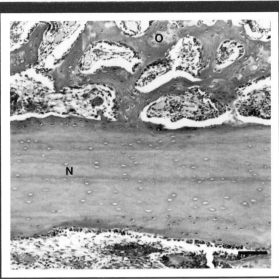

FIGURE 5.53
Cerebral infarction. *Top:* The necrotic brain tissue (**N**) liquefied and attracted swarms of macrophages (derived from blood monocytes and brain microglia) that are phagocytizing the debris. Note the sharp demarcation line between the necrotic tissue and the living tissue above it. This type of change can occur within 48 hours of infarction. **Bar** = 250 μm. *Bottom:* Detail showing macrophages loaded with myelin debris. **Bar** = 100 μm. (Courtesy of Dr. T.W. Smith, University of Massachusetts Medical Center, Worcester, MA.)

FIGURE 5.54
Regeneration of bone from the periosteum in a rabbit. Twenty-one days after a tibial fracture, the tibial cortex near the fracture is necrotic (**N**), as shown by the empty bone lacunae; microscopic osteophytes ("bone growths," **O**) develop beneath the periosteum, not visible in this photograph. The spaces between the branches of the osteophytes will later be filled with lamellae of new bone. **Bar** = 100 μm.

POTASSIUM

Intracellular potassium is about 40 times the normal serum value (150–160 mEq/L versus 3.5–5.0 mEq/L); this means that *a dying cell is a small "potassium bomb."* The danger is greatest for the heart because it responds to high potassium concentrations quite simply by stopping (a solution of potassium at 25 mEq/L is used to hold the heart still during cardiac surgery). A life-threatening flood of potassium can reach the heart from two sources: a myocardial infarct or massive necrosis somewhere else in the body.

Electrocardiographic changes begin to occur at potassium plasma values of about 6 mEq/L and are severe at 8 mEq/L. To understand this potassium overload it helps to know that 100 g of heart contain 250–293 mg of potassium (3); the adult body contains about 3600 mEq, about six times the lethal dose. About 300–600 mEq/L administered acutely can be lethal (112). During experimental ischemia, high potassium concentrations have actually been found in heart tissue spaces (105) and in coronary blood (102). An excess of extracellular potassium partially depolarizes the myocardial cells, first increasing and then decreasing ventricular conduction time (102). It has been postulated that the potassium gradient between normal and ischemic tissue creates an injury current that induces abnormal stimuli in the living, hyperexcitable tissue around infarcts (102), creating the risk of fatal arrythmia (70, 102, 177).

A massive and lethal dose of potassium can be released from body tissues after **severe burns** and even under iatrogenic circumstances:

- in **tourniquet shock,** a life-threatening con-

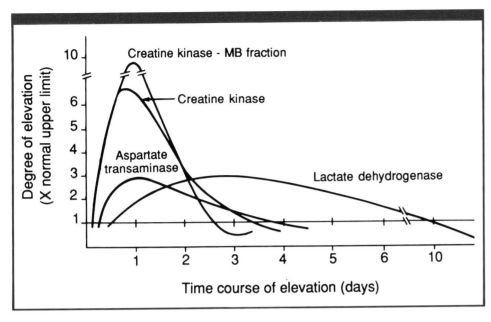

FIGURE 5.55
Time course of myocardial enzymes appearing in the blood after myocardial infarction. (Reproduced with permission from [255].)

dition that develops when a tourniquet is maintained on a limb for several hours and then released, suddenly restoring blood flow (125, 163, 232);

- after **embolectomy:** when an embolus causing ischemia of a lower limb is removed surgically; blood flow is restored, and cardiac arrest can follow (99);
- in the **tumor lysis syndrome,** a paradoxical result of successful chemotherapy for leukemias and other highly proliferative malignancies that become acutely necrotic as a result of the treatment (36, 180, 240); this group of tumors includes Burkitt's lymphoma, a malignant tumor that is very sensitive to X-rays and chemotherapy (p. 811) (5).

ENZYMES

As they leach out of dead cells *in vivo*, enzymes can find their way into the plasma, and when they do, they become invaluable clinically as signals that cellular injury and/or necrosis are occurring somewhere in the body. This phenomenon has given rise to the special field of **clinical enzymology** (138, 252) (Figure 5.55). Oddly enough, the brain is an exception: dead brain tissue does not seem to release into the blood any significant amount of large molecules. Correspondingly, despite the frequency of cerebral infarcts (which occur in 80 percent of strokes), no test for brain enzymes is currently available (181). Presumably the blood–brain barrier interferes with the passage of enzymes across the endothelium. *The specific type of mole-*

cule, enzyme, or isozyme found in the plasma can indicate the organ involved (prostate, heart, etc.) and can even suggest the extent, timing, and evolution of the damage. As might be expected, enzymes with smaller molecular weight are the first to escape.

Serious mistakes were made when it was not yet possible to distinguish similar enzymes originating from different tissues (isozymes). For example, the human heart and the human buttocks are very different, but both contain creatine kinase (CK). Years ago one of us was treated for myocardial infarction because of high plasma levels of this enzyme. It turned out later that the CK was coming from a poorly performed intramuscular injection.

The circulating enzymes rarely, if ever, cause any trouble. It may be relevant that 10 percent of plasma proteins are antiproteases. However, it is said that in severe acute pancreatitis, the heart, lungs, and kidneys may be affected (61, 140) and possibly also the brain (197a).

Proteolytic enzymes in the blood can have general effects if their concentration is high enough. Pulmonary edema may develop as a result of myocardial ischemia, but the mechanism (not fully understood) seems to involve activated platelets (87). The effect of intravenous papain in the rabbit was studied by Lewis Thomas of literary (and pathologic) fame: the ears become droopy because the matrix of the cartilage is digested away (Figure 5.56) (153).

MYOGLOBIN

Myoglobin escapes from dead myocardium and striated muscle just as hemoglobin escapes from

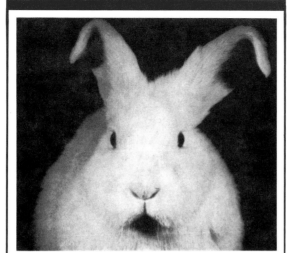

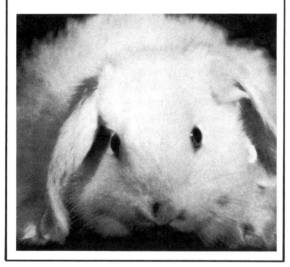

FIGURE 5.56 Illustrating the general effect of a proteolytic enzyme: two rabbits given 4 mg. of papain intravenously, 4 hours (*top*) and 16 hours (*bottom*) before the photograph was taken. Enzymatic degradation of the cartilage matrix throughout the body caused the ears to collapse. (Reproduced with permission from [153].)

red blood cells (22). When large amounts of myoglobin are released by damaged striated muscles, the condition is called **rhabdomyolysis;** it can be initiated by severe trauma or burns, strenuous exercise, potassium depletion (e.g., by severe exercise in hot climates), alcohol and drug abuse, and many other factors (120, 148). The molecule of myoglobin (molecular weight about 16,000) escapes through the glomerular filter; if the urine is acid (260), the myoglobin precipitates in the tubules forming casts (solid plugs), which may lead to renal failure.

URIC ACID

Uric acid becomes a problem in patients with malignancies that proliferate at a very high rate, especially leukemias (240), even in the absence of chemotherapy. Cellular purines are catabolized to xanthine and finally to uric acid; urate crystals

precipitate in the renal tubules and can lead to acute renal failure. Hyperuricemia is actually a facet of the tumor lysis syndrome.

Other examples of bioactive materials released by necrotic tissue: renal infarcts release a short-acting vasopressor agent (96). Excitotoxins were discussed earlier (p. 214). Toxic effects on the brain due to liver failure (hepatic encephalopathy) are due to several mechanisms, including the accumulation in the plasma of metabolic products that the liver failed to detoxify (75). Paradoxically, the slow destruction of the thyroid by an autoimmune process in Hashimoto's disease can lead to hyperthyroidism, which is attributed to the reabsorption of colloid.

Some 30 years ago it was believed that liver necrosis releases products toxic to the kidney (122); the current belief is that those experiments, carried out on dogs, were misleading due to the presence of bacteria in normal dog livers.

Disposal of circulating cellular proteins Enzymes and other cellular proteins that gain access to the plasma are eliminated via the kidney or slowly removed by the sinusoidal phagocytes of the liver, spleen, and bone marrow (p. 299). Occasionally some intracellular material is recognized as foreign by the immune system and gives rise to autoantibodies, but there is no clear evidence that they cause further disease.

Antibodies against heart tissue have been studied a great deal because of a mysterious syndrome that can appear 2–6 weeks after an infarct (pain, fever, leukocytosis, and a "pericardial rub" indicative of pericardial inflammation) (132). An autoimmune response was thought to be responsible, but the mechanism is still unknown. Antibodies against cardiolipin (a phospholipid) certainly do develop after myocardial infarction; in fact, high titers of these antibodies may be a marker for patients at increased risk for recurrent cardiovascular accidents (169).

Necrosis removes calcium from the plasma. So far we have emphasized the release of cell contents, but we should recall once again that necrosis absorbs calcium ions; if the necrosis is extensive, plasma calcium can drop low enough to cause tetany (p. 214). This is, in our opinion, the mechanism of hypocalcemia in severe muscle necrosis (rhabdomyolysis) (119). We have already mentioned the special mechanism of hypocalcemia in fat necrosis: the formation of calcium soaps from triglycerides (214).

Necrosis elicits local and general reactions, namely inflammation, fever, and humoral changes.

We will deal with these events in the chapter on inflammation.

TO SUM UP: Here ends our tale of cell injury and cell death. It was long, because it is involved in virtually every disease. There were many highlights: the concept that open cell wounds will heal, at the molecular level, much like open body wounds; the complex drama of ischemic cell death; the notions of programmed cell death, cell deletion, and cell suicide; the strange ritual of apoptosis; the different ways of cell death in different tissues. No topic shows more convincingly that the cell is the elementary patient.

References

Cell Injury and Cell Death; Necrosis

1. Acosta D, Puckett M, McMillin R. Ischemic myocardial injury in cultured heart cells: leakage of cytoplasmic enzymes from injured cells. In Vitro 1978;14:728–732.
2. Altekar W, Paul P, Nadkarni GB. Changes in tryptophan microenvironment in horse heart myoglobin due to γ-irradiation. Biochim Biophys Acta 1977;495:203–211.
3. Altman PL, Dittmer DS (eds). Respiration and circulation. Bethesda: Federation of American Societies for Experimental Biology, 1971.
4. Arends MJ, Morris RG, Wyllie AH. Apoptosis. The role of the endonuclease. Am J Pathol 1990;136:593–608.
5. Arsenau JC, Bagley CM, Anderson T, Canellos GP. Hyperkalaemia, a sequel to chemotherapy of Burkitt's lymphoma. Lancet 1973;1:10–14.
6. Aust SD, Morehouse LA, Thomas CE. Role of metals in oxygen radical reactions. J Free Radic Biol Med 1985;1:3–25.
7. Autor AP (ed). Pathology of oxygen. New York: Academic Press, 1982.
8. Azmi TI, O'Shea JD. Mechanism of deletion of endothelial cells during regression of the corpus luteum. Lab Invest 1984;51:206–217.
9. Ballard KJ, Holt SJ. Cytological and cytochemical studies on cell death and digestion in the foetal rat foot: the role of macrophages and hydrolytic enzymes. J Cell Sci 1968;3:245–262.
10. Bangham AD. Liposomes: realizing their promise. Hosp Pract 1992;27:51–62.
11. Bangham AD, Horne RW. Negative staining of phospholipids and their structural modification by surface-active agents as observed in the electron microscope. J Mol Biol 1964;8:660–668.
12. Barbe MF, Tytell M, Gower DJ, Welch WJ. Hyperthermia protects against light damage in the rat retina. Science 1988;241:1817–1820.
13. Barnes DM. Cells without growth factors commit suicide. Science 1988;242:1510–1511.
14. Barrett LA, McDowell EM, Harris CC, Trump BF. Studies on the pathogenesis of ischemic cell injury. XV. Reversal of ischemic cell injury in hamster trachea and human bronchus by explant culture. Beitr Pathol 1977;161:109–121.
15. Beal MF. Mechanisms of excitotoxicity in neurologic diseases. FASEB J 1992;6:3338–3344.
16. Beckman JS, Freeman BA. Antioxidant enzymes as mechanistic probes of oxygen-dependent toxicity. In: Taylor AE, Matalon S, Ward P (eds). Physiology of oxygen radicals. Bethesda: American Physiological Society, 1986, pp. 39–53.
17. Beckmann RP, Mizzen LA, Welch WJ. Interaction of Hsp 70 with newly synthesized proteins: implications for protein folding and assembly. Science 1990;248:850–854.
18. Bernelli-Zazzera A, Gaja G. Some aspects of glycogen metabolism following reversible or irreversible liver ischemia. Exp Mol Pathol 1964;3:351–368.
19. Berns MW, Aist J, Edwards J, et al. Laser microsurgery in cell and developmental biology. Science 1981;213:505–513.
20. Bessis M. Studies on cell agony and death: an attempt at classification. In: de Reuck AVS, Knight J (eds). Cellular injury. Ciba Foundation Symposium. London: J & A Churchill, Ltd, 1964, pp. 287–328.
21. Bessis M. La mort de la cellule. Triangle 1970;9:191–199.
22. Block MI, Said JW, Siegel RJ, Fishbein MC. Myocardial myoglobin following coronary artery occlusion. An immunohistochemical study. Am J Pathol 1983;111:374–379.
23. Bluemink JG. Cortical wound healing in the amphibian egg: an electron microscopical study. J Ultrastruct Res 1972;41:95–114.
24. Bond U, Schlesinger MJ. Ubiquitin is a heat shock protein in chicken embryo fibroblasts. Mol Cell Biol 1985;5:949–956.
25. Borkman RF, Lerman S. Fluorescence spectra of tryptophan residues in human and bovine lens proteins. Eye Res 1978;26:705–713.
26. Bouchardy B, Majno G. Histopathology of early myocardial infarcts. A new approach. Am J Pathol 1974;74:301–330.
27. Bowen ID. Laboratory techniques for demonstrating cell death. In: Davies I, Sigee DC (eds). Cell ageing and cell death. Cambridge: Cambridge University Press, 1984, pp. 5–40.
28. Bowen ID. Apoptosis or programmed cell death? Cell Biol Int 1993;17:365–380.
29. Bowen ID, Bowen SM. Programmed cell death in tumours and tissues. London: Chapman and Hall, 1990.
30. Bowen ID, Lockshin RA (eds). Cell death in biology and pathology. London: Chapman and Hall, 1981.
31. Bracken MB, Shepard MJ, Collins WF, et al. A randomized, controlled trial of methylprednisolone or naloxone in the treatment of acute spinal-cord injury. Results of the Second National Acute Spinal Cord Injury Study. N Engl J Med 1990;322:1405–1411.
32. Buckley IK. Phosphatides in the morphology of injured tissue. QJ Exp Physiol 1961;46:229–237.
32a. Burroughs M, Cabellos C, Prasad S, Tuomanen E. Bacterial components and the pathophysiology of injury to the blood-brain barrier: does cell wall add to t he effects of endotoxin in gram-negative meningitis? J Infect Dis 1992;165(suppl 1):S82–85.
33. Bus JS, Gibson JE. Lipid peroxidation and its role in toxicology. Rev Biochem Toxicol 1:125–149.
34. Carson DA, Ribeiro JM. Apoptosis and disease. Lancet 1993;341:1251–1254.
35. Carson DA, Seto S, Wasson DB, Carrera CJ. DNA strand breaks, NAD metabolism, and programmed cell death. Exp Cell Res 1986;164:273–281.
36. Cech P, Block JB, Cone LA, Stone R. Tumor lysis

syndrome after tamoxifen flare. N Engl J Med 1986;315:263–264.

37. Chan PH. The role of oxygen radicals in brain injury and edema. In: Chow CK (ed). Cellular antioxidant defense mechanisms, vol. III. Boca Raton: CRC Press, Inc., 1988, pp. 89–109.

38. Cheung JY, Bonventre JV, Malis CD, Leaf A. Calcium and ischemic injury. N Engl J Med 1986;314:1670–1676.

39. Chien KR, Abrams J, Pfau RG, Farber JL. Prevention by Chlorpromazine of ischemic liver cell death. Am J Pathol 1977;88:539–558.

40. Choi DW. Excitotoxic cell death. J Neurobiol 23:1261–1276.

41. Chopra J, Joist JH, Webster RO. Loss of 51Chromium, lactate dehydrogenase, and 111Indium as indicators of endothelial cell injury. Lab Invest 1987;57:578–584.

42. Chow CK (ed). Cellular antioxidant defense mechanisms, vols. II and III. Boca Raton: CRC Press, Inc., 1988.

43. Clements JA, Tierney DF. Alveolar instability associated with altered surface tension. In: Fenn WO and Rahn H (eds). Handbook of physiology, Section 3: Respiration. Washington, DC: American Physiology Society, 1965, pp. 1565–1583.

44. Collins VP. Cultured human glial and glioma cells. Int Rev Exp Pathol 1983;24:135–202.

45. Compton MM, Cidlowski JA. Rapid in vivo effects of glucocorticoids on the integrity of rat lymphocyte genomic deoxyribonucleic acid. Endocrinology 1986;118:38–45.

46. Corr PB, Gross RW, Sobel BE. Amphipathic metabolites and membrane dysfunction in ischemic myocardium. Circ Res 1984;55:135–154.

47. Costero I, Pomerat CM. Cultivation of neurons from the adult human cerebral and cerebellar cortex. Am J Anat 1951;89:405–468.

48. Craig EA. The heat shock response. CRC Crit Rev Biochem 1985;18:239–280.

49. Cross HR, Leu R, Miller MF. Scope of warmed-over flavor and its importance to the meat industry. In: St Angelo AJ, Bailey ME (eds). Warmed-over flavor of meat. Orlando: Academic Press, Inc, 1987, pp. 1–18.

50. Cutler RG. Antioxidants, aging, and longevity. In: Pryor WA (ed). Free radicals in biology, vol. VI. Orlando: Academic Press, Inc., 1984, pp. 371–428.

51. Cruveilhier J. Anatomie pathologique du corps humain. Paris: J.B. Baillière, 1829–1842.

52. Das DK, Engelman RM, Rousou JA, Breyer RH, Otani H, Lemeshow S. Role of membrane phospholipids in myocardial injury induced by ischemia and reperfusion. Am J Physiol 1986;251:H71–H79.

53. Davies I, Sigee DC (eds). Cell ageing and cell death. Cambridge: Cambridge University Press, 1984.

54. Délèze J. Calcium ions and the healing over of heart fibres. In: Taccardi B, Marchetti G (eds). International symposium on the electrophysiology of the heart. Oxford: Pergamon Press, 1965, pp. 147–148.

55. Del Maestro RF. An approach to free radicals in medicine and biology. Acta Physiol Scand [Suppl] 1980;492:153–168.

56. De Mello WC. Membrane sealing in frog skeletal-muscle fibers. Proc Natl Acad Sci USA 1973;70:982–984.

57. De Mello WC. Effect of intracellular injection of calcium and strontium on cell communication in heart. J Physiol 1975;250:231–245.

58. Demopoulos HB, Flamm ES, Pietronigro DD, Seligman ML. The free radical pathology and the microcirculation in the major central nervous system disorders. Acta Physiol Scand [Suppl] 1980;492:91–118.

59. Demopoulos HB, Flamm E, Seligman M, Pietronigro DD. Oxygen free radicals in central nervous system ischemia and trauma. In: Autor AP (ed). Pathology of oxygen. New York: Academic Press, 1982, pp. 127–155.

60. Draper HH, Dhanakoti SN, Hadley M, Piché LA. Malondialdehyde in biological systems. In: Chow CK (ed). Cellular antioxidant defense mechanisms, vol. II. Boca Raton: CRC Press, Inc., 1988, pp. 97–109.

61. Dubick MA, Mayer AD, Majumdar APN, Mar G, McMahon MJ, Geokas MC. Biochemical studies in peritoneal fluid from patients with acute pancreatitis. Relationship to etiology. Dig Dis Sci 1987;32:305–312.

62. Epstein JH. The pathological effects of light on the skin. In: Pryor WA (ed). Free radicals in biology, vol. III. New York: Academic Press, 1977, pp. 219–249.

63. Fahrbach SE, Truman JW. Mechanisms for programmed cell death in the nervous system of a moth. Ciba Found Symp 1987;126:65–81.

64. Farber E, Fisher MM (eds). Toxic injury of the liver, part A. New York: Marcel Dekker, Inc., 1979.

65. Farber E, Liang H, Shinozuka S. Dissociation of effects on protein synthesis and ribosomes from membrane changes induced by carbon tetrachloride. Am J Pathol 1971;64:601–622.

66. Farber JL. Reactions of the liver to injury. In: Farber E, Fisher MM (eds). Toxic injury of the liver, part A. New York: Marcel Dekker, Inc., 1979, pp. 215–241.

67. Farber JL. Calcium and the mechanisms of liver necrosis. Prog Liver Dis 1982;7:347–360.

68. Farber JL. Membrane injury and calcium homeostasis in the pathogenesis of coagulative necrosis. Lab Invest 1982;47:114–123.

69. Ferguson CC, Richardson JB. A simple technique for the utilization of postmortem tracheal and bronchial tissues for ultrastructural studies. Hum Pathol 1978;9:463–470.

70. Fisch C. Relation of electrolyte disturbances to cardiac arrhythmias. Circulation 1973;47:408–419.

71. Foote CS. Light, oxygen, and toxicity. In: Autor AP (ed). Pathology of oxygen. New York: Academic Press, 1982, pp. 21–44.

72. Foulks GN (ed). Noninfectious inflammation of the anterior segment. International Ophthalmology Clinics, vol. 23. Boston: Little, Brown and Company, 1983.

73. Frank L. Oxygen toxicity in eucaryotes. In: Oberley LW (ed). Superoxide dismutase. Boca Raton: CRC Press, 1985, pp. 1–43.

74. Frankel EN. Volatile lipid oxidation products. Prog Lipid Res 1982;22:1–33.

75. Fraser CL, Arieff AI. Hepatic encephalopathy. N Engl J Med 1985;313:865–873.

76. Frederiks WM, Fronik GM, Hesseling JMG. A method for quantitative analysis of the extent of necrosis in ischemic rat liver. Exp Mol Pathol 1984;41:119–125.

77. Freeman BA, Crapo JD. Free radicals and tissue injury. Lab Invest 1982;47:412–426.

78. Fretzin DF, Arias AM. Sclerema neonatorum and subcutaneous fat necrosis of the newborn. Pediatr Dermatol 1987;4:112–122.

79. Fridovich I. Oxygen radicals, hydrogen peroxide, and oxygen toxicity In: Pryor WA (ed). Free radicals in biology, vol. I. New York: Academic Press, 1976, pp. 239–277.

80. Fridovich I. Superoxide dismutase in biology and medicine. In: Autor AP (ed). Pathology of oxygen. New York: Academic Press, 1982, pp. 1–19.

81. Fulder SJ. The growth of cultured human fibroblasts treated with hydrocortisone and extracts of the medicinal plant panax ginseng. Exp Gerontol 1977;12:125–131.

82. Gahan PB. Cell senescence and death in plants. In:

Bowen ID, Lockshin RA (eds). Cell death in biology and pathology. London: Chapman and Hall, 1981, pp. 145–169.

83. Ganote CE, Vander Heide RS. Cytoskeletal lesions in anoxic myocardial injury. A conventional and high-voltage electron-microscopic and immunofluorescence study. Am J Pathol 1987;129:327–344.

84. Garcia JH, Conger KA, Lossinsky AS. The cellular pathology of ischemic stroke. In: Trump BF, Laufer A, Jones RT (eds). Cellular pathobiology of human disease. New York: Gustav Fischer, Inc., 1983, pp. 351–367.

85. Garcia JH, Yoshida Y, Chen H, et al. Progression from ischemic injury to infarct following middle cerebral artery occlusion in the rat. Am J Pathol 1993;142:623–635.

86. Gavrieli Y, Sherman Y, Ben-Sasson SA. Identification of programmed cell death in situ via specific labeling of nuclear DNA fragmentation. J Cell Biol 1992;119:493–501.

87. Gee MH, Flynn JT, Spath JA Jr. Pulmonary and coronary endothelial effects of acute myocardial ischemia in dogs. Am J Physiol 1982;242:H337–H348.

88. Glücksmann A. Cell deaths in normal vertebrate ontogeny. Biol Rev 1951;26:59–86.

89. Gobé GC, Axelsen RA. Genesis of renal tubular atrophy in experimental hydronephrosis in the rat. Role of apoptosis. Lab Invest 1987;56:273–281.

90. Goldblatt PJ, Trump BF, Stowell RE. Studies on necrosis of mouse liver in vitro. Alterations in some histochemically demonstrable hepatocellular enzymes. Am J Pathol 1965;47:183–208.

91. Goldman AS, Herold R, Piddington R. Inhibition of programmed cell death in the fetal palate by cortisol. Proc Soc Exp Biol Med 1981;166:418–424.

92. Gregoriadis G. The carrier potential of liposomes in biology and medicine. N Engl J Med 1976;295:704–710.

93. Grierson D. Nucleic acid and protein synthesis during fruit ripening. In: Davies I, Sigee DC (eds). Cell ageing and cell death. Cambridge: Cambridge University Press, 1984, pp. 189–202.

94. Grierson D, Maunders MJ, Slater A, et al. Gene expression during tomato ripening. Philos Trans R Soc Lond [Biol] 1986;314:399–410.

95. Grisham MB, McCord JM. Chemistry and cytotoxicity of reactive oxygen metabolites. In: Taylor AE, Matalon S, Ward P (eds). Physiology of oxygen radicals. Bethesda: American Physiological Society, 1986, pp. 1–18.

96. Grollman A. Pressor activity of circulating blood after focal infarction of the kidney in the rat. Proc Soc Exp Biol Med 1970;134:1120–1122.

97. Guilliermond A. La structure des cellules végétales a l'ultramicroscope. Protoplasma (Berl) 1932;16:454–477.

98. Guyton AC. Textbook of medical physiology, 7th ed. Philadelphia: WB Saunders Company, 1986.

99. Haimovici H. Metabolic complications of acute arterial occlusions. J Cardiovasc Surg 1979;20:349–357.

100. Halliwell B. Oxidants and human disease: some new concepts. FASEB J 1987;1:358–364.

101. Halliwell B, Gutteridge JMC. Iron as a biological pro-oxidant. ISI Atlas of Science:Biochemistry 1988;1:48–52.

102. Harris AS. Potassium and experimental coronary occlusion. Am Heart J 1966;71:797–802.

103. Heilbrunn LV. The dynamics of living protoplasm. New York: Academic Press, Inc., 1956.

104. Hendry JH, Scott D. Loss of reproductive integrity of irradiated cells, and its importance in tissues. In: Potten CS (ed). Perspectives on mammalian cell death. Oxford: Oxford University Press, 1987, pp. 160–183.

105. Hill JL, Gettes LS. Ischemia induced changes in interstitial potassium in in situ myocardium. Circulation 1977;56(suppl. III):III–108.

106. Hopwood D, Levison DA. Atrophy and apoptosis in the cyclical human endometrium. J Pathol 1976;119:159–166.

107. Ishida R, Akiyoshi H, Takahashi T. Isolation and purification of calcium and magnesium dependent endonuclease from rat liver nuclei. Biochem Biophys Res Commun 1974;56:703–710.

108. Itkonen P, Collan Y. Mitochondrial flocculent densities in ischemia. Digestion experiments. Acta Pathol Microbiol Immunol Scand A 1983;91:463–468.

108a. Itoh G, Tamura J, Suzuki M, Suzuki Y, Ideda H, Koike M, Nomura M, Jie T, Ito K. DNA fragmentation of human infarcted myocardial cells demonstrated by the Nick End Labeling method and DNA agarose gel electrophoresis. Am J Pathol 1995, 146:1325–1331.

109. Jennings RB, Shen AC, Hill ML, Ganote CE, Herdson PB. Mitochondrial matrix densities in myocardial ischemia and autolysis. Exp Mol Pathol 1978;29:55–65.

110. Judah JD, Ahmed, K, Mclean AEM. Possible role of ion shifts in liver injury. In: deReuck AVS, Knight J (eds). Cellular injury. Ciba Foundation Symposium. Boston: Little, Brown, 1964, pp. 187–204.

111. Kaltenbach JP, Kaltenbach MH, Lyons WB. Nigrosin as a dye for differentiating live and dead ascites cells. Exp Cell Res 1958;15:112–117.

112. Kaplan M. Suicide by oral ingestion of a potassium preparation. Ann Intern Med 1969;71:363–364.

113. Kauzmann W. Denaturation of proteins and enzymes. In: McElroy WD, Glass B (eds). A symposium on the mechanism of enzyme action. Baltimore: The Johns Hopkins Press, 1954, pp. 70–120.

114. Kerr JFR. Shrinkage necrosis: a distinct mode of cellular death. J Pathol 1971;105:13–29.

115. Kerr JFR, Bishop CJ, Searle J. Apoptosis. Recent Adv Histopathol 1984;12:1–15.

116. Kerr JFR, Harmon BV. Definition and incidence of apoptosis: an historical perspective. In: Tomei LD, Cope FO (eds). Apoptosis: the molecular basis of cell death. Cold Spring Harbor: Cold Spring Harbor Laboratory Press, 1991, pp. 5–29.

117. Kerr JFR, Searle J. Deletion of cells by apoptosis during castration-induced involution of the rat prostate. Virchows Arch Abt B Zellpathol 1973;13:87–102.

118. Kerr JFR, Wyllie AH, Currie AR. Apoptosis: a basic biological phenomenon with wide-ranging implications in tissue kinetics. Br J Cancer 1972;26:239–257.

119. Knochel JP. Serum calcium derangements in rhabdomyolysis. N Engl J Med 1981;305:161–163.

120. Knochel JP, Schlein EM. On the mechanism of rhabdomyolysis in potassium depletion. J Clin Invest 1972;51:1750–1758.

121. Koury MJ, Bondurant MC. Erythropoietin retards DNA breakdown and prevents programmed death in erythroid progenitor cells. Science 1990;248:378–381.

122. Kraus GE, Costa G. Systemic effects of massive hepatic necrosis. I. Acute effects of hepatic infarction on the kidneys. Arch Surg 1963;87:957–962.

122a. Kromer G, Petit P, Zamzami N, Vayassiere, Mignotte B. The biochemistry of programmed cell death. FASEB Journal 1995; 9:1277–1287.

123. La Claire JW. II: Inducement of wound motility in intact giant algal cells. Exp Cell Res 1983;145:63–69.

124. Lacy ER, Ito S. Microscopic analysis of ethanol damage to rat gastric mucosa after treatment with a prostaglandin. Gastroenterology 1982;83:619–625.

125. Larsson J, Bergström J. Electrolyte changes in muscle

tissue and plasma in tourniquet-ischemia. Acta Chir Scand 1978;144:67–73.

126. Lawrie RA. Meat science, 3rd ed. Oxford: Pergamon Press, 1979.

127. Ledda-Columbano GM, Coni P, Curto M, et al. Induction of two different modes of cell death, apoptosis and necrosis, in rat liver after a single dose of thioacetamide. Am J Pathol 1991;139:1099–1109.

128. Lefer AM, Tsao P, Aoki N, Palladino MA, Jr. Mediation of cardioprotection by transforming growth factor-β. Science 1990;249:61–64.

129. Lemasters JJ, Stemkowski CJ, Ji S, Thurman RG. Cell surface changes and enzyme release during hypoxia and reoxygenation in the isolated, perfused rat liver. J Cell Biol 1983;97:778–786.

130. Levi-Montalcini R, Aloe L. Mechanism(s) of action of nerve growth factor in tact and lethally injured sympathetic nerve cell in neonatal rodents. In: Bowen ID, Lockshin RA (eds). Cell death in biology and pathology. London: Chapman and Hall, 1981, pp. 295–327.

131. Li GC, Laszlo A. Thermotolerance in mammalian cells: a possible role for heat shock proteins. In: Atkinson BG, Walden DB (eds). Changes in eukaryotic gene expression in response to environmental stress. Orlando: Academic Press, 1985, pp. 227–254.

132. Liem KL, ten Veen JH, Lie KI, Feltkamp TEW, Durrer D. Incidence and significance of heartmuscle antibodies in patients with acute myocardial infarction and unstable angina. Acta Med Scand 1979;206:473–475.

132a. Lipton SA, Rosenberg PA. Excitatory amino acids as a final common pathway for neurologic disorders. New Engl J Med 1994;330:613–622.

133. Lockshin RA, Beaulaton J. Programmed cell death. Life Sci 1974;15:1549–1565.

134. Lockshin RA, Williams CM. Programmed cell death-IV. The influence of drugs on the breakdown of the intersegmental muscles of silkmoths. J Insect Physiol 1965;11:803–809.

135. Lockshin RA, Zakeri-Milovanovic Z. Nucleic acids in cell death. In: Davies I, Sigee DC (eds). Cell ageing and cell death. Cambridge: Cambridge University Press, 1984, pp. 243–268.

136. Loewenstein WR, Penn RD. Intercellular communication and tissue growth. II. Tissue regeneration. J Cell Biol 1967;33:235–242.

137. Lorch IJ, Danielli JF, Hörstadius S. The effect of enucleation on the development of sea urchin eggs. Exp Cell Res 1952;4:253–274.

138. Lott JA, Wolf PL. Clinical enzymology. New York: Field, Rich and Associates, Inc., 1986.

139. Lucy JA, Glauert AM. Structure and assembly of macromolecular lipid complexes composed of globular micelles. J Mol Biol 1964;8:727–748.

140. Lungarella G, Gardi C, de Santi MM, Luzi P. Pulmonary vascular injury in pancreatitis: evidence for a major role played by pancreatic elastase. Exp Mol Pathol 1985;42:44–59.

141. Machlin LJ, Bendich A. Free radical tissue damage: protective role of antioxidant nutrients. FASEB J 1987;1:441–445.

141a. Macklin CC. The pulmonary alveolar mucoid film and the pneumonocytes. Lancet 1954;1:1099–1104.

142. Majno G. Death of liver tissue: a review of cell death, necrosis, and autolysis. In: Rouiller Ch. The liver, vol. 2. New York: Academic Press, 1964:267–313.

142a. Majno G. Joris I. Apoptosis, oncosis, and necrosis: an overview of cell death. A J Pathol 1994 (in press).

143. Majno G, LaGattuta M, Thompson TE. Cellular death

and necrosis: chemical, physical and morphologic changes in rat liver. Virchows Arch Pathol Anat 1960;333:421–465.

143a. Martin DP, Johnson EM Jr. Programmed cell death in the peripheral nervous system. In: Tomei LD, Cope FO, eds. Apoptosis: the molecular basis of cell death. New York: Cold Spring Harbor Laboratory Press, 1991:247–261.

144. Martin LC, Johnson BK. Practical microscopy, 2nd ed. Brooklyn: Chemical Publishing Co, Inc., 1951.

145. Martin DP, Schmidt RE, DiStefano PS, Lowry OH, Carter JG, Johnson EM Jr. Inhibitors of protein synthesis and RNA synthesis prevent neuronal death caused by nerve growth factor deprivation. J Cell Biol 1988;106:829–844.

146. Marx JL. Oxygen free radicals linked to many diseases. Science 1987;235:529–531.

147. Matalon S, Nickerson PA. Alterations in mammalian blood-gas barrier exposed to hyperoxia. In: Taylor AE, Matalon S, Ward P (eds). Physiology of oxygen radicals. Bethesda: American Physiological Society, 1986, pp. 55–69.

148. Materson BJ, Preston RA. Myoglobinuria versus hemoglobinuria. Hosp Pract 1988;23:29–38.

149. Mathews-Roth MM. Carotenoid pigments and protection against photosensitization: how studies in bacteria suggested a treatment for a human disease. Perspect Biol Med 1984;28:127–139.

150. Mathews-Roth MM, Pathak A, Fitzpatrick TB, Harber LC, Kass EH. Beta-carotene as a photoprotective agent in erythropoietic protoporphyria. Trans Assoc Am Physicians 1970;83:176–184.

151. Mathieu JP. Optics, parts 1 and 2. Oxford: Pergamon Press, 1975.

152. Mayer LD, Hope MJ, Cullis PR. Vesicles of variable sizes produced by a rapid extrusion procedure. Biochim Biophys Acta 1986;858:161–168.

153. McCluskey RT, Thomas L. The removal of cartilage matrix, in vivo, by papain. Identification of crystalline papain protease as the cause of the phenomenon. J Exp Med 1958;108:371–384.

154. McConkey DJ, Hartzell P, Nicotera P, Orrenius S. Calcium-activated DNA fragmentation kills immature thymocytes. FASEB J 1989;3:1843–1849.

155. Mergner WJ, Costa M, Classen JB, Leventhal HJ. Plasma membrane and mitochondrial changes in cell injury. In: Mergner WJ, Jones RT, Trump BF (eds). Cell death. Mechanisms of acute and lethal cell injury, vol. 1. New York: Field & Wood Medical Publishers, Inc., 1990, pp. 87–109.

156. Mergner WJ, Jones RT, Trump BF (eds). Cell death. Mechanisms of acute and lethal cell injury, vol. 1. New York: Field & Wood Medical Publishers, Inc., 1990.

157. Mergner WJ, Jones RT, Trump BF. Introduction. In: Mergner WJ, Jones RT, Trump BF (eds). Cell death. Mechanisms of acute and lethal cell injury, vol. 1. New York: Field & Wood Medical Publishers, Inc, 1990, pp. 1–11.

158. Miller DL, Dillon J. An unusual abdominal mass in an elderly woman. N Engl J Med 1989;321:1613–1614.

159. Minotti, G, Aust SD. The role of iron in the initiation of lipid peroxidation. Chem Phys Lipids 1987;44:191–208.

159a. Morimoto RI, Sarge KD, Abravaya K. Transcriptional Regulation of Heat Shock Genes. J Biol Chem 1992; 267:

160. Morimoto RI, Tissières A, Georgopoulos C. The stress response, function of the proteins, and perspectives. In: Morimoto RI, Tissières A, Georgopoulos C (eds). Stress

proteins in biology and medicine. Cold Spring Harbor: Cold Spring Harbor Laboratory Press, 1990, pp. 1–36.

161. Morris RG, Hargreaves AD, Duvall E, Wyllie AH. Hormone-induced cell death. 2. Surface changes in thymocytes undergoing apoptosis. Am J Pathol 1984;115:426–436.

162. Mottet NK, Hammar SP. Ribosome crystals in necrotizing cells from the posterior necrotic zone of the developing chick limb. J Cell Sci 1972;11:403–414.

163. Mullick S. The tourniquet in operations upon the extremities. Surg Gynecol Obstet 1978;146:821–826.

164. Munro S, Pelham H. What turns on heat shock genes? Nature 1985;317:477–478.

165. Myers CE, McGuire WP, Liss RH, Ifrim I, Grotzinger K, Young RC. Adriamycin: the role of lipid peroxidation in cardiac toxicity and tumor response. Science 1977;197:165–167.

166. Nash G, Blennerhassett JB, Pontoppidan H. Pulmonary lesions associated with oxygen therapy and artificial ventilation. N Engl J Med 1967;276:368–374.

167. Nawroth PP, Stern DM, Kaplan KL, Nossel HL. Prostacyclin production by perturbed bovine aortic endothelial cells in culture. Blood 1984;64:801–806.

168. Nevalainen TJ, Anttinen J. Ultrastructural and functional changes in pancreatic acinar cells during autolysis. Virchows Arch B Cell Pathol 1977;24:197–207.

169. Norberg R, Ernerudh J, Hamsten A, Unander AM, Årfors L. Phospholipid antibodies in cardiovascular disease. Acta Med Scand Suppl 1987;715:93–98.

170. O'Connor TM, Wyttenbach CR. Cell death in the embryonic chick spinal cord. J Cell Biol 1974;60:448–459.

171. Oliveira-Castro GM, Loewenstein WR. Junctional membrane permeability. Effects of divalent cations. J Membrane Biol 1971;5:51–77.

172. Oppenheim RW, Maderdrut JL, Wells DJ. Cell death of motoneurons in the chick embryo spinal cord. VI. Reduction of naturally occurring cell death in the thoracolumbar column of Terni by nerve growth factor. J Comp Neurol 1982;210:174–189.

173. Ostro MJ (ed). Liposomes. New York: Marcel Dekker, Inc., 1983.

174. Ostro MJ (ed). Liposomes. From biophysics to therapeutics. New York: Marcel Dekker, Inc., 1987.

175. Ostro MJ. Liposomes. Sci Am 1987;256:102–111.

176. Palade GE. Membrane biogenesis: an overview. Methods Enzymol 1983;96:xxix-lv.

177. Parker JO, Chiong MA, West RO, Case RB. The effect of ischemia and alterations of heart rate on myocardial potassium balance in man. Circulation 1970;42:205–217.

178. Pekkala D, Heath IB, Silver JC. Changes in chromatin and the phosphorylation of nuclear proteins during heat shock of Achlya ambisexualis. Mol Cell Biol 1984;4:1198–1205.

179. Pepper MS, Spray DC, Chanson M, Montesano R, Orci L, Meda P. Junctional communication is induced in migrating capillary endothelial cells. J Cell Biol 1989;109:3027–3038.

180. Perry MC, Yarbro JW (eds). Toxicity of chemotherapy. Orlando: Grune & Stratton, 1984.

181. Pfeiffer FE, Homburger HA, Yanagihara T. Serum creatine kinase B concentrations in acute cerebrovascular diseases. Arch Neurol 1984;41:1175–1178.

182. Pilar G, Landmesser L. Ultrastructural differences during embryonic cell death in normal and peripherally deprived ciliary ganglia. J Cell Biol 1976;68:339–356.

183. Popescu MC, Swenson CE, Ginsberg RS. Liposome-mediated treatment of viral, bacterial, and protozoal

infections. In: Ostro MJ (ed). Liposomes. From biophysics to therapeutics. New York: Marcel Dekker, Inc., 1987, pp. 219–251.

184. Potten CS. Perspectives on mammalian cell death. Oxford: Oxford University Press, 1987.

185. Pryor WA (ed). Free radicals in biology, vol. I. New York: Academic Press, 1976.

186. Pryor WA. Free radical biology: xenobiotics, cancer, and aging. Ann NY Acad Sci 1982;393:1–23.

187. Puck TT. Radiation and the human cell. Sci Am 1960;202:142–153.

187a. Racusen LC. Alterations on human proximal tubule cell attachment in response to hypoxia: role of microfilaments. J Lab Clin Med 1994;123:357–364.

188. Reddy MK, Etlinger JD, Rabinowitz M, Fischman DA, Zak R. Removal of Z-lines and a-actinin from isolated myofibrils by a calcium-activated neutral protease. J Biol Chem 1975;250:4278–4284.

189. Riabowol KT, Mizzen LA, Welch WJ. Heat shock is lethal to fibroblasts microinjected with antibodies against hsp 70. Science 1988;242:433–436.

190. Rindfleisch E. Traité d'histologie pathologique. Paris: Baillière et Fils, 1873.

191. Ritossa F. A new puffing pattern induced by temperature shock and DNP in Drosophila. Experentia 1962;18:571–573.

192. Robaye B, Mosselmans R, Fiers W, Dumont JE, Galand P. Tumor necrosis factor induces apoptosis (programmed cell death) in normal endothelial cells in vitro. Am J Pathol 1991;138:447–453.

193. Sanderson AR. Quantitative titration, kinetic behaviour, and inhibition of cytotoxic mouse isoantisera. Immunology 1965;9:287–300.

193a. Sarge KD, Bray, AE, Goodson ML. Altered Stress response in testis. Nature 1995; 374:126.

194. Saunders JW. Death in embryonic systems. Science 1966;154:604–612.

195. Saunders JW, Fallon JF. Cell death in morphogenesis. In: Locke M (ed). Major problems in developmental biology. New York: Academic Press, 1966, pp 289–314.

196. Saunders JW, Gasseling MT, Saunders LC. Cellular death in morphogenesis of the avian wing. Dev Biol 1962;5:147–178.

197. Savill J, Dransfield I, Hogg N, Haslett C. Vitronectin receptor-mediated phagocytosis of cells undergoing apoptosis. Nature 1990;343:170–173.

197a. Schachenmayr W. Pankreatitis-assoziierte Gehirnbefunde: gibt es eine pankreatische encephalopathie? Pancreatitis-associated brain findings: does pancreatic encephalopathy exist? Verh Dtsch Ges Path 1987;71:280–283.

198. Schlesinger MJ. Heat shock proteins: the search for functions. J Cell Biol 1986;103:321–325.

199. Selye H. Prevention of various forms of metabolic myocardial necrosis by catatoxic steroids. J Mol Cell Cardiol 1970;1:91–99.

199a. Server AC, Mobley WC. Neuronal cell death and the role of apoptosis. In: Tomei LD, Cope FO, eds. Apoptosis: the molecular basis of cell death. New York: Cold Spring Harbor Laboratory Press, 1991;263–278.

200. Sessa G, Weissmann G. Phospholipid spherules (liposomes) as a model for biological membranes. J Lipid Res 1968;9:310–318.

201. Sessa G, Weissmann G. Incorporation of lysozyme into liposomes. A model for structure-linked latency. J Biol Chem 1970;245:3295–3301.

202. Shirazi Y, Mergner WJ. Phospholipids, phospholipases, and cell injury. In: Mergner WJ, Jones RT, Trump BF (eds). Cell death. Mechanisms of acute and lethal cell

injury, vol. 1. New York: Field & Wood Medical Publishers, Inc., 1990, pp. 201–220.

203. Skinner HA. The origin of medical terms, 2nd ed. Baltimore: The Williams & Wilkins Company, 1961.

204. Skipper HE, Perry S. Kinetics of normal and leukemic leukocyte populations and relevance to chemotherapy. Cancer Res 1970;30:1883–1897.

205. Small DM. Phase equilibria and structure of dry and hydrated egg lecithin. J Lipid Res 1967;8:551–557.

206. Small DM. Liquid crystals in living and dying systems. J Colloid Interface Sci 1977;58:581–602.

207. Smith LJ. The effect of methylprednisolone on lung injury in mice. J Lab Clin Med 1983;101:629–640.

208. Sobel MI. Light. Chicago: The University of Chicago Press, 1987.

209. Spacek J. Reoxygenation of anoxic human tissues. An application for electron microscopy and its limits. Virchows Arch [Cell Pathol] 1981;37:97–102.

210. Starke PE, Hoek JB, Farber JL. Calcium-dependent and calcium-independent mechanisms of irreversible cell injury in cultured hepatocytes. J Biol Chem 1986;261:3006–3012.

211. Steenbergen C, Hill ML, Jennings RB. Cytoskeletal damage during myocardial ischemia: changes in vinculin immunofluorescence staining during total in vitro ischemia in canine heart. Circ Res 1987;60:478–486.

212. Steenbergen C, Murphy E, Levy L, London RE. Elevation in cytosolic free calcium concentration early in myocardial ischemia in perfused rat heart. Circ Res 1987;60:700–707.

213. Stemerman MB, Colton C, Morell E. Perturbations of the endothelium. Prog Hemost Thromb 1984;7:289–324.

214. Stewart AF, Longo W, Kreutter D, Jacob R, Burtis WJ. Hypocalcemia associated with calcium-soap formation in a patient with a pancreatic fistula. N Engl J Med 1986;315:496–498.

215. Stoeckenius W. An electron microscope study of myelin figures. J Biophys Biochem Cytol 1959;5:491–500.

216. Szubinska B. "New membrane" formation in Amoeba proteus upon injury of individual cells. J Cell Biol 1971;49:747–772.

217. Szubinska B. Closure of the plasma membrane around microneedle in Amoeba proteus. An ultrastructural study. Exp Cell Res 1978;111:105–115.

218. Taylor AE, Matalon S, Ward P (eds). Physiology of oxygen radicals. Bethesda: American Physiological Society, 1986.

219. Taylor AE, Townsley MI. Assessment of oxygen radical tissue damage. In: Taylor AE, Matalon S, Ward P (eds). Physiology of oxygen radicals. Bethesda: American Physiological Society, 1986, pp. 19–38.

220. Teale FWJ, Weber G. Ultraviolet fluorescence of proteins. Biochem J 1959;72:15.

221. Thomas CE, Aust SD. Reductive release of iron from ferritin by cation free radicals of paraquat and other bipyridyls. J Biol Chem 1986;261:13064–13070.

222. Thomas CE, Aust SD. Release of iron from ferritin by cardiotoxic anthracycline antibiotics. Arch Biochem Biophys 1986;248:684–689.

223. Thomas CE, Morehouse LA, Aust SD. Ferritin and superoxide-dependent lipid peroxidation. J Biol Chem 1985;260:3275–3280.

224. Thorbecke GJ, Maurer PH, Benacerraf B. The affinity of the reticulo-endothelial system for various modified serum proteins. Br J Exp Pathol 1960;41:190–197.

225. Tipper DJ. Mode of action of β-lactam antibodies. Pharmac Ther 1985;27:1–35.

226. Tissières A, Mitchell HK, Tracy UM. Protein synthesis in salivary glands of Drosophila melanogaster: relation to chromosome puffs. J Mol Biol 1974;84:389–398.

227. Tomei LD, Cope FO (eds). Apoptosis: the molecular basis of cell death. Cold Spring Harbor: Cold Spring Harbor Laboratory, 1991.

227a. Tomei LD, Cope FO, (eds). Apoptosis II: the molecular basis of apoptosis in disease. New York: Cold Spring Harbor Laboratory Press, 1994.

228. Trump BF, Goldblatt PJ, Stowell RE. Studies on necrosis of mouse liver in vitro. Ultrastructural alterations in the mitochondria of hepatic parenchymal cells. Lab Invest 1965;14:343–371.

229. Trump BF, Goldblatt PJ, Stowell RE. Studies of mouse liver necrosis in vitro. Ultrastructural and cytochemical alterations in hepatic parenchymal cell nuclei. Lab Invest 1965;14:1969–1999.

230. Ts'o POP, Caspary WJ, Lorentzen RJ. The involvement of free radicals in chemical carcinogenesis. In: Pryor AW (ed). Free radicals in biology, vol. II. New York: Academic Press, 1977, pp. 251–303.

231. Turrens JF, Crapo JD, Freeman BA. Protection against oxygen toxicity by intravenous injection of liposome-entrapped catalase and superoxide dismutase. J Clin Invest 1984;73:87–95.

232. Van der Meer C, Valkenburg PW, Ariëns AT, van Benthem RMJ. Cause of death in tourniquet shock in rats. Am J Physiol 1966;210:513–525.

233. Venkatachalam MA, Weinberg JM. Structural effects of intracellular amino acids during ATP depletion. In: Hochachka PW, Lutz PL, Sick T, Rosenthal M, van den Thillart G. Surviving hypoxia. Mechanisms of control and adaptation. Boca Raton: CRC Press, 1993, pp. 473–493.

234. Virchow R. Cellular pathology as based upon physiological and pathological histology. 1859. (Translated from the Second German Edition by Frank Chance.) New York: Dover Publications, Inc., 1971, pp. 269–272.

235. Walker NI, Bennett RE, Kerr JFR. Cell death by apoptosis during involution of the lactating breast in mice and rats. Am J Anat 1989;185:19–32.

236. Walker NI, Gobé GC. Cell death and cell proliferation during atrophy of the rat parotid gland induced by duct obstruction. J Pathol 1987;153:333–344.

237. Walker NI, Harmon BV, Gobé GC, Kerr JFR. Patterns of cell death. Methods Achiev Exp Pathol 1988;13:18–54.

238. Wallevik K. Spontaneous denaturation as a possible initial step in the breakdown of serum albumin in vivo. Clin Sci Mol Med 1973;45:665–675.

239. Wallevik K. Spontaneous in vivo isomerization of bovine serum albumin as a determinant of its normal catabolism. J Clin Invest 1976;57:398–407.

240. Warrell RP, Jr, Bockman RS. Metabolic emergencies. In DeVita VT, Jr, Hellman S, Rosenberg SA (eds). Cancer: Principles and practice of oncology, 3rd ed. Philadelphia: JB Lippincott Company, 1989, pp. 1986–2003.

241. Webster DA, Gross J. Studies on possible mechanisms of programmed cell death in the chick embryo. Dev Biol 1970;22:157–184.

242. Weinstein JN. Liposomes in the diagnosis and treatment of cancer. In: Ostro MJ (ed). Liposomes. From biophysics to therapeutics. New York: Marcel Dekker Inc., 1987, pp. 277–338.

243. Welch WJ. The mammalian stress response: cell physiology and biochemistry of stress proteins. In: Morimoto RI, Tissières A, Georgopoulos C (eds). Stress proteins in biology and medicine. Cold Spring Harbor: Cold Spring Harbor Laboratory Press, 1990, pp. 223–278.

244. Welch WJ. How cells respond to stress. Sci Am 1993;268:56–64.

245. Welch WJ, Garrels JI, Thomas GP, Lin JJ-C, Feramisco JR. Biochemical characterization of the mammalian stress proteins and identification of two stress proteins as glucose- and Ca²⁺-ionophore-regulated proteins. J Biol Chem 1983;258:7102–7111.

246. Welch WJ, Mizzen LA. Characterization of the thermotolerant cell. II. Effects on the intracellular distribution of heat-shock protein 70, intermediate filaments, and small nuclear ribonucleoprotein complexes. J Cell Biol 1988;106:1117–1130.

247. Welch WJ, Suhan JP. Morphological study of the mammalian stress response: characterization of changes in cytoplasmic organelles, cytoskeleton, and nucleoli, and appearance of intranuclear actin filaments in rat fibroblasts after heat-shock treatment. J Cell Biol 1985;101:1198–1211.

248. Welch WJ, Suhan JP. Cellular and biochemical events in mammalian cells during and after recovery from physiological stress. J Cell Biol 1986;103:2035–2052.

249. Whetsell WO, Jr, Shapira NA. Neuroexcitation, excitotoxicity and human neurological disease. Lab Invest 1993;68:372–387.

250. White BC, Aust SD, Arfors KE, Aronson LD. Brain injury by ischemic anoxia: hypothesis extension—a tale of two ions? Ann Emerg Med 1984;13:127–132.

251. Wielckens K, Delfs T. Glucocorticoid-induced cell death and poly[adenosine diphosphate(ADP)-ribosylation: increased toxicity of dexamethasone on mouse S49.1 lymphoma cells with the poly(ADP)-ribosylation inhibitor benzamide. Endocrinology 1986;119:2383–2392.

252. Wilkinson JH. The principles and practice of diagnostic enzymology. Chicago: Year Book Medical Publishers, Inc., 1976.

253. Wilson SE, Bourne WM. Corneal preservation. Surv Ophthalmol 1989;33:237–259.

254. Winrow VR, McLean L, Morris CJ, Blake DR. The heat shock protein response and its role in inflammatory disease. Ann Rheum Dis 1990;49:128–132.

255. Wise BL, Cockayne S. Enzymes. In: Bishop ML, Duben-Von Laufen JL, Fody EP (eds). Clinical chemistry. Philadelphia: JB Lippincott Company, 1985, pp. 205–239.

256. Wyllie AH. Glucocorticoid-induced thymocyte apoptosis is associated with endogenous endonuclease activation. Nature 1980;284:555–556.

257. Wyllie AH, Morris RG, Smith AL, Dunlop D. Chromatin cleavage in apoptosis: association with condensed chromatin morphology and dependence on macromolecular synthesis. J Pathol 1984;142:67–77.

258. Young D, Lathigra R, Hendrix R, Sweetser D, Young RA. Stress proteins are immune targets in leprosy and tuberculosis. Proc Natl Acad Sci USA 1988;85:4267–4270.

259. Young RA, Elliott TJ. Stress proteins, infection, and immune surveillance. Cell 1989;59:5–8.

260. Zager RA. Studies of mechanisms and protective maneuvers in myoglobinuric acute renal injury. Lab Invest 1989;60:619–629.

261. Ziegler E. General pathology. New York: William Wood and Company, 1908.

262. Zivin JA, Choi DW. Stroke therapy. Sci Am 1991;265:56–63.

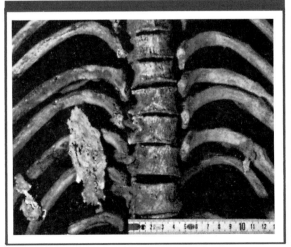

Pathologic Calcification

CHAPTER 6

From Plasma Calcium
to Apatite: Some Basic
Rules

Two Roads to
Pathologic Calcification

Growth and Fate of
Calcifications

The word *calcification* has a dry sound, but do not be misled; it is a dynamic process and extremely common. Some degree of pathologic calcification is found in every adult, be it in the arteries, in the kidney (59), or almost anywhere. Dead tissues are favorite targets for calcification, but even live cells and the extracellular matrix can calcify. The extent of calcification ranges from diffuse impregnations that only chemical analyses can detect, through granules that are visible microscopically as basophilic dots, to large stony masses that defy centuries and puzzle archaeologists (Figure 6.1). The topic is therefore broader than cellular pathology; we discuss it now because it is closely related to necrosis.

Why should calcium salts have the distinction of generating abnormal deposits? Why not sodium, potassium, or magnesium salts? If we include all forms of life, about 60 kinds of biominerals are known to exist (66). Noncalcific types of concretions do sometimes develop in humans, but calcification prevails because calcium homeostasis is always in precarious balance, easily upset to yield a precipitate of basic calcium phosphate, the mineral of bone. Pathologic calcification, in fact, is the price we pay for maintaining our skeleton, where more than 99 percent of body calcium is held (1). For this very reason, the mineral of bone and of most pathologic calcifications is basically the same, an analog of the naturally occurring mineral **hydroxyapatite,** $Ca_{10}(PO_4)_6(OH)_2$, which we will

call **apatite** for short. *The main structural difference between bone and pathologic calcifications is in the calcified substrate:* in bone the substrate is **osteoid,** a particular organic matrix, and in pathologic calcifications it can be almost any tissue structure, dead or alive, intra- or extracellular.

From Plasma Calcium to Apatite: Some Basic Rules

To understand calcification we must first understand how plasma calcium and phosphate relate to deposits of apatite.

FIGURE 6.1
Plaques of pleural calcification in a medieval leprosy patient buried in Denmark between 1175 and 1500 A.D. The mineral of such pathologic calcifications is the same as that of bone and persists accordingly. (Reproduced with permission from [72].)

What Triggers the Precipitation of Calcium Phosphate? Normally, total plasma calcium is 10 ± 1 milligrams per deciliter (mg/dl), and total phosphate is 3.5 ± 0.5 mg/dl. Less than half of the plasma calcium is ionized and physiologically active (Figure 6.2) (63), but it is generally agreed that the ionized fraction still represents a very high concentration of calcium. This is obvious to anyone who has tried to prepare a physiologic solution; when Ca^{2+} is added, even the slightest shift to alkalinity is enough to give a cloudy precipitate of calcium phosphate. Which brings out a basic rule: *calcium phosphate precipitates in an alkaline medium and is dissolved by acid.* To prove the latter point, leave a chicken thigh bone in vinegar for 3 or 4 weeks: you can tie it in a knot.

Until the 1970s it was dogma that the normal plasma concentration of ionized calcium is too low to allow the precipitation of calcium phosphate, but this concept has been challenged (90, 93). In the test tube, in the absence of proteins, even physiologic concentrations of calcium and phosphate may be sufficient to cause the precipitation of calcium phosphate. This precipitation does not generally occur in vivo, probably because calcification-inhibiting macromolecules are present.

Why do Apatite Crystals Proliferate? The first detectable mineral deposited *in vivo* during calcification is a poorly crystallized apatite, which perfects with age (20). (Apatite may be preceded by some short-lived intermediates such as octacalcium phosphate (20), but we need not be concerned with them here.) *Once the first apatite crystals appear, they continue to grow—crystal after crystal—by extracting more calcium and phosphate from the solution.*

If the experiment is done *in vitro*, starting with the normal plasma concentration of calcium, the tricky little crystals will go on proliferating until the concentration of calcium has dropped to one-third the normal level (56). In other words, the *plasma concentration of calcium appears to be supersaturated with regard to growing crystals of apatite* (19, 56, 75).

How does a Crystal Begin? Apatite crystals grow out of other crystal surfaces by a phenomenon called **secondary nucleation** (75, 78), which means that the surface of an apatite crystal—when exposed to a supersaturated solution—acts as a growth site for another crystal. Apatite crystals can also grow on the surface of a different material—not necessarily a crystal—which acts as a primary nucleus; this phenomenon is called **epitaxy.** A crude example of epitaxy is provided by a high school experiment: if a cord is suspended in a saturated solution of sugar that is allowed slowly to evaporate, beautiful crystals of sugar grow on the cord (10). Epitaxy contributes a great deal to pathologic calcifications because it does not require that the seeding surface be that of another crystal. As the cord-and-sugar experiment shows, almost any surface works as long as its atomic lattice is sufficiently similar to that of the crystal. There are many examples of epitaxy (75); apatite crystals can be seeded even by organic surfaces, as we will explain shortly.

MICROSCOPIC ASPECTS OF CALCIFICATION

It is fairly easy to recognize calcified structures in microscopic sections stained with hematoxylin and eosin: the basic rule is that *calcified structures are deeply basophilic or have at least a basophilic*

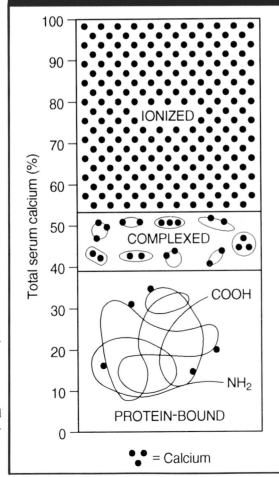

FIGURE 6.2
Total serum calcium consists of three fractions: ionized (the physiologically active fraction), protein-bound, and complexed (bound to several organic and inorganic anions). (Adapted from [63].)

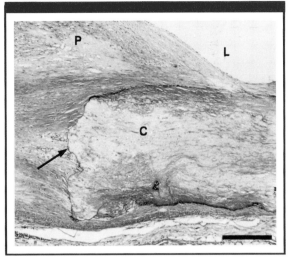

rim. Therefore, they will be deep blue or have a blue rim.

This basophilia is obvious but hard to explain. First of all, the basophilia is there whether the tissue sample has been decalcified or not. In other words, the basophilia has nothing to do with the mineral itself; it simply means that the calcified substrate has acquired negative charges, which bind the positively charged hematoxylin.

Another baffling fact is that a calcified mass always has a basophilic rim; but as the mass expands, the central part tends to lose its basophilia and to stain pink with eosin (Figure 6.3). This means that the traditional rule whereby calcifications are always basophilic is not entirely correct. After all, bone—the prototype of calcified structures—is eosinophilic overall. The mechanism of the basophilic change needs to be worked out.

Dead, calcified cells, single or in groups, are often seen in histologic sections. This raises a question: *did the cells die because they were calcified, or did they calcify because they were dead?* Both events can occur. Calcifications in live cells usually start in mitochondria; this effect is common in injured cells (Figures 6.4, 6.5). It is easily produced, even *in vitro*, simply by prolonged incubation of mitochondria in physiologic solutions (58). These organelles are naturally predisposed to accumulate calcium.

Why are mitochondria prone to calcification? Remember that the cell membrane pumps calcium *out*, so the concentration of calcium in the cytoplasm is 1,000–10,000 times lower than in the extracellular fluid. However, the mitochondrial membrane pumps calcium *into* the mitochondria, so these organelles have about ten times more free calcium than the extracellular fluid (p. 197). Whenever cytoplasmic calcium increases (e.g., because plasma calcium is abnormally high or because the cell membrane is damaged), *the mitochondria come to the rescue as active calcium traps* (4, 7, 46): the calcium that they pump in is taken out of solution and appears as granules or amorphous masses, probably of calcium phosphate. Calcified mitochondria cease to function. When too many mitochondria are calcified, the cell dies.

Some technical problems arise when calcified tissues are to be examined histologically. If the calcifications are of microscopic size, the tissues can be embedded and cut as usual, although the calcifications may nick the knife; larger calcifications must be decalcified in acid after fixation, just like bone. Of course, if microscopic sections are being made for the very

FIGURE 6.3 Wall of a human atherosclerotic artery. **L:** Lumen. **P:** Atherosclerotic plaque. **C:** A calcified mass developing in the media. The dark rim of the mass (**arrow**) is blue in the original. (Hematoxylin and eosin stain.) **Bar** = 500 μm.

purpose of studying the mineral deposits, exposure to acids must be avoided. Decalcification with a chelating agent (EDTA) is slow, but feasible. Histochemical methods are available to demonstrate either calcium or phosphate in the tissue sections.

Two Roads to Pathologic Calcification

With the preceding facts in mind, we are ready to understand that calcifications can be triggered *in vivo* by two mechanisms, one local, one general.

- In **dystrophic calcification,** by far the more common mechanism, *a local change or disturbance in the tissue favors the nucleation of apatite crystals. Plasma calcium and phosphate are normal.* (The ancient term *dystrophic* is supposed to remind us that there is a local disturbance or "dystrophy.")

- In **metastatic calcification,** the disturbance is body-wide. It occurs when *the plasma concentration of calcium (more rarely of phosphate) rises above a critical level,* whereby deposits of apatite crystals develop throughout the body. Because it is generalized, metastatic calcification can be lethal if the underlying metabolic defect is not removed. Virchow saw the widespread calcifications as secondary deposits comparable to those of malignant tumors, and therefore called them calcium "metastases."

DYSTROPHIC CALCIFICATION

Dystrophic calcification is always local, and plasma levels of calcium and phosphate are normal.

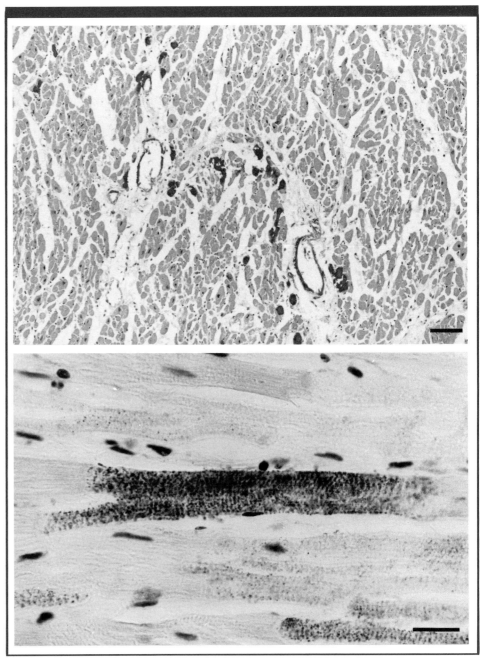

FIGURE 6.4
Top: Myocardium with metastatic calcifications (dark structures). From a case of hypercalcemia due to a parathyroid adenoma. Calcification affects myocardial cells as well as vascular walls. **Bar** = 100 μm. *Bottom:* Dystrophic calcification of mitochondria in a human heart near a recent infarct. **Bar** = 25 μm.

Calcification of Necrotic Tissue A classic example of dystrophic calcification is the calcification of necrosis. Even single dead endothelial cells can calcify, as was shown by injecting rats with tetracycline (48).

Tetracycline offers a simple and striking method for detecting ongoing calcification, normal (in bone and teeth) or pathologic. Whether it is injected or taken by mouth, it is somehow deposited in all structures that are becoming calcified. Although invisible per se, it has a beautiful gold autofluorescence in ultraviolet light.

Dead tissue, such as occurs in infarcts, is an excellent model for studying calcification. Enough calcium accumulates in myocardial infarcts to be visible histochemically (30) and sometimes grossly (Figure 6.6). Because the calcium is supplied by the blood in the surrounding live tissues, calcification begins at the periphery of the infarct. Within a day or two, the process is announced by a powdering of tiny basophilic granules of uneven size, no larger than nuclei, and long known as **calcospherites** (101) (Figure 6.7). The largest granules have a targetlike structure, which was recognized as early as 1857 (101). Calcospherites tend to grow and to coalesce: the result is an expanding calcified area with a basophilic rim and a rather eosinophilic center. Electron microscopy shows that the target structure of the calcospherites is due to concentric rings of apatite crystals (Figure 6.8).

The growth of calcospherites by successive waves is best explained by analogy with the famous **Liesegang rings,** known since the turn of the century (Figure 6.9) (39, 51, 91, 100). These systems of concentric rings can be produced by two reactants diffusing in a gel; they can be produced also with calcium and phosphate (22).

Calcification of the Aortic Valve Another example of the dystrophic mechanism is the calcification of the aortic valve (Figure 6.10). Notice a striking feature of this condition: the valve cusps do not simply "turn to stone"; they are also *enlarged* by rough, bulky, wartlike masses that are indeed as hard as stone. This tells us that calcification, under certain circumstances, seems to increase the volume of the calcified tissue. Considering that calcospherites—at a microscopic level—do grow by concentric expansion, the progressive thickening of the aortic valves could be the effect of crystal growth over a long time.

Histologically, the rock-hard aortic valves consist of calcium deposits in a mass of protein and lipid (59). What is this organic matrix? Is it some protein that seeped in from the plasma, and if so why? Did the lipid or the protein come first and the mineral later? Are we dealing with calcification triggered by proteolipids (79)?

Initiators of Dystrophic Calcification To explain a localized calcification (which occurs in spite of normal values of plasma calcium and phosphate) we need some local mechanism to set off the process by seeding apatite crystals. In theory, local calcification can be triggered in one of three ways (24): a local increase in the Ca × P product, exposure of nucleators (epitaxy), or removal of inhibitors. Examples of all three are known. However, *most crystal-seeding mechanisms assume that epitaxy is involved*; that is, an organic substrate has the property of binding calcium or phosphate in an orderly fashion, like a template, mimicking

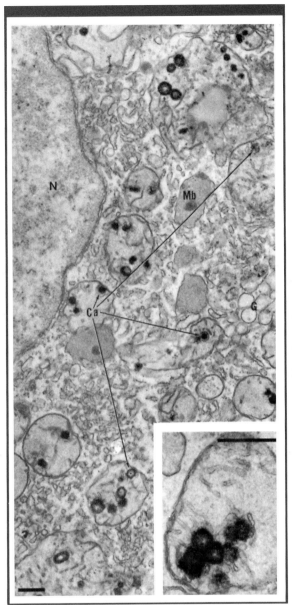

FIGURE 6.5 Part of a rat liver cell 16 hours after poisoning with carbon tetrachloride. **Ca:** Dark masses within mitochondria that represent calcification; some have a ringlike structure. **G:** Golgi apparatus. **Mb:** Microbody. **N:** Nucleus. **Bars** = 0.5 μm. (Reproduced with permission from [81].)

the crystalline surface of apatite and thereby triggering the birth of an apatite crystal. Perhaps each of the following mechanisms plays a role in initiating epitaxy in some circumstances.

- Phospholipids as initiators. *Phospholipids are amply proven to be nucleators (21, 25),* especially phosphatidyl serine, which is acidic and therefore able to bind calcium (Figure 6.11). This property of phospholipids would easily account for the prevalence of calcification in necrotic areas, where membrane phospholipids abound as ultramicroscopic vesicles. Such vesicles are especially common in atherosclerotic aortas (55, 88), from which source a proteolipid was ex-

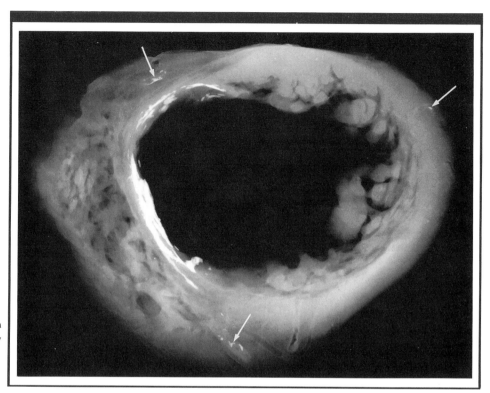

FIGURE 6.6
X-ray of a slice of heart, showing heavy calcification in an ancient infarct. Note also small calcifications in coronary arteries (**arrows**). (Courtesy of Dr. H.F. Cuénoud, University of Massachusetts Medical Center, Worcester, MA.)

tracted that actually caused nucleation of apatite *in vitro* (35) (**proteolipids** are integral membrane proteins that are soluble in organic solvents).

Here is the story of the matrix vesicles. Simple as they are, the membrane-bound vesicles so common in necrotic tissues raise a hot issue: are they related to the so-called extracellular "matrix vesicles" seen in normal enchondral ossification?

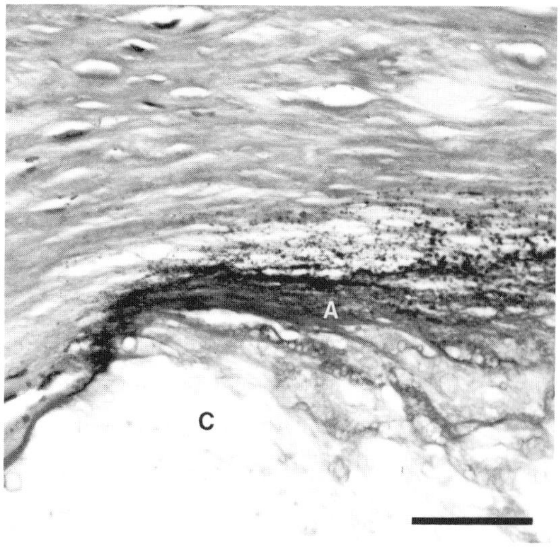

FIGURE 6.7
C: Calcified mass in the media of a human atherosclerotic artery. **A:** Basophilic rim where the calcification is advancing. The basophilic granules are calcospherites. **Bar** = 50 μm.

In the late 1960s, two research groups independently discovered 1000–2000 Å globules or vesicles in epiphyseal growth cartilage and proposed them as initiators of calcification in that system (2, 6, 14, 15). These matrix vesicles are thought to arise from local cells by a mechanism still under debate, perhaps by budding like viruses (6); the current concept is that calcium seeps into them and binds to the inner surfaces of their membranes by the phosphatidyl serine mechanism mentioned earlier; phosphatases in the membrane would then provide phosphate while also degrading pyrophosphate and ATP, which are crystal poisons (Figure 6.12). Vesicles of all sizes abound in necrotic tissues, including atherosclerotic arteries where many cells die leaving behind a magma of globules (55). Of course there is nothing specific about these "degenerative" vesicles; they are not necessarily the same as the "programmed" matrix vesicles of physiologically calcifying tissues. On the other hand, they might provide a protected environment in which the initial crystals form; they might also cause nucleation of apatite even without enzymatic intervention, by the surface mechanism shown in Figure 6.11 (6, 98).

Wherever the truth may lie, the beauty of these nondescript vesicular remains is that they may offer a link between normal and dystrophic calcification (5). The link would become a very tight one if it is true that the normal matrix vesicles arise not only by budding but also by death and fragmentation of chondrocytes (15).

- Elastic fibers as initiators. Elastic fibers are susceptible to calcification; they may calcify while the tissues around them do not (Figure 6.13). Several mechanisms have been proposed (56), including a progressive increase in carboxyl-bearing amino acids in the elastin molecule (62) and calcification of the microfibrils that surround the elastic fibers (50).
- Collagen fibrils as initiators. Collagen fibrils often calcify (84), for example, in poorly vascularized tissues such as tendons. Calcific deposits appear both around and within the fibrils; it has been proposed that there is a nucleation site within the fibril itself, where the quarter-staggered arrangement of the molecules leaves a space or "hole" (Figure 6.14) (10, 43).
- Role of denatured proteins. Denatured proteins have not yet been studied as nucleators of calcium phosphates, but, in necrotic tissues, it is almost certain that denatured proteins bind calcium and/or phosphate (p. 196).
- Role of GLA. GLA (gamma-carboxyglutamic acid), a fairly recent addition to the family of amino acids, is formed from glutamic acid by carboxylation in the presence of vitamin K (42). Its two adjacent carboxyls make it suitable for tightly binding calcium, calcium phosphates, and (via the calcium) phospholipids. GLA is found in the blood, in mineralized tissues, and in pathologic calcifications; a GLA-rich protein in bone is abundant enough to qualify for the name **osteocalcin** (47). In atherosclerotic plaques, a related GLA protein was found and named **atherocalcin** (65); osteocalcin was also present (64). Whether these proteins have a primary or a secondary role—or no role at all—remains to be seen.
- Role of phosphoproteins. Phosphoproteins are thought to play a role in normal and pathologic calcifications (87).
- Role of fatty acids. Fatty acids certainly bind calcium to form soaps (p. 214), but their role in physiological calcification is not clear (12) and perhaps nil (101).
- Bacteria as initiators. Some bacteria can be very efficient nucleators. Because bacteria

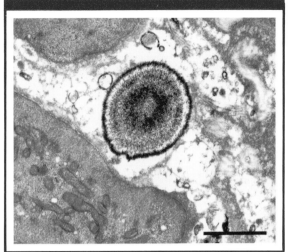

FIGURE 6.8 Typical target structure of a calcospherite in atherosclerosis (rat aorta). The target arrangement may be related to Liesegang rings (*see* Figure 6.9). Specimen not decalcified. **Bar** = 1 μm.

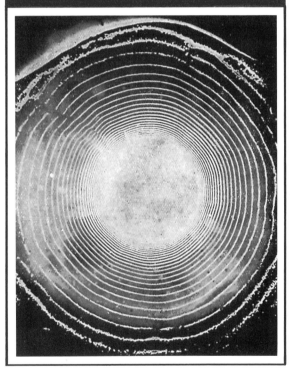

FIGURE 6.9 Example of a rhythmic chemical reaction: the Liesegang rings, as observed by Liesegang himself. A drop of 50% AgNo$_3$ is placed on a layer of gelatin containing 0.1% potassium bichromate. Precipitation occurs in concentric rings. (Reproduced with permission from [39].)

and mitochondria are related (p. 131) it is not too surprising that they should share also this bizarre property (96). It is the calcification of oral bacteria that produces **calculus,** that pernicious mineral periodically mined by dental hygienists (Figure 6.15). (We cannot resist mentioning the real meaning of *calculus:* it is Latin for "small stone." The Romans used pebbles for making simple "calculations.")

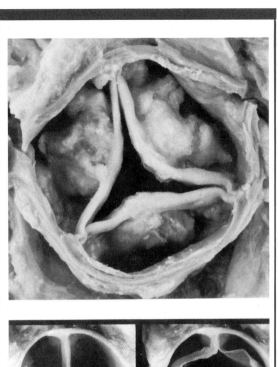

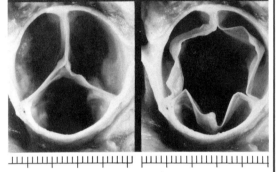

FIGURE 6.10
Top: Calcified aortic valve of an 80-year-old woman. Note that the tissue increases in volume as it calcifies. (Reproduced with permission from [33].) *Bottom:* Normal aortic valve viewed from above, in simulated closed (*left*) and open (*right*) positions. From a 33-year-old man. Scale in mm. (Reproduced with permission from [77].)

thought to be responsible for calcified masses that sometimes form around intrauterine devices (IUDs) (6, 45).

METASTATIC CALCIFICATION

The conditions that make metastatic calcification possible are **hypercalcemia** and, much more rarely, **hyperphosphatemia.** Hypercalcemia has many causes (Table 6.1). In hospitals it is seen most often in patients whose skeleton is rapidly destroyed by a malignant tumor, either metastatic or primary, such as multiple myeloma. Another classic but less common cause is hyperparathyroidism, which is due to functional tumors of the parathyroid glands (about 50,000 cases per year in the United States). For calcium metastases to develop, the critical value of plasma calcium is about 17 mg/dl (1); high plasma phosphate can also lead to metastatic calcification (102). Phosphate usually rises as a result of chronic renal failure when the glomerular filtration rate drops to 25 percent or less.

> A good rule of thumb is that the product of plasma calcium and phosphate in adults is normally 35–40 ; above 60 or 70, metastatic calcification occurs (94). The main clinical sign of hypercalcemia is severe muscular weakness—the opposite of hypocalcemia, which induces tetany.

Preferred Locations The so-called calcium metastases can appear almost anywhere as spotty deposits, but they have certain predilections. At first sight, a list of the tissues most afflicted by calcium metastases seems to make no sense at all:

- mucosa of the stomach
- kidneys and lungs
- cornea
- systemic arteries
- pulmonary veins

It was a member of the oral flora, *Bacterionema matruchotii* (Figure 6.16), that yielded the first phospholipid–protein complex capable of nucleating apatite *in vitro* (27, 35, 99). Actinomycetes are especially prone to calcify; they are

FIGURE 6.11
Diagram of a possible model of membrane-facilitated calcification. *Stage 1:* Calcium ions bind to two adjacent polar heads of phospholipid molecules (water is displaced in the process). *Stage 2:* Phosphate groups bind to the layer of calcium. *Stage 3:* The cycle of calcium and phosphate binding is repeated. *Stage 4:* By an internal rearrangement of the calcium and phosphate ions, a microcrystal develops (paracrystalline apatite). (Adapted from [97].)

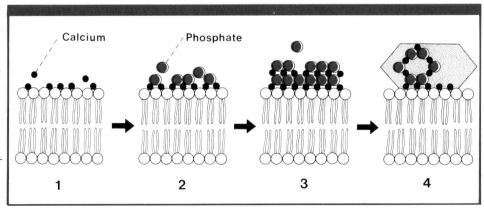

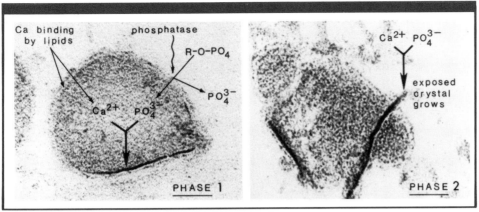

FIGURE 6.12
Scheme of the mineralization process operated by the matrix vesicles as it occurs in the growth plate cartilage of the rat. *Phase 1*: Intravesicular calcium concentration rises due to the affinity of calcium for the lipids of the inner membrane. Phosphatase in the membrane increases the local concentration of PO_4 in or near the vesicle. Thereby the Ca × PO_4 product in the vesicle is raised, initiating a mineral deposit near the membrane. *Phase 2*: Apatite crystals grow because the medium is supersaturated with respect to apatite. The growing crystals perforate the membrane. (Reproduced with permission from [3].)

It is quite a challenge to find a common feature among these disparate locations, but it does exist. The basic principle was recognized by Max Askanazy at the turn of the century (9, 92, 101). The law of Askanazy proposes that *calcium metastases favor those organs that lose acid* and therefore, presumably, harbor an internal alkaline compartment. Backing this principle are the following facts:

- The stomach secretes HCl, and the venous blood from the stomach does become more alkaline during the secretion of gastric juice (60).
- The renal tubules secrete acid urine.
- The lungs lose CO_2.
- The cornea loses CO_2 by diffusion (there is a carbonic anhydrase in the ciliary processes [67]), especially along the interpalpebral fissure where calcification is most common in association with renal failure (Figure 6.17).

Presumably, according to the same principle:

- The systemic veins are relatively spared because their blood is more acid (p. 242).
- The systemic arteries and pulmonary veins do calcify because they carry arterial blood in which carbonate is at its lowest (73, 101).
- There is also a tendency for heavier calcium deposition in the lining of the left side of the heart, where the blood is arterial (63, 73, 82).

Morphologic Findings The autopsy findings in cases of severe hypercalcemia are striking. Calcified tissues appear chalky. The gastric mucosa, for example, can appear strangely white: Virchow describes it as feeling like a rasp and grating under the knife, whereas the lung becomes "similar to a fine bathing sponge" (95), a very appropriate comparison because the alveolar walls become stiff with calcium deposits (Figure 6.18). Functionally the most damaging effect is **nephrocalcinosis,** calcification of the kidney (Figure 6.19), which causes retention of phosphate and secondary hyperparathyroidism, which in turn aggravates the

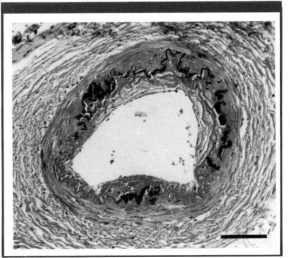

FIGURE 6.13
Selective calcification of the internal elastic lamina (black wavy line) in a human artery. The intima is thickened. **Bar** = 100 μm.

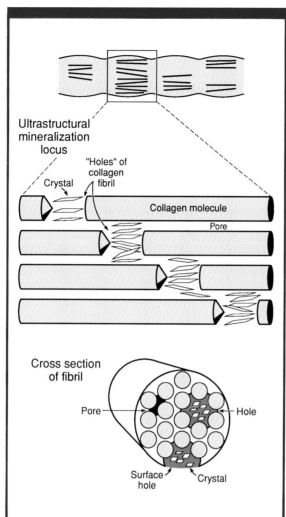

FIGURE 6.14
Pathologic calcification of the collagen fibrils is thought to begin in "holes" present in the fibrils, between the ends of the quarter-staggered molecules. (Adapted from [44].)

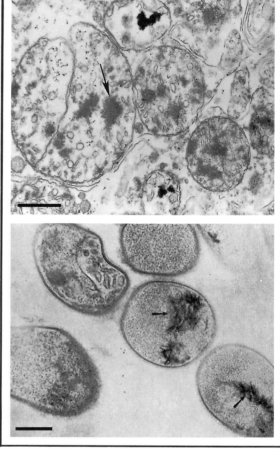

FIGURE 6.16
Calcification in mitochondria and bacteria. *Top:* Mitochondria incubated in physiologic concentrations of calcium and phosphate. **Arrow:** A type of density that contained calcium and phosphate when submitted to electron probe microanalysis. (Rat kidney cortex incubated in Earl's minimal essential medium plus Hank's BSS.) **Bar** = 0.5 μm. (Reproduced with permission from [58].) *Bottom:* Crystals of apatite (**arrows**) forming inside *Bacterionema matruchotii*, a large filamentous microorganism from the oral flora. Ultimately such bacterial calcifications lead to the formation of dental calculus. **Bar** = 0.5 μm. (Reproduced with permission from [99].)

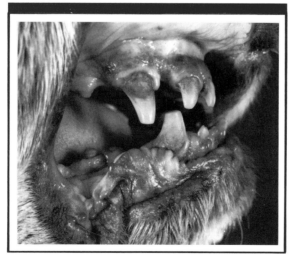

FIGURE 6.15
Bacterial calcification, as shown by dental calculus on the teeth of a 14-year-old dog. Similar calcified microbial plaques occur in humans. (Reproduced with permission from [31].)

hypercalcemia. In early stages it is reversible. Nephrocalcinosis should not be confused with nephrolithiasis (kidney stones).

Microscopically, mitochondria are the first cellular targets of hypercalcemia, especially in the heart and kidney. Deposits appear first as an amorphous mass and then as apatite needles (6, 69). Electron microscopy shows that calcified mitochondria appear at first in cells that are otherwise normal (16, 17); eventually the cells may die and become engulfed in mineral deposits.

TABLE 6.1

Hypercalcemia:
The Principal Causes

HYPERSECRETION OF PARATHYROID HORMONE (PTH) (→ INCREASED BONE RESORPTION)

primary (due to parathyroid hyperplasia or tumor)
secondary to renal failure (which causes retention of phosphate)
ectopic secretion of PTH by a malignant tumor (e.g., carcinoma of the lung)

DESTRUCTION OF BONE TISSUE

by a primary tumor of the bone marrow (e.g., multiple myeloma)
by diffuse skeletal metastases
by Paget's disease of bone (accelerated bone turnover)
by immobilization (immobility removes a stimulus to bone formation while resorption continues)

OTHER MECHANISMS

poisoning with vitamin A or D (in food faddists)
milk-alkali syndrome (from excess intake of both*)
thiazide diuretics
sarcoidosis (macrophages activate a vitamin D precursor)
uremia and dialysis (mechanism unclear, probably multiple)

*Randall, R.E., Jr., Strauss, M.B., McNeely, W.F.: The milk-alkali syndrome. Arch. Intern. Med., 107:163–181, 1961.
Adapted from Levine, M.M., and Kleeman, C.R. Hypercalcemia: Pathophysiology and treatment. Hosp. Pract., 22:93–110, 1987.

In hypercalcemia due to hyperparathyroidism, the entry of calcium into the cell is favored by the parathyroid hormone itself (18). Primary mitochondrial calcification has been seen also in normocalcemic animals after various insults (e.g., in aortic smooth muscle after adrenaline administration) (29). In striated muscle, metastatic calcium deposits occur mainly along the fibrils and in the sarcoplasmic reticulum (16).

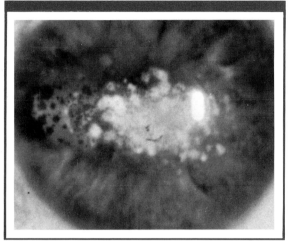

FIGURE 6.17
Calcification across the cornea in hypercalcemia (band keratopathy) attributed to local loss of CO_2. (Reproduced with permission from [52].)

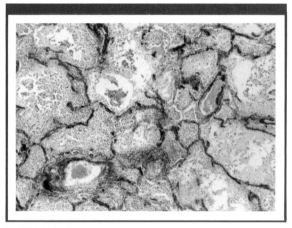

FIGURE 6.18
Lung tissue with diffuse calcification of the alveolar walls (dark network). The calcification was due to severe hypercalcemia caused by bone destruction secondary to multiple myeloma. (The alveoli are filled with cells; this is the pneumonia that eventually killed the patient.)

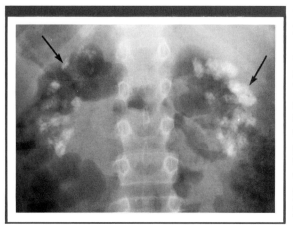

FIGURE 6.19
X-ray of a patient (boy aged 13) with bilateral renal calcifications. The opaque masses (**arrows**) represent the pattern of calcified pyramids. (Courtesy of Dr. A. Davidoff, University of Massachusetts Medical School, Worcester, MA.)

Basement membranes are another favorite site of metastatic calcification, but the mechanism is not as clear as for the mitochondria. Typical examples are seen in the lung (Figure 6.20) (34) and around the renal convoluted tubules (perhaps because this is where urine is being acidified) (28). Possibly the Ca^{2+} ions bind to the negative charges of glycosaminoglycans or other basement membrane components (remember that basement membranes are also known to bind silver ions, Ag^+) (p. 262).

Growth and Fate of Calcifications

Once started, calcifications tend to grow (84). Of this there are many examples. At the electron microscopic level, the calcospherites grow by successive waves (Figure 6.21). The advancing rim seems to destroy all microscopic detail, as if the forest of growing crystals had the effect of grinding up all the structures they encounter. Most obviously, calcified aortic valves swell to several times their original thickness (see Figure 6.10).

Presumably, the growth of calcifications reflects the ability of apatite crystals to proliferate by secondary nucleation. But apatite crystals can continue to proliferate in a physiologic concentration of calcium, so why do calcifications ever stop growing? In the skeleton, where apatite crystals have a surface estimated at 500,000 m², their growing frenzy is probably restrained by the organic matrix (23, 71); calcifications have no comparable barrier. We must assume that inhibitors come into play (37). Many have been described. Some are natural and have been found

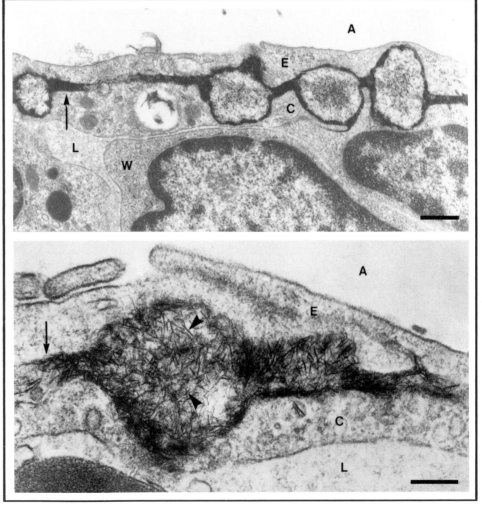

FIGURE 6.20
Calcification of the alveolar basement membrane in the lung of a rat, sacrificed 6 days after a single overdose of vitamin D by mouth. *Top:* The dystrophic calcification begins in the basement membrane and expands focally into a "rosary bead" pattern. **Bar** = 0.5 μm. *Bottom:* Detail showing the crystals of apatite (**arrowheads**). Although on electron micrographs these crystals appear as needles, they are in reality thin plates, 100–400 Å in length. **Bar** = 0.2 μm. **Arrows:** Basement membrane. **A**: Alveolar lumen. **E**: Alveolar epithelium. **C**: Capillary endothelium. **L**: Lumen of capillary. **W**: White blood cells. (Courtesy of Professor Y. Kapanci, University of Geneva, Switzerland.)

in the blood and urine (56, 83, 93). They include polyphosphates and macromolecules such as proteoglycans and heparin, but little is known of their behavior *in vivo*.

Macrophages and giant cells seem to be in no great hurry to attack and erode calcifications, although this may happen over months or years (13). Note that osteoclasts and macrophages are thought to be related (68)—which means that nibbling at calcifications, in theory at least, could well be included in the job description of macrophages. However, large dystrophic calcifications can persist throughout a person's life and never show a sign of their existence. Tuberculous lymph nodes, for example, become necrotic, calcify, and then remain visible on X-rays for a lifetime.

Sometimes a layer of osteoid is laid down over a pathologic calcification; then a little patch of real bone tissue develops, sometimes completed with real bone marrow—a case of double metaplasia that is not rare in the walls of atherosclerotic arteries. Metastatic calcifications can partially regress if the cause is corrected—for example, if a parathyroid adenoma is removed (89).

Prevention and treatment of calcifications can be attempted with bisphosphonates, which are related to pyrophosphates except that they have the structure P–C–P rather than P–O–P (Figure 6.22); remember that pyrophosphates are among the inhibitors of calcification. Bisphosphonates bind to the crystal surface and block its growth; by the same token they also prevent crystal dissolution. The P–C–P bond makes bisphosphonates resistant to all known enzymes. Their adoption for medical use was suggested by a curious analogy: they were used commercially to prevent scaling in water installations (38).

CALCIFICATION: LOOSE ENDS

Some types of calcification are difficult to explain or downright mysterious. Listed below are a few that are especially intriguing.

Non–Calcium Phosphate Deposits Not all calcifications are apatite or other calcium phosphates. In the kidney (28) and in the lung (74), for example, they sometimes consist of **calcium carbonate.** (Eggshells, by the way, are also made of carbonate.) Using special electron microscopic techniques, it is possible to analyze the atomic composition of microscopic and ultramicroscopic granules. These methods were applied to specimens of human breast

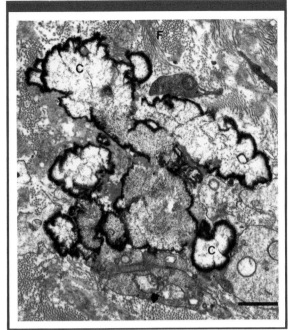

FIGURE 6.21 C: Foci of calcification (calcospherites) as seen by electron microscopy in a human atherosclerotic artery. F: Collagen fibers. The dark rims represent advancing fronts of apatite crystals. **Bar** = 1 μm.

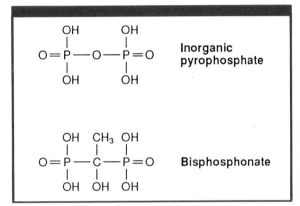

FIGURE 6.22 Comparing the formulae of inorganic pyrophosphate and bisphosphonate.

tissue that were surgically removed after mammography had shown them to contain "calcifications" associated with cancer. The radio-opaque nodules were then reported to contain calcium only, bound to some organic substrate, with little or no phosphate. Other concretions, more surprisingly, are noncalcifications containing Al, Fe, Mg, Si, Cu, Zn, Pb, Au, Ag, and other odd elements, alone or in combination (41); their significance is not known.

Arterial Calcifications The arteries of diabetics are especially prone to medial calcification (Figure 6.23); this serious problem is still unsolved. The same complication occurs in uremic patients undergoing dialysis (54). Several mechanisms

FIGURE 6.23 Calcified media (black circle) in a medium-sized artery from the thigh of a diabetic patient. The lumen is partially occluded by intimal thickening. **Bar** = 500 μm. (Reproduced with permission from [11].)

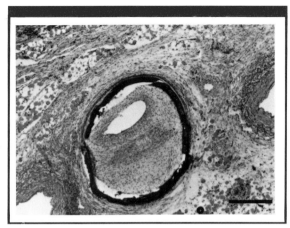

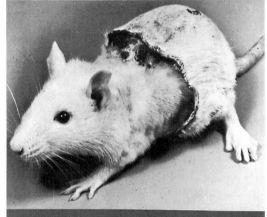

FIGURE 6.24 The phenomenon of calciphylaxis, illustrated by calcification of the skin of a rat. (Reproduced with permission from [85].)

"It is given to very few investigators in modern medicine to discover a new phenomenon, to describe it, and to characterize it. This Dr. Selye has done by his introduction of calciphylaxis as an entirely new biologic concept; one sure to have an impact on medicine comparable to that of the author's earlier concept of stress."
—Dr. Franklin C. McLean, The University of Chicago

continue to grow. This concept is an extension of the mechanism proposed to explain the different susceptibilities of arteries and veins to metastatic calcification (p. 237). Another major difference between right and left endocardium is that the transendothelial transport of lipid in early atherosclerosis is virtually limited to the valves on the left side; the subendocardial lipid deposit might be related to calcium deposition (32).

Calciphylaxis, A Strange Story Calciphylaxis is a bizarre laboratory phenomenon described in the rat and so named by the late endocrinologist Hans Selye (40, 85). It refers to the precipitous calcification of certain organs or tissues in rats that are pretreated with a hypercalcemic agent (called a **sensitizer**) and then injected with one of many possible substances called **challengers.** For example, a large dose of the sensitizer (vitamin D or analog, parathyroid hormone) is given by mouth or parenterally, which induces (presumably) a mild hypercalcemia; but no calcifications develop. Then, after a critical period of 24–48 hours, the challenger is given either locally or systemically; this induces rapid calcifications, even though the challenger alone would have had no significant effect. Some examples:

- A rat is given by mouth 1 mg of dihydrotachysterol; the next day the skin is challenged subcutaneously with an innocuous substance such as egg albumin. Promptly the injected skin calcifies, and after 23 days it is shed, revealing, says Selye, a newly formed skin underneath (Figure 6.24).
- After the use of the same sensitizer, an intravenous challenge with eggwhite produced an almost selective calcification of the pancreas, and egg yolk produced calcification of the whole spleen and of the Kupffer cells of the liver. The selectivity of the calcifications is astonishing.
- With the appropriate combination of sensitizer and challenger, Selye could predictably calcify either the right auricular appendage of the heart, or the thymus, the salivary glands, the two vagus nerves, or even the carotid body. None of these localizations is explained. Though they were firmly established on some 60,000 rats (85), their relevance to human diseases is not clear. The lesions of certain human diseases show analogies with calciphylactic changes, but

have been suggested, including the possibility that dialysis removes a calcification inhibitor.

The valves of the pulmonary artery never calcify whereas the aortic valves do. Nobody knows why.

We offer some speculations. The blood bathing the aortic valves is slightly more alkaline than that bathing the pulmonary valves: 7.45 versus 7.35 (86). This difference might be just enough to seed the first few apatite crystals, which would then

there is no hint that their mechanism could also be analogous (85).

Several cases recently published as calciphylaxis in renal failure and hyperphosphatemia are simply cases of metastatic calcification.

The term calciphylaxis (defense by calcium) is probably a misnomer; there is no evidence that this strange phenomenon has any defensive value except under artificial (40) experimental conditions. However, the overall lesson one can draw from these experiments is that *the administration of two successive drugs, each one harmless, may have unpredictable effects.*

Arthritis Due to Crystals of Apatite For reasons unknown, crystals of apatite can appear in joint spaces and cause inflammation (arthritis).

This peculiar phenomenon was discovered by investigating the joints of patients presumed to suffer from gout; it turned out that the crystals causing the damage were not sodium urate as expected, but calcium pyrophosphate dihydrate, a common product of intermediary metabolism (53). This "new" disease, called pseudo-gout or chondrocalcinosis, is now recognized as often asymptomatic and very common; it affects 5 percent of the adult population according to a study of autopsy cases (70). Later it was found that crystals of apatite are sometimes involved. Why should crystals inflame the joints? When phagocytized they can kill the phagocytic cell by perforating its lysosomes (p. 141). They may also adsorb and activate certain critical proteins specifically designed to trigger inflammation, such as those of the complement and kinin systems (to be discussed in Chapter 9). These properties are shared by several types of crystals, hence the unifying concept of crystal-induced diseases.

A Post Script on Apatite: Are Stones Our Ancestors? At the end of this chapter about live tissues turning to stone, it may be a shock to learn that stones may conceivably have something to do with the origins of life. We are referring to the fact that apatite crystals have a true enzymatic activity that cannot be destroyed by heat; they function as an ATPase. The paper reporting this fact in 1962 (61) went curiously unnoticed, perhaps because of its forbidding technical title. Yet this is sensational news, not only because stones are not supposed to be enzymes but also because it is fascinating to speculate that some of the early enzymes in evolution may have been the stones that were lying around. The same idea was proposed by another group 11 years later ("In The Beginning There Was Apatite") (76). Could it be true? We will leave the rest to the imagination of the reader.

TO SUM UP: if pathologic calcifications are the price we have to pay for our high levels of blood calcium and phosphate, necessary to maintain our skeleton, how high is the price? Overall not too high, but the answer will depend on who is asked. Small calcifications of the dystrophic type exist in virtually all people with normal blood calcium and phosphate; they are basically harmless, except for those that contribute to hardening the arteries and heart valves in atherosclerosis. In diabetics the arterial hardening is more severe. In individuals with high blood calcium or phosphate, metastatic calcifications can cause much damage—but then the underlying disease, such as bone cancer, may be the major problem. It is probably fair to say that *pathologic calcifications are never useful*, with the possible exception of those that develop in necrotic tuberculous lymph nodes: they might help to wall off the enemy.

References

Calcification

1. Albright F, Reifenstein EC Jr. The parathyroid glands and metabolic bone disease. Baltimore: The Williams & Wilkins Company, 1948.
2. Anderson HC. Electron microscopic studies of induced cartilage development and calcification. J Cell Biol 1967;35:81–101.
3. Anderson HC. Introduction to the second conference on matrix vesicle calcification. Metab Bone Dis Relat Res 1978;1:83–87.
4. Anderson HC. Calcification processes. Pathol Annu 1980;15:45–75.

5. Anderson HC. Calcific diseases. A concept. Arch Pathol Lab Med 1983;107:341–348.
6. Anderson HC. Matrix vesicle calcification: review and update. In: Peck WA (ed). Bone and mineral research/3: A yearly survey of developments in the field of bone and mineral metabolism. Amsterdam: Elsevier Science Publishers, 1985, pp 109–149.
7. Anderson HC. Calcific diseases: the role of membranes in pathological calcification. In: Ali SY (ed). Cell mediated calcification and matrix vesicles. Amsterdam: Excerpta Medica, 1986, pp 355–358.
8. Anderson HC. Mechanism of mineral formation in bone. Lab Invest 1989;60:320–330.

9. Askanazy M. Ueber Kalkmetastasen und progressive Knochenatrophie. In: Chemische und Medicinische Untersuchungen: Festschrift zur Feier des Sechzigsten Geburtstages von Max Jaffe. Braunschweig: Friedrich Vieweg und Sohn, 1901, pp 188–240.

10. Bachra BN. Nucleation in biological systems. In: Zipkin I (ed). Biological mineralization. New York: John Wiley & Sons, 1973, pp 845–881.

11. Banker BQ, Chester CS. Infarction of thigh muscle in the diabetic patient. Neurology 1973;23:667–677.

12. Berczi I. Fatty acids and soft tissue calcification. Exp Med Surg 1970;28:245–255.

13. Boivin G, Walzer C, Baud CA. Ultrastructural study of the long-term development of two experimental cutaneous calcinoses (topical calciphylaxis and topical calcergy) in the rat. Cell Tissue Res 1987;247:525–532.

14. Bonucci E. Fine structure of early cartilage calcification. J Ultrastruct Res 1967;20:33–50.

15. Bonucci E. Fine structure and histochemistry of "calcifying globules" in epiphyseal cartilage. Z Zellforsch 1970;103:192–217.

16. Bonucci E, Sadun R. An electron microscope study on experimental calcification of skeletal muscle. Clin Orthop 1972;88:197–217.

17. Bonucci E, Sadun R. Experimental calcification of the myocardium. Ultrastructural and histochemical investigations. Am J Pathol 1973;71:167–184.

18. Borle AB. Control, modulation, and regulation of cell calcium. Rev Physiol Biochem Pharmacol 1981;90:13–153.

19. Boskey AL. Current concepts of the physiology and biochemistry of calcification. Clin Orthop 1981;157:225–257.

20. Boskey AL. Overview of cellular elements and macromolecules implicated in the initiation of mineralization. In: Butler WT (ed). The chemistry and biology of mineralized tissues. Birmingham: Ebsco Media Inc, 1985, pp 335–343.

21. Boskey AL. Phospholipids and calcification: an overview. In: Ali SY (ed). Cell mediated calcification and matrix vesicles. Amsterdam: Excerpta Medica, 1986, pp 175–179.

22. Boskey AL. Hydroxyapatite formation in a dynamic collagen gel system: effects of type I collagen, lipids, and proteoglycans. J Phys Chem 1989;93:1628–1633.

23. Boskey AL. Noncollagenous matrix proteins and their role in mineralization. Bone Mineral 1989;6:111–123.

24. Boskey AL, Bullough PG. Cartilage calcification: normal and aberrant. Scan Electron Microsc 1984;II:943–952.

25. Boskey AL, Bullough PG, Posner AS. Calcium-acidic phospholipid-phosphate complexes in diseases and normal human bone. Metab Bone Dis Relat Res 1982;4:151–156.

26. Boyan BD, Swain LD, Boskey AL. Mechanisms of microbial calcification. In: ten Cate JM (ed). Recent advances in the study of dental calculus. Oxford: IRL Press, 1989, pp 29–35.

27. Boyan-Salyers BD, Boskey AL. Relationship between proteolipids and calcium-phospholipid-phosphate complexes in Bacterionema matruchotii calcification. Calcif Tissue Int 1980;30:167–174.

28. Caulfield JB, Schrag PE. Electron microscopic study of renal calcification. Am J Pathol 1964;44:365–381.

29. Cavallero C, Spagnoli LG, Di Tondo U. Early mitochondrial calcifications in the rabbit aorta after adrenaline. Virch Arch A Pathol Anat Histol 1974;362:23–39.

30. Chatelain P, Kapanci Y. Histological diagnosis of myocardial infarction: the role of calcium. Appl Pathol 1984;2:233–239.

31. Coignoul F, Cheville N. Calcified microbial plaque. Dental calculus of dogs. Am J Pathol 1984;117:499–501.

32. Eanes ED. Biophysical aspects of lipid interaction with mineral: liposome model studies. Anat Rec 1989;224:220–225.

33. Edwards WD. Applied anatomy of the heart. In: Brandenburg RO, Fuster V, Giulani ER, McGoon DC (eds). Cardiology: fundamentals and practice. Chicago: Year Book Medical Publishers, 1987, pp 47–112.

34. Eggermann J, Kapanci Y. Experimental pulmonary calcinosis in the rat. Ultrastructural and morphometric studies. Lab Invest 1971;24:469–482.

35. Ennever J, Creamer H. Microbiologic calcification: bone mineral and bacteria. Calcif Tissue Res 1967;1:87–93.

36. Ennever J, Vogel JJ, Riggan LJ. Calcification by proteolipid from atherosclerotic aorta. Atherosclerosis 1980;35:209–213.

37. Ferrans VJ, Boyce SW, Billingham ME, Jones M, Ishihara T, Roberts WC. Calcific deposits in porcine bioprostheses: structure and pathogenesis. Am J Cardiol 1980;46:721–734.

38. Fleisch H. Diphosphonates: history and mechanisms of action. Metab Bone Dis Relat Res 1981;3:279–288.

39. Freundlich H, Hatfield HS. Colloid and capillary chemistry. London: Methuen & Co. Ltd, 1926.

40. Gabbiani G, Tuchweber B, Selye H. Experimental ectopic calcification (calciphylaxis and calcergy). In: Zipkin I (ed). Biological mineralization. New York: John Wiley & Sons, 1973, pp 547–586.

41. Galkin BM, Frasca P, Feig SA, Holderness KE. Noncalcified breast particles. A possible new marker of breast cancer. Invest Radiol 1982;17:119–128.

42. Gallop PM, Lian JB, Hauschka PV. Carboxylated calcium-binding proteins and vitamin K. N Engl J Med 1980;302:1460–1466.

43. Glimcher MJ. A basic architectural principle in the organization of mineralized tissues. Clin Orthop 1968;61:16–36.

44. Glimcher MJ. On the form and function of bone: from molecules to organs. Wolff's Law revisited, 1981. In: Veis A (ed). The chemistry and biology of mineralized connective tissue. Amsterdam: Elsevier North Holland, Inc, 1981, pp 617–673.

45. Gonzalez ER. Calcium deposits on IUDs may play role in infections. JAMA 1981;245:1625–1626.

46. Greenawalt JW, Rossi CS, Lehninger AL. Effect of active accumulation of calcium and phosphate ions on the structure of rat liver mitochondria. J Cell Biol 1964;23:21–38.

47. Gundberg CM, Hauschka PV, Lian JB, Gallop PM. Osteocalcin: isolation, characterization, and detection. Methods Enzymol 1984;107:516–544.

48. Hansson GK, Schwartz SM. Evidence for cell death in the vascular endothelium in vivo and in vitro. Am J Pathol 1983;112:278–286.

49. Hasselbacher P. Crystal-protein interactions in crystal-induced arthritis. Adv Inflamm Res 1982;4:25–44.

50. Haust MD, Geer JC. Mechanism of calcification in spontaneous aortic arteriosclerotic lesions of the rabbit. Am J Pathol 1970;60:329–344.

51. Henisch HK. Crystals in gels and Liesegang rings. Cambridge: Cambridge University Press, 1988.

52. Hinzpeter EN, Naumann GOH. Cornea sclera. In: Naumann GOH, Apple DJ (eds). Pathology of the eye. New York: Springer-Verlag, 1986, pp 317–412.

53. Howell DS. Diseases due to the deposition of calcium pyrophosphate and hydroxyapatite. In: Kelley WN, Harris ED, Jr, Ruddy S, Sledge CB (eds). Textbook of

rheumatology, vol 2, 2nd ed. Philadelphia: WB Saunders Company, 1985, pp 1398–1416.

54. Ibels LS. The pathogenesis of metastatic calcification in uraemia. Prog Biochem Pharmacol 1980;17:242–250.

55. Kim KM. Calcification of matrix vesicles in human aortic valve and aortic media. Fed Proc 1976;35:156–162.

56. Kim KM. Pathological calcification. In: Trump BF, Arstila AU (eds). Pathobiology of cell membranes, vol III. New York: Academic Press, 1983, pp 117–155.

57. Kim KM. Role of membranes in calcification. Surv Synth Pathol Res 1983;2:215–228.

58. Kim KM. Nephrocalcinosis in vitro. Scanning Electron Microsc 1983;III:1285–1292.

59. Kim KM, Huang S-N. Ultrastructural study of calcification of human aortic valve. Lab Invest 1971;25:357–366.

60. Kivilaakso E, Fromm D, Silen W. Effect of the acid secretory state on intramural pH of rabbit gastric mucosa. Gastroenterology 1978;75:641–648.

61. Krane SM, Glimcher MJ. Transphosphorylation from nucleoside di- and triphosphates by apatite crystals. J Biol Chem 1962;237:2991–2998.

62. Lansing AI, Alex M, Rosenthal TB. Calcium and elastin in human arteriosclerosis. J Gerontol 1950;5:112–119.

63. Levine MM, Kleeman CR. Hypercalcemia: pathophysiology and treatment. Hosp Pract 1987;22:93–109.

64. Levy RJ, Gundberg C, Scheinman R. The identification of the vitamin K-dependent bone protein osteocalcin as one of the t-carboxyglutamic acid containing proteins present in calcified atherosclerotic plaque and mineralized heart valves. Atherosclerosis 1983;46:49–56.

65. Levy RJ, Lian JB, Gallop P. Atherocalcin, a t-carboxyglutamic acid containing protein from atherosclerotic plaque. Biochem Biophys Res Commun 1979;91:41–49.

66. Lowenstam HA, Weiner S. On biomineralization. New York: Oxford University Press, 1989.

67. Maren TH. Carbonic anhydrase: chemistry, physiology, and inhibition. Physiol Rev 1967;47:595–723.

68. Marks SC, Jr, Popoff SN. Bone cell biology: the regulation of development, structure, and function in the skeleton. Am J Anat 1988;183:1–44.

69. Matthews JL. Role of mitochondria in calcification. In: Ali SY (ed). Cell mediated calcification and matrix vesicles. Amsterdam: Excerpta Medica, 1986, pp 115–118.

70. McCarty DJ. Crystal deposition joint disease. Annu Rev Med 1974;25:279–288.

71. Menanteau J, Neuman WF, Neuman MW. A study of bone proteins which can prevent hydroxyapatite formation. Metab Bone Dis Relat Res 1982;4:157–162.

72. Moller-Christensen V, Weiss DL. One of the oldest datable skeletons with leprous bone-changes from the Naeslved Leprosy Hospital Churchyard in Denmark. Int J Lepr 1971;39:172–182.

73. Mulligan RM, Stricker FL. Metastatic calcification produced in dogs by hypervitaminosis D and haliphagia. Am J Pathol 1948;24:451–473.

74. Neff M, Yalcin S, Gupta S, Berger H. Extensive metastatic calcification of the lung in an azotemic patient. Am J Med 1974;56:103–109.

75. Neuman WF, Neuman MW. The chemical dynamics of bone mineral. Chicago: The University of Chicago Press, 1958.

76. Neuman WF, Neuman MW. In the beginning there was apatite. In: Zipkin I (ed). Biological mineralization. New York: John Wiley and Sons, 1973, pp 3–19.

77. Olson LH, Edwards WD, Tajik AJ. Aortic valve stenosis: etiology, pathophysiology, evaluation, and management. Curr Probl Cardiol 1987;12:459–508.

78. Posner AS, Betts F. Molecular control of tissue mineralization. In: Veis A (ed). The chemistry and biology of mineralized connective tissue. Amsterdam: Elsevier North Holland, Inc, 1981, pp 257–266.

79. Raggio CL, Boyan BD, Boskey AL. In vivo hydroxyapatite formation induced by lipids. J Bone Miner Res 1986;1:409–415.

80. Randall RE Jr, Strauss MB, McNeely WF. The milk-alkali syndrome. Arch Intern Med 1961;107:163–181.

81. Reynolds ES. Liver parenchymal cell injury. III. The nature of calcium-associated electron-opaque masses in rat liver mitochondria following poisoning with carbon tetrachloride. J Cell Biol 1965;25:53–75.

82. Roberts WC, Waller BF. Effect of chronic hypercalcemia on the heart. An analysis of 18 necropsy patients. Am J Med 1981;71:371–384.

83. Russell RGG, Robertson WG, Fleisch H. Inhibitors of mineralization. In: Zipkin I (ed). Biological mineralization. New York: John Wiley & Sons, 1973, pp 807–825.

84. Schoen FJ, Levy RJ, Nelson AC, Bernhard WF, Nashef A, Hawley M. Onset and progression of experimental bioprosthetic heart valve calcification. Lab Invest 1985;52:523–532.

85. Selye H. Calciphylaxis. Chicago: The University of Chicago Press, 1962.

86. Sherwood L. Human physiology. From cells to systems. St Paul: West Publishing Company, 1989.

87. Strawich E, Glimcher MJ. Phosphoproteins of mineralized tissues: the chemistry and biosynthesis of the phosphoproteins of dental enamel. In: Akeson WH, Bornstein P, Glimcher MJ (eds). Symposium on heritable disorders of connective tissue. San Diego, CA, May, 1980. St Louis: The CV Mosby Company, 1982, pp 173–191.

88. Tanimura A, McGregor DH, Anderson HC. Matrix vesicles in atherosclerotic calcification. Proc Soc Exp Biol Med 1983;172:173–177.

89. Taura S, Taura M, Imai H, Kummerow FA, Tokuyasu K, Cho-Simon BH. Ultrastructure of cardiovascular lesions induced by hypervitaminosis D and its withdrawal. Paroi Arterielle 1978;4:245–259.

90. Termine JD, Eanes ED. Calcium phosphate deposition from balanced salt solutions. Calcif Tissue Res 1974;15:81–84.

91. Tuur SM, Nelson AM, Gibson DW, et al. Liesegang rings in tissue. How to distinguish Liesegang rings from the giant kidney worm, Dioctophyma renale. Am J Surg Pathol 1987;11:598–605.

92. Urist MR. Biologic initiators of calcification. In: Zipkin I (ed). Biological mineralization. New York: John Wiley & Sons, 1973, pp 757–805.

93. Urist MR. Biochemistry of calcification. In: Bourne GH (ed). The biochemistry and physiology of bone, 2nd ed., vol IV. New York: Academic Press, 1976, pp 1–59.

94. Velentzas C, Meindok H, Oreopolous DG, et al. Visceral calcification and the Ca × P product. Adv Exp Mol Biol 1978;103:195–201.

95. Virchow R. Cellular pathology. Translated from the 2nd German Ed. by B Chance, 1859. Reproduced by Dover Publications, New York, 1971.

96. Vogel JJ. The microbial model in the study of calcification. In: Dickson GR (ed). Methods of calcified tissue preparation. Amsterdam: Elsevier Science Publishers BV, 1984, pp 607–621.

97. Vogel JJ. The membrane interface in biologic calcification. In: Ali SY (ed). Cell mediated calcification and matrix vesicles. Amsterdam: Excerpta Medica, 1986, pp 181–185.

98. Vogel JJ, Boyan-Salyers B, Campbell MM. Protein-

phospholipid interactions in biologic calcification. Metab Bone Dis Relat Res 1978;1:149–153.

99. Vogel JJ, Ennever J. The role of a lipoprotein in the intracellular hydroxyapatite formation in Bacterionema Matruchotii. Clin Orthop 1971;78:218–222.

100. Weiser HB. A textbook of colloid chemistry, 2nd ed. New York: John Wiley & Sons, Inc, 1949.

101. Wells HG. Chemical pathology, 5th ed. Philadelphia: WB Saunders Company, 1925.

102. Woodward SC. Mineralization of connective tissue surrounding implanted devices. Trans Am Soc Artif Intern Organs 1981;27:697–702.

Extracellular Pathology

The Extracellular World

We have spoken of the cell as the elementary patient; now we turn to the patient's environment to see what we can learn there about disease. But first we must clarify one point: cells relate to their environment much more closely than humans do. Cells are physically attached to the extracellular matrix by a variety of receptors for collagen, laminin, fibronectin, fibrin, and many other molecules, so that signals may be transmitted from the matrix to the cell and vice versa (24). For example, receptors of the integrin family link extracellular molecules with the cytoskeletal network. In this way, the "inert" extracellular matrix can affect cell attachment, shape, locomotion, and even gene expression (28, 29). As we mentioned earlier, it is everyday experience that cultured cells assume different phenotypes depending on the substrate on which they are grown (53).

At the submicroscopic level the extracellular spaces are a thick jungle of molecules; the four major components, best seen in loose connective tissue, are

- collagen fibers (non-branching)
- elastic fibers (branching)
- proteoglycans (a gel)
- basement membranes (sheets)

Extracellular pathology includes changes in quantity and quality of these normal components, as well as the appearance of abnormal materials. The mechanism may be a congenital defect (about 150 are known) (44) but most of extracellular pathology is acquired. By light microscopy some pathologic conditions are easily identified (such as excess collagen in a cirrhotic liver), but quite often the picture is that of a nondescript extracellular mass that cannot be identified without special histochemical stains. To describe such masses in a noncommittal way, microscopists have come up with a handy bit of jargon: "hyalin," which means "glassy." In other words, *hyalin is not a substance; it is an adjective.*

A common example: with advancing age, many arterioles become hyalinized, especially in the spleen and kidney (Figure 7.1). What is that hyalin material made of? In the cases illustrated it consists mainly of hyaluronic acid bound to a plasma protein, the third component of complement (C3), which must have seeped out of the lumen (8). Why C3 should behave in this manner is not clear. In many arterioles, plasma-derived lipid is mixed into this hyalin, presumably because the endothelium has become leaky: this seems to be the usual ailment of hyalinized arterioles.

FIGURE 7.1
Hyalinized arterioles. *Left:* Glomerular afferent arteriole from a renal biopsy in chronic diabetes. The media (smooth muscle layer) is largely replaced by a homogeneous hyalin mass. **Bar** = 10 μm. *Right:* Electron micrograph of a similar arteriole in a case of essential hypertension. The media is replaced by amorphous, basement-membranelike material (**x**). L: Lumen. **Bar** = 2 μm. (Reproduced with permission from [8].)

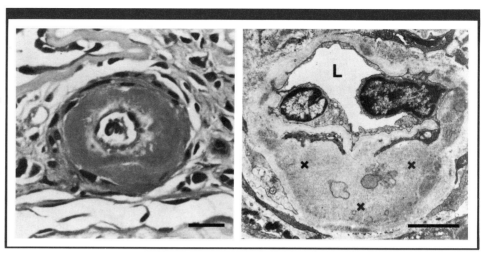

In other situations, hyalin masses may consist of fibrin, packed collagen or basement membrane (Figure 7.2), mucopolysaccharides (glucosaminoglycans), or an abnormal material called amyloid. *It is often important for the pathologist to identify the chemical nature of the hyalin because it may give a clue to a local or even a general disturbance,* acute or chronic. Amyloid, for example, may indicate one of a whole gamut of problems, ranging from an incidental finding to a death sentence.

Pathology of Collagen

Considering that collagen is probably the most abundant protein in the animal world and that it

FIGURE 7.2
Two hyalinized glomeruli (**arrows**) next to a normal one. This hyalin represents an overproduction of basement membrane. **Bar** = 100 μm.

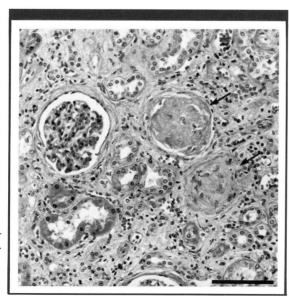

accounts for almost one-third of the mammalian body's proteins, its contribution to the daily worries of physicians is relatively modest. This makes sense because collagen is a pillar of life; it is responsible for holding the body together, skeleton included, and for healing injuries. It is clearly essential that such a vital protein be stable—and so it is. Full-blown, generalized abnormalities of collagen are rare: some are congenital, some are nutritional (e.g., scurvy), and others are toxic (e.g., osteolathyrism). Some of these diseases deserve to be examined in this book, if only because they offer elegant "clinico-molecular" correlations, including the possibility that some short people can be explained by shortened molecules (p. 250). As usual, some of the metabolic diseases of collagen provided clues to its biology (7, 9, 19, 22, 32–34, 43). Localized collagen-related problems are common and largely related to wound healing.

Only one type of collagen was known before 1969; now we know of over 15, numbered in order of discovery (9, 10, 31, 40). Each collagen molecule is made of three alpha-chains twisted in ropelike fashion; 25 different kinds of chains have been identified. A few details follow (Types I and III are listed consecutively because they are closely related).

- Type I is the principal fibrillar collagen, by far the most common. It provides tensile strength in tissues such as tendons and the cornea (Figure 7.3).
- Type III is made of thinner fibrils (Figure 7.3) and supports distensible organs such as blood vessels (when this collagen is defective, vessels tend to burst). *When new colla-*

gen is laid down, Type III tends to be deposited first, and is followed by Type I.

- Type II is also fibrillar but buried in cartilage, such as the hyaline cartilage of joints (Figure 7.3); correspondingly, when injected into susceptible rodents, it creates an immune response that affects the joints (50).
- Type IV is nonfibrillar; its molecules tend to aggregate by fours into X-shaped units (Figure 7.4) that join up to make the skeleton of the basement membranes (Figure 7.3).
- Types V, VI, IX, and XII tend to coat other collagen fibrils.

Fibroblasts share the capacity to secrete collagen with many other mesenchymal cells, especially smooth-muscle cells, but also with epithelia, which synthesize their own basement membranes.

The rope-shaped, fibrillar varieties of collagen are mainly responsible for tissue strength. The genesis of these "ropes" (the collagen fibers as seen by light microscopy) represented an evolutional production problem because their diameter is of the same order of magnitude as the cells themselves, and of course no cell is large enough to secrete such large objects. Nature solved the problem by having the cells secrete small precursors endowed with the power of self-assembly: a multistep process involving at least 13 enzymes and twice as many cofactors (Figure 7.5). The more complex a process is, the likelier it is to fail; thus, the pathology of collagen can fill a book, albeit a book of rare diseases. We will offer an overview, emphasizing the basic principles. It will be apparent that some accidents beset the immature collagen molecule inside the cell; others concern the free fiber.

Follow the sequence in Figure 7.5. The messenger RNA coding for collagen emerges from the nucleus and is translated by ribosomes into two types of pro–alpha chains, tipped by terminal polypeptides that are critical for the manufacture of the molecule. Then the immature molecule, advancing in membranous structures (rough ER and Golgi apparatus), undergoes **hydroxylation** of its proline and lysine residues, as well as **glycation,** whereby glucose and other carbohydrates are added. The chains are now ready for self-twisting in groups of three into a helix, which is secreted, at long last, as **procollagen**—still bearing its terminal peptides. Outside of the cell, this newly born molecule cannot self-assemble unless its two

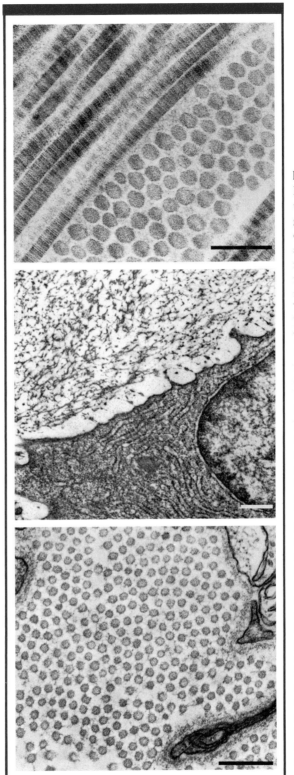

FIGURE 7.3
Four common types of collagen. *Top:* Type I, cut transversally and longitudinally (epineurium of a human nerve). *Center:* Type II, from rat hyaline cartilage. The fibrils are thinner and do not have a clearly visible banding pattern. *Bottom:* Type III (human endoneurium), cut transversally, shows fibrils with a smaller diameter than Type I. Parts of cells are included in this figure; they are covered with basement membrane, which contains collagen Type IV. **Bars** = 0.4 μm. (Courtesy of Prof. G.S. Montes, Department of Histology and Embryology, University of São Páulo Institute of Biomedical Sciences, Brazil.)

bunches of terminal peptides are clipped off by extracellular peptidases, which finally release the true elementary collagen molecule: **tropocollagen.** The tropocollagen molecules then self-assemble

FIGURE 7.4
Model of collagen Type IV. Four molecules are assembled by stable interactions, producing an X-shaped structure that is the backbone of basement membranes. (Reproduced with permission from [26].)

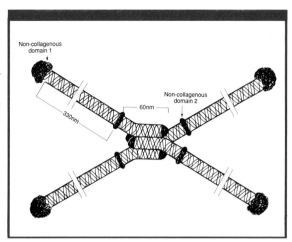

into *microfibrils,* which are promptly cross-linked with the help of another extracellular enzyme, lysyl oxidase. This enzyme, in the presence of copper and ascorbic acid (two critical conditions), converts some of the hydroxyl terminals to aldehydes, which are essential for creating links within and between adjacent molecules. The microfibrils then continue to self-assemble into larger units, the *fibrils,* which are visible by electron microscopy and show a characteristic cross-banding; their diameter is about 50 nm. The collagen fibers seen by light microscopy are bundles of these banded units.

Now we will run through this scheme again and see how it can go awry. Keep this fact in mind: *collagen defects can be inborn or acquired.* Inborn defects are well established only for the fibrillar collagens: Types I, II (40), III, and VII. Many errors are known or suspected for each of the steps in Figure 7.5; we will choose a few classic examples.

GENETIC DEFECTS

Another glance at Figure 7.5 will show you that in the elaborate sequence of collagen synthesis, which requires an hour or two (34), most of the modifications to the developing collagen molecule are posttranslational; this means that *congenital disease can arise from defects in two sets of genes: any of those that code for collagen, and any of those that code for the enzymes that are active in the post-translational events.* In either case, the result is defective fibers. Dozens of congenital human and animal diseases arise through these mechanisms (44, 49). Symptoms arise from those organs whose mechanical functions depend most heavily on collagen: the bones (50% of their dry weight is collagen), the joints (held in place by fibrous

ligaments), the skin (90% of its proteins are collagen), the large arteries (which have to withstand high internal pressure), the mitral valve (which is subjected to violent stresses at each heartbeat), and the eyes, especially the crystalline lens (which is held in place by a rim of collagen fibrils). Seen by electron microscopy, congenitally abnormal fibrils are somewhat disappointing: they can be a little too thick, a little too thin, or irregular, but they offer little help in differential diagnosis (54).

Several diseases of collagen have been known for centuries, because some of their manifestations are so striking that the patients were used for circus shows. A few of the molecular defects have been worked out (41). Traditionally, three main groups of congenital collagen diseases were recognized: the Marfan syndrome, osteogenesis imperfecta, and the Ehler–Danlos syndrome. Recent discoveries now place the Marfan syndrome among the congenital diseases of elastic fibers, even though elastin itself is not defective. The other two syndromes, which we will briefly describe, should be understood as constituting a spectrum of overlapping phenotypes due to different genetic defects that cause similar clinical abnormalities. Sometimes the defect leads to short individuals whose main problem lies in weak and brittle bones; this disease is **osteogenesis imperfecta.** It has been suggested that the short stature of these patients is ultimately linked to shortened collagen molecules (38). In other cases the genetic defect translates into patients suffering mostly from extremely loose joints (the "rubber people" of some circuses, "floppy babies," and "rubber puppies") and also from thin, lax skin that pulls into absurdly long folds; these are the key features of the 11 known varieties of the **Ehler–Danlos syndrome.** A map of relevant defects in the collagen molecule is being slowly assembled (39, 41, 42). Defects in the collagen polypeptide chains cause the assembled protein to be structurally incompetent and rapidly broken down, inside or outside the cell. It now seems that latent forms of these diseases are common, which would explain conditions that are apparently focal, such as "floppy mitral valves" (15), aortic aneurysms, and some forms of osteoarthritis. Even osteoporosis may be linked to an inborn defect of collagen (20, 40). Congenital collagen diseases may not be so rare after all.

We will sketch two typical clinical pictures to illustrate how a molecular defect can translate into a major human problem.

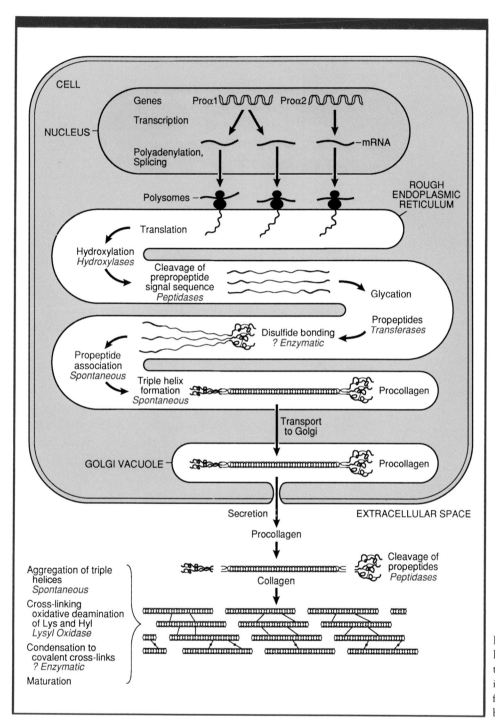

FIGURE 7.5
Biosynthesis of collagen Type I. Note the complex posttranslational processing: at every step there is a chance for congenital or accidental disturbance. (Adapted from [44].)

Osteogenesis Imperfecta This disease is also called brittle bone disease or Lobstein's disease after the same Lobstein who coined the term arteriosclerosis in 1833. Its prevalence is about 1 in 25,000 people, and it has a surprisingly wide range of severity, depending on the mutation in one of the two procollagen genes (over 70 mutations are known) (20). In some instances it is so severe that death occurs *in utero*; more fortunate individuals can lead normal lives by carefully avoiding mechanical stress (7); others are condemned to live with severe, progressive deformations of their long bones (Figure 7.6). Symptoms include "blue" (semitransparent) sclerae and opalescent teeth; both these tissues are rich in collagen Type I.

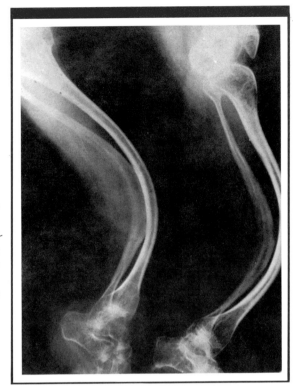

FIGURE 7.6 Osteogenesis imperfecta, a disease of the collagen molecule, as manifested in an adult. In this severe, progressive variant, the lower limbs are deformed. (Reproduced with permission from [19].)

Ehler–Danlos Syndromes These syndromes have two symptoms in common: a laxity of the joints, which can be spectacular (Figure 7.7), and an easily bruised skin (30). Although the skin is thin and hyperextensible (Figure 7.8), it can recoil because the elastic fibers are still there; all that is missing is the tethering effect of normal collagen fibers. The molecular defect is known for a few of the 11 known clinical phenotypes; it usually involves enzymes required for posttranslational processing of collagen Type I or III. The ultimate consequences include rupture of the aorta and other hollow organs such as the large bowel.

Dermatosparaxis: A Failure of Extracellular Assembly The collagen molecule is finally born when the procollagen molecule is assembled outside the cell (review this once again on Figure 7.5). But if the terminal peptides of procollagen are not removed, the nascent collagen molecules cannot assemble properly, and the mature collagen fibers are easily torn apart. This disturbance was the first proven collagen disease: it was discovered in calves by Belgian veterinarians (sheep are also affected) and named **dermatosparaxis**, from *derma*, "skin," and *sparássein*, "to tear" (Figure 7.9) (3, 14, 21). Originally, the gene of dermatosparaxis came to be selected because the heterozygous animals produce

a more tender flesh(!) (37), which is not surprising if you take a look at the state of the collagen fibrils in dermatosparaxis (52) (Figure 7.10). Homozygous animals are doomed.

ACQUIRED DEFECTS

If you had to design some way to produce weakened collagen fibers, your best bet would probably be to interfere with the cross-linking mechanisms within and between the fibrils. This is indeed what happens in real life, as a result of poor nutrition or toxic agents.

Deficient Hydroxylation We are now talking about **scurvy**, or vitamin C deficiency. Please refer once again to Figure 7.5: it will remind you that hydroxylation occurs *within* the fibroblast, as an early step in the genesis of the procollagen molecule. Historically, of course, scurvy was the curse of long voyages at sea; it reappeared in malnourished armies during World War I. The unfortunate sailors and soldiers who lost their teeth (Figure 7.11) and saw their old scars break down to gape as fresh wounds could not have guessed that their problem was essentially one of inadequate hydroxylation. *Vitamin C, a redox agent and a cofactor in many hydroxylation reactions, is also required for the hydroxylation of the proline and lysine of collagen.* Low hydroxylation of lysine leads to reduced cross-linking and thus to defective collagen fibers. The sailors' teeth fall out because the collagen in the periodontal ligament that holds the teeth in place has a short half-life: 1 day (in the rat) compared with 15 days for skin collagen (48); therefore, the tough bundles of old but normal periodontal collagen are fast replaced by defective ones. The breakdown of old scars is explained by a similar mechanism; we will learn later that collagen turnover in scars remains elevated long after the healing process is clinically terminated (p. 470). The subperiosteal bleeding seen in scurvy is probably due to the tearing of weakened tendon insertions; the general bleeding tendency may reflect a weakness of the microvascular basement membranes.

Defective Cross-Linking Several nutritional and toxic mechanisms interfere with the cross-linking of collagen. For example, copper-deficient swine, sheep and chicks can die literally of broken hearts or aortas—because lysyl oxidase requires copper as a cofactor. Among the toxic agents best known is a principle extracted from the sweet pea; in experimental animals it causes a most interesting condition, **osteolathyrism**, which taught us a great deal about collagen. During periods of starvation, people in India, Italy, and Spain once turned to a diet of chick peas (*Lathyrus sativus*), which caused neurologic problems (but no defect of collagen). While this form of poisoning—chick-pea lathyrism—was being worked out, it was accidentally discovered that the seeds of a related plant, the common sweet pea (*Lathyrus odoratus*), are also toxic but in a totally different way (22). The active principle of the sweet pea, BAPN (beta-aminopropionitrile), binds irreversibly to the enzyme lysyl oxidase, with the result that cross-linking is prevented, and correspondingly the mature collagen is extremely weak. Chicks poisoned with BAPN have extremely soluble collagen and therefore brittle and misshapen bones (11) (Figure 7.12) and brittle skin. This "osteo-lathyrism" did not help us understand chick-pea lathyrism, but it became widely used as a model of defective collagen cross-linking.

As a matter of fact, there have been some attempts to harness the specific toxicity of BAPN for therapeutic purposes. Many distressing human diseases are characterized by fibrosis: too much fibrous tissue, which implies too much collagen. Understandably, this led to the idea that a therapeutically induced collagen defect might bring some benefit (43). The choice fell mainly on BAPN and penicillamine, the latter because it chelates copper and also competes for the aldehyde radicals required for cross-linking of collagen and elastin. Animal experiments gave some hope, but in human patients the results were disappointing. Penicillamine was also used in a totally different context. Because it chelates copper, it can alleviate Wilson's disease, which is characterized by toxic cellular concentrations of free copper. The result: after several years, in some patients, the treatment produces faulty collagen (46) (Figure 7.13) and faulty elastin, clumps of which are then eliminated through the skin—a condition called **elastosis ulcerans serpiginosa** (4). Thus, the price for treating Wilson's disease was a subtype of lathyrism.

Interestingly, there is also a congenital metabolic disease that leads to a "toxic" defective cross-linking of collagen and elastin: **homocystinuria.** *Due to the lack of an enzyme, homocysteine accumulates in the blood and tissues; it interacts with the aldehydes formed by lysyl oxidase, and thus blocks the*

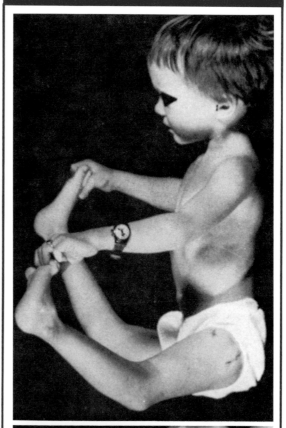

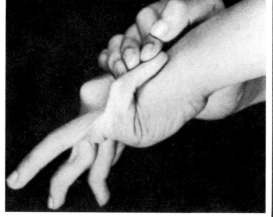

FIGURE 7.7
Joint laxity in a child affected by one type of Ehler–Danlos syndrome. Dislocated hips and hypermobile knee joints were noted at birth. (Reproduced with permission from [30].)

development of stable cross-links (32). In other words, homocysteine functions here much like penicillamine; the two molecules are actually similar. The clinical picture includes a dislocation of the crystalline lens (which is held in place by a crown of collagen fibers) and was once confused with the Marfan syndrome.

Excessive Cross-Linking Excessive cross-linking is a typical effect of aging and diabetes (p. 267). If a joint is immobilized experimentally, the cross-linking of the capsular collagen increases as if it

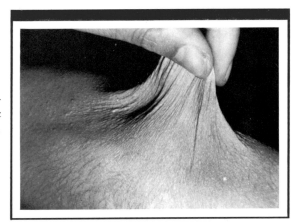

FIGURE 7.8
Abnormally stretchable skin from a case of Ehler–Danlos syndrome, probably Type I. Elastic fibers are present, but the tethering effect of collagen fibers is missing. (Reproduced with permission from [19].)

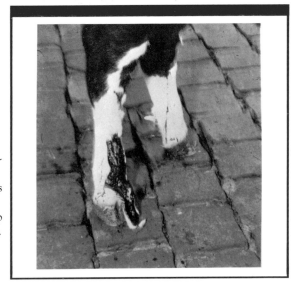

FIGURE 7.9
Dermatosparaxis (a disease of the collagen molecule). The skin of these calves has the consistency of wet blotting paper. The trauma of birth is sufficient to tear it and even to rip it off completely. (Reproduced with permission from [14].)

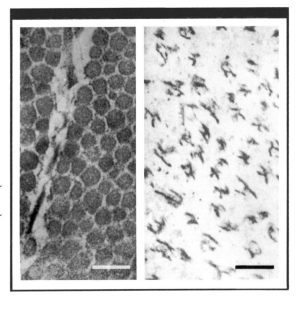

FIGURE 7.10
Dermatosparaxis. *Left:* Cross section of collagen fibers from the skin of a normal newborn lamb. *Right:* Collagen fibers from the skin of a dermatosparactic lamb. **Bar** = 0.2 μm. (Reproduced with permission from [52].)

had prematurely aged (1). We suspect that this mechanism contributes to the stiffness that develops so rapidly in joints immobilized by plaster casts.

Digestion by Enzymes As we stated earlier, collagen is a very stable protein, especially when highly cross-linked. Its half-life ranges from hours to years. Native collagen is practically unaffected by trypsinlike proteolytic enzymes unless it is denatured; in fact the collagen in meat can be utilized as food only because the acid pH of the stomach denatures it, preparing it for digestion by pepsin. However, native collagen can be digested by one family of highly specific enzymes, the **collagenases**. This exposes the collagen fibers to a whole set of possible mishaps, such as bacterial attack. Until 1962, the only known collagenases were bacterial; animal collagenases remained a mystery. It was obvious that collagenous structures (such as bone) could be removed as part of normal tissue turnover, but nobody had ever succeeded in demonstrating collagenase activity in any tissue. It was rationalized, quite correctly, that collagenases in tissues would be potentially dangerous, because if let loose they could reduce the body to a pile of jelly. Indeed, today we know that tissue collagenases do exist but they are kept in check by powerful inhibitors from the moment they are secreted (35); this is what makes these enzymes so difficult to find. Eventually they were discovered by an experiment *in vitro*, in which—by a fortunate technical accident—the inhibitors were left out (Figure 7.14) (12).

In pathology, the body's own collagenase is relevant mainly as an agent of collagen breakdown and turnover, such as occurs normally in wound healing, bone resorption, and receding gums. *Collagenase is thought to cause damage in at least two conditions: in* **osteoarthritis** *(degenerative arthritis), in which part of the problem is a breakdown of the hyalin cartilage matrix (collagen included) by endogenous enzymes; and in* **corneal diseases** *of many kinds, in which the precious corneal stroma is destroyed by collagenases.* These enzymes can be produced by bacteria, corneal fibroblasts, the corneal epithelium, and inflammatory cells; anticollagenase treatments have been devised (45).

Bacterial collagenase plays a major role in the pathogenesis of infection by the anaerobic, collagenase-producing *Clostridium histolyticum*, the agent of the fast-spreading and life-threatening gas

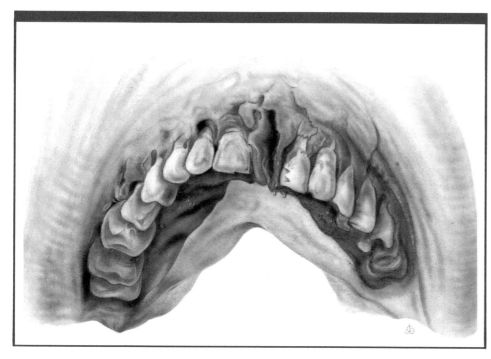

FIGURE 7.11
Effect of scurvy (avitaminosis C) on the gums and teeth. Lacking vitamin C, the fast-renewing collagen of the periodontal ligament is improperly hydroxylated, resulting in tooth mobility, tooth loss, bleeding, and periodontal infection. From the autopsy of a soldier who died of scurvy in 1919. (Redrawn with permission from [2].)

gangrene typical of wounds cantaminated with soil. In these infections, collagenase favors the spread of the bacteria by clearing their path in the connective tissue (*histo-lyticum* means "tissue-dissolving"). The first inkling that a specific collagenase must exist came from the histologic study of gas gangrene (27). This is a fine example to show how morphology, well interpreted, can point the way to biochemistry.

Calcification The price of aging includes a tendency of collagen to calcify (the same is true for elastin). Tendon collagen is especially at risk. The fibers become impregnated with apatite crystals—we might say fossilized—by a mechanism that was discussed earlier (p. 235).

Heat Shrinkage Heat shrinkage is a peculiar property of collagen fibers. When heated to 65°C, they shrink to about one-third their original length. This is why bacon strips shrink so drastically in the frying pan, and also how Amazonian natives used to shrink deboned human heads (25). The contracted fibers turn into a semitransparent mass called **gelatin** (34) (Figure 7.15). Gelatin is not only a familiar food; it is also sticky, and as such it was long used as carpenter's glue, a fact preserved in the name of its precursor, *collagen* ("generator of glue"; *colla* is Latin for "glue"). Leather is essentially dermal collagen made almost unshrinkable by tanning, a special type of cross-

linking (leather jackets should not shrink if boiled). The thick, hyalinized lumps seen microscopically in the track of the thermocautery (Figure 7.16) and around the paths of bullets represent thermally shrunken collagen (i.e., gelatin). The role of this phenomenon in skin burns, strangely enough, has not yet been investigated.

Alkaptonuria This rare disease, also called **ochronosis**, can be interpreted as collagen tanning *in vivo*. The patients lack homogentisic acid oxidase, without which homogentisic acid (a normal metabolite of tyrosine and phenylalanine) accumulates in large amounts. The result is dark urine and a darkening or "staining" of articular cartilage, which dies and breaks down causing progressive joint disease. It has been suggested that homogentisic acid is a natural tanning agent that denatures the collagen (23). It may also inhibit lysyl hydroxylase, thus modifying the collagen by yet another mechanism (37).

The Riddle of a Blistering Disorder *Epidermolysis bullosa* is the generic term for 10–14 genetic disorders of the skin and mucous membranes that have one ugly feature in common: the development of blisters after minor trauma. The medical complications can be dramatic: scarring between the fingers and toes, which can lead to digital fusion (Figure 7.17), contractures of joints, scarring of the corneas, chronic infection, and worse. Electron

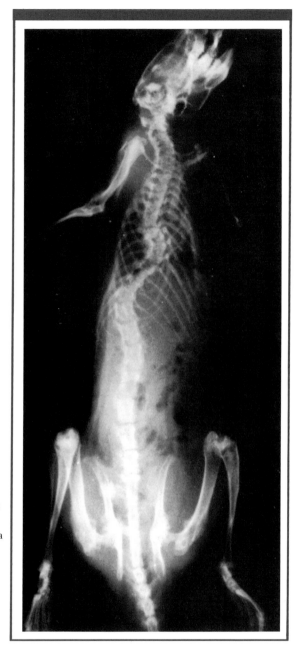

FIGURE 7.12
X-ray of a rat with experimental osteolathyrism: severe distortion of the spinal column, a result of inadequate cross-linking of collagen. (Reproduced with permission from [11].)

medicine is the term "collagen diseases" for a group of connective tissue diseases of autoimmune pathogenesis, such as systemic lupus erythematosus (SLE), rheumatoid arthritis, rheumatic fever, polyarteritis nodosa, dermatomyositis, and scleroderma. The misnaming dates from years—not so long ago—when collagen could be used to mean "connective tissue." It was essentially an accident. In 1942, the eminent pathologist Paul Klemperer realized that these conditions had something in common; he could not yet recognize the autoimmune mechanism, but he correctly identified the common thread as an inflammatory condition in the connective tissue, and thus proposed the name collagen diseases (really meaning connective tissue diseases) (18). The name spread like wildfire, and when Klemperer attempted to change it in 1950, it was too late (17). Just remember that in these "collagen diseases" the collagen is normal. Better yet, try not to use that term.

Pathology of Elastin

The arteries need to be elastic, the skin needs to be elastic, and all soft tissues need some recoil. Elastin is the answer. Fibroblasts and smooth-muscle cells produce most of it. As a protein, elastin is unusual (78, 84); it has received much

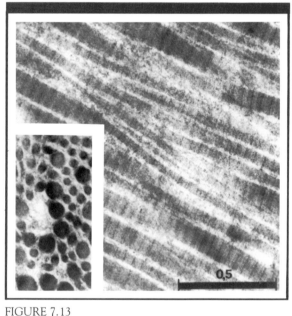

FIGURE 7.13
Collagen fibers of irregular thickness as seen by electron microscopy. *Inset:* Cross section. This was a side effect after 10 years of treatment for Wilson's disease with penicillamine. This drug, used clinically for chelating copper, is thought to interfere with cross-linking in both collagen and elastin. (Reproduced with permission from [46].)

microscopy shows that the blisters form just above or beneath the basement membrane; there is also a lack of anchoring fibrils, the fine filaments of collagen Type VII that tether the basement membrane to the dermis (Figure 7.18) (6, 13, 16). The blisters contain an excessive amount of collagenase that is structurally abnormal (5). Are we dealing here with disorders of collagen, collagenase, or some attachment protein(s)?

A final warning: some "collagen diseases" are not diseases of collagen. One of the classic misnomers in clinical

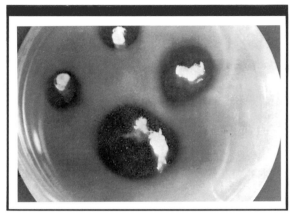

FIGURE 7.14
The discovery of collagenase. Fragments of tadpole tissue were placed on a layer of collagen gel (the opalescent area). The black regions around the explant show digestion of the gel by collagenase. By a stroke of good luck, the authors neglected to add serum or embryo extract to the culture medium, both of which contain a collagenase inhibitor that would have abolished the effect. (Reproduced with permission from [11].)

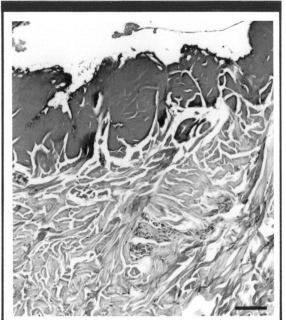

FIGURE 7.16
Thermal shrinkage of collagen along a cut made in human skin with an electrocautery. *Top:* Gelatinized fibers. *Bottom:* Normal collagen fibers. **Bar** = 100 μm.

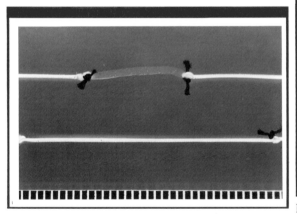

FIGURE 7.15
The phenomenon of thermal contraction of collagen. In these two rat-tail tendons, segments of equal length were marked with knots. In the upper tendon, the segment between the knots was briefly dipped in water at 80°C; it shrank to about one-third of its original size and became gelatinized in the process. The other tendon is a control. Scale in millimeters.

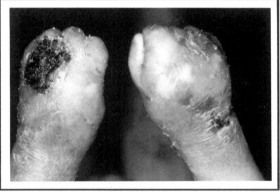

FIGURE 7.17
"Mitten deformity" in a case of epidermolysis bullosa, a clinical condition attributed to a defect in basement membranes. (Courtesy of Dr. E.A. Bauer, Division of Dermatology, Washington University School of Medicine, Seattle, WA.)

attention because it changes (for the worse) with age. Its resistance to chemical agents is astonishing. Until recently the standard method for extracting elastin from a piece of tissue was to autoclave the whole thing or to boil it in alkali, and the solid that was left was assumed to be elastin. Elastin also tends to persist in necrotic tissues after all other structures have disappeared.

Elastin shares with collagen the molecular feature of cross-linking as well as the cross-linking enzyme lysyl oxidase; for this reason it also shares some of collagen's pathology, namely the disturbances induced by cross-linking inhibitors such as those that occur in lathyrism, penicillamine treatment, and copper deficiency (p. 253).

One type of cross-link is specific to elastin. Two lysine residues on one chain join two others of an

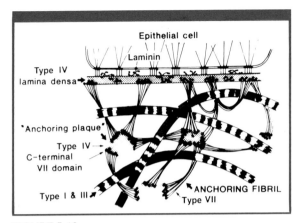

FIGURE 7.18

The complex interaction among four types of collagen beneath an epithelial cell. Anchoring fibrils (Type VII collagen) form loops, and fibrils of Types I and III pass through them. Malfunction of the anchoring fibrils results in epidermolysis (see Figure 7.17). (Reproduced with permission from [16].)

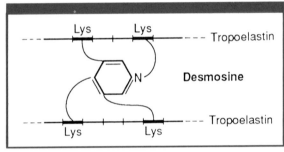

FIGURE 7.19

Desmosine, an amino acid unique to elastin. It develops from four lysine residues in two adjacent molecules of tropoelastin. (Adapted from [61].)

FIGURE 7.20
Arachnodactily (spider fingers) typical of Marfan syndrome, a congenital disease of fibrillin—a component of elastic fibers. (Reproduced with permission from [75].)

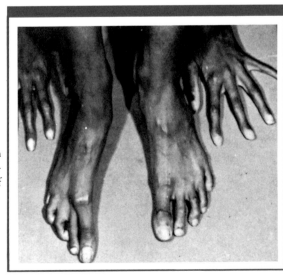

adjacent chain, and the four together form a new amino acid: desmosine or its isomer isodesmosine (Figure 7.19) (61). This amino acid is not reused when elastin is broken down, so the amount of desmosine excreted in the urine can be used to measure elastin turnover (63), much as urinary proline can be used as a marker of collagen turnover.

Compared with rubber threads of the same size, isolated elastic fibers can stretch at least five times more (55), but in the context of tissues they cannot reach that limit because they are intertwined with collagen fibers, which are virtually inextensible. Elastin also differs from rubber in that water is required for its recoil. Its molecule contains hydrophobic regions, which may be related to its tendency to bind lipids (81). It also binds fatty acids, and once it is thus complexed, it is much more susceptible to digestion by elastase (78). These features may play a role in atherosclerotic plaques, where elastin and lipids abound.

Diseases of elastin can be congenital or acquired and can cause the elastic fibers to be increased, decreased, or abnormal (56).

GENETIC DEFECTS

Congenital diseases affecting the elastic fibers are many but, except for Marfan syndrome, rare (56).

Marfan Syndrome One of the most common heritable disorders of connective tissue, Marfan syndrome affects about 1 in 10,000 people. It is typically represented by tall individuals with long, spidery fingers: "arachnodactily" (Figure 7.20). It has been suggested that President Lincoln and Paganini, two of history's tall men, were victims of Marfan syndrome, presumably in a mild form. President Lincoln's DNA is presently being studied (73). The clinical picture includes loose joints, a deformed spine, floppy mitral valves (leading to regurgitation), and eye troubles such as dislocation of the lens. The main threat to life is a sudden rupture of the aorta; histology of the aortic wall shows a thickened wall with defective elastin (Figure 7.21) and pools of metachromatic material (Figure 7.22) (80). After a great deal of work, the molecular defect was linked to two fibrillin genes on chromosomes 5 and 15 (67, 72, 82). The glycoprotein **fibrillin,** identified only in 1986, is a component of the microfibrils associated with elastin, and it happens to be especially abundant in the aorta, the periosteum, and the ligament that holds the lens in place: the tissues most

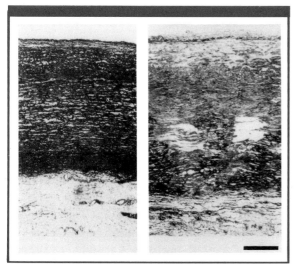

FIGURE 7.21
Example of elastin pathology: aortic wall in cystic medial necrosis (*right*) compared with the wall of a normal aorta (*left*). The pathogenesis of the elastin change in this condition is not understood. Verhoeff's elastic stain. **Bar** =1 mm. (Reproduced with permission from [62].)

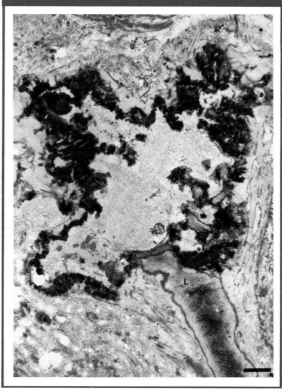

FIGURE 7.22
Faulty elastin in the wall of an artery in Marfan's syndrome. An elastic lamella (**L**) appears to break up into a disorganized mass. **Bar = 2** μm. (Reproduced with permission from [80].)

affected by Marfan syndrome (73). So, a century after it was described by a Paris pediatrician, Marfan syndrome is recognized as a disease of elastic fibers, which disturb these fibers without affecting the elastin molecule itself. It includes a wide spectrum of clinical manifestations (58a).

Cutis Laxa A congenital disease of the elastic fibers is cutis laxa, in which elastic fibers are too few. The skin lacks recoil and appears too large for the body; the face is typically droopy, recalling a bloodhound (Figure 7.23) (74), and the voice may be baritonal because the vocal cords lack tension. Our outward appearance depends a great deal on elastin.

ACQUIRED DEFECTS

Elastin is particularly sensitive to aging, as the cosmetic industry well knows, and elastogenesis in the skin is affected by sunlight, a problem not shared by collagen. The organs richest in elastin are the lungs, and the pathogenesis of emphysema is centered around the destruction of elastic fibers.

Aging Cross-linking increases with age in elastin as it does in collagen, which means that the arteries become progressively stiffer. The amount of calcium bound to the elastic fibers also increases with age. This has been attributed to a progressive increase in acidic amino acids (aspartic and

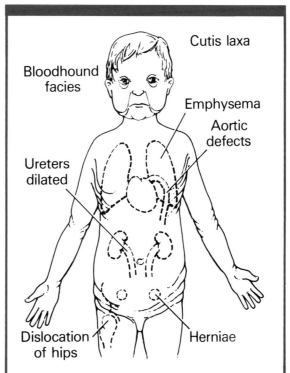

FIGURE 7.23
Multiple defects arising from the lack of normal elastin in cutis laxa. (Modified from [74].)

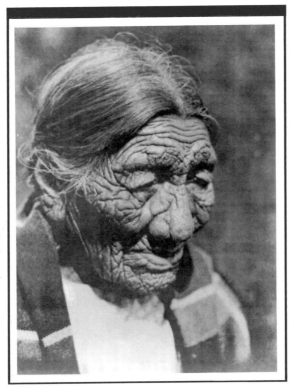

FIGURE 7.24 Portrait of a Cheyenne woman (Black Belly) taken by Edward S. Curtis at the turn of the century. The lumpy skin (solar elastosis) is a long-term effect of exposure to the sun. (Reproduced with permission from [57].)

dermatoheliosis (58, 60) but should really be called sun-worshipers' disease. At first the skin becomes finely wrinkled and loses its elasticity; eventually it becomes lumpy, coarsely wrinkled, and even criss-crossed by deep furrows (Figure 7.24). A classic example is the "redneck," which you might never recognize under the pompous name of *cutis rhomboidalis nuchae*. Microscopically, in all skin areas exposed to the sun, the dermis is thickened and contains seemingly amorphous pools of a basophilic hyalin. This material takes up dyes that normally stain elastic fibers, hence the name *elastosis*; in fact, by scanning electron microscopy, it corresponds to a dense matting of fine, abnormal elastic fibers (Figure 7.25) (83). It is believed that the dermal fibroblasts produce defective elastic fibers because they are damaged by the sun's rays. Note that the cells in the dermis do not live in total darkness: 50–75 percent of sunlight penetrates the epidermis. Experimentally, solar elastosis has been reproduced in hairless mice by exposure to UV light (76) or to X-rays (71).

glutamic), which could bind calcium (68, 69); but it may also depend on an intrinsic property of the elastin molecule, which can nucleate apatite crystals (78). In some atherosclerotic arteries the internal elastic lamina is specifically and strikingly calcified (Figure 6.13).

Solar Elastosis Among the acquired diseases of elastin, solar elastosis can affect almost everybody's face after the age of 30. It is also called

Digestion by Enzymes Elastin is extremely resistant to enzymes, even more so than collagen. However, it can be digested by the elastases. These enzymes are not as specific as collagenases; they also digest many other proteins. Elastases are present in the pancreatic juice, in the granules of neutrophils (66), and on the surfaces of macrophages (70). Elastases are produced by many bacteria, such as *Pseudomonas*; they can play a role in the infectious process by "opening up" the

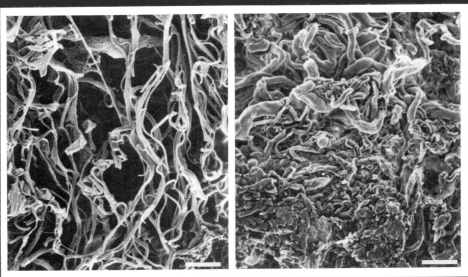

FIGURE 7.25
Elastin fibers obtained from samples of human dermis. (The collagen was destroyed by autoclaving.) *Left:* Normal skin. *Right:* Solar elastosis from the neck of a "redneck" (cutis rhomboidalis nuchae). Scanning electron micrographs. **Bars** = 25 μm. (Reproduced with permission from [83].)

connective tissue spaces and thus favoring bacterial spread. Many strains of *Clostridium histolyticum* produce elastase as well as collagenase (their name *histoLYTICUM* is well deserved). There is even a *Flavobacterium elastolyticum*. Some snake venoms, especially those of rattlesnakes and vipers, owe their local destructive properties to elastase. However, the elastase most relevant to human disease is endogenous: neutrophil elastase, the enzyme that leads to emphysema.

Emphysema. To understand emphysema, remember that the lung is subdivided into myriads of microscopic air spaces (the alveoli) that have the purpose of increasing the surface area avilable for gas exchanges. In emphysema the walls between the alveoli tend to break down, so that the air spaces become larger and larger, and the surface area available for gas exchanges is correspondingly reduced. The lung tissue is vanishing because it is being robbed of its critical elastin scaffolding, as a result of an imbalance between elastase and anti-elastase (called alpha-1-*antitrypsin*). The correlation between emphysema and alpha-1-antitrypsin, as mentioned earlier, is complex (59, 65), but the essentials are as follows. Alpha-1-antitrypsin, despite its name, is important primarily as an antielastase (it represents 90 percent of the antielastase activity of the blood). It is powerless against macrophage elastase but very effective against granulocyte elastase. In smokers, more granulocytes are attracted into the lungs, and there they release their enzymes, elastase included, either because they are activated or because they die. The enzymes cross the endothelial barrier (by transcytosis?), and the elastase attacks the functionally critical elastin framework of the alveoli. The elastase is, of course, more effective if the level of the plasma inhibitor is low (cigarette smoke itself renders the inhibitor ineffective). The final result is a breakdown of the alveolar walls: emphysema. The only enzyme that produces emphysema experimentally if instilled into the bronchi is elastase (66).

Pathology of Basement Membranes

Basement membranes are so thin that they remained ill-defined until the electron microscope came along (96, 97). They are thin indeed (less than 0.1 μm) but surprisingly tough. By electron microscopy, in damaged tissues, it is quite common to see that cells have been destroyed, whereas the basement membranes that supported them are still there. This ability to persist after cell damage has a definite survival value: it enables regenerating cells to grow back into the right places by creeping along a guiding surface (p. 22). The mechanical toughness of basement membranes is largely due to their skeleton of Type IV collagen, which consists of molecules arranged in a network (Figure 7.26)

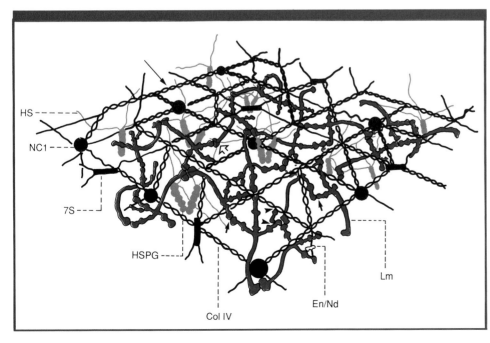

FIGURE 7.26
Molecular model of basement membrane. **HS**: Heparan sulfate chains. **NC1**: Globular (noncollagenous-1) domain of collagen IV. **7S**: N-terminal 7S domain of collagen IV. **HSPG**: Heparan sulfate proteoglycan. **Col IV**: Collagen IV. **En/Nd**: Entactin/nidogen. **Lm**: Laminin. **Long arrow**: Lateral associations of collagen. **Solid short straight arrows**: Laminin self-interactions. **Hollow arrow**: HS binding to laminin G domain. **Arrowheads**: Entactin/nidogen interactions with laminin and collagen. (Courtesy of Dr. P.D. Yurchenco, University of Medicine & Dentistry of New Jersey, Piscataway, NJ.)

(111). This collagenous structure is also their Achilles' heel: it makes them susceptible to destruction by collagenases, which are secreted by leukocytes, especially in the course of inflammation (p. 322, 402).

Basement Membranes as Molecular Traps All basement membranes contain highly charged, "sticky" molecules such as heparan sulfate and fibronectin. This explains their affinity for calcium and silver ions; the latter property is exploited to make them visible in histologic

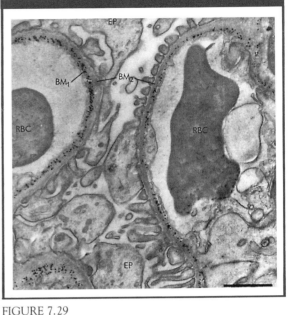

FIGURE 7.29

Affinity of basement membranes for silver nitrate (argyrophilia). Glomerulus of a normal rat that was made argyric upon weaning and then allowed to live for another 5 months without silver in the drinking water. **BM₁**: Oldest layer of basement membrane synthesized during silver treatment; note the peppering of silver granules (black dots). The younger layer free of silver (**BM₂**) lies beneath the epithelial cells (**EP**), indicating that these are the cells that synthesized it. **RBC**: Red blood cell. **Bar** = 1 μm. (Reproduced with permission from [92].)

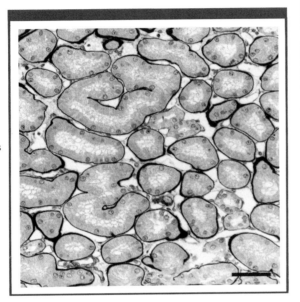

FIGURE 7.27 Basement membrane (thin black line) around kidney tubules demonstrated by means of silver impregnation. **Bar** = 50 μm. (Courtesy of Geneviève Leyvraz, Department of Pathology, University of Geneva, Switzerland.)

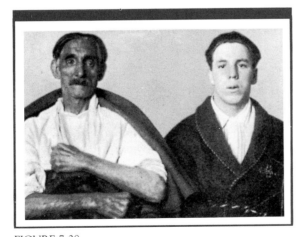

FIGURE 7.28

Left: Argyria in a man who worked for about 20 years in the manufacture of silver nitrate. His skin became a slaty-grey, hence the nickname of "blue men" for such individuals. *Right:* Normal man for comparison. (Reproduced with permission from [91].)

sections (Figure 7.27). The same property is displayed by basement membranes *in vivo*. So, try to imagine what might happen to people who absorb silver ions, for one reason or another, over several years. Not so long ago, patients who faithfully followed prescriptions of silver nitrate *per os* for several years, supposedly as a cure for gastric ulcer (85), became slowly grey as their basement membranes became impregnated with metallic silver. The same condition, known as **argyria** (90), can develop from industrial exposure (Figure 7.28) (91). It is easily reproduced in rats by adding silver nitrate to the drinking water and can be used for studying the slow growth of glomerular basement membranes (Figure 7.29) (92, 108), much as we use tree rings to study the growth of a tree (94). The silver-binding story may sound like a freak accident, but what binds silver may bind other molecules. *Basement membranes can act as reservoirs of growth factors.* This surprising development is well explained by the very nature of growth factors, which can be separated biochemically according to their affinity for heparin (87, 104). Thus growth factors, including angiogenic factors, happen to be stored ready for use precisely where they will be needed. We expect to hear about other molecules stored in basement membranes.

Pathologic Thickening Thickening of the basement membrane is fairly common, especially around capillaries and beneath epithelia. Perhaps it reflects a persistent, low-grade state of irritation of the cells that produce the basement membrane, be they epithelial or other. For example, in the bronchial mucosa of asthmatics, the subepithelial basement membrane can become thick enough to be visible by light microscopy, thus earning the name **lamina vitrea** (Figure 7.30); the bronchial epithelium of asthmatics is certainly in a chronic state of irritation (p. 524). The lamina vitrea seems to be harmless, but it is quite another matter when multiple thick layers of basement membrane are wrapped around capillaries; in such cases there must be some restriction of the lumen (95) although this effect has not been well studied. Just glance at two examples taken from tissues exposed to chronic, subtle injury, such as the skin of

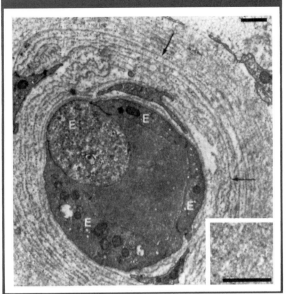

FIGURE 7.31 Multiple basement membranes (**arrows**) around a capillary of the dermis in a case of erythropoietic protoporphyria produced by long-wave UV light. **E**: Endothelial cells. *Inset: detail.* **Bars** = 1 μm. (Reproduced with permission from [88].)

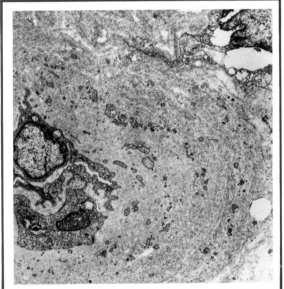

FIGURE 7.32 Thickening of the basement membrane in a ureteral capillary of a patient who abused the analgesic phenacetin. Severe restriction of the lumen. (Courtesy of M.J. Mihatsch, Institute for Pathology, Basel, Switzerland.)

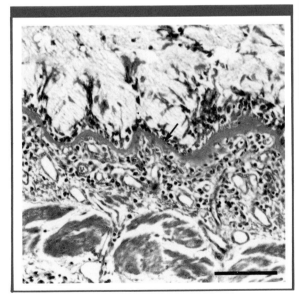

FIGURE 7.30 Thickening of the epithelial basement membrane (**arrow**) in a bronchus from a case of asthma. At the top is the lumen of the bronchus, filled with mucus and desquamated epithelial cells. In the connective tissue of the mucosa, many inflammatory cells are present. The thickening of the basement membrane is probably due to chronic irritation of the epithelial cells that produce it. **Bar** = 100 μm.

patients suffering from **porphyria,** a condition of abnormal sensitivity to sunlight (Figure 7.31), or the renal and perirenal tissues in individuals who abused the analgesic phenacetin (Figure 7.32) (88, 101).

The multilayered appearance of the pericapillary basement membrane was once explained by cycles of death and regeneration of pericytes, which are entirely wrapped in basement membrane. A more likely explanation is that endothelial cells are somehow turned on to form successive layers of basement membrane (97, 105, 106). What might turn them

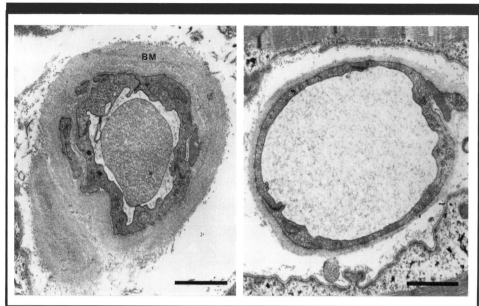

FIGURE 7.33
Left: Thickening of the pericapillary basement membrane (**BM**) in human diabetes. *Right:* Control. **Bars** = 1 μm. (Courtesy of Dr. J.R. Williamson, Washington University School of Medicine, St. Louis, MO.)

on remains unknown. Regarding the abuse of phenacetin, all we can say is that rats treated with analgesics can develop outright necrosis of the renal papilla (89). (Note: Multiple basement membranes around venules are a normal feature (110), but onion-skin arrangements such as illustrated in Figure 7.31 and 7.32 are clearly abnormal.)

A diffuse thickening of the pericapillary basement membranes is typical in diabetics (109) (Figure 7.33), which is puzzling in several respects. Why does it develop? Why does it select the capillary basement membranes? How does it affect the microcirculation? In diabetes the thickening around the glomerular capillaries can be extreme: irregular lumps of basement membrane material are large enough to be seen by light microscopy and to warrant a special name for this condition, **Kimmelstiel–Wilson glomerulosclerosis** (95).

The biochemical changes in the capillary basement membranes of diabetics are complex and not fully understood (102). In the glomerular basement membranes of diabetics the heparan sulfate component is reduced, which correlates well with the observed increase in glomerular permeability (96). Persistent hyperglycemia is harmful because it leads to cross-linking of proteins and thus to the formation of "advanced glycosylation end-products" (AGE, p. 267). The AGE in turn have a number of pernicious effects (Table 7.1). In rats the intravenous injection of glycosylated plasma proteins for 12 weeks caused glomerular changes similar to those of diabetes (100). Experimental diabetes induced in rats with streptozotocin (which selectively kills the pancreatic

---

TABLE 7.1

Possible Effects of Hyperglycemia on Capillary Basement Membrane (BM)

AGE* develop on and between BM macromolecules; this
- interferes with the self-assembly of BM
- reduces the susceptibility of BM to enzymatic degradation
- traps plasma proteins seeping into the BM
- decreases BM affinity for growth-modulating heparan sulfate proteoglycans

AGE bind to macrophage receptors; the activated macrophages release cytokines (TNF, IL-1, etc.) with multiple effects:
- stimulation of matrix synthesis
- hypertrophy/hyperplasia of endothelial/smooth muscle cells
- procoagulant changes of the endothelial surface

**Advanced glycosylation end-products.*
Adapted from (102).

beta cells) also produces the typical glomerular changes. In humans this lesion is at least partially reversible by control of the hyperglycemia (103). There is much evidence to show that diabetes affects the endothelium and the pericytes (p. 669).

Basement Membranes Are Not All Alike Basement membranes look alike but differ chemically. The first evidence for this was provided in 1933 by a Japanese pathologist, M. Masugi, who injected rats with anti–rat-kidney antibodies prepared by injecting rat kidney into rabbits (99). The result was a glomerular disease now known as **Masugi nephrotoxic nephritis,** characterized by antibody deposition all along the glomerular basement membranes. What did *not* happen to Masugi's rats was very interesting: *the basement membranes in other organs remained intact (93, 98).* Therefore, they must be chemically different.

A similar lesson is taught by a human autoimmune disease, best known as the **Goodpasture syndrome.** This disease depends on an antigen present only in the basement membranes of the glomeruli and of the alveolar capillaries (p. 529, 574).

> **Congenital diseases of the basement membrane.** *The best candidate for a congenital disease is the rare Alport syndrome (hereditary progressive glomerulopathy), in which the glomerular basement membrane is thinned, allowing the escape of red blood cells (hematuria). Renal insufficiency may follow. Recent studies of one family suggest a diffuse abnormality of all basement membranes (97). A primary basement membrane defect may also be at the root of the nephronopthisis syndrome, a cause of renal failure in the young: cystic dilatations appear in the medullary tubules, and the cortex becomes atrophic (86).*

Pathology of Proteoglycans

Proteoglycans are huge, feathery molecules shaped like test-tube brushes. The stem is a long molecule of hyaluronic acid (a **glycosaminoglycan,** formerly called mucopolysaccharide). Attached to this stem at regular intervals are **core proteins** bearing many chains of shorter glycosaminoglycans (e.g., chondroitin sulfate, keratan sulfate). Link proteins reinforce the attachment (Figure 7.34). Although typical of the connective tissue spaces, proteoglycans are also a component of basement membranes and of cell membranes, where their main functions relate to cell recognition, attachment, and growth control (123, 128).

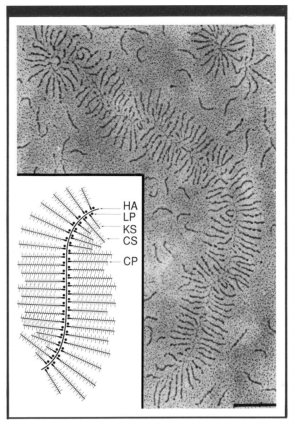

FIGURE 7.34 The feathery structure of a proteoglycan molecule seen with the electron microscope. (Reproduced with permission from [113].) *Inset:* Diagram of the molecular architecture. **HA:** Backbone of hyaluronic acid. **LP:** Link protein. **KS:** Keratan sulfate. **CS:** Chondroitin sulfate. **CP:** Core protein. (Reproduced with permission from [127].)

When woven into the connective tissue matrix, *proteoglycans bind vast amounts of fluid and are therefore responsible for holding interstitial water in place;* without them, all the water would flow into our legs, as actually happens when their fluid-carrying capacity is exceeded (p. 603). *They also bind a variety of other molecules, such as growth factors* (117, 128): a wonderful arrangement for keeping on hand, and in an inactive state, bioactive molecules that may be needed on short notice. The same arrangement is at work in mast cell granules: a core of proteoglycans binds inflammatory mediators, ready to be released within seconds (p. 329).

Proteoglycans are involved in the pathology of joints. They form the bulk of the matrix in articular cartilage where they are synthesized by the chondrocytes under the stimulus of mechanical loading. They are essential for the protection of cartilage against overload; under pressure, some of the water squeezes out and mixes with the synovial fluid, helping lubrication. When joint cartilage is underloaded, as happens when a limb is immobilized in a plaster cast, there is a sharp decrease in proteoglycan synthesis within a few days (112, 126).

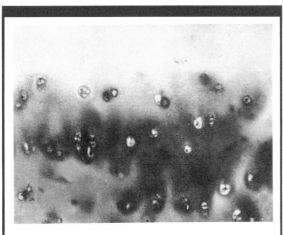

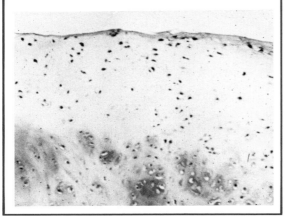

FIGURE 7.35
Top: Normal articular cartilage from the femoral head. The dark areas, red in the original, correspond to the dye Safranin-O and indicate a normal content of proteoglycans. *Bottom:* Similar cartilage in osteoarthrosis, showing extensive loss of proteoglycans. (Courtesy of the American Rheumatism Association, Atlanta, GA.)

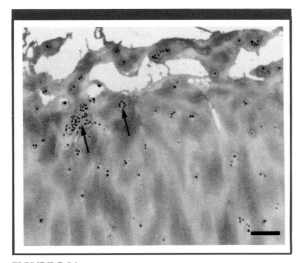

FIGURE 7.36
Breakdown of the extracellular matrix on the articular surface of a knee joint, in a case of degenerative arthritis. Bits of cartilage are flaking off; clusters of regenerating cells do develop (**arrows**) but a coordinated replacement of the lost cartilage does not occur. **Bar** = 100 μm. (From a biopsy, courtesy of Dr. Y. Kapanci, Department of Pathology, Geneva, Switzerland.)

Extracellular "Degeneration" of Cartilage The very common osteoarthritis (degenerative arthritis) begins with a reduction in the proteoglycan content of the articular cartilage (Figure 7.35). The mechanism is not clear (112, 118). Later the collagen fibers, which normally act as a scaffolding for the proteoglycans, are exposed and tend to separate like the hair of a brush, so that the normally shiny surface of the joint cartilage appears velvety (Figure 7.36). *This complex extracellular breakdown is one of the rare pathologic events that can properly be called "degenerative."*

> The term "degeneration" was widely used in pathology before the 1950s, when little was known about cell biology; it vaguely implied that some sort of breakdown was involved. For example, steatosis was called fatty degeneration, as if the droplets of fat were released by the breakdown of cellular structures. Today we know better. The label "degeneration" remains legitimate in rare instances, e.g. for the joint disease just mentioned in which there is a true breakdown of extracellular material, and for Wallerian degeneration, which refers to the breakdown of the axon separated from its cell of origin (p. 26). In neuropathology the term "degenerative" is applied—only as "a confession of ignorance" (115)—to diseases in which neurons disappear for no known reason, as in Alzheimer's disease.

Myxedema Myxedema ("mucous edema") is the traditional name for a special variety of edema due to an excess of proteoglycans or their building blocks. It is nonpitting (p. 608) and limited to a few conditions, one of which is **advanced hypothyroidism,** now rarely seen. Hyaluronic acid accumulates in the tissue spaces (with some organ preferences) and causes symptoms accordingly: puffy face, thick cold skin, hoarse voice, swollen tongue, and stiff joints. The metabolic disturbance appears to be a reduction in hyaluronic acid degradation (116, 122). Paradoxically, Grave's disease, which leads to **hyperthyroidism,** also leads to an excessive deposition of glycosaminoglycans; even more strangely, this happens only in the pretibial area (pretibial myxedema) (Figure 7.37) (120). Because the thyroid in Grave's disease is overstimulated by an autoimmune mechanism (p. 571), it is possible that some fibroblasts may be stimulated by a similar mechanism (121). But why just the pretibial fibroblasts? Studies *in vitro* have shown that fibroblasts can be stimulated by a factor in the blood of these patients, whereas fibroblasts obtained from the shoulder area remain indifferent

(114). This is a fine example of "homologous" cells from different parts of the body not being biologically identical.

Pathologic Changes Due to Glucose

Our quest for mechanisms of disease leads us to discuss a danger that faces many of our macromolecules, be they extra- or intracellular. *Proteins that have very long lives, such as collagen and hemoglobin, are subject to chronic attack from an unlikely source: glucose.* The mechanism is **nonenzymatic glycation** (formerly called glycosylation).

Our story begins once again with the food industry, which has long been aware of the "browning reaction". This reaction is essentially a nuisance: if milk is heated for a long time, sugar and proteins combine to form brown, bitter, burnt-tasting products called melanoidins (nothing to do with melanin, nor with the browning of fruit, which is due to different compounds, p. 103). This reaction contributes to the brown color and toughness of cooked meat (135). Only recently did it dawn upon nonfood scientists that the same reaction is involved in aging and especially in diabetes (131).

The reaction proceeds step by step without the help of enzymes, reversibly at first and then irreversibly. To begin, the aldehyde group of glucose reacts randomly with an amino group on a protein, giving rise to a ketoamine or Schiff base, which is unstable (Figure 7.38). This product quickly rearranges itself into a so-called Amadori product—still reversible. Now, if the protein persists in the body for months or years (or if food

is cooked longer), some of its Amadori products slowly dehydrate and rearrange themselves—again—into irreversible, brown, autofluorescent structures that Cerami and his group have called **advanced glycosylation end-products** or AGEs, a hint to their presumed role. Some of the AGEs can form cross-links between adjacent proteins, for instance, by condensation of two Amadori products (Figure 7.39) (129).

This sequence has enormous implications, especially for diabetes. *If we list all the long-term complications of diabetes* (better known since insulin therapy was introduced in 1922), *a link with long-lived proteins now seems obvious for all:* accelerated arteriosclerosis (hardening of arteries), cataract, neuropathy, microangiopathy, and stiffened joints (well illustrated in Figure 7.40 by the so-called prayer sign). In diabetes, collagen does indeed become more brown, more cross-linked, as if it were older (133, 134), and autofluorescent (136). The thickening of basement membranes

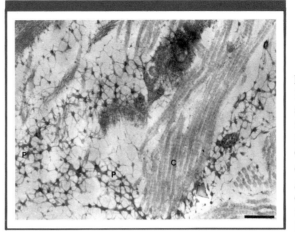

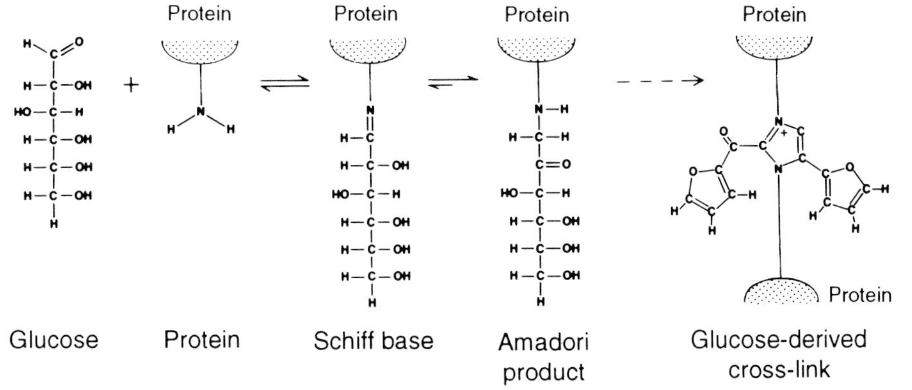

FIGURE 7.37 Electron microscopic view of myxedema: **P:** Proteoglycan. **C:** Collagen bundles. **Bar** = 0.5 μm. (Reproduced with permission from [120].)

FIGURE 7.38 Mechanism of non-enzymatic glycation, showing how two molecules of protein become cross-linked by glucose. (Reproduced with permission from [131].)

Glucose   Protein   Schiff base   Amadori product   Glucose-derived cross-link

FIGURE 7.39 Formation of cross-links in matrix protein due to advanced glycosylation end-products (AGEs). The vertical columns represent collagen or other interstitial proteins. From the top downward, the figure shows the formation of irreversible AGE products. The lower part shows how lipoproteins can also become cross-linked with matrix proteins. The latter process may explain why atherosclerosis is accelerated in diabetics. (Reproduced with permission from [129].)

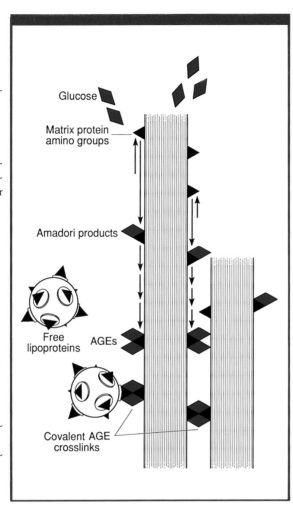

Glucose

Matrix protein amino groups

Amadori products

Free lipoproteins

AGEs

Covalent AGE crosslinks

5 percent of Hb is covalently linked to glucose and becomes chromatographically distinct as HbA_{1c}. In diabetes, HbA_{1c} is increased 2- or 3-fold; thus the concentration HbA_{1c} is now used as a convenient measure of overall glucose control (130, 134).

It is certainly a paradox that glucose, the principal cellular fuel, should also be an enemy of extracellular proteins. High glucose levels may even up-regulate the expression of Type VI collagen genes (137). All this may explain nature's efforts to keep blood glucose below 200 mg/dl (134).

Amyloid

The ways of disease are never-ending: one of them is to create deposits of a material called amyloid. This is a fascinating topic but not an easy one. We will therefore begin by offering a working definition of amyloid. The reader will find out by the end of this chapter that almost every part of this definition has exceptions, but it will be useful as a compass while we are zigzagging through this difficult territory.

The term **amyloid** *refers to a group of largely unrelated, pathologic, insoluble, extracellular, fibrous proteins that usually derive from precursors present in the blood, and have in common several properties:*

- *They are stained by the dye Congo red, and once so stained, they appear green in polarized light.*
- *They appear by electron microscopy as filaments 75–100 Å thick.*
- *By X-ray diffraction the polypeptide chains in the filaments do not run lengthwise but transversely back and forth, in the unusual beta or pleated-sheet pattern.*

Amyloidosis, the extracellular accumulation of amyloid, ranges from local microscopic deposits of no clinical significance to extensive, lethal infiltrations of vital organs (Figure 7.41). Because this massive form can arise as a side-effect of chronic inflammatory diseases, it was seen frequently in the past when tuberculosis and osteomyelitis were incurable. Massive amyloidosis is rare today, but many microscopic forms have been discovered. As a result, amyloidosis is recognized once again as one of the most prevalent pathologic processes, associated not only with chronic infections but also with chronic aseptic inflammatory diseases such as rheumatoid arthritis, with tumors, aging, old thrombi (180), and Alzheimer's disease. It also occurs in hereditary forms.

could also be related to protein trapping and cross-linking (129, 132). In fact, the structural modification of proteins could have almost limitless consequences (132).

In this light, diabetes can be seen as a natural model of accelerated aging, a hypothesis that can be tested—to some extent—*in vitro*: Cerami et al. found that the long, thin tendons of young rat tails become tougher if incubated with glucose, and clear solutions of bovine lens proteins become cloudy if glucose is added, suggesting a "cataract in the test tube" (131). All these findings also mean that *blocking AGE formation could offer new hope against damage to proteins.* There are some facts to support this hope, based on therapeutic tests with hydrazines, which bind to Amadori products and prevent them from progressing to AGEs (129, 131, 131a).

In the meantime, at least one glycation product has found practical uses: hemoglobin (Hb), which is constantly exposed to blood glucose during its relatively long 4-month life; even normally about

Only a few years ago amyloid was a total mystery. Today some key facts are clear; they add up to a very unpredictable story (152, 155).

THE AMYLOID SAGA

When amyloid is present in kilogram amounts, it is hard to miss, at least at autopsy; anatomists in the 1700s knew very well that sometimes the liver, the spleen, and other organs appear strangely swollen and firm, as if they had been infiltrated by some abnormal stiff material. In the mid-1800s the Viennese school described such organs as "lardaceous" (baconlike); but this, Virchow objected, meant only that the Viennese understood little about bacon—waxy was more accurate (236). In any event, it was clear that some abnormal hyalin material was infiltrating the tissues, and in 1853 Virchow took the view that it was probably an "animal cellulose," a tempting synthesis of the plant and animal kingdoms (237). In his day it was known that cellulose treated with sulfuric acid was converted into a carbohydrate called amyloid (starchlike), which turned blue with iodine (219). Virchow convinced himself that fresh "waxy" organs gave this reaction and concluded that the mysterious material was indeed an animal cellulose. In retrospect, the color change produced on fresh organs was not always willing to appear, and the term amyloid was a misnomer. However, Virchow did confirm that the abnormal material was often found in the organs of patients who had died of some wasting disease and even hypothesized that a precursor material should exist in the blood. Promptly the chemists objected that amyloid was albuminous, that is, a protein, not a carbohydrate, and right they were.

From then onward progress was slow because all the proteins called amyloid (as we now know) seem to be planned to complicate the lives of chemists as well as histologists: *amyloids are almost insoluble, they are inert (poorly reactive), refractory to most stains, and poorly antigenic.*

However, in 1922, a step forward took place: the accidental discovery that the dye Congo red stained amyloid rather selectively. This staining method did not reveal anything about the nature of amyloid, but it made the microscopic diagnosis of amyloid much easier. It is used to this day.

> The accidental discovery was made in a medical ward in Hamburg where Congo red was being used to study blood volume (145). In some patients the dye seemed to disappear faster, and a look at the records showed that all these patients suffered from

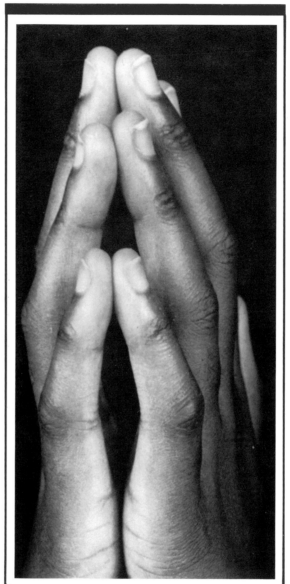

FIGURE 7.40
The "prayer sign" in diabetes. Pathologic cross-linking of collagen molecules results in stiff joints, including the inability to approximate the palmar surfaces. (Young woman of 17 with insulin-dependent diabetes for 14 years.) (Reproduced with permission from [138].)

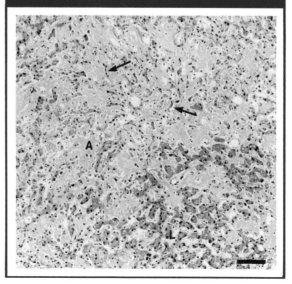

FIGURE 7.41
Amyloidosis of the liver. The cords of liver cells (**L**) are dissociated by masses of amyloid (**A**). Note the extreme atrophy of some liver cells (**arrows**). **Bar** = 100 μm.

amyloidosis. At the autopsy of one patient, the glomeruli on the cut surface of the kidney stood out as red dots, and the liver looked unusually red. The next step was obvious: try Congo red as a histologic stain. This story also tells us that wasting diseases must have been very common in 1922.

The Congo red method came with a bonus. Although the stained amyloid on tissue sections looked rather pale, yellowish, and unimpressive, under polarized light it shone bright green (163). This means that stained amyloid is dichroic, i.e., that the absorption of light passing through it varies with the plane of polarization of the light (183). Today this apple-green effect is still the best method for the microscopic diagnosis of amyloid. Furthermore, unstained amyloid was reported to be birefringent, indicating that despite its smooth, glassy appearance it had to be, at the ultramicroscopic level, a fibrillar material (163). This turned out to be perfectly accurate.

By the 1950s it was apparent that amyloid infiltration of various organs developed under sets of conditions that had nothing in common. The best that one could do was to separate the cases of generalized amyloidosis into two categories: cases in which there seemed to be no underlying disease at all, called **primary amyloidosis,** and cases in which there was an associated wasting disease (as Virchow and others had noticed), called **secondary amyloidosis.** Furthermore, many cases—but not all—pointed to some association with the immune response; for instance, amyloidosis was common in the hyperimmunized horses used for the commercial production of antisera, yet the amyloid itself was different from antibody proteins (i.e., gamma globulins) and it certainly was no antigen–antibody precipitate. Amyloid was also discovered in certain tumors or in isolated lumps with no relation to tumors; it appeared even in the pancreatic islets of aging individuals. No unifying theory seemed possible. Amyloid was a depressing topic.

Then came the electron microscope. In 1959, Cohen and Calkins contributed some important new facts. Amyloid was indeed fibrillar (154) (Figure 7.42), and fibrils were nonbranching, 75–100 Å in diameter, and made of two filaments twisted around each other. Another component, a doughnut-shaped pentagonal molecule, was usually associated with them (Figure 7.43) (147). But this newly discovered unity was itself a puzzle. How could the same types of fibrils be formed under such diverse clinical conditions?

Eventually chemistry came through. Amyloid, which had been so stubbornly insoluble, yielded to more drastic extraction methods with denaturing solvents, and eventually it turned out—somewhat embarrassingly—that the best solvent was distilled water (215). Thanks to the availability of purified amyloid, the material from two cases of primary amyloidosis was sequenced in 1971 by Glenner and colleagues at the National Institutes of Health (NIH). Surprise: *that particular type of amyloid turned out to have the same amino acid sequence as the light chains of gamma globulin molecules* (Figure 7.44) (175). This was a great step: it echoed the prediction of an eminent immunologist, who used to say that someday amyloid would turn out to be "gammyloid" (but not all amyloids are "gammyloids," as we will see).

However, every discovery raises new questions. If some amyloid fibrils were made of gamma globulin light chains, why did they aggregate into fibrils? One good place for studying the light chains of gamma globulins was the urine of patients with multiple myeloma, a tumor of the gamma globulin-secreting plasma cells. Apparently the malignant plasma cells produce not only gamma globulins but also an excess of one of their building blocks, the light chains. These are small enough to pass into the urine, where they have long been known as **Bence–Jones protein.** This protein deserves the distinction of a personal name because it has an unusual property: it precipitates if the urine is heated to 40–50°C but then redissolves at the boiling point. The precipitate of Bence–Jones proteins was examined: it was not fibrillar. Why not? Here lay an obvious challenge.

The elegant answer came again from NIH. If the Bence–Jones protein is submitted to mild digestion with a proteolytic enzyme (trypsin), it promptly turns into a cloudy precipitate made of fibrils that are stainable by Congo red and have the ultrastructure of amyloid (175). This was a major breakthrough; it meant that *amyloid could be obtained from a given protein by mild proteolytic digestion.* The path was now clear for the next step: if semidigested immunoglobulins could be turned into fibrils, the same result might be obtained with other proteins (173).

All this work was done *in vitro.* To explain amyloid as a disease, we need some mechanism to produce mild proteolytic digestion *in vivo.* The culprit is now thought to be the macrophage; therefore, the current working hypothesis to explain amyloid (or better, *some* amyloids) is that

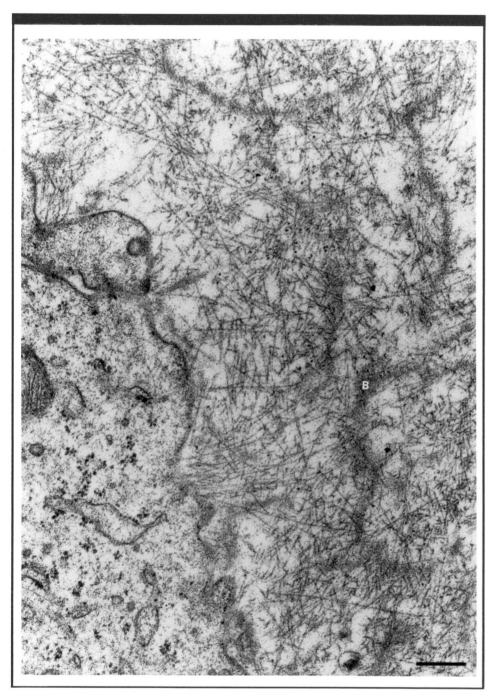

FIGURE 7.42
Experimental amyloidosis in the guinea pig. Renal peritubular deposit of typical amyloid fibrils: rigid, non-branching, diameter 70–100 Å, length indeterminate. **B**: Basement membrane. **Bar** = 0.5 μm. (Kindly provided by Dr. A.S. Cohen, Boston City Hospital, Boston, MA.)

the macrophages are capable of acting on various amyloid precursor proteins, converting them by partial digestion into fibrils that all look very much alike (164). This processing could be in part intracellular (225), but there is evidence that the responsible enzyme is an elastase that is present on the surface of macrophages and other cells. This means that the precursor protein might be processed just by contact with the right type of cell. Monocytes killed and lightly fixed with glutaralde-

hyde are of course not capable of phagocytizing, yet if they are incubated with an amyloid precursor protein, amyloid appears in the medium, suggesting that a surface enzyme has survived fixation (204). Other cell types may have such surface enzymes—for instance, lymphocytes (203).

X-ray diffraction (148, 167) shows that the polypeptide chains of amyloid are arranged perpendicular to the axis of the fibril in the beta or pleated-sheet pattern (Figure 7.45), which is

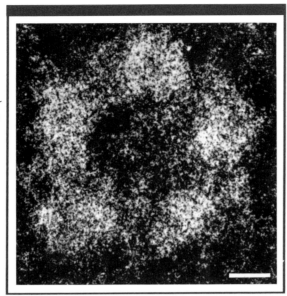

FIGURE 7.43
Ring-shaped component of human spleen amyloid, negatively stained with phosphotungstic acid. This enlargement clearly shows five globular subunits. **Bar** = 0.001 μm. (Reproduced with permission from [147].)

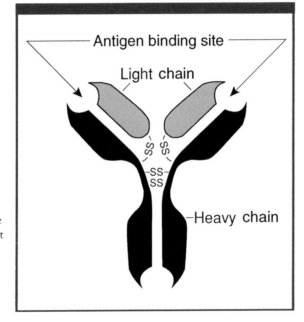

FIGURE 7.44
Diagram of an IgG molecule, emphasizing the light chains that are relevant to the genesis of amyloidosis. (Adapted from [186].)

Antigen binding site

Light chain

-SS-
-SS-
-SS-
-SS

Heavy chain

found in silk but is uncommon in vertebrates (148). In fact, amyloid has been described as an abortive effort of the vertebrates to rival the silkworms (171). Because this beta or pleated sheet structure is the basic characteristic of amyloid, it has been proposed that the many conditions that lead to amyloid deposition be unified under the name **beta fibrilloses** (171).

To visualize the pleating, it should be understood that the amyloid fibril is really a ribbon, as shown in Figure 7.45. Generally speaking, in filamentous proteins the polypeptide chains can assume two orderly arrangements, alpha and beta. The alpha

pattern is a helix; the beta pattern is a flat sheet or ribbon in which the polypeptide chain runs back and forth transversely (the so-called antiparallel arrangement). The ribbon is finely corrugated, that is, pleated longitudinally (238). In amyloid, two such ribbons are twisted together. The beta pleated sheet structure of amyloid is consistent with its resistance to digestion in vivo and in vitro, with its optical properties, and also with the staining by Congo red (174). In one type of amyloid (AA) there seems to be an associated, longitudinal, nonbeta component.

Who could ever have predicted that macrophages could process such widely different proteins to yield the same type of fibril?

Other pieces of the puzzle have now been added. To be amyloidogenic after proteolysis, proteins must contain beta pleated-sheet sequences that can be excised; thereafter, the segments chopped out must be able to self-assemble into ribbons. Some amyloids do not appear to require proteolysis: the precursor assembles by a natural tendency or even as a result of high concentration. Other mechanisms of fibrillogenesis may still be discovered.

GROSS AND MICROSCOPIC ASPECTS OF AMYLOIDOSIS

Mild deposits of amyloid escape the naked eye, but heavily infiltrated organs are pale, stiff, and waxy, just as Virchow insisted; after fixation the liver or spleen may be almost as hard as wood. Histologically, the connective tissue spaces are filled with an extraneous, insoluble, eosinophilic, hyaline material (150); the deposits have a strong tendency to infiltrate the vascular walls, especially the arterioles, recalling the fact that amyloid precursors come mostly from the blood (Figure 7.46). A small amount of highly sulfated glycosaminoglycans is incorporated in many and perhaps all amyloids (198, 206, 230, 231); perhaps it explains the occasional carbohydratelike reaction dear to Virchow.

The bulk of amyloid is extracellular; however, bundles of fibrils can be found in plasma cells, macrophages, hepatocytes, neurons, and other cells, either free or in lysosomes (168, 225, 241). Amyloid sometimes develops in deep indentations of the surfaces of macrophages, much as collagen arises from deep infoldings of fibroblasts. *The tissues infiltrated with amyloid do not seem to react;* somehow, the macrophages do not perceive the fibrils as foreign material to phagocytize. The tissue response is passive: cells are crowded out, undergo atrophy, and fade away. This effect can be extreme in the

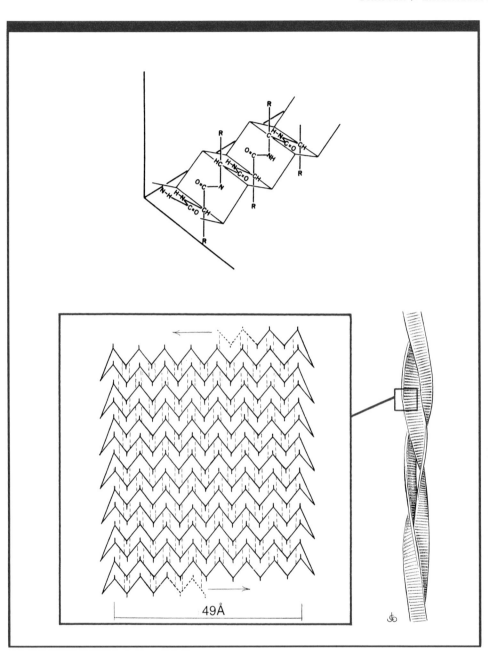

FIGURE 7.45
Molecular structure of amyloid fibrils. *Top*: Three-dimensional representation of a molecular chain in the beta conformation, showing the pleated sheet effect. (Reproduced with permission from [141].) *Bottom left*: Scheme of a "cross-beta" pleated sheet ribbon 49 Å in width. The long axis of the ribbon is from top to bottom. (Modified from [177].) *Bottom right*: Entire fibril, made of two intertwined ribbons. (Reproduced with permission from [159].)

spleen (Figure 7.47), and in the liver (Figure 7.41); however, the functional reserve of the liver is such that liver failure in amyloidosis is rare. Amyloidosis of the heart is the main cause of death in generalized amyloidosis. Amyloid deposits in the wall of the glomerular capillaries cause them to become, rather paradoxically, more permeable to protein; renal insufficiency is the second major cause of death by amyloidosis (Figure 7.48).

MAIN TYPES OF AMYLOID AND THEIR GENESIS

Each type of amyloidosis is an interesting experiment of nature. We cannot discuss every type

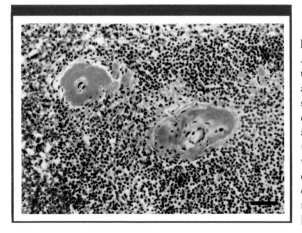

FIGURE 7.46
Amyloid deposition in two arterioles of the spleen. The media is hyalinized and destroyed. (Man aged 57 with AA amyloidosis.) (Reproduced with permission from [212].)

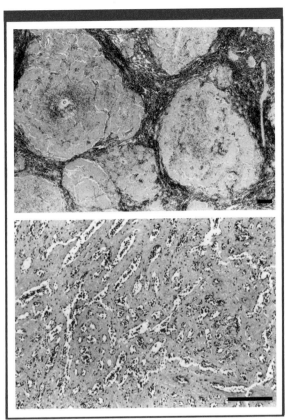

FIGURE 7.47
Two patterns of amyloid deposition in the human spleen. *Top:* "Sago spleen." Nodular deposition in the white pulp (AA amyloid). *Bottom:* "Lardaceous spleen." Diffuse deposition occurs in the red pulp (AL amyloid). The mechanisms leading to these patterns are not understood. **Bar** = 100 μm. (Reproduced with permission from [212].)

shown in the latest official classification (Table 7.2) (153, 190), but we can summarize the current status (151, 155, 171, 176, 177, 197, 200). There are local and generalized forms, all with different amyloid precursors all of which are defined. We will begin with the two best known generalized forms, which (like all amyloids) were saddled with rather skimpy names:

- **AL** (for **a**myloid/**l**ight chain, sometimes called *primary* or myeloma-related);
- **AA** (for amyloid A, so called because it was the first to be chemically characterized; also called *secondary*).

Amyloid AL This is the light-chain variety and as such it includes the cases due to multiple myeloma (201). The reader may notice a contradiction: if this is also called primary amyloidosis, how can it be secondary to myeloma? The reason is that in earlier days some patients with this form of amyloidosis seemed to have no physical disease at all. Then plasma electrophoresis came along and showed that these patients do indeed have an abnormality; the tracing shows a thick band of gamma globulins or of their light-chain fragment (Figure 7.49).

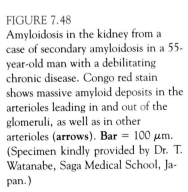

FIGURE 7.48
Amyloidosis in the kidney from a case of secondary amyloidosis in a 55-year-old man with a debilitating chronic disease. Congo red stain shows massive amyloid deposits in the arterioles leading in and out of the glomeruli, as well as in other arterioles (**arrows**). **Bar** = 100 μm. (Specimen kindly provided by Dr. T. Watanabe, Saga Medical School, Japan.)

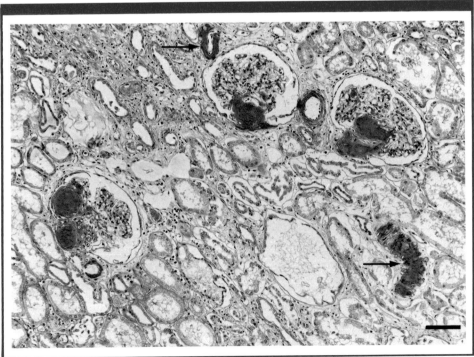

TABLE 7.2

The 1990 Guidelines for Nomenclature and Classification of Amyloid and Amyloidosis

AMYLOID PROTEIN[a]	PROTEIN PRECURSOR	PROTEIN TYPE OF VARIANT	CLINICAL
AA[b]	apoSAA		Reactive (secondary)
			Familial Mediterranean fever
			Familial amyloid nephropathy with urticaria and deafness (Muckle–Wells syndrome)
AL	Kappa, lambda (e.g., kIII)	Ak,A, (e.g., A K III)	Idiopathic (primary), myeloma or macroglobulinemia-associated
AH	IgG 1 (τ1)	Aτ1	
ATTR	Transthyretin	e.g., Met 30	Familial amyloid polyneuropathy (Portuguese)
		e.g., Met 111	Familial amyloid cardiomyopathy (Danish)
		TTR or Ile 122	Systemic senile amyloidosis
AApoAI	apoAI	Arg 26	Familial amyloid polyneuropathy (Iowa)
AGel	Gwlaolin	Asn 187[c] (15)	Familial amyloidosis (Finnish)
ACys	Cystatin C	Gln 68	Hereditary cerebral hemorrhage with amyloidosis (Icelandic)
AB	B protein precursor (e.g., BPP 695[d])	Gln 618 (22)	Alzheimer's disease, Down's syndrome, hereditary cerebral hemorrhage amyloidosis (Dutch)
AB$_2$M	B2-microglobulin		Associated with chronic dialysis
AScr	Scrapie protein, precursor 33–35[e] cellular form	Scrapie protein 27–30	Creutzfeldt–Jakob disease, etc.
		e.g., Leu 102	Gertsmann–Straussler–Scheinker syndrome
ACal	(Pro)calcitonin	(Pro)calcitonin	Medullary carcinoma of thyroid
AANF	Atrial natriuretic factor		Isolated atrial amyloid
AIAPP	Islet amyloid polypeptide		Islets of Langerhans, Diabetes type II, insulinoma

[a]Nonfibrillar proteins (e.g., protein AP, amyloid P-component) excluded.
[b]Abbreviations not explained in table: AA, amyloid A protein; SAA, serum amyloid A protein; apo, apolipoprotein; L, immunoglobulin light chain; H, immunoglobulin heavy chain.
[c]Amino acid positions in the mature precursor protein; the position in the amyloid fibril protein is given in parentheses.
[d]Number of amino acid residues.
[e]Molecular mass in kilodaltons.
From (190).

These excess plasma proteins are immunoglobulins, and as such they can only be manufactured by B-cells (plasma cells); the electrophoretic pattern suggests that all the B-cells producing this protein belong to the same clone. Conclusion: somewhere in the bone marrow of these patients a clone of plasma cells is busily producing immunoglobulin, but without proliferating out of control (i.e., without behaving—yet—

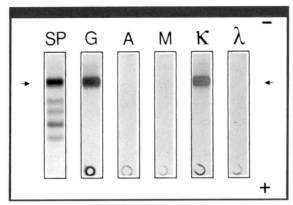

FIGURE 7.49
Electrophoresis of the serum from a 74-year-old woman with multiple myeloma. The small round well at the bottom of each strip is the point of application of the serum. All strips were overlaid with various antibodies, then the antigen-antibody complexes were stained with amido black. **SP**: Control strip overlaid with antibody against normal human serum. **G, A, M,** κ and λ: Strips overlaid with antibodies against IgG, IgA, IgM, and kappa or lambda light chains. The arrows indicate that the "myeloma protein" in this case is a monoclonal IgG with kappa light chains. No IgA or IgM is visible on the corresponding strips because the synthesis of these proteins is suppressed by the overproduced IgG. (Courtesy of Dr. R.B. Zurier, University of Massachusetts Medical School, Worcester, MA.)

like a malignant tumor of the marrow). These clinical conditions are referred to as B-cell dyscrasias or benign monoclonal gammopathies. Actually about 10 percent go on to develop malignant B-cell tumors, that is, myelomas. This means that it is not very proper to call them benign (199). Regarding those patients who do have myelomas, 6–15 percent also develop amyloidosis.

Interestingly, bone marrow from a patient with myeloma, cultured *in vitro*, produced amyloid. The malignant plasma cells were closely apposed to macrophages (164).

AL amyloid is always plasma cell amyloid (be it from benign or malignant plasma cells). Because it represents—in essence—fragments of antibody, no two cases of AL amyloid can be exactly alike.

Regarding prognosis: if the underlying disease is a benign gammopathy, the patient is condemned to die in 14 months or so of the amyloidosis itself; if the underlying disease is multiple myeloma, the prognosis is even worse: death is inevitable because of the tumor.

Amyloid AA This form corresponds to secondary amyloidosis, also called reactive amyloidosis (171). Its precursor in the blood is serum amyloid A (SAA).

Remember the term **reactive amyloidosis.** This form of amyloidosis is due to a general bodily reaction to chronic and wasting diseases, be they inflammatory or neoplastic—rheumatoid arthritis, chronic infections such as osteomyelitis and tuberculosis, and malignant tumors (especially renal cell carcinoma and Hodgkin's disease). Whatever the cause, the liver responds by changing its pattern of plasma protein synthesis (p. 491); the production of some proteins is reduced, and other proteins are secreted in vastly increased amounts. The latter go under the odd name of **acute-phase proteins.** The increased secretion of some of these can be explained; fibrinogen, for example, is necessary to make fibrin, and fibrin is necessary as a glue for injured vessels. For other proteins, however, the increase is baffling. Serum amyloid A, for example, has no known major function, and in the long run it may turn into deposits of amyloid A (it does not always do so). Medical students find this mechanism quite confusing, and they are not alone; what is the purpose of producing more SAA if it can lead to amyloidosis? We can only answer that the increase in SAA "must have" an overriding purpose that we do not yet comprehend.

Amyloid A was chemically defined by Benditt et al. in Seattle (143). Its circulating precursor (SAA) was discovered by searching for the target of antibodies against amyloid A. SAA is an apoprotein of high density lipoprotein (HDL) (144, 188)—another puzzle. Amyloid A can be produced experimentally in mice by the old and now classical method of injecting casein (210); obviously the mice produce amyloid A because they have a blood precursor homologous to human SAA.

Amyloid P (AP) Amyloid P is the pentagonal molecule mentioned earlier (Figure 7.42); *it does not occur alone but as a component (5–10 percent) of almost all other types of amyloid.* It is present under normal conditions in the basement membrane of glomerular capillaries, around small vessels of a few other sites (166), and in the microfibrils that surround elastic fibers (214), which means that *not all amyloid is pathologic.* Like amyloid A, which has its circulating precursor (SAA) belonging to the acute-phase reactants, amyloid P has its serum amyloid P (SAP) precursor in a pentagonal protein identical to AP. SAP is similar to another pentagonal plasma protein, the C-reactive protein ([p.492]) another acute-phase reactant, and also to the so-called hamster female protein. These proteins have been grouped into a family as **pentraxins** (from the Greek words for "five" and "berries").

Senile Amyloid (AS) Senile amyloid is much more prevalent than previously realized, especially in the heart and aorta (160). It is found in about one-third of all autopsies after the age of 70 and in 50 percent of all hearts after the age of 90. Its significance as a cause of death is not yet clear (160). In some cases its serum precursor is a protein confusingly called prealbumin although it has nothing to do with albumin. It transports thyroxin and retinol (vitamin A); hence its alternative name is **trans-thy-ret-in (TTR).**

Endocrine Amyloid (AE) Amyloid AE occurs, for instance, in the stroma of some thyroid tumors (in medullary carcinomas its precursor is calcitonin [213]) and especially in the islets of the pancreas, where it is associated with adult-onset diabetes (Figure 7.50) and with advancing age (208). The diabetes connection has produced new insights regarding both amyloid and diabetes (192–194).

It has been known since 1900 that many pancreatic islets are hyalinized, especially in diabetics; now it turns out that the hyalin is a special type of amyloid derived from an islet-associated polypeptide (IAPP), synthesized by normal beta cells and probably cosecreted with insulin. The story of IAPP is not yet completely worked out, but it appears that IAPP somehow opposes the action of insulin in peripheral tissues, thus explaining the pathogenesis of non–insulin-dependent diabetes. As time goes by, the deposition of amyloid in the islets may become a secondary cause of diabetes. The tendency of IAPP to polymerize spontaneously in the extracellular spaces is found only in a few species, such as human, cat, and raccoon (192, 194).

Iatrogenic Amyloidosis A recently discovered consequence of chronic hemodialysis, iatrogenic amyloidosis came to light because 10 percent of patients who had undergone hemodialysis for 5–10 years or longer developed the carpal tunnel syndrome, caused by a narrowing of the tunnel in the wrist where the medial nerve fits snugly along with nine tendons. Surgical release is

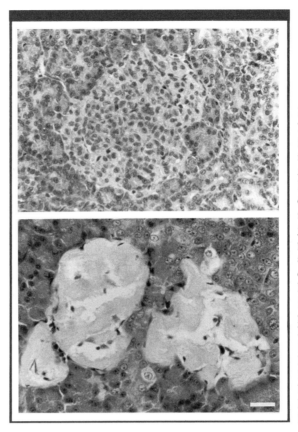

FIGURE 7.50
Top: Pancreatic islet from a normal cat. *Bottom:* Amyloid-laden islets from an aged cat with diabetes mellitus. The major protein component of islet amyloid in the diabetic cat and human is IAPP (islet amyloid polypeptide). **Bar** = 50 μm. (Courtesy of K. H. Johnson, D.V.M., Ph.D., University of Minnesota, St. Paul, MN.)

required. The amyloid that develops in the tunnel belongs to a specific type whose precursor is beta-2-microglobulin (155, 184, 227). The precursor protein is normally catabolized in the kidney—and these patients have no kidneys. The resulting high concentration of precursor seems to be the critical factor; amyloid fibrils can be obtained from normal beta-2-microglobulin also *in vitro.*

Heredofamilial Amyloidosis (AF) This amyloidosis is rare except in foci scattered around the world from Portugal to Brazil, Japan, England, and elsewhere—perhaps because a gene for it was spread by navigators (146). In most cases the amyloid consists of transthyretin (TTR) that is abnormal by a single amino acid; clinically the prevalent form of this disease is a polyneuropathy that appears around the age of 25–35 years (the delay is not well understood). Another rare hereditary form is familial Mediterranean fever, the only type of human amyloidosis that is treatable and preventable because the disease responds—for reasons unclear—to colchicine (149, 233, 240).

Beta Amyloid—Alzheimer's Disease Minuscule amounts of beta (or A4) amyloid are produced in Alzheimer's disease, but the literature on the subject is enormous, reflecting public concern over this disease. As longevity increases, so does the prevalence of Alzheimer dementia: 10 percent for ages 75–85 years and 20 percent after age 85, enough to occupy about half the beds of all nursing homes (191).

The brain changes of Alzheimer's disease are qualitatively similar to those of age without dementia, but they are much more severe (161, 172, 178, 179). In either situation the neuropathology is based on three types of lesions, two of which definitely contain amyloid:

- **Neurofibrillary tangles,** found inside neurons; they consist of filaments that react histochemically like amyloid, but their nature is still uncertain (Figure 7.51).
- **Senile plaques,** spherical lesions 100–200 μm in diameter that are made of a central core of amyloid wrapped in a tangle of abnormal, "degenerating" neurites and glial cells (Figure 7.52).
- **Congophilic angiopathy,** a pompous name meaning simply that an amyloid that is stainable with Congo red is present in the walls of certain cerebral arteries and arterioles (Figure 7.53).

The number of tangles and plaques correlates roughly with the degree of dementia.

A precursor has recently been found for brain amyloid: amyloid beta-protein precursor (APP) (224). It is a membrane protein that is expressed in many tissues besides brain; a fragment is clipped off APP and aggregates as amyloid. APP appears to be an important protein involved in the regulation of cell growth (195) and perhaps also in synaptic function (216). It is coded by a gene on chromosome 21 (223); this also happens to be the chromosome that is tripled in Down's syndrome, or trisomy 21, in which amyloid material is deposited at a very early age (222).

As the Alzheimer-amyloid story develops, new leads are being uncovered; they do not yet fit into a coherent story, but here are four tidbits.

- *Alzheimer patients and some normal, though aged, subjects have deposits of an APP fragment in the skin and gut: could it be that Alzheimer's disease is a systemic condition?*
- *APP is stored in the alpha granules of platelets; it is a growth factor and a potent protease inhibitor (234), all of which suggests a possible role in hemostasis and wound healing. Now we can understand earlier reports that thrombi sometimes stain with Congo red (181).*
- *Normal serum contains a protein that is antigenically similar to beta protein, and it is increased in patients with Down's syndrome. This would help us understand the deposits of amyloid in cerebral arteries (222).*
- *According to some reports, beta amyloid injected into animal brains is neurotoxic (216, 239).*

Localized (Tumorlike) Amyloidosis Occasionally a small lump is surgically removed, especially from the upper respiratory mucosa, and found to be not a tumor but a mass of amyloid. These peculiar "amyloidomas" are thought to be the end-stage of a cluster of plasma cells and macrophages that produced a mass of amyloid and then burned out, leaving behind the amyloid and a few telltale plasma cells (171).

Amyloid Bodies Amyloid bodies have long been known to exist in the normal prostate and elsewhere. They do deserve their name (starchlike) because they resemble starch granules in size and concentric structure. They contain various

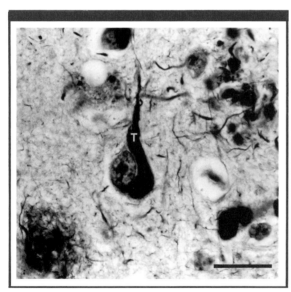

FIGURE 7.51
T: Neurofibrillary tangle, an intracellular disturbance of neurons possibly related to amyloid, in human cortex. With Bielschowsky's silver impregnation the tangle appears black and fills the cell. Like the senile plaques (lower left), the neurofibrillary tangles increase in number with age. **Bar** = 50 μm. (Courtesy of Dr. T.W. Smith, University of Massachusetts Medical Center, Worcester, MA.)

materials including fibrils made of beta pleated sheets (185), perhaps arising from residues of epithelial cells that continue to slough off and die in the lumen (142). They are of little pathologic significance.

DIAGNOSIS, PROGNOSIS, AND THERAPY OF AMYLOIDOSIS

Systemic amyloidosis can be discovered secondarily after the causal disease is recognized (e.g., myeloma). Clinical hints are a large liver or spleen, or proteinuria, especially in a patient suffering from chronic disease. An enlarged tongue carries the same message; **macroglossia** is caused by selective deposition of amyloid in the lingual muscles (Figure 7.54). Peculiar, but not uncommon, is the **carpal tunnel syndrome** already mentioned. *The final diagnosis of amyloid hinges on biopsy, staining with Congo red, and examination in polarized light.*

There is no blood test for amyloidosis. A group of imaginative British investigators proposed the following diagnostic method. Remember first that amyloid P (AP) occurs as a component of almost all amyloids; it also has a serum precursor called serum AP (SAP). Now, an intravenous injection of radioactively labeled SAP should localize wherever there is a deposit of amyloid, and so it does. One of the difficulties is to procure SAP; the method is not yet current (187).

The rectal mucosa has long been the biopsy site of choice for diagnosing amyloid, the rationale being that the gastrointestinal tract is commonly affected; also, the rectal mucosa provides several varieties of tissues (sometimes even a lymphatic nodule) with practically no pain and surprisingly little risk of infection. Needle aspiration of abdominal fat is a less traumatic alternative (158, 165). Congo red staining of a tissue sample followed by study in polarized light is still the best method; staining with thioflavin followed by study under ultraviolet light gives a yellow fluorescence, but this technique is less specific. Other methods exist (158).

Regarding prognosis, when amyloid is deposited in association with a malignant tumor (such as myeloma or renal cell carcinoma), the outcome is of course bleak on account of the primary lesion. However, the relentless deposition of amyloid can be lethal in itself; survival in primary amyloidosis is on the order of 12–14 months; death is due mainly to cardiac and renal failure (202). A few proven cases of regression after the primary cause

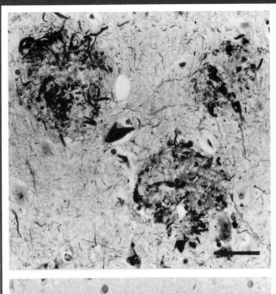
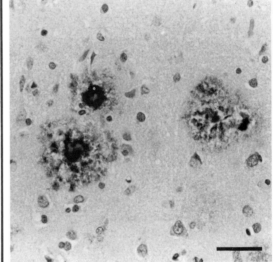

FIGURE 7.52 *Top:* Three senile plaques demonstrated with Bielschowsky's silver impregnation, which stains axons and dendrites black. The plaques consist of swollen, fragmented axons. *Bottom:* Senile plaques demonstrated with an immunoperoxidase stain for beta amyloid. A dark mass of amyloid is demonstrated in the center of three senile plaques. **Bars** = 100 μm. (Courtesy of Dr. T.W. Smith, University of Massachusetts Medical Center, Worcester, MA.)

was removed have been described (169); clinical improvement of renal function can also occur (162). Therapy with colchicine has had some success in protecting against renal amyloidosis associated with Mediterranean fever (240) and perhaps even causing it to regress (157, 220); colchicine also prolongs the survival in AL amyloidosis (155). The mechanism of colchicine therapy is not clear. Another therapeutic approach has been to attempt to denature the tough amyloid fibrils by administering large doses of dimethyl sulfoxide—with some success, although the mechanism is again unclear.

The rationale for trying colchicine in Mediterranean fever was quite unrelated to amyloidosis (182); its favorable effect on amyloid deposition was found by

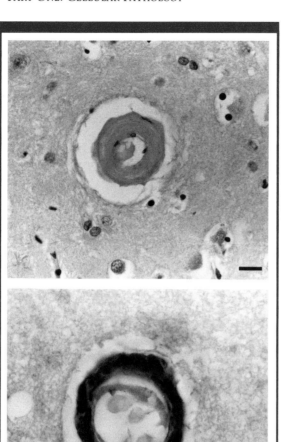

FIGURE 7.53 Amyloidosis of arterioles in the brain, the so-called congophilic angiopathy. *Top:* The arteriole is hyalinized. The clear space surrounding it is an artefact. *Bottom:* A similar arteriole demonstrated with an immunoperoxidase stain for beta amyloid. This type of amyloid deposition occurs spontaneously in old age, but it is exaggerated in Alzheimer's disease. **Bars** = 50 μm. (Courtesy of Dr. T. W. Smith, University of Massachusetts Medical Center, Worcester, MA.)

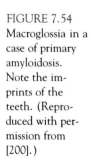

FIGURE 7.54 Macroglossia in a case of primary amyloidosis. Note the imprints of the teeth. (Reproduced with permission from [200].)

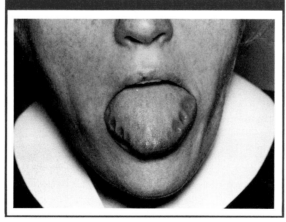

accident. It is interesting to speculate that colchicine disturbs phagocytosis and cell movements by interfering with the microtubular skeleton. Are the macrophages impaired by colchicine in their amyloidogenic activities?

AMYLOIDOSIS: LOOSE ENDS

There are still many open questions in the amyloid story. Where and why do the blood-borne precursors exit from the bloodstream? Why do they localize where they do? (Perhaps fibronectin helps as a "glue" [196]). Once the precursor is outside the blood vessels, why do the macrophages develop their "invertebrate" frenzy? What triggers them in some individuals and not in others? Why is it that in some cases the Bence–Jones proteins produce amyloid fibrils *in vitro* and in other cases not? What other components are involved in building the amyloid fibrils? And could it be, as has been proposed, that amyloidosis hinges also on an inadequate "amyloidolytic" capacity of the plasma (209) and possibly also of the macrophages (204)?

Another incomplete chapter is represented by the so-called **amyloid-enhancing factors;** they are extracts prepared from the spleen or liver of animals injected with casein and sacrificed during the preamyloidotic or amyloidotic stage (189, 211). Injected into animals already treated with casein, they can shorten the time of amyloid deposition to as little as 48 hours (140). Extracts of hamster (189) or human amyloid (235) are also effective. Recent work with mouse peritoneal macrophages suggests that the enhancing factor favors the second phase of amyloidogenesis, that is, not its production but its deposition in the tissues (226).

Among all the loose ends of amyloid, the most perplexing is the exciting story of amyloid and **prions:** *could amyloid be a parasite? This may sound preposterous, but read on.*

In the 1950s, Sigurdsson and collaborators in Iceland suggested that two demyelinating diseases of sheep and goats, visna and scrapie, were caused by "slow viruses" (228, 229). Thus was born the concept of slow infections, characterized by "neurodegenerative" noninflammatory changes in the central nervous system, a long incubation (months to decades), a short clinical course leading to death, pathology limited to a single organ, and natural host usually limited to a single species (217, 218). There are parallels in humans, notably Creutzfeldt–Jakob disease and kuru; the latter became widely known because it was originally transmitted by ritual cannibalism in New Guinea (170). The infectious agents in all four diseases were presumed to be viruses; in fact, visna turned out to be due to a retrovirus (217), but the infectious agents of the other slow infections remained elusive. Then a neurologist, S.B. Prusiner,

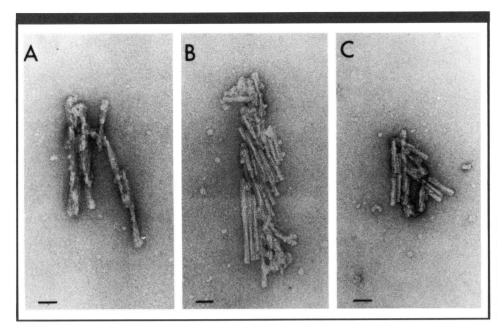

FIGURE 7.55
Electron microscopy of purified prion amyloid. **A**: Amyloid extracted from the brain of a scrapie-infected sheep. **B, C**: Amyloid obtained from human brains affected by Creutzfeldt–Jakob disease. **Bars** = 500 Å. (Reproduced with permission from [217].)

proposed that the agent was a new type of particle, which he named **prion** (a combination of protein and infectious). The astonishing property of prions is that they contain little or no nucleic acid (218): is this a new form of life? Moreover, the prions self-aggregate into rods that are indistinguishable from amyloid fibrils (Figure 7.55); they even stain with Congo red. That amyloid could be something alive was more than the experts could swallow; however, a prion protein was sequenced, its gene identified, and prions are here to stay. The prion protein is a transmembrane protein (207) which appears to be necessary for normal synaptic function (158a). According to Prusiner, it raises the possibility that "normal, necessary proteins may be converted into malignant, lethal molecules" (217, 232). A current hypothesis is that the normal prion protein is protease-sensitive; if it is accidentally converted into a protein-resistant form, this conversion is autocatalytic—and causes neurodegenerative disease (221). The protein-resistant form has a high content of beta-pleated sheet (146a), which is consistent with its propensity to form amyloid.

It is clear that most amyloids are unrelated to prions, but the enigmatic prions are obviously the beginning of something new—and rather frightening.

TO SUM UP: it is clear that we should no longer speak of amyloid but rather of amyloids. Which raises a basic question: why should there be so many amyloids? Why should so many and disparate polypeptides aggregate into fibrils of similar diameter, physical structure, and affinity for Congo red? Is there any purpose to this aggregation? If so, it is not apparent—for amyloid as we understand it is nothing but bad news.

References

Pathology of Collagen

1. Akeson WH, Amiel D, Mechanic GL, Woo SL-Y, Harwood FL, Hamer ML. Collagen cross-linking alterations in joint contractures: changes in the reducible cross-links in periarticular connective tissue collagen after nine weeks of immobilization. Connect Tissue Res 1977;5:15–19.
2. Aschoff L, Koch W. Skorbut. Eine pathologisch-anatomische Studie. Jena: Verlag Gustav Fischer, 1919.
3. Bailey AJ, Lapière CM. Effect of an additional peptide extension of the N-terminus of collagen from dermatosparactic calves on the cross-linking of the collagen fibers. Eur J Biochem 1973;34:91–96.
4. Bardach H, Gebhart W, Niebauer G. "Lumpy-bumpy" elastic fibers in the skin and lungs of a patient with a penicillamine-induced elastosis perforans serpiginosa. J Cutan Pathol 1979;6:243-252.
5. Bauer EA. Collagenase in recessive dystrophic epidermolysis bullosa. Ann NY Acad Sci 1985;460:311–320.
6. Briggaman RA, Wheeler CE. Epidermolysis bullosa dystrophica-recessive: a possible role of anchoring fibrils in the pathogenesis. J Invest Dermatol 1975;65:203–211.
7. Byers PH, Barsh GS, Holbrook KA. Molecular pathology in inherited disorders of collagen metabolism. Hum Pathol 1982;13:89-95.
8. Gamble CN. The pathogenesis of hyaline arteriosclerosis. Am J Pathol 1986;122:410–420.
9. Gay S, Gay RE. Connective tissue structure and function. In: Wyngaarden JB, Smith LH, Jr, Bennett JC (eds). Cecil textbook of medicine, 19th ed, vol 2. Philadelphia: WB Saunders Company, 1992, pp 1491–1496.

10. Gay S, Miller EJ. What is collagen, what is not. Ultrastruct Pathol 1983;4:365–377.
11. Gross J. Collagen biology: structure, degradation, and disease. Harvey Lect 1974;68:351–432.
12. Gross J, Lapière CM. Collagenolytic activity in amphibian tissues: a tissue culture assay. Proc Natl Acad Sci USA 1962;48:1014–1022.
13. Hanna W, Silverman E, Boxall L, Krafchik BR. Ultrastructural features of epidermolysis bullosa. Ultrastruct Pathol 1983;5:29–36.
14. Hanset R, Lapière CM. Inheritance of dermatosparaxis in the calf. J Heredit 1974;65:356–358.
15. Jeresaty RM. Mitral valve prolapse. New York: Raven Press, 1979.
16. Keene DR, Sakai LY, Lunstrum GP, Morris NP, Burgeson RE. Type VII collagen forms an extended network of anchoring fibrils. J Cell Biol 1987;104:611–621.
17. Klemperer P. The concept of collagen diseases. Am J Pathol 1950;26:505–519.
18. Klemperer P, Pollack AD, Baehr G. Diffuse collagen disease. Acute disseminated lupus erythematosus and diffuse scleroderma. JAMA 1942;119:331–332.
19. Krane SM. Genetic and acquired disorders of collagen deposition. In: Piez KA, Reddi AH (eds). Extracellular matrix biochemistry. New York: Elsevier, 1984, pp 413–463.
20. Kuivaniemi H, Tromp G, Prockop DJ. Mutations in collagen genes: causes of rare and some common diseases in humans. FASEB J 1991;5:2052–2060.
21. Lapière CM, Lenaers A, Kohn L. Procollagen peptidase: an enzyme excising the coordination peptides of procollagen. Proc Natl Acad Sci USA 1971;68:3054–3058.
22. Levene CI. Effect of lathyrogenic compounds on the cross-linking of collagen and elastin in vivo. In: Aldridge WN (ed). A symposium on mechanisms of toxicity. New York: St Martin's Press, 1971, pp 67–81.
23. Levene CI. Diseases of the collagen molecule. J Clin Pathol 31 (Suppl Roy Coll Pathol) 1978;12:82–94.
24. Madri JA, Basson MD. Extracellular matrix-cell interactions: dynamic modulators of cells, tissue and organism structure and function. Lab Invest 1992;66:519–521.
25. Majno G. The story of the myofibroblasts. Am J Surg Pathol 1979;3:535–542.
26. Martinez-Hernandez A, Amenta PS. The basement membrane in pathology. Lab Invest 1983;48:656–677.
27. Maschmann E. über Bakterienproteasen. IX. Mitteilung: Die Anaerobiase der Gasbranderreger. Biochem Z 1938;297:284–296.
28. McDonald JA. Receptors for extracellular matrix components. Am J Physiol 1989;257:L331-L337.
29. McDonald JA. Matrix regulation of cell shape and gene expression. Curr Opin Cell Biol 1989;1:995–999.
30. McKusick VA. Heritable disorders of connective tissue, 4th ed. St Louis: The CV Mosby Company, 1972.
31. Miller EJ, Gay S. Collagen: an overview. Methods Enzymol 1982;82:3–32.
32. Minor RR. Collagen metabolism. A comparison of diseases of collagen and diseases affecting collagen. Am J Pathol 1980;98:225–280.
33. Montes GS, Junqueira LCU. Biology of collagen. Rev Can Biol Exp 1982;41:143–156.
34. Nimni ME. Collagen: structure, function, and metabolism in normal and fibrotic tissues. Semin Arthritis Rheum 1983;13:1–86.
35. Pérez Tamayo R. Pathology of collagen degradation. A review. Am J Pathol 1978;92:507–566.
36. Piez KA, Reddi AH (eds). Extracellular matrix biochemistry. New York: Elsevier, 1984.
37. Pinnell SR, Murad S. Disorders of collagen. In: Stanbury JB, Wyngaarden JB, Fredrickson DS, Goldstein JL, Brown MS (eds). The metabolic basis of inherited disease, 5th ed. New York: McGraw-Hill Book Company, 1983, pp 1425–1449.
38. Prockop DJ. Osteogenesis imperfecta: phenotypic heterogeneity, protein suicide, short and long collagen. Am J Hum Genet 1984;36:499–505.
39. Prockop DJ. Genetic defects of collagen. Hosp Pract 1986;21:125–140.
40. Prockop DJ. Mutations in collagen genes as a cause of connective-tissue diseases. N Engl J Med 1992;326:540–546.
41. Prockop DJ, Kivirikko KI. Heritable diseases of collagen. N Engl J Med 1984;311:376–386.
42. Prockop DJ, Kuivaniemi H. Inborn errors of collagen. Rheumatology 1986;10:246–271.
43. Prockop DJ, Kivirikko KI, Tuderman L, Guzman NA. The biosynthesis of collagen and its disorders. Parts I and II. N Engl J Med 1979;301:13–23 and 77–85.
44. Pyeritz RE. Heritable defects in connective tissue. Hosp Pract 1987;22:153–168.
45. Ralph RA. Chemical burns of the eye. In: Duane TD, Jaeger EA (eds). Clinical ophthalmology, vol 4. Philadelphia: Harper & Row, 1985, pp 1–25.
46. Reymond JL, Stoebner P, Zambelli P, Beani JC, Amblard P. Penicillamine induced elastosis perforans serpiginosa: an ultrastructural study of two cases. J Cutan Pathol 1982;9:352–357.
47. Shields GS, Coulson WF, Kimball DA, Carnes WH, Cartwright GE, Wintrobe MM. Studies on copper metabolism. XXXII. Cardiovascular lesions in copper-deficient swine. Am J Pathol 1962;41:603–621.
48. Sodek J. A comparison of the rates of synthesis and turnover of collagen and non-collagen proteins in adult rat periodontal tissues and skin using a microassay. Arch Oral Biol 1977;22:655–665.
49. Stanbury JB, Wyngaarden JB, Fredrickson DS, Goldstein JL, Brown MS (eds). The metabolic basis of inherited disease, 5th ed. New York: McGraw-Hill Book Company, 1983.
50. Stuart JM, Townes AS, Kang AH. Type II collagen-induced arthritis. Ann NY Acad Sci 1985;460:355–362.
51. Takebayashi S, Kubota I, Takagi T. Ultrastructural and histochemical studies of vascular lesions in Marfan's syndrome, with report of 4 autopsy cases. Acta Pathol Jpn 1973;23:847–866.
52. Uitto J, Lichtenstein JR. Defects in the biochemistry of collagen in diseases of connective tissue. J Invest Dermatol 1976;66:59–79.
53. Vernon RB, Angello JC, Iruela-Arispe ML, Lane TF, Sage EH. Reorganization of basement membrane matrices by cellular traction promotes the formation of cellular networks in vitro. Lab Invest 1992 66:536–547.
54. Vogel A, Holbrook KA, Steinmann B, Gitzelmann R, Byers PH. Abnormal collagen fibril structure in the gravis form (type I) of Ehlers-Danlos syndrome. Lab Invest 1979;40:201–206.

Pathology of Elastin

55. Alberts B, Bray D, Lewis J, Raff M, Roberts K, Watson JD. Molecular biology of the cell. New York: Garland Publishing, Inc, 1989.
56. Bader, L. Disorders of elastic tissue: a review. Pathology 1973;5:269–289.
57. Curtis ES. Portraits from North American Indian life. New York: Promontory Press, 1972.

58. Fitzpatrick TB, Eisen AZ, Wolff K, Freedberg IM, Austen KF. Update: dermatology in general medicine. New York: McGraw-Hill Book Company, 1983.

58a. Francke U, Furthmayr H. Marfan's syndrome and other disorders of fibrillin. N Engl J Med 1994;330:1384–1385.

59. Gadek JE, Pacht ER. The protease-antiprotease balance within the human lung: implications for the pathogenesis of emphysema. Lung (Suppl) 1990;552–564.

60. Gilchrest BA. Skin and aging processes. Boca Raton: CRC Press, Inc, 1984.

61. Halme T. Elastin and collagen of human ascending aorta. Academic dissertation. Turku, Finland, 1987.

62. Halme T, Savunen T, Aho H, Vihersaari T, Penttinen R. Elastin and collagen in the aortic wall: changes in the Marfan syndrome and annuloaortic ectasia. Exp Mol Pathol 1985;43:1–12.

63. Harel S, Janoff A, Yu SY, Hurewitz A, Bergofsky EH. Desmosine radioimmunoassay for measuring elastin degradation in vivo. Am Rev Respir Dis 1980;122:769–773.

64. Holton JB, Ireland JT (eds). Inborn errors of skin, hair and connective tissue. Baltimore: University Park Press, 1975.

65. Janoff A. Elastases and emphysema. Current assessment of the protease-antiprotease hypothesis. Am Rev Respir Dis 1985;132:417–433.

66. Janoff A, Sloan B, Weinbaum G, Damiano V, Sandhaus RA, Elias J, Kimbel P. Experimental emphysema induced with purified human neutrophil elastase: tissue localization of the instilled protease. Am Rev Respir Dis 1977;115:461–478.

67. Kainulainen K, Pulkkinen L, Savolainen A, Kaitila I, Peltonen L. Location on chromosome 15 of the gene defect causing Marfan syndrome. N Engl J Med 1990;323:935–939.

68. Lansing AI, Alex M, Rosenthal TB. Calcium and elastin in human arteriosclerosis. J Gerontol 1950;5:112–119.

69. Lansing AI, Roberts E, Ramasarma GB, Rosenthal TB, Alex M. Changes with age in amino acid composition of arterial elastin. Proc Soc Exp Biol Med 1951;76:714–717.

70. Lavie G, Zucker-Franklin D, Franklin EC. Elastase-type proteases on the surface of human blood monocytes: possible role in amyloid formation. J Immunol 1980;125:175–180.

71. Ledoux-Corbusier M, Achten G. Elastosis in chronic radiodermatitis. An ultrastructural study. Br J Dermatol 1974;91:287–295.

72. Lee B, Godfrey M, Vitale E, Hori H, Mattei M-G, Sarfarazi M, Tsipouras P, Ramirez F, Hollister DW. Linkage of Marfan syndrome and a phenotypically related disorder to two different fibrillin genes. Nature 1991;352:330–334.

73. McKusick VA. The defect in Marfan syndrome. Nature 1991;352:279–281.

74. Newbold PCH. Inborn errors of skin. In: Holton JB, Ireland JT (eds). Inborn errors of skin, hair and connective tissue. Baltimore: University Park Press, 1975, pp 3–14.

75. Pinnell SR, Murad S. Disorders of collagen. In: Stanbury JB, Wyngaarden JB, Frederickson DS, Goldstein JL, Brown MS (eds). The metabolic basis of inherited disease, 5th ed. New York: McGraw-Hill Book Company, 1983.

76. Poulsen JT, Staberg B, Wulf HC, Brodthagen H. Dermal elastosis in hairless mice after UV-B and UV-A applied simultaneously, separately or sequentially. Br J Dermatol 1984;110:531–538.

77. Prockop DJ, Kuivaniemi H. Inborn errors of collagen. Rheumatology 1986;10:246–271.

78. Rucker RB, Tinker D. Structure and metabolism of arterial elastin. Int Rev Exp Pathol 1977;17:1–47.

79. Stanbury JB, Wyngaarden JB, Frederickson DS, Goldstein JL, Brown MS (eds). The metabolic basis of inherited disease, 5th ed. New York: McGraw-Hill Book Company, 1983.

80. Takebayashi S, Kubota I, Takagi T. Ultrastructural and histochemical studies of vascular lesions in Marfan's syndrome, with report of 4 autopsy cases. Acta Pathol Jpn 1973;23:847–866.

81. Tokita K, Kanno K, Ikeda K. Elastin sub-fraction as binding site for lipids. Atherosclerosis 1977;28:111–119.

82. Tsipouras P, Del Mastro R, Sarfarazi M, et al. Genetic linkage of the Marfan syndrome, ectopia lentis, and congenital contractural arachnodactyly to the fibrillin genes on chromosomes 15 and 5. N Engl J Med 1992;326:905–909.

83. Tsuji T. The surface structural alterations of elastic fibers and elastotic material in solar elastosis: a scanning electron microscopic study. J Cutan Pathol 1984;11:300–308.

84. Urry DW. What is elastin; what is not. Ultrastruct Pathol 1983;4:227–251.

Pathology of Basement Membranes

85. Boersma D, Baker BL. Sites of deposition of silver in argyria. With special reference to the axillary glands. Arch Dermatol Syph 1948;57:1009–1012.

86. Cohen AH, Hoyer JR. Nephronophthisis. A primary tubular basement membrane defect. Lab Invest 1986;55:564–572.

87. Folkman J, Klagsbrun M, Sasse J, Wadzinski M, Ingber D, Vlodavsky I. A heparin-binding angiogenic protein—basic fibroblast growth factor—is stored within basement membrane. Am J Pathol 1988;130:393–400.

88. Gschnait F, Wolff K, Konrad K. Erythropoietic protoporphyria—submicroscopic events during the acute photosensitivity flare. Br J Dermatol 1975;92:545–557.

89. Harper GS, Axelsen RA. Salicylate-induced renal papillary necrosis in the Gunn rat. The role of bilirubin. Lab Invest 1982;47:258–264.

90. Hill WR, Pillsbury DM. Argyria. The pharmacology of silver. Baltimore: Williams & Wilkins Company, 1939.

91. Hunter D. The diseases of occupations. London: The English Universities Press Ltd, 1969.

92. Kurtz SM, Feldman JD. Experimental studies on the formation of the glomerular basement membrane. J Ultrastruct Res 1962;6:19-27.

93. Mackay IR, Burnet FM. Autoimmune diseases. Springfield, IL: Charles C Thomas, 1963.

94. Majno G. Ultrastructure of the vascular membrane. In: Hamilton WF, Dow P (eds). Handbook of physiology, sect 2, vol III. Washington, DC: American Physiological Society, 1965, pp 2293–2375.

95. Makino H, Yamasaki Y, Haramoto T, Shikata K, Hironaka K, Ota Z, Kanwar YS. Ultrastructural changes of extracellular matrices in diabetic nephropathy revealed by high resolution scanning and immunoelectron microscopy. Lab Invest 1993;68:45–55.

96. Martin GR, Rohrbach DH, Terranova VP, Liotta LA. Structure, function, and pathology of basement membranes. In: Wagner BM, Fleischmajer R, Kaufman N (eds). Connective tissue diseases. Baltimore: Williams & Wilkins, 1983, pp 16–30.

97. Martinez-Hernandez A, Amenta PS. The basement membrane in pathology. Lab Invest 1983;48:656–677.

98. Masugi M. Über das Wesen der spezifischen Veränderungen der Niere und der Leber durch das Nephro-

toxin bzw. das Hepatotoxin. Zugleich ein Beitrag zur Pathogenese der Glomerulonephritis und der eklamptischen Lebererkrankung. Beitr Pathol Anat 1933;91: 82–112.

99. McCluskey RT, Vassalli P. Experimental glomerular diseases. In: Rouiller C, Muller AF (eds). The kidney: morphology, biochemistry, physiology, vol II. New York: Academic Press, 1969, pp 83–198.

100. McVerry BA, Fisher C, Hopp A, Huehns ER. Production of pseudodiabetic renal glomerular changes in mice after repeated injections of glucosylated proteins. Lancet 1980;1:738–740.

101. Mihatsch MJ, Torhorst J, Amsler B, Zollinger HU. Capillarosclerosis of the lower urinary tract in analgesic (phenacetin) abuse. An electron-microscopic study. Virchows Arch A Pathol Anat Histol 1978; 381:41–47.

102. Mullarkey CJ, Brownlee M. Biochemical basis of microvascular disease. In: Pickup JC, Williams G (eds). Textbook of diabetes, vol 2. Oxford: Blackwell Scientific Publications, 1991, pp 534–545.

103. Raskin P, Pietri AO, Unger R, Shannon WA. The effect of diabetic control on the width of skeletal-muscle capillary basement membrane in patients with type I diabetes mellitus. N Engl J Med 1983;309:1546–1550.

104. Rogelj S, Klagsbrun M, Atzmon R, et al. Basis fibroblast growth factor is an extracellular matrix component required for supporting the proliferation of vascular endothelial cells and the differentiation of PC12 cells. J Cell Biol 1989;109:823–831.

105. Vracko R. Basal lamina layering in diabetes mellitus. Evidence for accelerated rate of cell death and cell regeneration. Diabetes 1974;23:94–104.

106. Vracko R. Basal lamina scaffold—anatomy and significance for maintenance of orderly tissue structure. Am J Pathol 1974;77:314–346.

107. Wagner BM, Fleischmajer R, Kaufman N (eds). Connective tissue diseases. Baltimore: Williams & Wilkins, 1983.

108. Walker F. Basement-membrane turnover in man. J Pathol 1972;107:123–125.

109. Williamson JR, Kilo C. Basement-membrane thickening and diabetic microangiopathy. Diabetes 1976;25 (Suppl 2): 925–927.

110. Yen A, Braverman IM. Ultrastructure of the human dermal microcirculation: the horizontal plexus of the papillary dermis. J Invest Dermatol 1976;66:131–142.

111. Yurchenco PD, O'Rear J. Molecular and cellular aspects of basement membranes. In: Rohrbach DH, Timpl R (eds). Monographs in cell biology. New Yoork: Academic Press, 1992 (in press).

Pathology of Proteoglycans

112. Brandt KD, Radin E. The physiology of articular stress: osteoarthrosis. Hosp Pract 1987;22:103–126.

113. Buckwalter JA, Rosenberg L. Structural changes during development in bovine fetal epiphyseal cartilage. Collagen Rel Res 1983;3:489–504.

114. Cheung HS, Nicoloff JT, Kamiel MB, Spolter L, Nimni ME. Stimulation of fibroblast biosynthetic activity by serum of patients with pretibial myxedema. J Invest Dermatol 1978;71:12–17.

115. Cotran

116. DeMartino GN, Goldberg AL. A possible explanation of myxedema and hypercholesterolemia in hypothyroidism: control of lysosomal hyaluronidase and cholesterol esterase by thyroid hormones. Enzyme 1981;26:1–7.

117. Gordon MY, Riley GP, Watt SM, Greaves MF. Compartmentalization of a haematopoietic growth factor (GM-CSF) by glycosaminoglycans in the bone marrow microenvironment. Nature 1987;326:403–405.

118. Hamerman D. The biology of osteoarthritis. N Engl J Med 1989;320:1322–1330.

119. Ingbar SH, Braverman LE (eds). Werner's the thyroid: a fundamental and clinical text, 5th ed. Philadelphia: JB Lippincott Company, 1986.

120. Kobayasi T, Danielsen L, Asboe-Hansen G. Ultrastructure of localized myxedema. Acta Derm Venereol (Stockh) 1976;56:173–185.

121. Kohn LD. Connective tissue. In: Ingbar SH, Braverman LE (eds). Werner's the thyroid: a fundamental and clinical text, 5th ed. Philadelphia: JB Lippincott, 1986, pp 816–839.

122. Kohn LD. Connective tissue. In: Ingbar SH, Braverman LE (eds). Werner's the thyroid: a fundamental and clinical text, 5th ed. Philadelphia: JB Lippincott, 1986, pp 1128–1130.

123. Kresse H, Cantz M, von Figura K, Glössl J, Paschke E. The mucopolysaccharidoses: biochemistry and clinical symptoms. Klin Wochenschr 1981;59:867–876.

124. Makita Z, Radoff S, Rayfield EJ, Yang Z, Skolnik E, Delaney V, Friedman EA, Cerami A, Vlassara H. Advanced glycosylation end products in patients with diabetic nephropathy. N Engl J Med 1991;3:836–842.

125. Morris JH. The nervous system. In: Cotran RS, Kumar V, Robbins SL (eds). Robbins pathologic basis of disease, 4th ed. Philadelphia: WB Saunders Company, 1989, pp 1385–1449.

126. Palmoski M, Perricone E, Brandt KD. Development and reversal of a proteoglycan aggregation defect in normal canine knee cartilage after immobilization. Arthritis Rheum 1979;22:508–517.

127. Rosenberg L. Structure of cartilage proteoglycans. In: Burleigh PMC, Poole AR (eds). Dynamics of connective tissue macromolecules. Amsterdam: North-Holland Publishing Company, 1975, pp 105–128.

128. Trelstad RL. Glycosaminoglycans: mortar, matrix, mentor. Lab Invest 1985;53:1–4.

Nonenzymatic Glycation

129. Brownlee M, Cerami A, Vlassara H. Advanced glycosylation end products in tissue and the biochemical basis of diabetic complications. N Engl J Med 1988;318: 1315–1321.

130. Bunn HF, Gabbay KH, Gallop PM. The glycosylation of hemoglobin: relevance to diabetes mellitus. Science 1978;200:21–27.

131. Cerami A, Vlassara H, Brownlee M. Glucose and aging. Sci Am 1987;256:90–96.

132. Cohen MP. Nonenzymatic glycation: a central mechanism in diabetic microvasculopathy? J Diabetic Complications 1988;2:214-217.

133. Hamlin CR, Kohn RR, Luschin JH. Apparent accelerated aging of human collagen in diabetes mellitus. Diabetes 1975;24:902–904.

134. Kennedy L, Baynes JW. Non-enzymatic glycosylation and the chronic complications of diabetes: an overview. Diabetologia 1984;26:93–98.

135. Lawrie RA. Meat science, 3rd ed. Oxford: Pergamon Press, 1979.

136. Monnier VM, Kohn RR, Cerami A. Accelerated browning of collagen in diabetic humans. Diabetes 1982;31:28a.

137. Muona P, Jaakola S, Zhang R-Z, Pan T-C, Pelliniemi L, Risteli L, Chu M-L, Uitto J, Peltonen J. Hyperglycemic

glucose concentrations up-regulate the expression of type VI collagen in vitro. Am J Pathol 1993;142:1586–1597.

138. Rosenbloom AL, Silverstein JH, Lezotte DC, Richardson K, McCallum M. Limited joint mobility in childhood diabetes mellitus indicates increased risk for microvascular disease. N Engl J Med 1981;305:191–194.

139. Ruderman NB, Williamson JR, Brownlee M. Glucose and diabetic vascular disease. FASEB J 1992;6:2905–2914.

139a. Vlassara H, Bucala R, Striker L. Pathogenic effects of advanced glycosylation: biochemical, biological, and clinical implications for diabetes and aging. Lab Invest 1994;70:138–151.

Amyloid

140. Axelrad MA, Kisilevsky R, Willmer J, Chen SJ, Skinner M. Further characterization of amyloid-enhancing factor. Lab Invest 1982;47:139–146.

141. Barrow GM. Physical chemistry. New York: McGraw-Hill, 1966.

142. Beems RB, Gruys E, Spit BJ. Amyloid in the corpora amylacea of the rat mammary gland. Vet Pathol 1978;15:347–352.

143. Benditt EP, Eriksen N. Chemical classes of amyloid substance. Am J Pathol 1971;65:231–252.

144. Benditt EP, Eriksen N. Amyloid protein SAA is associated with high density lipoprotein from human serum. Proc Natl Acad Sci USA 1977;74:4025–4028.

145. Bennhold H. Über die Ausscheidung intravenös einverleibter Farbstoffe bei Amyloidkranken. Verh Dtsch Ges Inn Med 1922;34:313-315.

146. Benson MD. Hereditary amyloidosis—disease entity and clinical model. Hosp Pract 1988;23:165–181.

146a. Beyreuther K, Masters CL. Catching the culprit prion. Nature 1995;370:419–420.

147. Bladen HA, Nylen MU, Glenner GG. The ultrastructure of human amyloid as revealed by the negative staining technique. J Ultrastruct Res 1966;14:449–459.

148. Bonar L, Cohen AS, Skinner MM. Characterization of the amyloid fibril as a cross-beta protein. Proc Soc Exp Biol Med 1969;131:1373–1375.

149. Castaño EM, Frangione B. Human amyloidosis, Alzheimer disease and related disorders. Lab Invest 1988;58:122–132.

150. Chopra S, Rubinow A, Koff RS, Cohen AS. Hepatic amyloidisis. A histopathologic analysis of primary (AL) and secondary (AA) forms. Am J Pathol 1984;115:186–193.

151. Cohen AS. An update of clinical, pathologic, and biochemical aspects of amyloidosis. Int J Dermatol 1981;20:515–530.

152. Cohen AS. General introduction and a brief history of amyloidosis. In: Marrink J, van Rijswijk MH (eds). Amyloidosis. The Netherlands: Martinus Nijhoff, 1986, pp 3–19.

153. Cohen AS. Amyloidosis. Bull Rheum Dis 1991;40:1–12.

154. Cohen AS, Calkins E. Electron microscopic observations on a fibrous component in amyloid of diverse origins. Nature 1959;183:1202–1203.

155. Cohen AS, Connors LH. The pathogenesis and biochemistry of amyloidosis. J Pathol 1987;151:1–10.

156. Cohen AS, Rubinow A, Anderson JJ, Skinner M, Mason JH, Libbey C, Kayne H. Survival of patients with primary (AL) amyloidosis. Colchicine-treated cases from 1976 to 1983 compared with cases seen in previous years (1961 to 1973). Am J Med 1987;82:1182–1190.

157. Cohen AS, Rubinow A, Kayne H, Libbey C, Skinner M, and Mason J. The life span of patients with primary (AL) amyloidosis and the effect of colchicine treatment. In: Glenner GG, Osserman EF, Benditt EP, Calkins E, Cohen AS, Zucker-Franklin D (eds). Amyloidosis. New York: Plenum Press, 1986, pp 559–565.

158. Cohen AS, Skinner M. The diagnosis of amyloidosis. In: Cohen AS (ed). Laboratory diagnostic procedures in the rheumatic diseases, 3rd ed. Orlando: Grune & Stratton, Inc, 1985, pp 377–399.

158a. Collinge J, Whittington MA, Sidle KCL, Smith CJ, Palmer MS, Clarke AR, Jefferys JGR. Prion protein is necessary for normal synaptic function. Nature 1994;370:295–297.

159. Cooper JH. Selective amyloid staining as a function of amyloid composition and structure. Lab Invest 1974;31:232–238.

160. Cornwell GG III, Murdoch WL, Kyle RA, Westermark P, Pitkänen P. Frequency and distribution of senile cardiovascular amyloid. A clinicopathologic correlation. Am J Med 1983;75:618–623.

161. Dickson DW, Kress Y, Crowe A, Yen S-H. Monoclonal antibodies to Alzheimer neurofibrillary tangles. 2. Demonstration of a common antigenic determinant between ANT and neurofibrillary degeneration in progressive supranuclear palsy. Am J Pathol 1985;120:292–303.

162. Dikman SH, Kahn T, Gribetz D, Churg J. Resolution of renal amyloidosis. Am J Med 1977;63:430–433.

163. Divry P, Florkin M. Sur les propriétés optiques de l'amyloïde. CR Soc Belg Biol 1927;97:1808–1810.

164. Durie BGM, Persky B, Soehnlen BJ, Grogan TM, Salmon SE. Amyloid production in human myeloma stem-cell culture, with morphologic evidence of amyloid secretion by associated macrophages. N Engl J Med 1982;307:1689–1692.

165. Duston MA, Skinner M, Shirahama T, Cohen AS. Diagnosis of amyloidosis by abdominal fat aspiration. Analysis of four years' experience. Am J Med 1987;82:412–414.

166. Dyck RF, Lockwood CM, Kershaw M, McHugh N, Duance VC, Baltz ML, Pepys MB. Amyloid P-component is a constituent of normal human glomerular basement membrane. J Exp Med 1980;152:1162–1174.

167. Eanes ED, Glenner GG. X-ray diffraction studies on amyloid filaments. J Histochem Cytochem 16:673–677.

168. Eriksson L, Westermark P. Intracellular neurofibrillary tangle-like aggregations. A constantly present amyloid alteration in the aging choroid plexus. Am J Pathol 1986;125:124–129.

169. Fitchen JH. Amyloidosis and granulomatous ileocolitis. Regression after surgical removal of the involved bowel. N Engl J Med 1975;292:352–353.

170. Gajdusek DC. Unconventional viruses and the origin and disappearance of kuru. Science 1977;197:943–960.

171. Glenner GG. Amyloid deposits and amyloidosis. The beta-fibrilloses. Parts I and Part II. N Engl J Med 1980;302:1283–1292, 1333–1343.

172. Glenner GG. Alzheimer's disease: multiple cerebral amyloidosis. In Katzman R. (ed). Banbury report 15. Biological aspects of Alzheimer's disease. Cold Spring Harbor, NY: Cold Spring Harbor Laboratory, 1983, pp 137–144.

173. Glenner GG, Eanes ED, Bladen HA, Linke RP, Termine JD. Beta-pleated sheet fibrils. A comparison of native amyloid with synthetic protein fibrils. J Histochem Cytochem 1974;22:1141–1158.

174. Glenner GG, Eanes ED, Page DL. The relation of the properties of congo red-stained amyloid fibrils to the beta-conformation. J Histochem Cytochem 1972;20:821–826.

175. Glenner GG, Ein D, Eanes ED, Bladen HA, Terry W, Page DL. Creation of "amyloid" fibrils from Bence Jones proteins in vitro. Science 1971;174:712–714.

176. Glenner GG, Osserman EF, Benditt EP, Calkins E, Cohen AS, Zucker-Franklin D (eds). Amyloidosis. New York: Plenum Press, 1986.

177. Glenner GG, Page DL. Amyloid, amyloidosis, and amyloidogenesis. Int Rev Exp Pathol 1976;15:1–92.

178. Glenner GG, Wong CW. Alzheimer's disease: initial report of the purification and characterization of a novel cerebrovascular amyloid protein. Biochem Biophys Res Commun 1984;120:885–890.

179. Glenner GG, Wong CW. Amyloid research as a paradigm for Alzheimer's disease. In: Glenner GG, Osserman EF, Benditt EP, Calkins E, Cohen AS, Zucker-Franklin D (eds). Amyloidosis. New York: Plenum Press, 1986, pp 693–701.

180. Goffin YA, Gruys E, Sorenson GD, Wellens F. Amyloid deposits in bioprosthetic cardiac valves after long-term implantation in man. A new localization of amyloidosis. Am J Pathol 1984;114:431–442.

181. Goffin YA, Rickaert F. Histotopographic evidence that amyloid deposits in sclerocalcific heart valves and other chronic lesions of the cardiovascular system are related to old thrombotic material. Virchows Arch [Pathol Anat] 1986;409:61–77.

182. Goldfinger SE. Colchicine for familial Mediterranean fever. N Engl J Med 1972;287:1302.

183. Goldstein DJ. Detection of dichroism with the microscope. J Microsc 1969;89 (Pt. 1):19–36.

184. Gorevic PD, Casey TT, Stone WJ, DiRaimondo CR, Prelli FC, Frangione B. Beta-2 microglobulin is an amyloidogenic protein in man. J Clin Invest 1985;76:2425–2429.

185. Gueft B. The x-ray diffraction pattern of prostatic corpora amylacea. Acta Pathol Microbiol Scand 1972;Sect. A, 80 (Suppl. 233):132–134.

186. Halpern GM. L'immunoglobuline E, 20 ans après. Méd Hyg 1985;43:1074–1092.

187. Hawkins PN, Lavender JP, Pepys MB. Evaluation of systemic amyloidosis by scintigraphy with ^{123}I-labeled serum amyloid P component. N Engl J Med 1990;323:508–513.

188. Hoffman JS, Ericsson LM, Eriksen N, Walsh KA, Benditt EP. Murine tissue amyloid protein AA. NH$_2$-terminal sequence identity with only one of two serum amyloid protein (ApoSAA) gene products. J Exp Med 1984;159:641–646.

189. Hol PR, Snel FWJJ, Niewold TA, Gruys E. Amyloid-enhancing factor (AEF) in the pathogenesis of AA-amyloidosis in the hamster. Virchows Arch (Cell Pathol) 1986;52:273–281.

190. Husby G, Araki S, Benditt EP, et al. The 1990 guidelines for nomenclature and classification of amyloid and amyloidosis. In: Natvig JB, Førre F, Husby G, et al. (eds). Amyloid and amyloidois 1990. Dordrecht: Kluwer Academic Publishers, 1991, pp 7–11.

191. Jenike MA. Alzheimer's disease. Sci Am Med 1990;13:1–5.

192. Johnson KH, O'Brien TD, Betsholtz C, Westermark P. Islet amyloid, islet-amyloid polypeptide, and diabetes mellitus. N Engl J Med 1989a;321:513–518.

193. Johnson KH, O'Brien TD, Hayden DW, et al. Immunolocalization of islet amyloid polypeptide (IAPP) in pancreatic beta cells by means of peroxidase-antiperoxidase (PAP) and protein A-gold techniques. Am J Pathol 1988;130:1–8.

194. Johnson KH, O'Brien TD, Jordan K, Westermark P. Impaired glucose tolerance is associated with increased islet amyloid polypeptide (IAPP) immunoreactivity in pancreatic beta cells. Am J Pathol 1989b;135:245–250.

195. Katzman R, Saitoh T. Advances in alzheimer's disease. FASEB J 1991; 5:278–286.

196. Kawahara E, Shiroo M, Nakanishi I, Migita S. The role of fibronectin in the development of experimental amyloidosis. Evidence of immunohistochemical codistributibution and binding property with serum amyloid protein A. Am J Pathol 1989;134:1305–1314.

197. Kisilevsky R. Amyloidosis: a familiar problem in the light of current pathogenetic developments. Lab Invest 1983;49:381–390.

198. Kisilevsky R. Heparan sulfate proteoglycans in amyloidogenesis: an epiphenomenon, a unique factor, or the tip of a more fundamental process? Lab Invest 1990;63:589–591.

199. Kyle RA. "Benign" monoclonal gammopathy. A misnomer? JAMA 1984;251:1849–1854.

200. Kyle RA, Bayrd ED. Amyloidosis: review of 236 cases. Medicine 1975;54:271–299.

201. Kyle RA, Greipp PR. Amyloidosis (AL). Clinical and laboratory features in 229 cases. Mayo Clin Proc 1983;58:665–683.

202. Kyle RA, Greipp PR, Garton JP, Gertz MA. Primary systemic amyloidosis (AL): comparison of melphalan-prednisone vs. colchicine treatment in 101 cases. In: Glenner GG, Osserman EF, Benditt EP, Calkins E, Cohen AS, Zucker-Franklin D (eds). Amyloidosis. New York: Plenum Press, 1986, pp 545–557.

203. Lavie G. Further studies on the mechanism of action of surface associated proteolytic enzymes on lymphocytes and monocytes which degrade SAA precursor to AA-like products. In: Glenner GG, Osserman EF, Benditt EP, Calkins E, Cohen AS, Zucker-Franklin D (eds). Amyloidosis. New York: Plenum Press, 1986, pp 217–223.

204. Lavie G, Zucker-Franklin D, Franklin EC. Degradation of serum amyloid A protein by surface-associated enzymes of human blood monocytes. J Exp Med 1978;148:1020–1031.

205. Lavie G, Zucker-Franklin D, Franklin EC. Elastase-type proteases on the surface of human blood monocytes: possible role in amyloid formation. J Immunol 1980;125:175–180.

206. Linker A, Carney HC. Presence and role of glycosaminoglycans in amyloidosis. Lab Invest 1987;57:297–305.

207. Lopez CD, Yost CS, Prusiner SB, Myers RM, Lingappa VR. Unusual topogenic sequence directs prion protein biogenesis. Science 1990;248:226–229.

208. Maloy AL, Longnecker DS, Greenberg ER. The relation of islet amyloid to the clinical type of diabetes. Hum Pathol 1981;12:917–922.

209. Maury CPJ, Teppo A-M. Mechanism of reduced amyloid-A-degrading activity in serum of patients with secondary amyloidosis. Lancet 1982;2:234–237.

210. Miura K, Takahashi Y, Shirasawa H. Immunohistochemical detection of serum amyloid A protein in the liver and the kidney after casein injection. Lab Invest 1985;53:453–463.

211. Niewold TA, Hol PR, van Andel ACJ, Lutz ETG, Gruys E. Enhancement of amyloid induction by amyloid fibril fragments in hamster. Lab Invest 1987;56:544–549.

212. Ohyama T, Shimokama T, Yoshikawa Y, Watanabe T. Splenic amyloidosis: correlations between chemical types of amyloid protein and morphological features. Mod Pathol 1990;3:419–422.

213. O'Leary TJ, Levin IW. Secondary structure of endocrine amyloid: infrared spectroscopy of medullary carcinoma of the thyroid. Lab Invest 1985;53:240–242.

214. Pepys MB, Baltz ML, de Beer FC, et al. Biology of serum amyloid P component. Ann NY Acad Sci 1982; 389:286–298.

215. Pras M, Schubert M, Zucker-Franklin D, Rimon A, Franklin EC. The characterization of soluble amyloid prepared in water. J Clin Invest 1968;47:924–933.

216. Price DL, Walker LC, Martin LJ, Sisodia SS. Amyloidosis in aging and Alzheimer's disease. Am J Pathol 1992;141:767–772.

217. Prusiner SB. Prions and neurodegenerative diseases. N Engl J Med 1987;317:1571–1581.

218. Prusiner SB, DeArmond SJ. Prions causing nervous system degeneration. Lab Invest 1987;56:349–363.

219. Puchtler H, Sweat F. A review of early concepts of amyloid in context with contemporary chemical literature from 1839 to 1859. J Histochem Cytochem 1966;14:123–134.

220. Ravid M, Robson M, Kedar I. Prolonged colchicine treatment in four patients with amyloidosis. Ann Intern Med 1977;87:568–570.

221. Roberts GW, Collinge J. Playing clue with prion disease. Lab Invest 1991;65:607–609.

222. Rumble B, Retallack R, Hilbich C, et al. Amyloid A4 protein and its precursor in Down's syndrome and Alzheimer's disease. N Engl J Med 1989;320:1446–1452.

223. St. George-Hyslop PH, Tanzi RE, Polinsky RJ, et al. The genetic defect causing familial Alzheimer's disease maps on chromosome 21. Science 1987;235:885–890.

224. Selkoe DJ. Deciphering Alzheimer's disease: the amyloid precursor protein yields new clues. Science 1990;248:1058–1060.

225. Shirahama T, Cohen AS. Intralysosomal formation of amyloid fibrils. Am J Pathol 1975;81:101–116.

226. Shirahama T, Miura K, Ju S-T, Kisilevsky R, Gruys E, Cohen AS. Amyloid enhancing factor-loaded macrophages in amyloid fibril formation. Lab Invest 1990; 62:61–68.

227. Shirahama T, Skinner M, Cohen AS, et al. Histochemical and immunohistochemical characterization of amyloid associated with chronic hemodialysis as beta-2-microglobulin. Lab Invest 1985;53:705–709.

228. Sigurdsson B. Rida, a chronic encephalitis of sheep with general remarks on infections which develop slowly and some of their special characteristics. Br Vet J 1954; 110:341–354.

229. Sigurdsson B, Pálsson PA. Visna of sheep. A slow, demyelinating infection. Br J Exp Pathol 1958;39:519–528.

230. Snow AD, Kisilevsky R, Stephens C, Anastassiades T. Characterization of tissue and plasma glycosaminoglycans during experimental AA amyloidosis and acute inflammation. Qualitative and quantitative analysis. Lab Invest 1987;56:665–675.

231. Snow AD, Willmer J, Kisilevsky R. Sulfated glycosaminoglycans: a common constituent of all amyloids? Lab Invest 1987;56:120–123.

232. Stahl N, Prusiner SB. Prions and prion proteins. FASEB J 1991;5:2799–2807.

233. Stone MJ. Amyloidosis: a final common pathway for protein deposition in tissues. Blood 1990;75:531–545.

234. Van Nostrand WE, Schmaier AH, Farrow JS, Cunningham DD. Protease nexin-II (amyloid β-protein precursor): a platelet a-granule protein. Science 1990; 248:745–748.

235. Varga J, Flinn MSM, Shirahama T, Rodgers OG, Cohen AS. The induction of accelerated murine amyloid with human splenic extract. Virchows Arch (Cell Pathol) 1986;51:177–185.

236. Virchow R. Cellular pathology. Translated from the 2nd German ed. by B Chance, 1859. Reproduced by Dover Publications, New York, 1971.

237. Virchow R. Ueber eine im Gehirn und Rückenmark des Menschen aufgefundene Substanz mit der chemischen Reaction der Cellulose. Virchows Arch [Pathol Anat] 1854;6:135–138.

238. Walton AG, Blackwell J. Biopolymers. New York: Academic Press, 1973.

239. Yankner BA, Dawes LR, Fisher S, Villa-Komaroff L, Oster-Granite ML, Neve RL. Neurotoxicity of a fragment of the amyloid precursor associated with Alzheimer's disease. Science 1989;245:417–420.

240. Zemer D, Pras M, Sohar E, Modan M, Cabili S, Gafni J. Colchicine in the prevention and treatment of the amyloidosis of familial Mediterranean fever. N Engl J Med 1986;314:1001–1005.

241. Zucker-Franklin D, Franklin EC. Intracellular localization of human amyloid by fluorescence and electron microscopy. Am J Pathol 1970;59:23–42.

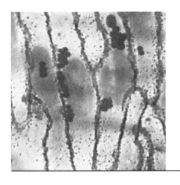

LOCAL INJURY AND INFLAMMATION

Introduction to Inflammation

CHAPTER 8

A Working Definition

Inflammation: The Evolution of a Concept

Exploring the "Reticulo-endothelial System"

Inflammation: A Pictorial Overview

With inflammation we step into a real-life drama, traditionally interpreted as the microscopic equivalent of warfare against true or perceived invaders, with its cellular heroes, villains, casualties, suicides, and even victims of friendly fire. About ten types of cells are involved. The setting is a battlefield in which real blood is shed, and the pace may be frantic or sluggish, but the action is always highly programmed, with messages flying in all directions. This makes cellular pathology sound rather static in retrospect, but of course it was essential for understanding the performers on the battlefield.

A Working Definition

Let us begin with a working definition and then examine its parts.

Inflammation is a response to injury of vascularized tissues. Its purpose is to deliver defensive materials (blood cells and fluid) to a site of injury. It is not a state but a process.

First we want to know why we have a special response to injury, and why this response should be the delivery of blood-borne materials.

We must step back and examine the threats posed by a local injury such as a wound. The basic problems caused by injury are three (Figure 8.1):

some vessels are severed, some tissue is destroyed, and the door is open to bacteria. The first problem, bleeding, is quite critical, but it is quickly, almost instantly, brought under control by the local mechanisms of hemostasis, which we will explain later (p. 612). The second problem, loss of tissue, is less urgent; the loss will be compensated in due time (days, weeks) by regeneration while local scavenger cells clear up the debris. The third problem, infection, is critical, but for this task the local defenses are not adequate. The local antibacterial "national guard," spread out in the tissues, amounts to a few sleepy macrophages scattered among the fibroblasts. They are not enough to ward off sudden bacterial attacks. The reason for this inadequacy is that it would be extremely expensive, biologically speaking, to

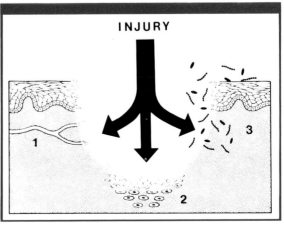

FIGURE 8.1
Injury to bacteria-laden surfaces creates three problems:
1. Vessels bleed.
2. Cells are destroyed. 3. Microbial invaders penetrate.

maintain fully alert defenses everywhere in the body. Nature has solved the problem by concentrating most of the defensive forces in the blood, where they circulate in inactive mode; then, wherever a problem arises, they are delivered—and activated. The delivery and the battle that ensues are the essence of inflammation.

The defensive materials supplied by the inflammatory response are basically two: **leukocytes,** some of which are specialized for fighting bacteria, and **plasma,** which contains defensive proteins of many kinds, including (a) proteins that coat foreign materials and make them easier to phagocytize (**opsonins**), (b) a group of about 20 proteins (cumulatively known as **complement**) that can be assembled locally to build a bacteria-perforating machine, and (c) **antibodies** that will bind to the surfaces of bacteria and other parasites. Because all these materials (cells and fluid) occupy space, the inflamed part of the body swells, and because the local blood vessels dilate in order to speed up the delivery, the inflamed part becomes red and hot. The name inflammation—evoking fire—is well deserved.

This mustering of forces that is inflammation is not as simple as it sounds because the cells and fluid must be **extravasated,** that is, transferred out of the vessels without interrupting the blood flow itself, which is the lifeline of all tissues as well as the source of the defensive materials. Just consider: the circulating white blood cells, which must be delivered to the extravascular space, are larger than the red blood cells, which must be kept inside the vessels. We do not know of any plumbing created by

humans that could solve this tricky problem. Inflammation manages to gather locally its needed supplies of cells and fluid by providing all the cells involved, including the microvascular endothelium and the leukocytes traveling in the blood vessels, with specific instructions in the form of chemical messengers: the *mediators of inflammation.* Some mediators, for example, will instruct the endothelium to become leaky; others will tell the leukocytes to stop and emigrate. The earliest mediators to appear on the scene of an injury are produced by the injured tissue itself. Note the perfect feedback loop: *the defense reaction is triggered by the products of the aggression* (Figure 8.2).

The mixture of leukocytes and plasma that accumulates in the tissues is called inflammatory exudate or simply **exudate.** When the exudate is rich with cells it becomes creamy and its name becomes **pus.** Pus requires a special introduction, because in the nonmedical world it tends to be misunderstood. Let it be clear: despite its repulsive reputation *pus is a very noble substance.* It is composed of leukocytes that have given up their lives to phagocytize bacteria. They have rushed to a site of infection in response to an ancestral call: they are attracted not only by products of injury but also by substances produced by invading bacteria. A wound that produces a lot of pus can be looked upon in two ways: it is heavily infected, and its inflammatory response is excellent.

Inflammation lasts as long as required to eliminate the cause and to repair the damage. With time it usually changes in character; vascular dilatation tends to subside and the redness correspondingly

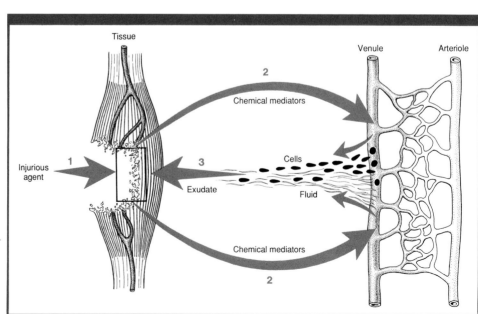

FIGURE 8.2
The basic feedback principle of inflammation. Injured tissue (1) releases chemical mediators (2) that diffuse to neighboring blood vessels and trigger an exudate of cells and fluid (3): the first step in the repair process.

abates; the amount of fluid lost may decrease and so the swelling subsides; in the meantime the cell population changes to a predominance of mononuclear cells. The process may last hours or years.

We have portrayed inflammation primarily as an antibacterial response, but let it be clear that *inflammation operates against all invaders:* fungi, worms, viruses, and other parasites. It just so happens that bacteria far outnumber the other aggressors, so that evolution has patterned the cellular responses especially against bacteria.

Now we return to our working definition of inflammation and comment on another feature. If inflammation is a reaction of vascularized tissues to injury, what happens when nonvascularized tissues are injured?

If injury selectively hits a tissue devoid of blood vessels, such as the cornea, the damaged tissue responds very simply by regenerating, if it can do so. In practice, however, an inflammatory response will occur in the surrounding vascularized tissues. Two mechanisms explain this phenomenon: (a) the injury may involve several tissues (e.g., trauma may affect the articular cartilage and the bone beneath it), and (b) the avascular injured tissue produces chemical messages that elicit inflammation in the surrounding tissues. A classic example: a scratch in the cornea, which has no vessels, induces an inflammatory response (redness and pain) in the sclera.

INFECTION VERSUS INFLAMMATION

Laymen tend to equate infection and inflammation. Please do not join the crowd. It is true that bacterial infection usually brings about inflammation, but the words infection and inflammation represent very different concepts. **Inflammation** is a reaction; **infection** simply means "contamination with microorganisms." There can be infection without inflammation, for example, in a severely immunosuppressed patient. There can also be inflammation without infection: remember that inflammation is triggered by products of tissue injury, and thus that any aseptic injury will trigger inflammation. A classic example is a myocardial infarct. The purpose of such programmed inflammation without infection is a semiphilosophical problem; we shall come to it on p. 420.

Inflammation is also one of the effector arms of the immune response. In a nutshell: the immune response produces (a) cells that are programmed to attack specific targets and (b) antibody molecules that are shaped to bind to specific targets. In general, wherever encounters occur between cells and their targets and between antibodies and their targets, mediators are released that elicit inflammation. Inflammation is thereby "borrowed" by the immune response as a nonspecific but very effective ally in destroying its selected targets. This is a wonderful arrangement, but it comes at a price: it so happens that the immune response often reacts excessively to innocuous targets, such as pollen, or selects inappropriate targets, such as normal tissues in autoimmune disease. Inflammation is triggered anyway. The result: in the case of pollen, a nuisance such as hay fever; in the case of autoimmune disease, serious disorders such as rheumatoid arthritis. *Under these conditions, inflammation becomes a disease,* and antiinflammatory measures, which could be deadly when inflammation is performing its proper antibacterial function, become therapeutic.

TERMINOLOGY OF INFLAMMATION

The suffix *-itis* usually means inflammation of that organ or tissue (appendic-itis, mening-itis, pleur-itis). The terms **acute** and **chronic** have been defined on p. 7: briefly, the two terms are used loosely to mean events that evolve over *hours and days* versus *weeks, months, or years;* "acute" in a clinical setting means "coming sharply to a climax." **Injury** means damage: that is, the effect of an injurious agent. **Local injury** is damage inflicted to a limited part of the body as opposed to **systemic injury,** such as poisoning, cooling, dehydration, or whole-body irradiation. The term **exudate** always refers to the product of inflammation, namely the extravasated mixture of protein-rich fluid and cells; *it is opposed to* **transudate,** *the ultrafiltrate of plasma that arises from normal vessels.* The term *inflammatory infiltrate* or simply **infiltrate** is often used for a swarm of inflammatory cells from an exudate as seen under the microscope. The ancient terms *phlogistic* and *antiphlogistic* are still used to mean "inflammatory" and "antiinflammatory"; they come from the Greek *phlox* for "flame."

Inflammation: The Evolution of a Concept

Because local injury is part of everyday life, inflammation is probably the most common aspect of tissue pathology and has always been perceived as a central issue in the practice of medicine. It has inspired theories that have had enormous impact

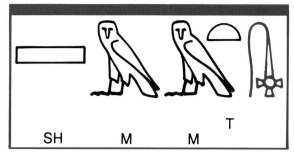

FIGURE 8.3
One of the ancient Egyptian words for inflammation: SH-M-M-T, conventionally pronounced "shememet." The first four hieroglyphs stand for the consonants indicated. The last sign, called a "determinative," is not to be pronounced; it indicates the general meaning of the preceding word. In this case it represents a brazier filled with oil, with a flame arising from it and a trail of smoke curling downward. (Reproduced with permission from [31].)

(Figure 8.3). The reader may wonder how any particular word of a dead language can be translated by our current term inflammation; but in fact, several of the ancient terms so translated refer most definitely to what we call inflammation because they relate to heat, to redness, or to an actual flame (31, 32).

Today we know that inflammation is a life-saving reaction, usually to infection. In ancient times, however, when the concept of bacterial infection did not exist, a swollen red finger was interpreted as meaning that the finger was "sick with inflammation." Inflammation was thought to be the disease—and was treated accordingly. How could one fight inflammation? Simple. The ancient Greeks argued, quite plausibly, that the redness is due to an excess of red blood. All excesses being bad, according to Greek culture, the obvious treatment was to draw blood. Such was the antiinflammatory therapy championed by the Hippocratic physicians and perpetuated by their heirs for some 2300 years. Bloodletting became the treatment of choice for any case of inflammation; eventually, blood was drawn even if no redness was visible, not only because this procedure seemed helpful as a form of drainage—removal of bad humors—but also because inflammation was thought to be at the root of most diseases (31). In Western medicine this aberrant therapy became extraordinarily popular because it seemed to make such good sense. The fashion continued well into the nineteenth century: Napoleon's wounded soldiers were bled of their last few ounces of blood on the battlefield to prevent inflammation of their wounds. Such is the power of theory.

The Romans went along with Greek theory, but they made one everlasting contribution. Cornelius Celsus, a writer of the first century, compiled a

on medical treatment; some bad ones have killed many more people than the good ones have saved. It has also inspired great discoveries; for example, the concept of bacterial infection, which was discovered in 1867 by the surgeon Joseph Lister, later Lord Lister, while studying inflamed wounds (30).

INFLAMMATION AS A DISEASE

A red eye, a hot and swollen finger, a wound that is surrounded by reddened skin and exuding pus are impressive sights: no healer of any era could fail to notice them. Accordingly, words for inflammation are found in the most ancient medical texts—Egyptian, Mesopotamian, Greek, and Chinese. The oldest known are the Egyptian papyri, which reach as far back as 2700 B.C.

FIGURE 8.4
The four cardinal signs of inflammation were codified by Celsus in the first century A.D. This is how they appeared much later in a codex of the tenth century. (Reproduced with permission from [31].)

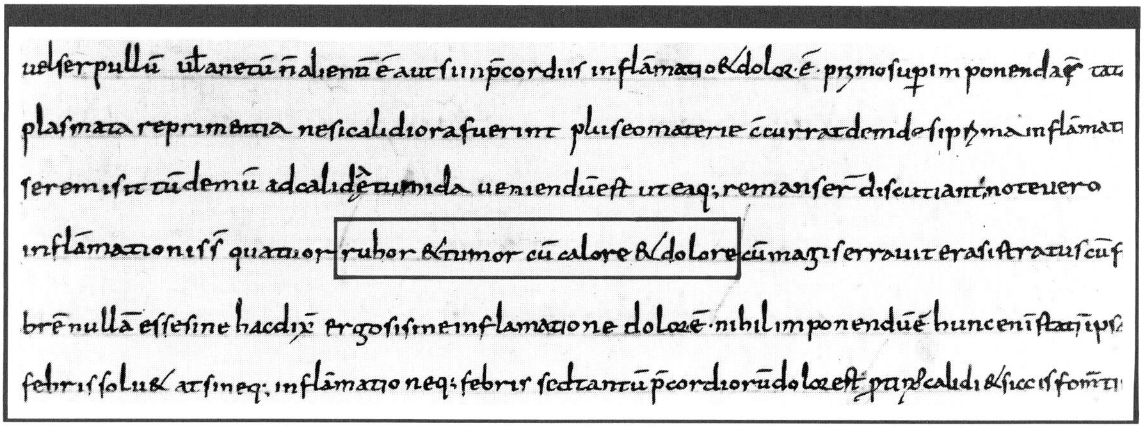

large encyclopedia; in the section on medicine (*De medicina*) he wrote: "*Notae vero inflammationis sunt quatuor: rubor et tumor cum calore et dolore,*" meaning "Truly the signs of inflammation are four, redness and swelling with heat and pain" (Figure 8.4). To this day, nobody has improved upon this definition of acute inflammation, which has been recited by medical students century after century and still appears on the National Board exams, though not in Latin.

INFLAMMATION AS A USEFUL REACTION

The thought that inflammation might be useful emerged as a speculation in the 1700s (40, p. 148); it was spelled out unmistakably by John Hunter, a Scottish surgeon and naturalist endowed with tremendous insight and a genius for research. Hunter had tended hundreds of festering war wounds. His famous treatise *On the Blood, Inflammation and Gunshot Wounds*, published in 1794, contains this nugget: "Inflammation in itself is not to be considered as a disease, but as a salutary operation, consequent either to some violence or some disease" (25, p. 249). "Some violence" or "some disease" was his masterly intuition for "injured tissue" and "bacteria."

In the days of John Hunter, the microscope was used by few scientists. It had the reputation of being more a toy than a tool; its images were considered difficult to distinguish from artefacts and were therefore viewed with suspicion (33). Half a century later, Rudolf Virchow, the father of modern pathology and a firm believer in the microscope, published his revolutionary *Cellular Pathology* (1859). By his time it had become fashionable to study pus under the microscope, and it was well known that pus contained "pus corpuscles," the emigrated leukocytes. Virchow portrayed them as he saw them (Figure 8.5) and noted their similarity to white blood cells, but he added that "it will probably still require a number of years" before anyone could decide whether they migrated from the blood into the pus or from the pus into the blood (47, p. 182).

Actually, Virchow had not quite done his homework: the emigration of leukocytes from blood vessels had been clearly described by the Frenchman H. Dutrochet in 1824 (16), and the origin of the pus globules from "blood corpuscles perforating the capillaries" had been established in 1846 by an Englishman, Augustus Waller, who also described the "Wallerian degeneration" of resected nerves

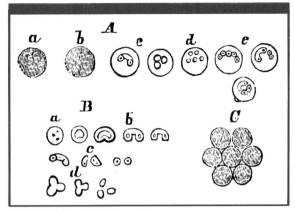

FIGURE 8.5
Pus corpuscles (leukocytes), as illustrated by Virchow in 1859. The darker ones (**Aab, C**) are fresh; all others have been treated with acetic acid, then a standard procedure for making tissues more transparent (stains were not yet used). The multilobed nucleus of the neutrophils is clearly shown in **Ac–e**, but Virchow was noncommittal as to the origin of the pus corpuscles, except for stating that "colorless blood-cells are so like pus corpuscles as easily to be mistaken for them." (Reproduced with permission from [47].)

(17, 40). Dutrochet and Waller having been forgotten, diapedesis had to be rediscovered in 1867 by one of Virchow's most famous pupils, Julius Cohnheim. At that time the thin histologic sections that we now take for granted did not exist. Like many of his contemporaries, including Waller, Cohnheim did his microscopic work on cumbersome but transparent living membranes such as the mesentery or the tongue of the frog (Figure 8.6): this limitation turned out to be a major advantage, because blood flow in living tissues offered the opportunity to observe dynamic events, such as diapedesis. One day, as he was studying a preparation of frog mesentery, Cohnheim observed a sequence of events that gave inflammation a whole new meaning (12). He noticed that the arterioles in the irritated tissue became wider and more blood filled all the vessels; flow at first was faster, then it slowed, and eventually white blood cells emigrated out into the tissues (diapedesis) while plasma also leaked out. Now the four cardinal signs stated by Celsus could be explained in scientific terms: the redness and heat were due to increased blood flow, the swelling to the exudation of cells and fluid, and the pain would follow. Cohnheim was understandably elated.

This was a big step forward. Little does it matter that Cohnheim was not the first to see diapedesis (he acknowledges it in a footnote that reads very

mesoderm of transparent invertebrates. Then, in his words:

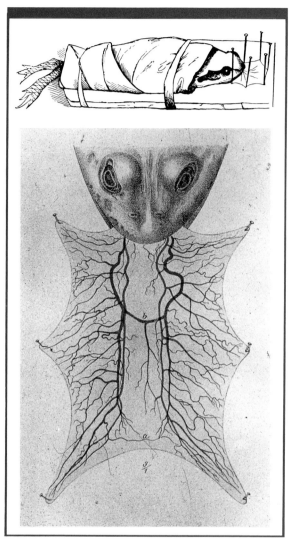

> *One day when the whole family had gone to a circus to see some extraordinary performing apes, I remained alone with my microscope, observing the life in the mobile cells of transparent star-fish larvae, when a new thought suddenly flashed across my brain. It struck me that similar cells might serve in the defence of the organism against intruders. Feeling that there was in this something of surpassing interest, I felt so excited that I began striding up and down the room and even went to the seashore to collect my thoughts. I said to myself that, if my supposition was true, a splinter introduced into the body of a star-fish larva, devoid of blood vessels or of a nervous system, should soon be surrounded by mobile cells as is observed in a man who runs a splinter into his finger. This was no sooner said than done. There was a small garden in our dwelling, in which we had a few days previously organized a "Christmas tree" for the children on a little tangerine tree; I fetched from it a few rose thorns and introduced them at once under the skin of some beautiful star-fish larvae as transparent as water. I was too excited to sleep that night in the expectation of the result of my experiment, and very early the next morning I ascertained that it had fully succeeded. This experiment formed the basis of the phagocyte theory, to the development of which I devoted the next twenty-five years of my life. (36)*

Nobody could have done more with rose thorns and starfish larvae. This seminal experiment was soon confirmed by another masterly observation, this time on a tiny transparent crustacean, *Daphnia*, the water flea (Figure 8.7) (34, 35, p. 82). The structure of this little creature is essentially that of an intestinal tube and a skin, separated by a space or coelom. Metchnikoff noticed that sometimes a rod-shaped microorganism, *Monospora*, escaped from the intestinal tube into the surrounding space, causing the animal to die. At other times the invading *Monospora* was attacked and engulfed by free-floating cells, and in these cases the animal survived. Once again, the phagocytes were proven to be defensive cells.

Metchnikoff had no medical training, but when he learned of Cohnheim's findings on inflammation and diapedesis he suddenly grasped the link: *the purpose of inflammation was to deliver phagocytes to a site of injury.* Fortunately he was not discouraged by a passing visitor, Professor Virchow, who politely advised him that the current theory of inflammation was quite the opposite: leukocytes were engaged in spreading bacteria(!) (36).

much like "oops": Professor Virchow, now partially updated, had just given him the reference to Waller): Cohnheim's was the first comprehensive theory of inflammation.

STARFISH AND PHAGOCYTES

Although Cohnheim did see the leukocytes emigrate, he had no idea what their functions could be out in the tissues. For that critical step we must skip to Messina, in Sicily, in 1882. The Russian zoologist Ilya Metchnikoff had just settled in Messina to escape turmoil in his native country. He had no job and worked at his home on the seaside, supported by his wealthy wife; the beach was a generous source of microscopic subjects for someone who knew where to look. In 1880 he discovered and named phagocytosis by studying the fate of carmine particles introduced into the

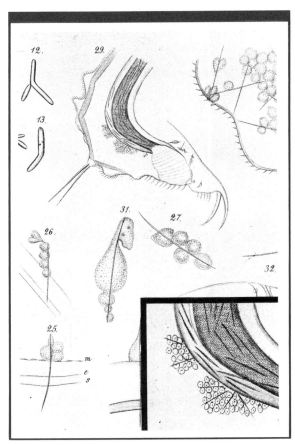

FIGURE 8.7

The defensive function of leukocytes as illustrated by Metchnikoff in 1884 from observations on the water flea, *Daphnia magna*. **29:** Abdominal portion of a Daphnia. The intestinal lumen contains many rodlike spores of a primitive fungus that Metchnikoff called *Monospora bicuspidata*. Inset: Some of the spores have found their way into the wall of the intestine; others have emerged into the abdominal cavity where they are surrounded by leukocytes. **31,27:** Other spores surrounded by leukocytes. (Reproduced with permission from [35].)

ENTER ANTIBODIES

Then came another explosive novelty: in 1890 Behring and Kitasato discovered antidiphtheric toxin. Antibodies suddenly appeared on the medical scene, and a new theory of inflammation was launched: *the purpose of inflammation was to bring antibodies, not cells, to the site of infection.* This caused much bitterness to Metchnikoff, who was then working at the Pasteur Institute in Paris, and much energy was wasted by scientists of the two opposing sides, largely German versus French. The battle died away when it became obvious, as so often happens in the history of science, that both sides were right. The defensive purpose of inflam-

mation hinges on phagocytes *and* on antibodies: cells and fluid, as stated in our definition. In 1908 Metchnikoff shared the Nobel prize with Paul Ehrlich, a member of the antibody faction (23).

ENTER THE RETICULOENDOTHELIAL SYSTEM

A few years after Metchnikoff received the Nobel prize, his favorite cell, the macrophage, received the ultimate accolade. Metchnikoff had already used the expression "system of macrophages," but an eminent German pathologist, Ludwig Aschoff, seized upon it and proposed an even broader generalization: *all the phagocytic cells in the body can be considered as part of a "diffuse organ" with many functions, including defense.* He called this organ the reticuloendothelial system (RES) (3). We will now review it because it turned out to be even more important to survival than Aschoff had predicted: it plays a key role in orchestrating local and general defenses, including the immune system.

Exploring the "Reticuloendothelial System"

The reticuloendothelial system or RES (forgive this archaic name—we will discuss it shortly) was at first considered to be just a system of phagocytic cells. Now it is known to have many functions other than phagocytosis. Still, finding the sites where phagocytosis normally takes place is the simplest way to map the RES; so we will use phagocytosis as a guide.

To map the diffuse RES organ, Aschoff and his collaborators chose a number of colored materials (solutions of dyes and suspensions of particulate pigments), injected them either locally or intravenously, and found out which cells picked them up. They soon realized that almost any cell in the body will phagocytize if pushed to do so, and therefore decided to include only the most actively phagocytic cells in the RES. (Today the accepted term for these most active cells is **professional phagocytes.**) They also noticed that the most active "provinces" (their word) of the RES were the liver, spleen, and bone marrow.

The members of the RES family have changed somewhat since the time of Aschoff. The fibroblasts and endothelium have been thrown out as nonprofessional phagocytes, and other cells have been admitted (Figure 8.8). The members of the

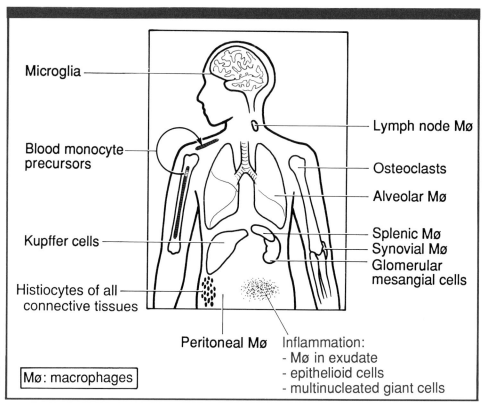

FIGURE 8.8

Types of cells considered to belong to the reticuloendothelial system (mononuclear phagocyte system). (Adapted from [41].)

modern RES cells have a great deal in common, even their ancestry. It is now believed that a single cell type—the monocyte—is born in the bone marrow, is distributed throughout the body, and then differentiates, depending on where it lands, into cells as disparate as the microglia, the osteoclasts, and the Kupffer cells of the liver. Phagocytosis is no longer thought to be the sole act of the RES. The monocyte/macrophage has a mind-boggling series of functional properties: it is involved in the immune response, tumor cell control, hematopoiesis, coagulation, and much else (29). Of course, the importance of the RES has skyrocketed, even though it remains an "invisible organ," hidden inside all other organs.

In view of these developments, a committee of experts renamed the RES in 1972 as MPS (*mononuclear phagocyte system*) (46). Because both names are currently used, we will use them both until evolution dictates the survival of the fittest. In the meantime, the name RES was applied to a society and a journal, and a book published on the RES reaches the size of an encyclopedia (18).

By the way: there should be some feeling of frustration among the polymorphs, which are not admitted to the RES/MPS despite their exemplary phagocytic properties. The reason: they are biologically quite different, as we will see (p. 320). Phagocytosis alone is not enough of a passport for membership in the RES/MPS club.

The provinces of the phagocytic system can be conveniently mapped, as Aschoff did, by injecting phagocytizable materials that are also colored; thus, each and every phagocyte will acquire its own label from one or another material. We now offer you a guided tour through these classic experiments; much is to be learned in the process, because the RES/MPS is a pillar of the body's defenses. Just remember that no single material method can reveal all the phagocytes: one group or another will be excluded by every experiment. Predictably, the size of the labeling particles makes a difference: intravenously injected suspensions of colloidal pigments that cannot cross the endothelium will label only those phagocytes that line the bloodstream; solutions of dyes that can cross the endothelium will also label the phagocytes that lie outside the vessels. Therefore, both types of experiments are essential for understanding inflammation; they also illustrate what happens to foreign particles (including bacteria) in the blood or in the tissues.

MAPPING THE RES WITH AN INTRAVENOUS INJECTION OF COLLOIDAL PARTICLES

The beauty of this experiment is that it shows us the fate of foreign particles traveling in the bloodstream. Carbon black is the prototype of colloidal suspensions; its particles are 300 Å or more in diameter (the order of magnitude of lipoproteins) and cannot be transcytosed by the endothelium. Although they are much smaller than bacteria, they are picked up by the same cells that pick up bacteria.

> *Ordinary India ink should not be used for these experiments because its shellac promotes clotting (20). A special "biological" suspension of carbon suspended in a gelatin solution is commercially available (26).*

Three drops of carbon black suspension (0.3 ml) are enough to give the skin and mucosae of a 300-g albino rat an ominous grey hue, but the discoloration fades away under the eyes of the experimenter, and in 5–10 minutes the normal pink color returns. Inspection of the internal organs after 15 minutes is absolutely striking. The novice will probably expect all organs to be grey. Not at all: the liver and spleen are jet black, and all other organs are normal. If a long bone is opened, its marrow will also appear blackened, though not as intensely as the liver and spleen. The carbon black accumulates in the liver, spleen, and bone marrow because these organs have special, wide capillaries called **sinusoids** that are partially lined with flat macrophages (Figure 8.9). In ruminants also the capillaries of the lung are capable of performing some phagocytosis (9, 10, 49).

So we have learned that the RES/MPS has a special "province:" a set of phagocytes lining the finest blood vessels in the liver, spleen, and bone marrow, and in ruminants also in the lung.

This particular province of phagocytes is called upon whenever some particulate foreign material is carried by the blood. There is no official name for it, which is regrettable, because we will often need to mention this sector of the RES/MPS. We will therefore adopt the rarely used but excellent name **littoral phagocytes;** littoral means "on the beach" (*litus* is Latin for "shore," referring to the "shores" of the bloodstream). *This system of littoral phagocytes includes about 90 percent of all mononuclear phagocytes (11, p. 247) and is therefore the largest segment of the RES/MPS; it functions as the filter of the blood.*

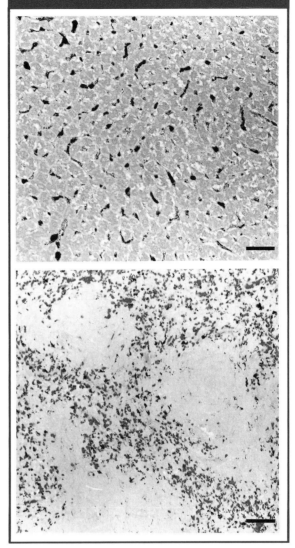

FIGURE 8.9
Littoral (or sinusoidal) phagocytes of the liver and spleen, in a rat injected 1 hour earlier with a colloidal suspension of carbon black. *Top:* Liver. The dots and streaks correspond to single Kupffer cells loaded with carbon. No carbon is picked up by the hepatocytes. *Bottom:* Spleen. The clear areas correspond to lymph follicles, because lymphocytes are not phagocytic. The dots represent phagocytes in the red pulp. Stain: Eosin only. **Bars =** 50 μm.

An alternative name for the littoral phagocytes is sinusoidal phagocytes. We find littoral more pictorial.

The littoral phagocytes of different organs do not have identical properties; for example, the spleen more easily recognizes those particles that are coated with immunoglobulin, of which it recognizes the "free end" (the so-called Fc portion). This may explain why the removal of the spleen can be followed by fulminating pneumococcal sepsis: the liver's littoral phagocytes are not efficient in recognizing immunoglobulin-coated bacteria (21, 44).

Quantitative studies of the blood of rats injected intravenously with carbon show that, depending on the dose, most of the circulating carbon is removed in less than an hour (Figure

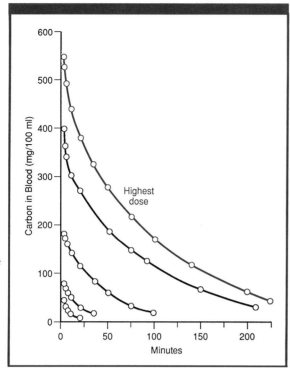

FIGURE 8.10
Rate of clearance of carbon black from the blood. Low doses are cleared faster. (Reproduced with permission from [6].)

8.10) (5, 6). In general, the clearance of colloidal particles from the blood depends on their number (Figure 8.10), size, and nature. *Larger particles, including bacteria, are cleared faster than smaller particles* (11). Repeated intravenous injections lead to decreased uptake (6). This has been referred to as a "blockade of the RES" as if the diminished rate of clearance were due to overstuffing the phagocytes; in fact, it is more likely that repeated flooding of the plasma with foreign particles depletes it of phagocytosis-promoting proteins (opsonins) (42).

The speed with which the RES/MPS clears the blood is amazing. In laboratory animals the liver alone clears about 80 percent of colloidal foreign material in a single passage; in fact, this rate can be used for measuring blood flow through the liver (7, 42).

We now discuss some lessons from these experiments with particles injected into the bloodstream.

FATE OF INDIGESTIBLE MATERIAL

Indigestible material stored in the littoral phagocytes is there for life. There is no way out of the RES/MPS—except for some *inhaled* particles. When the littoral macrophages die, they may well spill their carbon into the bloodstream, but some

other littoral macrophages will pick it up and repeat the cycle.

The only province of the RES/MPS that does have a way out is represented by the alveolar macrophages, which are transported out by the ciliary conveyor belt (rats swallow about two million alveolar macrophages per hour) (9). Other monocytes/macrophages are probably lost into the gut, but neither group of cells can get rid of significant amounts of materials injected intravenously. Evolution has not prepared the RES/MPS for this housecleaning task.

There was a time not long ago—in the early days of radiology—when thorotrast, a suspension of radioactive(!) thorium dioxide particles, was injected intraarterially to visualize arterial branches. It accumulated in the RES/MPS and damaged especially the liver (Figure 8.11). Its long-term effects included cancer.

MEDICAL USES FOR LITTORAL PHAGOCYTES

Littoral phagocytes can be exploited for diagnosis or therapy. Colloidal sulfur technetium, a radioactive particle with a very short half-life, can be used to visualize the RES. Some parasites such as *Leishmania* have chosen the littoral phagocytes as a biological niche: they have found a way to survive inside them after being phagocytized. One way to hit them is to inject a colloidal drug intravenously; the littoral phagocytes take it up, and that is the end of the parasite (p. 212).

RELATION OF LYMPH NODES TO THE RES

Lymph nodes are certainly full of phagocytes, but remember that these are strategically placed to clear the *lymph*. The phagocytes in the lymph nodes line the lymphatics, not the blood vessels; therefore, in theory, an intravenous injection of carbon black should not label the lymph nodes at all. However, after an intravenous injection of carbon black some faint outlines of blackened vessels can be seen in the lymph nodes (Figure 8.12) (27) and in Peyer's patches of the intestine, another lymphatic organ (Figure 8.13) (37, 43, 51). Close study showed that this does not represent phagocytosis. The retention of particles is due to venular leakage of a special kind.

The blackened vessels are the famous high-endothelial venules, which are the doorway for lymphocyte recycling. The lymphocytes in the blood recognize this special endothelial surface, stick to it,

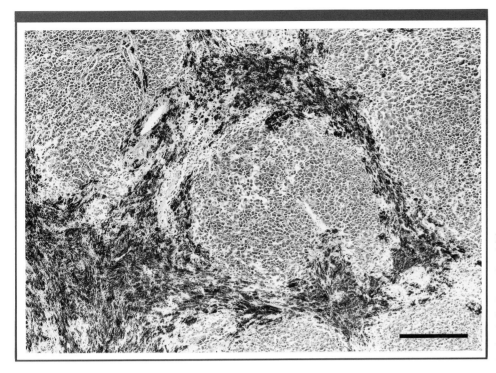

FIGURE 8.11
The scarred liver of a patient who died many years after an arteriography performed with an intra-arterial injection of thorotrast. The scars appear dark due to countless macrophages loaded with thorotrast. Autopsy performed in 1940. **Bar** = 500 μm.

crawl across the endothelium, and float away in the lymph, which will carry them back to the blood. As they perform their diapedesis across the endothelium of the high-endothelial venules, a few of the injected carbon particles can sneak across with them and then remain trapped against the basement membrane.

BACTERIA IN THE BLOODSTREAM

The littoral phagocytes probably save our lives on a daily basis. Any bacteria that find their way into the bloodstream—and this must happen all the time—are promptly removed, as can be shown experimentally (Figure 8.14). The simple act of chewing is said to cause bacteremia, bacteria being forced into the vessels of the pocket between tooth and gum. A door wide open to bacteria is created when a tooth is pulled (4). Using very sensitive culture methods, Fiore-Donno has cultivated as many as 32 varieties of oral bacteria from the bloodstream after tooth extractions (Fiore-Donno G, Faculty of Dental Medicine, Geneva, Switzerland; personal communication). Normally, this invasion is quickly overwhelmed by the littoral phagocytes.

Individuals with defective heart valves are especially prone to developing bacterial endocarditis, probably because bacteria circulating in the bloodstream become easily attached to injured surfaces. For patients with such defects, even the simple procedure of tooth scaling can release into the blood enough bacteria to cause endocarditis, unless antibiotics are used prophylactically.

MAPPING THE RES/MPS WITH A LOCAL INJECTION OF COLLOIDAL PARTICLES

This is, in essence, what tattoo artists do when they inject carbon black or other colloidal pigments into the skin. The particles are taken up by the local macrophages, which are reinforced by blood monocytes attracted there by the trauma. These cells store the indigestible particles in their residual bodies until they die; at that time the debris will be taken up by other macrophages. A few particles will be swept into the lymphatics, especially during the trauma of tattooing, and will end their journey in the nearest filter: the regional lymph node. As a matter of fact, the filtering function of the lymph nodes was discovered by Virchow when performing the autopsy of a soldier who had a colored tattoo on the arm; the red cinnabar had persisted in the lymph node for nearly 50 years (47, pp. 218–220).

The lesson of this experiment is that *material injected into the tissues can find its way into the local lymphatic vessels and reach the regional lymph nodes.* This pathway is exploited in vaccination: the antigen is carried to the "antibody factory" in the lymph nodes.

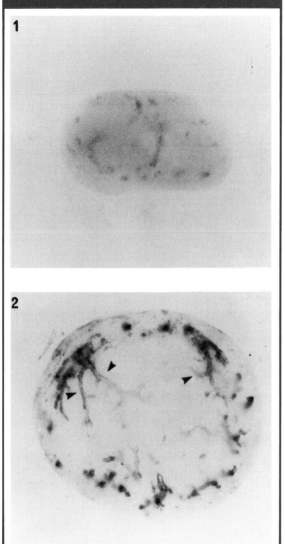

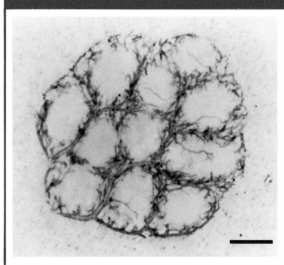

FIGURE 8.13
Peyer's patch of a rat. The high-endothelial venules have been labeled in black by a hefty dose of carbon black injected intravenously 2 hours earlier. The labeling of the venules is due to carbon particles leaking out during the emigration of lymphocytes. **Bar** = 1 mm. (Courtesy of Dr. G.I. Schoefl, The John Curtin School of Medical Research, The Australian National University, Canberra.)

FIGURE 8.12
A special variety of vascular labeling in normal and acutely inflamed lymph nodes. *Top:* Normal mouse popliteal lymph node after a single intravenous injection of 0.1 ml of carbon black/100g body weight. There is some faint labeling of the venules, especially of the high-endothelial variety, due to leakage of carbon black accompanying lymphocyte diapedesis. *Bottom:* Mouse popliteal lymph node labeled with carbon black 12 hours after an injection of endotoxin in the footpad (which caused the lymph node to become acutely inflamed). Note the heavier labeling of the venules (**arrowheads**), representing an increased transendothelial traffic of lymphocytes. (Courtesy of Dr. M. C. Kowala [27]).

MAPPING THE **RES/MPS** WITH SOLUBLE DYES INJECTED INTRAVENOUSLY

A favorite dye for this RES/MPS mapping experiment is Evans blue, which can also be used in humans to determine plasma volume. The dye binds to plasma albumin, so the result is much the same as that of injecting blue albumin. Water-soluble materials such as Evans blue, when injected intravenously, are taken up by all the macrophages in the body except those that lie beyond a blood–tissue barrier.

Trypan blue and Evans blue are traditionally used for this type of experiment simply because blue contrasts nicely with the color of the skin of albino rats; there is nothing magic about the blueness.

Do proteins cross the endothelium? Although the endothelium has the reputation of being a semipermeable barrier that is impermeable to protein, it is a fact that virtually all plasma proteins can be ferried across (however slowly) by transcytosis. This is true even for the large lipoprotein particles, which can be found in the tissue spaces. Furthermore, albumin is also taken up by specific receptors on the endothelial surface and then transcytosed (19, 39).

Over a few days a white rat or rabbit injected with Evans blue slowly turns blue because all the phagocytes in the skin and connective tissues pick

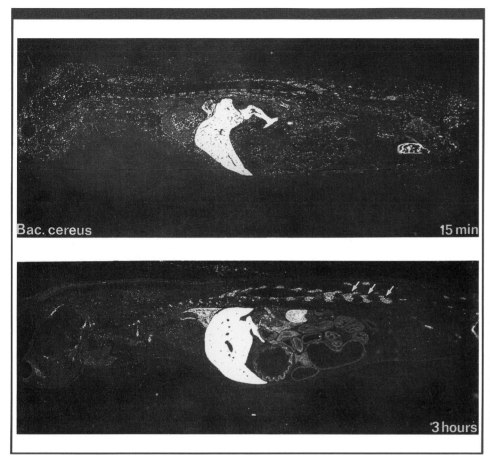

FIGURE 8.14
Autoradiograph of sections of two mice injected with radioactive bacilli (*Bacillus cereus*) 15 minutes and 3 hours before sacrifice. Note the high concentration of radioactivity in the organs that contain littoral phagocytes: the liver, spleen, and bone marrow (vertebrae, **arrows**). (Reproduced with permission from [8].)

up molecules of blue albumin emerging from the microcirculation. The circulating albumin–blue complex is not recognized as extremely foreign by the littoral phagocytes, and its clearance is accordingly slower than that of carbon black (the clearance has not been studied in detail [24], but the dye probably remains in the circulation for more than 1 day). Of course, the littoral phagocytes are also blue; and once again, undigestible materials cannot escape from the RES/MPS: the animals will remain blue as long as they live.

It should be clear at this point that an intravenous injection of Evans blue demonstrates more macrophages than carbon black. Besides the littoral phagocytes it demonstrates all the phagocytes in the connective tissue spaces *except those that lie behind blood–tissue barriers.* These are the blood–brain, blood–nerve, and blood–testis barriers and presumably also the blood–skin barrier (15). At autopsy, the blue body of the rat or rabbit contrasts sharply with the bright white color of the brain and nerves (Figure 8.15).

The blood–skin barrier is intriguing. The evidence for such a barrier is the presence in the superficial capillaries of the dermis of the same marker that is present in brain capillaries (the P-glycoprotein or multidrug-resistance protein, p. 936). However, the skin does become blue in the Evans blue experiment; the role of this barrier is not yet clear.

In summary: to demonstrate the *littoral phagocytes* in the liver, spleen, and bone marrow, inject carbon black intravenously; to demonstrate the *phagocytes in the lymph nodes*, inject carbon black in the lymphatics (or in the tissues drained by those lymph nodes); to demonstrate *all phagocytes in the body* with one method is impossible, but Evans blue injected intravenously will eventually reach *all macrophages except those beyond the blood–tissue barriers.*

SOME HIGHLIGHTS OF RES/MPS PHYSIOLOGY

- *The role of blood flow.* It stands to reason that the littoral phagocytes can take up

FIGURE 8.15
The fate of foreign materials carried by the bloodstream of a rat. *Left:* If the particles are too large to cross the normal endothelium (e.g., bacteria, or carbon black in the form of biological India ink), they are phagocytized by the littoral phagocytes in the liver, spleen, and bone marrow. In the lymph nodes (not shown) very little uptake occurs, and not by phagocytosis. *Right:* If the particles can be transported across normal endothelium (e.g., Evans blue dye, which binds to albumin), they will cross the endothelium throughout the body except where a blood–tissue barrier exists (in the brain, nerves, testes, and skin). While in the bloodstream, these particles also are picked up by littoral phagocytes; once outside the vessels, they are picked up by interstitial macrophages. Note: the red color in this illustration shows organs that would be blue after an IV injection of Evans blue.

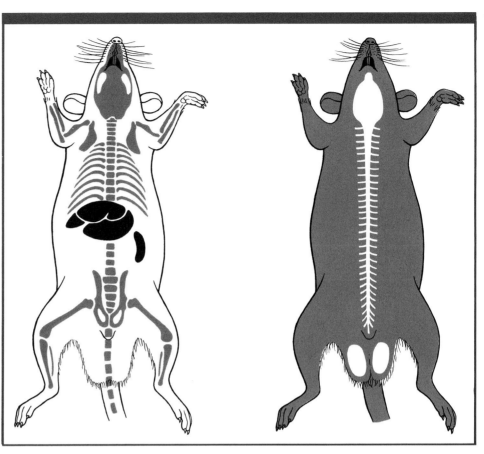

only what is delivered to them; therefore, in shock, when blood flow is poor, clearance is decreased (2).

- A few drugs and hormones such as small doses of steroids can increase phagocytosis (2).
- The system of littoral phagocytes can be a nuisance when it removes particles or molecules—such as artificial red blood cells or enzymes for enzyme-deficient children—that the physician would like to circulate as long as possible. Recently it was discovered that the RES can be tricked: macromolecules such as enzymes are camouflaged with long, wavy molecules of polyethylene glycol. These "hairy" molecules become almost invisible to the RES because the so-called hairs, which are constantly in motion, tend to hide the surface sites that are usually recognized by the phagocytes (38).

THE SYSTEM OF PHAGOCYTES COMES OF AGE

Metchnikoff, who viewed his macrophages primarily as "big eaters" and named them accordingly,

would be aghast to find out that phagocytosis is no longer seen as their main function. The insights of cell biology have proven the macrophages to be secretory cells capable of manufacturing some 100 products—enough to compete with the liver cells (Table 8.1). Their local and general powers are mind-boggling: they can "present antigens" to lymphocytes and thereby initiate the immune response; they can stimulate the formation of new vessels and induce fibroblasts to produce collagen fibers; they can cause blood to clot and secrete cytokines that induce fever and sleep; in individuals with severe infections or malignant tumors they can even induce the miserable condition called *cachexia*, whereby the whole body withers away (they do so by secreting a factor called *cachexin* or *tumor necrosis factor*). And for a final bow, macrophages can swallow bacteria and become scavengers to clean up the place.

TO SUM UP: The most obvious of all bodily defenses, inflammation, was explained in the late 1800s by means of simple experiments performed *in vivo*, on starfish and daphniae, and on transpar-

TABLE 8.1

Products of Macrophages: A Partial List*

Enzymes
Lysozyme
Plasminogen activator
Collagenase
Elastase
Angiotensin convertase
Acid proteases
Acid lipases
Acid nucleases
Acid phosphatases
Acid glycosidases
Acid sulfatases
Arginase
Lipoprotein lipase
Phospholipase A_2
Cytolytic proteinase

Inhibitors of enzymes
α-2 Macroglobulin
α-1 Antiprotease
α-1 Antichymotrypsin
Lipocortin (macrocortin)

Coagulation factors
Factors II, V, VII, IX, X
Thromboplastin
Prothrombin
Thrombospondin
Fibrinolysis inhibitor
Plasminogen activator

Components of complement
C_1, C_2, C_3, C_4, C_5
Factors B, D, H, I
Properdin

Growth factors and other proteins
Colony-stimulating factors
Angiogenesis factor
Platelet-derived growth factor
Fibroblast growth factor
Erythropoietin
Transforming growth factors
Growth inhibitors
Apolipoprotein E
Tumor necrosis factor
Interleukins 1, 3, 6, 8, 10, 12
Interferons alpha, beta
Serum amyloids A, P
Transferrin
Ferritin
Haptoglobin
Macrophage Inflammatory Proteins
Fibronectin

Reactive oxygen intermediates
Superoxide anion (O_2^-)
Hydrogen peroxide (H_2O_2)
Hydroxyl radical ($OH\cdot$)
Hypohalous acids

Lipid mediators
Prostaglandins
Prostacyclin
Thromboxanes
Platelet-activating factor

Small molecules
Purines
Pyrimidines
Glutathione
Nitric oxide

Adapted from (1, 22, 50).

ent mammalian tissues. These experiments led to the discovery of phagocytosis, and then to the discovery of an invisible organ, the system of phagocytes. In the hierarchy of bodily defenses this system ranks even higher than inflammation; its champion is the macrophage, a dull-looking but amazing creature, the oldest and thus the most experienced of the ten types of cells that participate in inflammatory responses. We will further learn to appreciate it as the mastermind of chronic inflammation and of the immune response.

Inflammation: A Pictorial Overview

Before we dissect the process of inflammation, as we have to do in order to explain it, we will present a few snapshots to show what inflammation looks like in real life. The illustrations should speak for themselves. Each one raises a number of questions, to be addressed in pages to come.

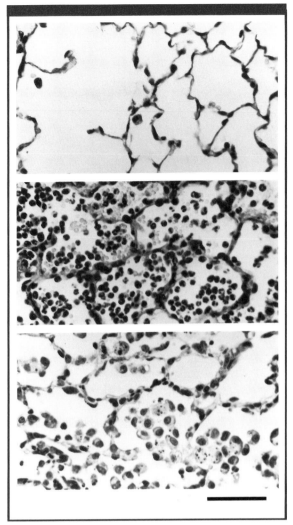

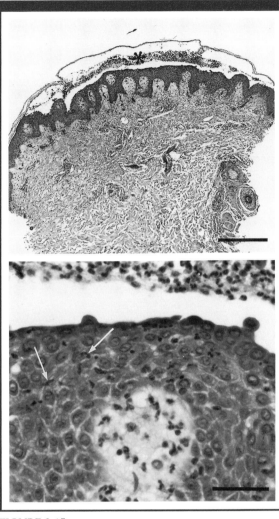

FIGURE 8.16

Acute inflammation in the lung produced experimentally by dripping a biological irritant (C5a desArg, a side product of complement activation) into a bronchus. *Top:* Normal rabbit lung with a few "resident" alveolar macrophages. *Middle:* 6 hours after irritation: the alveoli are filled with exudate, i.e. neutrophils in a protein-rich fluid (this condition of alveolar filling is known as *pneumonia* or *pneumonitis*). *Bottom:* 24 to 48 hours later the neutrophils are replaced by macrophages, a sequence typical of acute inflammation. Once the irritant has disappeared, the exudate can be cleared out in a few days. In the lung, inflammatory exudate gathers at first within the thickness of the alveolar walls, but these are very tight spaces; soon the exudate spills out into the alveoli, as shown here. There is no visible damage to the lung tissue; this mild inflammatory response is entirely reversible. **Bar** = 50 μm. (Reproduced with permission from [28].)

FIGURE 8.17

A pustule. Pustules are caused by bacteria in or on the epidermis. The bacteria attract an army of neutrophils, which emigrate from vessels in the dermis, crawl up into the epidermis, and form a droplet of pus (the familiar pimple) beneath the horny layer. This process illustrates the power of bacterial chemotactic messages. Biopsy of skin pustule. *Top:* **Arrow:** layer of cornified cells; **asterisk** = pus (a collection of leukocytes); **E** = epidermis; **D** = dermis. **Bar** = 500 μm. *Bottom:* detail **Arrows:** leukocytes crawling upwards; **asterisk** = pus. **Bar** = 50 μm. (Preparation courtesy of Dr. A.B. Ackerman.)

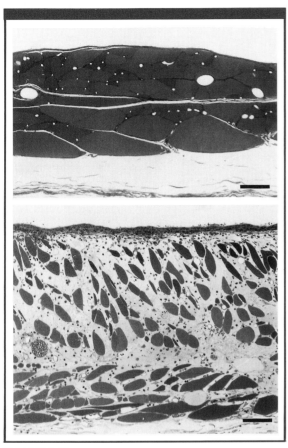

FIGURE 8.18

Acute inflammation in a striated muscle. Top: Control normal rat muscle. The muscle fibers, seen in cross section, are tightly packed (the vessels are open and empty because the tissue was fixed by perfusion). *Bottom:* Similar muscle after 2 days of exposure to an aseptic irritant (a piece of rat liver, not shown). The space between the muscle fibers represents edema; the cells free in this space indicate that this edema is inflammatory. The muscle fibers have shrunk (mechanism unclear). The number of fibroblasts seems normal, suggesting that the inflammation has not lasted long enough to stimulate their proliferation; they require 2–3 days to become visibly increased. **Bars** = 100 μm.

The main point: inflamed tissue becomes swollen with exudate, with some damage to the local parenchymal cells. If this inflammatory process were allowed to continue for another few days, the edema would be partly replaced by fibrous tissue.

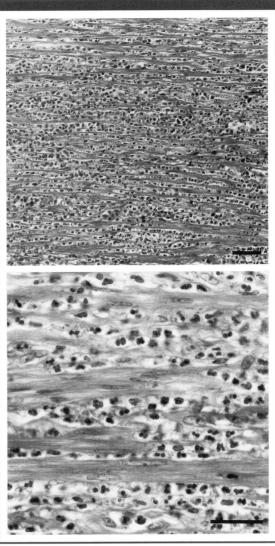

FIGURE 8.19

Acute appendicitis. The appendix becomes inflamed when bacteria contained in the lumen penetrate into the mucosa and spread centrifugally into the muscular and serosal layers. *Top:* The muscular wall of the appendix: a dramatic view of smooth muscle tissue overrun by an army of leukocytes chasing an invisible horde of bacteria. *Bottom:* A higher power shows that the cells packed between the muscle fibers are granulocytes (neutrophils), recognizable by their multilobed nucleus. **Bars** = 50 μm. In this and in most other bacterial infections the inflammatory response is obvious, but the bacteria are difficult to see unless special stains are used.

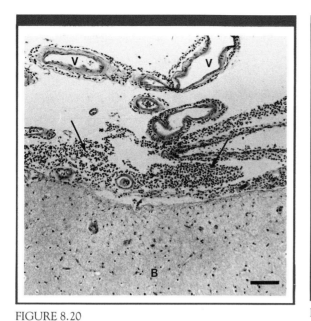

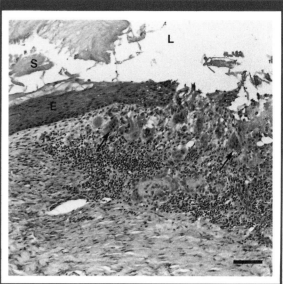

FIGURE 8.20

Meningococcal meningitis. Another example of bacteria attracting swarms of leukocytes (**arrows**). Bacteria are not
visible at this enlargement. The thin fibrous strands
containing blood vessels (**V**) belong to the arachnoid
(meningeal structure). Beneath it, the brain tissue (**B**) in
this section is normal, but sometimes its outer layer does
become inflamed. **Bar** = 250 μm. (Courtesy of Dr. T. W.
Smith, University of Massachusetts Medical Center,
Worcester, MA.)

FIGURE 8.21

Chronic aseptic inflammation in the skin around an epidermal
cyst that broke open. Epidermal cysts (wens) are common;
they are spheres lined by epidermis with its horny layer
inward, which explains why they are filled with
desquamated cornified cells. Most of these cysts derive from
hair follicles, a few arise by traumatic displacement of
epidermal cells. When they break open, their aseptic
content spills into the connective tissue and becomes a
persistent irritant: it attracts a population of macrophages,
some of which become multinucleated giant cells. All these
cells contribute to phagocytize and eliminate the foreign
material. **L** = Lumen of the cyst; **E** = Epidermal lining; S
= epithelial squames contained in the cyst. To the right the
cyst is broken; the exposed content induced an intense,
chronic inflammatory reaction. **Arrows:** Foreign body giant
cells, a response to the dead keratinized cells. **Bar** = 100
μm.

The main points: chronic inflammatory exudates contain
mostly mononuclear cells. Foreign bodies induce the formation of giant cells.

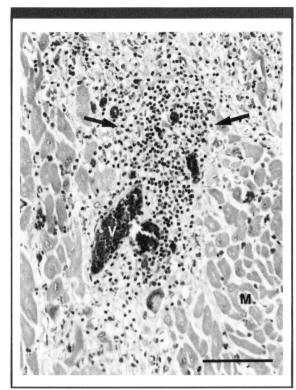

FIGURE 8.22

Chronic, focal inflammation of the heart (myocarditis). **M** = heart muscle (myocardium); **asterisk** = focus of inflammation, consisting mainly of lymphocytes; **V** = congested venule. **Bar** = 50 μm.

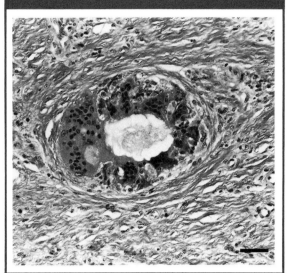

FIGURE 8.23

Chronic granulomatous inflammation. When the irritant consists of tiny "quanta" dispersed in the tissues and difficult to eliminate, the inflammatory response consists mainly of clusters of macrophages called granulomas, gathered around each "quantum" of the irritant. Multi-nucleated cells are often present. This granuloma was caused by urate crystals in a case of gout. **Bar** = 9 μm.

FIGURES 8.24–8.29 *Inflammation around dead tissue.* This is a common setting of inflammation, because masses of tissue often die of inadequate blood flow (the process called infarction). Dying and dead tissue, even if aseptic, is an irritant and elicits acute inflammation, which becomes chronic and ends with the removal of the mass and the formation of a scar; this removal process is called "organization." To illustrate this sequence we simulated an infarct by implanting a piece of sterile rat liver into the abdominal cavity of another rat. Under these conditions the implant is promptly wrapped up by the omentum, a thin connective tissue membrane that hangs like an apron from the transverse colon. The omentum is highly vascularized and sets up an inflammatory response. Six stages are shown; *each stage is represented by a topographic view (top) and by a higher power (bottom).* **Bars** = 200 μm. On the opposite page, a diagram explains the main features of the topographic view.

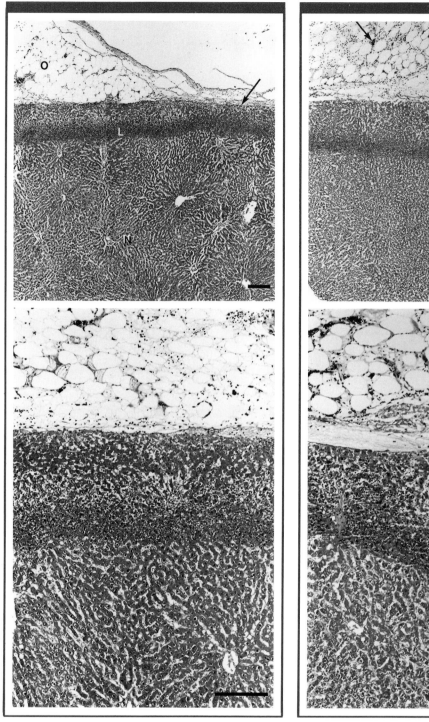

FIGURE 8.24
Stage: 1 day

FIGURE 8.25
Stage: 2 days

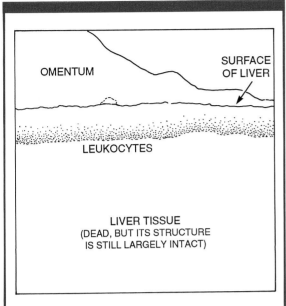

DIAGRAM OF FIGURE 8.24 (top)
Stage: 1 day

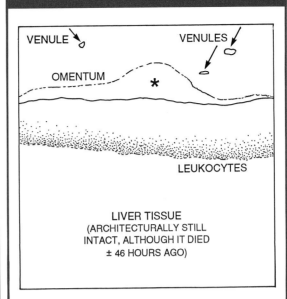

DIAGRAM OF FIGURE 8.25 (top)
Stage: 2 days

FIGURE 8.24

Top: The liver implant, which by now is ne-
crotic (**N**), is covered by the omentum (**O**) to which it is
firmly glued by a layer of fibrin not visible at this enlargement. **Arrow:** Surface of the liver. The dark horizontal layer represents a cemetery of leukocytes: the blood
vessels of the omentum, irritated by materials seeping
from the dying tissue, have supplied swarms of leukocytes
that penetrated into the liver implant. Note that all the
leukocytes die very nearly at the same depth, probably
where they run out of oxygen. *Bottom:* The leukocytes (**L**)
appear as dots between the necrotic, coagulated liver
cords.

FIGURE 8.25

Top: The omentum is visibly inflamed: it is peppered with
inflammatory cells, and its venules are congested (**arrows**);
they are the source of the emigrating leukocytes. *Bottom:* In
the space between omentum and liver (**asterisk**) the
thready material is fibrin, a polymer of a protein supplied by
the blood as fibrinogen; it serves as a glue between the
omentum and the dead tissue.

The main points: tissues that are dying or died recently
attract leukocytes—which are doomed to die frustrated,
because they find no bacteria to phagocytize. The
omentum is rich in vessels, which are key to its defensive
function.

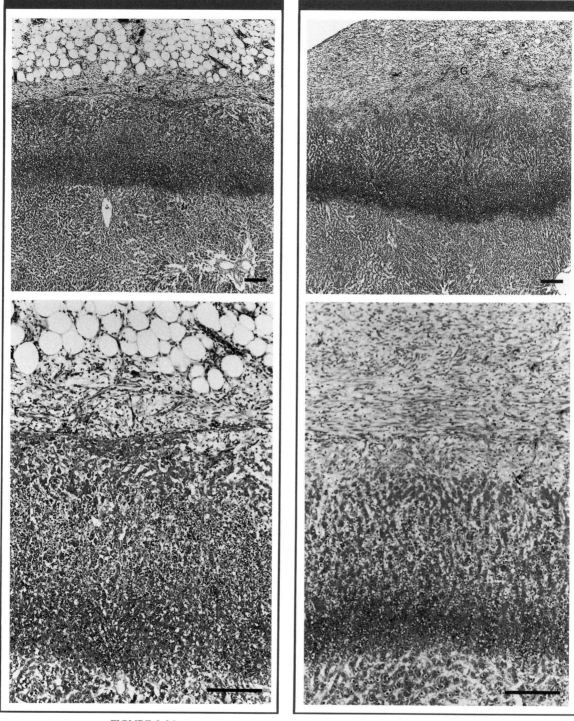

FIGURE 8.26
Stage: 3 days

FIGURE 8.27
Stage: 7 days

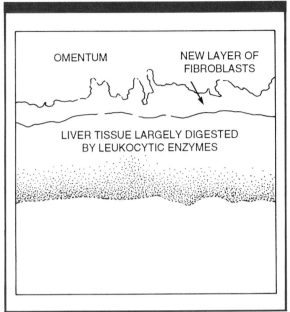

DIAGRAM OF FIGURE 8.26 (top)
Stage: 3 days

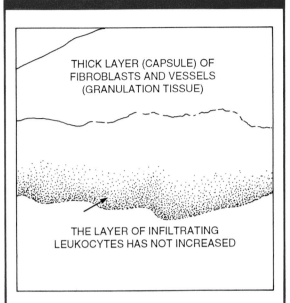

DIAGRAM OF FIGURE 8.27 (top)
Stage: 7 days

FIGURE 8.26

Top: The salient novelty is the proliferation of fibroblasts (**F**), which are now forming a new layer between the omentum and the dead tissue. This layer is the beginning of what will become "granulation tissue." The fibroblasts are supplied by the omentum as a component of the inflammatory response. The dark band of leukocytes is still there: new waves of leukocytes are probably still arriving.
Bottom: The zone of fibroblast proliferation (**F**) contains streaks of nuclei (**arrows**), which represent budding capillaries originating from the omentum.

FIGURE 8.27

Top: The layer of fibroblasts has evolved into a thick layer of "young" connective tissue called *granulation tissue* (young because it is rich in cells and sprouting vessels) (**G**). This newly formed tissue behaves as a temporary organ, which (in this particular example) is responsible for removing the necrotic mass. *Bottom:* Detail showing how the granulation tissue begins to erode the surface of the necrotic mass (compare with the figure at left). This erosion is accomplished mainly by the phagocytic activity of macrophages, not well recognizable at this enlargement.

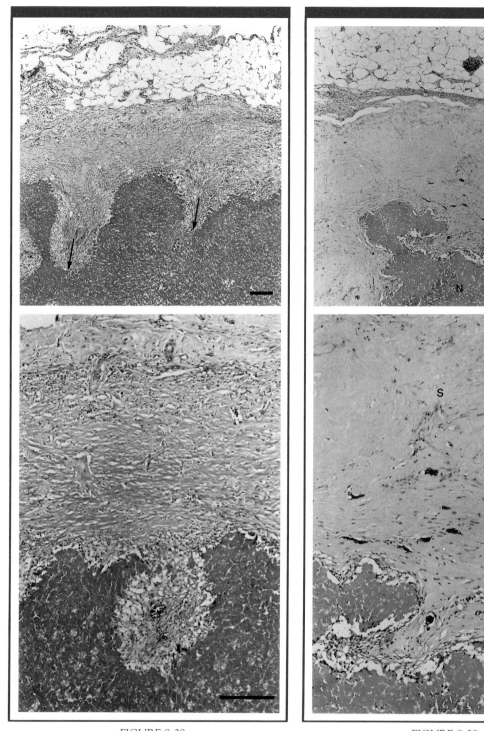

FIGURE 8.28
Stage: 1 month

FIGURE 8.29
Stage: 13 months

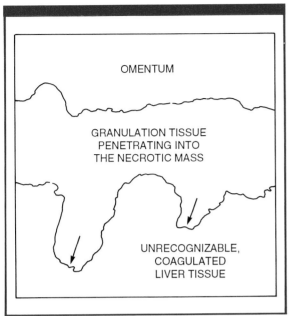

DIAGRAM OF FIGURE 8.28 (top)
Stage: 1 month

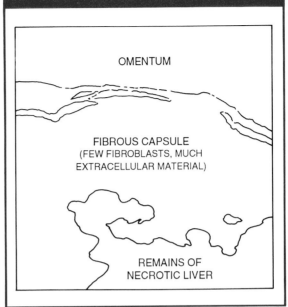

DIAGRAM OF FIGURE 8.29 (top)
Stage: 13 months

FIGURE 8.28

Top: It is now obvious that the granulation tissue (**G**) is invading and reabsorbing (**arrows**) the necrotic mass. Note that this mass no longer contains a layer of leukocytes: it is fully coagulated (denatured) and has ceased to emit chemical messages that attract leukocytes. Its removal is entirely dependent on the granulation tissue. *Bottom:* Note the number of cells in the granulation tissue in comparison with Figure 8.29.

FIGURE 8.29

Top: The granulation tissue appears clearer because it has lost most of its cells and capillaries and has acquired more collagen fibers. It has become a fibrous scar. The persistence of some necrotic material (**N**) at this late stage suggests that not much reabsorption is occurring, as might also be guessed from the structural change of the granulation tissue. Surprisingly, the outlines of liver tissue are still recognizable. Special stains would show that the necrotic mass is partly calcified. *Bottom:* The loss of cells in the former granulation tissue is obvious (compare with the figure at left).

The main point: granulation tissue—when its defensive (or reabsorptive) function is accomplished—matures into a fibrous scar. In this experiment, what was once one cubic centimeter of dead liver tissue has become a pinhead of mummified, calcified material wrapped in a fibrous capsule. A job well done.

References

1. Adams DO, Hamilton TA. Phagocytic cells: Cytotoxic activities of macrophages. In: Gallin JI, Goldstein IM, Snyderman R (eds). Inflammation. Basic principles and clinical correlates. New York: Raven Press 1988: 471–492.

2. Altura BM. Relationship of reticuloendothelial cell function to microcirculatory blood flow and low-flow states. In: Altura BM, Saba TM (eds). Pathophysiology of the reticuloendothelial system. New York: Raven Press, 1981, pp. 159–208.

3. Aschoff L. Lectures on pathology. New York: Paul B. Hoeber, Inc., 1924.

4. Baltch AL, Schaffer C, Hammer MC, et al. Bacteremia following dental cleaning in patients with and without penicillin prophylaxis. Am Heart J 1982;104:1335–1339.

5. Benacerraf B. Quantitative aspects of phagocytosis. In: Brauer RW (ed). Liver function. A symposium on approaches to the quantitative description of liver function. Washington: American Institute of Biological Sciences, 1958:205–234.

6. Biozzi G, Benacerraf B, Halpern BN. Quantitative study of the granulopectic activity of the reticulo-endothelial system. II. A study of the kinetics of the granulopectic activity of the R.E.S. in relation to the dose of carbon injected Relationship between the weight of the organs and their activity. Br J Exp Pathol 1953;34:441–457.

7. Biozzi G, Benacerraf B, Halpern BN, Stiffel C, Hillemand B. Exploration of the phagocytic function of the reticulo-endothelial system with heat denatured human serum albumin labeled with I^{131} and application to the measurement of liver blood flow, in normal man and in some pathologic conditions. J Lab Clin Med 1958;51:230–239.

8. Bonventre PF, Nordberg BK, Schmiterlöw CG. An autoradiographic study of radioactively labelled Bacillus cereus in the mouse. Acta Pathol Microbiol Scand 1961;51:157–163.

9. Brain JD. Physiology and pathophysiology of pulmonary macrophages. In: Reichard SM, Filkins JP (eds). The reticuloendothelial system. A comprehensive treatise, vol. 7B, Physiology. New York: Plenum Press, 1985: 315–337.

10. Brain JD. Macrophages in the respiratory tract. In: Fishman AP, Fisher AB (eds). Handbook of physiology. Section 3: The respiratory system, vol. 1. Bethesda: American Physiological Society, 1985: 447–471.

11. Buchanan JW, Wagner HN Jr. Regional phagocytosis in man. In: Reichard SM, Filkins JP. (eds). The reticuloendothelial system. A comprehensive treatise, vol. 7B, Physiology. New York: Plenum Press, 1985:247–270.

12. Cohnheim J. Ueber Entzündung und Eiterung. Virchows Arch Pathol Anat Physiol Klin Med 1867;40:1–79.

13. Cohnheim J. Untersuchungen ueber die embolischen Processe. Berlin: Verlag von August Hirschwald, 1872.

14. Cohnheim J. Lectures in general pathology, 2nd ed, vol. 1 (translated from the 2nd German edition). London: The New Sydenham Society, 1889.

15. Cordon-Cardo C, O'Brien JP, Casals D, et al. Multidrug-resistance gene (P-glycoprotein) is expressed by endothelial cells at blood-brain barrier sites. Proc Natl Acad Sci USA 1989;86:695–698.

16. Dutrochet MH. Recherches anatomiques et physiologiques sur la structure intime des animaux et des végétaux, et sur leur motilité. Paris: JB Baillière, 1824.

17. Florey HW. General pathology. Philadelphia: W.B. Saunders Company, 1970.

18. Friedman H, Escobar M, Reichard SM (series eds). The reticuloendothelial system: A comprehensive treatise. New York: Plenum Press, 1980–1988.

19. Ghinea N, Eskenasy M, Simionescu M, Simionescu N. Endothelial albumin binding proteins are membrane-associated components exposed on the cell surface. J Biol Chem 1989;264:4755–4758.

20. Halpern BN, Benacerraf B, Biozzi G. Quantitative study of the granulopectic activity of the reticulo-endothelial system. I: The effect of the ingredients present in India ink and of substances affecting blood clotting in vivo on the fate of carbon particles administered intravenously in rats, mice and rabbits. Br J Exp Pathol 1953;34:426–440.

21. Hamburger MI, Fields TR, Gerardi EN, Bennett RS. Assessment of reticuloendothelial system function in man using receptor specific probes. Adv Inflamm Res 1983;5:67–85.

22. Henson PM, Henson JE, Fittschen C, Kimani G, Bratton DL, Riches DWH. Phagocytic cells: degranulation and secretion. In: Gallin JI, Goldstein IM, Snyderman R (eds). Inflammation: Basic principles and clinical correlates. New York: Raven Press, 1988, pp. 363–390.

23. Hirsch JG, Hirsch BI. Metchnikoff's life and scientific contributions in historical perspective. In: Karnovsky ML, Bolis L (eds). Phagocytosis—past and future. New York: Academic Press, 1982:1–12.

24. Hunsaker WG. Determination of Evans Blue in avian plasma by protein precipitation and extraction. Proc Soc Exp Biol Med 1965;120:747–749.

25. Hunter J. A treatise on the blood, inflammation, and gun-shot wounds. London: John Richardson, 1794.

26. Joris I, Cuénoud HF, Doern GV, Underwood JM, Majno G. Capillary leakage in inflammation. A study by vascular labeling. Am J Pathol 1990;137:1353–1363.

27. Kowala MC. Acute inflammation of the lymph node. Ph.D. thesis, The Australian National University, 1982.

28. Larsen GL, Henson PM. Mediators of inflammation. Annu Rev Immunol 1983;1:335–359.

29. Lasser A. The mononuclear phagocytic system: a review. Hum Pathol 1983;14:108–126.

30. Lister J. On a new method of treating compound fracture, abscess, &c, with observations on the conditions of suppuration (Lancet, 1:326, 357, 387, 507; 2:95; 1867). In: The collected papers of Joseph, Baron Lister, 2 vols. Oxford: Clarendon Press, 1909:1–36.

31. Majno G. The healing hand. Man and wound in the ancient world. Cambridge: Harvard University Press, 1975.

32. Majno G. Inflammation and infection: historic highlights. In: Majno G, Cotran RS, Kaufman N (eds). Current topics in inflammation and infection. Baltimore: Williams & Wilkins, 1982:1–17.

33. Majno G, Joris I. The microscope in the history of pathology. Virchows Arch Abt A Pathol Anat 1973;360:273–286.

34. Metchnikoff E. Ueber eine Sprosspilzkrankheit der Daphnien. Beitrag zur Lehre über den Kampf der Phagocyten gegen Krankheitserreger. Virchows Arch Pathol Anat Physiol Klin Med 1884;96:177–195.

35. Metchnikoff E. Lectures on the comparative pathology of inflammation (translated from the French by FA Starling and EH Starling, MD), 1893. (Reproduced by Dover Publications, Inc., New York, 1968).

36. Metchnikoff O. Life of Elie Metchnikoff 1845–1916. Boston: Houghton Mifflin Company, 1921.

37. Nopajaroonsri C, Luk SC, Simon GT. The passage of

intravenously injected colloidal carbon into lymph node parenchyma. Lab Invest 1974;30:533–538.

38. Pool R. PEG-treated enzymes are nearly invisible to the immune system. Science 1990;248:305.

39. Predescu D, Simionescu M, Simionescu N, Palade GE. Binding and transcytosis of glycoalbumin by the microvascular endothelium of the murine myocardium: evidence that glycoalbumin behaves as a bifunctional ligand. J Cell Biol 1988;107:1729–1738.

40. Rather LJ. Addison and the white corpuscles: An aspect of nineteenth-century biology. London: Wellcome Institute of the History of Medicine, 1972.

41. Roitt IM. Essential immunology, 6th ed. Oxford: Blackwell Scientific Publications, 1988.

42. Saba TM. Physiology and physiopathology of the reticuloendothelial system. Arch Intern Med 1970;126:1031–1052.

43. Schoefl GI. Structure and permeability of venules in lymphoid tissue. In: Société Française de Microscopie Electronique: Septième Congrès International de Microscopie Électronique, Grenoble, 1970:589–590.

44. Traub A, Giebink GS, Smith C, et al. Splenic reticuloendothelial function after splenectomy, spleen repair, and spleen autotransplantation. N Engl J Med 1987;317:1559–1564.

45. Unanue ER. Macrophages, antigen presenting cells and the phenomena of antigen handling and presentation. In: Paul WE (ed). Fundamental immunology, 3rd ed (in press).

46. van Furth R, Cohn ZA, Hirsch JG, Humphrey JH, Spector WG, Langevoort HL. The mononuclear phagocyte system: a new classification of macrophages, monocytes, and their precursor cells. Bull WHO 1972;46:845–852.

47. Virchow R. Cellular pathology (translated from the 2nd German edition by B. Chance), 1859. Reproduced by Dover Publications, New York: 1971.

48. Waller A. Microscopic examination of some of the principal tissues of the animal frame, as observed in the tongue of the living frog, toad, &c. The London, Edinburgh and Dublin Philosophical Magazine and Journal of Science 1846;3:271–287.

49. Warner AE, Brain JD. Intravascular pulmonary macrophages: a novel cell removes particles from blood. Am J Physiol 1986;250:R728–R732.

50. Wolpe SD, Cerami A. Macrophage inflammatory proteins 1 and 2: members of a novel superfamily of cytokines. FASEB J 1989;3:2565–2573.

51. Yamaguchi K, Schoefl GI. Blood vessels of the Peyer's patch in the mouse: II. In vivo observations. Anat Rec 1983;206:403–417.

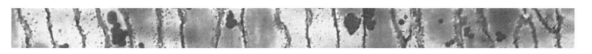

Inflammation: The Actors and Their Language

CHAPTER 9

> The Actors of Inflammation
>
> Mediators: The Chemical Language of Inflammation

On a battlefield we would expect to find three types of populations: the aggressors, the defenders, and the local people as innocent bystanders. In a focus of inflammation the setting is quite similar. The aggressor is not always apparent microscopically: it might be an invisible toxic chemical or a virus (even bacteria, as we saw in Chapter 8, are not very obvious). So the defending cells tend to dominate the field, at least visually; they belong to ten families (Table 9.1), and keep in touch by means of chemical messages, the mediators of inflammation, which include agents lethal for attacking cells. As for the local population of parenchymal cells, it is caught in the crossfire and suffers, sometimes more, sometimes less; on the whole it has little to say regarding the battle, but it does voice its concern by producing a few chemical messages of its own.

TABLE 9.1

Inflammation: The Cellular Actors

CELL TYPE	MAJOR FUNCTIONS
Neutrophils	Typical of *acute* inflammation; not found in normal tissues; first line of defense against bacteria; *end cells*
Eosinophils	Can kill worms; intervene in immune reactions
Monocytes/ Macrophages (Mφ)	Monocytes are precursors of tissue macrophages, key cells of *chronic* inflammation; synthesize dozens of mediators; bactericidal; *long-lived*
Platelets	Essential for upkeep of normal endothelium; play key roles in blood clotting, hemostasis, thrombosis; source of mediators in injured tissues
Endothelium	Mediates exchanges of fluid and cells between blood and tissues
Fibroblasts	Intervene during healing; become plasma cells; produce collagen; can modulate to myofibroblasts
Mast Cells/ Basophils	Related but not identical cells; functions not clear; are loaded with histamine and can produce many other mediators; key role in anaphylaxis.
T lymphocytes	Intervene in immune responses; secrete cytokines; kill cells
B Lymphocytes	Intervene in immune responses; become plasma cells; produce antibodies
NK cells	Perform selective cell killing independent of the immune response

The Actors of Inflammation

To pursue our military metaphor we should speak of the "soldiers" of inflammation: we prefer to adopt a more peaceful tone, and consider inflammation as a play with a cast of ten main characters. Each type of inflammatory cell is specialized in some way, and therefore not all are called upon at every inflammatory occasion; plasma cells do not appear unless antibody formation is involved, eosinophils participate only in certain settings, and so on. *All ten cell types are normally quiescent and become activated in the inflammatory focus; all have subtypes; and all ten can produce inflammatory mediators.*

It is essential to know, at least in outline, what each cell type is programmed to do, so a short biography of each one follows. Whole volumes are available for those who may want to know more (29).

(1) NEUTROPHILS: THE BACTERICIDAL SPECIALISTS

The neutrophil, a leukocyte normally found only in blood and bone marrow, seems to have been

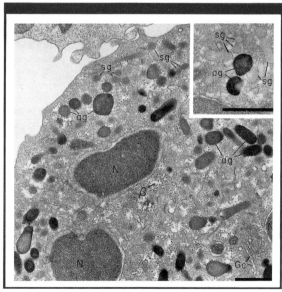

FIGURE 9.1

Part of a human neutrophil reacted for peroxidase. The cytoplasm is loaded with granules. The pale ones, negative for peroxidase, are the specific granules (**sg**). The darker, positive granules are the azurophilic granules (**ag**). Note the abundant supplies of beta particles of glycogen (**β**). **Gc:** Golgi cisternae. **N:** Lobes of the nucleus. **Bar** = 1 μm. **Inset bar** = 0.5 μm. (Reproduced with permission from [6].)

designed by evolution as a bacteria-killing machine (Figure 9.1). It cannot multiply, and its life is one of the shortest on record: 12–20 hours in the bloodstream (48), which means that not all neutrophils will ever live to experience their moment of bactericidal glory. However, we must assume that many get to make their kill somewhere, even under normal conditions, because when the number of leukocytes in human blood drops below 1000–500/mm^3 (neutropenia) from the normal 4000–11,000/mm^3 bacterial infection immediately becomes a threat.

When they float freely, neutrophils are spherical and a little larger than red blood cells, which means that every time a neutrophil is swept into a capillary (about twice a minute: once in the lung, once in a peripheral capillary), it must endure a squeeze. Like all other leukocytes, but unlike many bacteria, they can only crawl, not swim. This is why they do a poor job against bacteria in waterlogged (edematous) tissue.

Much of the bactericidal equipment of the neutrophils is stored in some 2000 granules of at least three types; the primary and secondary are so called because they appear in that order during cellular maturation. The **primary** (also called **azurophil**) **granules** are rather similar to lysosomes. The **secondary** (also called **specific**) **granules** are the most numerous and quite specialized; they are also the first to be "spent" during phagocytosis (88), which means that their content is most likely to be spilled into the cell's surroundings. Perhaps this priority has something to do with restoring an aseptic environment, because the specific granules contain three antibacterial proteins: **lactoferrin, lysozyme,** and **cobalophilin** (also called vitamin B$_{12}$ binding protein) (Table 9.2).

With a life of less than a day in the bloodstream, the neutrophils would have little use for synthetic equipment; in fact, like all granulocytes, they have very little endoplasmic reticulum (however, if stimulated, they can synthesize cytokines: see Table 9.2). They have few mitochondria but prominent glycogen reserves (Figure 9.2), from which they draw energy for their movements when they venture out into poorly oxygenated areas of injury, as required by their job description.

Why their nuclei are subdivided into two to five lobes connected by a thread is not known, but the multilobed nuclei are excellent markers for recognizing neutrophils in tissue sections (Figure 9.3). When a neutrophil dies, the various lobes of its nucleus can flow into a single one, making it

TABLE 9.2

Possible Secretory Products of Neutrophils

(R: rabbit, H: human, O: other species)

Azurophil granules	Specific granules	Other granule types	Membranes
Peroxidase (R, H)		Acid phosphatase (R, H)	Acid phosphatase (R, H)
Acid phosphatase (R, H)		Heparitinase (H)	5′-Nucleotidase (H)
β-Glucosaminidase (R, H)	Alkaline phosphatase (R)	β-Glucosaminidase (R, H)	Alkaline phosphatase (H)
5′-Nucleotidase (R, H)	Histaminase (H)	α-Mannosidase (R, H)	Neutral α-glucosidase (H)
Arylsulfatase (R, H)			Ribonuclease? (H)
α-Fucosidase (H)			Leucyl-β-naphthylaminidase (H)
Neuraminidase? (H)	(*Intracellular, site uncertain:* cytokines [42a]: IL-1, IL-6, IL-8, IFN-alpha, TNF, G-CSF, GM-CSF)		
Esterase (H)			
Cathepsin A? (R)			
Cathepsin D? (R, H)			
Cathepsin E? (R)			
Cathepsin F? (O)			
Cathepsin G? (acid) (O)			
Collagenolytic cathepsin (R, O)		Collagenolytic cathepsin? (R)	Elastase (*de novo synthesis*) (H)
Elastase (H)		Elastase? (H)	
Cathepsin G (neutral) (H)	Collagenase (R, H)	Gelatinase (H)	Plasminogen activator? (*de novo synthesis*) (H)
Histonase (H)			
Lysozyme (R, H)	Lysozyme (R, H)		
Phospholipase A (R)	Vitamin B$_{12}$ binding protein (H)		
Cationic proteins (R, H)	Laminin receptor (H)	Laminin receptor (H)	Phospholipase (H)
Bactericidal/permeability-inducing protein (R, H)	C3bi receptor (H)		
Defensins (R, H)	fMet-Leu-Phe receptor (H)		
Glycosaminoglycans (R, H)	Lactoferrin (R, H)	Glycosaminoglycans (R, H)	Platelet activating factors (PAFs)
Chondroitin sulfate (H)	Cytochrome b$_{245}$ (H)		Prostaglandins Leukotrienes
Heparin sulfate (H)	Flavoproteins (H)		

Reproduced with permission from (29) with some items added.

difficult to recognize the cell as a former granulocyte (p. 208).

Neutrophils are programmed to crawl out of the vessels and into the tissue spaces in response to many chemical calls, originating from bacteria, injured tissues, or other inflammatory cells. Because they are primarily bacteria killers they pour out by billions at sites of infection by certain bacteria; if they are concentrated enough the exudate becomes pus. For this reason the neutro-

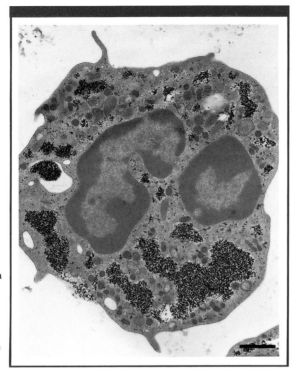

FIGURE 9.2 Human neutrophil stained with silver proteinate to demonstrate glycogen (the black, granular material). **Bar** = 1 μm.

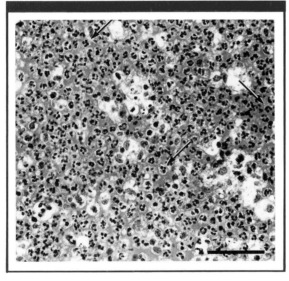

FIGURE 9.3 Collection of pus, photographed in a dental abcess. The prevalent cell, the neutrophil, is clearly recognized by the multilobed structure of the nucleus (**arrows**). **Bar** = 50 μm.

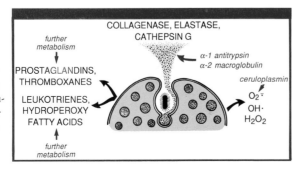

FIGURE 9.4 Principal mediators arising from an activated neutrophil and their principal inhibitors. (Adapted from [82].)

phil is usually portrayed as a single-minded, kamikaze-type cell that is programmed to chase bacteria, kill them, and die. This is basically true. However, in order to kill, the neutrophil must be activated and undergo an "oxygen burst" (p. 408); in the process it releases enzymes and other proteins, prostaglandins, and bactericidal oxygen-derived free radicals. Therefore *the neutrophil can also be construed as a secretory cell* (Figure 9.4). Interestingly, *the secretion of enzymes begins as soon as the neutrophil is summoned by a chemotactic call* (p. 354), which amounts to salivating in response to a dinner invitation. The overall result of neutrophil secretion is best seen in pus, which is so rich in enzymes that it functions as a natural tenderizer capable of destroying any component of dead tissue, from collagen to nuclei; even normal tissues can be damaged (p. 532).

The same activities that make the neutrophil a secretory cell also make it a *potentially harmful cell*: what kills a bacterium can also kill a friendly body cell. In fact, much of the injury that occurs during inflammation can be attributed to the neutrophils.

Note: despite their tremendous appetite for bacteria, the neutrophils tend to shun other objects. They take to scavenging as a low priority; for this reason Metchnikoff called them *microphages* (51), a name that has not survived.

Surprisingly, it is not yet clear how and where the neutrophils normally end their lives. Many are thought to be taken up by the spleen or to break up in the capillaries of the lung; others are probably lost in the mouth and the gut. In inflammatory foci, spent or obsolete neutrophils are phagocytized by macrophages (p. 426), probably as a result of a surface change that labels them as obsolete. One might think that swallowing a neutrophil loaded with enzymes might be hazardous, but the macrophage is none the worse for its meal: the neutrophil's enzymes are probably denatured in the death process.

In essence: the profile of the neutrophil is that of a short-lived bactericidal cell that can neither multiply nor modulate. Normally it is found only in the blood and in the bone marrow; its presence in tissues signals two possible acute events: invasion by bacteria or some other parasite, and/or tissue injury.

(2) Eosinophils: The Worm Killers

The eosinophil seems to have evolved—like the neutrophil—in response to invaders, but to larger invaders, especially worms (Figure 9.5) (5,17,31,32,73,84). *In vitro* it can kill, for example, a worm (*Schistosoma mansoni*) and a protozoan (*Trypanosoma cruzi*) responsible for two of the world's major tropical diseases. In relatively worm-free societies the eosinophil may be a frustrated cell. Although it has some similarities to the neutrophil, the differences are great. It is much better equipped with mitochondria and endoplasmic reticulum and correspondingly has a much longer life span, perhaps 4 days in the blood, and weeks (for reasons unknown) in the tissues. It can phagocytize and kill bacteria, but it does so much less efficiently than the neutrophil; on the other hand, when stimulated, the oxygen burst of the eosinophil lasts longer and produces twice the amount of superoxide anion (O_2^-) than that of the neutrophil (74).

In the blood there are only 2 or 3 eosinophils for 55 neutrophils; but *in the tissues, where there are no neutrophils at all, eosinophils are scattered almost everywhere, especially where mast cells abound* (72), as in the mucosa of the gastrointestinal tract (could they be waiting for worms?). Their granules are larger and fewer (about 200, roughly one-tenth of the neutrophil's endowment) and are probably modified peroxisomes rather than lysosomes (5).

Eosinophil granules contain several cationic (or positively charged) proteins (60), a fact that fits with their affinity for the acid stain eosin (*eosin*ophils). Why should they be cationic? It took a long time to find out that this property has a purpose; *it makes these proteins toxic by enabling them to bind with critical, negatively charged molecules on the surface of other cells*, a strategy presumably aimed at parasites. The so-called **major basic protein** (MBP) takes up more than half of each granule, in the form of a crystalloid mass (Figure 9.6); it can kill worms as well as normal mammalian cells (Figure 9.7) (23). Another cationic protein, **eosinophil cationic protein** (ECP), is said to create pores in cell membranes; it is harmless against bacteria but kills schistosoma larvae (60). At least three of the eosinophil cationic proteins can behave as neurotoxins; injected into the cerebral ventricles they cause selective death of the cerebellar Purkinje cells (Figure 9.8) (22).

When and where do the eosinophils accumulate in disease? This should tell us something about their functions. In the blood, hypereosinophilia is a common effect of allergy and of parasitic infestation. In the tissues, a few eosinophils can be found in any acute inflammatory focus, along with

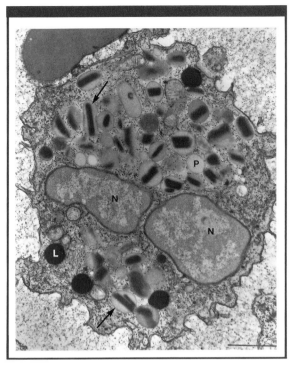

FIGURE 9.5
Human eosinophil. **N:** Typical bilobed nucleus. **Arrows:** Specific granules with dense central crystal. **P:** Primary granule, devoid of crystal. **L:** Lipid body. **Bar** = 1.4 μm. (Reproduced with permission from [17].)

the neutrophils, but they seem to be incidental. Large numbers are found in lesions due to parasites, in relation to some immune responses, in relation to angiogenesis, in healing wounds, and in some tumors (e.g., Hodgkin's disease). Eosinophils have a special relationship with mast cells, which secrete several eosinophil chemotac-

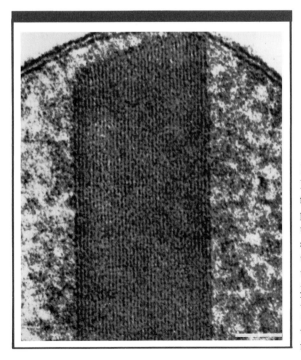

FIGURE 9.6
Part of a granule from a rat eosinophil, seen by electron microscopy; showing part of the typical central crystal of major basic protein. **Bar** = 0.05 μm. (Reproduced with permission from [52].)

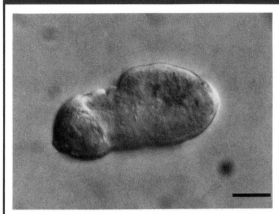

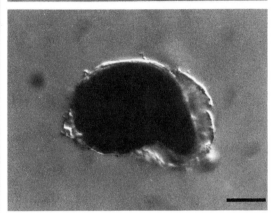

FIGURE 9.7
Top: Normal larva of *Schistosoma mansoni.* *Bottom:* After incubation with eosinophil major basic protein (MBP) the larva is damaged, as shown by the detached and ballooning membrane. **Bars** = 50 μm. (Reproduced with permission from [32].)

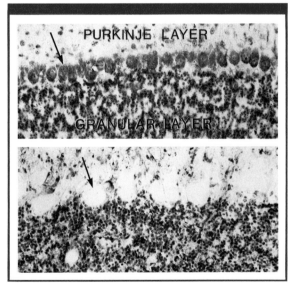

FIGURE 9.8
Destructive power of eosinophil cationic protein (ECP). *Top:* Cerebellum of a normal guinea pig; note the normal layer of Purkinje cells (**arrow**). *Bottom:* Seven days after an intraventricular injection of 0.3 micrograms of ECP; the Purkinje cells have disappeared, leaving empty spaces. **Bar** = 100 μm. (Reproduced with permission from [22].)

tic factors, whereas major basic protein causes mast cells to release histamine.

> It has been noticed that eosinophils contain enzymes that could be used for shutting off inflammation: histaminase, arylsulfatase (which inactivates leukotrienes), and a phospholipase that could inactivate the powerful platelet activating factor (32)— hence the suggestion that "the eosinophil can undo what the mast cell has done" (66). But before this can become a slogan, more data are needed (32).

It is clear that eosinophils can do a lot of damage.

- Asthma is always accompanied by an intense eosinophilic infiltration of the bronchi. MBP can paralyze the cilia of the bronchial epithelium (*ciliostasis,* 14), and cationic proteins have been demonstrated in damaged bronchial epithelium and in the sputum (72). Furthermore, the characteristic spasm of bronchial muscle can be correlated with the tendency of eosinophils to produce the spasmogenic leukotrienes LTC$_4$ and LTE$_4$ rather than the leukotactic LTB$_4$ produced by neutrophils (32,72).

- The idiopathic *hypereosinophilic syndrome* is characterized by infiltration by eosinophils of many organs, including the heart; the result is a fibrosis that can be life-threatening, and eosinophil cationic proteins can be demonstrated in the tissue (32). Since 1989, a syndrome of hypereosinophilia and myalgia (muscle pain) has been described in individuals ingesting products that contain the "dietary supplement" L-tryptophan (16).

- Here is a teaser: the destructive major basic protein is contained in the placenta and in the plasma of pregnant women (78). It is tempting to speculate that this destructive protein may relate to the ability of fetal trophoblastic cells to invade the uterine wall (47).

- **Charcot-Leyden crystals** are microscopic, bypyramidal, hexagonal protein crystals (Figure 9.9) that have been known since the 1800s to be associated with eosinophils in the sputum of asthmatics. They can be obtained *in vitro* from eosinophils and also from basophils; they are made of phospholipase C from the cell membrane (17,72).

In essence: the eosinophil is loaded with powerful antiparasitic cytotoxins, which can also be misdirected and cause tissue damage, as happens in asthma. It has a mast cell connection, in that it can be summoned by several chemotaxins produced by mast cells: hence its presence in allergic lesions, in which mast cells are a key factor. This points to a primordial alliance between these two cells, originally intended to fight worms and other large parasites (p. 525). But worms apart, we still do not know why we should be grateful for the existence of the eosinophil.

(3) MACROPHAGES: THE MASTER MINDS

Monocytes and macrophages must be dealt with together because they represent two phases of the same cell—a circulating phase and a tissue phase, respectively (Figure 9.10). Monocytes are born in the bone marrow; they circulate, in humans, for about 6 days (77), then migrate into the tissues and settle there as macrophages, quite turned off until they are activated by some local challenge. Macrophages found in tissues are also called *histiocytes*.

From the point of view of evolution, monocytes/macrophages derive from the ancestral invertebrate macrophage; this is the cell that Metchnikoff saw at work in his starfish larvae, and that evolved into the many phagocytic and multi-talented cells of the vertebrate RES/MPS, as we know from Chapter 8. The biology of macrophages (often abbreviated Mϕ) is the subject of impressive handbooks, including a Manual of Macrophage Methodology (36), and an enormous literature, growing by about 4,000 papers per year (40,75).

There is something stately and professional about the macrophages. In inflammation they make their appearance as a second wave, to finish what the neutrophils had started, and then they take over. On the whole, they can phagocytize the same bacteria as the neutrophils, although not always as effectively; however, they are better equipped to handle hard-to-kill intracellular bacteria such as *Mycobacterium tuberculosis*. We have already alluded to the awesome capabilities of the macrophage besides phagocytosis: they include initiating the immune response, angiogenesis, fibrosis, clotting, scavenging, secreting a wide variety of proteins, inducing fever and other general responses. It is regrettable for the human observer, especially for a novice, that *the omnipotent macrophage has no obvious morphologic marker unless it has phagocytized something obvious.* Fortunately, histochemical markers do exist.

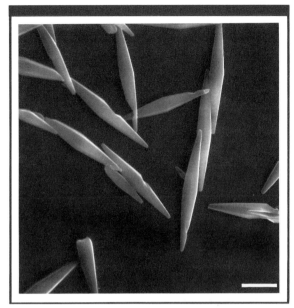

FIGURE 9.9
Charcot-Leyden crystals of phospholipase obtained from human eosinophils, seen by scanning electron microscopy. These protein crystals are commonly found in the sputum of asthmatics and are visible by light microscopy. **Bar** = 25 μm. (Reproduced with permission from [72].)

*The most specific but cumbersome methods for identifying macrophages are a histochemical stain for nonspecific esterase and surface markers (antigens) for subsets of macrophages. For example, the alveolar macrophages have a surface marker not present in resident peritoneal macrophages (76). Circulating monocytes are less heterogeneous but do have **subsets** (56) that vary in their response to chemotactic agents (20). The variations are probably due to microenvironmental effects and/or to maturation. Neutrophils are more uniform, but "fast" and "slow" sets have been described; there are also subsets of eosinophils (63).*

Exactly how long macrophages live nobody knows, but it is probably months (40). Because

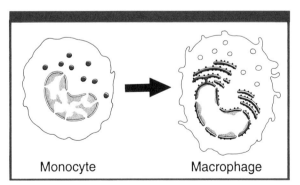

FIGURE 9.10
When a monocyte (left) migrates out of the vessels and becomes a resident macrophage (right), it becomes larger but downgrades its level of activity; peroxidase (red), present in the monocyte's granules, is restricted in the resident macrophage to the nuclear envelope and to the endoplasmic reticulum. (Adapted from [76].)

they multiply, their individual life span matters little.

FUNCTIONS

Macrophage activation can be a confusing topic because macrophages are capable of being turned on in two ways: a quick, short-term and a slow, long-term activation.

- **Quick activation** (better called **stimulation**) is a burst of activity triggered in second or minutes, usually by phagocytosis. It causes exocytosis of lysosomal enzymes and the secretion of oxygen-derived free radicals. This is the equivalent of the respiratory burst of the neutrophils (p. 406) except that it is less dramatic: macrophages consume less than half the amount of oxygen and produce only 20 percent as much hydrogen peroxide as neutrophils (64).

- **Slow activation** is akin to hypertrophy; it implies changes in macrophages that occur over days (and therefore could not occur with neutrophils because they do not live long enough). In the 1960s, G.B. Mackaness noticed that peritoneal macrophages of mice injected intravenously with *Listeria* (a facultative intracellular parasite) became more effective against other bacteria as well; they were larger, more ruffled, contained more granules, and had *in vitro* a much greater propensity to stick and spread over surfaces (Figure 9.11) (45). We now know that such macrophages, dubbed **angry macrophages,** also have a much more powerful respiratory burst and greater bactericidal and/or tumoricidal ability than resting macrophages. Histochemical studies have shown that the activation to angry macrophage is a multistep process, each step being defined by a particular set of surface markers and enzymatic content while given functions increase or decrease (2, 76).

The principal agents of this long-term activation are **lymphokines,** especially interferon gamma produced by lymphocytes (40), which means that this type of activation is to be expected mainly in infections and in immune responses. Macrophages can probably also stimulate themselves. When exposed to endotoxin, a powerful lipopolysaccharide produced by gram-negative bacteria, they produce tumor necrosis factor (TNF), which activates macrophages *in vitro* (40). Autostim-

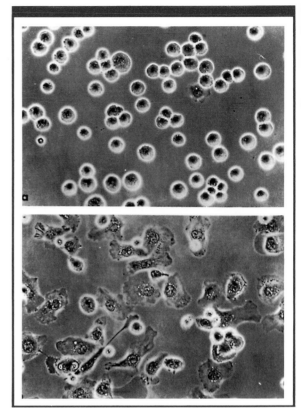

FIGURE 9.11
Structural and functional changes in activated macrophages. *Top:* Normal mouse macrophages obtained from the peritoneum; after 1 hour of incubation over a glass slide, they still retain their rounded shape, failing to attach and spread. *Bottom:* Activated peritoneal macrophages from mice vaccinated with BCG and obtained by injecting into the peritoneum a suspension of BCG. After incubation for only 15 minutes, they have become attached and spread. (Reproduced with permission from [46].)

ulation would be an advantage because the macrophages could become "angry" immediately, without having to wait for several days—the time it would take for the immune response to develop and for lymphocytes to produce their interferon gamma.

Studies of macrophage activation have shown that a suspension of absolutely resting macrophages is not easily obtained. A classic way to obtain macrophages is to irritate the peritoneal cavity "slightly" with a mild substance such as glycogen. Today it is clear that macrophages answering this call, however gentle it may be, are partially activated, or primed (that is, ready to respond more intensely if stimulated) (41). Another established method for separating macrophages (for example, from the peritoneal fluid of a rat) is to place a drop of the peritoneal fluid on a glass or plastic surface: the macrophages adhere to it and spread (Figure 9.11), and the other cells can be washed away. However, adherence leads to partial activation (42). Alveolar macrophages can be obtained by bronchial lavage, a fairly uncomfortable procedure (15).

Besides activation, the macrophages can respond to external stimuli by undergoing either of two striking adaptations: they can become stuffed with lipid and become **foam cells,** the villains of atherosclerosis, or they can fuse with each other and become **giant cells,** the sometime heroes of chronic inflammation. Both changes deserve special treatment elsewhere (p. 87 and 449).

There is a dark side to the macrophages. Activated macrophages can be dangerous, just like neutrophils. In the lung, for example, they can attack the elastin scaffolding with their elastase (8,86). One of their most powerful products, **tumor necrosis factor** (TNF), can destroy tumors under certain conditions (p. 351), but it also can

be secreted in doses large enought to kill the host—hence TNF is also called **cachectin**. The syndrome of septic shock is caused by endotoxin, but that is largely because endotoxin stimulates macrophages to oversecrete TNF and other cytokines (p. 701). Macrophages can cause trouble also by becoming reservoirs for infectious agents, including the AIDS virus (40).

In essence: Unlike the single-minded, short-lived neutrophil, the macrophage is a highly versatile, long-lived cell with a multitude of biological properties that make it the mastermind of inflammation, especially in the chronic stage (Figure 9.12). Like the neutrophil, it can become dangerous.

(4) PLATELETS
The platelets are stiff little discs, passively dragged around in the bloodstream (Figure 9.13). Their most obvious roles are intravascular: they maintain the integrity of the endothelium, by a mechanism

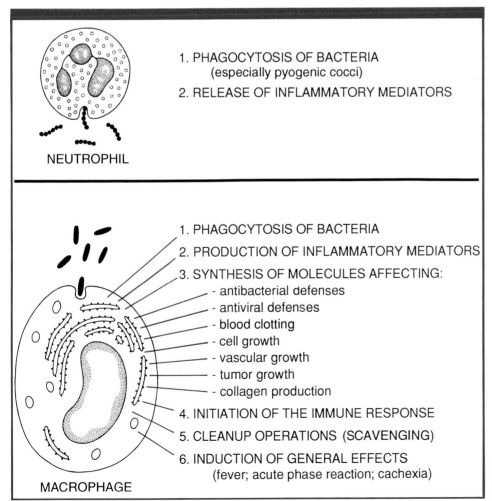

NEUTROPHIL

1. PHAGOCYTOSIS OF BACTERIA
   (especially pyogenic cocci)
2. RELEASE OF INFLAMMATORY MEDIATORS

MACROPHAGE

1. PHAGOCYTOSIS OF BACTERIA
2. PRODUCTION OF INFLAMMATORY MEDIATORS
3. SYNTHESIS OF MOLECULES AFFECTING:
   - antibacterial defenses
   - antiviral defenses
   - blood clotting
   - cell growth
   - vascular growth
   - tumor growth
   - collagen production
4. INITIATION OF THE IMMUNE RESPONSE
5. CLEANUP OPERATIONS (SCAVENGING)
6. INDUCTION OF GENERAL EFFECTS
   (fever; acute phase reaction; cachexia)

FIGURE 9.12
Basic functions of granulocytes and macrophages.

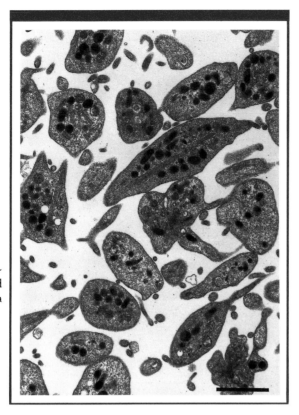

FIGURE 9.13
Normal rat platelets, isolated and spun down into a pellet. Note the abundant granular content. **Bar** = 0.2 μm. (Reproduced with permission from [9].)

trated platelets produces a tremendous inflammatory response (9). But then, the platelets are unable to crawl out of the blood vessels, as the leukocytes do: so how can they reach the extracellular spaces where inflammation is raging, and use their arsenal of helpful molecules? The answer seems to be very simple: wherever injury occurs, millions of vessels are severed and bleed; the platelets rush to plug those leaks, and within a matter of seconds or minutes they break up, releasing their load. In other words, despite the fact that they cannot actively emigrate from the blood vessels, they are the very first to supply mediators where they are urgently needed. (Platelet activation is discussed on p. 613).

In essence: platelets, small as they are, are essential (a) for the daily upkeep of the blood vessels, (b) for blood clotting and hemostasis, and (c) for the instant delivery of mediators to injured tissues.

(5) ENDOTHELIAL CELLS

Endothelial cells are critical to inflammation because they are the barrier that must be crossed by the two components of the inflammatory exudate, plasma and leukocytes. Rivers of ink continue to flow around this dull-looking, flat cell, which was once thought to be as passive as a cellophane sheet (65,68,70). The revolution began when it became possible to grow endothelial cells of various kinds *in vitro*. Please take note that the supposedly dull endothelial cells enjoy—among other distinctions—the privilege of a

yet unknown (in the absence of platelets the endothelium falls apart) (30); they plug gaps in the endothelium; they are essential for stopping hemorrhage (p. 613); and they take part in blood clotting. However, *the platelets are also loaded with at least 19 types of molecules that can play a number of useful roles in inflammation* (54,83,87) (Figure 9.14). In fact, a subcutaneous injection of concen-

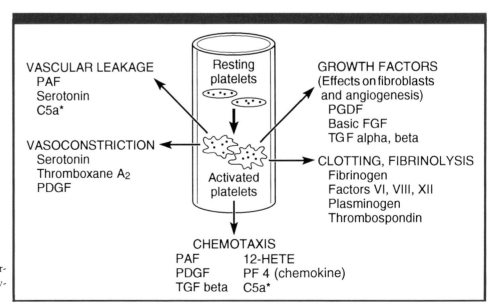

FIGURE 9.14
The platelets are loaded with molecules that are actual or potential inflammatory mediators. *C5a is generated secondarily by proteolytic cleavage of complement component C5.

VASCULAR LEAKAGE
PAF
Serotonin
C5a*

Resting
platelets

GROWTH FACTORS
(Effects on fibroblasts
and angiogenesis)
PGDF
Basic FGF
TGF alpha, beta

VASOCONSTRICTION
Serotonin
Thromboxane A$_2$
PDGF

Activated
platelets

CLOTTING, FIBRINOLYSIS
Fibrinogen
Factors VI, VIII, XII
Plasminogen
Thrombospondin

CHEMOTAXIS
PAF   12-HETE
PDGF   PF 4 (chemokine)
TGF beta   C5a*

specific morphologic marker: the rod-shaped Weibel-Palade bodies, which are loaded with a specific protein (the von Willebrand factor) involved in clotting and other important functions. Nobody can claim to be growing endothelial cells *in vitro* without proving that they carry this passport—the Weibel-Palade bodies.

We will discuss the endothelium in action when we analyze the various phases of inflammation; however, we must record here three endothelial dogmas relevant to inflammation:

- *The endothelium is the largest endocrine organ,* weighing perhaps as much as one kilogram (68). Endothelial cells secrete a great variety of molecules (69).
- *The endothelium can be activated:* if stimulated by cytokines or other agents, the endothelial cells respond instantly by producing prostaglandins or in a few hours by secreting adhesion molecules and other proteins (61).
- *What is true for one set of endothelial cells may not be true for another.* The properties of endothelial cells vary a great deal along the vascular tree and from organ to organ.

The permeability of the endothelium in the microcirculation is discussed on p. 596 and p. 369.

(6) FIBROBLASTS

Fibroblasts, once thought to be rather monotonous fibermakers, turn out to be quite dynamic: they can respond to chemotactic stimuli and move around (62); they can also modulate into contractile cells (p. 472). On the other hand, they have lost their status as the sole synthesizers of collagen, elastin, and glucosaminoglycans; it is now clear that these molecules can be produced also by smooth muscle cells and endothelium.

(7) MAST CELLS AND BASOPHILS

Although mast cells live in tissues and basophils in the blood, these two types of cells must be mentioned together because they are very similar in structure and function; they both arise from bone marrow precursors (26,43,71) but—unlike the monocyte/macrophage tandem—the basophils are *not* precursors of the mast cells. Whenever we make general statements about mast cells, we should often say "mast cells and basophils."

There are, however, some clear-cut differences between the two cell types (26): basophils are smaller, their nucleus is multilobed, they live only days as compared to months (27,71), and the response to activators are not identical to those of mast cells (26).

By light and by electron microscopic standards, mast cells and basophils are spectacular; they are stuffed with large granules programmed to release histamine and other inflammatory mediators in such amounts that the whole animal (human or other) can die of it in minutes. In fact we will discuss them in more detail in the section on anaphylaxis, a syndrome of generalized mast cell release. Yet we are not sure about their normal function.

Mast cells were described around 1876 by a medical student who developed a passion for the newly available aniline dyes, which were being tested on tissues by his older cousin Carl Weigert, a famous pathologist. The young man soon noticed that some leukocytes stain with basic dyes, as do the mast cells (he called these **basophils***), others stain with acid dyes such as eosin (he called them* **eosinophils***), and still others stain with neither (* **neutrophils***). The medical student was Paul Ehrlich, who later originated the concept of receptors; it was he who shared the Nobel prize with Metchnikoff in 1908. After Ehrlich's work, interest in mast cells and basophils faded away for decades for the simple reason that their granules are almost invisible with the routine hematoxylin–eosin stain.*

In the 1930s the granules of mast cells and basophils were found to contain the anticoagulant heparin, a highly acidic, sulfated glycosaminoglycan: its negative charge explains the basophilia of the granules, and some years later it was realized that histamine and other molecules were bound to the heparin (67). Today the macromolecular matrix of the mast cell and basophil granules can actually be conceived as a cation exchange resin to which positively charged molecules are reversibly attached (Figure 9.15) (50). Held in this manner are histamine, several proteases, and chemotactic factors; in rats and mice, but not in humans, histamine is joined by serotonin.

Mast cells are notoriously heterogeneous with respect to structure, mediator content, granule proteoglycan, and most important, response to drugs (Figure 9.16, 9.17) (7,24, 25, 26,80). Two major types have been identified: the **connective tissue mast cells (TC)** and the **mucosal mast cells (MC)** (Figures 9.15 and 9.16). Mucosal mast cells

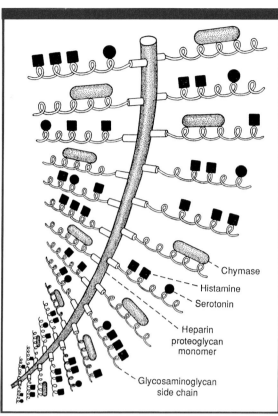

FIGURE 9.15 Artist's view of a heparin molecule in a mast cell granule. The long axis is a protein, to which are attached (in featherlike fashion) glycosaminoglycan molecules. To the latter are bound (in noncovalent fashion) histamine, serotonin, and proteolytic enzymes (chymases of multiple types). (Adapted from [3,50].)

Chymase

Histamine

Serotonin

Heparin proteoglycan monomer

Glycosaminoglycan side chain

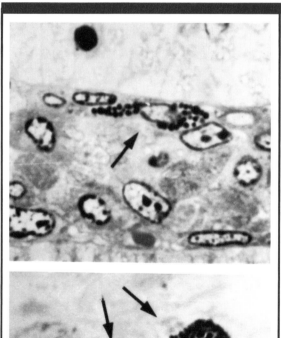

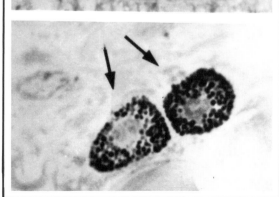

FIGURE 9.16 Diffferent aspects of mucosal mast cells (top) and connective tissue mast cells (bottom). Duodenal submucosa and tongue of the rat; toluidine blue stain. (Reproduced with permission from [19].)

are smaller and more mobile, have fewer granules and less histamine, and have shorter life-spans than those of the connective tissue (19); in the rat, they fail to respond to a powerful degranulator (a substance called 48/80) and also to a powerful protector against degranulation (disodium cromoglycate). These differences may be clinically important with regard to the treatment of allergies (p. 517) (7).

Whatever their regional distribution (connective tissues, mucosae), mast cell populations, when studied histochemically, are a mixture of two subsets: MC/TC, which contain tryptase and chymase, and MC/T, which contain tryptase only (25).

The one great act of mast cells and basophils is degranulation and release of granule content (18). Because "exploded" mast cells are often seen in traumatized tissues, pathologists tend to see mast cells as fragile bags of granules ready to burst if prodded (Figure 9.18); in contrast, mast cell experts see degranulation as a biochemical response. Both views are probably right. One typical form of degranulation is mediated by an immunologic mechanism, which leads to anaphylaxis (p. 513). The details of degranulation vary, but the overall result is that the membranes surrounding the granules fuse to form tubes and the granules are extruded (18,38). In rats the whole process takes about 2 minutes, in humans it spreads over 15 to 40 minutes. How long it takes for an individual mast cell to replace its granules is not clear. Fawcett found (21) that all the mast cells in the peritoneum of a rat can be destroyed (not just degranulated) by an intraperitoneal injection of distilled water; this procedure appears drastic but is surprisingly well tolerated by the other peritoneal cells. Under these conditions a new set of mast cells slowly reappears over 6 weeks (21), presumably supplied by bone marrow precursors.

When they degranulate, the mast cells release many mediators besides histamine (and serotonin in rodents) such as platelet activating factor and various cytokines (28,33), including the powerful tumor necrosis factor alpha: no other cell type is known to contain a *preformed* supply of this cytokine (26,34). *Different types of mast cells produce different mediators* (35).

Mast cells can be coaxed into phagocytizing (50), but perhaps more significant is the ability of mast cell granules to perform another type of uptake: they can somehow adsorb from the

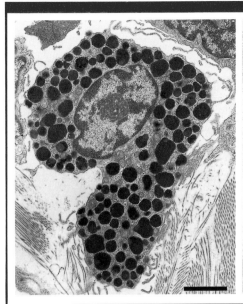 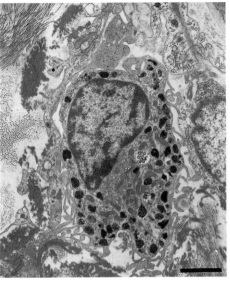

FIGURE 9.17
Two main types of human mast cells. *Left:* TC type (tryptase positive, chymase positive) found in the skin; it is analogous to the rodent "typical" or connective tissue type mast cells. *Right:* T-type (tryptase positive) mast cell from the lung, analogous to the rodent "atypical" or mucosal type. In the latter, the granules are fewer and smaller. **Bars** = 2 μm. (Reproduced with permission from [13].)

bloodstream and concentrate certain molecules such as metals, toxins, and enzymes (24,67). Selye called this phenomenon "mastopexy," presumably without realizing that this is also the name of a surgical operation on the female breast, which may explain why his term never caught on.

Mast cells can be induced to multiply and even to form tumors; in fact, mast cell tumors (mastocytomas) have been useful as sources of mast cells in bulk for chemical study.

> *Normal mast cells multiply in response to a T-cell lymphokine (53) now named interleukin 3. During parasitic infestations, this growth factor appears in the blood and even in the urine (71). There are conditions, called mastocytoses, that are excesses of mast cells, and can be localized, systemic (to the skin, as in urticaria pigmentosa), or generalized. Some of the symptoms of mastocytosis reflect an exaggerated release of histamine, such as skin eruptions, diarrhea, and flushes (58). Mast cells also appear in swarms in certain immune responses of the poison ivy type (p. 550), but their presence is not essential (27). Strains of mast-cell–deficient mice exist (26,55), but these animals have other problems as well, which makes them an imperfect model.*

In essence: mast cells are beautiful, but their functions are still rather mysterious. Perhaps they should be seen as triggers of the acute inflammatory response, a function for which they are perfectly equipped. Mast cells also have an eosinophil connection: this may be an important lead to their evolutionary meaning (p. 525).

Whatever they do, they must be important: estimates of their total mass in humans vary a great deal, but 100 g is conservative (79).

(8,9) T AND B LYMPHOCYTES

T and B lymphocytes are the agents of the immune system, and as such they have held the scientific and medical limelight for the past 30 years. An immunologist might have a fit at seeing that we deal with them here in only a few paragraphs. Our reason was stated in the preface: we assume that the reader has some background in immunology.

On the microscope stage, lymphocytes appear

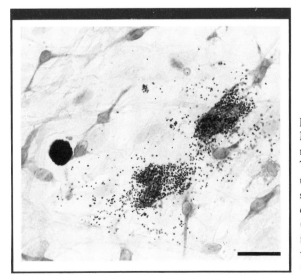

FIGURE 9.18
Mast cells in the rat mesentery. Two have degranulated, presumably during dissection; one (left) is in a resting state. Cresyl violet stain. **Bar** = 25 μm.

to be the least interesting of all cells. They are the smallest leukocytes, about as large as a red blood cell, and have so little cytoplasm that they look like plain nuclei in histologic sections. Their granules are tiny and rare; Ehrlich missed them altogether and branded the lymphocytes "physiologically inferior to the polymorphonuclear leukocytes" (37). Until the 1940s they were known only as "cells typical of chronic inflammation".

In human blood, lymphocytes make up 33 percent of the leukocytes; of these, 70–75 percent are T cells, 10–15 percent B cells, and 10 percent NK cells. Alas, none of these types can be distinguished from the others under the light microscope, so the only way to label them is to use immunochemical methods based on antibodies that recognize specific surface markers. Another difficulty in identifying lymphocytes is their ability to become much larger when undergoing the so-called blast transformation, which is a combination of hypertrophy and hyperplasia; the so-called *blasts* look distressingly similar to macrophages. The B cells, however, reveal their identity when they become elegant plasma cells, the antibody secretors (Figure 9.19).

> *Incidentally, rat blood swarms with lymphocytes (86% of their white blood cells). We have no explanation.*

The presence of lymphocytes in histologic sections of tissues normally devoid of these cells is suggestive of a local immune response (i.e., some antigenic material is or has been handled there). What the lymphocytes are actually doing in a given inflammatory focus can only be inferred from the enormous literature on lymphocyte functions: they might be

- processing antigens
- secreting antibodies (*)
- secreting cytokines that give orders to any of the ten cell types involved in inflammation, and thus
- activating cells
- recruiting leukocytes from the blood
- causing local cells to multiply
- causing other cells to secrete cytokines
- causing mast cells to degranulate
- causing vessels to leak
- killing cells (*)
- modulating collagen production by fibroblasts
- inducing bone marrow cells to proliferate
- inducing fever and other general effects
- or doing nothing at all, if they are not activated.

Only two functions (*) can be recognized on histologic sections, especially the first: *the presence of plasma cells (modified B lymphocytes) always indicates antibody synthesis.* Notice that one item is conspicuously missing in the list above: phagocytosis.

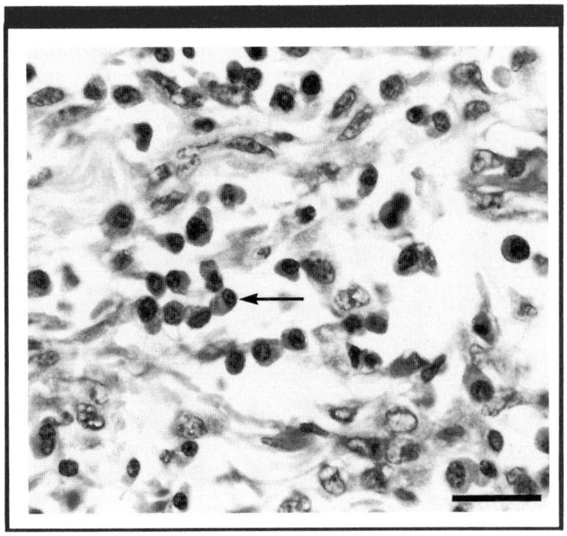

(10) NATURAL KILLER CELLS

Natural killer cells (NK cells) are also known as **large granular lymphocytes** (LGL). They were identified as late as 1973 by their ability to kill tumor cells without previous sensitization (57). These amazing cells are programmed to kill other cells, such as tumor cells (unfortunately not all) and especially virus-infected cells. Therefore they accumulate in virus-infected organs (49).

How the NK cells choose their targets is not yet clear. By comparison, killer T-lymphocytes attack cells that are duly labelled as targets by the presence of antigen on their surface, combined with an "identity marker", a surface protein of the MHC family (p. 559). NK cells do not take these cues. However, recent evidence has shown that NK cells tend to kill targets that express *low* levels of certain MHC molecules; this suggests that these surface markers may be delivering to the NK cells a *negative* signal, by telling them to spare that target (85). This is the so-called "missing self" hypothesis of cell killing.

Because NK cells can eliminate virus-infected cells without the help of the immune response, they are vitally important as an early defense against virus infections (the immune system needs several days for mobilizing its own counterattack).

FIGURE 9.19 Typical plasma cells in a nasal polyp. **Arrow:** Plasma cell showing the paranuclear halo, which corresponds to the Golgi apparatus. **Bar** = 25 μm.

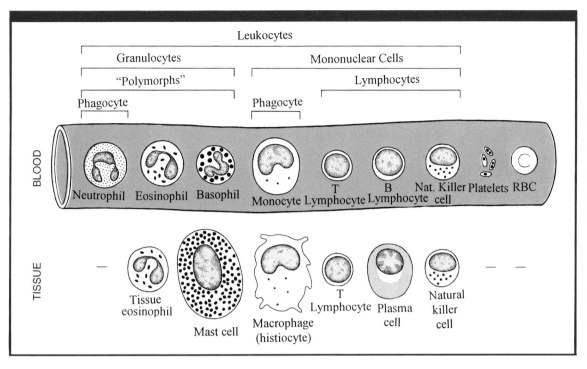

FIGURE 9.20 Nomenclature of the inflammatory cells. Most of the blood-borne inflammatory cells have a counterpart in the tissues; only the neutrophils and the platelets do not. The red blood cell is added for scale (diameter 7 μm.). *Top:* alternate names often employed for particular groups of inflammatory cells.

They may represent a primitive immune system that evolved after the macrophages but before the T-cell system (39). Their role in inflammation—when unrelated to viruses—is still under study.

TO SUM UP: Ten types of cells collaborate to preserve us against infections and to repair injuries. Figure 9.20 is a synopsis of the blood-borne inflammatory cells. It should help newcomers review the overlapping terms *leukocyte, polymorph,* and *phagocyte.* This figure also shows that most blood-borne inflammatory cells have a counterpart in the normal extravascular spaces, with two exceptions: neutrophils and platelets. Only two inflammatory cells are significantly phagocytic: neutrophils and macrophages. One cell type most active in chronic inflammation, the fibroblast, is generally believed to derive only from connective tissue fibroblasts and not from the blood. However, a recent paper seems to explode this dogma: hidden in the circulating "monocyte" population is a small but significant fraction of undifferentiated stem cells that emigrate into areas of injury and behave as fibroblasts (9a). If confirmed, this finding will open new vistas: it implies that the cellular components of the blood can produce whole new connective tissue (albeit without blood vessels).

The circulating fibroblast precursors can be identified by immunochemical means: they stain positively for collagen, vimentin, and the protein CD34 which is a surface marker for bone marrow stem cells. In mammals, *the circulating blood also contains other stem cells derived from the bone marrow and capable of producing all types of blood cells (hematopoiesis).* They, too, can be identified by marker proteins, including CD34 (44a.).

All these cells speak a chemical language, which we will now examine.

Mediators: The Chemical Language of Inflammation

Although learning a language is never painless, the language that cells use in the emergency of inflammation is full of interesting twists. It may be the oldest language on earth. Insects use it in their stings (a very effective means of communication), as does the nettle. Bacteria use messenger peptides that resemble our own (217). The language comes in some 12 dialects (Table 9.3), Vertebrate cells seem to be fluent in all (plus the language of the aggressors), but no human can make that claim. People who speak "prostaglandin" have a strong accent when they speak free radicals, and those who speak "complement" are barely understandable to anyone else. We will do our best to steer you along a Berlitz-type path; for the faint of

TABLE 9.3
Families of Chemical Mediators
of Inflammation

ENDOGENOUS MEDIATORS

1. Vasoactive amines (histamine, serotonin)
2. Kinin system products (e.g., bradykinin)
3. Peptides from various sources (e.g., substance P)
4. Complement system by-products (e.g., anaphylatoxins)
5. Clotting system products (plasmin, fibrinopeptides); fibrinolytic system products (fibrin fragments)
6. Arachidonic acid metabolites (eicosanoids)
   - Cyclooxygenase products (prostaglandins, thromboxanes)
   - Lipoxygenase products (leukotrienes, HETEs, HPETEs)
   - Non-enzymatic products (chemotactic lipids)
7. Platelet-activating factors (PAFs)
8. Cytokines (e.g., interleukins, tumor necrosis factor; chemokines)
9. Growth factors (e.g., platelet-derived growth factor)
10. Lysosomal enzymes (e.g., collagenase)
11. Oxygen-derived free radicals (e.g., HO·)
12. Nitric oxide (NO) and other small molecules

EXOGENOUS MEDIATORS

13. Chemotactic factors (e.g., fMLP)
14. Anti-leukocytic factor (leukocidin)
15. Macrophage activator (endotoxin)
16. Enzymes and other bacterial products

Valy Menkin, who proposed this concept in the 1930s (182,183) was largely ignored.

What is a mediator of inflammation? In today's definition, *a mediator is any molecule that is generated in a focus of inflammation and modulates the inflammatory response in some way.* According to this definition, molecules generated by aggressor parasites should also be considered as mediators; we will consider them last (as *exogenous mediators*) because they are a disparate and untidy group that includes frankly injurious agents.

The classic definition of mediator in physiologic processes is much more strict. According to an eminent pharmacologist, an endogenous material can be accepted as a mediator in a physiopathologic phenomenon if (a) it is found in tissues in appropriate amounts, (b) it can be released by the stimulus that produces the phenomenon, (c) it has the same universality in various species as the phenomenon itself, (d) it is destroyed in the place of release, and (e) it can be blocked by inhibitors (214).

The endogenous mediators, these chemical messages that spread back and forth in a focus of inflammation, belong to very different chemical families (see Table 9.3). Some act like local hormones, binding to a specific receptor and elicit a specific response. To this category of mediators belong histamine, serotonin, prostaglandins, leukotrienes, and cytokines. Others do not bind to receptors and can be considered messengers only in a broad sense: they "make a difference." Lysosomal enzymes are an example. Still others, such as free radicals, mediate inflammation simply by causing damage.

Today we have to deal with hundreds of endogenous mediators filling dozens of books and several specialized journals (29). We humans tend to visualize the cells in inflamed tissues as being overwhelmed by a cacophony of conflicting orders (Figure 9.21), but the cells themselves seem to have no problem in deciding what to do. The difficulty in interpretation is entirely ours.

Autacoid *has been proposed as an alternative term for inflammatory mediator. It comes from the Greek* autós + ákos, *meaning "self-drug," and may be more appropriate because many of the "inflammatory" mediators are just endogenous drugs that can be secreted under circumstances other than inflammation and that have noninflammatory effects (e.g., prostaglandin E1 stimulates bone formation). By definition, autacoids are supposed to be pharmacologically active molecules that are secreted locally*

heart, the tables, the "bottom lines," and the summary figures may be enough.

We acknowledge one major difficulty: the size of the dictionary. In the blissful ignorance of the 1920s only one endogenous messenger was known, histamine, with only one target, blood vessels. Nobody dared think then that *all* aspects of inflammation were driven by chemical signals;

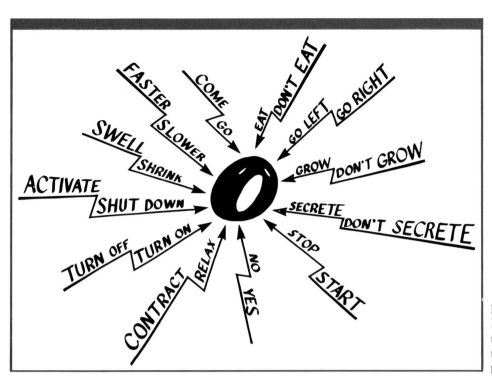

FIGURE 9.21
In inflamed tissues, each cell is submitted to a myriad of contradictory messages. How it chooses the appropriate response remains a mystery.

and are neither neurotransmitters nor hormones. We accept the basic concept, but the distinction is not sharp: prostaglandins should be typical autacoids, yet prostacyclin can circulate like a hormone. (The term autacoid, by the way, was proposed in 1916 as an improvement over the then new term "hormone" proposed by Starling. The latter term was considered inappropriate because it means "the exciting substance" whereas not all hormones excite (127, 142,231).

How do cells respond to inflammatory mediators? Considering that *any function of any cell is a potential target for any one of the mediators,* the number of possible effects is appalling. Fortunately, not all effects are significant. **Motion** and **secretion** are common responses to mediators: for example, vascular smooth muscle cells contract or relax, venular endothelial cells contract, leukocytes move in given directions and phagocytize certain targets, and many cell types secrete prostaglandins, cytokines, or other mediators.

Following are some basic facts about endogenous mediators of inflammation.

- *For every mediator there are one or more inhibitors.* Without an inhibitive mechanism, the inflammatory exudate would become an enormous pool of messages that could seep into the bloodstream (via the lymphatics or by reabsorption into the venules) and raise havoc everywhere. This

is what actually happens in anaphylaxis and in septic shock.

- *Mediators have short lives,* seconds or minutes, and their effects do not last much longer (minutes to an hour or so). Therefore, month-long and year-long chronic inflammations must be sustained by a well-orchestrated production and/or succession of mediators.

- *Endogenous mediators are supplied by the plasma, the leukocytes, and the local tissues,* that is, not only by the inflammatory cells but probably by all tissue cells. This is a recent discovery. When inflammation takes place in a parenchyma such as a gland or striated muscle, it certainly makes sense that the epithelial cells and the muscle fibers would have "their say." *Some parenchymal cells are known to speak out in terms of cytokines or prostaglandins;* to quote Sir John Vane, 1982 Nobel laureate for his work in this field, "mammalian cells seem to disgorge prostaglandins at the slightest provocation" (203).

- *Virtually all mediators are two-edged swords.* They can cause trouble both locally and generally. For example, histamine release can cause hives, itching, swelling, and even choking if the swelling occurs in the larynx. The simultaneous release of virtually all inflammatory mediators into the blood stream is the underlying mechanism of septic shock.

- *The effects of any mediator can vary from tissue to tissue and from species to species;* we must therefore be very cautious with generalizations. For example, histamine constricts large arteries and dilates small ones, but not uniformly in all species (107,232). This variance justifies the use of the noncommittal term **vasoactive,** which implies that a given mediator may vasodilate, vasoconstrict, or increase vascular permeability.

We will now briefly describe all but one of the categories of mediators without implying any "pecking order" except that those in the first category are usually the first to appear during inflammation. The remaining category, oxygen-derived free radicals, is discussed elsewhere (p. 182).

Vasoactive Amines

The two amines histamine and serotonin (Figure 9.22) are especially important because—unlike most other mediators—*they are available from performed supplies.* Histamine is stored in the granules of the mast cells and basophils and serotonin in the granules of platelets (as well as in the mast cells of rodents). Correspondingly, *histamine and serotonin are among the first mediators to be released during inflammation.* They seem to play little or no role in chronic inflammation.

The value of preformed mediators is easy to understand. If a defensive action is suddenly required, it is useful to have a store of mediators on hand. But why only two? We can reason as follows. Mediators are potent molecules, which means that they can be toxic in low doses. Consider histamine. When mast cells throughout the body liberate their histamine, the result is anaphylactic shock, one of the fastest ways to die (p. 519). In adults, 0.33 mg of intravenous histamine will drop pulse and blood pressure to dangerously low levels (245); and the skin alone contains about 100 times that critical dose (239). It seems that evolution has wisely equipped us with large supplies of only two ready-made mediators while many other can be produced on short order, in even less than one minute.

Histamine

Histamine is found in virtually all tissues, in spinach and tomatoes, in wine, in the hairs of gypsy-moth caterpillars (228), and most prominently in the stingers of the nettle, where its function correlates with offense rather than defense (it discourages mammals that may have an appetite for nettles) (p. 524). It can also be synthesized by many tissues, including granulation tissue, the new, young connective tissue that is produced in chronic inflammation. In mammals it is found primarily in mast cells, bound to heparin, in platelets, in the gastric mucosa, and in the brain as a neurotransmitter (229). *In acute inflammation, histamine produces pain plus three major "vasoactive" effects, all related to cellular contraction:*

- *contraction of smooth muscle,*
- *arteriolar dilatation, and*
- *venular leakage (i.e., increased permeability) due to endothelial contraction.*

Therefore the overall effect of histamine injected into the skin is a wheal that looks very much like a mosquito bite.

Students are baffled by drugs that contract *and* dilate vessels. So are we. Whether the vessels respond by contracting or relaxing must depend on dosage and on the physiology of the receptors, but the mechanism is incompletely understood (232,234,235). On the whole, *histamine tends to contract large arteries and to dilate small ones:* thus, the systemic effect of its release is either hypertension or hypotension, depending on the prevalent effect, which varies with the species. In humans there are two syndromes of acute histamine poisoning: anaphylaxis (although histamine is not the only culprit; p. 519) and a variety of fish poisoning, namely scombroid poisoning (p. 526). The dramatic drop in blood pressure caused by histamine is due to arteriolar dilatation, aggravated by the loss of blood volume due to widespread venular leakage.

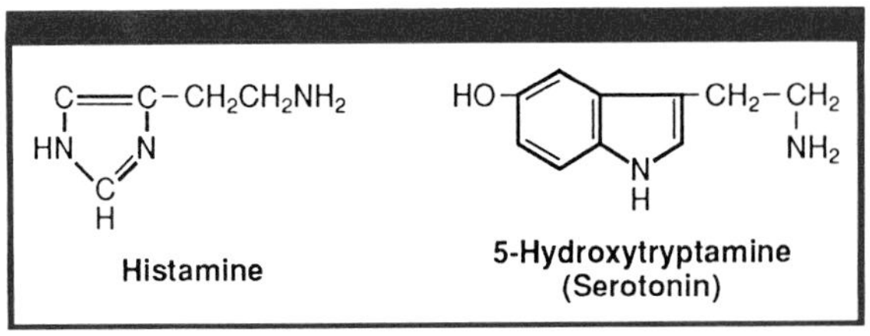

Histamine in low doses is said to attract eosinophils, but it is not leukotactic for neutrophils. However, histamine causes endothelial cells to redistribute, to their surface, the content of the Weibel–Palade bodies; this content includes the adhesion protein GMP-140, which induces leukocytes to stick (150). There are histamine receptors on all leukocytes, but their

FIGURE 9.22 Formulae of histamine and serotonin (5-hydroxytryptamine, 5-HT).

Histamine

5-Hydroxytryptamine (Serotonin)

significance in vivo is not known (110). Three to four hours after a local injection of histamine, and probably of any permeability-increasing mediator, there will be a mild local infiltration of leukocytes (p. 419).

SEROTONIN

Serotonin, or 5-hydroxytryptamine (5-HT) (136, 198) is distributed much like histamine, except that only in rodents do the mast cells carry it. It is contained in platelets (Figure 9.14), in the mucosa of the gut, in enterochromaffin cells, and in the central nervous system. On the whole *its basic vascular effects are similar to those of histamine: venular leakage (i.e. increased vascular permeability)—arterial contraction, and arteriolar dilatation, but with a greater tendency to induce contraction (vasospasm), as implied by its name* (serotonin means "serum substance that increases pressure").

Serotonin also has a property that histamine lacks: *it stimulates fibroblasts* (105). A good way to remember these disparate effects of serotonin is to picture the plight of individuals who carry a serotonin-secreting tumor. Those tumors, called carcinoids, derive from chromaffin cells in the gut or in the lung; they produce serotonin and other vasoactive substances and because they are structured like endocrine glands their secretion is poured into the blood. The patients suffer from acute flushes of the skin, and at autopsy there is a fibrosis of the endocardium on the right side

(Figure 9.23) but not on the left because serotonin is inactivated by the pulmonary endothelium.

Serotonin is rapidly destroyed by monoamine oxidase, present in many cells including monocytes and the endothelium.

VASOACTIVE PEPTIDES

Peptide mediators come from many sources, but they share one feature: they are bits of existing proteins, and have to be cleaved off by appropriate enzymes. Of course these enzymes are normally inactive; thus the genesis of these mediators begins with the activation of the corresponding enzymes.

THE KININ SYSTEM

Kinins (the prototype is bradykinin) are extraordinarily potent vasoactive peptides that are normally carried in the blood in inactive form as parts of plasma molecules called **kininogens** (Figure 9.24). The kinins can be cleaved from the kininogens by specific proteases: the **kallikreins,** which are present in the blood and urine as well as in various body fluids and tissues (188). Obviously, the plasma kallikrein must circulate as an inactive precursor, prekallikrein. Plasma prekallikrein is activated in relation to blood clotting, namely when the plasma protein that initiates the clotting cascade—the Hageman factor—is activated by contact with collagen or

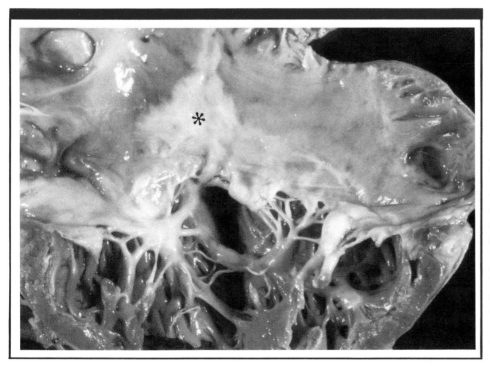

FIGURE 9.23
Plaque of fibrosis (*) in the right atrium of the heart in a case of carcinoid tumor with liver metastases. The fibrosis is an effect of serotonin and bradykinin secreted by the tumor and conveyed to the right side of the heart. The left side of the heart is rarely affected, because the causal agents are inactivated as they pass through the lungs. (Courtesy of Dr. F.J. Schoen, Harvard Medical School, Brigham and Women's Hospital, Boston, MA.)

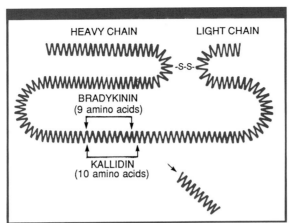

BRADYKININ
(9 amino acids)

KALLIDIN
(10 amino acids)

FIGURE 9.24
Showing how two vasoactive kinins (bradykinin and kallidin) are cleaved from the molecule of high molecular weight kininogen. (Adapted from [168].)

with any other negatively charged surface. This means that *when blood clots abundant kinins are produced,* mainly bradykinin (Figure 9.25).

We have just mentioned a pivotal factor carried by the blood, the **Hageman factor.** *We recommend that the reader contemplate figure 9.25, which conveys this important message:* nature has endowed the Hageman factor with the power of activating four systems involved in the inflammatory response:

- *i the* **kinin system,** *which produces vasoactive kinins*
- *the* **clotting system,** *which produces fibrin*
- *the* **fibrinolytic system,** *which produces plasmin, which breaks down the fibrin*
- *the* **complement system,** *which has many inflammatory functions*

The last three will be discussed later.

The kallikreins have no monopoly on kinin release; kininogen can also be cleaved nonspecifically by neutrophil enzymes and by plasmin (124, 168). This reminds us of a general principle. *Plasmin and leukocyte proteases are always floating around in an inflammatory focus, and one of their effects is to generate bradykinin,* either directly or by cleaving the Hageman factor, which activates the clotting cascade (192).

The major component of the kinin family is the nonapeptide bradykinin. *Its effects are very similar to those of histamine: increased vascular permeability* (by contraction of venular endothelial cells, p. 376), *vasodilatation* or *vasoconstriction,* depending on the circumstances, *and burning pain.* As an **algogen** (pain inducer) bradykinin is even more powerful than histamine and serotonin; wasps and hornets use all three in their sting (128). All these effects are intense and immediate, quite out of line with the name bradykinin, which implies slow moving (the name was chosen when it was found that strips of gut, exposed to bradykinin *in vitro,* respond with a slow contraction). Instilled into the nose, *bradykinin reproduces the symptoms of a common cold with sore throat* (208).

Because the plasma carries substrate and proenzyme (kininogen and prekallikrein) in amounts large enough for a massive release of kinins, a powerful inactivating system is at hand: *the kininases cut the half-life of circulating active kinin to less than one minute* (128). Any remaining kinin is

FIGURE 9.25
Diagram illustrating the multiple roles of the Hageman factor, activated by contact with a negatively-charged surface. Thanks to the proximity of high molecular weight kininogen (HMWK) it can activate the kinin as well as the coagulation cascade; it also activates the fibrinolytic and the complement cascades. Note the feedback activation from activated kallikrein.

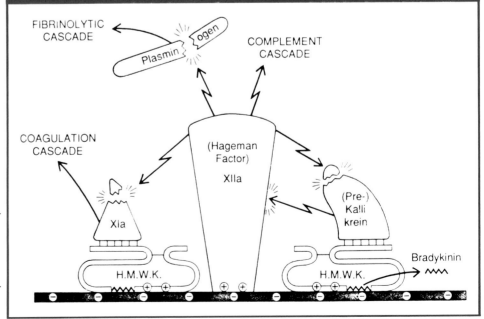

inactivated by a single passage through the lung, thanks to the **angiotensin-converting enzyme** (ACE, or kininase II), which is located on the endothelial surface. Paradoxically, this same enzyme (which inactivates the kinins) activates angiotensin I by cleaving it to angiotensin II, one of the most powerful vasoconstrictors known (221).

This homeostatic mechanism is disrupted in respiratory failure. Local acidosis increases the production of kinins as hypoxia impairs the inactivation mechanism; the result is an excess of local bradykinin, with local and possibly also general effects (172, 193).

Bradykinin was discovered during a homely experiment: a few ml of urine, injected intravenously into anesthetized dogs, lower blood pressure (127, 140) because it contains kallikrein. Later, various organ extracts were found to have a similar effect, especially those of pancreas (kallikréas in Greek, hence the name kallikrein). Tested in vitro these tissue kallikreins cleave the same substrate, kininogen, to form a decapeptide, kallidin.

Note: **Histamine-type mediators** is a convenient term for referring to a group of mediators that dilate arterioles and cause venular leakage: histamine, serotonin, bradykinin and the anaphylatoxins, and three products of activated complement (C3a, C4a, and C5a).

OTHER PEPTIDES

Peptides produced by the digestion of fibrin increase vascular permeability and are also mild vasoconstrictors (96). Peptides of this kind should appear wherever fibrin appears, which includes most types of inflammation: fibrin formation and fibrin digestion are activated at the same time. We suspect that peptides produced by the self-digestion of dead cells (autolysis) have similar effects, but surprisingly they have not been tested.

There are about twenty vasoactive peptides other than the kinins (223, 226), including vasopressin, the angiotensins, the neurokinins, somatostatin, endothelium-derived relaxing factor (EDRF) (230), the endothelins—powerful vasoconstrictors (94)—, and VIP—which happens to stand for vasoactive intestinal peptide. Some are related to hypertension or shock. **Substance P** *is especially relevant to inflammation (199); it resembles bradykinin, is released by the endings of sensory C fibers, degranulates mast cells, and may be involved in the pathogenesis of the so-called triple response (p. 366). Because many of these polypeptides are neuropeptides, they have been implicated in the little understood field of "neurogenic inflammation" (165, 226).*

Cytokines are a special group of polypeptide mediators; they will be considered further.

COMPLEMENT: A SIMPLIFIED VERSION

Judged by power and by complexity, complement is the star of inflammatory mediators. Basically, *complement is a machine for poking holes into cells. It circulates in the blood stream disassembled into about 20 proteins; when it assembles itself, it also generates—as by-products—some powerful inflammatory mediators.*

This is enough to convey that complement is a very intricate topic (218). Eminent scientists have spent their lives on it. Presumably Nature made it so complicated for purposes of control. The basic concept, however, is simple (190). Many parasites, especially bacteria, can be killed if they are perforated (a very human approach). However, just poking little holes in their surfaces would accomplish little because lipid membranes self-heal very fast. A better plan is to perforate them with stiff little tubes or plugs that create persisting leaks: this is the ultimate purpose of complement (Figure 9.26). The little ring-shaped plugs, called membrane attack complexes (MACs), are self-

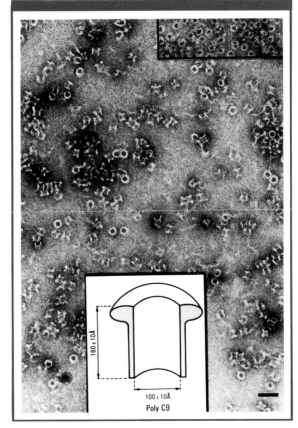

FIGURE 9.26 Electron microscopic image of free "membrane attack complexes" formed by C9 polymerized *in vitro.* Viewed from the top they appear as rings with a 100 Å internal diameter; viewed from the side they are rectangular. **Bar** = 0.05 μm. *Upper inset:* complement lesions on rabbit erythrocytes (internal diameter about 100 Å). *Lower inset:* schematic drawing of "poly C9". (Reproduced with permission from [204].)

assembled mainly from 12 to 18 identical molecules that circulate in the plasma under the name of C9.

There is a bonus in this complicated assembly mechanism. Remember that complement is typically needed for killing invaders, which must also be fought off with inflammation. Well, as the proteins of complement are activated by enzymatic action, they release small fragments that fly off and trigger or enhance the main functions of inflammation, such as summoning leukocytes, causing exudation of plasma, and assisting phagocytosis.

It follows, of course, that if complement is extremely useful, it is also extremely dangerous. If it were activated in the wrong circumstance, it would perforate and kill any cell at all. *Evolution has taken care of this problem by creating a machine that circulates disassembled in many pieces* that can be fitted together only under highly controlled circumstances with inhibitors at every step. The system is so complex than only the experts have memorized it all, and we will outline only the essentials, enough to appreciate this marvel of Nature.

Vocabulary of Complement—and Some Helpful Hints Consider that the plug-shaped MAC is not thrust into the target cell like an arrowhead, but created within the membrane, at a site selected by the first component of complement (C1). The nine basic pieces required for triggering the assembly of the MAC are numbered in the order in which they settle on the target membrane—with the exception of C4, which was named before it was understood. *So the order, alas, really is 1 → 423 → 56789* (followed by more C9 to make up the ring). We clustered these numbers to point out that the nine components actually form three little heaps: 1 by

itself, 423 nearby, and 56789 near 423. Those components that are activated by proteolysis are split into a large piece (b), which takes part in further reactions, and a small piece (a), which flies off as a mediator. (Beware: *a* does not mean "activated" as it does in the clotting cascade. This is not our fault.)

THE ENCOUNTER COMPLEMENT-BACTERIUM

A typical scenario could begin as follows: a colony of *E. coli* sets up an inflammatory reaction in the skin (coli endotoxin is a powerful inflammatory agent). Plasma seeps out of the vessels and with it come all the complement components, so the bacteria find themselves exposed to the still-disassembled complement. *Now there are two possibilities:* the plasma may or may not contain antibodies against the bacteria.

Let us assume the more likely hypothesis. Because *E. coli* are common infecting agents antibodies are present in the plasma, and so complement activation follows the so-called **classical pathway.** The antibodies promptly coat the bacteria, but no harm ensues, because antibodies alone usually cause no damage to their target; their role is only to label the target (in this case, bacteria) as antigens. How do circulating antibodies reach the bacteria? Remember that we are on a battlefield: the bacteria have set up an inflammatory response, whereby the vessels are leaking, and the tissue spaces are soaked with plasma. At this point, then, visualize the bacterial surfaces bristling with antibody molecules, say of the immunoglobin (IgG) type: these molecules are shaped like Ys, and they are attached by their two branches, with the stems (called Fc segments) sticking out.

Now, suspended in the plasma is also C1, a marvelous molecule shaped like a flower (its six petals are unusual because they resemble collagen). If a molecule of C1, hovering above the bacterial surface, meets two Fc segments that are spaced just right, it becomes activated (Figure 9.27); then the next three components are activated as a chain reaction (C2, C3, C4) and settle onto the bacterial surface nearby (the actual order, remember, is C423). These three molecules become involved simply because they are present in the mixture of plasma proteins. Activated C3 and C4 give off the fragments C3a and C4a, which are mediators of inflammation (anaphylatoxins). At this stage *we can visualize the first assembly (C1 + antibody molecules) sitting on the bacterial surface, surrounded by little piles of C234* (more precisely C2, 3b, 4b) (Figure 9.28).

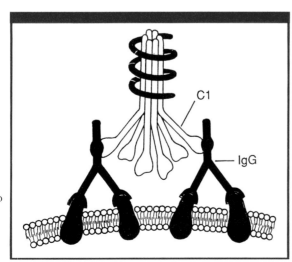

FIGURE 9.27
How C1, the first component of complement, is activated by contact with the Fc portion of two precisely spaced IgG molecules. (Adapted from [91].)

C1

IgG

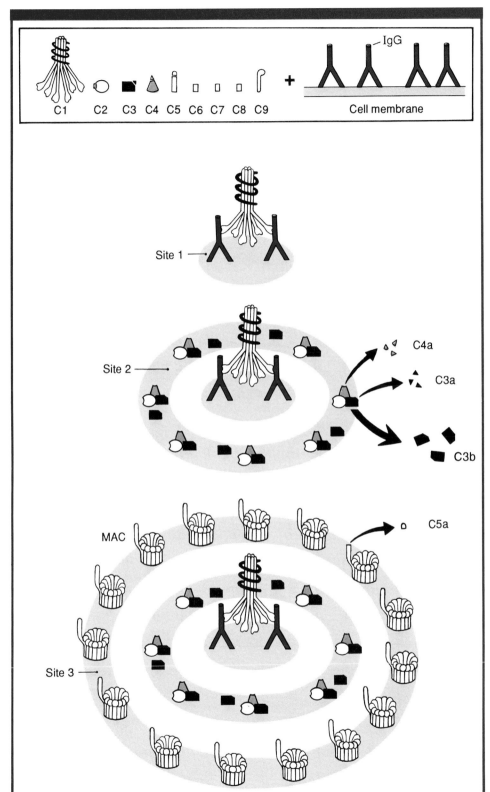

FIGURE 9.28
Geography of complement activation on the surface of a cell to be destroyed. The diagram emphasizes that three sites are involved. *Site 1* is chosen by C1 when it meets two appropriately spaced immunoglobulin molecules; C1 then activates C4, C2, and C3, which form an enzyme complex that settles nearby on the cell membrane *(Site 2)*. Note that some molecules of C3b also settle singly on the cell membrane, where they perform as opsonins. The enzyme complex C234 now acts on other complement molecules floating around, and modifies them in such a way that they assemble into membrane attack complexes *(Site 3)*. At sites 2 and 3, anaphylatoxins are released (C3a, C4a, C5a), whereby inflammation is induced.

Note: *some additional C3b fragments settle on the bacterial membrane on their own, as shown in Figure 9.28. Their function is to make the bacterium more appetizing for the phagocytes. More details follow.*

Each little pile of C234 acts as an enzyme and splits any C5 that may be floating by. The smaller fragment (C5a) flies off to become the most powerful of the three anaphylatoxins. The larger fragment (C5b) settles onto the nearby bacterial surface and performs an amazing feat: it develops into a stiff rod by lining up with C6, C7, and C8 (which also happen to be floating by). The rod has a hydrophobic head that is thrust into the bacterial membrane: *perforation has begun.* The rod formed by C5b678 *acts like a shoehorn for C9,* the last arrival, which can be visualized as an egg-shaped molecule (205). When C9 hits the shoehorn it becomes activated and straightens out into a rigid stick that enlarges the hole. More C9 molecules (as many as 19) bump into the settled C9, straighten out and begin to form a circular palisade. In the end the completed MAC looks like a short tube with a handle made up of C5b678 (Figure 9.29). The entire MAC can therefore be summed up as C5b678+999999999999. Milliseconds from the start, the mission is accomplished. The whole sequence—as visualized on a perforated cell membrane—has involved three types of complement sites, which we can imagine as set in three concentric areas (Figure 9.28): the C1 site in the center, surrounded by a ring of C234 sites (many more than C1 sites) and by an outer ring of C5b6789 sites (many more than C234 sites). The perforations can be demonstrated by electron microscopy (Figure 9.26). Some cells, including blood cells and the endothelium, carry a membrane glycoprotein called *protectin* or CD59 that acts as a partial shield against the thrust of the MACs (184).

The principle of perforating membranes by means of a plug is not unique to complement; several killer cells of the immune system perforate their targets by a similar mechanism. However, leukocytes can kill without assembling MAC-like pores; one such agent is tumor necrosis factor (see below).

A few details: the rod-shaped, four-molecule assembly C5b678 (without C9) causes some leakage from the bacterium but not enough to kill it. The size of the MACs varies somewhat depending on the number of C9 molecules that participate. Regarding the "dosage" of MACs required for a kill, a single MAC hit is said to be lethal to red blood cells, but nucleated cells perforated by MACs have defenses that they can mobilize; in one experiment the cells somehow got rid

of the MACs in about 2 minutes (210). If a purified solution of C9 is incubated, it polymerizes into typical tubular assemblies (Figure 9.26) (205); this takes 3 days at 37°C, but just 10 minutes in the presence of the C5b678 complex, which acts, as expected, as an accelerator of C9 polymerization (233).

Let us now return to the mechanism of complement activation, and consider the *second alternative: the coli bacilli attack a host that has no anti-coli antibodies.* Clearly, complement can not be activated as we just described, because that mechanism required a carpet of antibody molecules coating the bacteria. Still, complement is not defeated: it is simply activated by another route, called the **alternative** or **properdin pathway** (143). Bacterial surfaces can themselves attract C3b (a small amount is always present in the plasma); this C3b then activates C3 in a special manner that causes it to interact with five proteins (B, D, P (properdin), H, and I), which also circulate in plasma. The final result is the activation of the typical cascade, amputated of its early components C1, C4, and C2. Note the most important feature of this alternative pathway for survival: *complement attacks bacteria even when they are "seen" for the first time, without the benefit of antibodies.*

The discovery of the alternative pathway took place in sad circumstances. In the early 1950s, Dr. Louis Pillemer—a "tormented genius" (212)—was sure that he had discovered an important new type of antibacterial defense, independent of antibody and therefore nonspecific; it involved a protein that activated complement "in midstream" without using up the early components C1, C4, and C2 (but C3 was essential) (201). He called it properdin, suggesting an enzyme that intervened before (pro) the loss (perdo, "I lose [from the solution, by consumption]") of C3 (212). Pillemer met with a storm of opposition and ridicule; when he suddenly died of a barbiturate overdose, at the hight of the controversy, the properdin story was certainly involved (173, 212). Shortly thereafter his views were vindicated: the discovery of complement activation in guinea pigs that genetically lacked C4 proved that there was, indeed, an alternative pathway.

The inflammatory effects of complement derive from two sources. (a) The small fragments C3a, C4a and C5a. They have similar effects and are called **anaphylatoxins** because they cause mast cell degranulation, which—if extensive—leads to anaphylactic shock (the shock is due to massive loss of plasma by a generalized increase in vascular permeability; p. 519). The anaphylatoxins also attract and activate leukocytes and stimulate other cells to produce mediators; for example, C5a causes the leukocytes to release prostaglandins (154). There is evidence that anaphylatoxins can also increase vascular permeability directly (i.e., not via the mast cells) (242).

The biological potency of the three anaphylatoxins is C5a > C3a > C4a, dropping by a factor of roughly 100 from one peptide to the next (this is why C5a is often mentioned above). However, C3a is generated in 15-fold molar excess over C5a (104).

(b) Another important proinflammatory effect is due to C3b, which settles on cell membranes and prepares them for phagocytosis by the leukocytes, which have C3b receptors (C3b gets swallowed in the process). This prophagocytic effect is called **opsonization** (p. 401); it means that the bacterium is perforated *and* prepared to be phagocytized.

The bacterium, incidentally, loses its *milieu intérieur* through the many MAC perforations, dies, and is eventually scavenged. Bacteria that are resistant to complement attack, such as Gram-positive bacteria and some strains of Gram-negative bacteria, seem to be protected by a coat of filamentous molecules that keep the MACs at a distance from the cell membrane (Figure 9.30) (161). Viruses can also be killed by MACs if they are duly coated with complement (Figure 9.31) (240).

In certain conditions complement can also become activated in the plasma, that is, in a fluid phase. This could be a disaster for any cell exposed to free-floating MACs, but these are promptly deactivated by a providential plasma inhibitor known as Protein S (103, 190).

PATHOLOGY OF COMPLEMENT

As may be expected, the complement sequence is sometimes activated inappropriately. For example, in autoimmune diseases based on the antibody mechanism, the problem is that antibodies label a "friendly" structure, and complement, their blind accomplice, destroys it. This is what happens to the neuromuscular plaques in myasthenia gravis (p. 575) (222). In immunologic diseases based on the formation of antigen–antibody complexes (e.g., in the wall of arteries; p. 536), the complexes themselves do no harm. Arteritis develops because the complexes activate complement. Traumatized and necrotic tissues activate complement even if no bacteria are involved; whether this is good or bad is not clear (p. 420). The plastic membranes used for hemodialysis and those of cardiopulmonary bypass

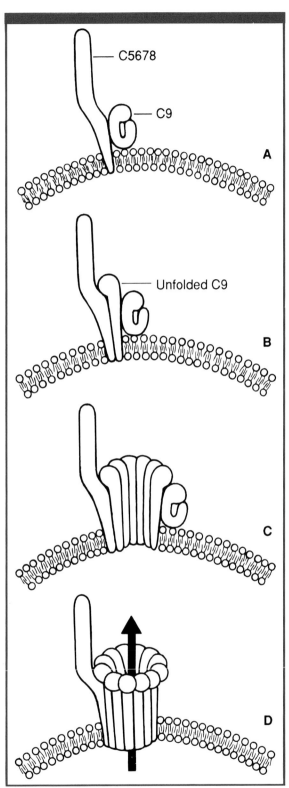

FIGURE 9.29 Development of the complement-derived Membrane Attack Complex (MAC). **A:** a rod-shaped structure formed by four complement components (5b, 6, 7 and 8 [C5678 on the figure]). The hydrophobic end of this complex stabs the cell membrane, and then comes in contact with a folded molecule of C9. **B:** The molecule of C9 is induced to unfold and to penetrate into the cell membrane; the long C5b678 complex appears to act as a "shoehorn." Now another molecule of unfolded C9 comes in contact with the previous one, and it is also induced to unfold, as shown in **C.** The process is repeated until a complete tubular structure is formed **D** . (Adapted from [206].)

pumps can activate complement too and therefore lead to hemolysis; they can also activate leukocytes that will be trapped in the lung and cause damage (adult respiratory distress syndrome or ARDS) (111, 147, 224).

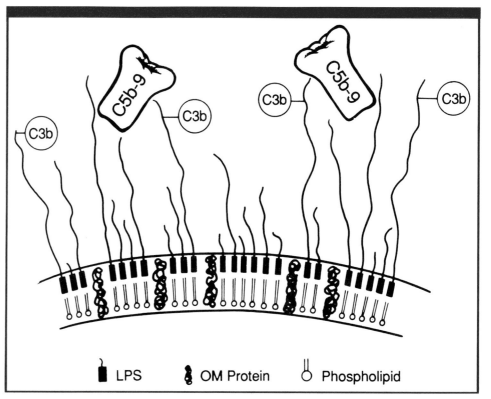

FIGURE 9.30
Why certain bacteria are not harmed by the MAC of complement. Complement is activated when C3b becomes attached to the side chains of endotoxin molecules (LPS for lipopolysaccharide). Steric hindrance by the long endotoxin molecules prevents the MAC from reaching the bacterial wall; the MAC is eventually shed. (Adapted from [161].)

*Congenital deficiencies of a complement component are rare and can be troublesome, but they are not usually lethal because the bodily defenses against microorganisms are so redundant. C3 deficiency causes increased susceptibility to pyogenic infections, in keeping with the loss of the C3b opsonin, but it is something of a shock to find that the lack of C9 is usually asymptomatic (215). The most important congenital deficiency is the lack of the inhibitor to C1 (C1 esterase inhibitor): as a result of physical or even emotional trauma these patients suffer acute episodes of edema of the skin and mucosae, which can be fatal if it affects the airways (**angioneurotic edema** or better **angioedema**) (125, 197). The kinin and clotting systems also appear to be involved in the pathogenesis of angioedema.*

Has the reader wondered how complement earned its peculiar name? In 1896 Bordet found that specific antisera against vibrios, if heated, could not destroy their targets (the vibrios were coated with antibody, but heating had destroyed complement); however, lysis took place if a little "complement" of nonspecific fresh serum was added (139, 176).

THE CLOTTING AND FIBRINOLYTIC CASCADES

Blood becomes a solid clot when the soluble protein fibrinogen turns into a network of fibrin filaments (Figure 9.32). Opposing processes in Nature are often linked: indeed, the dissolution of clots (**fibrinolysis**) is linked with clot formation. The two processes combined generate inflammatory mediators by several mechanisms.

- By-products of polymerization: to aggregate into fibrin, the fibrinogen molecule must lose two couples of peptides, fibrinopeptides A and B (Figure 9.33), which are chemotactic and increases vascular permeability (219).
- Destruction of the polymer occurs at the same time. As fibrinogen aggregates, the opposite (fibrinolytic) system is also activated, and **plasmin,** a proteolytic enzyme, breaks down the fibrin filaments. The resulting *fibrin degradation products* increase vascular permeability by releasing histamine from mast cells (135).
- Plasmin, the key enzyme of fibrinolysis, as a protease can release inflammatory peptides from substrates other than fibrin, such as kininogen (to release kinins) and C3 (to release the anaphylatoxin C3a) (225).

Plasmin also has a feedback loop (Figure 9.25): it activates a critical molecule, the Hageman factor, which reactivates the whole clotting cascade, plus the fibrinolytic and kinin cascades (Figure 9.34).

MEDIATORS DERIVED FROM PHOSPHOLIPIDS

As words of a chemical language, the mediators derived from phospholipids could not be better placed: the dictionary, so to say, is built into the cell membrane, ready to be spoken out. Bits of phospholipids can be released as messages within seconds, almost as if they had been preformed. This family of lipid mediators includes derivatives of arachidonic acid (eicosanoids) and the platelet activating factors (PAFs).

THE EICOSANOIDS

Éikosi is Greek for "twenty," and these molecules derive from the 20-carbon arachidonic acid, which can be processed along two pathways: the **cyclooxygenase pathway,** first to be discovered, which leads to the prostaglandins and thromboxanes, and the **lipoxygenase pathway,** which produces the leukotrienes (Figure 9.35). *Each type of cell—if appropriately stimulated—generates its own particular choice of eicosanoids.* For example, endothelium responds to stimulation by producing prostacyclin, whereas platelets go the way of thromboxanes. The stimulus may be injury or another mediator: for example, interleukin-1 prods endothelial and smooth muscle cells to secrete prostacyclin (PGI_2) (216).

Prostaglandins The prostaglandins owe their name to a misunderstanding.

> *In 1930 two gynecologists at Columbia University noticed that during artificial insemination the uterus sometimes contracted violently, sometimes relaxed (98). Later research proved the existence of a contracting agent thought to come from the prostate; it actually comes from the seminal vesicles. To this day the prostaglandins have retained important gynecologic connections, for instance, the initiation of labor by uterine contraction and the control of bleeding (98).*

It is now clear that *all mammalian cells, from brain to fat, from skin to stomach, produce prostaglandins if duly stimulated* (187).

A simplified scheme of prostaglandins and other arachidonic acid derivatives is shown in Figure 9.35. Leaving details to specialized treatises, we will only summarize the effects of prostaglandins that are relevant to inflammation. The most important prostaglandins in this respect are two: PGE_2 (produced, e.g., by stimulated macrophages) (106) and PGI_2, also called prostacyclin (produced e.g., by vascular tissues).

> *Prostacyclin is just another prostaglandin, but it deserved a special name because it is extremely potent*

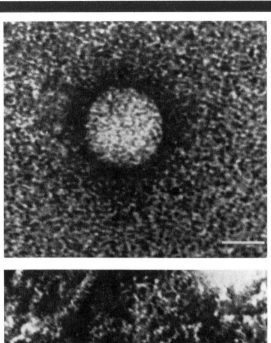
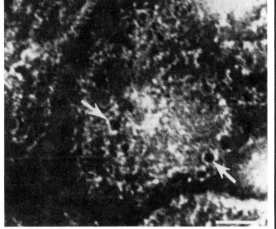

FIGURE 9.31 Scanning electron microscopic view of a virus exploded by complement. *Top:* Normal particle of murine leukemia virus. *Bottom:* The arrows point to several holes produced by complement. **Bars** = 500 Å. (Reproduced with permission from [114].)

> *and because it is the only prostaglandin to escape immediate inactivation as it passes through the lung. It therefore qualifies as a hormone, as opposed to an autacoid (186).*

The principal effect of PGE_2 and PGI_2 is vasodilatation; they can therefore increase the exudation of fluid and the supply of leukocytes (157) by increasing flow through vessels that are already leaky but without increasing permeability or causing diapedesis (p. 415) (152).

Prostaglandins of the PGE series are intensely *hyperalgesic:* that is, they make the skin hypersensitive to painful stimuli. Yet, no prostaglandins cause pain directly. PGE_2 is also one of the most potent agents for producing *fever* (152).

Prostaglandins are not chemotactic, in fact they tend to oppose leukocyte activities.

In essence, the prostaglandins contribute to all four cardinal signs of inflammation listed by Cornel-

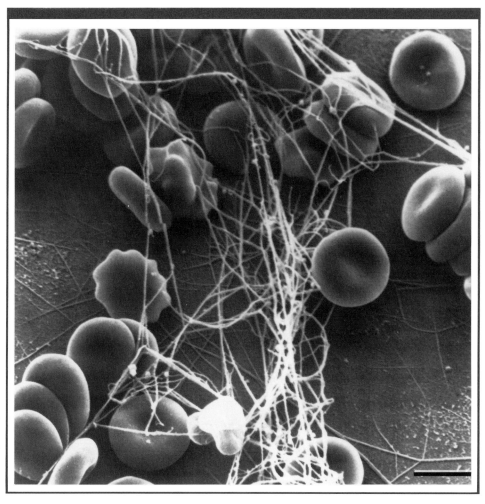

FIGURE 9.32
Scanning electron micrograph of a developing blood clot: red blood cells enmeshed in a network of fibrin filaments. **Bar** = 5 μm. (Courtesy of Dr. M.J. Karnovsky, Harvard Medical School, Boston, MA.)

FIGURE 9.33
Polymerization of fibrinogen to fibrin. The first step is accomplished by the enzyme thrombin. The fibrinopeptides A and B are clipped off and join the pool of inflammatory mediators; the fibrinogen molecule is then converted to fibrin monomer, which self-assembles into filaments of fibrin. (Adapted from [126].)

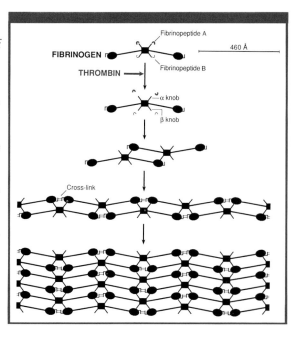

ius Celsus, *rubor et tumor cum calore et dolore*: by increasing blood flow they favor *rubor* and *calor*; they increase the *dolor* if some other agent causes pain and the *tumor* if some other agent causes vascular leakage. Besides increasing pain, their main effects are vascular. Overall, *the main role of prostaglandins in inflammation could be that of guaranteeing an ample supply of blood* (i.e., cells and fluid for the exudate) despite local controlling factors (138).

But then, to remind us that nothing is absolutely clear-cut, *PGE₁ is a typical antiinflammatory agent:* it counteracts histamine, serotonin, and other mediators (137, 209).

We might add that prostaglandins are metabolized in minutes, but "the effects of PGE₂ greatly outlast its presence" (243), perhaps by an hour or two. Drugs that inhibit prostaglandin synthesis are the best proof that prostaglandins are involved in inflammation. The drugs include aspirin, corticoids and non-steroidal inhibitors such as indomethacin (Figure 9.35).

Thromboxanes These mediators have received much attention thanks largely to the platelets because thromboxane A2 (produced by platelets) is a potent platelet aggregator and vasoconstrictor, two properties that suggest an important role in bleeding vessels. Also, there is a classic opposition between platelets, which metabolize arachidonic acid in the direction of thromboxanes, and endothelium, which metabolize it to produce prostacyclin, with diametrically opposite effects.

Leukotrienes Just like their relatives the prostaglandins, the leukotrienes were first identified through their effect on smooth muscle.

> *Perfused lungs, challenged with snake venom, release into the perfusing medium a substance that, when applied to strips of smooth muscle, caused a slow, persistent contraction. It was named slow-reacting substance (SRS). Later it was found that anaphylactic challenge of the lungs yielded a similar material, SRS-A (SRS of anaphylaxis). In 1979 the agent was identified as a metabolite of arachidonic acid and the name leukotriene was adopted for this class of compounds (148).*

This brief history points out three characteristics of the leukotrienes: they play a special role in lung pathology, they can be generated by an allergic mechanism, and they can cause smooth muscle spasm.

The leukotrienes (Figure 9.35) are generated from arachidonic acid by an enzyme, 5-lipoxygenase, which is present in only a few cells (174, 175). Hence *the leukotrienes, unlike the prostaglandins, are produced by few cell types*: all the leukocytes (as the name implies), including some subsets of lymphocytes; mast cells; and perhaps human bronchial epithelium. The stimulus can be allergic, as in the antigenic challenge of mast cells, but endotoxin and certain hormones are also effective.

Regarding inflammation, a few facts about the leukotrienes are important.

- Leukotriene B_4 is one of the most potent chemotactic substances known; applied to human skin it draws neutrophils into the epidermis, producing microscopic abscesses similar to those found in psoriasis (Figure 9.36) (108).
- Other lipid chemotactic factors (in addition to LTB$_4$) are produced by the lipoxygenase pathway: they are called HPETEs and HETEs (for hydro-peroxy- or hydroxy-eicosa-tetraenoic acid derivatives) (Figure 9.35).

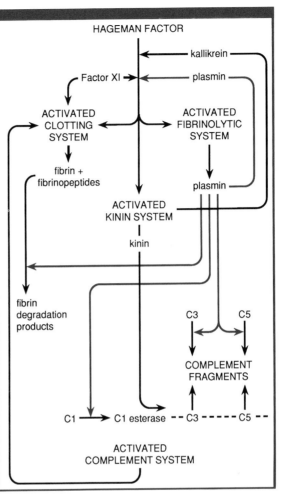

FIGURE 9.34 "The tangled web": an appropriate name for the bewildering network of interactions of the clotting, fibrinolytic, kinin, and complement systems. Note the prominent role of the Hageman factor. (Adapted from [220].)

- Leukotrienes C_4, D_4, and E_4 cause leakage from the venules (148, 162).
- The same leukotrienes C_4, D_4 and E_4 cause a combination of vasospasm and vasodilatation, but the tendency to spasm prevails, hence their role in the bronchospasm of asthma and possibly of the coronary arteries (151).

PLATELET ACTIVATING FACTORS

Platelet activating factors (PAFs) are unforgettable, not just because of their splashy name, but also because, as mediators, they can do almost everything: just glance at Figure 9.37. Their direct effects include everything needed to induce inflammation with the possible exception of vasodilatation. The PAFs also illustrate the extraordinary economy of nature: *they are made from leftovers of eicosanoid production.*

Consider the basic structure of a PAF (Figure 9.38): it is a classic phospholipid. It has the typical glycerol backbone and the usual long-chain fatty

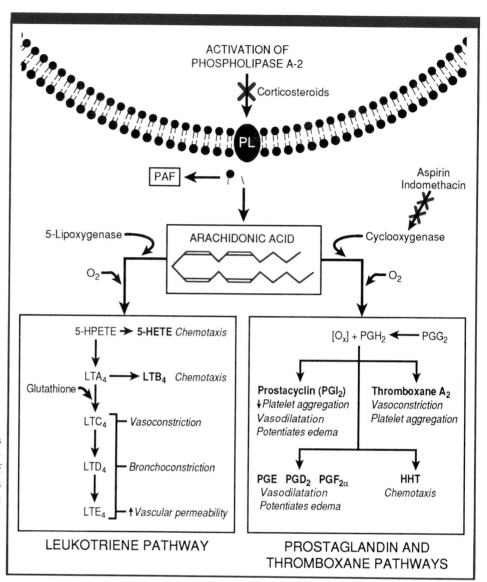

FIGURE 9.35
Arachidonic acid and its metabolites relevant to inflammation. **PL** = phospholipase. Notice that the splitting of each phospholipid molecule generates two sets of mediators: the larger part of the molecule becomes PAF (platelet activating factor) whereas arachidonic acid gives rise to leukotrienes, prostaglandins, and thromboxanes. (Adapted from [115].)

acid in position A, but it has an unusually short chain in position B. The original long-chain fatty acid in position B, arachidonic acid, was snipped out by a phospholipase and then replaced with a two-carbon chain, a critical substitution for producing PAF. This means that two potent sets of mediators have been produced for the price of one: arachidonic acid became available for producing an eicosanoid, and the rest of the phospholipid molecule was turned into PAF.

The first inkling of PAF was found around 1970. Basophils from a rabbit sensitized against an antigen were exposed in vitro to the same antigen, in the presence of platelets. It was noticed that the platelets around the basophils clumped—a sign of activation, hence the name platelet activating factor. An alter-

native but unpronounceable name for PAF is acetyl-glyceryl-ether-phosphorylcholine (AGEPC) (155).

When the PAF molecule was identified it turned out to have many variants, depending on slight changes in the fatty acid chains; this is why we now speak of PAFs in the plural. It was confirmed that PAFs are released primarily in allergic reactions from a limited number of cells: all the leukocytes (basophils and their cousins the mast cells, neutrophils, eosinophils, monocytes/macrophages, NK cells), endothelium, platelets, mesangial cells, and some epithelial cells (202, 246).

Because they are not water-soluble, PAFs are carried to their target organ bound to albumin. They do dissolve in lipoproteins, in which they are found in surprisingly large amounts (97).

When PAFs are injected into the skin, they cause immediate blanching followed by vascular leakage (at molar concentrations 100–10,000 times lower than any other autacoid, including histamine), accumulation of leukocytes and burning pain, and eventually a red flare, perhaps due to histamine release. When injected intravenously, they cause, as their name promises, instant aggregation of platelets and leukocytes, which embolize the lungs (Figure 9.39) while the number of circulating leukocytes and platelets, understandably, drops (180).

After all this buildup, it is somewhat sobering to conclude that the role of PAFs as presently understood is limited to acute allergic reactions. Their effects help explain the air hunger (bronchial constriction) and the immediate drop in circulating leukocytes typical of anaphylactic shock. Yet there is no indication that the PAFs, despite their amazing versatility, are put to use in ordinary, nonallergic inflammation. Time will tell.

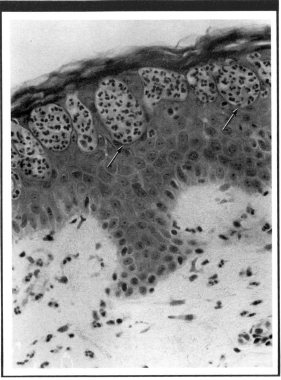

FIGURE 9.36 Chemotactic effect of leukotriene B$_4$. Photomicrograph from a skin biopsy, 24 hours after topical application of 100 ng of LTB$_4$. The granulocytes attracted by the mediator have collected in intraepidermal microabcesses (**arrows**). (Courtesy of Dr. R.D.R. Camp, Guy's and St. Thomas's Hospitals, University of London, London, United Kingdom.)

CYTOKINES AND CHEMOKINES

Cytokines are polypeptide messages secreted by many, and perhaps all, cell types in response to appropriate stimuli; they bind to specific receptors and therefore act as hormones, performing at the autocrine, paracrine, and endocrine level. **Chemokines** (short for chemotactic cytokines) are a special family of cytokines characterized by a common molecular feature—small proteins with two disulfide bridges formed by four cysteine residues—and by their ability to attract and activate leukocytes, even very specific types, such as subsets of T lymphocytes. Over 20 are known; they are produced, in acute and in chronic inflammation, by activated macrophages and by a large variety of other cells, including epithelia and chondrocytes (227a) which means that *parenchymal "bystander cells" also participate in the production of inflammatory mediators.* Some were previously known under other names, such as Platelet Factor 4 (PF4) or Interleukin 8 (140a).

Although the study of cytokines is currently booming, a concise synthesis of their pathophysiology is nowhere to be found, and for a good reason: *they are much more complicated in their effects than the "old" mediators of inflammation,* such as histamine. For example, interleukin-1 (IL-1) induces the entire spectrum of acute *and* chronic

inflammation, including leukocyte accumulation, yet it is not chemotactic. Furthermore, the effects of a given cytokine depend on the presence of other cytokines, and one cytokine may induce another: IL-2, for example, induces IL-1 (167). Another major difference from histamine-type mediators: cytokines have important general effects, such as fever.

In inflammation, the most relevant cytokines (165) are IL-1, IL-2, and IL-6; tumor necrosis factor (TNF) alpha and beta; interferon (IFN) alpha, beta, and gamma; and transforming growth factor (TGF) beta. Plastic, slow-release pellets loaded with any one of these cytokines produce distinctive effects. IL-1 alpha and beta and TNF beta result in acute followed by chronic inflammation (129); the least effect is produced by IFN gamma, which tends to *inhibit* cell proliferation (hence attempts to use it against cancer).

Although most of the stimuli that lead to cytokine secretion arise in the course of an immune response, it should be noted that cytokines are also produced in the absence of immune reaction; for example, macrophages stimulated with silica produce IL-1 (216).

The first cytokines to be identified were lymphocyte products that function as chemical mediators of the

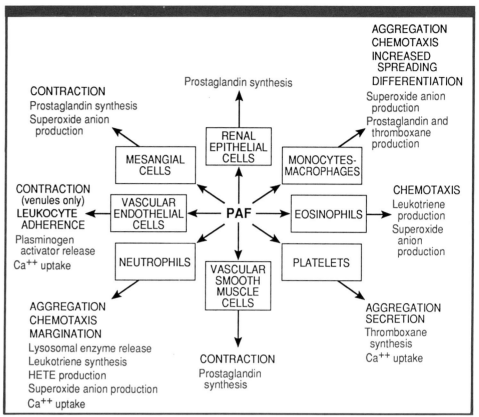

FIGURE 9.37
Versatility of platelet activating factor as an inflammatory mediator. (Adapted from [202].)

immune response and were therefore called lymphokines. Then came monokines, produced by macrophages. Eventually, it was realized that the same molecules could be secreted by a great variety of cells, from epidermis to smooth muscle, as a result of stimuli that were not necessarily a part of the immune response. In fact, cultured keratinocytes secrete IL-1 without any apparent stimulus (121). So the overall name cytokines was adopted. By international agreement in 1986, any new cytokine to be discovered and sequenced receives the name interleukin followed by a number (123). We are presently at interleukin-15. Although numerical names are somewhat inhuman, they do have a justification: the alternative would be to name the cytokines by their effects, which are far too many. However, a few cytokines with especially striking properties retain their maiden names: the interferons, the colony-stimulating factors, and the tumor necrosis factors.

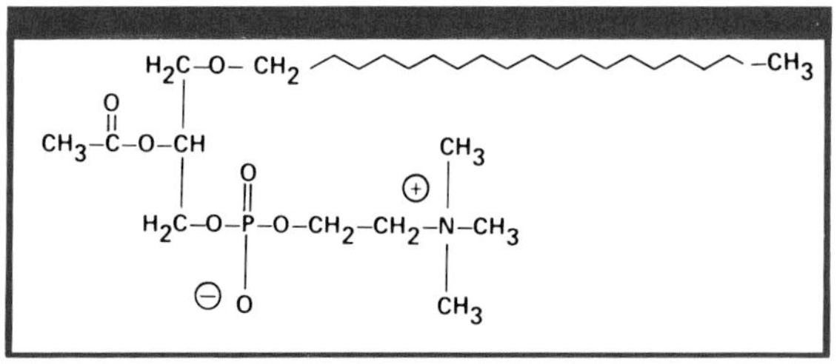

The current explosion of cytokine research is explained by the multiple relevance of the many cytokine molecules.

- They are key mediators of inflammation, both acute and chronic.
- They are key mediators of immune responses.
- They are ultimately responsible for much of the damage in autoimmune diseases and in immunopathology altogether.
- When they are lacking, immunosuppression may develop.
- They are a major link in the pathogenesis of shock.
- Some have great promise as therapeutic agents.

The interested reader is referred to specialized monographs (112, 140a, 166) or to the latest textbook of immunology (89) for details in this

FIGURE 9.38
Structural formula of PAF. A typical phospholipid molecule, characterized by two fatty acids attached to a glycerol backbone, the third carbon being occupied by a phosphate group bound to choline. Critical features are the long-chain fatty acid in position A and the very short chain in position B (acetyl).

area. There are at least 50 cytokines at the time of this writing. We have chosen here to point out two major cytokines that have overlapping local as well as general effects (90, 121).

INTERLEUKIN-1

Interleukin-1 (IL-1) has so many effects that it was discovered and named independently half a dozen times (119, 120). Its first name (in the 1940s) was "endogenous pyrogen." It took some 30 years to realize that all the disparate effects were due to a single agent.

IL-1 (alpha and beta) is produced by monocytes and macrophages and an assortment of other cells including NK cells, smooth muscle, and some epithelia. Injected locally, IL-1 increases vascular permeability and causes leukocyte emigration (116, 117). Its general effects, listed in Figure 9.40, seem to reach every corner of the body. Notice the familiar clinical symptoms that accompany "dis-ease": fever, sleepiness, and loss of appetite. Muscle aches may also be due to IL-1-mediated muscle breakdown (92), but this was not confirmed with recombinant IL-1; the effect may have been due to a contaminant, perhaps tumor necrosis factor (120).

Some of the general effects are clearly beneficial (e.g., leukocytosis), and others are puzzling. For example, the ability to induce PGE_2 and collagenase secretion by macrophages in the joints looks like a mechanism that is certain to cause arthritis; the production of IL-1 by gingival epithelium can activate the adjacent osteoclasts, causing bone loss and receding gums. More problems of this nature are raised by tumor necrosis factor.

TUMOR NECROSIS FACTOR

Tumor necrosis factor (TNF), also called cachectin, is so powerful that it was perceived even in the 1800s (100, 194, 195).

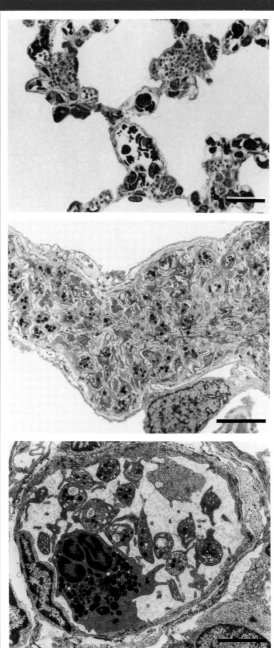

FIGURE 9.39 Platelet-aggregating effect of PAF in a rabbit lung fixed 30 seconds after an intravenous infusion of PAF. *Top:* Alveolar capillaries are stretched by large platelet aggregates. **Bar** = 25 μm. *Center:* Alveolar capillary filled with aggregated platelets. **Bar** = 5 μm. *Bottom:* Leukocytes participate in the platelet aggregates produced by PAF. **Bar** = 5 μm. (Reproduced with permission from [181].)

In the late 1800s it was observed that occasional cancers regressed when the patient suffered a concurrent bacterial infection. A few courageous physicians attempted to induce infections in their cancer patients. Some regressions were obtained, but the risk was great, so a New York surgeon, William B. Coley, turned to killed bacteria. The name **Coley's toxin** *was applied to a mixture of killed Streptococcus pyogenes and Serratia marcescens, which were reported to induce some complete regressions (Figure 9.41) (113). As late as 1934 there was no other medical treatment for cancer. Then came radio- and chemotherapy, and Coley's toxins were relegated to*

the controversial; they might have been forgotten entirely if Coley's daughter had not collected his and other similar records (191). But experimental work continued: tumor-bearing mice were challenged with bacteria or culture filtrates. Eventually, endotoxin was found to produce hemorrhagic necrosis in certain mouse tumors, especially if the mice had been "primed" with an infection by Bacillus Calmette-Guérin (BCG), an attenuated Mycobacterium tuberculosis used for vaccinating humans against tuberculosis (109, 185). It was in the serum of these mice that TNF was first discovered; further work

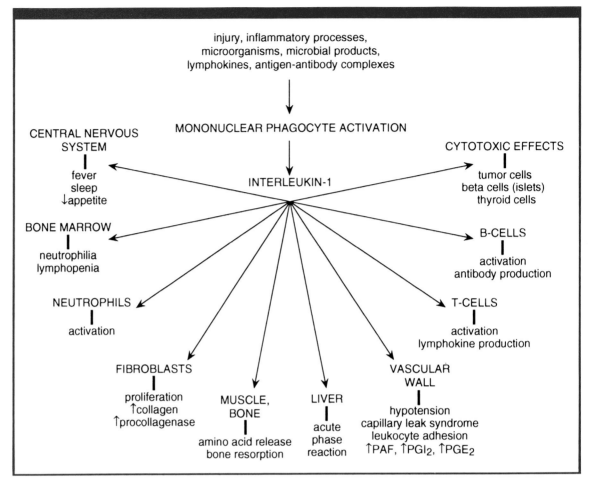

injury, inflammatory processes,
microorganisms, microbial products,
lymphokines, antigen-antibody complexes

MONONUCLEAR PHAGOCYTE ACTIVATION

CENTRAL NERVOUS
SYSTEM

fever
sleep
↓appetite

INTERLEUKIN-1

CYTOTOXIC EFFECTS

tumor cells
beta cells (islets)
thyroid cells

BONE MARROW

neutrophilia
lymphopenia

B-CELLS

activation
antibody production

NEUTROPHILS

activation

T-CELLS

activation
lymphokine production

FIBROBLASTS

proliferation
↑collagen
↑procollagenase

MUSCLE,
BONE

amino acid release
bone resorption

LIVER

acute
phase
reaction

VASCULAR
WALL

hypotension
capillary leak syndrome
leukocyte adhesion
↑PAF, ↑PGI$_2$, ↑PGE$_2$

FIGURE 9.40
Main biological
effects of
Interleukin-1.
(Reproduced
with permission
of the New En-
gland Journal of
Medicine from
[119].)

showed that the hemorrhagic necrosis in the tumors
was not produced by the endotoxin but by the TNF
that the macrophages secreted under the stimulus of
endotoxin (Figure 9.42). Note: TNF was discovered
again in relation to sleeping sickness, another fascinating story (p. 810).

One now speaks of TNF alpha and beta: the
beta form was previously known as lymphotoxin, a
product of activated T lymphocytes. The two
molecules are structurally related and bind to the
same receptors, and their biological effects are
indistinguishable. TNF consists of subunits with a
molecular weight of 17 kD (101).

The story of TNF actually deserves more than
casual mention because it includes two mind-
boggling developments: TNF turned out to be
largely responsible for the cachexia caused by malignant tumors (p. 810) and for the major manifestations
of septic shock (p. 701). The macrophages and
surely some other cells seem to be capable of
betrayal—suicidal betrayal.

When they were first discovered, the properties

of TNF raised high hopes for tumor therapy. When
39 types of tumor cells were exposed to TNF in
vitro, about 30 percent were killed, but the choice
of targets seemed capricious: some were sarcomas,
some were carcinomas. Normal cells were spared.
TNF injected intravenously killed the same tumors
that were affected in vitro (99).

As to the mechanism of TNF killing, the cells
exposed to TNF become much more sensitive to its
toxic effect if they are previously treated with an
inhibitor of protein synthesis—and the reader may
recall what this suggests: cells that commit suicide and
die by apoptosis seem to require a burst of protein
synthesis before they die (p. 203). Indeed, the cells
killed by TNF undergo the structural and biochemical
changes of apoptosis (Figure 9.43) (171). Normal
cells exposed to TNF in vitro are stimulated in a
variety of ways (102, 170), but mysteriously, they
are not killed at the doses that kill tumor cells.

When TNF is injected intravenously to tumor-
bearing animals, the typical effect—hemorrhagic

necrosis—is spectacular. The mechanism may be related—in part—to the fact that TNF induces apoptosis in cultured endothelial cells; furthermore, TNF has microvascular effects (such as fibrin thrombi), which preclude its therapeutic use (158). After all, TNF is a major mediator of septic shock.

When TNF is injected into the skin, it induces acute inflammation (116). When infused subcutaneously, it induces acute and then chronic inflammation; in high doses massive necrosis develops, suggesting a direct toxic effect (200). A single intravenous injection in mice produces a "vascular leak syndrome" and necrosis of the villi in the small bowel (213). In human pathology TNF is currently turning up as a link in the pathogenesis of various diseases such as cerebral malaria (145) and graft-versus-host disease (p. 565). Alas, TNF is not a magic bullet that hits tumors only. Clinical trials have been very disappointing (100).

LYSOSOMAL ENZYMES

Lysosomal enzymes find their way into an area of injury by two mechanisms: (a) by spilling from dying cells (including leukocytes), (b) by secretion from leukocytes. Oddly enough, leukocytes begin to "drool" their enzymes as soon as they perceive a chemotactic stimulus, because they are activated by chemotactic stimuli. They also spill enzymes during phagocytosis (p. 404). *Lysosomal enzymes can hydrolyze any cellular or extracellular material.* In so doing, they generate more mediators because some products of hydrolysis have functional effects: proteases in particular cleave kininogen to produce bradykinin; they also cleave C3 and C5 to yield chemotactic fragments, or fibrin to yield active "split products".

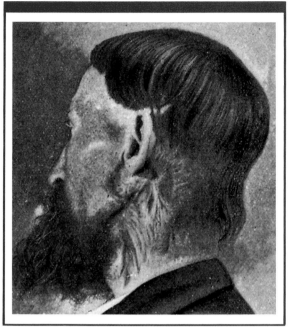

FIGURE 9.41.
Infection cured this patient of a malignant tumor, one of the cases that inspired William B. Coley (1893) to try infection as a cure for malignancy. This patient was operated on five times in three years for a "round-celled sarcoma of the neck" at age 31. "At the last operation it was found impossible to remove all of the tumor, and the case was considered hopeless. Two weeks after the operation a severe *(spontaneous)* attack of erysipelas occurred, followed by a second attack shortly after the first had subsided. . . . The sarcoma entirely disappeared, the wound rapidly healed, and the patient was seen . . . by myself seven years afterward, at which time this photograph was taken." (Reproduced with permission from [113].)

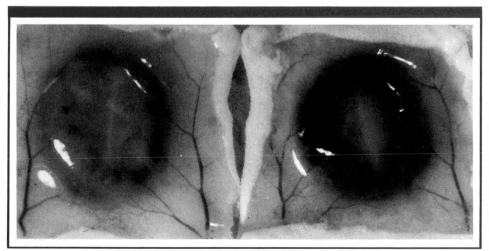

FIGURE 9.42
Effect of TNF. *Left:* A tumor growing in the subcutaneous tissue of a mouse; the feeding vessels are somewhat enlarged. *Right:* A similar tumor 6 hours after an intravenous injection of TNF. The vessels are somehow damaged, bleed, and the tumor undergoes necrosis. (Reproduced with permission from [195].)

FIGURE 9.43
Stages of apoptosis induced by TNF in cells of a monocyte-like line (U937). The target cells emit buds and eventually appear to burst. The process requires 1 or 2 hours from stage A (normal cell binding TNF) to stage D. **Bar** = 10 μm. (Adapted from [171].)

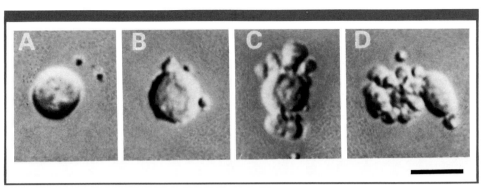

As sources of secondary mediators, proteases are especially important. Wherever proteases are on the loose, inflammatory mediators appear. Proteases can also stimulate mitosis and differentiation; there is even a human leukemia line that can be stimulated by trypsin to mature *in vitro* (227).

> *A practical example of proteases as a nuisance: some individuals who wear* **contact lenses** *complain of irritation of the cornea (keratitis). In some cases this is due to infection by bacteria that secrete a protease; this protease, besides its direct effect on the cornea, activates the omnipotent Hageman factor and releases kinins, which are powerful inflammatory mediators (164).*

Inhibitors of free proteases are mainly alpha-1-antitrypsin and alpha-2-macroglobulin.

NITRIC OXIDE AND OTHER SMALL MOLECULES

A potent vasodilator originally called *endothelium-derived relaxing factor* (EDRF) is now known to be nitric oxide (NO). This tiny mediator, derived from the amino acid L-arginine, has several other physiologic roles including that of neurotransmitter (186a). It opposes platelet aggregation and is therefore important in vascular pathology. It is also produced by activated macrophages as a *bactericidal agent*, hence its right to be listed among the inflammatory mediators. We have already mentioned that other normal neurotransmitters can play a role in injuries of nervous tissue as "excitotoxins" (214).

EXOGENOUS MEDIATORS OF INFLAMMATION

If we included under this heading all the substances released by bacteria and other parasites in inflammatory foci, a book would not suffice. We will consider only a few bacterial products that are of special interest relative to the inflammatory process. For example, some bacteria produce true inflammatory mediators, such as chemotactic agents.

Why should bacteria, or any other parasite, produce inflammatory mediators? It is obviously against their interest. It probably happened because the vertebrates' parasites were around long before the vertebrates, and became set in their basic metabolic pathways. Eons later, when the vertebrates came along their cells learned to "sniff out" minute amounts of the parasites' products and to respond to them by inflammation (236).

The best example of exogenous mediator is the typical bacterial tetrapeptide **fMLP** produced by *E. coli* (179). Mammalian tissues respond to it with a wave of leukocytes; in other words, fMLP acts as a powerful chemotactic agent (p. 387). fMLP stands for formyl-methionyl-leucyl-phenylalanine. In prokaryotic cells, *N*-formylated methionyl peptides are released as signal peptides from newly synthesized proteins and then diffuse around. Therefore, a whiff of fMLP says to a leukocyte: *"warning—live bacteria nearby."*

Another example: *Streptococcus faecalis* cannot mate in peace in the tissues because leukocytes are attracted by its sex pheromones (132).

The most formidable bacterial mediator is **endotoxin,** a product of gram-negative bacteria. When introduced into the tissues, it triggers inflammation; if it is released into the blood, it activates all the inflammatory mechanisms at once. The catastrophic result is septic shock. *Yet we have slowly come to realize that endotoxin does not "do" most of this damage;* it induces macrophages to secrete cytokines, and these are the real culprits.

> *Most bacterial toxins are best considered as injurious agents rather than inflammatory mediators. They can generate an inflammatory response indirectly, by killing or damaging cells (156, 177) or by triggering immunologic mechanisms (241).*

We also know of a few bacterial *antiinflammatory* mediators, such as the leukocyte-killing **leuko-**

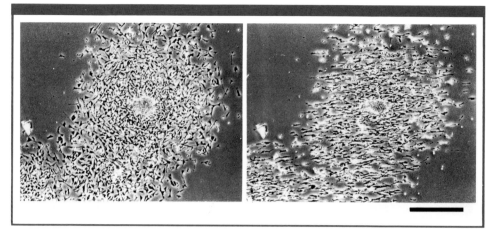

FIGURE 9.44
Cultured fibroblasts before and after 90 minutes of exposure to an electric field of 400 mV/mm. This field strength is only about three times higher than the field strength measured in guinea pig wounds. **Bar** = 500 μm. (Reproduced with permission from [134].)

cidin produced by staphylococci (244). Bacteria have also evolved several antioxidant defenses, which can protect them against the oxygen-derived offensive weapons of the leukocytes (149).

One of the marvels of evolution is the pharmacologic cunning of stinging insects: bees, wasps, and hornets borrow pain-producing mammalian inflammatory mediators with which they lace their stings. The painful cocktail includes histamine, serotonin, and bradykinin, plus the histamine liberator acetylcholine. A similar combination is found in some snake poisons (146). We will learn later the fascinating technique used by the nettle (p. 524) (133). The conclusion may sound like a pun—but truly what we are witnessing in all these cases is the exogenous use of endogenous mediators.

MEDIATORS: LOOSE ENDS

We have avoided discussing the effects that the various mediators have on each other: this topic is important, but our knowledge is still fragmentary.

A curious development in the field of mediators is that they are now referred to as **biological response modifiers** and are discussed in a journal by that name, together with a variety of other endogenous products. The reason, it seems, is purely practical: mediators obviously have biological effects, and for this reason they are tested as drugs for possible clinical use.

An editorial in the first issue of the Journal of Biological Response Modifiers (196) includes under that name "immunoaugmenting, immunomodulating, and immunorestorative agents; interferon and interferon inducers; lymphokines; cytokines; thymic factors; antitumor and antilymphoid cell antibodies . . . ; tumor antigens" and much else. The common theme seems to be any endogenous molecule that has a biological effect.

Are all the inflammatory messages necessarily soluble, extracellular, or even chemical? Probably not. (a) Electrical stimuli were once thought to play a role in chemotaxis and thrombosis, but the topic has disappeared from the literature (144). However, it is still thought that the arrangement of fibroblasts in wounds may have something to do with injury potentials. Figure 9.44 shows that fibroblasts do respond to electrical fields of a magnitude that can be expected from injury potentials in vivo (134, 238). Electrical stimuli are currently used to assist bone repair (93). (b) Heat may play a role in directing the motion of leukocytes, if the phenomenon of thermotaxis can be confirmed (p. 391). (c) Intracellular messages are exchanged across junctions or by direct contact; in this manner, the news of a wound should travel some distance within the epidermis, and there is some evidence that this may actually happen. Knowledge in this area is just beginning to develop. (d) The extracellular matrix provides many clues to the cells in contact with it; this is a recurring theme that we will encounter again in discussing haptotaxis, the tendency of cells to move toward surfaces offering greater adhesion (p. 391).

TO SUM UP: An overview of the plasma- and cell-derived mediators is provided in Figures 9.45 and 9.46, and Table 9.4 summarizes the mediators according to their effects.

The tremendous degree of redundancy in the system has traumatized many a student. There are two ways to justify it. First, by the bland statement that inflammation is a life-saving reaction and must be triggered unfailingly. Second, when we say that many mediators have the same effects, we are only speaking of effects known to us; the redundancy may be only apparent.

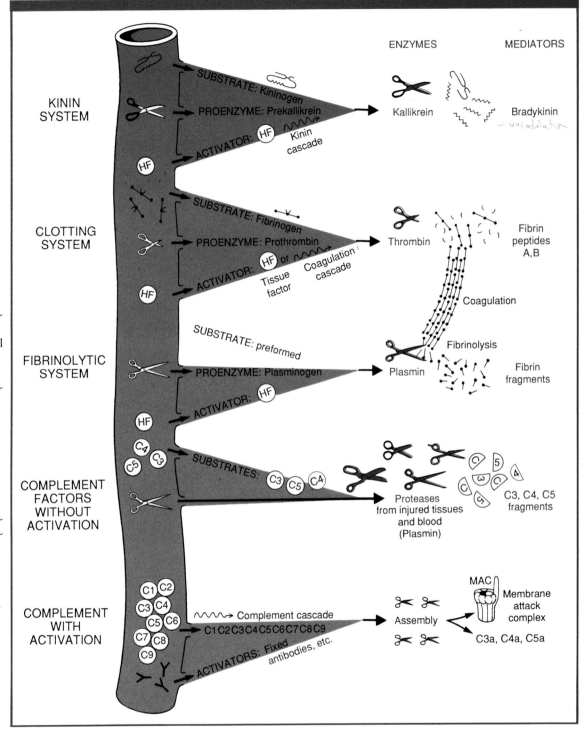

FIGURE 9.45 Overview of the plasma-derived inflammatory mediators. A damaged blood vessel (which could be of any kind) is shown as containing the inactive precursors of five mediators. The vessel allows plasma to escape through five leaks, and for each one of these, the activation of an inflammatory mediator is illustrated. The various types of scissors represent proteolytic enzymes; note that enzymes are always involved in generating the mediators. **HF** =Hageman Factor.

Overall, it is well to remember that the mediators are not summoned to perform in a standard sequence; *different pathologic conditions at different stages and in different organs call for different mediator cocktails*, even though we do not always understand the mechanism. This fact is important to remember for therapeutic purposes: some in-flammations may call for aspirin, others may be made worse by aspirin. Here are some guidelines:

- Histamine and serotonin are the earliest mediators of acute inflammation, being present for the first hour or so (remember the mosquito bite); then other mediators take over.

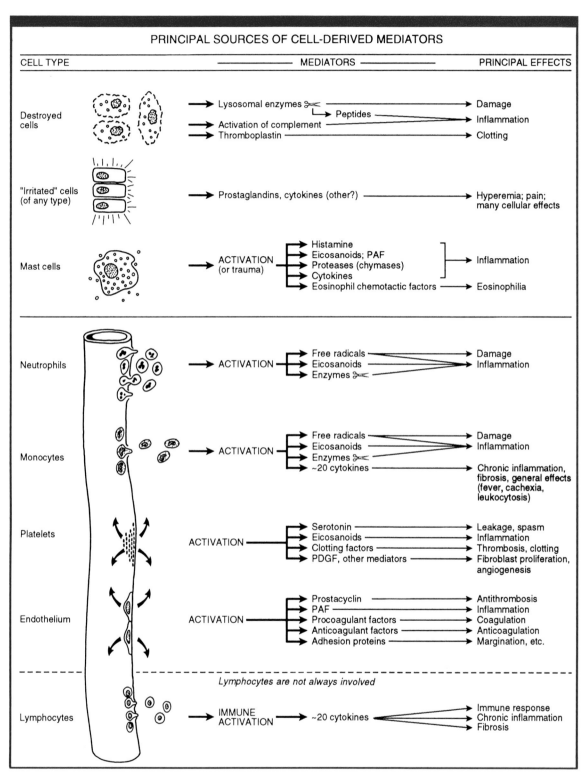

PRINCIPAL SOURCES OF CELL-DERIVED MEDIATORS

| CELL TYPE | ——————— MEDIATORS ——————— | PRINCIPAL EFFECTS |

Destroyed cells
→ Lysosomal enzymes → Damage
↳ Peptides → Inflammation
→ Activation of complement
→ Thromboplastin → Clotting

"Irritated" cells (of any type)
→ Prostaglandins, cytokines (other?) → Hyperemia; pain; many cellular effects

Mast cells
→ ACTIVATION (or trauma)
→ Histamine
→ Eicosanoids; PAF
→ Proteases (chymases)
→ Cytokines → Inflammation
→ Eosinophil chemotactic factors → Eosinophilia

Neutrophils
→ ACTIVATION
→ Free radicals → Damage
→ Eicosanoids → Inflammation
→ Enzymes

Monocytes
→ ACTIVATION
→ Free radicals → Damage
→ Eicosanoids → Inflammation
→ Enzymes
→ ~20 cytokines → Chronic inflammation, fibrosis, general effects (fever, cachexia, leukocytosis)

Platelets
ACTIVATION
→ Serotonin → Leakage, spasm
→ Eicosanoids → Inflammation
→ Clotting factors → Thrombosis, clotting
→ PDGF, other mediators → Fibroblast proliferation, angiogenesis

Endothelium
ACTIVATION
→ Prostacyclin → Antithrombosis
→ PAF → Inflammation
→ Procoagulant factors → Coagulation
→ Anticoagulant factors → Anticoagulation
→ Adhesion proteins → Margination, etc.

Lymphocytes are not always involved

Lymphocytes
→ IMMUNE ACTIVATION → ~20 cytokines
→ Immune response
→ Chronic inflammation
→ Fibrosis

FIGURE 9.46 Overview of the cell-derived inflammatory mediators and their major effects. The cells capable of supplying mediators are mainly leukocytes and platelets, but many and perhaps all tissue cells can be induced to participate.

For example, if the pleura of the rat is irritated with 1 percent kaolin, at 20 minutes the exudation is mediated mainly by kinins, histamine, and serotonin; at 3 hours mainly by prostaglandins and possibly kinins (153). There are other such examples (159).

- The dominant mediators vary from organ to organ and depend on the type of inflammation (allergic or not). For example:
- Mechanical trauma breaks up mast cells (his-

TABLE 9.4
Main Roles and Main Sources of Inflammatory Mediators

VASODILATION
Histamine, serotonin	Mast cells, platelets
Prostaglandins	Probably all cells

IMMEDIATE VASCULAR
LEAKAGE
Histamine, serotonin	Mast cells, platelets
Brakykinin	Plasma precursor
Leukotrienes C_4, D_4, E_4	Leukocytes, mast cells
PAF	Membrane phospholipids
C5a, C3a, C4a	Plasma precursors
Proteases	Lysosomes, neutrophils, plasma precursors (*), damaged cells

DELAYED VASCULAR
LEAKAGE
Cytokines (IL-1, TNF, IFN-γ)	Macrophages, mast cells,lymphocytes, NK cells

CHEMOTAXIS
Leukotriene B_4, HETEs	Leukocytes, mast cells
C5a, C3a, C4a	Plasma precursors
PAF	Membrane phospholipids of few cell types
Chemokines	Macrophages, neutrophils, other cell types
Bacterial products	Bacterial metabolism

PAIN
Bradykinin	Plasma precursor
[Prostaglandins, by lowering pain threshold]	Probably all cells

OPSONINS
C3b	Plasma precursor
Mannose-binding protein (***)	Plasma

TISSUE DAMAGE
Free radicals	Activated leukocytes
Leukocytic enzymes	Leukocyte regurgitation
Lysosomal enzymes	Damaged cells
Bacterial products	Bacteria

(*) *Proteases originating from the clotting (thrombin), fibrinolytic (plasmin) and complement (C3, C4, C5) cascades.*

(**) *(211)*

(***) *(169)*

mine) and spills blood, producing plasma-derived mediators such as bradykinin, and serotonin from platelet thrombi.

- Infection offers a special challenge to complement, and there is also a role for exogenous bacterial mediators (chemotactic agents, endotoxin).
- Chronic inflammation is a favorite ground for monokines—and for lymphokines if immunologic mechanisms are involved (antihistamines are no help!).
- Wound healing is largely driven by growth factors; it has very little to do with histamine-type mediators or with prostaglandins (178).
- Nasal allergies release histamine, leukotrienes (163), and kinins (208).
- In the bronchi, there is a tendency to produce leukotrienes, in the joints (arthritis) prostaglandins and IL-1.
- Remember Sir John Vane's dictum: *virtually all cells, when irritated by injury or even by inflammation, are ready to disgorge prostaglandins.*

References

Inflammation: The Actors

1. Adams DO, Hamilton TA. The cell biology of macrophage activation. Annu Rev Immunol 1984;2:283–318.
2. Adams DO, Hamilton TA. Phagocytic cells: cytotoxic activities of macrophages. In: Gallin JI, Goldstein IM, Snyderman R (eds). Inflammation. Basic principles and clinical correlates. New York: Raven Press 1988:471–492.
3. Austen KF. Biologic implications of the structural and functional characteristics of the chemical mediators of immediate-type hypersensitivity. Harvey Lect 1979;73:93–161.
4. Austen KF. The heterogeneity of mast cell populations and products. Hosp Pract 1984;19:135–146.
5. Bainton DF. Phagocytic cells: developmental biology of neutrophils and eosinophils. In: Gallin JI, Goldstein IM, Snyderman R (eds). Inflammation. Basic principles and clinical correlates. New York: Raven Press 1988:265–280.
6. Bainton DF, Friedlander LM, Shohet SB. Abnormalities in granule formation in acute myelogenous leukemia. Blood 1977;49:693–704.
7. Befus AD, Bienenstock J, Denburg JA (eds). Mast cell differentiation and heterogeneity. New York: Raven Press, 1986.
8. Brain JD. Toxicological aspects of alterations of pulmonary macrophage function. Annu Rev Pharmacol Toxicol 1986;26:547–565.
9. Braunstein PW Jr, Cuénoud HF, Joris I, Majno G. Platelets, fibroblasts, and inflammation. Tissue reactions to platelets injected subcutaneously. Am J Pathol 1980;99:53–66.
9a. Bucala R, Spiegel LA, Chesney J, Hogan M, Cerami A. Circulating fibrocytes define a new leukocyte subpopulation that mediates tissue repair. Molec Med 1994 1:71–81.
10. Buchanan JW, Wagner HN Jr. Regional phagocytosis in man. In: Reichard SM, Filkins JP (eds). The reticuloendothelial system. A comprehensive treatise. Vol. 7B Physiology. New York: Plenum Press, 1985:247–270.
11. Capron M, Capron A, Joseph M, Verwaerde C. IgE receptors on phagocytic cells and immune response to schistosome infection. Monogr Allergy 1983;18:33–44.
12. CIBA, 1956
   (REFERENCE TO FOLLOW)
13. Craig SS, Schechter NM, Schwartz LB. Ultrastructural analysis of human T and TC mast cells identified by immunoelectron microscopy. Lab Invest 1988;58:682–691.
14. Dahl R, Venge P, Fredens K. Eosinophils. In: Barnes PJ, Rodger IW, Thomson NC (eds). Asthma: Basic mechanisms and clinical management. London: Academic Press 1988:115–129.
15. Daniele RP, Dauber JH. Collection and enrichment of human alveolar macrophages. In: Herscowitz HB, Holden HT, Bellanti JA, Ghaffar A (eds). Manual of Macrophage Methodology. New York: Marcel Dekker, Inc., 1981:23–30.
16. Duffy J. The lessons of eosinophilia-myalgia syndrome. Hosp Pract 1992;27:65–88.
17. Dvorak AM, Ackerman SJ, Weller PF. Subcellular morphology and biochemistry of eosinophils. In: Harris JR (ed). Blood cell biochemistry, vol. 2. New York: Plenum Publishing Company, 1991:237–344.
18. Dvorak AM, Schulman ES, Peters SP, MacGlashan DW, Newball HH, Schleimer RP, Lichtenstein LM. Immunoglobulin E-mediated degranulation of isolated human lung mast cells. Lab Invest 1985;53:45–56.
19. Enerback L. Mast cell heterogeneity: the evolution of

the concept of a specific mucosal mast cell. In: Befus AD, Bienenstock J, Denburg JA (eds). Mast cell differentiation and heterogeneity. New York: Raven Press, 1986:1–26.
20. Falk W, Leonard EJ. Human monocyte chemotaxis: migrating cells are a subpopulation with multiple chemotaxin specificities on each cell. Infect Immun 1980;29:953–959.
21. Fawcett DW. An experimental study of mast cell degranulation and regeneration. Anat Rec 1955;121:29–51.
22. Fredens K, Dahl R, Venge P. The Gordon phenomenon induced by the eosinophil cationic protein and eosinophil protein X. J Allergy Clin Immunol 1982;70:361–366.
23. Frigas E, Loegering DA, Gleich GJ. Cytotoxic effects of the guinea pig eosinophil major basic protein on tracheal epithelium. Lab Invest 1980;42:35–43.
24. Galli SJ. New approaches for the analysis of mast cell maturation, heterogeneity, and function. Fed Proc 1987;46:1906–1914.
25. Galli SJ. New insights into "the riddle of the mast cells": microenvironmental regulation of mast cell development and phenotypic heterogeneity. Lab Invest 1990;62:5–33.
26. Galli SJ. New concepts about the mast cell. N Engl J Med 1993;328:257–265.
27. Galli SJ, Dvorak AM, Dvorak HF. Basophils and mast cells: morphologic insights into their biology, secretory patterns, and function. Prog Allergy 1984;34:1–141.
28. Galli SJ, Wershil BK, Gordon JR, Martin TR. Mast cells: immunologically specific effectors and potential sources of multiple cytokines during IgE-dependent responses. Ciba Found Symp 1989;147:53–73.
29. Gallin JI, Goldstein IM, Snyderman R. Inflammation: Basic Principles and Clinical Correlates, 2nd ed. New York: Raven Press, 1992.
30. Gimbrone MA, Aster RH, Cotran RS, Corkery J, Jandl JH, Folkman J. Preservation of vascular integrity in organs perfused in vitro with a platelet-rich medium. Nature 1969;222:33–36.
31. Gleich GJ. Current understanding of eosinophil function. Hosp Pract 1988;23:137–160.
32. Gleich GJ, Adolphson CR. The eosinophilic leukocyte: structure and function. Adv Immunol 1986;39:177–253.
33. Gordon JR, Burd PR, Galli SJ. Mast cells as a source of multifunctional cytokines. Immunol Today 1990;11:458–464.
34. Gordon JR, Galli SJ. Mast cells as a source of both preformed and immunologically inducible TNF-a/cachectin. Nature 1990;346:274–276.
35. Gurish MF, Austen KF. Different mast cell mediators produced by different mast cell phenotypes. Ciba Found Symp 1989;147:36–52.
36. Herscowitz HB, Holden HT, Bellanti JA, Ghaffar A (eds). Manual of macrophage methodology. New York: Marcel Dekker, Inc., 1981.
37. Hirsch JG, Hirsch BI. Paul Ehrlich and the discovery of the eosinophil. In: Mahmoud AAF, Austen KF, Simon AS (eds). The eosinophil in health and disease. New York: Grune & Stratton, 1980:3–23.
38. Ishizaka K (ed). Mast cell activation and mediator release. Basel S. Karger, 1984.
39. Janeway CA. A primitive immune system. Nature 1989;341:108.
40. Johnston RB Jr. Monocytes and macrophages. N Engl J Med 1988;318:747–752.
41. Johnston RB Jr, Kitagawa S. Molecular basis for the

enhanced respiratory burst of activated macrophages. Fed Proc 1985;44:2927–2932.

42. Kelley JL, Rozek MM, Suenram CA, Schwartz CJ. Activation of human blood monocytes by adherence to tissue culture plastic surfaces. Exp Mol Pathol 1987;46:266–278.

43. Kirshenbaum AS, Kessler SW, Goff JP, Metcalfe DD. Demonstration of the origin of human mast cells from CD34+ bone marrow progenitor cells. J Immunol 1991;146:1410–1415.

44. LeRoith D, Roth J. Evolutionary origins of messenger peptides: materials in microbes that resemble vertebrate hormones In: Falkmer S, Hakanson R, Sundler F (eds). evolution and tumour pathology of the neuroendocrine system. New York: Elsevier Science Publishers, 1984:147–164.

44a. Levitt D, Mertelsmann R. (eds.) Hematopoietic Stem Cells. New York, Marcel Dekker, Inc. 1995.

45. Mackaness GB. The mechanism of macrophage activation. In: Mudd S (ed). Infectious agents and host reactions. Philadelphia: W.B. Saunders Company, 1970:61–75.

46. Mackaness GB. The monocyte in cellular immunity. Semin Hematol 1970;7:172–184.

47. Maddox DE, Kephart GM, Coulam CB, Butterfield JH, Benirschke K, Gleich GJ. Localization of a molecule immunochemically similar to eosiniphil major basic protein in human placenta. J Exp Med 1984;160:29–41.

48. Malech HL. Phagocytic cells: egress from marrow and diapedesis. In: Gallin JI, Goldstein IM, Snyderman R (eds). Inflammation. Basic principles and clinical correlates. New York: Raven Press, 1988:297–308.

49. McIntyre KW, Welsh RM. Accumulation of natural killer and cytotoxic T large granular lymphocytes in the liver during virus infection. J Exp Med 1986;164:1667–1681.

50. Metcalfe DD, Kaliner M, Donlon MA. The mast cell. CRC Crit Rev Immunol 1981;3:23–74.

51. Metschnikoff E. Sur la lutte des cellules de l'organisme contre l'invasion des microbes. Ann Instit Pasteur 1887;1:321–336.

52. Miller F, DeHarven E, Palade GE. The structure of eosinophil leukocyte granules in rodents and in man. J Cell Biol 1966;31:349–362.

53. Nabel G, Galli SJ, Dvorak AM, Dvorak HF, Cantor H. Inducer T lymphocytes synthesize a factor that stimulates proliferation of cloned mast cells. Nature 1981;291:332–334.

54. Nachman RL, Weksler BB. The platelet as an inflammatory cell. In: Weissmann G (ed). The cell biology of inflammation. Amsterdam: Elsevier/North-Holland Biomedical Press, 1980:145–162.

55. Nakano T, Kanakuba Y, Nakahata T, Matsuda H, Kitamura Y. Genetically mast cell-deficient W/W^v mice as a tool for studies of differentiation and function of mast cells. Fed Proc 1987;46:1920–1923.

56. Noga SJ, Normann SJ, Weiner RS. Isolation of guinea pig monocytes and Kurloff cells: characterization of monocyte subsets by morphology, cytochemistry, and adherence. Lab Invest 1984;51:244–252.

57. Oldham RK. Natural killer cells: artifact to reality: an odyssey in biology. Cancer Metastasis Rev 1983;2:323–336.

58. Parwaresch MR., Horny H-P, Lennert K. Tissue mast cells in health and disease. Pathol Res Pract 1985;179:439–461.

59. Pennington DG, Streatfield K, Roxburgh AE. Megakaryocytes and the heterogeneity of circulating platelets. Br J Haematol 1976;34:639–653.

60. eters MS, Rodriguez M, Gleich GJ. Localization of human eosinophil granule major basic protein, eosinophil cationic protein, and eosinophil-derived neurotoxin by immunoelectron microscopy. Lab Invest 1986;54:656–662.

61. Pober JS, Cotran RS. The role of endothelial cells in inflammation. Transplantation 1990;50:537–544.

62. Postlethwaite AE, Kang AH. Fibroblasts. In: Gallin JI, Goldstein IM, Snyderman R (eds). Inflammation. Basic principles and clinical correlates. New York: Raven Press 1988:577–597.

63. Prin L, Charon J, Capron M, Gosset P, Taelman H, Tonnel AB, Capron A. Heterogeneity of human eosinophils. II. Variability of respiratory burst activity related to cell density. Clin Exp Immunol 1984;57:735–742.

64. Reiss M, Roos D. Differences in oxygen metabolism of phagocytosing monocytes and neutrophils. J Clin Invest 1978;61:480–488.

65. Ryan US. Endothelial Cells, Vols I, II, III. Boca Raton: CRC Press, Inc., 1988.

66. Samter M. Eosinophils—nominated but not elected. N Engl J Med 1980;303:1175–1176.

67. Selye H. The mast cells. Washington: Butterworths, 1965.

68. Simionescu M. Receptor-mediated transcytosis of plasma molecules by vascular endothelium. In: Simionescu N, Simionescu M (eds). Endothelial cell biology in health and disease. New York: Plenum Press, 1988:69–104.

69. Simionescu N, Simionescu M (eds). Endothelial cell biology in health and disease. New York: Plenum Press, 1988.

70. Simionescu N, Simionescu M (eds).. Endothelial cell dysfunction. New York: Plenum Press, 1992.

71. Siraganian RP. Mast cells and basophils. In: Gallin JI, Goldstein IM, Snyderman R (eds). Inflammation. Basic principles and clinical correlates. New York: Raven Press, 1988:513–542.

72. Slifman NR, Adolphson CR, Gleich GJ. Eosinophils: biochemical and cellular aspects. In: Middleton E Jr, Reed CE, Ellis EF, Adkinson NF Jr, Yunginger JW (eds). Allergy Principles and Practice, 3rd ed. St. Louis: The C.V. Mosby Company, 1988:179–205.

73. Spry CJF. Eosinophils. Oxford: Oxford University Press, 1988.

74. Tauber AI, Goetzl EJ, Babior BM. Unique characteristics of superoxide production by human eosinophils in eosinophilic states. Inflammation 1979;3:261–272.

75. Unanue ER. Machrophages, antigen presenting cells and the phenomena of antigen handling and presentation. In: Paul WE (ed). Fundamental immunology, 3rd ed. (in press).

76. van Furth R. Phagocytic cells: development and distribution of mononuclear phagocytes in normal steady state and inflammation. In: Gallin JI, Goldstein IM, Snyderman R (eds). Inflammation. Basic principles and clinical correlates. New York: Raven Press, 1988:281–295.

77. van Furth R, Raeburn JA, van Zwet TL. Characteristics of human mononuclear phagocytes. Blood 1979;54:485–500.

78. Wasmoen TL, McKean DJ, Benirschke K, Coulam CB, Gleich GJ. Evidence of eosinophil granule major basic protein in human placenta. J Exp Med 1989;170:2051–2063.

79. Wasserman SI. The mast cell and the inflammatory response. In: Pepys J, Edwards AM (eds). The mast cell. Bath: The Pitman Press, 1979:9–20.

80. Weidner N, Austen KF. Evidence for morphologic diversity of human mast cells. An ultrastructural study of mast cells from multiple body sites. Lab Invest 1990;63:63–72.

81. Weissmann G, Korchak HM, Perez HD, Smolen JE, Goldstein IM, Hoffstein ST. Leukocytes as secretory organs of inflammation. In: Weissmann G, Samuelsson B, Paoletti R (eds). Advances in inflammation research, vol. 1. New York: Raven Press, 1979:95–112.

82. Weissmann G, Smolen JE, Korchak HM. Release of

inflammatory mediators from stimulated neutrophils. N Engl J Med 303:27–34, 1980

83. Weksler BB. Platelets. In: Gallin JI, Goldstein IM, Snyderman R (eds). Inflammation. Basic principles and clinical correlates. New York: Raven Press, 1988:543–557.

84. Weller PF. The immunobiology of eosinophils. N Engl J Med 1991;324:1110–1118.

85. Welsh RM, Vargas-Cortes M. Natural killer cells in viral infection. In: Lewis CE, McGee JO'D (eds). The Natural Killer Cell. Oxford: IRL Press, 1992:107–150.

86. Werb Z, Gordon S. Elastase secretion by stimulated macrophages. Characterization and regulation. J Exp Med 1975;142:361–377.

87. White JG. Platelet secretory granules and associated proteins. Lab Invest 1993;68:497–498.

88. Wright DG. The neutrophil as a secretory organ of host defense. In: Gallin JI, Fauci AS (eds). Advances in host defense mechanisms. vol. 1, Phagocytic cells. New York: Raven Press, 1982:75–110.

Inflammation: The Chemical Language

89. Abbas AK, Lichtman AH, Pober JS. Cellular and molecular immunology, 2nd ed. Pennsylvania: W.B. Saunders Company, 1994.

90. Akira S, Hirano T, Taga T, Kishimoto T. Biology of multifunctional cytokines: IL 6 and related molecules (IL 1 and TNF). FASEB J 1990;4:2860–2867.

91. Alberts B, Bray D, Lewis J, Raff M, Roberts K, Watson JD. Molecular Biology of the Cell. New York: Garland Publishing, Inc., 1989.

92. Baracos V, Rodemann HP, Dinarello CA, Goldberg AL. Stimulation of muscle protein degradation and prostaglandin E2 release by leukocytic pyrogen (interleukin-1). N Engl J Med 1983;308:553–558.

93. Bassett CAL, Jackson SF. A critique of medical uses of weak pulsing electromagnetic fields. In: Chiabrera A, Nicolini C, Schwan HP (eds). Interactions between electromagnetic fields and cells. New York: Plenum Press, 1985:569–579.

94. Battistini B, D'Orleans-Juste P, Sirois P Biology of disease endothelins: circulating plasma levels and presence in other biologic fluids. Lab Invest 1993;68:600–628.

95. Beer DJ, Matloff SM, Rocklin RE. The influence of histamine on immune and inflammatory responses. Adv Immunol 1984;35:209–268.

96. Belew M, Gerdin B, Porath J, Saldeen T. Isolation of vasocative peptides from human fibrin and fibrinogen degraded by plasmin. Thromb Res 1978;13:983–994.

97. Benveniste J, Nunez D, Duriez P, Korth R, Bidault J, Fruchart J-C. Preformed PAF-acether and lyso PAF-acether are bound to blood lipoproteins. FEBS Lett 1988;226:371–376.

98. Bergström S. The prostaglandins: from the laboratory to the clinic. In: Les Prix Nobel en 1982. The Nobel Foundation, 1983:127–148.

99. Beutler B. The tumor necrosis factors: cachectin and lymphotoxin. Hosp Pract 1990;25:45–56.

100. Beutler B. Tumor Necrosis Factors: The molecules & their emerging role in medicine. New York: Raven Press, 1992.

101. Beutler B, Cerami A. Cachectin and tumour necrosis factor as two sides of the same biological coin. Nature 1986;320:584–588.

102. Beutler B, Cerami A. The biology of cachectin/TNF—a primary mediator of the host response. Annu Rev Immunol 1989;7:625–655.

103. Bhakdi S, Roth M. Fluid-phase SC5b-8 complex of human complement: generation and isolation from serum. J Immunol 1981;127:576–580.

104. Bitter-Suermann D. The anaphylatoxins. In: Rother K, Till GO (eds). The complement system. Berlin: Springer-Verlag, 1988:367–395.

105. Boucek RJ, Speropoulos AJ, Noble NL. Serotonin and ribonucleic acid and collagen metabolism of fibroblasts in vitro. Proc Soc Exp Biol Med 1972;140:599–603.

106. Brune K, Kälin H, Schmidt R, Hecker E. Regulation of prostaglandin release from macrophages. In: Weissmann G, Samuelsson B, Paoletti R (eds). Advances in inflammation research, Vol. 1. New York: Raven Press, 1979:467–475.

107. Burn JH, Dale HH. The vaso-dilator action of histamine, and its physiological significance. J Physiol (Lond) 1926;61:185–214.

108. Camp R, Jones RR, Brain S, Woollard P, Greaves M. Production of intraepidermal microabscesses by topical application of leukotriene B4. J Invest Dermatol 1984;82:202–204.

109. Carswell EA, Old LJ, Kassel RL, Green S, Fiore N, Williamson B. An endotoxin-induced serum factor that causes necrosis of tumors. Proc Natl Acad Sci USA 1975;72:3666–3670.

110. Casale TB, Wescott S, Rodbard D, Kaliner M. Characterization of histamine H-1 receptors on human mononuclear cells. Int J Immunopharmacol 1985;7:639–645.

111. Chenoweth DE, Cooper SW, Hugli TE, Stewart RW, Blackstone EH, Kirklin JW. Complement activation during cardiopulmonary bypass. Evidence for generation of C3a and C5a anaphylatoxins. N Engl J Med 1981;304:497–503.

112. Clemens MJ. Cytokines. Oxford: BIOS Scientific Publishers Ltd., 1991.

113. Coley WB. The treatment of malignant tumors by repeated inoculations of erysipelas: with a report of ten original cases. Am J Med Sci 1983;105:487–511.

114. Cooper NR, Welsh RM Jr. Antibody and complement-dependent viral neutralization. Springer Semin Immunopathol 1979;2:285–310.

115. Cotran RS, Kumar V, Robbins SL. Robbins pathologic basis of disease, 4th ed. Philadelphia: W.B. Saunders Company, 1989:56.

116. Cybulsky MI, Chan MKW, Movat HZ. Acute inflammation and microthrombosis induced by endotoxin, interleukin-1, and tumor necrosis factor and their implication in gram-negative infection. Lab Invest 1988;58:365–378.

117. Cybulsky MI, Movat HZ, Dinarello CA. Role of interleukin-1 and tumour necrosis factor$_{-x}$ in acute inflammation. Ann Inst Pasteur Immunol 1987;138:505–512.

118. Dale HH, Richards AN. The vasodilator action of histamine and of some other substances. J Physiol 1918;52:110–165.

119. Dinarello CA. Interleukin-1 and the pathogenesis of the acute-phase response. N Engl J Med 1984;311:1413–1418.

120. Dinarello CA. Biology of interleukin 1. FASEB J 1988;2:108–115.

121. Dinarello CA. Cytokines: interleukin-1 and tumor necrosis factor (cachectin). In: Gallin JI, Goldstein IM, Snyderman R (eds). Inflammation. Basic principles and clinical correlates. New York: Raven Press, 1988:195–208.

122. Dinarello CA, Cannon JG, Wolff SM, et al. Tumor necrosis factor (cachectin) is an endogenous pyrogen and induces production of interleukin 1. J Exp Med 1986;163:1433–1450.

123. Dinarello CA, Mier JW. Lymphokines. N Engl J Med 1987;317:940–945.

124. Dittman B, Wimmer R, Mindermann R, Ohlsson K. The effect of human granulocyte proteinases on kininogens. Adv Exp Med Biol 1979;120B:297–304.

125. Donaldson VH. The challenge of hereditary angioneurotic edema. N Engl J Med 1983;308:1094–1095.

126. Doolittle RF. Fibrinogen and fibrin. Sci Am 1981;245:126–135.

127. Douglas WW. Autacoids. Introduction. In: Goodman LS, Gilman A (eds). The Pharmacological basis of therapeutics, 4th ed. London: Collier-MacMillan Limited, 1970: 620–621.

128. Douglas WW. Polypeptides—angiotensin, plasma kinins, and other vasoactive agents; prostaglandins. In: Goodman LS, Gilman A (eds). The pharmacological basis of therapeutics, 4th ed. London: Collier-MacMillan Limited, 1970:663–676.

129. Dunn CJ. Cytokines as mediators of chronic inflammatory disease. In: Kimball ES (ed). Cytokines and inflammation. Boca Raton: CRC Press, 1991:1–33.

130. Dvorak AN, Schulman ES, Peters SP, et al. Immunoglobulin E-mediated degranulation of isolated human lung mast cells. Lab Invest 1985;53:45–56.

131. Eichler O, Farah A (eds). Handbook of experimental pharmacology. vol. 18, Pt. 1. Histamine and antihistaminics. New York: Springer-Verlag, 1966.

132. Ember JA, Hugli TE. Characterization of the human neutrophil response to sex pheromones from Streptococcus faecalis. Am J Pathol 1989;134:797–805.

133. Emmelin N, Feldberg W. The mechanism of the sting of the common nettle (Urtica Urens). J Physiol 1947;106:440–455.

134. Erickson CA, Nuccitelli R. Embryonic fibroblast motility and orientation can be influenced by physiological electric fields. J Cell Biol 1984;98:296–307.

135. Eriksson M, Saldeen K, Saldeen T, Strandberg K, Wallin R. Fibrin-derived vasoactive peptides release histamine. Int J Microcirc: Clin Exp 1983;2:337–345.

136. Erspamer V. Half a century of comparative research on biogenic amines and active peptides in amphibian skin and molluscan tissues. Comp Biochem Physiol 1984;79C:1–7.

137. Fantone JC, Kunkel SL, Ward PA, Zurier RB. Suppression by prostaglandin E_1 of vascular permeability induced by vasoactive inflammatory mediators. J Immunol 1980;125:2591–2596.

138. Forrest MJ, Jose PJ, Williams TJ. The role of the complement-derived polypeptide C5a in inflammatory reactions. In: Higgs GA, Williams TJ (eds). Inflammatory mediators. London: MacMillan, 1985:99–115.

139. Frank MM. The complement system in host defense and inflammation. Rev Infect Dis 1979;1:483–501.

140. Frey EK, Kraut H, Werle E. Das Kallikrein-Kinin-System und Seine Inhibitoren. Stuttgart: F Enke Verlag, 1968.

140a. Furie MB, Randolph GH. Chemokines and tissue injury. Am J Pathol 1995;146:1287–1301.

141. Gallin JI, Goldstein IM, Snyderman R. Inflammation: Basic principles and clinical correlates, 2nd ed. New York: Raven Press, 1992.

142. Goodman LS, Gilman A (eds). The pharmacological basis of therapeutics, 3rd ed. New York: MacMillan, 1965.

143. Gordon DL, Hostetter MK. Complement and host defence against microorganisms. Pathology 1986; 18:365–375.

144. Grant L. The sticking and emigration of white blood cells in inflammation. In: Zweifach BW, Grant L, McCluskey RT (eds). The inflammatory process, 2nd ed., vol. 2. New York: Academic Press, 1973:205–249.

145. Grau GE, Fajardo LF, Piguet P-F, Allet B, Lambert P-H, Vassalli P. Tumor necrosis factor (cachectin) as an essential mediator in murine cerebral malaria. Science 1987;237:1210–1212.

146. Habermann E. Chemistry, pharmacology, and toxicology of bee, wasp, and hornet venoms. In: Bücherl W, Buckley EE (eds). Venomous animals and their venoms. Vol. III, Venomous invertebrates. New York: Academic Press, 1971:61–93.

147. Hakim RM, Breillatt J, Lazarus JM, Port FK. Complement activation and hypersensitivity reactions to dialysis membranes. N Engl J Med 1984;311:878–882.

148. Hammarström S. The leukotrienes. In: Litwak G (ed). Biochemical actions of hormones, vol. XI. New York: Academic Press, 1984:1–23.

149. Hassett DJ, Cohen MS. Bacterial adaptation to oxidative stress: implications for pathogenesis and interaction with phagocytic cells. FASEB J 1989;3:2574–2582.

150. Hattori R, Hamilton KK, Fugate RD, McEver RP, Sims PJ. Stimulated secretion of endothelial von Willebrand factor is accompanied by rapid redistribution to the cell surface of the intracellular granule membrane protein GMP-140. J Biol Chem 1989;264:7768–7771.

151. Higgs GA, Moncada S. Leukotrienes in disease. Implications for drug development. Drugs 1985;30:1–5.

152. Higgs GA, Moncada S, Vane JR. Eicosanoids in inflammation. Ann Clin Res 1984;16:287–299.

153. Hori Y, Jyoyama H, Yamada K, Takagi M, Hirose K, Katori M. Time course analyses of kinins and other mediators in plasma exudation of rat kaolin-induced pleurisy. Eur J Pharmacol 1988;152:235–245.

154. Hugli TE. Structure and function of the anaphylatoxins. Springer Semin Immunopathol 1984;7:193–219.

155. Humphrey DM, McManus LM, Satouchi K, Hanahan DJ, Pinckard RN. Vasoactive properties of acetyl glyceryl ether phosphorylcholine and analogues. Lab Invest 1982;46:422–427.

156. Issekutz AC, Megyeri P, Issekutz TB. Role for macrophage products in endotoxin-induced polymorphonuclear leukocyte accumulation during inflammation. Lab Invest 1987;56:49–59.

157. Issekutz AC, Movat HZ. The effect of vasodilator prostaglandins on polymorphonuclear leukocyte infiltration and vascular injury. Am J Pathol 1982;107:300–309.

158. Jäättelä M. Biologic activities and mechanisms of action of tumor necrosis factor-a/cachectin. Lab Invest 1991; 64:724–742.

159. Johnston MG, Hay JB, Movat HZ. The role of prostaglandins in inflammation. Curr Top Pathol 1979; 68:259–287.

160. Johnston RB Jr. Monocytes and macrophages. N Engl J Med 1988;318:747–752.

161. Joiner KA, Frank MM. Mechanisms of bacterial resistance to complement-mediated killing. In: Jackson GG, Thomas H (eds). The pathogenesis of bacterial infections. Berlin: Springer-Verlag, 1985:122–136.

162. Joris I, Majno G, Corey EJ, Lewis RA. The mechanism of vascular leakage induced by leukotriene E_4. Endothelial contraction. Am J Pathol 1987;126:19–24.

163. Kaliner M, Wasserman SI, Austen, KF. Immunologic release of chemical mediators from human nasal polyps. N Engl J Med 1973;289:277–281.

164. Kamata R, Yamamoto T, Matsumoto K, Maeda H. A serratial protease causes vascular permeability reaction by activation of the Hageman factor-dependent pathway in Guinea pigs. Infect Immun 1985;48:747–753.

165. Kimball ES. Involvement of cytokines in neurogenic inflammation. In: Kimball ES (ed). Cytokines and inflammation. Boca Raton: CRC Press, 1991:169–189.

166. Kimball ES (ed). Cytokines and inflammation. Boca Raton: CRC Press, 1991.

167. Kovacs EJ. Control of IL-1 and TNFa production at the level of second messenger pathways. In: Kimball ES (ed). Cytokines and inflammation. Boca Raton: CRC Press, 1991: 89–107.

168. Kozin F, Cochrane CG. The contact activation system of plasma: biochemistry and pathophysiology. In: Gallin JI, Goldstein IM, Snyderman R (eds). Inflammation: Basic principles and clinical correlates. New York: Raven Press, 1988:101–120.

169. Kuhlman M, Joiner K, Ezekowitz RAB. The human mannose-binding protein functions as an opsonin. J Exp Med 1989;169:1733–1745.

170. Kunkel SL, Remick DG, Strieter RM, Larrick JW. Mechanisms that regulate the production and effects of tumor necrosis factor-a. CRC Crit Rev Immunol 1989;9:93–117.

171. Larrick JW, Wright SC. Cytotoxic mechanism of tumor necrosis factor-a. FASEB J 1990;4:3215–3223.

172. Larsen GL, Henson PM. Mediators of inflammation. Annu Rev Immunol 1983;1:335–359.

173. Lepow IH. Louis Pillemer, properdin, and scientific controversy. J Immunol 1980;125:471–478.

174. Lewis RA, Austen KF. Leukotrienes. In: Gallin JI, Goldstein IM, Snyderman R (eds). Inflammation: Basic principles and clinical correlates. New York: Raven Press, 1988:121–128.

175. Lewis RA, Austen KF, Soberman RJ. Leukotrienes and other products of the 5-lipoxygenase pathway. Biochemistry and relation to pathobiology in human diseases. N Engl J Med 1990;323:645–655.

176. Loos M. Bacteria and complement—A historical review. Curr Topics Microbiol Immunol 1985;121:1–5.

177. Lubran MM. Bacterial toxins. Ann Clin Lab Sci 1988;18:58–71.

178. Lundberg C, Gerdin B. The inflammatory reaction in an experimental model of open wounds in the rat. The effect of arachidonic acid metabolites. Eur J Pharmacol 1984;97:229–238.

179. Marasco WA, Phan SH, Krutzsch H, Showell HJ, Feltner DE, Nairn R, Becker EL, Ward PA. Purification and identification of formyl-methionyl-leucyl-phenylalanine as the major peptide neutrophil chemotactic factor produced by Escherichia coli. J Biol Chem 1984;259:5430–5439.

180. McManus LM, Pinckard RN. Kinetics of acetyl glyceryl ether phosphorylcholine (AGEPC)-induced acute lung alterations in the rabbit. Am J Pathol 1985;121:55–68.

181. McManus LM, Pincard RN, Hanahan DJ. Acetyl glyceryl ether phosphorylcholine (AGEPC) in allergy and inflammation. In: Theoretical and clinical aspects of allergic diseases symposium Oct. 12–14. Stockholm: Skandia Group, 1982:165–182.

182. Menkin V. Newer Concepts of Inflammation. Springfield: Charles C. Thomas, 1950.

183. Menkin V. Modern views on inflammation. Int Arch Allergy Appl Immunol 1953;4:131–168.

184. Meri S, Waldmann H, Lachmann PJ. Distribution of protectin (CD59), a complement membrane attack inhibitor, in normal human tissues. Lab Invest 1991;65:532–537.

185. Michie HR, Manogue KR, Spriggs DR, et al. Detection of circulating tumor necrosis factor after endotoxin administration. N Engl J Med 1988;318:1481–1486.

186. Moncada S, Korbut R, Bunting S, Vane JR. Prostacyclin is a circulating hormone. Nature 1978; 273:767–768.

186a. Moncad S, Higgs EA. Endogenous nitric oxide: physiology, pathology and clinical relevance. Eur J Clin Invest 1991;21:361–374.

187. Moncada S, Radomski MW. The problems and the promise of prostaglandin influences in atherogenesis. Ann NY Acad Sci 1985;454:121–130.

188. Movat HZ. The kinin system and its relations to other systems. Curr Top Pathol 1979;68:111–134.

189. Müller-Eberhard HJ. The significance of complement activity in shock. In: Proceedings of a symposium on recent research developments and current clinical practice in shock: The cell in shock. A scope publication. Upjohn 1975:35–38.

190. Müller-Eberhard HJ. The membrane attack complex. Springer Semin Immunopathol 1984;7:93–141.

191. Nauts HC. The Beneficial Effects of Bacterial Infections on Host Resistance to Cancer. End Results in 449 Cases. Monograph No. 8, 2nd ed. New York: Cancer Research Institute, Inc., 1980.

192. Newball HH, Revak SD, Cochrane CG, Griffin JH, Lichtenstein LM. Activation of human Hageman factor by a leukocytic protease. Adv Exp Med Biol 1979;120B:139–151.

193. O'Brodovich HM, Stalcup SA, Pang LM, Lipset JS, Mellins RB. Bradykinin production and increased pulmonary endothelial permeability during acute respiratory failure in unanesthetized sheep. J Clin Invest 1981;67:514–522.

194. Old LJ. Tumor necrosis factor (TNF). Science 1985;230:630–632.

195. Old LJ. Tumor necrosis factor. Sci Am 1988;258:59–75.

196. Oldham RK. Journal of biological response modifiers: why another journal? J Biol Resp Modif 1982;1:1–2.

197. Oltvai ZM, Wong ECC, Atkinson JP, Tung KSK. C1 inhibitor deficiency: molecular and immunologic basis of hereditary and acquired angioedema. Lab Invest 1991;65:381–388.

198. Page IH. The discovery of serotonin. Perspect Biol Med 1976;20:1–8.

199. Pernow B. Substance P. Pharmacol Rev 1983;35:85–141.

200. Piguet PF, Collart MA, Grau GE, Sappino A-P, Vassalli P. Requirement of tumour necrosis factor for development of silica-induced pulmonary fibrosis. Nature 1990; 344:245–247.

201. Pillemer L, Blum L, Lepow IH, Ross OA, Todd EW, Wardlaw AC. The properdin system and immunity: I. Demonstration and isolation of a new serum protein, properdin, and its role in immune phenomena. Science 1954;120:279–285

202. Pinckard RN, Ludwig, JC, McManus LM. Platelet-activating factors. In: Gallin JI, Goldstein IM, Snyderman R (eds). Inflammation: Basic principles and clinical correlates. New York: Raven Press, 1988:139–167

203. Piper P, Vane J. The release of prostaglandins from lung and other tissues. Ann NY Acad Sci 1971;180:363–385.

204. Podack ER. Assembly of transmembrane tubules (poly perforins) on target membranes by cloned NK and TK cells: comparison to poly C9 of complement. In: Hoshino T, Koren HS, Uchida A (eds). Natural killer activity and its regulation. Amsterdam: Excerpta Medica, 1984:101–106.

205. Podack ER, Tschopp J. Circular polymerization of the ninth component of complement. J Biol Chem 1982; 257:15204–15212.

206. Podack ER, Tschopp J. Membrane attack by complement. Mol Immunol 1984;21:589–603.

207. Proud D, Reynolds CJ, Lacapra S, Kagey-Sobotka A, Lichtenstein LM, Naclerio RM. Nasal provocation with bradykinin induces symptoms of rhinitis and a sore throat. Am Rev Respir Dis 1988;137:613–616.

208. Proud D, Togias, A, Naclerio RM, Crush SA, Norman PS, Lichtenstein LM Kinins are generated in vivo following nasal airway challenge of allergic individuals with allergen. J Clin Invest 1983;72:1678–1685.

209. Pullman-Mooar S, Laposata M, Lem D, Holman RT, Leventhal LJ, DeMarco D, Zurier RB. Alteration of the cellular fatty acid profile and the production of eicosanoids in human monocytes by gamma-linolenic acid. Arthritis Rheum 1990;33:1526–1533.

210. Ramm LE, Whitlow MB, Koski CL, Shin ML, Mayer MM. Elimination of complement channels from the plasma membranes of U937, a nucleated mammalian cell line: temperature dependence of the elimination rate. J Immunol 1983;131:1411–1415.

211. Rampart M, Van Damme J, Zonnekeyn L, Herman AG. Granulocyte chemotactic protein/interlueukin-8 induces plasma leakage and neutrophil accumulation in rabbit skin. Am L Pathol 1989;135:21–25.

212. Ratnoff WD. A war with the molecules: Louis Pillemer and the history of properdin. Perspect Biol Med 1980;23:638–657.

213. Remick DG, Kunkel RG, Larrick JW, Kunkel SL. Acute in vivo effects of human recombinant tumor necrosis factor. Lab Invest 1987;56:583–590.

214. Rocha e Silva M. A brief history of inflammation. In: Vane JR, Ferreira SH (eds). Inflammation. Handbook of experimental pharmacology, vol. 50/I. Berlin: Springer-Verlag 1978:6–25.

215. Rosen FS, Alper CA. Genetic deficiencies of the complement system. Clin Immunol Allergy 1985;5:371–377.

216. Rossi V, Breviario F, Ghezzi P, Dejana E, Mantovani A. Prostacyclin synthesis induced in vascular cells by interleukin-1. Science 1985;229:174–176.

217. Roth J, Leroith D, Collier ES, Watkinson A, Lesniak MA. The evolutionary origins of intercellular communication and the Maginot lines of the mind. Ann NY Acad Sci 1986;463:1–11.

218. Rother K, Till GO (eds). The complement system. Berlin: Springer-Verlag, 1988.

219. Ryan GB. Inflammation. Mediators of inflammation. Beitr Pathol 1974;152:272–291.

220. Ryan GB, Majno G. Inflammation (A Scope Publication). Kalamazoo, MI: The Upjohn Company, 1977

221. Ryan JW, Ryan US. Biochemical and morphological aspects of the actions and metabolism of kinins. In: Pisano JJ, Austen KF (eds). Chemistry and biology of the Kallikrein-Kinin system in health and disease, Fogarty Int Center Proc, No. 27. Washington, DC: US Government Printing Office, 1976:315–333.

222. Sahashi K, Engel AG, Lambert EH, Howard FM Jr. Ultrastructural localization of the terminal lytic ninth complement component (C9) at the motor end-plate in myasthesia gravis. J Neuropathol Exp Neurol 1980;39:160–172.

223. Said SI. Vasoactive peptides. State-of-the-art review. Hypertension 1983;5 (Suppl I):I-17–I-26.

224. Salama A, Hugo F, Heinrich D, et al. Deposition of terminal C5b-9 complement complexes on erythrocytes and leukocytes during cardiopulmonary bypass. N Engl J Med 1988;318:408–414.

225. Saldeen T. The fibrinolytic system in inflammation. In: Higgs GA, Williams TJ (eds). Inflammatory Mediators. London: MacMillan 1985:87–97.

226. Saria A, Lundberg JM. Neurogenic inflammation. In: Higgs GA, Williams TJ (eds). inflammatory mediators. London: MacMillan 1985:73–85.

227. Scher W. The role of extracellular proteases in cell proliferation and differentiation. Lab Invest 1987;57:607–633.

227a. Selvan RS, Butterfield JH, Krangel MS. Expression of multiple chemokine genes by a human mast cell leukemia. J Biol Chem 1994;269:13893–13898.

228. Shama SK, Etkind PH, Odell TM, Canada AT, Finn, AM, Soter NA. Gypsy-moth-caterpillar dermatitis. N Engl J Med 1982;306:1300–1301.

229. Steinbusch HWM, Mulder AH. Localization and projections of histamine-immunoreactive neurons in the central nervous system of the rat. In: Ganellin CR, Schwartz J-C (eds). Frontiers in Histamine Research. Oxford: Pergamon Press, 1985:119–130.

230. Stuart-Smith K, Vanhhoutte PM. Epithelium-derived relaxing factor. In: Agrawal DK, Townley RG (eds). Airway Smooth Muscle: Modulation of Receptors and Response. Boca Raton: CRC Press, 1990:129–145.

231. Thorgeirsson G. Endothelial autacoids. Acta Med Scand 1985;217:453–456.

232. Toda N. Heterogeneous responses to histamine in blood vessels. In: Vanhoutte PM (ed). Vasodilatation. New York: Raven Press, 1988:531–535.

233. Tschopp J, Podack ER, Müller-Eberhard HJ. The membrane attack complex of complement: C5b-8 complex as accelerator of C9 polymerization. J Immunol 1985;134:495–499.

234. Tsuru H. Heterogeneity of the vascular effects of bradykinin. In: Vanhoutte PM (ed). Vasodilatation. New York: Raven Press, 1988: 479–482.

235. Vanhoutte PM, Cohen RA, Van Nueten JM. Serotonin and arterial vessels. J Cardiovasc Pharmacol 1984;6 (suppl 2):S421–S428.

236. Ward PA, Lepow IH, Newman LJ. Bacterial factors chemotactic for polymorphonuclear leukocytes. Am J Pathol 1968;52:725–736.

237. Warren JS, Ward PA, Johnson KJ. Tumor necrosis factor: a plurifunctional mediator of acute inflammation. Mod Pathol 1988;1:242–247.

238. Weaver JC, Astumian RD. The response of living cells to very weak electric fields: the thermal noise limit. Science 1990;247:459–462.

239. Weissmann G. Mediators of inflammation. New York: Plenum Press, 1974.

240. Welsh RM Jr, Lampert PW, Burner PA, Oldstone MBA. Antibody-complement interactions with purified lymphocytic choriomeningitis virus. Virology 1976;73:59–71.

241. Wilder RL. Proinflammatory microbial products as etiologic agents of inflammatory arthritis. Rheum Dis Clin North Am 1987;13:293–306.

242. Williams T, Jose PJ. Mediation of increased vascular permeability after complement activation. J Exp Med 1981;153:136–153.

243. Willis AL. The eicosanoids: an introduction and an overview. In: Willis AL (ed). CRC Handbook of Eicosanoids: Prostaglandins and Related Lipids vol. 1. Boca Raton: CEC Press Inc., 1987:3–46.

244. Woodin AM, Wieneke AA. Leukocidin, tetraethylammonium ions, and the membrane acyl phosphatases in relation to the leukocyte potassium pump. J Gen Physiol, 1970;56:16–32.

245. Yurt RW. Role of the mast cell in trauma. In: Dineen P, Hildick-Smith G (eds). The Surgical Wound. Philadelphia: Lea & Febiger, 1981:37–62.

246. Zhou W, Chao W, Levine BA, Olson MS Evidence for platelet-activating factor as a late-phase mediator of chronic pancreatitis in the rat. Am J Pathol 1990;137:1501–1508.

247. Zurier RB. Prostaglandin E_1: is it useful? J Rheumatol 1990;17:1439–1441.

The Four Cardinal Signs of Inflammation

CHAPTER 10

> ### Mechanisms of Redness and Heat
>
> ### Inflammatory Swelling: Mechanisms of Vascular Leakage

Having reviewed the actors of inflammation and their language, we can now view the play: redness and swelling with heat and pain (*rubor et tumor cum calore et dolore*).

Mechanisms of Redness and Heat

The Greeks, who believed there was "too much blood" in inflamed tissues, were three times right. There are in fact three reasons for the vessels to contain more blood than normal (hyperemia): (1) *the inflow of blood is increased*, (2) *the outflow is hampered*, and (3) *the capillary network is completely filled* whereas many capillaries are normally empty. The increased inflow and filling of all capillaries explain the hotter skin. The slower outflow explains the purplish hue: the tissues have more time to extract oxygen from the blood, which becomes **cyanotic** (p. 600) (Figure 10.1).

It is a stirring experience to watch these vascular events in live tissues under the microscope. Cohnheim marveled over them in 1867, in the mesentery of the living frog (4). Note that he did not need to injure the mesentery; it became inflamed on its own due to the trauma of exposure. Here is what he saw:

> *The first thing you notice in the exposed vessels is a dilatation which occurs chiefly in the arteries, then in the veins, and least of all in the capillaries. With the dilatation which is gradually developed, but which during the space of fifteen to twenty minutes has usually attained considerable proportions (often exceeding twice the original diameter) there immediately sets in the mesentery an acceleration of the bloodstream, most striking again in the arteries. . . . Yet this acceleration never lasts long; after half an hour or an hour . . . it invariably gives place to a decided retardation, the velocity of the stream falling more or less below the normal. (6).*

The dilatation of the arterioles (small arteries) is the cumulative effect of vasoactive mediators (histamine and many others) and probably also of nervous impulses.

What happens when arterioles dilate? Physiology teaches us that the arterioles are the resistance vessels of the arterial tree. Under normal conditions they bring about the largest drop in blood pressure (from ~85 to 30 mm Hg), which means that their upstream effect is to provide the heart pump with a resistance while their downstream effect is that of floodgates: they protect the capillaries from the high arterial pressure. *If all the arterioles throughout the body were to dilate at the same time, the arterial blood pressure would drop precipitously* (this is what happens in anaphylactic shock). In inflammation they dilate only in a limited area, so that systemic arterial pressure is not affected. However, *downstream from the dilated arterioles, flow accelerates and capillary pressure rises*: the floodgates are open, and capillaries that are normally empty

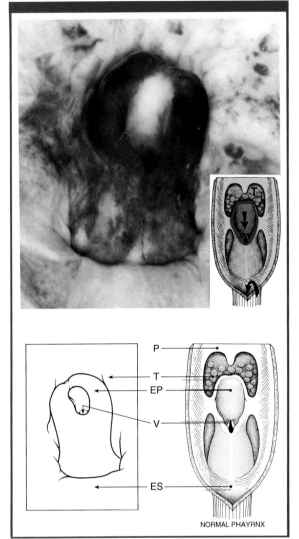

FIGURE 10.1

See color plate 8. A black-and-white rendition of the inflammatory *rubor*. This craterlike structure is the acutely inflamed epiglottis of a 7-year-old child who died of asphyxia. Such infections are usually caused by *Haemopjilus influenzae*; the epiglottis swells and becomes "cherry-red." Stridor (harsh sound during respiration) is a warning and should be treated as an emergency. Approx. 2×. *Bottom:* Diagram of top figure and scheme of the epiglottis as seen from behind the soft palate looking forward: **P** = Soft palate, **T** = root of the tongue, **EP** = epiglottis, **V** = vocal cords, **ES** = entrance to the esophagus. (Courtesy of Dr. F.J. Krolikowski, Medical Examiner, Commonwealth of Massachusetts.)

are filled by the incoming tide, enough to give the gross impression of a blush. Indeed this is what does happen when people blush. Blood flow can increase as much as tenfold (22).

Capillary dilatation is minimal, but the venules become distended. The cause can be guessed from

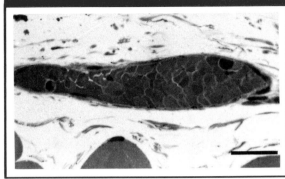

FIGURE 10.2
Congested venule in an acutely inflamed muscle. The vessel is filled with compacted red blood cells; under normal circumstances about half of the space in the lumen should be occupied by plasma. The tissue surrounding the venule is edematous, presumably from plasma lost by this and other leaky venules. **Bar** = 25 μm.

Figure 10.2, which portrays a typical venule in an inflamed area. This venule contains only blood cells, no plasma. Normally, blood cells make up about 44 percent of the total blood volume. Thus, 56 percent should be plasma, yet little or no plasma is left in "inflamed" venules. Where did it go? Light microscopy cannot clearly show it, but the walls of these venules have become leaky: plasma has escaped through tiny, almost submicroscopic gaps between endothelial cells. The semi-solid cylinder of red blood cells that now fills the lumen opposes a much greater resistance to flow (Figure 10.3). The increased resistance raises the pressure upstream, and the lumen expands. Now flow becomes slower, as Cohnheim observed. All this happens within a few minutes. The leakiness of venules will be explained later.

Notice how these venular changes fit the overall plan: the increased flow from the arterioles, fighting against an obstacle in the leaky venules, leads to greater exudation of fluid—which is one of the two basic purposes of inflammation: to deliver fluid and cells to the site of injury.

To better understand the "redness", we will resort to a simple experiment on human skin: the so-called *triple response*.

THE TRIPLE RESPONSE OF THE SKIN

The mechanisms of arterial dilatation were worked out in the skin, the most accessible organ, as early as the 1920s by the pioneer studies of a British clinician, Sir Thomas Lewis (38). His experiments, though extremely simple, were a landmark because they led to discover the first inflammatory mediator, histamine, cautiously referred to in those days as substance H. You can try his basic experiment as you read these lines. Take a ruler, and pull one of its corners rather firmly along the skin of your forearm (Figure 10.4). A three-step reaction will follow:

1. A red line appears within seconds (vasodilatation).
2. A red flare appears after 15–30 seconds, spreading all around the line to a distance of several centimeters (again vasodilatation).
3. The red line becomes a wheal (a transient swelling of the skin, such as is produced by the sting of a nettle). This takes a little longer, 1–3 minutes, because it is due to vascular leakage, which requires time. At first the wheal is red; as it swells further, it tends to pale.

The triple response is explained as follows. The trauma caused by the ruler breaks up or somehow degranulates the mast cells in the dermis; the mast cells spill their histamine, which causes local vasodilatation (red line) followed by vascular leakage (wheal). As to the flare, it is not conceivable that histamine could diffuse several centimeters in a matter of seconds. Sir Thomas found that it is due to an axon reflex, as explained in Figure 10.5 (3, 59). He tried the triple response experiment in accident victims in whom the sensory nerve leading to the test area had been severed; for the first 5 days after the nerve was cut, the flare did develop; then it disappeared, coincidentally with the slow breakdown of the severed axons.

The triple response helps us understand the redness of the skin around an injury (look for the

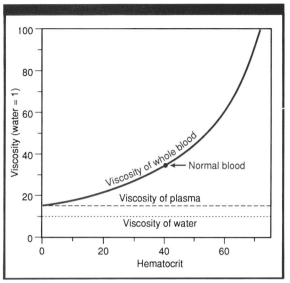

FIGURE 10.3
The viscosity of the blood rises sharply as the hematocrit increases. This explains the slow flow in leaky venules of inflammatory foci: the plasma has leaked out, and the hematocrit inside the venule approaches 100 percent. (Reproduced with permission from [17].)

flare around your next mosquito bite). As to the meaning of the response itself: it increases local blood flow and may therefore have a protective effect (38).

The triple response is reduced in diabetics, presumably because of the diabetic neuropathy (27). Whether it occurs also in internal organs is not clear (22); however, it has been proposed that the bronchial spasm of asthma is due to an axon reflex, which in this case would be obnoxious. The bronchial epithelium, damaged by eosinophil products, exposes C fibers, which generate an axon reflex leading to bronchial spasm and hypersecretion of mucus (1).

HEAT AND PAIN

The heat of inflamed skin is due to the increased perfusion of the tissues with blood, and so the

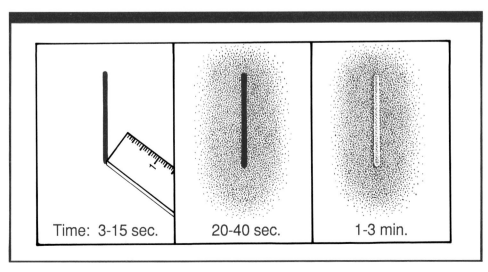

FIGURE 10.4
The "triple response" of Lewis, produced by firmly stroking the skin with a blunt object. First a red line appears; then a red flare develops along the red line; eventually the red line turns into a wheal.

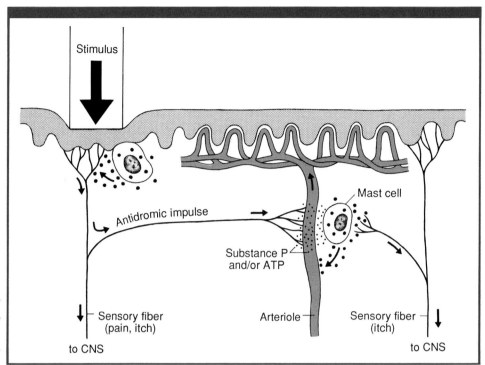

FIGURE 10.5
Mechanism of the triple response shown in Figure 10.4. The stimulation of a sensory fiber and the mast cell degranulation initiate an impulse; by an antidromic pathway the impulse reaches an arteriole, where the nerve endings release substance P and/or ATP. This causes mast cells to degranulate, producing further sensory and vasomotor effects. (Adapted from [3].)

temperature can never be higher than that of blood. It follows that *calor* can develop only in the skin, which is normally cool. Inflamed inner organs cannot become hotter because they are already as hot as they can be. Does the increased temperature of the skin have any significance? It has been shown that leukocytes maintained in a thermal gradient *in vitro* move toward warmer temperatures (**thermotaxis**) (34); but whether this is actually helpful *in vivo* is not known. However, in discussing fever, we will mention several potentially beneficial effects of higher temperatures; for example, leukocytes move faster. It is therefore possible that the *calor* of inflamed skin may have a survival value.

The pain occurs when specialized nerve-fiber endings are stimulated by mediators, especially bradykinin (remember that many insects use bradykinin to make their stings painful).

> A standard test for pain mediators (**algogens**) in humans is to raise a blister on the forearm with the ancient blistering agent cantharidin (prepared from the dried, crushed body of a beetle), cut off the epidermis, and drip the substance to be tested on the denuded dermis. This test shows that bradykinin is about 50 times more potent than histamine or serotonin in eliciting pain (14).

It is possible that tissue pressure may enhance the pain, but there is no good evidence of correlation between tissue swelling and pain; noninflammatory edema is painless. Prostaglandins sensitize the nerve endings to the effects of bradykinin and other algogens (47). Once again, *aspirin reduces the pain of inflammation by cutting off the supply of prostaglandins.* This explains why aspirin is of no help in many types of noninflammatory pain (47).

> **Itching** *is probably not the same modality as pain, but little is known about it. Histamine is certainly involved: a small intradermal dose of histamine causes itching, a larger dose pain. Proteases are also involved (1a, 13). How itching powder works (cowhage, the spicules of a tropical fruit) is still not clear (1a, 13).*

CAN THERE BE ACUTE INFLAMMATION WITHOUT REDNESS?

Not really, except for one special case: on a slice of lung, seen at autopsy, a focus of acute inflammation (bronchopneumonia) appears whitish because that is the color of fibrin and leukocytes that fill the alveoli (Figure 10.6). In chronic inflammation, however, redness is often lacking.

CAN THERE BE ACUTE INFLAMMATION WITHOUT PAIN?

Certainly. In internal organs, such as the lung, inflammation is painless unless it reaches the serosal lining, as proven by the phenomenon of "walking pneumonia": you can have a focus of acute inflammation in a lung and walk around feeling sick but without realizing that your problem is pneumonia. Many dermatologic inflammatory conditions cause redness with little or no pain. In our experience, the purple-red erythema of Lyme disease is painless to the point of escaping notice. Perhaps a special mixture of mediators is involved.

TO SUM UP: **Rubor** represents good news, more blood supplies for the defenses; **dolor** is incidental, although it may help by pointing to an area of trouble; **calor** is limited to inflammation in the skin, where it may have a protective value. We now turn to the **tumor**.

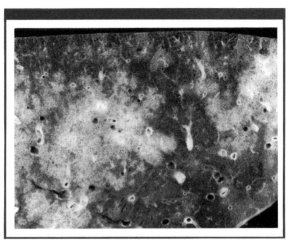

FIGURE 10.6
Slice of human lung showing foci of bronchopneumonia: an inflammatory condition in which the air spaces are replaced by white blood cells and fibrin. A combination of these produces the whitish discoloration of the lung's cut surface. Natural size.

Inflammatory Swelling: Mechanisms of Vascular Leakage

We must now explain the inflammatory swelling. During the first day or two of acute inflammation, the swelling is due overwhelmingly to excess fluid. The basic mechanism was proposed by Cohnheim in 1873 when he ventured a guess beyond the resolving power of his microscope: *plasma escapes from the blood vessels, which have somehow become leaky* (5). In terms of pathophysiology, the situation is actually a little more complex:

- *Leaks in the microcirculation* are indeed present.
- *Filtration pressure has increased* due to arteriolar dilatation, whereby the loss of fluid through the leaks is enhanced.
- *Reabsorption of fluid into the bloodstream is impaired* because plasma proteins have escaped into the extracellular spaces where they tend to neutralize the osmotic pressure of the plasma in the vessels.

The key factor in the genesis of the swelling is vascular leakage. So we must now agree on the meaning of the convenient term *leaky*—which, incidentally, does not exist in Latin languages.

Vascular Leakage as a Plumbing Problem The loss of fluid occurs in the vessels of the microcirculation, where the vascular walls are thinnest: capillaries and venules, which consist of endothelium and basement membrane, plus a few cells hugging the endothelium, called pericytes. These spidery cells were beautifully demonstrated by Zimmerman in 1923 (Figure 10.7) (63); when grown in culture they appear to "give orders" to the endothelial cells (Figure 10.8) (50). The permeability barrier in all blood vessels is the

endothelium; the basement membrane (thin but tough) lends mechanical support. What happens if these layers of the vascular wall are damaged?

- If the endothelial layer alone is interrupted, the permeability barrier is lost and plasma leaks out, but the basement membrane remains and holds the vessel together; it acts temporarily as a coarse filter until the endothelium is repaired. Blood cells rarely escape by breaking through (Figure 10.9).
- If the basement membrane alone is destroyed (by enzymes), the vessel tends to break apart: for example, if collagenase is injected into the skin of a rat, it produces extensive hemorrhage. This shows the mechanical role of the basement membrane.

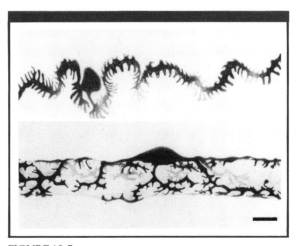

FIGURE 10.7
Pericytes, impregnated (blackened) with silver as illustrated by K. W. Zimmermann in 1923. *Top:* Pericyte stretched along capillaries of the human tongue (actual length about 0.15 mm). *Bottom:* Pericytes on a postcapillary venule in cat heart. **Bar** = 5 μm. (Reproduced with permission from [63].)

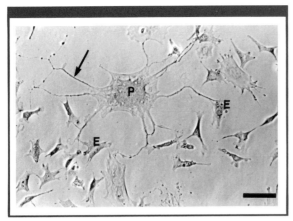

FIGURE 10.8
A pericyte (**P**) apparently "giving orders" to endothelial cells (**E**). Phase contrast photograph from a co-culture of bovine pericytes and endothelial cells. Grown under these conditions, in a matter of days, the pericytes extend thin processes (**arrow**) that contact endothelial cells, apparently inhibiting endothelial cell proliferation by inducing the synthesis of transforming growth factor beta. **Bar** = 10 μm. (Reproduced with permission from [50].)

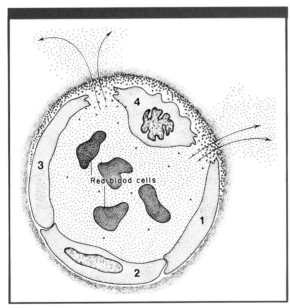

FIGURE 10.9
Behavior of endothelium and basement membrane in a venule responding to a histamine-type (permeability-increasing) mediator. **1, 2, 3, 4:** Endothelial cells. Cell 4 has contracted, thereby creating a gap on either side. Plasma proteins (**small dots**) escape through these gaps and succeed in crossing the basement membrane. Particles of carbon black injected intravenously (**heavy dots**) are too large to negotiate the basement membrane; they are retained on it and form a black deposit ("vascular labeling" phenomenon). (Adapted from [40].)

- If both layers are destroyed, the result is not leakage but hemorrhage.

Loss of the pericytes alone occurs in the diabetic retinal vessels, for unknown reasons. The microscopic outpouchings of the capillaries (capillary aneurysms) in the diabetic retina are thought to reflect the loss of support by the pericytes.

METHODS FOR DEMONSTRATING VASCULAR LEAKAGE

The basic principle for demonstrating vascular leakage is the same that civil engineers use when they look for a leak in a septic tank: they pour fluorescein into the tank and see where the fluorescence turns up. In fact, intravenous fluorescein is used by ophthalmologists for demonstrating leaky vessels in the retina.

However, the study of leaky vessels includes a refinement not available for testing septic tanks. In experimental animals, two kinds of colored materials can be used, with different but complementary results: *a soluble dye* such as Evans blue and *colloidal particles* such as India ink. These are the same two sets of colored materials used for mapping the RES/MPS (p. 297). The critical difference is the size of the colored particles (Figure 10.10).

With Soluble Dyes This classic method is often referred to as **bluing,** notwithstanding the fact that red dyes can also be used (37, 44). As seen on the shaved skin of a white rabbit, the result is striking. If 3 ml of a 1 percent solution of trypan blue or Evans blue are injected intravenously, the rabbit shows little change, except that within hours and days it slowly acquires a blue-gray tinge. However, if the skin is slightly irritated in one area, that area will turn bright blue in 2–3 minutes (Figure 10.11).

This test is very sensitive because albumin, which carries the blue dye (p. 81), is among the smallest plasma proteins: just what is needed for detecting fine leaks.

In the skin, the severity of the leakage is roughly proportional to the diameter of the blue spot, which is better seen by dissecting off the skin and examining its underside (Figure 10.12) (48). It is also possible to extract and quantitate the amount of extravasated dye (33). The bluing test is currently used experimentally not only for measuring the ability of given compounds to increase vascular permeability but also for testing the effectiveness of antiinflammatory drugs. The leakage of protein can also be quantitated using intravenous injections of ^{125}I-labeled albumin (49).

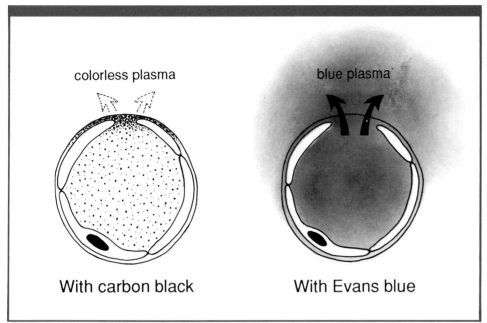

colorless plasma

blue plasma

With carbon black

With Evans blue

FIGURE 10.10
Principles underlying two methods for demonstrating vascular leakage. The diagram shows two microscopic leaky vessels with a gap between two endothelial cells. *Left:* vascular labeling (using particles that cannot cross the basement membrane). *Right:* "bluing", using dyes that combine with albumin; the albumin-dye complex leaks out into the extravascular space, but the vessel itself is not labeled.

The bluing test is simple and sensitive, and it does demonstrate the general area in which vessels are leaking, but it does not indicate precisely which vessels are leaking (Figure 10.13, top). To do this we must inject into the blood some colored material that can be trapped in the wall of the leaking vessels.

With Colloidal Suspensions (Vascular Labeling)
The principle is quite simple (Figure 10.9): We choose this method when we want to pinpoint individual leaky vessels, that is, vessels that have a leaky endothelium and an intact basement membrane. Knowing that histamine produces leaky vessels, we can prepare a rat with a subcutaneous injection of histamine. Experience has shown that the basement membrane retains particles larger than 200–300 Å (the exact figure probably varies from site to site), so we can inject intravenously a colloidal suspension such as carbon black (biological India ink), which consists of particles about 300 Å in diameter. As the carbon-loaded plasma rushes out of the endothelial gaps, the suspended particles remain trapped against the basement membrane, much as coffee piles up on a filter (Figure 10.9). Within a minute or so the deposit can be dense enough to be seen by light microscopy or even by the naked eye. In contrast with the dense blue spot obtained with trypan blue, one can see a fine design of blackened vessels in the skin and especially in the more vascular striated muscle. *The main advantage over the bluing method is*

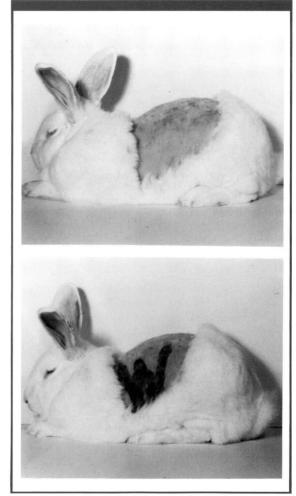

FIGURE 10.11
See color plate 9. An experiment demonstrating the speed of the permeability-increasing response. *Top:* a white rabbit with back and flanks shaved, 1 minute after an intravenous injection of trypan blue. A "W" (for Worcester) has been painted on the skin with xylene, a very mild irritant. Comparison with the photograph below will show that the outline of the W is just beginning to appear. *Bottom:* The same rabbit 5 minutes later. Trypan blue leaked out of the vessels only where the skin had been irritated.

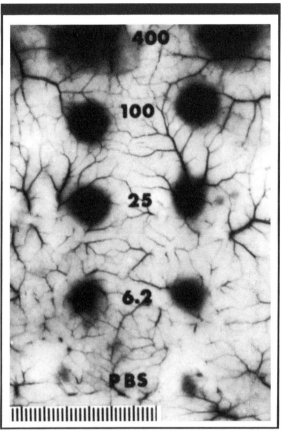

FIGURE 10.12
Bluing method
for measuring in-
creased vascular
permeability.
The undersurface
of guinea pig
skin after an in-
travenous injec-
tion of Evans
blue and in-
tradermal injec-
tions of brady-
kinin (doses ex-
pressed in
nanograms).
PBS: Phosphate-
buffered saline.
Scale in mm.
(Reproduced
with permission
from [48].)

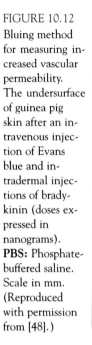

that each leaky vessel remains permanently marked, so it is easy to determine precisely where the leakage is occurring. This can be important; the type of leaking vessel (arteriole, capillary, or venule) can give a clue as to the causal agent. Another advantage is the possibility of injecting intrave- nously *two different pigments at different times.* This double labeling—for example, black and blue— demonstrates exactly which vessels were leaking at each time point (Figure 10.13).

Vascular labeling occurs during the first few minutes after the intravenous injection of carbon black; after that time the concentration of colloidal carbon particles in the plasma drops precipitously, due to clearance by the RES/MPS (p. 297).

Tissues with labeled vessels can be studied in ordinary histologic sections; in addition, tissues shaped as membranes (such as skin, mesentery, and some muscles) can be fixed, made semitrans- parent by soaking them in glycerin, and studied "in bulk" under the microscope (Figure 10.13). In this way the entire microcirculatory tree is laid out, and the topography of leakage can be seen in detail.

What becomes of the labeled vessels? The insoluble material piled up against the basement membrane is slowly phagocytized by the endothelium and by the pericytes, and some may gradually find its way out into the tissues; but, basically, the vessels remain tattooed for life (7).

NATURAL MARKERS OF LEAKY VESSELS

Vessels develop leaks all the time, in bruises and insect bites, and are labeled in a natural way by natural "marker particles" that exist in the bloodstream—namely, chylomicrons and the larg- er lipoproteins. Wherever there is an endothelial gap, the basement membrane retains these parti- cles and the blood vessel remains labeled with lipid (39). We once had the opportunity to demonstrate that a cup of heavy cream (with chocolate) produces in an adult human, after 4 hours, enough chylomicrons to label leaky vessels (Figure 10.14). Incidentally, this mechanism does not explain the accumulation of lipid in arteries in atherosclerosis. In this disease lipoproteins are actively picked up by the endothelium and transferred into the wall of the artery; gaps do not seem to play an important role (p. 655).

A corollary to vascular labeling: *circulating bacteria tend to localize in inflamed tissues.* This is an old observation (16, 45); the mechanism is probably the same as that of vascular labeling: bacteria escape through endothelial gaps. This principle can be extended to explain the development of bone infection (osteomyelitis) in the metaphyses of growing children: an electron microscopic study of the metaphyses in growing rats has shown that the capillaries in this zone are riddled with large gaps, through which even red blood cells can escape; carbon black injected intravenously pro- duces a grossly visible black band of labeling in this area (18). We will see later that injured tissues tend to retain also circulating cancer cells (p. 803).

Detection of Leaky Vessels in Histologic Sec- tions When we look for leaky vessels in a microscopic section of acutely inflamed tissue, we are not much better off than Cohnheim because the endothelial gaps are usually very small, of the order of one micrometer. However, anyone can diagnose increased permeability indirectly, on purely morphologic grounds. One good lead is **edema,** the presence of excess fluid in the tissue spaces. Edema is not always inflammatory, but *if it is accompanied by inflammatory cells* it is likely to reflect inflammatory vascular leakage. Another

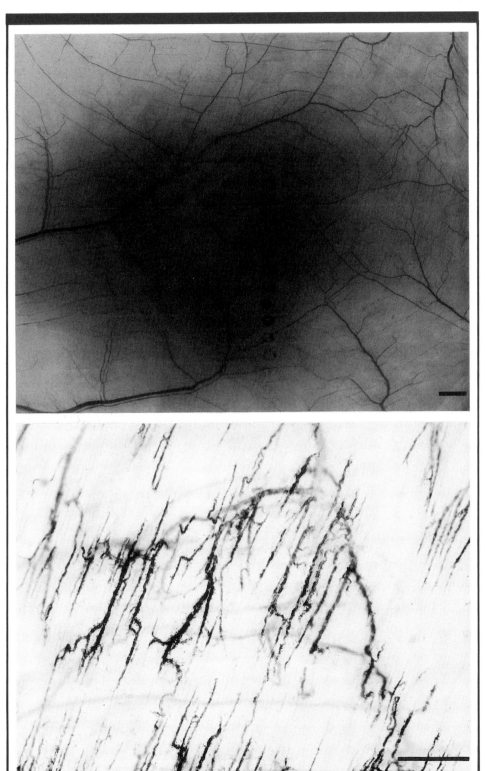

FIGURE 10.13
See color plate 10. Contrasting two methods for demonstrating vascular leakage. Cremaster muscles 30 minutes after a local injection of histamine; whole mounts, transilluminated. *Top:* "Bluing" by an intravenous injection of the dye Trypan blue (chemically similar to Evans blue). The dye is not retained within the walls of the leaky vessels. **Bar** = 1000 μm. (Preparation by Dr. G.I. Schoefl; from (52a). *Bottom:* Vascular labeling identifies individual leaky vessels. The horizontal unlabeled vessel is an arteriole. (This preparation also illustrates double labeling, with carbon black followed by Monastral blue; see text.) **Bar** = 500 μm.

hint is the presence of **fibrin** filaments in the extracellular spaces (Figure 10.15). Fibrin is a polymer of fibrinogen, a rod-shaped molecule about 460 Å long that cannot escape in bulk unless the endothelium is leaky. In other words, words, the presence of fibrin means that the building block, fibrinogen, must have escaped from leaky blood vessels. Indeed, if enough fibrin has formed, the diagnosis of leaky vessels can be made even with the naked eye.

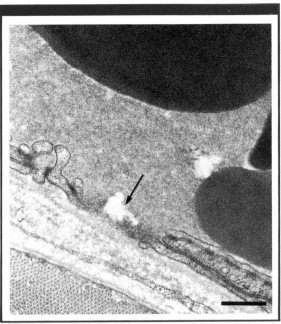

FIGURE 10.14
"Natural" vascular labeling in a man. Part of a venule from a biopsy of striated muscle. **Arrow:** a chylomicron, which lies against the basement membrane in a gap between two endothelial cells. **Bar** = 0.5 μm.

vessels and study them in tissue sections. This approach would be informative, but it could not provide a topographic overview of the changes. Imagine how frustrating it would be to work out the damage in the wires of a telephone exchange by studying a cross section of the whole system. It would make more sense to leave the damaged wires intact and to examine them in their proper context. The same is true for the circulatory network: damaged (and especially labeled) vessels are best studied either in living, transparent tissues, or in fixed tissues examined as a whole after they have been made transparent by glycerin. Several of our illustrations (Figures 10.13, 10.16, 10.17, 10.20) were obtained by photographing a thin striated muscle cleared in glycerin; in this manner arterioles, capillaries and venules are easily identified.

The method: In the rat, each testicle is contained in a thin bag of striated muscle, the cremaster, which is continuous with the abdominal internal oblique muscle. An inflammatory mediator injected into the skin of the scrotum diffuses into the cremaster; carbon black (biological India ink) is then injected intravenously, and leaky vessels in the cremaster become labeled. Because the carbon black is cleared very quickly from the blood stream (thanks to the littoral phagocytes, p. 299) vascular labeling can occur only within the first 1–2 minutes after the intravenous injection. The cremaster is then excised, fixed, cleared in glycerin, and examined by transillumination (42).

TYPES OF VASCULAR LEAKAGE

So far we have established, by bluing and vascular labeling, that inflammation entails microvascular leakage. But which vessels are involved, and why do they leak?

To answer these questions experimentally, the conventional approach would be to challenge a vascularized tissue in several ways, then to label the

FIGURE 10.15
Deposition of fibrin (**F**) in acutely inflamed, edematous connective tissue. **C:** Collagen. **Arrows:** Scattered inflammatory cells. The structural patterns are adequate for distinguishing collagen (thick, wavy bundles) from fibrin (fine meshwork); special stains could distinguish them also by color. **Bar** = 50 μm.

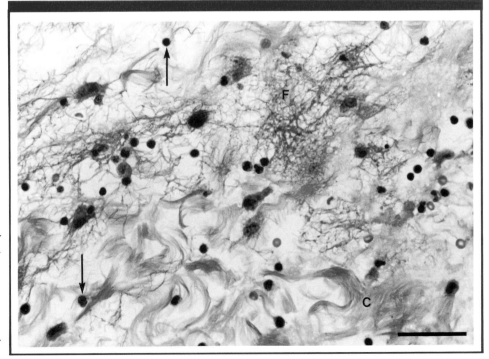

This approach demonstrates at least three mechanisms of microvascular leakage: *leakage by direct injury, histamine-type leakage,* and *late capillary leakage.*

1) Leakage by Direct Injury of Vessels This is self explanatory: a crude physical or toxic insult destroys endothelial cells in all types of vessels: arterioles, capillaries, and venules. The escape of fluid begins immediately and continues until the vessels are repaired or plugged, which takes about one day.

This sequence is easily demonstrated. In an anesthetized rat, we inject subcutaneously in the scrotum a drop of a locally injurious agent, such as acetone. Ten minutes later, by which time vascular damage has occurred, we inject carbon black intravenously to label the vessels that are leaking at that time; an hour later we sacrifice the rat, and examine the underside of the skin at the injected site, as well as the underlying cremaster. Result: *all types of vessels are labeled: arterioles, capillaries and venules* (39) (Figure 10.16). Electron microscopy of all the labeled vessels shows dying or dead endothelial cells breaking up over an intact basement membrane (7). Over the next day or two, these vessels will be lined by new cells gliding along the basement membrane; failing this, the damaged vessels will be plugged by platelets and "condemned."

Note: direct injury, if severe, causes vessels to leak immediately; however, if it is mild, the cellular damage to the endothelium may take some time to develop and the affected vessels may not leak until several hours later (the sunburn is a classic example). We will discuss this phenomenon shortly.

2) Leakage Induced by Histamine-Type Mediators. This variety of leakage is also immediate; it is induced by a group of mediators that are preformed in the tissues (such as histamine) or produced within the first minute or so (bradykinin, PAF, leukotrienes). Although these mediators belong to entirely different chemical families, their mode of action is shared: if we inject a permeability-increasing mediator of this group into the skin, and label the leaky vessels with carbon black, we find that *vascular leakage is restricted almost exclusively to the venules.* The specificity of these mediators for the venules is striking (Figures 10.13, 10.18); the capillaries and arterioles are spared (Figure 10.18). The leakage persists for 20–30 minutes. We refer to this mechanism as *histamine-type vascular leakage* (42).

This specificity of histamine for the venules demolishes a dogma at least 60 years old, whereby histamine was supposed to increase *capillary* permeability (54). Physiologists, with notable exceptions (20), have been slow in accepting this singular behavior of the venules. Many continue to speak of the "capillary effect" of histamine, even though the astonishing fact is that *capillaries are specifically spared* not only by histamine but also by other mediators that have been tested: serotonin, bradykinin, PAF, and LTE_4 (reviewed in [31]). To this day, *we do not know a single physiologic chemical mediator that can immediately increase or modify capillary permeability.*

Why are the Capillaries Spared? We can only answer that nature must have some good reasons for protecting the capillary from histamine-type mediators, but we do not know them. We did once speculate that leaky capillaries would soon become clogged with blood cells; however, this line of reasoning collapsed when we realized that Nature had in store a planned variety of capillary leakage (see next section). The reverse question, "how are the venules selected?" is easier to answer: using histamine complexed with ferritin (which is visible by electron microscopy), Heltianu et al. (19) showed that venular endothelium has more histamine receptors than endothelium in other parts of the microvascular tree.

Mechanism of Venular Leakage Minutes after the local injection of a mediator, transmission electron microscopy shows small gaps here and there between endothelial cells of the venules; the gaps are only 1–2 μm in diameter, as if two endothelial cells had pulled apart and become disconnected at one limited spot (Figures 10.18, 10.19) (31, 41). Some gaps are plugged by a platelet, others by a red blood cell that has been sucked in by the escaping plasma. In so doing, the red blood cells demonstrate their extraordinary plasticity: whereas in blood smears they look deceptively like stiff little coins, in reality they behave much more like "plastic bags filled with syrup" (we owe this analogy to the late Dr. Eugene M. Landis, the first physiologist to measure capillary pressure). It is not unusual to see a single red blood cell sucked into two adjacent gaps, presumably about to be torn apart.

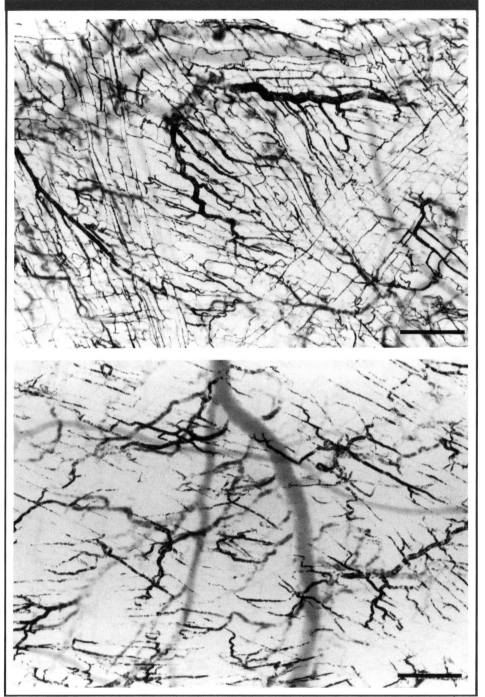

FIGURE 10.16
Illustration of the contrast between direct vascular injury and histamine-induced vascular leakage. Preparations of cremaster muscle seen by transillumination. *Top:* Cremaster muscle labeled with carbon black immediately after a local injection of acetone, which caused direct vascular injury. The labeling pattern shows that virtually all the blood vessels—arterioles, venules, and capillaries—have become leaky. *Bottom:* Vascular labeling with carbon black immediately after a local injection of histamine. Leaky vessels are shown in black. From their branching structure it is obvious that they are venules. **Bars** = 500 μm.

If the same venule is challenged twice at an interval of 20–40 minutes, as can be done in a living preparation under the microscope, gaps seem to develop each time in the same places *(15).*

How do the gaps develop? Electron microscopy shows that the cells on either side of a gap bulge into the lumen, and their nucleus shows unusual, tight infoldings (Figure 10.19). This is strong evidence of cellular contraction. Whenever a contractile cell shortens (be it striated muscle, myocardium, or other), its nucleus is thrown into folds rather like an accordion (31, 43). We can therefore conclude that *venular gaps develop because adjacent endothelial cells contract and pull apart* at a limited point. This behavior has been confirmed *in vitro,* for instance by exposing endothelial cells to histamine and thrombin (2, 35,

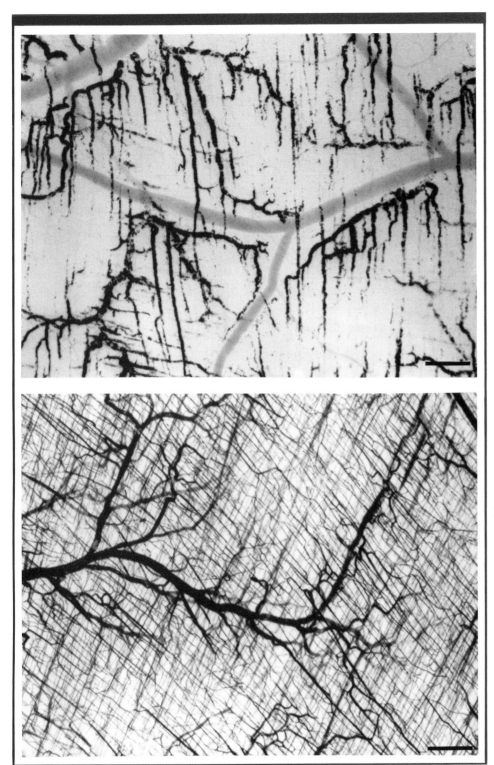

FIGURE 10.17
Two rat cremasters shown at the same enlargement, demonstrating that a vast number of vessels (capillaries) are not caused to leak with histamine-type mediators. *Top:* Black, branching structures are labeled venules, 1 hour after a local injection of serotonin and an intravenous injection of carbon black. *Bottom:* Cremaster of normal rat, in which the entire vasculature has been injected with a mixture of carbon black and gelatin. By comparing this photograph with the top one, we can see that most vessels are not induced to leak. **Bars** = 250 μm. (Reproduced with permission from [41].)

36). Correspondingly, *some drugs that inhibit leakage are also inhibitors of smooth muscle contraction (31)*.

An alternative explanation of the endothelial gaps has been proposed: the mechanism could be a contraction of the pericytes (46). Proof of this hypothesis is lacking, whereas there is overwhelming proof of endothelial contraction, both in vivo (32) and in vitro (2).

3) Late Capillary Leakage This type of leakage begins to occur 12–18 hours after the challenge;

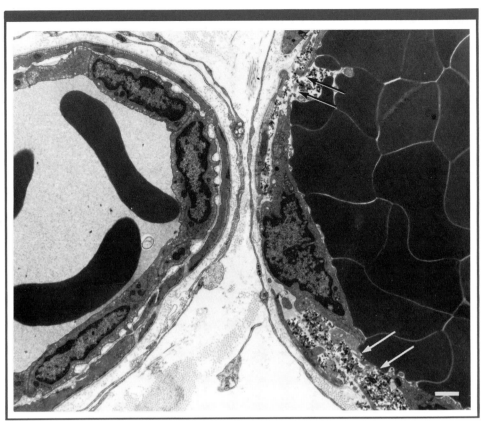

FIGURE 10.18
Arteriole (left) and venule (right) of a guinea pig 12 minutes after a local injection of histamine and an intravenous injection of carbon black. In the venule, two endothelial gaps have developed (**arrows**); escaping carbon particles are trapped in the venular wall. Because plasma has leaked out, the red blood cells are compacted ("stasis"). Note the contrast with the arteriole, whose endothelium did not become leaky: the arteriolar lumen contains a normal amount of plasma. **Bar** = 1 μm.

typically, *it occurs in a focus of inflammation that persists long enough.* It affects specifically the capillaries, and ceases—as far as we know today—within 72 hours of the stimulus.

This form of vascular leakage was observed recently, in a study of inflammation around dead tissue (28). We undertook this study because most of the previous work on vascular leakage had focussed on the immediate effect of *purified mediators* injected into the skin—an experimentally clean but biologically very unnatural situation. What type of leakage would occur in a "dirty" but natural situation, such as inflammation around an infarct?

To find the answer, we turned once again to the rat. We placed a striated muscle in contact with a piece of dying tissue (such as rat liver). Then we injected carbon black i.v. to label leaky vessels at varying time periods. Up to 3–4 hours the muscle showed venular leakage, as expected. But after 12–18 hours, more and more capillaries were found to leak, and by 48 hours the leakage was almost purely capillary (Figure 10.20); after that point it ceased abruptly.

This capillary leakage was mystifying, because none of the histamine-type mediators that in-

crease vascular permeability is known to affect the capillaries. Besides, electron micrographs of the leaky capillaries showed no evidence of endothelial contraction; the endothelial cells looked merely plump and "activated". Even more mystifying was the observation that the increased capillary permeability could not be due to materials leaching out of the dead tissue, because it occurred also in inflammatory reactions set up by sterile glass or teflon beads. We concluded that *the capillary leakage is brought about by the persisting inflammatory response,* not by the initial injury.

This chain of events is not entirely understood, but cytokines, especially IL-1, TNF- and IFN-gamma, seem to be a part of the answer. Experiments on cultured endothelial cells have shown that several cytokines rearrange the cytoskeleton in such a way that the endothelial sheet suffers a long-lasting increase in permeability (51, 52, 56). We can therefore postulate the following sequence: injury → inflammation → macrophage activation → secretion of cytokines → endothelial activation → vascular leakage. *The delay of the "late" vascular leakage may be due to the time it takes for macrophage and endothelial activation.* Endotoxin injected into the skin increases *capillary*

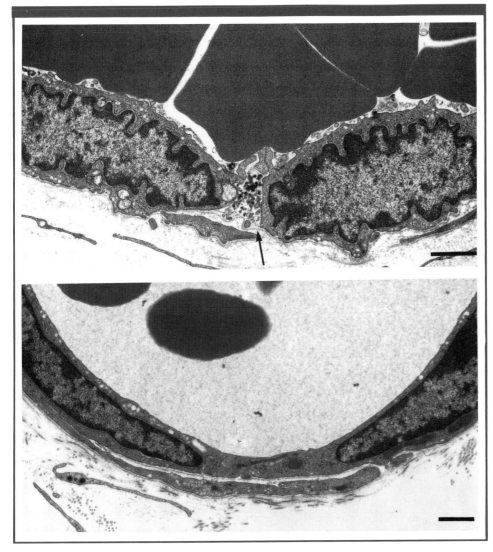

FIGURE 10.19

Top: Venule in the abdominal muscle of a guinea pig, 11 minutes after an intradermal injection of LTE$_4$ and an intravenous injection of carbon black. Endothelial contraction has caused the cells to become thicker and the nuclear membranes to fold. Between the endothelial cells is a gap filled with carbon particles. **Arrow:** Basement membrane. Note the packed red blood cells in the lumen, a consequence of plasma loss. *Bottom:* Wall of a normal venule in the abdominal muscle of a guinea pig. **Bars** = 1 μm. (Reproduced with permission from [31].)

permeability with a delay of about 8 hours (62); endotoxin is a powerful inducer of cytokine synthesis by macrophages.

There is no doubt that endothelial activation leads to endothelial leakage (11, 12) and that several cytokines are involved (52). In fact, the intravenous injection of IL-2 induces a generalized "capillary leak syndrome" (p. 892). However. we still cannot understand why the leakage should concern specifically the capillaries. Our current hypothesis is that persistent hyperemia causes the capillaries to expand and to become leaky in the process (29).

THE TIME-COURSE OF VASCULAR LEAKAGE

Inflammation can last as long as years. Over such a lengthy period, vascular leakage is sustained by several mechanisms; physicians need to know them because several can be opposed by specific drugs

(Figure 10.21). To the naked eye—in rats as well as in people—vascular leakage in a given lesion appears to be a continuum; there is no evidence of successive phases. However, to visualize the mechanisms that might be operative at any given time, the following facts should be kept in mind:

- *Direct injury* causes leakage that starts immediately and continues until the damaged vessels are repaired or closed. In some infections, a steady release of bacterial products may continue to damage the vessels until the infection is overcome.
- *Histamine-type mediators* are released in the earliest phases: mast cell histamine at time zero, platelet serotonin shortly thereafter, while PAF and leukotrienes are secreted mainly from leukocyte membranes.
- *Cytokines* (especially IL-1, TNF- and IFN-

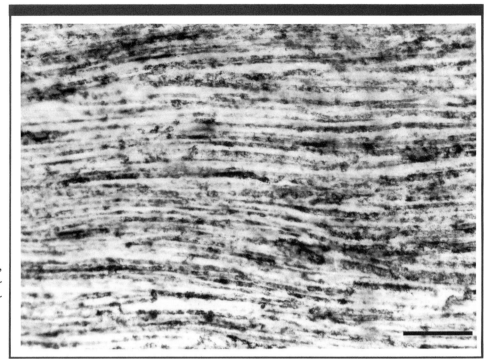

FIGURE 10.20
Late capillary leakage in aseptic inflammation: cremaster muscle of a rat, 48-hour stage. The leaky vessels, labeled with carbon black, form a pattern of parallel lines: in striated muscles the capillaries run primarily along the muscle fibers, hence this parallel pattern indicates capillary leakage. **Bar** = 500 μm.

gamma) intervene as soon as they can be secreted by activated cells, possibly as early as 2 hours, certainly within 6–12 hours (52).

- *Neutrophils* contribute to maintain vascular leakage as long as they are present, as can be demonstrated in neutrophil-depleted animals (62).
- *Vasodilatation by prostaglandins* increases blood flow and therefore tends to exaggerate vascular leakage due to any mechanism.
- *Leaky sprouts of regenerating vessels* contrib-

ute their share of leakage in chronic inflammation (p. 431). Exception: in some allergic reactions involving mast cell degranulation a "second wave" of inflammation is clinically well known; it is probably due to the activation of proteases contained in the spilled mast cell granules (p. 517).

How long does the leakage last? Basically, as long as there are gaps in the endothelium. On a free surface such as the skin the loss of fluid may continue indefinitely, but whenever inflammation

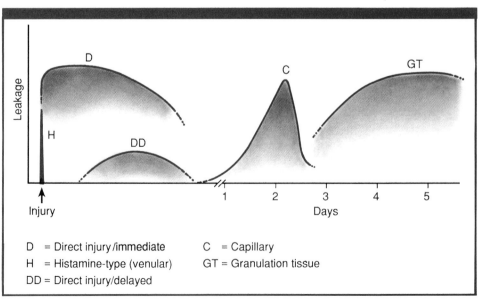

FIGURE 10.21
Five possible sources of vascular leakage in a focus of inflammation lasting several days. Immediately after the injury, there is a short burst of histamine-type leakage (**H**) superimposed on the fluid loss from direct vascular injury (**D**). Some types of injury are followed by a delayed manifestation of direct injury (**DD**). A phase of capillary leakage follows (**C**), possibly due to cytokines. Last, when granulation tissue develops (**GT**), its leaky capillaries contribute fluid to the exudate.

D = Direct injury/immediate
H = Histamine-type (venular)
DD = Direct injury/delayed

C = Capillary
GT = Granulation tissue

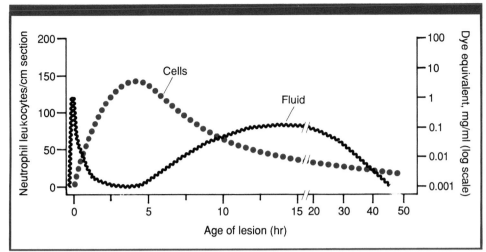

FIGURE 10.22
Example of "delayed capillary leakage:" biphasic fluid exudation (**wavy line**) obtained by painting xylene on guinea pig skin; chloroform, benzene, and many other irritants have a similar effect. Note that the neutrophil response (**dotted line**) follows a different curve. (Adapted from [55].)

occurs in a closed space such as a joint or deep within the body *a limiting factor is tissue pressure,* which increases until it equilibrates with the blood pressure in the microcirculation (p. 417). This is why inflammation causes much more swelling where the skin is loose, as in the eyelid.

THE CASE OF THE SUNBURN (DELAYED CAPILLARY LEAKAGE DUE TO MILD DIRECT INJURY)

In experimental animals, if a mild injury is produced in the skin, and the ensuing leakage is studied by the "bluing" method, it is often found that the leakage is biphasic (61) (Figure 10.22). This applies to injuries produced by ultraviolet light, X rays, mild heat (7, 9, 53), toxins (8, 24), infection, and a variety of chemicals (10). Even a triphasic course has been observed (61). The late phase usually begins after 2–3 hours or longer, and lasts a few hours. It can even develop without an apparent early phase: everyone knows that *overexposure to the sun during the morning is followed by a sunburn at night.* In some cases the leaky vessels were studied and turned out to be capillaries (9, 24).

What is the pathogenesis of this so-called "delayed-prolonged" vascular leakage? It is probably *not* related to chemical mediators, and certainly not to histamine, because anti-histamines have no effect; PAF does induce a biphasic

leakage, but it takes place within the time span of one hour (21). Electron microscopy shows no sign of endothelial contraction, but it does show evidence of endothelial damage (7, 8). The most likely conclusion (58) is that this form of delayed leakage represents *a slow-developing form of direct injury* (23), e.g., by sunlight in sunburns. If this is true, then this "delayed capillary leakage" is probably not related to the "late capillary leakage" that we observed after 12–48 hours.

TO SUM UP: Vascular leakage is a central feature of inflammation. It is necessary, because the fluid has many useful features (to be discussed later). Some of the leakage is part of the injury and therefore accidental; some is purposeful, as part of the inflammatory reaction, and caused by several mechanisms of which the best understood is endothelial contraction in the venules. Whether the later, cytokine-related phase of capillary leakage is only incidental to endothelial activation—or "purposeful"—we do not know. To close, we would like to share with the reader an admirable example of natural economy. It once seemed quite mysterious that a single molecule such as histamine could have two effects as different as *smooth muscle contraction* and *increased vascular permeability.* Now we realize that they are obtained by one and the same mechanism: cellular contraction.

References

1. Barnes PJ. Asthma as an axon reflex. Lancet 1986;1: 242–245.
1a. Berhard, JD (ed.), Itch: Mechanisms and management of pruritus. McGraw-Hill, Inc. 1994.
2. Boswell CA, Joris I, Majno G. The concept of cellular

tone: reflections on the endothelium, fibroblasts and smooth muscle cells. Perspect Biol Med 1992.
3. Burnstock G. Autonomic neuroeffector junctions — reflex vasodilatation of the skin. J Invest Dermatol 1977;69:47–57.

4. Cohnheim J. Über Éntuzündung und Eiterung. Virchows Arch Pathol Ana Physiol Klin Med 1867;40:1–79.

5. Cohnheim J. Neue Úntersuchungen über die Entzündung. Berlin: A. Hirschwald, 1873.

6. Cohnheim J. Lectures on general pathology, vol. 1 (translated from the 2nd German edition). London: New Sydenham Society, 1889:248.

7. Cotran RS. The delayed and prolonged vascular leakage in inflammation. II. An electron microscopic study of the vascular response after thermal injury. Am J Pathol 1965;46:589–620.

8. Cotran RS. Studies on inflammation. Ultrastructure of the prolonged vascular response induced by Clostridium oedematiens toxin. Lab Invest 1967a;17:39–60.

9. Cotran RS. Delayed and prolonged vascular leakage in inflammation. III. Immediate and delayed vascular reactions in skeletal muscle. Exp Mol Pathol 1967b;6:143–155.

10. Cotran RS, Majno G. The delayed and prolonged vascular leakage in inflammation. I. Topography of the leaking vessels after thermal injury. Am J Pathol 1964;45:261–281.

11. Cotran RS, Pober JS. Effects of cytokines on vascular endothelium: their role in vascular and immune injury. Kidney Int 1989;35:969–975.

12. Cotran RS, Pober JS, Gimbrone MA Jr, et al. Endothelial activation during interleukin 2 immunotherapy: a possible mechanism for the vascular leak syndrome. J Immunol 1987;139:1883–1888.

13. Denman T. A review of pruritis. J Am Acad Dermatol 1986 14:375–392.

14. Garcia Leme J. Bradykinin-system. In: Vane JR, Ferreira SH, eds. Inflammation. Berlin: Springer-Verlag, 1978:464–522.

15. Gawlowski DM, Ritter AB, Duran WN. Reproducibility of microvascular permeability responses to successive topical applications of bradykinin in the hamster cheek pouch. Microvasc Res 1982:24:354–363.

16. Ginsburg I, Gallis HA, Cole R.M, Green I. Group A streptococci: localization in rabbits and Guinea pigs following tissue injury. Science 1969;166:1161–1163.

17. Guyton AC. Textbook of medical physiology. Philadelphia: WB Saunders, 1986.

18. Ham KN, Hurley JV, Ryan GB, Storey E. Localization of particulate carbon in metaphyseal vessels of growing rats. Aust J Exp Biol Med Sci 1965;43:625–638.

19. Heltianu C, Simionescu M, Simionescu N. Histamine receptors of the microvascular endothelium revealed in situ with a histamine-ferritin conjugate: characteristic high-affinity binding sites in venules. J Cell Biol 1982;93:357–364.

20. Horan KL, Adamski SW, Ayele W, Langone JJ, Grega GJ. Evidence that prolonged histamine suffusions produce transient increases in vascular permeability subsequent to the formation of venular macromolecular leakage sites. Proof of the Majno-Palade hypothesis. Am J Pathol 1986;123:570–576.

21. Humphrey DM, McManus LM, Satouchi K, Hanahan DJ, Pinckard RN. Vasoactive properties of acetyl glyceryl ether phosphorylcholine and analogues. Lab Invest 1982;46:422–427.

22. Hurley JV. The sequence of early events. In: Vane JR and Ferreira SH, eds. Inflammation. Berlin: Springer-Verlag, 1978: 26–67.

23. Hurley JV, Ham N, Ryan G.B. The mechanism of the delayed prolonged phase of increased vascular permeability in mild thermal injury in the rat. J Pathol Bacteriol 1967;94:1–12.

24. Hurley JV, Jago MV. Delayed and prolonged vascular leakage in inflammation: the effects of dehydromonocrotaline on blood vessels in the rat cremaster. Pathology 1976;8:7–20.

25. Hurley JV, Ryan GB. A delayed prolonged increase in venular permeability following intrapleural injections in the rat. J Pathol Bacteriol 1967;93:87–99.

26. Hurley JV, Spector WG. Delayed leucocytic emigration after intradermal injections and thermal injury. J Pathol Bacteriol 1961;82:421–429.

27. Hutchison KJ, Johnson BW, Williams HTG, Brown GD. The histamine flare response in diabetes mellitus. Surg Gynecol Obstet 1974;139:566–568.

28. Joris I, Cuénoud HF, Doern G.V, Underwood JM, Majno G. Capillary leakage in inflammation. A study by vascular labeling. Am J Pathol 1990;137:1353–1363.

29. Joris I, Cuénoud HF, Underwood JM, Majno G. Capillary remodeling in acute inflammation: a form of angiogenesis. FASEB J 1994;6:A938.

30. Joris I, DeGirolami U, Wortham K, Majno G. Vascular labelling with Monastral blue B. Stain Technol 1982;57:177–183.

31. Joris I, Majno G, Corey EJ, Lewis RA. The mechanism of vascular leakage induced by leukotriene E_4. Endothelial contraction. Am J Pathol 1987;126:19–24.

32. Joris I, Majno G, Ryan GB. Endothelial contraction in vivo: a study of the rat mesentery. Virchows Arch Abt B Zellpath 1972;12:73–83.

33. Judah JD, Willoughby DA. A quantitative method for the study of capillary permeability: extraction and determination of Trypan blue in tissues. J Pathol Bacteriol 1962;83:567–572.

34. Kessler JO, Jarvik LF, Fu TK, Matsuyama SS. Thermotaxis, chemotaxis and age. Age 1979;2:5–11.

35. Killackey JJF, Johnston MG, Movat HZ. Increased permeability of microcarrier-cultured endothelial monolayers in response to histamine and thrombin. Am J Pathol 1986;122:50–61.

36. Laposata M, Dovnarsky DK, Shin HS. Thrombin-induced gap formation in confluent endothelial cell monolayers in vitro. Blood 1983;62:549–556.

37. Lewis PA. The distribution of Trypan-red to the tissues and vessels of the eye as influenced by congestion and early inflammation. J Exp Med 1916;23:669–676.

38. Lewis T. The blood vessels of the human skin and their responses. London: Shaw & Sons, 1927.

39. Majno G. Mechanisms of abnormal vascular permeability in acute inflammation. In: Thomas L, Uhr JW, Grant L, eds. Injury, inflammation and immunity. Baltimore: Williams & Wilkins, 1964:58–93.

40. Majno G. The healing hand. Man and wound in the ancient world. Cambridge: Harvard University Press, 1975.

41. Majno G, Palade GE. Studies on inflammation. I. The effect of histamine and serotonin on vascular permeability: an electron microscopic study. J Biophys Biochem Cytol 1961;11:571–605.

42. Majno G, Palade GE, Schoefl GI. Studies on inflammation. II. The site of action of histamine and serotonin along the vascular tree: a topographic study. J Biophys. Biochem Cytol 1961;11:607–626.

43. Majno G, Shea SM, Leventhal M. Endothelial contraction induced by histamine-type mediators. An electron microscopic study. J Cell Biol 1969;42:647–672.

44. McClellan RH, Goodpasture EW. A method of demonstrating experimental gross lesions of the central nervous system. J Med Res 1923;44:201–206.

45. Menkin V. Studies on inflammation. VII. Fixation of bacteria and of particulate matter at the site of inflammation. J Exp Med 1931;53:647–660.

46. Miller FN, Sims DE. Contractile elements in the regulation of macromolecular permeability. Fed Proc 1986;45:84–88.

47. Moncada S, Ferreira SH, Vane JR. Pain and inflammatory mediators. In: Vane JR, Ferreira SH, eds. Inflammation. Berlin: Springer-Verlag, 1978: 588–616.

48. Movat H.Z. The kinin system and its relation to other systems. Curr Top Pathol 1979;68:111–134.

49. Movat HZ, Cybulsky MI, Colditz IG, William Chan MK, Minarello CA. Acute inflammation in Gram-negative infection: endotoxin interleukin 1, tumor necrosis factor, and neutrophils. FASEB 1987;46:97–104.

50. Orlidge A, D'Amore PA. Inhibition of capillary endothelial cell growth by pericytes and smooth muscle cells. J Cell Biol 1987;105:1455–1462.

51. Pober JS, Cotran RS. Cytokines and endothelial cell biology. Physiol Rev 1990a;70:427–451.

52. Pober JS, Cotran RS. The role of endothelial cells in inflammation. Transplantation 1990b;50:537–544.

52a. Ryan GB, Majno G. Inflammation. A SCOPE monograph. Kalamazoo, Mich.: Upjohn, 1977.

53. Sevitt S. Early and delayed oedema and increase in capillary permeability after burns of the skin. J Pathol Bacteriol 1958;75:27–37.

54. Spector WG. Substances which affect capillary permeability. Pharmacol. Rev., 10:475–505, 1958.

55. Steele R.H, Wilhelm D.L. The inflammatory reaction in chemical injury. III. Leucocytosis and other histological changes induced by superficial injury. Br J Exp Pathol 1970;51:265–279.

56. Stolpen AH, Guinan EC, Fiers W, Pober JS. Recombinant tumor necrosis factor and immune interferon act singly and in combination to reorganize human vascular endothelial cell monolayers. Am J Pathol 1986;123:16–24.

57. Wasi S, Movat H.Z. Phlogistic substances in neutrophil leukocyte lyosomes: their possible role *in vivo* and their *in vitro* properties. Curr Top Pathol 1979;68:213–237.

58. Wells F.R, Miles A.A. Site of the vascular response to thermal injury. Nature, 200:1015–1016, 1963.

59. Westerman RA, Magerl FW, Szolcsanyi J, et al. Vasodilator axon reflexes. In: Vanhoutte, PM, ed. Vasodilatation. New York: Raven Press, 1988: 107–112.

60. Wilhelm DL. Chemical mediators. In: Zweifach BW, Grant L, McCluskey RT, eds. The inflammatory process, vol. II, 2nd ed. New York: Academic Press, 1973a:251–301.

61. Wilhelm D.L. Mechanisms responsible for increased vascular permeability in acute inflammation. Agents Action 1973b;3:297–306.

62. Yi Eunhee S, Ulich Thomas R. Endotoxin, interleukin-1, and tumor necrosis factor cause neutrophildependent microvascular leakage in postcapillary venules. Am J Pathol 1992;140: 659–663.

63. Zimmerman KW. Der feinere Bau der Blutcapillaren. Z Anat Entwicklungsgeschichte 1923;69:29–109.

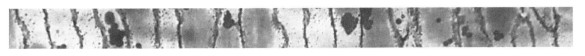

The Leukocyte's Call To Action: Five Steps to Phagocytosis

CHAPTER 11

Chemotaxis

Activation

Margination

Diapedesis

Recognition and Attachment

Phagocytosis

Bacterial Killing: Metabolic Aspects of Phagocytosis

The purpose of inflammation, as we defined it, is to convey fluid and cells to a site of injury. Fluid is delivered first, in a matter of seconds; cells take a little longer (minutes) because they cannot just pour out of the vascular system. Indeed, before a circulating leukocyte can capture a bacterium that is lurking in the tissue spaces, no less than five events must take place: the leukocyte must be summoned to the area of injury by a proper call (*chemotaxis*), and switch to a higher metabolic level (*activation*); then it must stick to the endothelial surface (*margination*), crawl through the endothelium (*diapedesis*), recognize the intruder and become attached to it (*recognition–attachment*). These five steps tend to telescope. Chemotaxis, for example, overlaps with margination: conveniently, some of the chemotaxins also increase the stickiness of the endothelium and/or of the leukocytes so that a trap is added to the call. *Chemotaxis is also coupled with activation*, so that a leukocyte can land upon its prey fully prepared to kill it. For convenience, we will discuss these steps separately.

Chemotaxis

All free cells, from bacteria to amoebae and spermatozoa, have the privilege of moving toward a chemical attractant (chemotaxin) (48, 136, 169, 177, 182). This directional movement is called **chemotaxis.** Bacteria have the extra advantage of **negative chemotaxis:** besides being able to swim toward amino acids and sugars (Figure 11.1) (3, 107), they also can swim *away* from phenol, a disinfectant (1, 90, 156). No example of negative chemotaxis has been proven in mammalian cells; but the ability to answer a call is given also to some cells that are usually fixed (29), including fibroblasts, endothelium, smooth muscle, and tumor cells (p. 797). In inflamed tissues, chemotaxis explains the orderly maneuvers of all cells, free and fixed.

On the broad biological scene, chemotaxis enables free cells to pursue food, to escape danger, or even to meet their sexual counterparts; in fact, chemotaxis was discovered by studying the fertilization of ferns. This is but one of many basic discoveries that cell biology owes to botanists;

FIGURE 11.1
Photomicrograph showing that *Escherichia coli* are attracted by chemical stimuli. The capillary tube contained aspartate (2 ≤ 10^{-3}M). **Bar** = 50 μm. (Reproduced with permission from [128].)

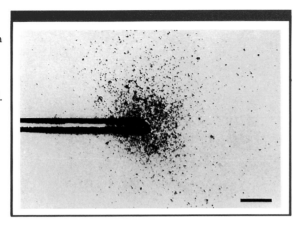

earlier discoveries include the nucleus and the very notion of cell.

> It was 1884 when Wilhelm Pfeffer showed that the antherozoids of the male fern, trapped in a fine glass tube, would migrate toward higher concentrations of malic acid (123, 177). Four years later a German ophthamologist, Theodor Leber, followed the lead and began implanting capillary tubes into the corneas or anterior chambers of rabbit eyes. In those days the cornea was a favorite tool for experimental pathology: as a transparent tissue, easily excised and studied directly under the microscope, it offered better visibility than the thick tissue slices of the time. Leber found that capillary tubes loaded with bacteria or extracts of putrefying tissues attracted leukocytes, and concluded that chemotaxis was the force drawing leukocytes into an inflammatory focus. Metchnikoff, who had just discovered phagocytosis, promptly incorporated this new phenomenon into his own theory of inflammation (108).

The next major advance came almost a century later, in 1962, when it became possible to study chemotaxis quantitatively thanks to a simple, ingenious Australian device: the **Boyden chamber** (Figure 11.2) (23). This is essentially a small vertical plastic cylinder subdivided into an upper and a lower compartment by a filter; the upper chamber is filled with a suspension of leukocytes, the lower with the chemotactic solution to be tested. After 30 minutes at 37°C the filter is removed and examined microscopically: the number of leukocytes that can be counted, either in the thickness of the filter as seen in cross sections or on the lower surface, gives a measure of the chemotactic response (Figure 11.3).

> To use the Boyden chamber properly it is essential to distinguish between chemotaxis and **chemokinesis**. The latter is simply accelerated motion of cells, without any directional preference in response to a chemical stimulus. It can mimic chemotaxis. Suppose that some chemical accelerated the random leukocyte motion in the neighborhood of a leukocyte "trap" such as a porous surface. More leukocytes would end up being trapped simply because they moved around more, even though the porous surface exerted no attraction. The accepted control for this possible artefact when using the Boyden chamber is to mix the chemotaxin with the leukocytes in the upper chamber and count how many cells become trapped in the filter by accelerated random motion. This procedure shows that many chemotaxins are also chemokinetic; after all, chemokinesis could also be beneficial in a focus of inflammation.

Studies *in vitro* show that neutrophils moving up a chemotactic gradient crawl at a speed of about 30 μm per minute, almost 2 mm per hour (182) and in a reasonably straight line (Figure 11.4); monocytes are a little slower (62, 122).

CHEMOTACTIC AGENTS (CHEMOTAXINS)

If we had to guess the sources of leukotactic stimuli, knowing that leukocytes must be summoned into infected lesions, we would probably suggest three appropriate sources: bacterial prod-

FIGURE 11.2
Schematic diagram of the Boyden chamber (*right*) showing two compartments separated by a porous filter (*left*). Migrating cells cross the filter and appear on the underside; they can be quantitated by several methods. (Reproduced with permission from [58].)

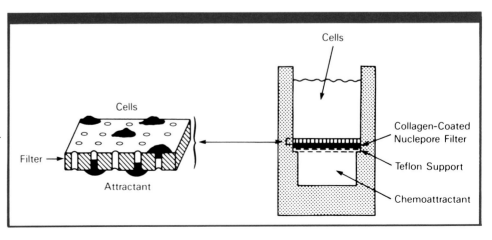

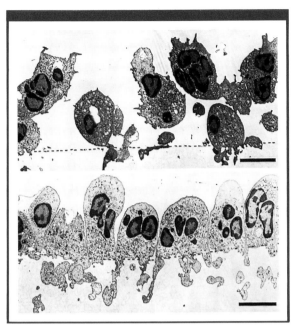

FIGURE 11.3
Behavior of neutrophils on a 0.45 μm pore filter in the Boyden chamber. The surface of the filter is indicated by a dotted line. *Top:* Condition of "activated random migration." A chemotactic agent is present on both sides of the filter in equal concentrations. *Bottom:* Chemotactic agent is present only below the filter. **Bars = 5 μm.** (Reproduced with permission from [101].)

ucts, injured tissues, and spilled blood. All three guesses would be correct.

Most chemotaxins are peptides (95) and attract neutrophils as well as macrophages, but there are examples of specific attraction, especially for eosinophils.

Bacterial chemotaxins The chemotactic effect of pyogenic bacteria is easily seen *in vitro* (Figure 11.4). It is of course suicidal for bacteria to attract leukocytes, but they do it anyway.

There may be an evolutionary explanation for the apparent indifference of bacteria to being eaten by leukocytes. The metabolic pathways of bacteria originated about 3.6 billion years ago; multicellular creatures appeared only 700 million years ago (55). The exposure of bacteria to vertebrate leukocytes is therefore a late and, overall, rare event: death by exposure to leukocytes does not make a dent in any bacterial population.

The story of bacterial chemotaxins includes two highlights: endotoxin and f-Met-Leu-Phe (fMLP), which we have already encountered as an exoge-

nous mediator of inflammation. **Endotoxin** is a lipopolysaccharide (LPS) built into the outer membrane of gram-negative bacteria. We will have a great deal more to say about it because it is a major factor in the pathogenesis of shock by gram-negative sepsis (p. 700). *An extraordinary feature of this complex molecule is that it is biologically pernicious, potent in picogram doses, and yet it is barely toxic.* It may not even deserve its name. According to the facts now available, it induces macrophages and other cells to produce large amounts of cytokines such as tumor necrosis factor (TNF) and interleukin-1 (IL-1). It is the cytokines that are responsible for the adverse biological effects.

Endotoxin does have two direct biological effects, but they cannot really be called "toxic": it activates the alternative pathway of complement (109a) and the coagulation cascade (52, 165).

One of the indirect effects of endotoxin is chemotaxis (32, 37). An intracutaneous injection of endotoxin causes an influx of neutrophils with a peak at 2 hours, a little later than after an injection of TNF or IL-1, presumably because the endotoxin effect requires two steps: stimulation of macrophages and secretion of TNF and IL-1.

Studies of bacterial chemotaxins have been very fruitful and have led to the discovery of the prototype chemoattractant, f-Met-Leu-Phe. The potency of various chemotaxins is compared in Figure 11.5.

Cultures of growing E. coli *are powerfully chemotactic with regard to leukocytes; the attraction*

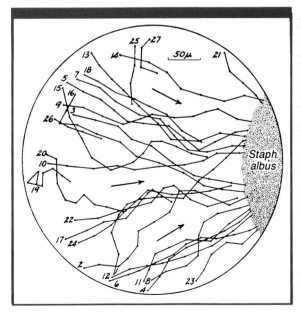

FIGURE 11.4
Microscopic field showing that leukocytes are attracted by a mass of staphylococci. The starting points of 27 leukocytes are indicated by numbers. Most of the cells head directly toward the staphylococci; after 30 minutes 17 had made contact. (Reproduced with permission from [105].)

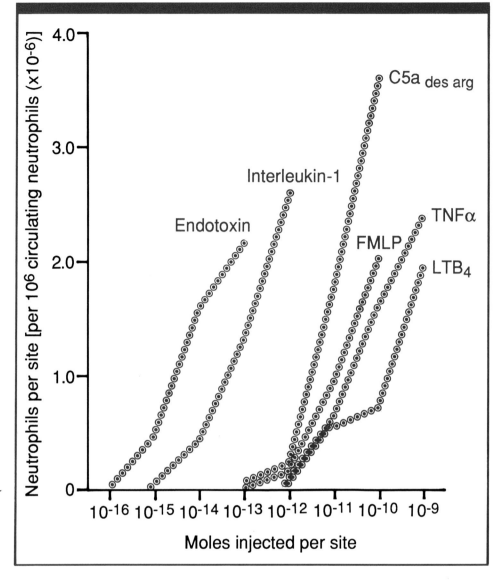

FIGURE 11.5
Effectiveness of six inflammatory agents in causing neutrophil emigration into rabbit skin. Endotoxin is considerably more powerful than leukotriene B_4 or the complement-derived chemotaxin C5a des Arg. (Adapted from [110].)

was found to depend on a mixture of relatively small polypeptides (137). Following this lead, it has been possible to pinpoint the chemical structure of these peptides that is critical for chemotaxis, and thus to synthesize dozens of chemotactic di-, tri-, and tetrapeptides. Today the most widely used chemotactic peptide is the potent fMLP or f-Met-Leu-Phe, active even in dilutions of 10^{-11} (14). Hundreds of similar peptides are now commercially available for experimental purposes.

Phagocytes have membrane receptors that are specific for fMLP and other chemotaxins (143). A huge reserve of chemotactic receptors is stored in the membranes of the so-called specific granules of the neutrophils (Figure 11.6) (49). When these granules fuse with the plasma membrane of the neutrophil, the chemotactic response is enhanced because the cell surface is then equipped with many more receptors.

As mentioned earlier, the characteristic structure of fMLP and its relatives exists for a reason: prokaryotic cells initiate protein synthesis with formyl-methionyl t-RNA (in contrast to the methionyl-tRNA of eukaryotic cells); thus, the attractants produced by growing E. coli can be interpreted as the N-formylated peptides released from newly synthesized protein by an expanding bacterial population (136). Obviously the leukocytes have evolved an ability to recognize this telltale signal: the smell of an active bacterium.

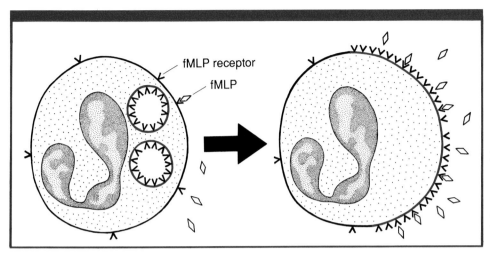

FIGURE 11.6
Illustrating how receptors stored on the inner surface of leukocyte granules can be transferred to the surface of the cell and increase its responsiveness to a chemotactic stimulus. (Adapted from [50].)

Chemotaxins derived from clotted blood Fresh blood, of course, is not chemotactic; but when it clots, it sends out three sets of chemotaxins. Clotting will be explained in detail later, but for now we can say that a clot is formed when red blood cells become trapped in a mesh of fibrin, which is an insoluble protein. Fibrin develops as follows: a cascade of plasma enzymes is activated, leading to the formation of the enzyme *thrombin;* thrombin attacks a plasma protein called *fibrinogen,* snipping off four peptides, whereby fibrinogen is converted into a molecule that self-aggregates into filaments of *fibrin.* All three of the molecules just mentioned are related to chemotaxis:

- thrombin itself is a potent chemoattractant for monocytes (13);

- one of the peptides that thrombin cleaves off fibrinogen is yet another chemotaxin;

- eventually fibrin is broken down by another proteolytic enzyme, *plasmin,* and the so-called *fibrin split products* are chemotactic.

This list of clot-derived chemotaxins could be longer, but the point is that *clotting blood attracts leukocytes.*

> It was found long ago that if fibrin is digested with trypsin in vitro, *a fraction of the resulting peptides—containing 5–14 amino-acid residues—is chemotactic (145); and it is likely that similar fibrin fragments are produced in vivo.*

Chemotaxins derived from complement As we have seen, the activation of complement releases a number of proinflammatory by-products. These include chemotactic molecules—namely, small fragments of C3, C4, and especially C5—another wonderful arrangement, because complement alone is ineffective against many thick-walled bacteria. Calling in the leukocytes is good strategy.

Complement chemotaxins can be produced even if complement is not activated: C3, C4 and C5 can be cleaved nonspecifically by a variety of other proteolytic enzymes that are always available in a focus of inflammation (plasmin from the fibrinolytic cascade, proteases from lysosomes of injured tissues, and leukocytic enzymes) (54). The result of this nonspecific cleavage of C3, C4, and C5 is a soup of chemotactic peptides (66, 67, 169).

Chemotaxins secreted by live cells When duly stimulated, leukocytes secrete chemotactic polypeptides (cytokines and chemokines [p. 349]). The most versatile cells are the lymphocytes, which can produce lymphokines chemotactic for at least six types of cells, including basophils and fibroblasts (136). Eventually it may turn out that any inflammatory cell, when properly stimulated, can summon any other by means of chemotactic messages.

For example, when alveolar macrophages ingest bacteria or particles, they summon neutrophils (47); when neutrophils are busy ingesting foreign material such as crystals of monosodium urate in a gouty joint, they summon other neutrophils (143).

A powerful lipid chemotaxin is also produced by stimulated cells: leukotriene B_4 (Figure 9.36).

Chemotaxins derived from injured tissues The partial digestion of interstitial materials such as collagen (126), elastin (140), and fibronectin (114) generates chemotaxins—another helpful arrangement, because it means that products of interstitial damage can summon leukocytes.

The chemotactic effect of dying or dead cells is a simple story in retrospect, but for a time it was utterly confusing. It is perfectly obvious *in vivo* that leukocytes rush toward dead tissue and crawl into it as far as they can (Figures 8.24 and 8.25). The confusion began when the chemotactic effect was sought *in vitro*. We will present the reader with the puzzle as it originated in 1953.

> *An eminent scientist (62) published a paper showing that dead tissue was not chemotactic in vitro. His test objects were liver and muscle autolyzed aseptically for 3–24 hours. He concluded that chemotaxis could not play much of a role in disease, and so interest in chemotaxis sagged for a while (167). Then a French hematologist, Marcel Bessis, showed very dramatically that when a single leukocyte was killed under the microscope by a laser beam, other leukocytes converged on it "like sharks . . . upon one of their number which has blood escaping from a wound" (18, 178). Bessis actually coined the term necrotaxis. How can these opposite findings be reconciled?*

The answer: *WHILE* cells are dying, they release or produce chemotaxins; but when this terminal outburst is over, no more messages are sent and so the necrotic lump ceases to attract the "sharks" (p.440) (99). Today nobody really doubts that dying and dead cells liberate "necrotaxins" and other inflammatory mediators, although the chemical nature of these messages (polypeptides?) has not been investigated. It is in fact an axiom of general pathology that *dying tissue in vivo elicits an intense, transient, acute inflammatory reaction.* The mechanisms are many (p. 437).

> **Sundry chemotaxins** *(177). It was an ancient custom to dress wounds with flour, and in modern times it turns out that starch is chemotactic. Perhaps the starch granules in flour helped by attracting more leukocytes. Other chemotaxins include PDGF,* **lectins** *(32), exogenous* **cyclic AMP** *(169), and, oddly enough,* **neuropeptides** *such as beta-endorphin and mood-modifying drugs such as the benzodiazepines (valium). Why would mono-cytes have receptors for valium? Could they really represent a link in a "psycho-immuno-endocrine network altering the behavior of the whole organism" (129)?*

MECHANISMS OF CHEMOTAXIS

How can a cell, small as it is, recognize a chemical gradient in its medium? In theory, there should be two possibilities (183): a cell might be able to compare concentrations of a substance at two points in time, in quick succession, which would require some sort of memory (*temporal mechanism*); or it might be able to compare concentrations along two points of its own surface (*spatial mechanism*) (Figure 11.7).

Flagellated bacteria are thought to use the

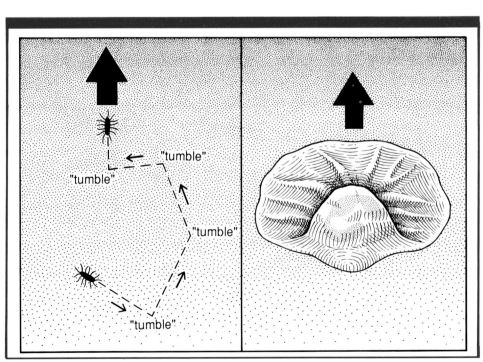

FIGURE 11.7
Two mechanisms of chemotaxis. *Left:* Motile bacteria move about by short, seemingly random "darts" interrupted by "tumbles". They advance along a gradient by prolonging the darts in the favorable direction, as if they had a memory of the concentration from which they have last moved. *Right:* Responsive eukaryotic cells move toward a favorable stimulus because they can sense the gradient of that stimulus along their body.

temporal mechanism. They swim in a zigzag fashion: short straight runs interrupted by "tumbles" when at which point they change direction randomly. When submitted to a chemical gradient, creating a choice between a "favorable" and "unfavorable" direction, they continue to swim and tumble in random fashion—but they prolong the straight runs in the favorable direction. The net effect is movement in the favorable direction. This means that the chemical change on the surface of the bacterium somehow translates into longer bursts of swimming up or down the gradient (90, 98, 156).

Leukocytes are thought to use the spatial mechanism. This would mean that they are able to recognize a 1 percent concentration gradient along the 10 μm of their own bodies (38, 89).

Other Kinds of Directional Stimuli   Chemotaxis means only that cells can answer the call of chemical stimuli; they also take physical clues. The term **haptotaxis** was coined to describe their ability to move toward surfaces that offer greater adhesion (27) (*hapto* is Greek for "I fasten"). **Thermotaxis** can be demonstrated with leukocytes *in vitro*; they tend to move toward a source of heat (45, 78, 86). Little is known about the relevance of this phenomenon to pathology. Parasitic worms display thermotaxis, which may play a role in host–worm relations (109).

Negative Chemotaxis Although there are no accepted examples of leukocyte repulsion regarding mammalian cells, there are inhibitors of chemotaxis. Plasma and serum usually contain several factors that deactivate either the leukocytes or the chemotaxins (159). For example, chemotactic factor inactivator (CFI) (74) and cell-directed inhibitor (CDI), present in normal serum, increased in 70 percent of patients with malignant tumors, resulting in a leukotactic defect (169). Another endogenous inhibitor is prostaglandin A_1 (127).

Activation

A cell responding to a chemotactic stimulus is "turned on" in many more ways than directed motion (143). Within less than 5 seconds after the chemotaxins have bound to the cell's surface receptors, Ca^{2+} and Na^+ rush in and the concentration of cAMP rises, while cytosolic pH drops; the

cell swells, reorganizes its cytoskeleton, assuming a roughly triangular shape, and becomes polarized in the direction of the stimulus (Figure 11.8). In 5–10 seconds it begins to send out pseudopodia or a lamellipodium (Figure 11.9), in which Ca^{2+} reaches its highest concentration (133), and the chemotactic receptors begin to cluster at the front end (49). Superoxide is also generated from the cell's outer membrane while arachidonic acid is released.

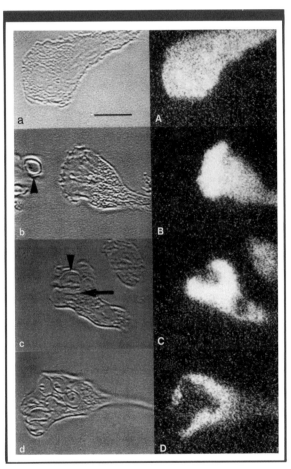

FIGURE 11.8
Displacements of intracellular free calcium in a human neutrophil during chemotaxis and phagocytosis. **a:** Unstimulated neutrophil that is already polarized (it has a head and a tail). **A:** Calcium distribution in the same neutrophil: white areas represent the highest concentration. **b:** Neutrophil migrating toward an opsonized zymosan particle (**arrowhead**). **B:** Calcium distribution in the same cell. Calcium is migrating to the lamellipodium. **c:** Neutrophil engulfing a zymosan particle. **C:** Calcium distribution. **d, D:** Neutrophil that has ingested several zymosan particles. High regional calcium appears to be important for oxidative metabolism, chemotaxis, phagocytosis, and degranulation. **Bar** = 10 μm. (Reproduced with permission from [133].)

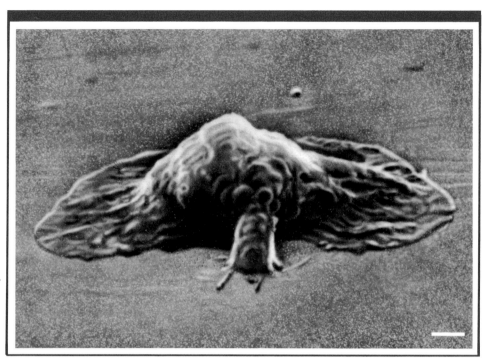

FIGURE 11.9
Scanning electron micrograph of a granulocyte moving away from the observer on a glass surface. Notice the tail end (uropod) and the extremely thin, advancing lamellipodium. **Bar** = 1 μm. (Reproduced with permission from [19].)

The biochemical mechanism of leukocyte activation is partly worked out. When the receptor for the chemotaxin is occupied, phospholipase C is activated by a G protein to produce IP$_3$ and diacylglycerol; PIP$_2$ hydrolysis leads to increased membrane permeability to calcium (144).

This burst of hyperactivity is short-lived: degranulation and superoxide production do not persist beyond 2–5 minutes and the same is true for increased intracellular Ca^{2+} and cAMP (144). How this shutdown occurs is not entirely clear. Chemotaxins, like all mediators, are quickly inactivated; it is also well established that after prolonged exposure to high concentrations of chemotaxins the leukocytes cease to respond (**deactivation**) (182).

A curious feature of activated leukocytes is that they also become "stickier," probably because of the observed loss of surface negative charges. This may make it easier for them to crawl ahead in their slippery environment. The stickiness is also manifested toward other leukocytes as a tendency to aggregate (70) (Figure 11.10). Therefore, *agents that activate neutrophils also cause neutropenia when injected intravenously (61)*, obviously because the clumps of leukocytes are trapped in the lungs. Does this have a survival value? We suspect that leukocyte aggregation has some profound meaning, but it escapes us. A similar phenomenon can be observed in the starfish: a clumping of this creature's amoebocytes is a standard reaction to injury (Figure 11.11).

Margination

Given the existence of signals (chemotaxins) summoning the leukocytes out into the tissues, how do these signals work? The leukocytes are circulating at high speed, and can perceive the call for only a second or two as they whiz through the microcirculation. Nature's answer is to make them stick to the walls of venules. After they are thus trapped, they can come to a full stop, pay heed to the chemotactic call, and crawl out of the vessel. This process is called *margination* because the leukocytes (*in vivo* and in tissue sections) assume marginal positions in the vessels.

LEAVING THE MAINSTREAM

The stratagem of summoning the cells by making them stickier is wonderful, but one can argue that it should not work: the leukocytes are the largest formed elements of the blood; as such they should be carried along in midstream (42, 113), where stickiness would have no effect. This "sorting" rule applies to the gravel in mountain streams: larger stones come to lie in the middle of the bed, smaller pebbles pile up on the shores. However, biophysicists who explored the microcirculation found an answer: several mechanisms conspire to force the leukocytes against the walls of the venules. The four principal mechanisms can be summarized as follows.

- *In the smallest venules, where cells have just emerged from capillaries, special flow conditions prevail* (Figure 11.12). There the large, spherical leukocytes tend to advance more slowly than the smaller, disc-shaped red blood cells; as the red blood cells overtake and pass by the leukocytes, they tend to push them to the sides (139).

- *Whenever a capillary feeds into the side of a venule,* like a tributary into a river, *the cells in the capillary blood are swept by laminar flow along the wall of the venule* (Figure 11.12).

- *In low-flow conditions, red blood cells tend to aggregrate and form rouleaux.* Now rouleaux become the largest elements of the blood, so they occupy the center of the stream and push the leukocytes to the side (Figures 11.12, 11.13) (113). If inflammation persists long enough to trigger an increased erythrocyte sedimentation rate (p. 492), the tendency to form rouleaux is much increased.

- *As wall shear stress decreases* (as should happen in the venules), models show that *the leukocytes tend to move away from the center and toward the periphery* (113).

ROLLING AND STICKING: ROLE OF ADHESION MOLECULES

Margination is partly a physiologic phenomenon. In a normal person there is a pool of marginated neutrophils estimated at 60 to 300 percent of the total number of circulating neutrophils (60); there are similar reserves of monocytes and lymphocytes. These marginated leukocytes are loosely attached to the endothelium and roll along it but do not proceed to diapedesis. When living vessels are examined under the microscope, many leukocytes are seen rolling along the intima of the veins without stopping to emigrate. This suggests that *there are two types of margination: a loose adhesion that is conducive to rolling, and a tight sticking that is preliminary to emigration* (Figure 11.14).

Endothelial cells have a baseline stickiness for leukocytes in normal conditions, which is demonstrable in vitro by pouring suspensions of leukocytes over cultures of endothelial cells. (30, 31, 121).

It was long suspected that some sort of molecular glue is involved in margination, but

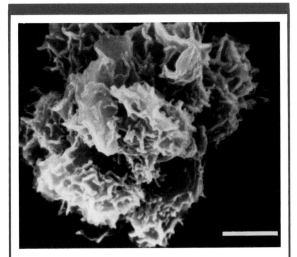

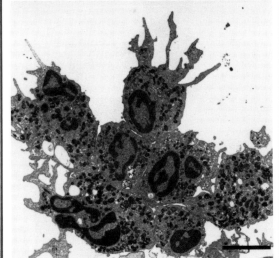

FIGURE 11.10
An example of neutrophil aggregation: these human neutrophils were stimulated with a chemotactic factor (fMLP) and stirred; 1 minute later they were fixed. *Top:* Scanning electron micrograph shows a cluster of aggregated neutrophils with obvious ruffles, evidence of activation. *Below:* Transmission electron micrograph of a similar cluster. The ruffles are obvious on the free surfaces. **Bars** = 5 μm. (Reproduced with permission from [70].)

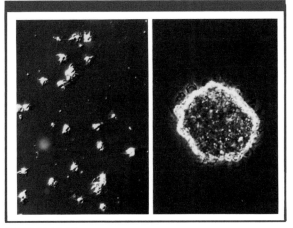

FIGURE 11.11
Cell aggregation as it occurs with amoebocytes from a starfish. *Left:* Dispersed amoebocytes. *Right:* Mass of amoebocytes that have aggregated upon contact with the glass. The phenomenon requires 15–20 minutes. Nomarski optics. (Reproduced with permission from [12].)

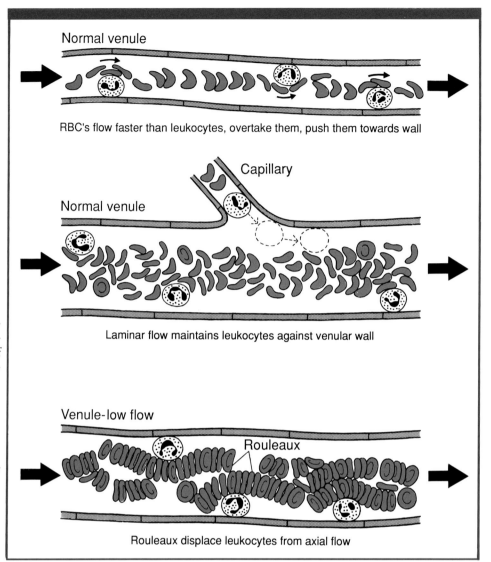

Normal venule

RBC's flow faster than leukocytes, overtake them, push them towards wall

Capillary

Normal venule

Laminar flow maintains leukocytes against venular wall

Venule-low flow

Rouleaux

Rouleaux displace leukocytes from axial flow

FIGURE 11.12
Under normal and near-normal conditions, leukocytes emerging from capillaries are pushed toward the walls of the venules. Three mechanisms contribute. *Top:* In the smallest venules the red blood cells flow faster than the leukocytes, overtake them, and in so doing push them toward the wall. *Center:* Leukocytes reaching a venule from a tributary capillary are swept along the wall of the venule by laminar flow. *Bottom:* In conditions of low flow, red blood cells tend to aggregate into rouleaux, and these larger structures tend to occupy the center, displacing the leukocytes toward the periphery.

none could be seen with the electron microscope. In recent years a variety of approaches has led to a breakthrough: over 12 adhesion molecules have been identified and cloned; they belong to three families: selectins, integrins and immunoglobulin-related (Table 11.1) (59). The field has become extremely complex and plagued with synonyms, but some basic facts are clear (Figure 11.15) (92):

1) *The inflammatory trapping of leukocytes by adhesion molecules is actually a variant of a normal phenomenon,* the homing of lymphocytes in different tissues: this involves the trapping action of specific endothelial adhesion molecules (addressins) in the high-endothelial venules, combined with the presence of appropriate ligands (homing receptors) on the lymphocytes (106, 147). The

mechanism of leukocyte trapping in inflammation is due to receptor-ligand interactions between endothelium and leukocytes in the *microcirculation,* but it seems that any endothelial cell can be stimulated to express adhesion molecules: most of the studies on adhesion molecules have been carried out on cultures of large-vessel endothelium.

2) *Rolling and sticking are indeed different phenomena, governed by different adhesion molecules.* This was proven *in vitro* by experiments of almost artistic beauty: imagine a suspension of leukocytes being washed, at known shear rates, over a lipid bilayer in which known adhesion molecules are incorporated (92). In this system the role of a given protein can be verified by inactivating it with a specific antibody.

TABLE 11-1

Endothelial Adhesion Molecules

MOLECULE	STRUCTURE	NORMAL LOCALIZA-TION	STIMULATED LOCALIZATION IN ENDOTHELIUM	LIGAND ON LEUKOCYTE	POSSIBLE FUNCTION
GMP-140	Selectin	Platelet α granule; Endothelial Weibel-Palade body	Redistributed to surface by histamine, thrombin	Unknown	Rapid neutrophil adhesion
ELAM-1	Selectin	Not present	TNF/IL-1 induced; Endothelial selective	Unknown	Early (4-6 h) neutrophil adhesion
ICAM-1	Immuno-globulin	Endothelium, fibroblasts, lymphocytes	Upregulated by TNF, - IL-1 IFN-τ	LFA-1	Neutrophil and lymphocyte adhesion
ICAM-2	Immuno-globulin	Endothelium, fibroblasts, lymphocytes	Not upregulated by cytokines	LFA-1	Lymphocyte adhesion
INCAM-110/ VCAM-1	Immuno-globulin	Endothelium, follicular dendritic cells, certain epithelia	Upregulated by TNF, IL-1	VLA-4	Lymphocyte and mono-cyte adhesion

Reproduced with permission from (35).

3) *Rolling is related to the selectin GMP-140* (GMP stands for granule membrane protein) also called CD62 or PADGEM (for platelet-activation-dependent granule external membrane protein). This protein is present on the membranes of the platelets and of the endothelium, and in the Weibel-Palade bodies typical of endothelial cells (79). Inflammatory mediators such as histamine or thrombin cause the Weibel-Palade bodies to supply more of this protein to the luminal surface of the endothelium (51, 63). The ligands for this selectin are "sticky sugars" on the leukocytes (148).

4) *Sticking occurs when two related INTEGRINS on the surface of the neutrophils are somehow activated* by chemoattractants, a process that takes place in minutes. These integrins (130) are already present on the normal neutrophil surface (Figure 11.16) but need to be made more avid for their ligand, perhaps by a change in configuration (157); once activated they bind to a preexisting ligand on the endothelium (an immunoglobulin-related mole-

cule called ICAM-1), and the leukocyte comes to a dead stop. *Without the leukocyte integrins no diapedesis can occur.* (The names of these integrins: LFA-1 and Mac-1, of the CD11/CD18 group shown in Figure 11.16).

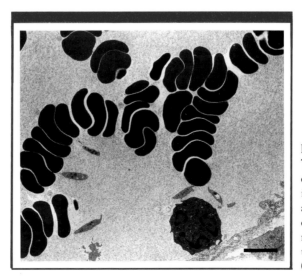

FIGURE 11.13
Typical rouleaux of red blood cells in a venule of an acutely inflamed omentum. Note marginating neutrophil. **Bar** = 0.5 μm.

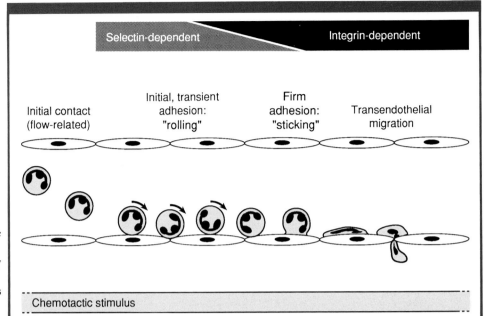

FIGURE 11.14
Four steps in the process of leukocyte extravasation. First, leukocytes must be pushed toward the endothelium by flow-related forces; thereafter rolling and sticking are controlled by various adhesion molecules: selectins and integrins. (Adapted from [141].)

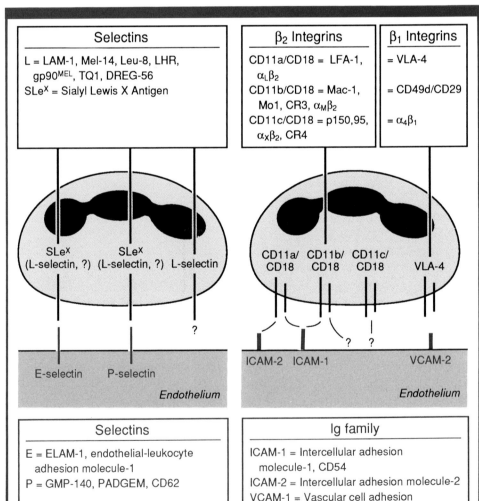

FIGURE 11.15
An attempt to make some order the current status of leukocytic and endothelial adhesion molecules. The two main groups, selectins and integrins, are represented in the sequence in which they are thought to intervene (rolling followed by sticking). The names in the boxes merely indicate synonyms. In the scheme at the right, the three endothelial adhesion molecules (ICAM-2, ICAM-1, and VCAM-1) are constitutively expressed. The diagram concerns neutrophils as well as monocytes. (Adapted from [59].)

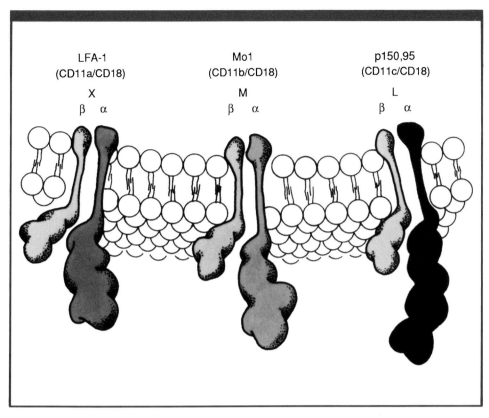

LFA-1	Mo1	p150,95
(CD11a/CD18)	(CD11b/CD18)	(CD11c/CD18)
X	M	L
β α	β α	β α

FIGURE 11.16
Schematic representation of the leukocyte adhesion molecules of the CD11/CD18 family. Each transmembrane glycoprotein is a heterodimer consisting of a distinctive higher molecular weight α subunit, noncovalently associated with an identical lower molecular weight β subunit. (Adapted from [152].)

In vitro the integrin-activating effect of the chemoattractants is very fast: by pretreating leukocytes or endothelial cells with fMLP, C5a, LTB$_4$ and PAF, it was shown that stickiness peaked at 2 minutes (153). Cytokines such as TNF and IL-1 are also effective (157).

5) *A second wave of margination and diapedesis occurs when the endothelium, activated by inflammatory cytokines, has had time to synthesize more adhesion proteins* and to express them on its surface (124). The maximal effect is reached in 4–6 hours. The role of cytokines in inducing the endothelium to express adhesion proteins was discovered by M. Bevilacqua and colleagues at Harvard (21). These simple and elegant experiments were carried out by growing endothelial cells *in vitro*, and then overlaying them with leukocytes (Figure 11.17). Pretreatment of the cultures with Interleukin-1 increased endothelial stickiness. The effect peaked at 4–6 hours, was reversible, and prevented by inhibitors of protein synthesis. Similar effects were obtained with Tumor Necrosis Factor and endotoxin (35, 138). In this manner the first endothelial-leukocyte adhesion molecule was identified and labeled ELAM-1. (Tab. 11.1).

Now let us return to real life, and draw up a simplified version of what might happen in a focus of injury. Histamine is released by damaged mast cells, and it induces the nearby venular endothelial cells to transfer some of the sticky selectin GMP-140 from the Weibel-Palade bodies to the endothelial surface. The leukocytes, which have several hydrodynamic reasons for bumping into the venular endothelium (Figure 11.12), begin to roll along it. Now chemotaxins come into play (from bacteria if infection is involved, from activated complement, from platelets, etc.); they seep into the venules, activate the CD11/CD18 integrins on the rolling leukocytes, and put on the brakes: the leukocytes remain stuck to the endothelial surface. The next step will be emigration. As hours go by, the endothelium is activated by cytokines, produces adhesion molecules, and more leukocytes are recruited to the scene.

Why Are the Leukocytes Larger than the Capillaries? At this point in our description of leukocyte "trapping" by activated adhesion molecules, we should stop to consider the time-frame of these events (100). In the capillaries of the skin or

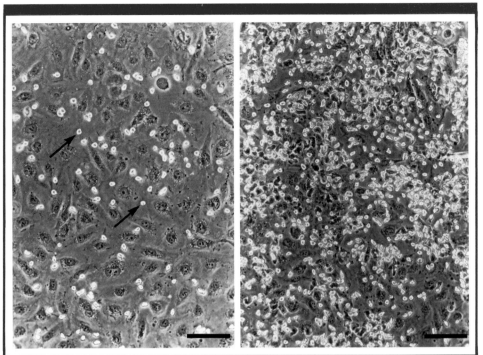

FIGURE 11.17
Monolayers of human endothelium incubated with a suspension of human polymorphonuclear leukocytes for 10 minutes, then washed. *Left:* Control experiment with untreated endothelium. After washing, only scattered leukocytes (**arrows**) have remained attached. *Right:* This endothelium was pretreated with interleukin-1 for 4 hours. The cytokine has greatly increased the adhesiveness of the endothelial cells for the leukocytes. **Bars** = 100 μm. (Reproduced with permission from [21].)

muscle, the velocity of blood flow, measured for red blood cells, is such that an average red blood cell would flash by in about half a second. This would be a very short time for a chemotaxin to diffuse into the blood and activate the leukocyte integrins. Evolution seems to have solved this problem in two ways: (a) *By trapping the leukocytes in the venules and slowing them down by making them roll; this should give them ample time (minutes?) to perceive a chemotactic call.* (b) *By slowing down the leukocytes even farther upstream, as they squeeze through the capillaries.* In the normal lung, leukocytes studied *in vivo* have been found to remain trapped in capillaries as long as 20 or 40 minutes (60, 94, 155). *Perhaps Nature made the leukocytes much larger than the capillary lumen for this very reason: that they would have more time to receive their marching orders.*

The concept that the leukocytes are reached by chemotaxins upstream from the venules was confirmed by experiment: two chemotaxins, fMLP and LTB$_4$, applied by micropipette to a venule in the hamster cheek pouch, had no visible effect; applied to the capillaries upstream, they caused margination in the corresponding venule (111).

ADHESION MOLECULES AND DISEASE

Adhesion molecules intervene in the pathogenesis of a variety of settings:

- *Chronic inflammation.* Predictably, adhesion proteins are important players in chronic inflammation: the glycoprotein ELAM-1—which binds neutrophils, monocytes, and some lymphocytes—is chronically expressed in rheumatoid arthritis; ICAM-1 appears to be involved in the damage caused by *cerebral malaria,* by binding parasitized erythrocytes and thereby stopping the microcirculation (17).

- *Gram-negative sepsis.* When the blood is contaminated with gram-negative bacteria, endotoxin induces ELAM-1 on endothelial cells throughout the vascular system; by this mechanism leukocytes are inappropriately recruited, and the result, as we will see, may be multiple organ failure (120).

- *Leukocyte Adhesion Deficiencies.* Some patients, fortunately few, lack the beta-2 integrin molecule; their condition is known as Leukocyte Adhesion Deficiency (LAD) type 1 (7). Depending on the severity of the defect, some of the patients are identified at birth, while others can survive to adulthood. The signs include *delayed separation of the umbilical cord,* necrotizing infections with inadequate pus formation, and granulocytosis (Figure 11.18) (7). Normally, the dried-up stump of the umbilical cord attracts leukocytes and falls off in 7–10 days, severed by the leukocytic enzymes (Figure 11.19). In LAD patients, the leukocytes in the umbilical circulation are condemned to circulate perpetually without stopping for a chemotactic call, the essential prelude to diapedesis and to the enzymatic surgery of the umbilical stump.

As if these patients did not have enough trouble, one of the normal CD11/CD18 integrins (Mac-1) turns out to be also the receptor for C3b, the complement-derived opsonin. This means that the lack of Mac-1 leads to impaired leukocyte adhesion plus a phagocytosis defect. In LAD type 2, the leukocytes lack the ligand for an endothelial selectin (50).

- *Arteriosclerosis.* One of the very first steps in arteriosclerosis is the sticking and emigration of monocytes (80), apparently trapped by adhesion molecules (33) (p. 657).
- *Tumor metastases.* Tumor cells circulating in the blood may express adhesion molecules (which will cause them to halt in given organs) or be trapped by them (4).
- *The other side of the coin: anti-adhesion molecule therapy* has proven effective in a number of experimental models, especially in reducing inflammation as well as vascular plugging by leukocytes (p. 699), but this type of therapy is of course a two-edged sword: it can be dangerous to depress inflammation (60).

Diapedesis

No photograph taken through the light microscope can adequately portray diapedesis: a white blood cell, drawn by an ancestral call, sneaks out of a venule through an invisible hole. In histologic sections the event can only be guessed: some leukocytes are marginating, others are lying within the venular wall, others yet are free outside (Figure 11.20). It is no wonder that diapedesis was discovered in living tissues. Electron microscopy, however, succeeds in bringing the event to life: marginating leukocytes can be seen either astride of an intercellular junction (perhaps they can sniff the chemotaxins coming through it), or forcing it open, and squeezing through (Figure 11.21). The first electron micrographs of diapedesis were provided in 1960 by Vincent T. Marchesi, an

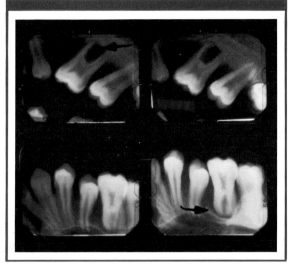

FIGURE 11.18 X-rays of the jaws in a 12-year-old child affected by leukocyte adhesion deficiency. **Arrows** point to severe bone loss due to infection. The gums were inflamed and deep peridontal pockets had formed. (Reproduced with permission from [6].)

American medical student working in Oxford with Lord Florey (103, 104). They showed that the leukocyte fits very tightly into its narrow passage; little fluid escapes around it, as can be shown by loading the plasma with visible colloidal particles. Interestingly, *the leukocyte digs its own way out;* it does not seem to use the endothelial gaps previously induced by permeability-increasing mediators. This can be rationalized. Endothelial gaps are created for a purpose: to deliver the fluid part of the exudate. If they were immediately plugged by leukocytes, this purpose would be defeated.

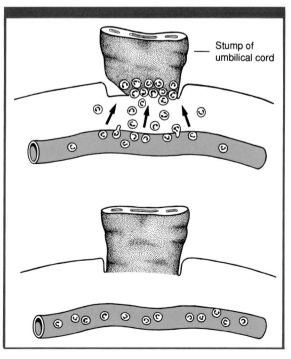

FIGURE 11.19 The "umbilical cord phenomenon" in leukocyte adhesion deficiency. *Top:* Normal situation: within 7–10 days the necrotic stump of the umbilical cord, acting as an irritant, attracts leukocytes and is cut off by their enzymes. *Bottom:* In leukocyte adhesion deficiency the leukocytes cannot emigrate, and the umbilical stump is retained.

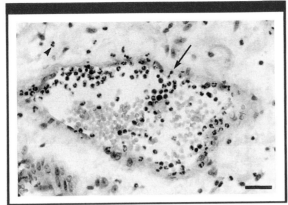

FIGURE 11.20

See color plate 11. Diapedesis in histologic sections can only be guessed. A venule in the wall of an acutely inflamed colon. Neutrophils are recognizable by their nucleus subdivided into 2-3 lobes (**arrowhead**). Some are adherent to the endothelium, trapped within the thickness of the vascular wall (**arrow**) or free outside. **Bar = 25 μm.**

As soon as the leukocytes have crossed the endothelium, they run into an obstacle: the basement membrane (Figure 11.21). Many are deflected by it and squeeze laterally into the narrow subendothelial space, where they stop for some time—about 30 minutes (115)—as if waiting for something to happen (141). Eventually they burst out into the extravascular spaces: do they manage it by sheer violence, or do they nibble at the basement membrane with some enzyme? They probably use both means. Remember that chemotaxins in high enough concentrations activate leukocytes while they attract them. Activation includes secretion of enzymes, and leukocytes are equipped with collagenase—which can break down the basement membrane. Monocytes produce a surface elastase (91), and neutrophil elastase can attack basement membranes (9).

FIGURE 11.21 Margination of a neutrophil (**A**) followed by 5 stages of diapedesis (**B–F**). In **B** and **C** the emigrating neutrophil is temporarily held up by the basement membrane. In **D** and **E** the emigrating cells are monocytes. In **F** the neutrophil has reached the extravascular space. The reason for the high electron density of the neutrophils is not known. From the inflamed omentum of a rat. **Bars = 2 μm.**

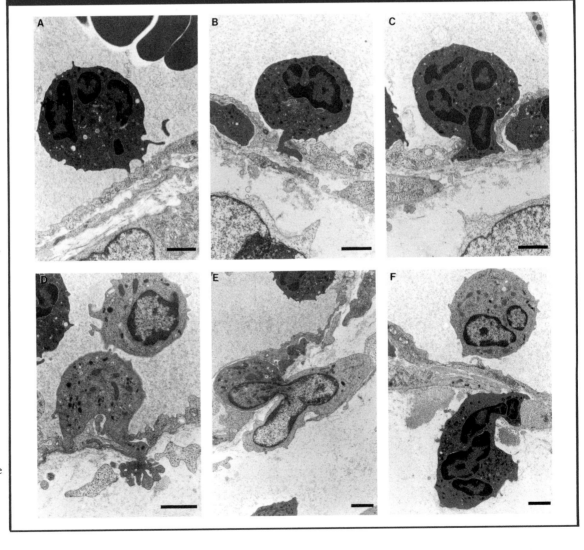

An episode of diapedesis leaves the basement membrane in shambles. This was shown by an ingenious experiment (76) based on the principle of vascular labeling. In a normal rat, if the venules are labeled in black by a local injection of histamine followed by an intravenous injection of carbon black, the outlines of the blackened venules are sharp (see Figure 10.17). If the experiment is repeated 4 hours after a local injection of serum, which causes a burst of diapedesis, the torn-up basement membranes are unable to hold the carbon, which spills out as a cloud of black fuzz (Figure 11.22). It is not known how long it takes for the basement membrane to be repaired.

The whole process of diapedesis takes 3–9 minutes according to one study (56), 11–49 minutes according to another (115). As soon as the leukocytes are out of the venule, they crawl toward their target by hauling themselves along collagen fibers or other tissue structures. If they fall into a fluid-filled cavity, such as the peritoneum or a joint, they float aimlessly unless a random collision brings them in contact with the archetypal enemy, a bacterium.

Why does diapedesis occur from the venules? A moment's thought suggests that the use of capillaries for diapedesis would be disastrous (100). Monocytes and granulocytes are about twice as wide as most capillaries and have a tight squeeze every time they pass through them (p. 686). Because the process takes 3–9 minutes, every single leukocyte that emigrated from a capillary would cause a 3–9 minute traffic jam; blood flow in that capillary would stop, defeating the very purpose of inflammation. By contrast, the leukocytes can marginate in the venules at their leisure while blood continues to flow past—however slowly—and to supply more leukocytes for margination.

There is one exception to venular diapedesis: *in the lung, the leukocytes emigrate from the alveolar capillaries* (94). However, the layout of these capillaries is unique. The alveolar capillaries are extremely short, averaging 8 μm (71), and form a very tight gridlike network, as is beautifully shown with plastic casts (Figure 11.23) (26). This layout means that many leukocytes can stick here and there in the grid without stopping the red-cell traffic. It is calculated that even if half of all the leukocytes in the blood were trapped in the human lung, only 10 percent of the alveolar capillary segments would be blocked (71).

Diapedesis can occur without inflammation. Arteriosclerosis begins with the diapedesis of monocytes and a few lymphocytes into the arterial wall (80). Cells of malignant tumors perform diapedesis as well as reverse diapedesis, crawling in and out of blood vessels.

Recognition and Attachment

After the leukocyte has been lured into the extravascular world, it must identify what to attack, and then stick to the target (149). How it does so is not entirely clear to us, but it is certainly clear to the leukocyte, which moves about in crowded quarters and knows enough to push aside a normal red blood cell, for example, but to seize an aged one. The clue to recognition must be subtle cell-surface differences, including charge, hydrophilic properties, and molecular structure.

Opsonization If the surface of the target is prepared (*opsonized*) by plasma proteins, phagocytosis is made easier, though some targets can be taken up without this coating (Figure 11.24).

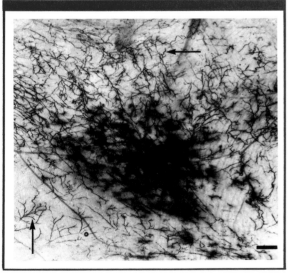

FIGURE 11.22
Demonstrating how the basement membranes are torn by diapedesis. Rat cremaster muscle. One hour before this tissue was fixed, histamine was injected locally, and carbon black was injected intravenously. Typical venular labeling developed as expected (**arrows**) except in the central zone: here, diapedesis had been induced 5 hours previously with an injection of serum. The black mass is carbon that spilled out of the basement membranes. **Bar** = 1 mm. (Reproduced with permission from [75].)

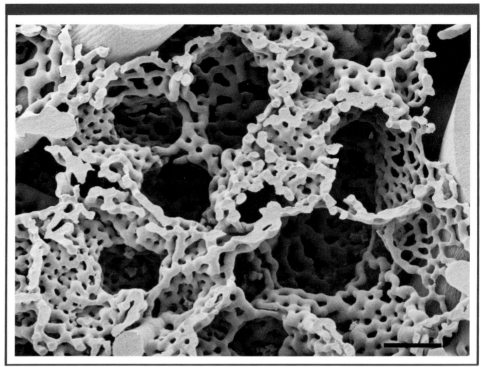

FIGURE 11.23
Demonstrating why leukocytes do not cause traffic jams in alveolar capillaries of the lungs. The capillary network is so richly branched that many capillaries are as long as they are wide (about 8 mm). Muscle capillaries are about 100 times longer. (Rat lung capillaries injected with plastic; the tissue has been removed.) **Bar** = 25 μm. (Courtesy of Drs. L. Fisher and P. H. Burri, University of Berne, Switzerland.)

Opsonization (149, 164, 166) was discovered in 1903. Two Englishmen, Wright and Douglas, noticed that serum contains factors that coat bacteria and make them more palatable for the leukocytes; they called them opsonins (ópson is Greek for "prepared food").

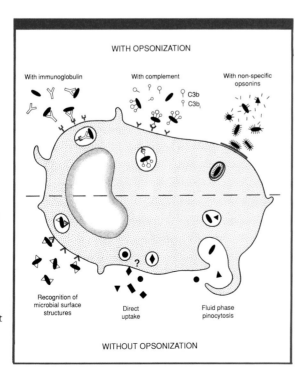

FIGURE 11.24
A macrophage can phagocytize by at least six pathways: three require opsonization, three do not. The small oval objects represent bacteria. (Adapted from [2].)

There are three types of opsonins (Figure 11.23):

- **IgG antibody** This is the most important opsonin, which means that whenever a bacterium is encountered for the *first* time, an important defense mechanism will be lacking. However, life exposes us to so many subclinical infections that some antibody-opsonin is usually available. IgG antibody works like a ligand: the Fab part of the globulin (see Figure 7.44) binds to the surface of the microorganism while the Fc portion sticks out and fits into the membrane receptors of the phagocyte.

- **C3b fragment of complement** Being a fragment of C3, C3b is set free when complement is activated. Like IgG, C3b has a tail end that fits into a receptor on the surfaces of phagocytic cells.

- **Nonspecific opsonins** Several proteins have opsonic properties (164), for example, Hageman factor, fibronectin (somewhat debated), and perhaps C-reactive protein.

Phagocytosis without opsonization In some situations, however, opsonization is not needed. Consider an alveolar macrophage: the dust that it is supposed to clean up must be phagocytized in the absence of serum—and so it is, quite avidly (119). In this regard, the macrophage lives up to the prowess of its distant ancestor, the ameba, which takes all of its meals, presumably, without the benefit of having them labeled dinner. Neutrophils do the same but with less enthusiasm. The molecular mechanism is not clear (166). Better understood is the uptake of nonopsonized bacteria, another feat of the macrophage: certain sugars on the surface of the phagocyte are recognized by a receptor on the bacterial surface, or vice versa (53). Also, of course, very small particles, of the order of magnitude of proteins, can be taken in accidentally by the macrophage in the course of pinocytosis. This has been called piggy-back phagocytosis.

Reverse opsonization Reverse opsonization modifies the surface of the phagocyte, which amounts to whetting the appetite rather than spicing the meal. Because phagocytosis is facilitated by conditioning the surface of the target, it would be strange if there were no way to condition the surface of the phagocyte. Such is the function of the tetrapeptide **tuftsin,** which is incorporated in IgG1 molecules (44) and is cleaved off in two steps, in the spleen and on the surface of phagocytic cells (53, 112, 112a). Tuftsin stimulates phagocytosis, motility, cytotoxicity, and other leukocytic functions.

Phagocytosis

After a target has been recognized and seized by a phagocyte it must be ingested to be eliminated. Transmission electron microscopy gives the impression that two pseudopods emerge from the surface of the phagocyte and surround the target like a pair of arms (Figure 11.25), but in three dimensions the event looks different. Usually, a circular ridge rises around the attached particle, grows to form a cup, and develops into a crater (Figure 11.26) (116). Eventually the crater closes up, the apposed plasma membranes fuse, and the particle finds itself in an intracellular vacuole (phagosome).

Then the digestion process begins. As seen in phagocytes that have been fixed and stained, this event appears utterly bland; somehow the phagocyte looses its granules (it is said to become "degranulated"), and the phagocytized bacteria may or may not die. In reality, what happens in living cells is truly dramatic. It has been recorded in a movie that every biologist should see (68).

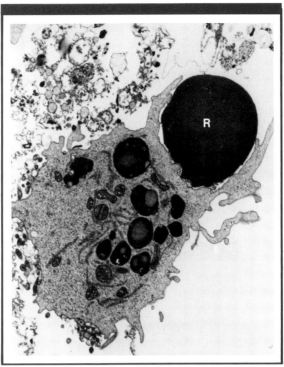

FIGURE 11.25
Phagocytosis of a red blood cell (**R**): The phagocyte here shown is a cloned NK cell engulfing a red blood cell coated with antibody. Note that the granules have moved toward the contact site. In this two-dimensional view the phagocyte appears to "throw two arms" around its prey but compare it with the three-dimensional crater seen by scanning electron microscopy (Fig. 11.26). (Reproduced with permission from [125].)

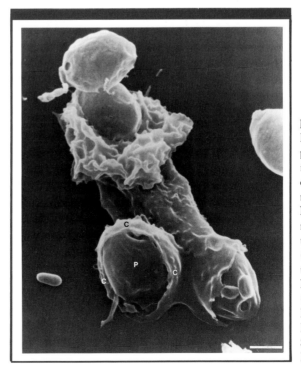

FIGURE 11.26
Human neutrophil phagocytizing foreign particles: a three dimensional view. Note how the membrane rises to form a cup (**C**) surrounding the particle (**P**). **Bar** = 2 μm. (Courtesy of Dr. M.J. Karnovsky, Harvard Medical School, Boston MA.)

How Granulocytes Loose Their Granules In the early 1960s James Hirsch and Gordon Archer recorded on film the behavior of granulocytes phagocytizing various types of particles (8, 68). In each sequence, a cell creeps toward its immobile target until it engulfs it in a pocket of cytoplasm. Eventually the pocket closes up and becomes a phagosome. In the meantime, in a matter of seconds, the cell's granules move to the pocket, fuse with it, and eject their enzymes into it. This is literally an explosive event: the granules pop one by one like ammunition, until the phagocyte is degranulated. Two representative frames are shown in Figure 11.27. The specific granules are the first to be expended (180), perhaps because of their high content of antibacterial molecules.

> *Movies of phagocytosis had been taken before, but by the more "hi-tech" time-lapse method, whereby the popping event, which lasts only one-tenth of a second, was regularly missed. Hirsch and Archer took the movie by the ordinary and cheaper method, which produced a slow but complete recording.*

An important detail: *the popping of granules begins to occur even before the particule is completely engulfed.* This can be seen also on electron micrographs (Figure 11.28). The result is that some of the extruded enzymes leak out into the tissue spaces, a messy event known by the colorful name of **regurgitation while feeding** (which helps us understand why the inflammatory exudate is rich in hydrolytic enzymes).

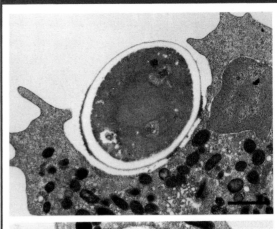
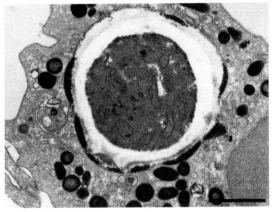

FIGURE 11.28

Human neutrophils phagocytizing opsonized yeast. Section reacted for peroxidase: the peroxidase-positive, electron-dense azurophil granules stand out against the peroxidase-negative specific granules. *Top:* The neutrophil has recognized the yeast cell and is about to engulf it. Already at this early stage, enzymes of the azurophil granules are present at the surface of the yeast cell. *Bottom:* Detail of a yeast cell fully enclosed in a phagocytic vacuole. Note the massive release of granule contents. **Bars** = 1 μm. (Reproduced with permission from [11].)

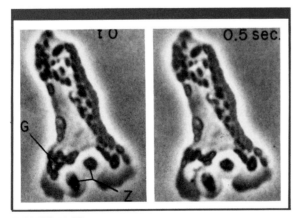

FIGURE 11.27

Two frames from a historical movie showing the bursting of the granules (**G**) during phagocytosis. Chicken leukocytes phagocytizing a particle of zymosan (**Z**). *At time 0:* Two granules are intact. *At .5 seconds:* they have burst, leaving a clear space. (Reproduced with permission from [68].)

Frustrated Phagocytosis This colorful term fits the following situation: when a phagocyte runs into a large, flat surface that it recognizes as foreign, it "attempts" to phagocytize it by lying on it; it pops its granules against it but of course is never be able to take it in (Figure 11.29) (65). The frustration, however, may be only in the mind of the beholder; the phagocyte can cause plenty of damage to this type of prey without swallowing it. This is the very principle of a killing mechanism known in immunology as ADCC (p. 527).

Surface Phagocytosis Surface phagocytosis is a mechanism for relieving frustrated phagocytes

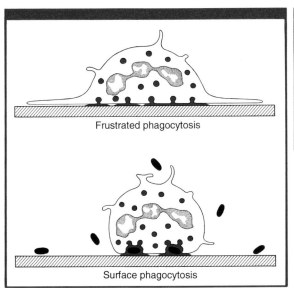

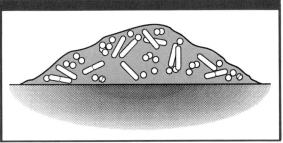

FIGURE 11.30
Bacteria attached to a surface may evade the attack of leukocytes by burying themselves in a mucous "biofilm" (slime). (Adapted from [57].)

FIGURE 11.29

Top: Frustrated phagocytosis. A phagocyte spreads over a large foreign body as if attempting to engulf it, and empties its granules against it (exocytosis). The enzymes seep out into the surroundings. *Bottom:* Surface phagocytosis. A phagocyte can easily ingest bacteria trapped against a surface but cannot ingest free-floating bacteria unless it collides with them accidentally.

Phagokinesis *is a curious* in vitro *phenomenon: as cells that are growing on a surface coated with gold particles move about, they clean up the particles by phagocytizing them; they leave a clear track that makes it possible to follow their wanderings (5) (Figure 11.31).*

(142, 179). Imagine a phagocyte hopelessly chasing around a slippery particle without being able to grab it (recalling the popular game of trying to bite an apple floating on water). The chase can end only if the particle is backed against a resistant surface; filaments of fibrin may perform this function in inflammatory foci.

Surface phagocytosis can be demonstrated by an elegant experiment: phagocytes are incubated with encapsulated pneumococci (notoriously slippery) in a rotating tube; after 30 minutes, few of the phagocytes contain bacteria because it was hard for them to phagocytize while floating. If a piece of filter paper or strands of fibrin are added to the mixture, after 30 minutes many more bacteria have been ingested (142).

Phagocytosis Frustrated by Slime Phagocytes sometimes encounter a third type of surface problem. Some bacteria are able to attach themselves to a surface, such as a catheter, and then coat themselves with a layer of slime (Figure 11.30). This makes them almost inaccessible to phagocytes. Perhaps we should call this **frustrated surface phagocytosis.** This phenomenon explains why physicians are reluctant to insert catheters, and why surgeons are always worried about foreign bodies.

Bacterial Killing: Metabolic Aspects of Phagocytosis

Phagocytosis of bacteria is a prelude to bacterial killing. Bacteria engulfed by neutrophils or macrophages can be destroyed by two mechanisms: oxygen-dependent (thanks to oxygen-derived free radicals) and oxygen-independent (22). The latter mechanism reminds us that leukocytes are often called upon to kill bacteria in injured tissues, in which the oxygen supply is low. The two mechanisms are almost equally powerful, but the oxygen dependent mechanism has a slight edge (162).

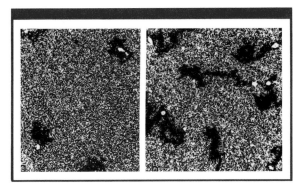

FIGURE 11.31

Two scenes of phagokinesis. *Left:* Cultured capillary endothelial cells deposited on a surface covered with gold particles. *Right:* Similar setting except that the cells have been stimulated with the supernatant from a culture of tumor cells. As the cells move about, they pick up gold particles. (Courtesy of Dr. B.R. Zetter, Harvard Medical School, Boston MA.)

OXYGEN-DEPENDENT ANTIBACTERIAL MECHANISMS

Phagocytosis was once considered a purely physical phenomenon based on surface tensions, and there may be some truth in this concept (164). Yet in 1933 it was shown that oxygen uptake increases during phagocytosis (81). The topic attracted little interest for 26 years until Anthony Sbarra and Manfred Karnovsky returned to it during a study of host–parasite relations (83, 134). They discovered some startling facts: granulocytes incubated with polystyrene particles phagocytized them equally well under aerobic or anaerobic conditions. The phagocytizing cells did show an increased oxygen uptake (Figure 11.32); but they continued to phagocytize if they were poisoned with cyanide, which uncouples oxidative phosphorylation. In other words, the extra oxygen uptake did not represent mitochondrial respiration. The energy for phagocytosis seemed to derive from glycolysis because poisoning with iodoacetate or fluoride did inhibit the uptake of particles. This last finding made good sense, at least for the leukocytes. Because these cells are often called on to perform in traumatized areas where the circulation is impaired, it is certainly convenient that they should be able to engulf bacteria in the absence of oxygen by drawing energy from their built-in supply of glycogen. But then why would phagocytizing leukocytes need more oxygen? The increased uptake can be huge, over 50 times the normal (10).

The answer came two years later. Stimulated (activated) phagocytes release H_2O_2 (hydrogen peroxide) and *superoxide anion* (O_2^-), and these molecules are further metabolized into highly toxic oxidants, so *the purpose of the respiratory burst is not to provide energy, but to produce lethal oxidants as antibacterial agents* (10,46, 82).

The enzyme responsible for the increased oxygen uptake (NADPH oxidase) is built into the cell membrane; its NADPH binding site projects into the cytosol. But its products are released outside of the cell, and therefore into phagosomes, as required for killing bacteria (a phagosome is lined with internalized cell membrane). In a resting cell the enzyme remains dormant, but when activated it catalyzes the one-electron reductions of oxygen at the expense of NADPH:

$$O_2 + NADPH \rightarrow O_2^- + NADP+ + H^+$$

It is no mean feat of histochemistry that superoxide, which lasts only milliseconds, can be demonstrated on electron micrographs (Figure 11.33) (25), but we find it even more astonishing that the generation of oxygen-derived free radicals is accompanied by the emission of *light* (photons), so that a standard method for measuring the activation of leukocytes is to monitor their chemoluminescence. Most of the O_2^- promptly reacts with itself, producing oxygen and hydrogen peroxide:

$$2O_2^- + 2H+ \rightarrow H_2O_2 + O_2$$

At the same time, glucose is metabolized via the hexose monophosphate (HMP) shunt in order to regenerate the NADPH (this explains why Sbarra and Karnovsky found that during phagocytosis the catabolism of glucose via the HMP shunt is greatly accelerated). Today, the expression *respiratory burst* refers to the four events: increased oxygen uptake, increased catabolism of glucose via the HMP shunt, release of H_2O_2, and release of O_2^-.

Up to this point we have H_2O_2 and superoxide radical, neither of which is very effective at killing bacteria, but they are used as starting materials for producing the really effective antiseptics, which belong to two categories: *oxidizing radicals* and *oxidized halogens*.

The best-known oxidized radical is the hydroxyl radical (OH·), which is produced by a metal-catalyzed reaction, the Haber–Weiss reaction (p. 185):

$$O_2^- + H_2O_2 \xrightarrow{Fe^{++}or Cu^{++}} OH\cdot + OH^- + O_2$$

Hydroxyl radical is formed and released not only in the phagocytic vacuole but also around the

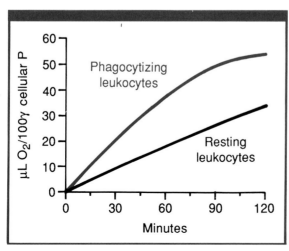

FIGURE 11.32 The respiratory burst induced by phagocytosis: respiration of guinea pig peritoneal cells (80% neutrophils) at rest and during phagocytosis. The particles to be phagocytized were introduced at zero time. (Adapted from [134].)

pronged myeloperoxidase—H_2O_2—halide system, more simply known as the *Klebanoff system*, works inside the phagosome as follows (Figure 11.34):

- myeloperoxidase is supplied by fusion of the phagosome with a primary granule.
- H_2O_2 is supplied mostly by the oxygen burst occurring in the phagosome membrane (which really represents activated cell membrane) by means of the NADPH-oxidase; some H_2O_2 can also be contributed by the bacterium in the phagosome.
- Halide is supplied by the cell; it can be Cl^-, I^-, or Br^-.

The basic reaction is the following:

$$H^+ + Cl^- + H_2O_2 \xrightarrow{\text{myeloperoxidase}} HOCl + H_2O$$

All this being said, it is fascinating to realize that the phagocytes have been using two of our basic commercial antiseptics for millions of years (174): *hydrogen peroxide*, an ancient household disinfectant, and *hypochlorite*, the "chlorine" of swimming pools and the antiseptic of the household detergent *Clorox*.

OXYGEN-INDEPENDENT ANTIBACTERIAL MECHANISMS

Several lines of evidence show that leukocytes can also kill bacteria by mechanisms unrelated to oxygen metabolism (41, 146). Ground up, leukocytes still have some antibacterial effects. Leuko-

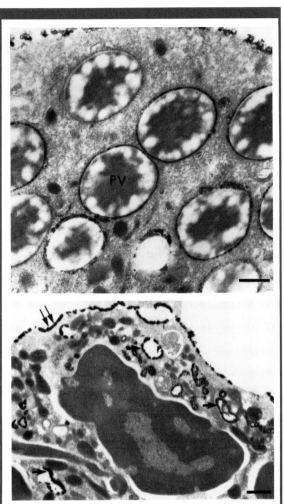

FIGURE 11.33

Electron micrographs of activated neutrophils treated by a histochemical method to show the sites of H_2O_2 generation. The black precipitate represents the reaction product. *Top:* Neutrophil activated by phagocytosis of polystyrene spheres. Reaction product on the cell surface and on the membranes of phagocytic vacuoles (**PV**). (Reproduced with permission from [24].) *Bottom:* Neutrophil stimulated with phorbol myristate acetate. **Arrows:** Reaction product on surface and on surface-derived membranes. **Bars** = 0.5μm. (Reproduced with permission from [82].)

activated phagocyte, because all the reagents are available there.

The prototype of the oxidized halogens is hypochlorite (**HOCl**), which can only be generated with the collaboration of myeloperoxidase (MPO), an enzyme present in the azurophil (primary) granules. Thus, the antiseptic power of the hypochlorite can only be exploited in the phagocytic vacuole, in which MPO conspires with two other reactants to produce a variety of toxic agents, including hypochlorite (87). This three-

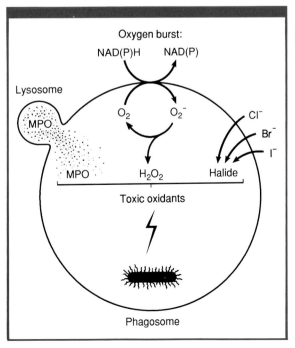

FIGURE 11.34
The Klebanoff system, an oxygen dependent antibacterial weapon of phagocytes, has three components: myeloperoxidase (MPO) supplied by lysosomes; H_2O_2 supplied by the oxygen burst (some H_2O_2 may be supplied by the bacterium itself), and a halide. The interaction of these three components supplies toxic oxidants.

cytes that are congenitally unable to produce oxygen bursts can still kill some bacteria. Each type of phagocyte has its own mix of antibacterial molecules (41). These are in part enzymatic: proteases, phospholipases, nucleases, and lysozyme, which is powerful against a few gram-positive bacteria. Many other antibacterial mechanisms such as the cationic proteins are nonenzymatic. Especially effective against gram-negative bacteria is a cationic protein that kills bacteria by increasing their permeability (BPI for bacterial permeability-increasing protein). Its possible mechanism of action is shown in Figure 11.35. *Defensins* (93) are small cytotoxic proteins. Other cytotoxic proteins are contained in eosinophils; one of them, the eosinophil cationic protein (ECP), is a pore-forming molecule (p. 323). *Lactoferrin* acts mainly as an iron-binding protein, depriving bacteria of iron as a growth factor; persons congenitally lacking in neutrophil lactoferrin may be prone to infections.

TRIGGERS OF PHAGOCYTE ACTIVATION

The respiratory burst can be induced by phagocytosis (135) as well as by the stimulation of surface receptors, for example by chemotaxins or phorbol myristate acetate, the primal activator (p. 61). The experimental use of this agent is, of course, highly artificial, but it is extremely effec-

tive and has been invaluable for working out the details of leukocyte activation.

It is possible experimentally to trigger each one of the various leukocyte functions separately (chemotaxis, phagocytosis, the oxygen burst, etc.) but it is more important to note that these responses are biologically integrated and that they occur together in inflammation (65): a leukocyte that has been summoned by chemotaxis is also preparing for phagocytosis and bacterial killing.

Reversibility of activation. Granulocytes stimulated by phagocytosis cannot be stopped in their tracks: in this respect they quite justify their kamikaze reputation. However, if they are chemically stimulated *in vitro* (e.g., by fluoride) the respiratory burst can be reversed by washing away the fluoride. (36).

TO SUM UP: Inflammation is designed for gathering fluid and cells at a site of injury. It does so by mechanisms that are triggered in seconds or minutes (such as the device for making venules leak, which is marvellously simple), backed up by slower mechanisms that come into play in a matter of hours. Obviously, the recruitment of cells is more complicated, because it requires more steps than creating little leaks in blood vessels; but note its strategic feature: although the drafted leuko-

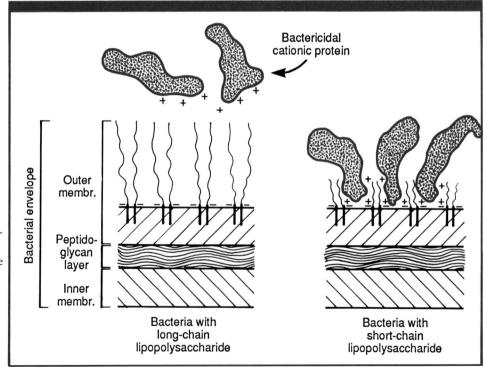

FIGURE 11.35
Bactericidal cationic proteins are among the oxygen-independent bactericidal systems of neutrophils. This scheme shows how these proteins are thought to interact with negative charges on the surface of gram-negative bacteria; the interaction is more effective when the polysaccharide chains of the lipopolysaccharide are short. (Adapted from [40].)

cytes may take hours to reach their bacterial prey, *they are switched on as soon as they perceive their chemotactic call.* This means that by the time they hit upon the bacteria, they are in full gear. If the bacteria had eyes they would perceive a terrifying sight: as the leukocytes are hauling themselves along the connective tissue fibers and closing in, following their sniff, they are swelling, huffing and puffing (their respiration is greatly increased), reaching out with long arms, drooling acid juices, and emitting sparks (real photons). What magnificent killing machines.

References

1. Aaronson S. Chemical communication at the microbial level, vol. 1. Boca Raton: CRC Press, 1981.
2. Adams DO, Hamilton TA. Phagocytic cells: cytotoxic activities of macrophages. In: Gallin, JI., Goldstein IM, Snyderman R, eds. Inflammation: basic principles and clinical correlates. New York: Raven Press, 1988: 471–492.
3. Adler J. Chemoreceptors in bacteria. Science 1969;166: 1588–1597.
4. Albelda SM. Role of integrins and other cell adhesion molecules in tumor progression and metastasis. Lab Invest 1993;68:4–17.
5. Albrecht-Buehler G. The phagokinetic tracks of 3T3 cells. Cell 1977;11:395–404.
6. Anderson DC, Schmalsteig FC, Finegold MJ, et al. The severe and moderate phenotypes of heritable Mac-1, LFA-1 deficiency: their quantitative definition and relation to leukocyte dysfunction and clinical features. J Infect Dis 1985;152:668–689.
7. Anderson DC, Springer TA. Leukocyte adhesion deficiency: an inherited defect in the Mac-1, LFA-1, and p150,95 glycoproteins. Annu Rev Med 1987;38:175–194.
8. Archer GT, Hirsch JG. Motion picture studies on degranulation of horse eosinophils during phagocytosis. J Exp Med 1963;118:287–294. (Available from Rockefeller University Press, Film Service, 222 East 70th Street, New York, NY 10021.)
9. Arsenis C, Kuettner KE, Schwartz DE Degradation of intact basement membranes by human neutrophil elastase. A model for enzyme degradation of intact collagenous matrices. In: Sen A, Thornhill T, eds. development and diseases of cartilage and bone matrix. New York: Alan R. Liss, 1987:45–54.
10. Babior BM. The respiratory burst of phagocytes. J Clin Invest 1984;73:599–601.
11. Baggiolini M. Phagocyte activation and its modulation by drugs. In: Glynn LE, Houck JC, Weissmann, G Handbook of inflammation, vol. 5. Amsterdam: Elsevier, 1985:117–121.
12. Bang FB. Disease processes in seastars: a Metchnikovian challenge. Biol Bull 1982;162:135–148.
13. Bar-Shavit R, Kahn A, Fenton JW II, Wilner GD. Chemotactic response of monocytes to thrombin. J Cell Biol 1983;96:282–285.
14. Becker EL. The formylpeptide receptor of the neutrophil. A search and conserve operation. Am J Pathol 1987;129: 16–24.
15. Becker EL, Naccache PH, Showell HJ, Sha'afi RI. Synthetic chemotactic peptides as initiators of multiple biologic functions of the neutrophil: the role of calcium. In: Gross E, Meienhofer J, eds. Peptides. Structure and biological function. Proceedings of the Sixth American Peptide Symposium. Rockford, Pierce Chemical Company, 1979:743–748.
16. Berenberg JL, Ward PA Chemotactic factor inactivator in normal human serum. J Clin Invest, 1973;52:1200–1206.
17. Berendt AR, Simmons DL, Tansey J, Newbold CI, Marsh K. Intercellular adhesion molecule-1 is an endothelial cell adhesion receptor for plasmodium falciparum. Nature 1989;341:57–59.
18. Bessis M. Studies on cell agony and death: an attempt at classification. In: deReuck, AVS, Knight, J, eds. Ciba Foundation Symposium on Cellular Injury. London: J & A Churchill, 1964:287–328.
19. Bessis M, Boisfleury AD. Les mouvements des leucocytes étudiés au microscope électronique à balayage. Nouv Rev Fr Hématol 1971;11:377–400.
20. Bessis M, Burte B. Chimiotactisme après destruction d'une cellule par microfaisceaux Laser. C R Soc Biol (Paris) 1964;158:1995–1997.
21. Bevilacqua MP, Pober JS, Wheeler ME, Cotran RS, Gimbrone MA Jr. Interleukin-1 activation of vascular endothelium. Effects on procoagulant activity and leukocyte adhesion. Am J Pathol 1985;121:393–403
22. Boxer GJ, Curnutte JT, Boxer LA. Polymorphonuclear leukocyte function. Hosp Pract 1985;20:69–90.
23. Boyden S. The chemotactic effect of mixtures of antibody and antigen on polymorphonuclear leucocytes. J Exp Med 1962;115:453–466.
24. Briggs RT, Drath DB, Karnovsky ML, Karnovsky MJ. Localization of NADH oxidase on the surface of human polymorphonuclear leukocytes by a new cytochemical method. J Cell Biol 1975;67:566–586.
25. Briggs RT, Robinson JM, Karnovsky ML, Karnovsky MJ. Superoxide production by polymorphonuclear leukocytes. A cytochemical approach. Histochemistry 1986; 84:371–378.
26. Caduff JH, Fischer LC, Burri PH Scanning electron microscope study of the developing microvasculature in the postnatal rat lung. Anat Rec 1986;216:154–164.
27. Carter SB. Principles of cell motility: the direction of cell movement and cancer invasion. Nature 1965;208: 1183–1187.
28. Castellot JJ, Karnovsky MJ, Spiegelman BM. Differentiation-dependent stimulation of neovascularization and endothelial cell chemotaxis by 3T3 adipocytes. Dev Biol 1982;79:5597–5601.
29. Caterina MJ, Devreotes PN. Molecular insights into eukaryotic chemotaxis. FASEB J 1991;5:3078–3085.
30. Charo IF, Yuen C, Goldstein IM. Adherence of human polymorphonuclear leukocytes to endothelial monolayers: effects of temperature, divalent cations, and chemotactic factors on the strength of adherence measured with a new centrifugation assay. Blood 1985;65:473–479.
31. Charo IF, Yuen C, Perez HD, Goldstein IM. Chemotactic peptides modulate adherence of human polymorphonuclear leukocytes to monolayers of cultured endothelial cells. J Immunol 1986;136:3412–3419.
32. Colditz IG, Movat HZ. Kinetics of neutrophil accumulation in acute inflammatory lesions induced by chemotaxins and chemotaxinigens. J Immunol 1984;133:2169–2173.
33. Collins T. Endothelial nuclear factor-kB and the initiation of the atherosclerotic lesion. Lab Invest 1993;68: 499–508.

34. Cotran RS. New roles for the endothelium in inflammation and immunity. Am J Pathol 1987;129:407–413.

35. Cotran RS, Pober JS. Cytokine-endothelial interactions in inflammation, immunity, and vascular injury. J Am Soc Nephrol 1990;1:225–235.

36. Curnutte JT, Babior BM, Karnovsky ML. Fluoride-mediated activation of the respiratory burst in human neutrophils. A reversible process. J Clin Invest 1979;63:637–647.

37. Cybulsky MI, McComb DJ, Movat HZ. Neutrophil leukocyte emigration induced by endotoxin. Mediator roles of interleukin 1 and tumor necrosis factor a. J Immunol 1988;140:3144–3149.

38. Devreotes PN, Zigmond SH. Chemotaxis in eukaryotic cells: a focus on leukocytes and Dictyostelium. Annu Rev Cell Biol 1988;4:649–686.

39. Eckert R. Bioelectric control of ciliary activity. Locomotion in the ciliated protozoa is regulated by membrane-limited calcium fluxes. Science 1972;176:473–481.

40. Elsbach P, Weiss, J. Oxygen-independent bactericidal systems of polymorphonuclear leukocytes. Adv Inflam Res 1981;2:95–113.

41. Elsbach P, Weiss, J. Phagocytic cells: oxygen-independent antimicrobial systems. In: Gallin JI, Goldstein IM, Snyderman R, eds. Inflammation: Basic principles and clinical correlates. New York: Raven Press, 1988:445–470.

42. Fåhraeus R. The suspension stability of the blood. Physiol Rev 1929;9:241–274.

43. Figdor CG, van Kooyk Y. Regulation of cell adhesion. In: Harlan JM, Liu DY, eds. Adhesion: Its role in inflammatory disease. New York: WH Freeman, 1992:151–182.

44. Fridkin M, Najjar VA. Tuftsin: its chemistry, biology, and clinical potential. Crit Rev Biochem Mol Biol 1989;24:1–40.

45. Fu TK, Kessler JO, Jarvik LF, Matsuyama SS. Philothermal and chemotactic locomotion of leukocytes. Method and results. Cell Biophys 1982;4:77–95.

46. Gabig TG, Babior BM. Oxygen-dependent microbial killing by neutrophils. In: Oberley, LW, ed. Superoxide Dismutase, vol. 2. Boca Raton: CRC Press, 1982:1–13.

47. Gadek JE, Hunninghake GW, Zimmerman RL, Crystal G. Regulation of the release of alveolar macrophage-derived neutrophil chemotactic factor. Am Rev Respir Dis 1980;121:723–733.

48. Gallin JI, Quie PG. Leukocyte Chemotaxis: methods, physiology, and clinical implications. New York: Raven Press, 1978.

49. Gallin JI, Seligmann BE Mobilization and adaptation of human neutrophil chemoattractant fMet-Leu-Phe receptors. Fed Proc 1984;43:2732–2736.

50. Gallin JI. Phagocytic cells: disorders of functions. In: Gallin JI, Goldstein IM, Snyderman R, eds. Inflammation: basic principles and clinical correlates. New York: Raven Press, 1988:493–511.

51. Geng J-G, Bevilacqua MP, Moore KL, McIntyre TM, Prescott SM, Kim JM, Bliss GA, Zimmerman GA, McEver RP. Rapid neutrophil adhesion to activated endothelium mediated by GMP-140. Nature 1990;343:757–760.

52. Ghosh S, Latimer D, Gray B.M Harwood RJ, Auduro A. Endotoxin-induced organ injury. Crit Care Med 1993;21:S19–S24.

53. Goldman R, Bar-Shavit Z. Phagocytosis—modes of particle recognition and stimulation by natural peptides. In: Karnovsky ML, and Bolis L, eds. Phagocytosis — past and future. New York: Academic Press, 1982:259–285.

54. Goldstein IM. Complement: biologically active products. In: Gallin JI, Goldstein IM, Snyderman R, eds. Inflammation. basic principles and clinical correlates. New York: Raven Press, 1988:55–74.

55. Gould SJ. Wonderful life: The burgess shale and the nature of history. New York: WW Norton, 1989.

56. Grant L. The sticking and emigration of white blood cells in inflammation. In: Zweifach BW, Grant L, McCluskey RT, eds. The inflammatory process. New York: Academic Press, 1965:197–244.

57. Gristina AG, Oga M, Webb LK, Hobgood C.D. Adherent bacterial colonization in the pathogenesis of osteomyelitis. Science 1985;228:990–993.

58. Grotendorst GR, Martin GR. Cell movements in wound-healing and fibrosis. Rheumatology 1986;10:385–403.

59. Harlan JM, Liu DY, eds. Adhesion: its role in inflammatory disease. New York: WH Freeman, 1992.

60. Harlan JM, Winn RK, Vedder NB, Doerschuk CM, Rice CL. In vivo models of leukocyte adherence to endothelium. In: Harlan JM, and Liu DY, eds. Adhesion: its role in inflammatory disease. New York: WH Freeman, 1992:117–150.

61. Harlan JM. Leukocyte-endothelial interactions. Blood 1985;65:513–525.

62. Harris H. Chemotaxis of monocytes. Br J Exp Pathol 1953;34:276–279.

63. Hattori R, Hamilton KK, Fugate RD, McEver RP, Sims PJ. Stimulated secretion of endothelial von Willebrand factor is accompanied by rapid redistribution to the cell surface of the intracellular granule membrane protein GMP-140. J Biol Chem 1989;264:7768–7771.

64. Hebbel RP, Yamada O, Moldow CF, Jacob HS, White JG, Eaton JW. Abnormal adherence of sickle erythrocytes to cultured vascular endothelium. Possible mechanism for microvascular occlusion in sickle cell disease. J Clin Invest 1980;65:154–160.

65. Henson PM, Henson JE, Fittschen C, Kimani G, Bratton DL, Riches DWH. Phagocytic cells: degranulation and secretion. In: Gallin JI, Goldstein, IM, Snyderman R, eds. Inflammation: basic principles and clinical correlates. New York: Raven Press, 1988;363–390.

66. Hill JH, Ward PA. The phlogistic role of C3 leukotactic fragments in myocardial infarcts of rats. J Exp Med 1971;133:885–900.

67. Hill JH, Ward PA. C3 leukotactic factors produced by a tissue protease. J Exp Med 1969;130:505–518.

68. Hirsch JG. Cinemicrophotographic observations on granule lysis in polymorphonuclear leucocytes during phagocytosis. J Exp Med 1962;116:827–834.

69. Hirsch JG. Phagocytosis and degranulation. A 16mm silent movie. (Available from the Film Service Department, The Rockefeller University, York Avenue and E 66th Street, New York City, NY 10021.)

70. Hoffstein ST, Friedman RS, Weissmann G. Degranulation, membrane addition, and shape change during chemotactic factor-induced aggregation of human neutrophils. J Cell Biol 1982;95:234–241.

71. Hogg JC. Neutrophil kinetics and lung injury. Physiol Rev 1987;67:1249–1295.

72. Hoover RL, Karnovsky MJ, Austen KF, Corey EJ, Lewis RA. Leukotriene B$_4$ action on endothelium mediates augmented neutrophil/endothelial adhesion. Proc natl acad sci USA 1984;81:2191–2193.

73. Hunninghake GW, Gallin JI, Fauci AS. Immunologic reactivity of the lung. The in vivo and in vitro generation of a neutrophil chemotactic factor by alveolar macrophages. Am Rev Respir Dis 1978;117:15–23.

74. Hunt JD, Ward PA. Chemotactic factor inactivator release from rat leukocytes. Inflammation 1979;3:203–214.

75. Hurley JV. Acute inflammation: the effect of concurrent leucocytic emigration and increased permeability on

particle retention by the vascular wall. Br J Exp Pathol 1964;45:627–633.

76. Hurley JV. Acute inflammation. Baltimore: Williams and Wilkins, 1972.

77. Hynes R.O. Integrins: a family of cell surface receptors. Cell 1987;48:549–554.

78. Jarvik LF, Matsuyama SS, Kessler JO, Fu T.-K, Tsai SY, Clark EO. Philothermal response of polymorphonuclear leukocytes in dementia of the Alzheimer type. Neurobiol Aging 1982;3:93–99.

79. Johnston GI, Cook RG, McEver RP. Cloning of GMP-140, a granule membrane protein of platelets and endothelium: sequence similarity to proteins involved in cell adhesion and inflammation. Cell 1989; 56:1033–1044.

80. Joris I, Zand T, Nunnari JJ, Krolikowski FJ, Majno G. Studies on the pathogenesis of atherosclerosis. I. Adhesion and emigration of mononuclear cells in the aorta of hypercholesterolemic rats. Am J Pathol 1983;113:341–358.

81. Karnovsky ML. Metabolic basis of phagocytic activity. Physiol Rev 1962;42:143–168.

82. Karnovsky MJ, Robinson JM, Briggs RT, Karnovsky ML. Oxidative cytochemistry in phagocytosis: the interface between structure and function. Histochem J 1981;13:1–22.

83. Karnovsky ML, Sbarra AJ. Metabolic changes accompanying the ingestion of particulate matter by cells. Am J Clin Nutr 1960;8:147–155.

84. Kay AB, Pepper DS, Ewart MR. Generation of chemotactic activity for leukocytes by the action of thrombin on human fibrinogen. Nature New Biol 1973; 243:56–57.

85. Keller H.U, Borel JF, Wilkinson PC, et al. Reassessment of Boyden's technique for measuring chemotaxis. J Immunol Met 1972;1:165–168.

86. Kessler JO, Jarvik LF, Fu TK, Matsuyama SS. Thermotaxis, chemotaxis and age. Age 1979;2:5–11.

87. Klebanoff SJ. Phagocytic cells: products of oxygen metabolism. In: Gallin JI, Goldstein IM, Snyderman R, eds. Inflammation: basic principles and clinical correlates. New York: Raven Press, 1988:391–444.

88. Lasky LA. The homing receptor (LECAM 1/L Selectin): a carbohydrate-binding mediator of adhesion in the immune system. In: Harlan JM, and Liu DY, eds. Adhesion: Its role in inflammatory disease. New York: WH Freeman, 1992:43–63.

89. Lauffenburger D, Farrell B, Tranquillo R, Kistler A, Zigmond S. Gradient perception by neutrophil leucocytes, continued. J Cell Sci 1987A;88:415–416.

90. Lauffenburger DA, Rivero M, Kelly F, Ford R, DiRienzo J. Bacterial chemotaxis. Cell flux model, parameter measurement, population dynamics, and genetic manipulation. Ann NY Acad Sci 1987b;506:281–295.

91. Lavie G, Zucker-Franklin D, Franklin EC. Elastase-type proteases on the surface of human blood monocytes: possible role in amyloid formation. J Immunol 1980;125:175–180.

92. Lawrence MB, Springer TA. Leukocytes roll on a selectin at physiologic flow rates: distinction from and prerequisite for adhesion through integrins. Cell XXXX;65:859–873.

93. Lehrer RI, Ganz T, Selsted ME. Defensins: endogenous antibiotic peptides of animal cells. Cell 1991;64:229–230.

94. Lien DC, Henson PM, Capen RL, et al. Neutrophil kinetics in the pulmonary microcirculation during acute inflammation. Lab Invest 1991;65:145–159.

95. Lynn WS, Somayajulu RSN, Sahu S, Selph J. Characterization of chemotactic agents produced in experimental pleural inflammation. In: Gallin JI, Quie, PG, eds.

Leukocyte chemotaxis: methods, physiology, and clinical implications. New York: Raven Press, 1978:299–306.

96. MacGregor RR, Macarak EJ, Kefalides NA. Comparative adherence of granulocytes to endothelial monolayers and nylon fiber. J Clin Invest 1978;61:697–702.

97. MacGregor RR, Spagnuolo PJ, Lentnek AL. Inhibition of granulocyte adherence by ethanol, prednisone, and aspirin, measured with an assay system. New Eng J Med 1974;291:642–646.

98. Macnab RM, Koshland DE Jr. The gradient-sensing mechanism in bacterial chemotaxis. Proc Natl Acad Sci USA 1972;69:2509–2512.

99. Majno G. Interactions between dead cells and living tissue. In: deReuck AVS, Knight J, eds. Ciba Foundation Symposium on Cellular Injury. London: J & A Churchill, 1964:87–105.

100. Majno G. The capillary then and now: an overview of capillary pathology. Mod Pathol 1992;5:9–22..

101. Malech HL, Root RK, Gallin JI. Structural analysis of human neutrophil migration. J Cell Biol 1977;75:666–693.

102. Marchesi VT. The site of leucocyte emigration during inflammation. Q J Exp Physiol 1961;46:115–118

103. Marchesi VT, Florey HW. Electron micrographic observations on the emigration of leucocytes. Q J Exp Physiol 1960;45:343–348.

104. Marlin SD, Springer TA. Purified intercellular adhesion molecule-1 (ICAM-1) is a ligand for lymphocyte function-associated antigen 1 (LFA-1). Cell 1987;51:813–819.

105. McCutcheon M, Wartman WB, Dixon HM. Chemotropism of leukocytes in vitro. Arch Pathol 1934;17:607–614.

106. McEver RP. Leukocyte interactions mediated by selectins. Thromb. Haemost 1991;66:80–87.

107. Mesibov R, Adler J. Chemotaxis toward amino acids in Escherichia coli. J Bacteriol 1972;112:315–326.

108. Metchnikoff E. Lectures on the comparative pathology of inflammation. Translated from the French by FA Starling, EH Starling, 1892. New York: Dover Publications, 1968.

109. Mok M, Abraham D, Grieve RB, Thomas CB. Thermotaxis in third and fourth-stage Dirofilaria immitis larvae. J Helminthol 1986;60:61–64.

110. Movat HZ, Cybulsky MI. Neutrophil emigration and microvascular injury. Role of chemotaxins, endotoxin, interleukin-1 and tumor necrosis factor alpha. Pathol Immunopathol Res 1987;6:153–176.

111. Nagai K, Katori M. Possible changes in the leukocyte membrane as a mechanism of leukocyte adhesion to the venular walls induced by leukotriene B$_4$ and fMLP in the microvasculature of the hamster cheek pouch. Int J Microcirc Clin Exp 1988;7:305–314.

112. Najjar VA, Nishioka K. "Tuftsin": a natural phagocytosis stimulating peptide. Nature 1970;228:672–673.

112a. Najjar VA. Tuftsin, a natural activator of phagocyte cells: an overview. In: Najjar VA, Fridkin M. (eds). Antineoplastic, immunogenic and other effects of the tetrapeptide tuftsin: a natural macrophage activator. New York: The New York Academy of Sciences, 1983:1–11.

113. Nobis U, Pries AR, Cokelet GR, Gaehtgens P. Radial distribution of white cells during blood flow in small tubes. Microvasc Res 1985;29:295–304.

114. Norris DA, Clark RAF, Swigart LM, Huff JC, Weston WL, Howell SE. Fibronectin fragment(s) are chemotactic for human peripheral blood monocytes. J Immunol 1982; 129:1612–1618.

115. Oda T, Katori M, Hatanaka K, Yamashina S. Five steps in leukocyte extravasation in the microcirculation by

chemoattractants. Mediators of inflammation 1992;1: 403–409.

116. Orenstein JM, Shelton E. Membrane phenomena accompanying erythrophagocytosis. A scanning electron microscope study. Lab Invest 1977;36:363–374.

117. Orredson SU, Knighton DR, Scheuenstuhl H, Hunt TK. A quantitative *in vitro* study of fibroblast and endothelial cell migration in response to serum and wound fluid. J Surg Res 1983;35:249–258.

118. Pabst R, Binns RM. Heterogeneity of lymphocyte homing physiology: several mechanisms operate in the control of migration to lymphoid and nonlymphoid organs *in vivo*. Immunol Rev 1989;108:83–109.

119. Parod RJ, Brain JD. Immune opsonin-independent phagocytosis by pulmonary macrophages. J Immunol 1986;136:2041–2047.

120. Paulson JC. Selectin/carbohydrate-mediated adhesion of leukocytes. In: Harlan, JM, and Liu, DY, eds. Adhesion: Its role in inflammatory disease. New York: WH Freeman, 1992:19–42.

121. Pawlowski NA, Abraham EL, Pontier S, Scott WA, Cohn ZA. Human monocyte-endothelial cell interaction *in vitro*. Proc Natl Acad Sci USA 1985;82:8208–8212.

122. Payling Wright G. Introduction to pathology. Boston: Little, Brown, 1958.

123. Pfeffer W. Locomotorische richtungs-bewegungen durch chemische Reize. Ber Dtsch Bot Ges 1883;1:524–533.

124. Pober JS. Cotran RS. Cytokines and endothelial cell biology. Physiol Rev 1990;70:427–451.

125. Podack ER. Molecular assemblies in complement—and lymphocyte-mediated cytolysis. In: Steinman RM, and North RJ, eds. Mechanisms of host resistance to infectious agents, tumors and allografts. New York: The Rockefeller Press, 1986.

126. Postlethwaite AE, Kang AH. Collagen and collagen peptide-induced chemotaxis of human blood monocytes. J Exp Med 1976;143:1299–1307.

127. Rabson AR, Anderson R, Glover A, Lomnitzer R. Inhibitory effect of prostaglandin A₁ on neutrophil motility. Br J Exp Pathol 1978;59:298–304.

128. Ramsey SW, Adler J. Chemoreceptors in bacteria. Science 1969;166:1588–1597.

129. Ruff MR, Pert CB, Weber RJ, Wahl LM, Wahl SM, Paul SM. Benzodiazepine receptor-mediated chemotaxis of human monocytes. Science 1985;229:1281–1283.

130. Ruoslahti E, Pierschbacher MD. New perspectives in cell adhesion: RGD and integrins. Science 1987;238:491–497.

131. Ryan GB, Hurley JV. The chemotaxis of polymorphonuclear leucocytes towards damaged tissue. Br J Exp Pathol 1966;47:530–536.

132. Savage DC, Fletcher M, eds. Bacterial Adhesion: Mechanisms and physiological significance. New York: Plenum Press, 1985.

133. Sawyer DW, Sullivan JA, Mandell GL. Intracellular free calcium localization in neutrophils during phagocytosis. Science 1985;230:663–666.

134. Sbarra AJ, Karnovsky ML. The biochemical basis of phagocytosis. I. Metabolic changes during the ingestion of particles by polymorphonuclear leukocytes. J Biol Chem 1959;234:1355–1362.

135. Sbarra AJ, Selvaraj RJ, Paul BB, Thomas GB, Cetrulo CL, Louis FJ, Mitchell GW Jr. Biochemical aspects of phagocytic cells: relationship between metabolic activities and physiological function. In: Altura BM, Saba TM, eds. Pathophysiology of the reticuloendothelial system. New York: Raven Press, XXXX:19819–19829.

136. Schiffmann E, Gallin JI. Biochemistry of phagocyte chemotaxis. Curr Top Cell Regulation, 1979;15:203–261.

137. Schiffmann E, Showell HV, Corcoran BA, Ward PA, Smith E, Becker EL. The isolation and partial characterization of neutrophil chemotactic factors from Escherichia coli. J Immunol 1975;114:1831–1837.

138. Schleimer RP, Rutledge BK. Cultured human vascular endothelial cells acquire adhesiveness for neutrophils after stimulation with interleukin 1, endotoxin, and tumor-promoting phorbol diesters. J Immunol 1986;136:649–654.

139. Schmid-Schönbein GW, Usami S, Skalak R, Chien S. The interaction of leukocytes and erythrocytes in capillary and postcapillary vessels. Microvasc Res 1980;19:45–70.

140. Senior RM, Griffin GL, Mecham RP. Chemotactic activity of elastin-derived peptides. J Clin Invest, 1980;66:859–862.

141. Smith CW. Transendothelial migration. In: Harlan JM, Liu DY, eds. Adhesion: its role in inflammatory disease. New York: WH Freeman, 1992:83–115.

142. Smith MR, Wood WB Jr. Surface phagocytosis. Further evidence of its destructive action upon fully encapsulated pneumococci in the absence of type-specific antibody. J Exp Med 1958;107:1–12.

143. Snyderman R, Pike MC. Chemoattractant receptors on phsgocytic cells. Annu Rev Immunol 1984;2:257–281.

144. Snyderman R, Uhing RJ. Phagocytic cells: stimulus-response coupling mechanisms. In: Gallin JI, Goldstein IM, Snyderman R, eds. Inflammation: basic principles and clinical correlates. New York: Raven Press, 1988:309–323.

145. Spector WG. The role of some higher peptides in inflammation. J Patho. Bacteriol 1951;63:93–110.

146. Spitznagel JK. Antibiotic proteins of human neutrophils. J Clin Invest 1990;86:1381–1386.

147. Springer TA Adhesion receptors of the immune system. Nature 1990;346:425–434.

148. Springer TA, Lasky LA. Sticky sugars for selectins. Nature 1991;349:196–197.

149. Stossel TP. Phagocytosis. New Eng J Med 1974;290:717–723, 774–780, and 833–839.

150. Streeter PR, Rouse BTN, Butcher EC. Immunohistologic and functional characterization of a vascular addressin involved in lymphocyte homing into peripheral lymph nodes. J Cell Biol 1988;107:1853–1862.

151. Till G, Ward PA. Two distinct chemotactic factor inactivators in human serum. J Immunol 1975;114:843–847.

152. Todd RF, Simpson PJ, Lucchesi BR. Anti–inflammatory properties of monoclonal anti-Mol (CD11b/CD18) antibodies *in vitro* and *in vivo*. In: Springer TA, Anderson DC, Rosenthal AS, Rothlein R, eds. Leukocyte adhesion molecules. New York: Springer-Verlag, 1988:125–137.

153. Tonnesen MG. Neutrophil-endothelial cell interactions: mechanisms of neutrophil adherence to vascular endothelium. J Invest Dermatol, 1989;93 (suppl. 2):53S–58S.

154. Tonnesen MG, Smedly LA, Henson PM. Neutrophil-endothelial cell interactions. Modulation of neutrophil adhesiveness induced by complement fragments C5a and C5a des arg and formyl-methionyl-leucyl-phenylalanine *in vitro*. J Clin Invest 1984;74:1581–1592.

155. Tonnesen MG, Worthen GS, Lien DC, Henson PM. Interaction of leukocytes with the vascular endothelium. In: Ryan, US, ed. Endothelial Cells, vol. 2. Boca Raton: CRC Press, 1988:193–211.

156. Tsang N, Macnab R, Koshland DE Common mechanism for repellents and attractants in bacterial chemotaxis. Science 1973;181:60–63.

157. Vadas MA, Gamble JR, Smith WB. Regulation of

myeloid blood cell-endothelial interaction by cytokines. In: Harlan, JM, Liu, DY, eds. Adhesion: its role in inflammatory disease. New York: WH Freeman, 1992: 65–81.

158. VanDeWater L, III. Phagocytosis. In: McDonagh, J, ed. Plasma fibronectin: structure and function. New York: Marcel Dekker, 1985:175–196.

159. Van Epps DE, Williams RC. Serum inhibitors of leukocyte chemotaxis and their relationship to skin test energy. In: Gallin JI, Quie, PG, eds. Leukocyte chemotaxis: methods, physiology, and clinical implications. New York: Raven Press, 1978:237–253.

160. Van Houten J. Two mechanisms of chemotaxis in Paramecium. J Comp Physiol 1978;127:167–174.

161. Van Houten J. Membrane potential changes during chemokinesis in Paramecium. Science 1979;204: 1100–1103.

162. Vel WAC, Namavar F, Verweij AMJJ, Pubben ANB, MacLaren DM. Killing capacity of human polymorphonuclear leukocytes in aerobic and anaerobic conditions. J Med Microbiol 1984;18:173–180.

163. Vicker MG, Lackie JM, Schill W. Neutrophil leucocyte chemotaxis is not induced by a spatial gradient of chemoattractant. J Cell Sci 1986;84:263–280.

164. von Oss C.J Phagocytosis as a surface phenomenon. Annu Rev Microbiol 1978;32:19–39.

165. Vukajlovich SW, Hoffman J, Morrison D.C. Activation of human serum complement by bacterial lipopolysaccharides: structural requirements for antibody independent activation of the classical and alternative pathways. Mol Immunol 1987;24:319–331.

166. Walters MN-I, Papadimitriou JM. Phagocytosis: a review. CRC Crit Rev Toxicol 1978;5:377–421.

167. Ward PA. Overview. In: Gallin JI, Quie, PG, eds. Leukocyte chemotaxis: methods, physiology, and clinical implications. New York: Raven Press, 1978: 405–411.

168. Ward PA. Chemotactic factors generated from the complement system. Protides Biol Fluids 1967;15:487–490.

169. Ward PA, Becker EL. Biology of leukotaxis. Rev. Physiol Biochem Pharmacol 1977;77:125–148.

170. Ward PA, Chapitis J, Conroy MC, Lepow IH. Generation by bacterial proteinases of leukotactic factors from human serum, and human C3 and C5. J Immunol 1973;110:1003–1009.

171. Ward PA, Hill JH. C5 chemotactic fragments produced by an enzyme in lysosomal granules of neutrophils. J Immunol 1970;104:535–543.

172. Ward PA, Newman LJ A neutrophil chemotactic factor from human C'5. J Immunol 1969;102:93–99.

173. Ward PA, Remold HG, David JR. The production by antigen-stimulated lymphocytes of a leukotactic factor distinct from migration inhibitory factor. Cell Immunol 1970;1:162–174.

174. Weiss SJ. Tissue destruction by neutrophils. New Eng J Med 1989;320:365–376.

175. Weissman IL, Butcher EC, Rouse RV, Scollay RG. Cell-cell interactions in the establishment and maintenance of lymphoid tissue architecture. In: Sercarz E, Cunningham AJ, eds. Strategies of immune regulation. New York: Academic Press, 1980:77–94.

176. White MV, Kaliner MA. Histamine. In: Gallin JI, Goldstein IM, and Snyderman R, eds. Inflammation: basic principles and clinical correlates. New York: Raven Press, 1988:169–193.

177. Wilkinson PC. Chemotaxis and inflammation, 2nd ed. Edinburgh: Churchill Livingstone, 1982.

178. Wilkinson PC, Lackie JM. The adhesion, migration and chemotaxis of leucocytes in inflammation. Curr Top Pathol 1979;68:47–88.

179. Wood WB Jr. White blood cells v. bacteria. Sci Am 1951;184:48–52.

180. Wright DG, Gallin JI. Secretory responses of human neutrophils: exocytosis of specific (secondary) granules by human neutrophils during adherence in vitro and during exudation in vivo. J Immunol 1979;123:285–294.

181. Yuli I, Oplatka A. Cytosolic acidification as an early transductory signal of human neutrophil chemotaxis. Science 1987;235:340–342.

182. Zigmond SH. Ability of polymorphonuclear leukocytes to orient in gradients of chemotactic factors. J Cell Biol 1977;75:606–616.

183. Zigmond SH. Chemotaxis by polymorphonuclear leukocytes. J Cell Biol 1978;77:269–287.

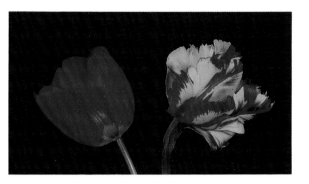

PLATE 1

Another disease that favored propagation: the tulip at the right is infected with a virus of the mosaic type. These Rembrandt or broken tulips are less hardy but much coveted; in Holland in the early 1600s they caused an outbreak of social tulipomania. Tiger lilies are a similar example of beautiful disease.

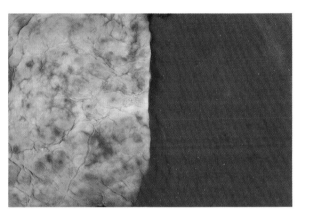

PLATE 2

Close-up view of two livers, placed next to each other and reproduced here in natural size. Left: Fatty liver with early cirrhosis in an alcoholic. Right: Normal liver as a control.

PLATE 3

Four common pigments seen in microscopic sections of animal tissues. A-D: hematoxylin and eosin stain. A: myocardial cells with lipofuscin granules (wear-and-tear pigment) collected in the space free of fibrils at either pole of the nucleus. Bar = 25 um. B: black granules of hematin (formol pigments), a fixation artifact. The pigments have formed over red blood cells because it derives from their hemoglobin. Bar = um. C: clusters of bilirubin crystals in necrotic tissue, at the edge of the spleen infarct. Arrowhead: one of the several cholesterol crystals, as often seen in necrotic tissue. The nuclei at right belong to mainly macrophages surrounding the infarcts. Bar = 100 um.

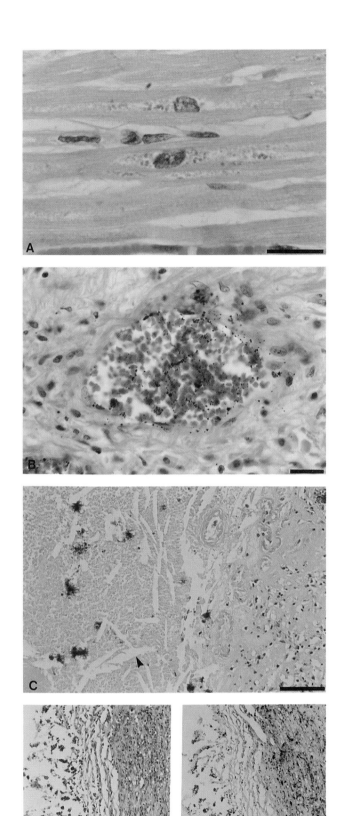

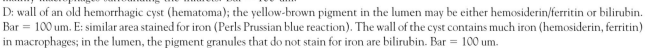

D: wall of an old hemorrhagic cyst (hematoma); the yellow-brown pigment in the lumen may be either hemosiderin/ferritin or bilirubin. Bar = 100 um. E: similar area stained for iron (Perls Prussian blue reaction). The wall of the cyst contains much iron (hemosiderin, ferritin) in macrophages; in the lumen, the pigment granules that do not stain for iron are bilirubin. Bar = 100 um.

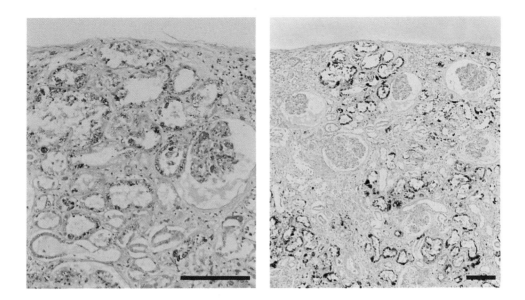

PLATE 4
Hemosiderosis in a human kidney, due to chronic low-grade hemolysis caused by a metallic prosthetic cardiac valve (St. Jude valve). Left: The dark (brown) deposits in the tubules represent hemosiderin derived from reabsorbed hemoglobin. Hematoxylin and eosin stain. Right: Same deposits for iron (Perls Prussian blue reaction). Bars = 200 um.

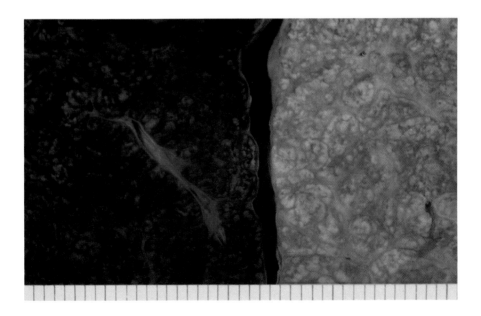

PLATE 5
Two slices of the same cirrhotic liver, from a case of hemochromatosis. Right: Fresh, untreated tissue. The rusty color betrays the presence of iron pigments (hemosiderin, ferritin). Lighter dots represent areas of regenerating liver. Left: Similar slice after a histochemical reaction from iron. The resulting Prussian blue shows that iron is everywhere, in the stroma as well as in the liver cells. Scale in mm.

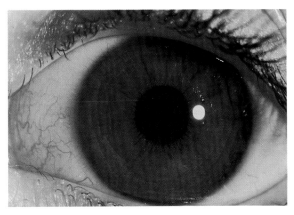

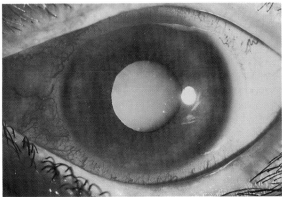

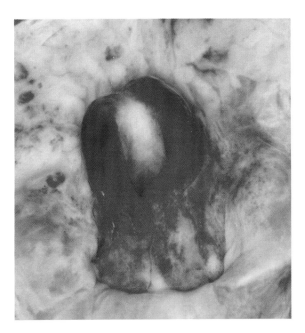

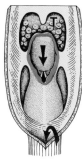

PLATE 6

A normal human eye and an eye with a cataractous lens. The whiteness of the necrotic lens, due to protein denaturation, is common to most necrotic tissues. (Courtesy of Dr. J. Babel, Geneva, Switzerland.)

PLATE 8

Inflammatory RUBOR: the acutely inflamed epiglottis of a 7-year-old child who died of asphyxia. Such infections are usually caused by Haemophilus influenzea; the epiglottis swells and becomes cherry red. Stridor (harsh sound during respiration) is a warning and should be treated as an emergency. Approx. 2x Below: anatomical scheme of the epiglottis, as seen from behind the soft palate, looking forward. T = root of the tongue; straight arrow = entrance to the airway; curved arrow = entrance to the esophagus. (Courtesy of Dr. F.J. Krolikowski, Medical Examiner Commonwealth of Massachusetts.)

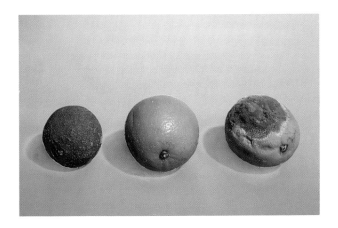

PLATE 7

The notion of dry and moist gangrene illustrated with oranges. Center: normal orange. Left: an orange that became dehydrated over several weeks at room temperature; it sustained no fungal or bacterial growth. A similar sequence applies to the umbilical cord. Right: moist gangrene. This orange became infected before it had time to dry, and is now being overgrown with fungi and bacteria.

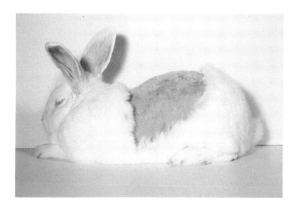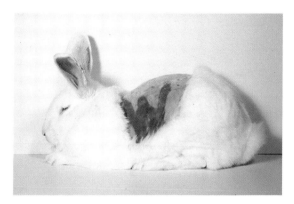

PLATE 9

Experiment demonstrating the speed of the permeability - increasing response. Left: White rabbit with shaven back and flanks, 1 minute after an intravenous injection of trypan blue. The letter W (for Worcester) has been painted on the skin with xylee, a very mild irritant. Comparison with the following photograph will show that the W is just beginning to appear. Right: The same rabbit 5 minutes later. Trypan blue leaked out of the vessels only where the skin has been irritated.

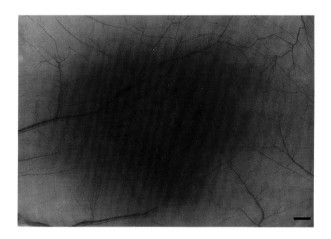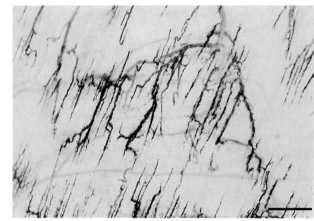

PLATE 10

Contrasting two methods for demonstrating vascular leakage. Cremaster muscles 30 minutes after a local injection of histamine; whole mounts, transilluminated. *Left*: "Bluing" by an intravenous injection of the dye Trypan blue (chemically similar to Evans blue). The dye is not retained within the walls of the leaky vessels. Bar = 1000 μm. (Preparation by Dr. G.I. Schoefl; from (52a). *Right*: Vascular labeling identifies individual leaky vessels. The horizontal unlabeled vessel is an arteriole. (This preparation also illustrates double labeling, with carbon black followed by Monastral blue; see text.) Bar = 500 μm.

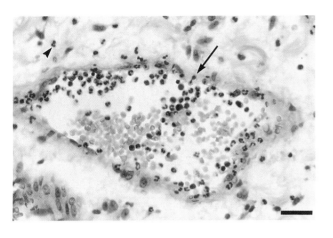

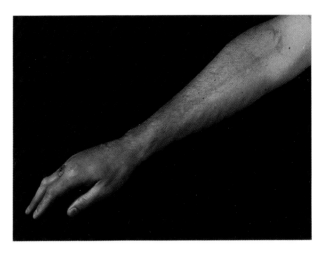

PLATE 11
Diapedesis in histologic sections can only be guessed. A venule in the wall of an acutely inflamed colon. Neutrophils are recognizable by their nucleus subdivided into 2-3 lobes (arrowhead). Some are adherent to the endothelium, trapped within the thickness of the vascular wall (arrow) or free outside. Bar = 25 um.

PLATE 12
Example of non-infectious lymphangitic streak. Arm of a 32-year-old man, 36 hours after uprooting without gloves a stem of poison ivy. Note the red streak running from the wrist to the elbow crease. The hand is swollen and a blister has appeared. (Courtesy of Mr. R.J. Madison.)

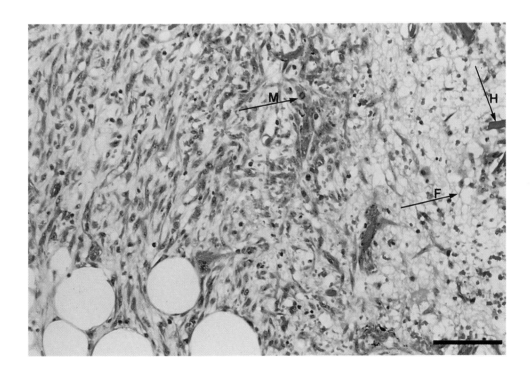

PLATE 13
Typical young granulation tissue surrounding a 5-day-old experimental hematoma (3 ml of blood were injected in the adipose tissue of a rat). The granulation tissue consist mainly of activated fibroblasts, forming a wall around the hematoma (just out of sight at the right). F = fibrin filaments; H = crystal of hemoglobin; M = mitosis, probably in a fibroblast. Bar = 100 um.

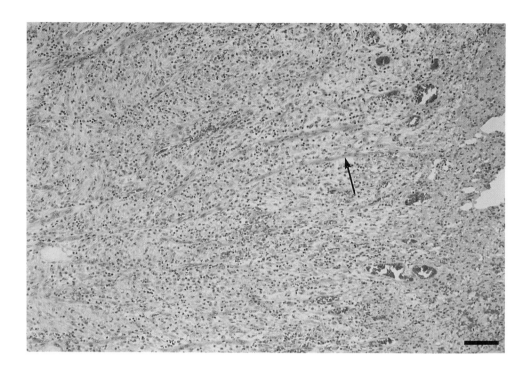

PLATE 14

Granulation tissue from a case of empyema of the pleura in a 30-year-old man. The pleura had been infected 3 weeks previously, and the inner surface of the chest wall had become coated with a layer of granulation tissue about 8 mm thick. The layer facing the cavity and exuding pus is at the right. Overall the cellular population consists mainly of fibroblasts, macrophages (not distinguishable here), and other inflammatory cells). Arrow: newly formed capillary. Bar = 100 um.

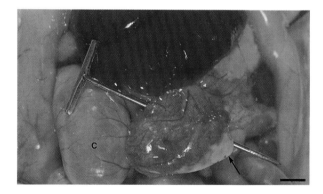

PLATE 15

Abdominal cavity of a rat 2 days after implantation of a fragment of sterile, fresh liver. The implant has inflamed the omentum, which has wrapped it up. A small area of white, necrotic liver is still visible at lower right (arrow). C: cecum. Bar = 5 mm.

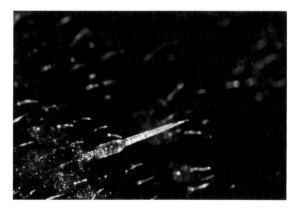

PLATE 16

Stringing hair on the leaf of a nettle, a plant of the genus Urtica, ready to inflict urticaria by injecting a sophisticated mix of inflammatory mediators. (About 25x).

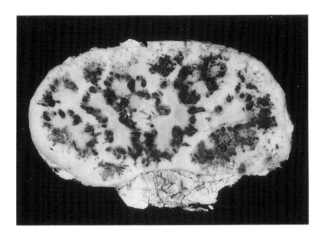

PLATE 17
Acutely rejected human kidney. The vessels are dilated and thrombosed; the parenchyma is white due to coagulation necrosis. Slightly reduced.

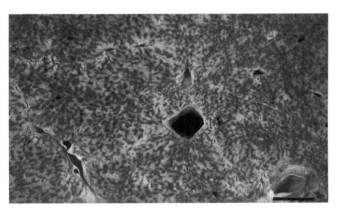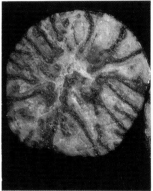

PLATE 18
The nutmeg liver typical of chronic congestion. The liver is filled with blood (hence the dark red background) and studded with yellow dots and streaks corresponding to the centers of the lobules. The steatosis responsible for the yellow discoloration is caused by anorexia. Scale in mm. Inset: the polished surface of a nutmeg justifies the comparison.

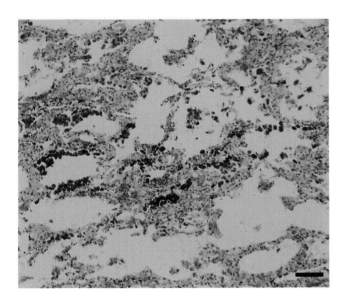

PLATE 19
Human lung with two typical changes of chronic passive congestion: (1) macrophages loaded with hemosiderin (the dark brown cells), (2) fibrosis of the alveolar walls, many of which are greatly thickened. Bar = 100 um.

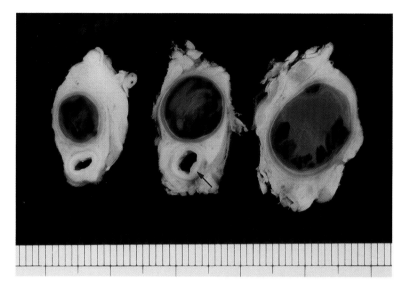

PLATE 20
Occluding thrombi in the popliteal and femoral veins. The thrombi are mixed (red and white). Note that the artery (arrow) is speared. From a patient who died of adenocarcinoma of the stomach. Scale in mm.

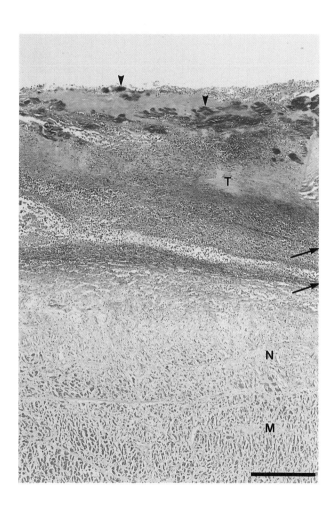

PLATE 21
An infected thrombus on the inner surface of the heart (left ventricle). Such thrombi may give rise to septic emboli. T = thrombus, almost free of red blood cells, and consisting mainly of platelets and fibrin; arrowheads point to colonies of bacteria, appearing as bluish clouds. M = myocardium, N = necrotic myocardium; this layer may have been killed by bacterial toxins and/or by deprivation of oxygen and nutrients by the overlying thrombus. The layer between arrows corresponds to the endocardium (former inner lining of the heart). Bar = 500 um.

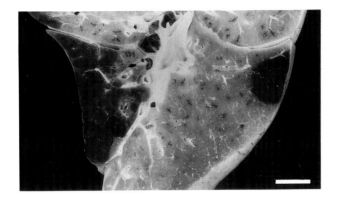

PLATE 22
Slice of human lung showing two recent infarcts still at the red stage. On a chest X-ray they would have appeared roughly as triangles with the base on the pleura. Bar = 2 cm.

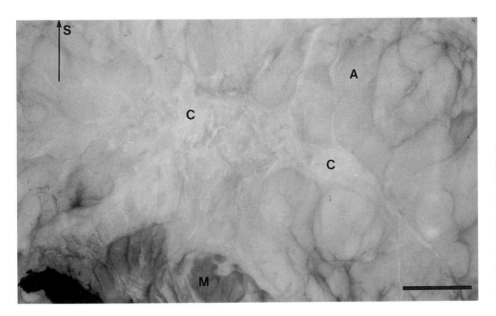

PLATE 23
Cross section of a carcinoma of the breast (C) infiltrating adipose tissue (A). Some of its extensions reach toward the skin (S) and toward the underlying muscle (M). The fine yellowish streaks within the main mass of the tumor are epithelial cords. Bar = 10 mm. (Courtesy of Miss T.M. Turner, University of Massachusetts, Worcester, MA.)

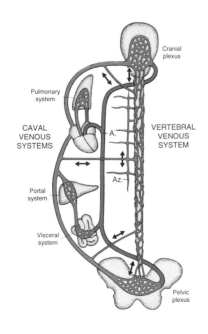

PLATE 24
Batsonís vertebral venous system: overall view. Notice how malignant cells released from a carcinoma in the pelvic region could reach the skull without ever passing through the caval system or the lungs. A: Aorta. Az: Azygos vein.

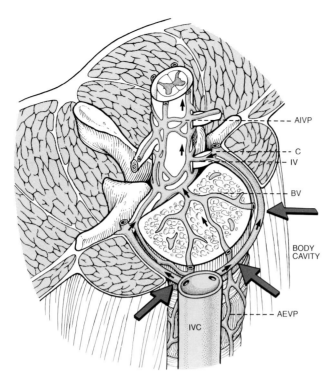

PLATE 25

Batson's vertebral venous system: detail. Note that the veins of the anterior external venous plexus are exposed to the pressure existing within the body cavity. If metastatic tumor cells are traveling in these veins, a sudden rise in abdominal pressure can squeeze them into deeper veins, and from there they can travel all the way up to the cranial plexus. AIVP = anterior internal venous plexus; C = connection of caval and vertebral systems via the lumbar vein; IV = intervertebral vein; BV = basivertebral vein; AEVP = anterior external venous plexus.

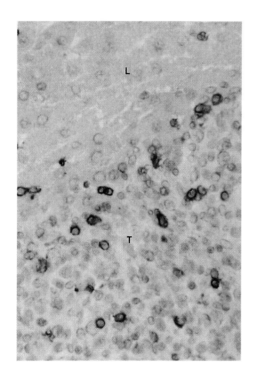

PLATE 26

NK cells infiltrating a tumor (T) growing in a rat liver (L). The NK cells (dark brown) are demonstrated with a powerful monoclonal antibody (3.2.3 prepared by Dr. J.C. Hiserodt). This tumor is a mammary adenocarcinoma that happens to be NK resistant. Immunoperoxidase stain. (Courtesy of Dr. J.C. Hiserodt, Pittsburgh, PA.)

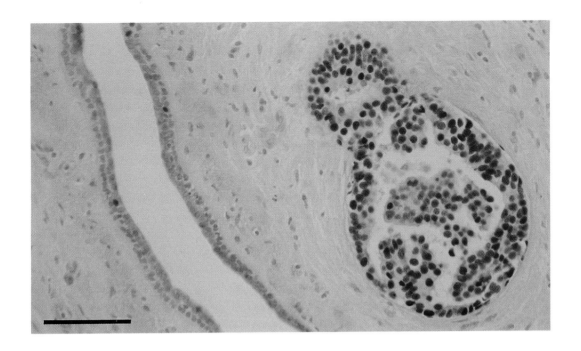

PLATE 27

Human breast; demonstration of estrogen receptors by immunohistochemistry. On the left is a normal duct; very few nuclei show a positive reaction. On the right is an atypical intraductal hyperplasia; many cells are estrogen receptor positive. This suggests that increased local sensitivity to estrogen may play a role in the pathogenesis of this condition. L = Lumen. Bar = 100 u. (Courtesy of Dr. M.E. Bur, Baystate Medical Center, Springfield, MA.)

The Inflammatory Exudate

CHAPTER 12

Dynamics of Exudation

Functions of the
Inflammatory Exudate

Types of Exudate

What Becomes of the
Inflammatory Exudate?

Exudate is the distinctive product of the inflammatory response. It is a well-programmed mixture of cells and fluid. Up to this point we have explained how these two components of the exudate are conveyed to site of injury, where the alarm has sounded. Now we are ready to step back and view the process of exudation as a whole.

Dynamics of Exudation

Both the escape of fluid and the exudation of cells are based on a mixture of biological responses and physical mechanisms. They also affect each other.

The extravasation of fluid Acute inflammation throws off the equilibrium of fluid exchanges at the level of the microcirculation. For those readers who need a reminder of the forces involved in this equilibrium (Starling's law), Table 12.1 contains the raw figures. In essence: under normal conditions, the biological filter of the microcirculation (the endothelium of the capillaries and venules) behaves more or less like a semipermeable membrane, allowing the escape of water and electrolytes but retaining most of the plasma proteins (this is an oversimplification, but it will do for our present purposes). Therefore, the exchanges between blood and tissue depend on hydrostatic and osmotic forces acting on both sides of the endothelium. Normally the main force driving fluid OUT of the vessels is the hydrostatic pressure of the blood; the main force driving fluid BACK INTO THE BLOOD is the colloidal osmotic pressure of the plasma proteins. (Table 12.1 also conveys the notion that the extravascular hydrostatic pressure is negative: we will return to this astonishing fact in discussing edema [p. 597]).

In acute inflammation all elements of this equilibrium are perturbed. The semipermeable membrane is riddled with leaks. Furthermore, the main force driving fluid out of the vessels is increased (because the arterioles are dilated, which increases capillary pressure); and the main force driving fluid back into the blood is decreased, because some plasma proteins are escaping into the tissue spaces, and create there an osmotic pressure that competes with that of the plasma remaining in the vessel (Figure 12.1). This means that the loss of fluid and protein through the endothelial leaks is exaggerated by the dilatation of the arterioles; thus, inflammatory mediators that dilate arterioles—but do not increase vascular permeability—will still increase the loss of fluid (26). This effect can be measured (Figure 12.2).

There is, in principle, no limit to the amount of exudate that can seep out of an inflamed *body surface*, such as a wound; but when exudation occurs in the tissue spaces, the tissues are distended, and the corresponding increase in tissue

TABLE 12.1
Forces Involved in Filtration and Reabsorption Along the Capillary and Venule

AT THE ARTERIAL END OF THE CAPILLARY	MM HG	AT THE VENULAR END OF THE CAPILLARY	MM HG
Forces tending to move fluid outward:		**Force tending to move fluid inward:**	
Capillary pressure	30.0	Plasma colloid osmotic pressure	28.0
Negative interstitial free fluid pressure	5.3	Total Inward Force	28.0
Interstitial fluid colloid osmotic pressure	6.0	**Forces tending to move fluid outward:**	
Total Outward Force	41.3	Capillary pressure	10.0
Forces tending to move fluid inward:		Negative interstitial free fluid pressure	5.3
Plasma colloid osmotic pressure	28.0	Interstitial fluid colloid osmotic pressure	6.0
Total Inward Force	28.0	Total Outward Force	21.3
Summation of forces:		**Summation of forces:**	
Outward	41.3	Inward	28.0
Inward	28.0	Outward	21.3
Net Outward Force	13.3	Net Inward Force	6.7

Adapted from (10)

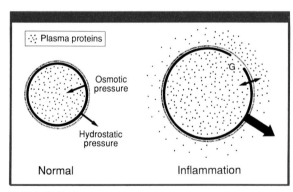

FIGURE 12.1
Schematic cross-section of two capillaries or venules, represented as membranes impermeable to plasma protein molecules (dots). *Left:* The normal condition. The two main opposing forces causing filtration and reabsorption (**arrows**) are balanced. *Right:* In inflammation, the membrane is interrupted by gaps (**G**); proteins escape, so that intra- and extravascular osmotic pressures tend to cancel each other; intravascular hydrostatic pressure is greatly increased (*heavy arrow*). Result: inflammatory edema.

pressure opposes further exudation. In a dog's knee that is experimentally inflamed by injected urate crystals (a sort of artificial gout), the joint pressure rises to a level approaching diastolic pressure (Figure 12.3).

The turnover of extractable (i.e., unbound) exudate proteins was measured in rabbit skin after burns produced with the ill-famed vesicant war gas nitrogen mustard. In one-day lesions the total renewal of the extractable proteins required about 8 hours; in three- and five-day lesions, about 35 hours (12).

The neutrophil—mononuclear cell sequence As we have mentioned, one of the constant features of inflammation is that the neutrophils arrive first at the scene of injury; then come the mononuclear cells (monocytes/macrophages, and lymphocytes). The sequence has few exceptions. It can be demonstrated in a human volunteer by applying two "skin windows" at a 12-hour interval (Figure 12.4). Another classic method is to inject a very mild irritant, such as glycogen, into the peritoneal cavity of a rat and then count, at various time intervals, the neutrophils and the mononuclear

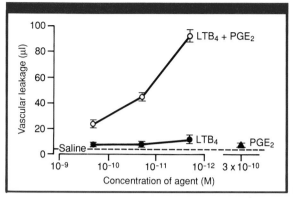

FIGURE 12.2
Demonstrating that vasodilators increase vascular leakage. Leukotriene B$_4$—injected alone into the skin of a rabbit—causes very little vascular leakage; if it is injected together with a powerful vasodilator (prostaglandin E$_2$) the loss of fluid is greatly increased. (Adapted from [53].)

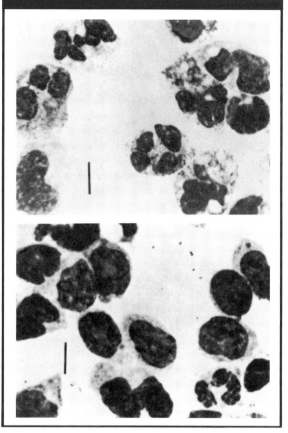

FIGURE 12.4
The sequence neutrophils–monocytes illustrated by the method of the "skin window." An area of skin 3 mm wide is scarified, and a coverslip is taped over it. *Top:* After 3 hours the predominant cell type on the coverslip is the neutrophil. *Bottom:* After 12 hours, the monocyte is predominant. **Bars** = 10 μm. (Reproduced with permission from [41].)

cells in the peritoneal fluid. Again, the two curves peak about 12 hours apart (Figure 12.5). The lymphocytes tend to follow the monocyte pattern (Figure 12.6).

It is easy to understand that the macrophages need to take over, but the mechanism that brings about this change is just beginning to be worked out. The old theory that "the neutrophils recruit the monocytes" is not entirely wrong, but it is probably irrelevant; because if the neutrophils are experimentally eliminated from the circulating blood, the monocytes emigrate on schedule (28). The current view is that *the endothelium begins to recruit more mononuclear cells than neutrophils*. It does so by expressing a different pattern of endothelium-leukocyte adhesion molecules; this shift must depend, in turn, on *a change in the chemotaxins* produced in the inflammatory focus; especially significant in this regard are the

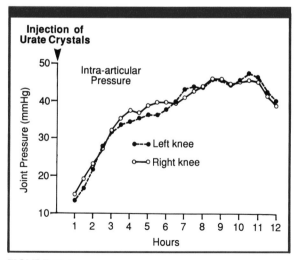

FIGURE 12.3
Experiment illustrating tissue pressure in acute inflammation. Intraarticular pressure of two joints (dog knees) inflamed by injection of urate crystals. The curves rise to a level approaching diastolic blood pressure. The joint space can be taken to represent an "enlarged interstitial space." (Reproduced with permission from [31].)

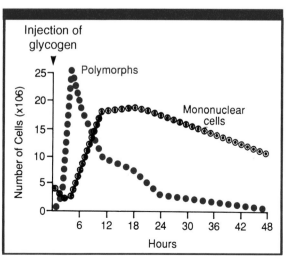

FIGURE 12.5
The cellular sequence of a typical acute inflammatory response, illustrated by injecting a mild irritant (glycogen) into the rat peritoneum. An early neutrophil response is followed by a more protracted mononuclear response. (Adapted from [22].)

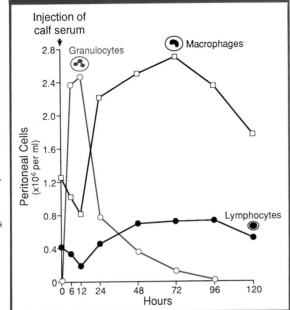

FIGURE 12.6
Changing numbers of granulocytes, macrophages, and lymphocytes in the mouse peritoneal cavity, which has been irritated by an injection of calf serum. (Reproduced with permission from [47].)

chemotactic cytokines (*chemokines*) which are specific for subsets of leukocytes, including monocytes (44a). Remember also that when inflammation becomes chronic, the venular endothelial cells come to resemble—in structure and function—the "high-endothelium venules" of lymphatic tissue, vessels that are specialized in recruiting lymphocytes (p. 430).

The overall picture is still sketchy, but data are accumulating fast, mostly from studies of endothelium grown in vitro. For example, endothelial cells are exposed to histamine in vitro, they begin to release a chemotaxin for neutrophils within 1

minute (5). When endothelial cells are exposed to interleukin-1, a macrophage product, they express ELAM-1 and ICAM-1, which bind mainly neutrophils, and VCAM-1, which binds selectively to monocytes and lymphocytes (37); they also secrete a monocyte chemoattractant protein called MCP-1/JE (42). As usual, nothing is simple: cytokine-stimulated endothelial cells also secrete an inhibitor of leukocyte adhesion (51).

The mononuclear cell population expands also because once emigrated, *the monocytes (macrophages) and lymphocytes are able to multiply*, whereas the neutrophils quickly die off and disappear.

Note that the neutrophil-monocyte sequence can be modulated: if the causal agent continues to call for neutrophils, as in an acute staphylococcal infection, the total number and percentage of neutrophils can remain high (22). In some long-lasting infections the outpouring of neutrophils continues for weeks and months.

Correlation between escaping fluid and cells It is fairly easy to measure the time course of local accumulation of fluid and cells—for example, in the skin of a rabbit after a standard injection of live *E. coli* (Figure 12.7). As the figure shows, the curves are almost parallel. Fluid begins to pour out of the vessels immediately after injury; the leukocytes appear after a slight delay because they need some time to crawl out of the vessels (9, 19, 32). Some red blood cells, too, tend to escape across the leaky endothelium.

Incidentally, why should an injection of E. coli increase vascular permeability? Because the endotoxin

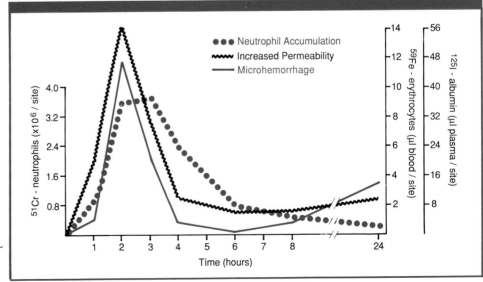

FIGURE 12.7
Time course of inflammatory events in the skin of a rabbit after intradermal injection of live *E. coli* (2 × 10⁷). Vascular permeability increases immediately and is promptly followed by microhemorrhage and extravasation of neutrophils. (Reproduced with permission from [32].)

on the surface of these gram-negative bacteria activates complement; and when this happens, permeability-increasing molecules are released (p. 345).

Do the venules become leaky as a result of diapedesis? We know that diapedesis tears up the basement membrane; it would not be surprising if persistant diapedesis also wore down the interendothelial junctions. Certainly the epithelium of the gut is disrupted by the transmigration of leukocytes: the tight junctions are damaged and an increased permeability to ions has been shown (33). Besides diapedesis, the very presence of leukocytes should play a role in fluid exudation. Remember that leukocytes answering a chemotactic stimulus are partially activated: therefore they might increase permeability by secreting enzymes, eicosanoids, PAF, cytokines, or free radicals, and there is some evidence that they do (29, 54, 55).

A bizarre development: it has been reported that rabbits that made leukopenic with nitrogen mustard do not respond to the permeability-increasing mediator C5a desArg, a breakdown product of C5a (24, 49). Perhaps the nitrogen mustard makes the vessels insensitive to permeability agents? Not so, because they still respond to histamine and bradykinin. We must conclude, rather surprisingly, that in certain conditions, "no leukocytes, no leakage."

Vascular leakage of any kind seems to be followed by a mild delayed episode of leukocyte emigration (Figure 12.8) (21), as if a plasma factor had become activated out in the tissues.

The mechanism is not clear, but here is a possibility: exudate includes the plasma protein Hageman factor, which is activated by collagen fibers. Activated Hageman factor triggers no less than four enzyme cascades, all of which produce chemotactic factors (p. 338).

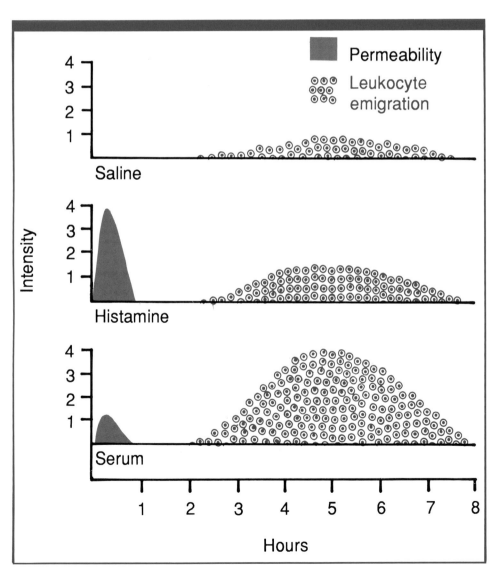

FIGURE 12.8
Examples of delayed leukocyte emigration, mainly of neutrophils, in rat skin after a local injection of vascular permeability-increasing agents such as normal saline, histamine, and serum. (Adapted from [20].)

Functions of the Inflammatory Exudate

Assuming that the exudate was designed by evolution as an anti-parasitic and especially anti-bacterial fluid, we can rationalize a defensive function for all its main components. The mere bulk of fluid may be helpful by diluting bacterial toxins (although the associated swelling should tend to diminish tissue oxygenation by increasing the distance between capillaries). The leukocytes phagocytize bacteria and debris, while delivering chemical commands to all other cells; if an immune response is required, the macrophages initiate it, while also orchestrating general effects such as fever. The proteins of the exudate assist in the antibacterial fight by providing opsonins, antibodies, and the killing mechanism called complement; as to the fibrin network, even though there is no proof that it acts as a bacterial trap as tradition maintains, it probably does hamper bacteria in a different way: by providing leukocytes with a surface against which they can better trap their prey (*surface phagocytosis*).

But then, what is the purpose of the exudate when there are no parasites to eliminate? Why, for example, should a myocardial infarct trigger acute inflammation?

The answer, we believe, lies once again in the evolutionary significance of inflammation as a primarily antibacterial response. The doubling time of common pathogenic bacteria is of the order of 20 minutes. The number of bacteria required to produce clinical infection is about 10^5 per gram of tissue (much less for beta-hemolytic streptococcus [13a]); a single bacterium could reach that number in just 6 hours. Therefore, it is essential to destroy the colony as soon as possible. The sooner the bacteria are attacked, the better. This is true also for antibiotic treatment (2) (Figure 12.9). Once bacteria have penetrated a tissue, there is a grace period of 2–4 hours during which the course of the infection can be influenced most successfully; after 6 hours the beachhead is well-entrenched and treatment is more difficult. The leukocytes seem to have learned that lesson long ago: if they waited for a call coming directly from the infectious agents, it might be too late.

Therefore, *an efficient antibacterial defense program requires that the acute inflammatory response be triggered BEFORE the bacteria reveal their presence.* Indeed, as we have seen, inflammation is triggered instantly by the products of tissue damage. The price to pay is that any kind of tissue damage, infected or not, infarcts included, will induce an immediate acute inflammatory response. So the activated bactericidal neutrophils invading an infarct find "nothing to do"; they just rush in because they follow a program, dictated by chemical messages. In infarcts of the heart's left ventricle the neutrophils probably make matters worse: their enzymes tenderize the dead tissue and make it more prone to burst under the pressure from within the ventricle.

However, it would be presumptuous to conclude that the inflammatory response from infarcts is totally useless. All infarcts must be reabsorbed (organized) anyway, and inflammation is needed for that purpose. The first wave of inflammatory cells may be wasted, but the second phase will perform an essential function.

Types of Exudate

The inflammatory exudate is not a standardized mixture: its major components (leukocytes, fluid, fibrin, red blood cells) appear in varying proportions. The differences among various exudates can be appreciated with the naked eye, and they can give important hints about the inflammatory response.

Pus A *purulent exudate, or more simply pus, is an exudate rich in cells;* its high cell content gives it a creamy, whitish look. Pus is typical of infections by

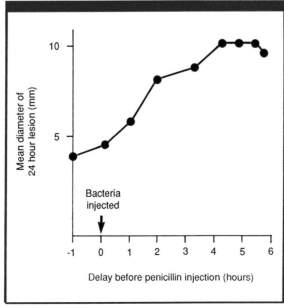

FIGURE 12.9
Effect of delaying antibiotic therapy after injection. Staphylococci were injected in the skin, and the size of the resulting lesion was measured 24 hours later. Penicillin was injected at various times during the 24 hours. As can be seen, the later the penicillin injection, the larger the lesion. (Adapted from Burke, [2].)

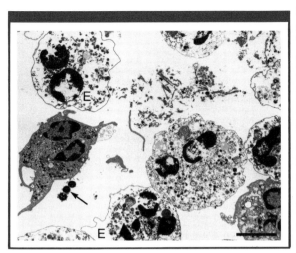

FIGURE 12.10
Electron microscopic aspect of pus from a subcutaneous infection of a guinea pig with *Staphylococcus aureus*. Most of the leukocytes are dead or dying as shown by cellular edema, nuclear changes, and cell debris. One live neutrophil has three bacteria (**arrow**) attached to it. **Bar** = 5 μm.

strongly chemotactic bacteria such as staphylococci (Figure 12.10). It follows that the formation of pus (suppuration) denotes a healthy and vigorous response. This fact was recognized in antiquity, however dimly: "creamy pus" was considered good news and was known as *pus bonum et laudabile*, good and laudable pus, in contrast to relatively thin, bloody pus of rapidly progressing infections.

Pus is acidic. Compared with plasma (Table 12.2) it has higher concentrations of two intracellular ions, potassium and phosphate, presumably from dead cells. The levels of potassium

correlate with hemolysis and are high enough to activate neutrophils (58), perhaps a useful feature. The protein content of pus is lower than that of plasma because every exudate is mixed with transudate (defined on p. 604): ultrafiltration is increased because blood flow is increased. Proteolytic activity is high, which may account for the low immunoglobulin and complement levels (48). The proteolytic or "digestive" activity of pus was also noticed in antiquity from the fact that suppuration of bruised wounds tends to dissolve and remove necrotic debris (30). The cell count in pleural pus has given figures of the order of 10^8 cells/ml (95% neutrophils, 60–90% alive) (48). Interestingly enough, bacterial counts in pus from several sources have been of the same order, which means that pus provides roughly one neutrophil per bacterium, a generous but not a wasteful supply.

Hemorrhagic exudates A hemorrhagic exudate contains—besides leukocytes—enough red blood cells to be grossly blood-stained. It implies vascular damage and therefore points to an infection of a destructive nature. (Incidentally, a hemorrhagic exudate in a serosal [peritoneal, pericardial, or pleural] cavity may also indicate invasion by a malignant tumor.)

Serous exudates A serous exudate is a protein-containing fluid that resembles serum. Serum is the thin, slightly yellowish fluid that is extruded by a blood clot as it retracts; it differs from plasma because it lacks fibrinogen and contains platelet factors and products of the activated clotting cascade. A serous exudate implies that few leuko-

TABLE 12.2

Chemistry of Human Pus

Assay	Units	Value	Range	Normal plasma values
pH	pH	**6.17**	5.5–6.8	7.35–7.45
Osmolality	mOsm/kg H₂O	402	207–535	280–296
Sodium	mEq/L	119	92–134	135–145
Potassium	mEq/L	**18.5**	10–33.5	3.5–5.0
Chloride	mEq/L	87.9	60–109	100–108
Calcium	mg/dl	6.2	2.8–9.3	8.5–10.5
Phosphate	mg/dl	**14.5**	6.2†–28.2	3.0–4.5
Protein[a]	g/L	29.9	± 12.6	60–84

Adapted from (1).
[a]*From* (48).
† *Originally published as 62, which we take to be an error.*

TABLE 12.3
Comparison of Exudate and Transudate Protein Content

Condition	Specific Gravity	Average protein concentration in pleural fluids (g%)			
		Total Protein	Fibrin	Serum Globulin	Serum Albumin
Acute pleurisy (exudate)	1021	4.59	0.047	2.00	2.54
Hydrothorax (transudate)	1014	1.77	0.009	0.61	1.16

Adapted from (35)

cytes have been summoned. An example is the content of a blister after a mild burn. Large serous exudates can develop in the pleural spaces as a result of chronic low-grade inflammation; it is important to distinguish them from transudates due to a hydrodynamic disturbance such as heart failure, because the therapy is obviously different. The basic difference is that transudates contain less protein (Table 12.3).

> Seroma, *a pocket filled with clear, sterile fluid, is a postoperative complication; the term appears almost exclusively in the surgical literature (38, 44). Seromas develop in several surgical settings, and correspondingly the fluid may not always be quite the same. For example, a seroma can develop in the free tissue space created when surgery (e.g., mastectomy) requires the undermining of a large skin flap; in this case the fluid is mainly lymph. Seromas can also develop around a tubular Dacron graft inserted along an artery; suggested causes include "weeping" of fluid across the Dacron, a serous inflammatory reaction, and a collection of lymph escaping from severed lymphatics. In any event, seromas should be removed by needle aspiration because they are a good culture medium for bacteria.*

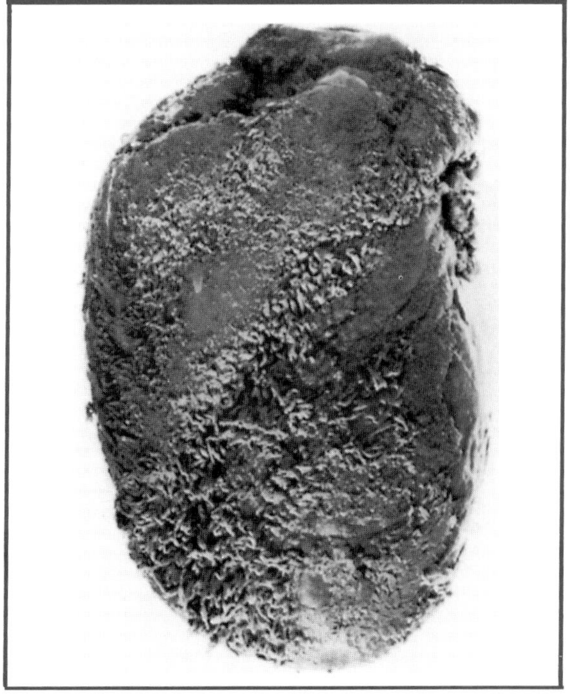

Fibrinous exudates Microscopic amounts of fibrin are found in all acutely inflamed tissues, but an exudate is called fibrinous when fibrin deposition is the dominant feature. Fibrin is essentially a blood clot without blood cells, thus it appears to the naked eye as a whitish material that might be compared to wet paper: a bland but unmistakable sight. When a thick fibrinous deposit coats the heart (*pericarditis*) it becomes furry, presumably because the heartbeat rubs it into threads (Figure 12.11); on the acutely inflamed peritoneum it looks rather like wet cotton wool (Figure 12.12). The presence of a fibrin coat on the heart or lung can be inferred clinically by a rubbing sound, due to the fact that the serosal surfaces are no longer smooth and slippery. The rub of an inflamed pleura was noticed even by the Hippocratic physicians, by placing an ear to the chest (30). Histologically, a thick fibrin deposit appears as an eosinophilic mass (Figure 12.13); it cannot persist indefinitely, because macrophages recognize it as abnormal and destroy it. (Thick fibrin deposits can last as long as years only when they are formed in aneurysms [pathologic outpouchings of arteries] where they escape phagocytosis; under such conditions the fibrin layer becomes as firm as leather).

The mechanism of fibrin formation seems clear.

FIGURE 12.11 A human heart covered by a layer of fibrin. This is *fibrinous pericarditis*, once known as *cor villosum* ("hairy heart"). The shaggy aspect of the fibrin deposit is thought to be due to the beating action of the heart. (Reproduced with permission from [8].)

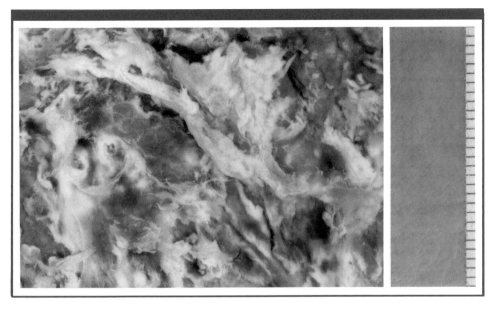

FIGURE 12.12
Left: Fibrin on the peritoneal surface. Compare this ragged coating with the smooth surface of the normal peritoneum (*right*). From a case of acute peritonitis. Photograph take under fluid. Scale in mm.

Any plasma that seeps out of the vessels into tissue spaces contains the monomer fibrinogen as well as the protein Hageman factor, which is capable of triggering the clotting system. The Hageman factor is activated by contact with collagen, which is plentiful in the tissue spaces (p. 338). Activated macrophages may help clotting by producing procoagulant factors (16).

It is important to recognize fibrin because it signals trouble, as injury, inflammation, or both. Its monomer, fibrinogen, is normally retained by the endothelial barrier; the small amount that normally seeps into the tissues has presumably crossed the endothelium by pinocytosis. Therefore, fibrin in the tissue spaces means that plasma proteins have escaped from leaky blood vessels.

You might think that such thin-walled vessels, caught in the high pressure of inflamed connective tissue, would be squeezed flat. Not so. By a wonderful arrangement, the lymphatics are not compressed as the tissues swell: they open up. Their outer walls are anchored to connective tissue fibers; when the tissue swells, the fibers are placed under tension, and the lymphatic is pulled open (Figure 12.14) (40). There is a limit to this mechanism: if the swelling is too great, the lymphatic is pulled apart and becomes nonfunctional.

The rising tissue pressure is transmitted to the lymph; values as high as 120 cm of water have been measured in the lymphatics of the ankle, after scalding the foot of anesthetized dogs (control values were close to zero) (7, 57). Of course,

What Becomes of the Inflammatory Exudate?

The excess fluid and some of the cells of the exudate find their way into the lymphatic vessels (lymphatics for short).

Visualize these as branching tubes, a little wider than blood capillaries, lined with overlapping endothelial cells architectured to function as one-way valves. Lymphatics are present in most tissues endowed with blood vessels; their normal function is to suck in and drain away about 10 per cent of the transudate oozing out of the blood capillaries, the remainder being reabsorbed by the venules.

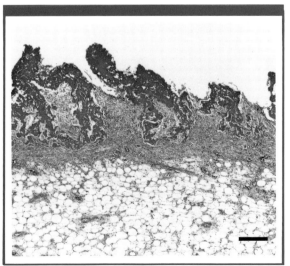

FIGURE 12.13
Histology of fibrinous pericarditis. The adipose tissue (lower half) corresponds to the epicardium. Above it is a layer of granulation tissue exuding lumps of fibrin (dark eosinophilic material). The nature of the irritant in this condition is not known. **Bar** = 250 μm.

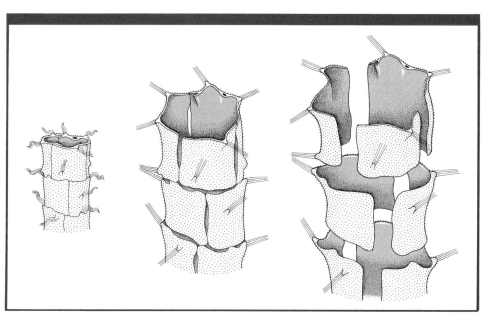

FIGURE 12.14

Effect of edema on a lymphatic capillary. *Left:* Normal condition; note the anchoring fibrils attached to the outer surfaces of the endothelial cells. *Center:* With moderate edema, the anchoring fibrils are stretched, causing slits to appear between the endothelial cells (a helpful development). *Right:* If the edema is severe, the endothelial cells are pulled apart and the lymphatic ceases to function as a draining tube. (Normal lymphatic adapted from [27].)

the lymph draining from an inflammatory focus is not normal; its protein content approaches that of exudate (and therefore of plasma) and therefore may even clot. This is a rare event. We have observed it only in lymphatics draining a focus of acute inflammation accompanied by extensive tissue destruction (Figure 12.15): dead cells release a clotting factor, thromboplastin (p. 618). It is more important to remember that the lymph draining a focus of acute inflammation, infectious or not, contains irritating materials that can inflame not only the nodes to which the lymph is conveyed (*lymphadenitis*) but also the lymphatics themselves (*lymphangitis*), as we will now explain.

THE LYMPHANGITIC STREAK

The sight of a lymphangitic streak is alarming even to the non-initiated. Imagine a hand or foot swollen by an acute case of poison ivy or by infection; after a day or two a tender, warm red streak 1–2 cm wide arises from the proximal side of the swelling and creeps toward the elbow or knee, in a matter of hours (Figure 12.16).

It is essential to understand the genesis of this phenomenon. The streak is a halo of inflammation

FIGURE 12.15
The rounded structure is a lymphatic vessel draining a territory that is acutely inflamed and teeming with bacteria (*necrotizing fasciitis*). The lymphatic is greatly dilated; its lumen has become progressively plugged by concentric layers of fibrin. **Bar** = 100 μm.

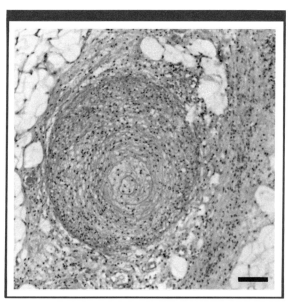

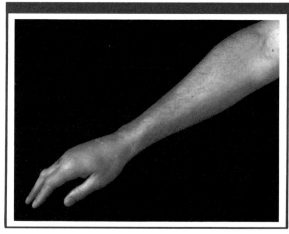

FIGURE 12.16
See color plate 12. Example of noninfectious lymphangitic streak. Arm of a 32-year-old man, 36 hours after uprooting, without gloves, a stem of poison ivy. Note the streak running from the wrist to the elbow crease. The hand is swollen and a blister has appeared. (Courtesy of Mr. R.J. Madison).

that develops around the main lymphatic trunks when the lymph (drained from a focus of acute inflammation) contains high concentrations of irritants, including inflammatory mediators (25), bacteria, or both. In the skin the telltale sign is the lymphangitic streak. Because this complication is common in severe infections (in which it *may* indicate that bacteria are swarming in the lymph) the appearance of a lymphangitic streak is usually treated—almost as a reflex—with antibiotics. However, it is important to remember that *a lymphatic streak can arise also from aseptic lesions,* in which cases it represents no threat at all; it just means that the lymph is loaded with inflammatory mediators (which the lymph node can easily handle) (11). We have seen lymphatic streaks develop from noninfected poison ivy lesions and from the red patch of a positive tuberculin test. Which amounts to saying that the clinical alarm reaction, and the "antibiotic reflex", must be kept under control.

LYMPHADENITIS

The river of lymph drained from an inflammatory focus is channelled to the nearest lymph nodes, which are filled with macrophages and therefore behave as very effective filters. The nodes may become inflamed, swollen, and painful—depending on the amount of irritating material—but their filtering capacity is so high that even if bacteria are present they are likely to be trapped. In one classic experiment, the popliteal lymph node of a dog was perfused (through an afferent lymphatic) with 5 ml of a culture medium containing 600 million bacteria per ml. After 80 minutes, cultures of the lymph draining out of the node showed that filtration had been 99 percent complete: "An efficiency so great as to make it fairly certain that in a part kept at rest [to minimize lymph flow] early in an infection, practically no microorganisms would escape the nodes in the line of drainage" (4). And if any did escape into the efferent lymph, and therefrom into the blood stream, they would run into another extremely efficient filter—the littoral phagocytes (p. 299).

Lympho-venous anastomoses. There is evidence that some lymph—under high pressure—may find its way into small veins through lympho-venous anastomoses. Peripheral connections between blood and lymph are probably not open normally, but they seem to exist as "safety valves" that open during emergencies, certainly after the ligature of large lymphatic ducts, and perhaps during exercise (46). Under

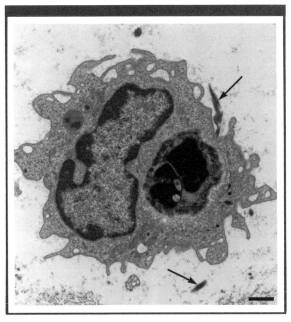

FIGURE 12.17 Macrophage that just engulfed a polymorph; the nuclear lobes are still recognizable. Note the wisps of fibrin (**arrows**). From a focus of acute inflammation in rat skin. **Bar** = 1 μm.

normal conditions, connections between blood and lymph have been demonstrated (functionally) in the lymph nodes (57).

THE END OF THE SHOW

While the fluid part of the exudate is drained away by the lymphatics, the fibrin is identified by local macrophages as "something that should not be

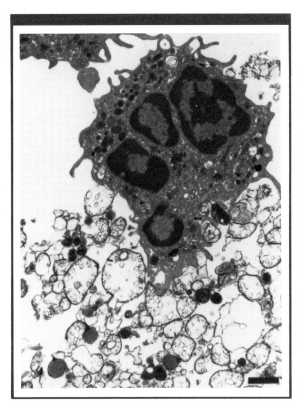

FIGURE 12.18 The destructive power of activated neutrophils. This human neutrophil sits over the debris of endothelial cells it has destroyed. It had been stimulated by a combination of endotoxin and chemotactic factors and then placed over a monolayer of cultured human endothelium. **Bar** = 1 μm. (Reproduced with permission from [17].)

there" and is removed. What happens to the inflammatory cells is only partly understood. The neutrophils die of programmed cell death and are scavenged by the macrophages (Figure 12.17) (43). Only a few macrophages and fibroblasts and perhaps some lymphocytes may become permanent local residents; all the others will somehow disappear.

If damaged parenchymal cells are able to regenerate, little or no trace will remain of the inflammatory drama; if regeneration is incomplete or lacking, a fibrous patch—called a scar—will be the permanent memento.

TO SUM UP: Nobody would doubt that inflammatory exudation is a marvellous and life-saving phenomenon. But then, we should not forget that parenchymal cells—in the tissues when inflammation rages—must take a dim view of the exudate. To them it must be an acid, corrosive, hypertonic, asphyxiating medium, thick with proteolytic enzymes only partially controlled by plasma antiproteases (56). The trigger-happy activated neutrophils, spewing enzymes and oxygen metabolites, must be especially dangerous neighbors (34, 50) (Figure 12.18). These side-effects of the exudate come to the foreground when inflammation involves tissues very sensitive to hydrolysis, such as articular cartilage, or to anoxia, such as the nervous system. In essence, a war—even if defensive—comes at a price.

References

1. Bryant RE. Pus: friend or foe? In: Root RK, Trunkey DD, Sande, MA, eds. New surgical and medical approaches in infectious diseases. New York: Churchill Livingstone, 1987:31–48.
2. Burke JF. The effective period of preventive antibiotic action in experimental incisions and dermal lesions. Surgery 1961;50:161–168.
3. Cybulsky MI, Movat HZ. Experimental bacterial pneumonia in rabbits: polymorphonuclear leukocyte margination and sequestration in rabbit lungs and quantitation and kinetics of ^{51}Cr-labeled polymorphonuclear leukocytes in E. coli-induced lung lesions. Exp Lung Res 1982;4:47–66.
4. Drinker CK, Field ME, Ward HK. The filtering capacity of lymph nodes. J Exp Med 193459:393–407.
5. Farber HW, Weller PF, Rounds S., Beer DJ, Center DM. Generation of lipid neutrophil chemoattractant activity by histamine-stimulated cultured endothelial cells. J Immunol 1986;137:2918–2924.
6. Field M, Rao MC, Chang .B. Intestinal electrolyte transport and diarrheal disease (second of two parts). N Engl.J Med 1989;321:879–883.
7. Field ME, Drinker CK, White JC. Lymph pressures in sterile inflammation. J Exp Med 1932;56:363–370.
8. Florey HW. General pathology, 4th ed. London: Lloyd-Luke (Medical Books), 1970:29.
9. Forrest MJ, Jose PJ, Williams TJ. The role of the complement-derived polypeptide C5a in inflammatory reactions. In: Higgs GA, Williams TJ, eds. Inflammatory mediators. New York: MacMillan, 1985:99–115.
10. Guyton AC. Textbook of medical physiology, 7th ed. Philadelphia: WB Saunders, 1986: 358.
11. Hall JG, Sinnett HD. The endolymphatic perfusion of lymph nodes with toxic materials. Br J Exp Pathol 1989;70:283–292.
12. Harada S, Dannenberg AM Jr, Kajiki A, Higuchi K, Tanaka F, Pula P.J. Inflammatory mediators and modulators released in organ culture from rabbit skin lesions produced in vivo by sulfur mustard. II. Evans blue dye experiments that determined the rates of entry and turnover of serum protein in developing and healing lesions. Am J Pathol 1985;121:28–38.
13. Harlan JM, Liu DY, eds.. Adhesion: its role in inflammatory disease. New York: WH Freeman, 1992.
13a. Heggers JP Variations on a theme. In Heggers JP, and Robsonn MC *Quantitative Bacteriology: Its Role in the Armamentarium of the Surgeon.* Boca Raton: CRC Press, 1991:15–23.
14. Heimberger H. Färbeversuche am capillarendothel und die lymphräume des papillarkörpergewebes. Zeitschr fd ges exp Med 1926;51:17–23.
15. Heimberger H. Verhalten auf reizung mit galvanischem strom. Zeitschr fd ges exp Med 1927;55:112–123.
16. Helin H. Macrophage procoagulant factors—mediators of inflammatory and neoplastic tissue lesions. Med Biol 1986;64:167–176.
17. Henson PM, Henson JE, Fittschen C, Kimani G, Bratton DL, Riches DWH. Phagocytic cells: degranulation and secretion. In: Gallin JI, Goldstein, IM, Snyderman R, eds. Inflammation: basic principles and clinical correlates. New York: Raven Press, 1988: 363–390.
18. Henson PM, Johnston RB Jr. Tissue injury in inflammation. Oxidants, proteinases, and cationic proteins. J Clin Invest 1987;79:669–674.
19. Higgs GA, Williams TJ, eds.. Inflammatory mediators. New York: MacMillan, 1985: 99–115.
20. Hurley JV. Substances promoting leukocyte emigration. Ann NY Acad Sci 1964;116:918–935.
21. Hurley JV. Acute inflammation. Baltimore: Williams and Wilkins, 1972.
22. Hurley JV, Ryan GB, Friedman A. The mononuclear response to intrapleural injection in the rat. J Pathol Bacteriol 1966;91:575–587.
23. Issekutz AC. Quantitation of acute inflammation in the skin: recent methodological advances and their application to the study of inflammatory reactions. Surv Synth Pathol Res 1983;1:89–110.
24. Issekutz TB, Issekutz AC, Movat HZ. The in vivo quantitation and kinetics of monocyte migration into acute inflammatory tissue. Am J Pathol 1981;103:47–55.
25. Johnston MG, Hay JB, Movat HZ. Kinetics of prostaglandin production in various inflammatory lesions, measured in draining lymph. Am J Pathol 1979;95:225–238.
26. Kopaniak MM, Hay JB, Movat HZ. The effect of hyperemia on vascular permeability. Microvasc Res 1978;15:77–82.
27. Leak LV, Burke JF. Ultrastructural studies on the lymphatic anchoring filaments. J Cell Biol 1968;36:129–149.
28. Leibovich SJ, Ross R. The role of the macrophage in

wound repair. A study with hydrocortisone and antimacrophage serum. Am J Pathol 1975;78:71–100.

29. Lundberg C, Lebel L, Gerdin B. Inflammatory reaction in an experimental model of open wounds in the rat. The role of polymorphonuclear leukocytes. Lab Invest 1984; 50:726–732.

30. Majno G. The healing hand: man and wound in the ancient world. Cambridge: Harvard University Press, 1975.

31. McCarty DJ. Short-term drug control of crystal-induced inflammation. In: Vane JR, Ferreira SH, eds. Anti-inflammatory drugs. (Handbook of Experimental Pharmacology, vol. 50/II). Berlin: Springer-Verlag, 1979:92–107.

32. Movat HZ, Cybulsky M.I. Neutrophil emigration and microvascular injury. Role of chemotaxins, endotoxin, interluekin-1 and tumor necrosis factor alpha. Pathol Immunopathol Res 1987;6:153–176.

33. Nash S, Stafford J, Madara JL. The selective and superoxide-independent disruption of intestinal epithelial tight junctions during leukocyte transmigration. Lab Invest 1988;59:531–537.

34. Okrent DG, Lichtenstein AK, Ganz T. Direct cytotoxicity of polymorphonuclear leukocyte granule proteins to human lung-derived cells and endothelial cells. Am Rev Respir Dis 1990;141:179–185.

35. Payling Wright G. An introduction to pathology, 3rd ed. Boston: Little, Brown, 1961:114.

36. Paz RA, Spector WG. The mononuclear-cell response to injury. J Pathol Bacteriol 1962;84:85–103.

37. Pober JS, Cotran RS. Cytokines and endothelial cell biology. Physiol Rev 1990;70:427–451.

38. Pricolo VE, Potenti F, Soderberg CH. Effect of perigraft seroma fluid on fibroblast proliferation in vitro. Ann Vas Surg 1991;5:462–466.

39. Pullinger BD, Florey HW. Some observations on the structure and functions of lymphatics: their behaviour in local oedema. Br J Exp Pathol 1935;16:49–61.

40. Pullinger BD, Florey HW. Proliferation of lymphatics in inflammation. J Pathol Bacteriol 1937;45:157–170.

41. Rebuck JW. Inflammatory cell dynamics in man. In: Reichard SM., Filkins JP, eds. The reticuloendothelial system. New York: Plenum Press, 1985:271–288.

42. Rollins BJ, Yoshimura T, Leonard EJ, Pober JS. Cytokine-activated human endothelial cells synthesize and secrete a monocyte chemoattractant, MCP-1/JE. Am J Pathol 1990;136:1229–1233.

43. Savill JS, Wyllie AH, Henson JE, Walport MJ, Henson PM, Haslett C. Macrophage phagocytosis of aging neutrophils in inflammation. Programmed cell death in the neutrophil leads to its recognition by macrophages. J Clin Invest 1989;83:865–875.

44. Shaw JHF, Rumball EM. Complications and local recurrence following lymphadenectomy. Br J Surg 1990; 77:760–764.

44a. Springer, TA Traffic signals for Lymphocyte Recirculation and Leukocyte Emigration: The Multistep Paradigm. Cell 1994;2:76,301–314.

45. Steele RH, Wilhelm DL. The inflammatory reaction in chemical injury. III. Leucocytosis and other histological changes induced by superficial injury. Br J Exp Pathol 1970;51:265–279.

46. Threefoot SA. Lymphovenous anastomoses. In: Földi M, Casley-Smith, JR, eds.. Lymphangiology. Stuttgart: FK Schattauer, 1983:177–184.

47. van Furth R. Mononuclear phagocytes in inflammation. In: Vane JR, Ferreira SH, eds. Inflammation. Berlin: Springer-Verlag, 1978:68–108.

48. Waldvogel FA. Pathophysiological mechanisms in pyogenic infections: two examples—pleural empyema and acute bacterial meningitis. In: Majno G, Cotran, RS, Kaufman N, eds. Current topics in inflammation and infection. Baltimore: Williams & Wilkins, 1982:115–122.

49. Wedmore CV, Williams TJ. Control of vascular permeability by polymorphonuclear leukocytes in inflammation. Nature 1981;289:646–650.

50. Weiss SJ. Tissue destruction by neutrophils. N Engl J Med 1989;320:365–376.

51. Wheeler ME, Luscinskas FW, Bevilacqua MP, Gimbrone MA Jr. Cultured human endothelial cells stimulated with cytokines or endotoxin produce an inhibitor of leukocyte adhesion. J Clin Invest 1988;82:1211–1218.

52. Wilhelm DL. Chemical mediators. In: Zweifach BW, Grant L, McCluskey RT, eds. The inflammatory process, vol. II, 2nd ed. New York: Academic Press, 1973:251–301.

53. Williams TJ. Factors that affect vessel reactivity and leukocyte emigration. In: Clark, RAF., Henson PM., eds. The molecular and cellular biology of wound repair. New York: Plenum Press, 1988:115–147.

54. Williams TJ, Jose PJ, Forrest MJ, Wedmore CV, Clough GF. Interactions between neutrophils and microvascular endothelial cells leading to cell emigration and plasma protein leakage. KROC Found. Ser 1984;16:195–208.

55. Williamson LM, Sheppard K, Davies JM, Fletcher J. Neutrophils are involved in the increased vascular permeability produced by activated complement in man. Br J. Haematol 1986;64:375–384.

56. Woessner JF Jr, Dannenberg AM Jr, Pula PJ, et al. Extracellular collagenase, proteoglycanase and products of their activity, released in organ culture by intact dermal inflammatory lesions produced by sulfur mustard. J Invest Dermatol 1990;95:717–726.

57. Yoffey JM, Courtice FC. Lymphatics, lymph and the lymphomyeloid complex. London: Academic Press, 1970.

58. Zimmerli W, Gallin JI Pus potassium. Inflammation 1988;12:37–43.

Chronic Inflammation

CHAPTER 13

General Aspects

Granulomatous
Inflammation

Fibrosis

I f its cause is not removed, inflammation becomes chronic and can persist for months, years, a lifetime. The process shifts to a simmering mode; of the four cardinal signs, the two that relate to "flames," redness and heat, are toned down, but swelling and pain remain.

General Aspects

The microscope usually tells us what is going on. First of all, it can tell us why the inflammatory response has not turned itself off by showing that the offending agent is still there. In chronic inflammation the agent is usually a parasite, bacterial or other, though it may be a sterile agent such as necrotic tissue, a foreign body, or an oily or crystalline substance that is difficult to eliminate, such as the urate crystals of gout (Figure 8.23). The cause can also be an antigen that is not directly visible microscopically, as in rheumatoid arthritis and other autoimmune diseases; but we suspect such causes from the nature of the cells that are involved in the response. The microscope also shows us that two major histologic changes have taken place in the inflamed tissues, as explained below.

HISTOLOGIC EVIDENCE OF CHRONIC INFLAMMATION

(a) Mononuclear cells (macrophages and lymphocytes) have become predominant in the tissues (Figure 13.1), and (b) a new type of connective tissue (granulation tissue) has formed; we have already illustrated its genesis in our panoramic overview of inflammation (Figures 8.24–8.29).

(A) THE SHIFT TO MONONUCLEAR CELLS

The fact that macrophages and lymphocytes have taken over reflects the need for cells that are specialized in tasks of which the neutrophils are incapable (incidentally, the expression "mononuclear cells" is technically not correct: the

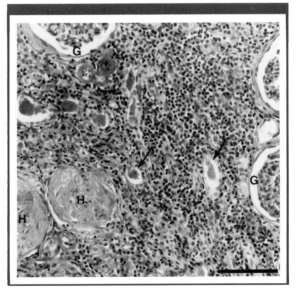

FIGURE 13.1
Typical example of chronic inflammation in the kidney cortex: chronic pyelonephritis. The culprits (bacteria) are not visible, but they elicited a diffuse infiltrate of mononuclear cells. **Arrows:** remnants of tubules that were destroyed either by bacteria or by the inflammatory infiltrate. **H:** Hyalinized glomeruli belonging to nephrons that have ceased to function. **G:** Normal glomeruli. **Bar** = 100 μm.

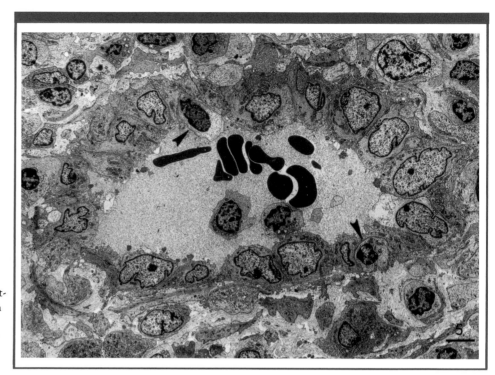

FIGURE 13.2
Large postcapillary venule in the synovium from a case of rheumatoid arthritis. Note the thickened ("activated") endothelium and two emigrating lymphocytes (**arrowheads**). Both features recall the high-endothelial venules of normal lymph nodes. **Bar** = 5 μm. (Reproduced with permission from [14].)

neutrophils also have one nucleus, albeit shaped into two or more lobes). The most versatile among the exudate cells are the macrophages. Once they reach the battleground the macrophages begin to phagocytize, become activated and secrete cytokines that summon and activate other cells (27). If bacteria are present, the macrophages phagocytize them and then present bacterial antigens to the surrounding lymphocytes, thereby initiating an immune response. The latter is a mechanism for dealing with antigens. It operates in two ways: by making antibodies (B lymphocytes turned into plasma cells are in charge of this) and by killing cells that are antigenic, such as virus-infected cells (a special subset of T lymphocytes performs this task).

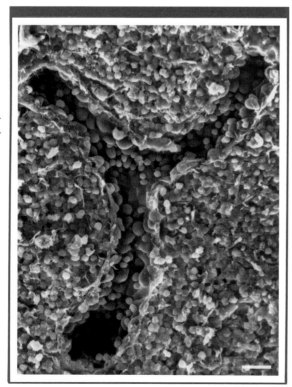

FIGURE 13.3
A high-endothelial venule: scanning electron micrograph showing the cut surface of a mouse lymph node. Note many lymphocytes attached to the plump endothelial cells; nonadherent blood elements were removed by perfusion before fixation. **Bar** = 50 μm (Reproduced with permission from [51].)

The local recruitment of lymphocytes and other leukocytes is aided by a clever trapping mechanism. The venules in a focus of chronic inflammation develop an unusually thick endothelium (Figure 13.2) (29) and come to resemble the so-called "high-endothelial venules" of the lymphatic organs (Figure 13.3). The similarity turns out to be also functional: just as the high-endothelial venules of lymphatic organs are specialized for trapping circulating lymphocytes, which then exit into the tissue spaces, the venules in chronically inflamed tissues recruit lymphocytes for the inflammatory focus (1,3,6–8,15,30,54). The recruitment mechanisms are similar but not identical (15,33). The expression of new adhesion molecules by the endothelium was discussed in the previous chapters.

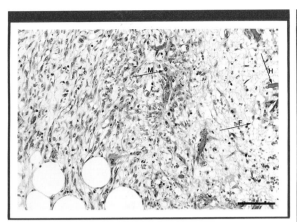

FIGURE 13.4
See color plate 13. Typical young granulation tissue surrounding a 5-day-old experimental hematoma (3 ml of blood were injected in the adipose tissue of a rat). The granulation tissue consists mainly of activated fibroblasts, forming a wall around the hematoma (just out of sight at the right). **F** = fibrin filaments; **H** = crystal of hemoglobin; **M** = mitosis, probably in a fibroblast. **Bar** = 100 μm.

(B) GRANULATION TISSUE

The development of granulation tissue is another key event in chronic inflammation. To understand it, remember that inflammation takes place in the extravascular spaces, that is, in the connective tissue (even in epithelial organs such as the liver, the epithelia lie in a delicate stroma or "bed" of connective tissue). After a day or two of inflammation, the connective tissue cannot remain indifferent to the battle that is being fought within it: it receives chemical messages conveyed by inflammatory mediators, and responds by producing new fibroblasts, new fibers, new blood vessels: in short, new tissue.

Granulation tissue is different from ordinary connective tissue because it is packed with cells, at first mainly activated fibroblasts, macrophages, and a sprinkling of other inflammatory cells; collagen fibers are scanty (Figure 13.4). As this population grows, new capillaries are needed, and capillary sprouts begin to appear. The newly-formed capillary sprouts are leaky because the endothelial cells are not yet well connected (Figure 13.5) (40,41); this explains the somewhat edematous, "juicy" aspect of granulation tissue compared with ordinary connective tissue. The genesis of new vessels will be taken up later (p. 468 and 755).

Granulation tissue can grow to a considerable volume; for example, when it surrounds a pocket of pus (as in an abscess) it can form a layer 10–12 mm thick (Figure 13.6). In such cases the inner

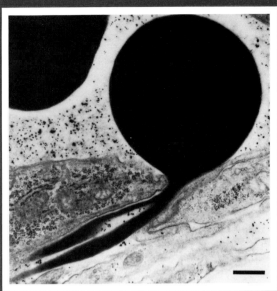

FIGURE 13.5
Red blood cell squeezing out of a regenerating capillary through a junction between two endothelial cells. This electron micrograph illustrates the excessive permeability of newly formed capillaries in granulation tissue, as well as the great plasticity of the red blood cells. **Bar** = 0.5 μm. (Reproduced with permission from [40].)

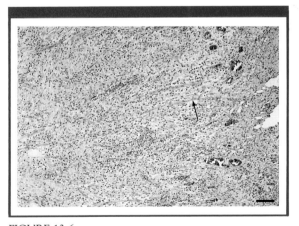

FIGURE 13.6
See color plate 14. Granulation tissue from a case of empyema of the pleura in a 30-year old man. The pleura had been infected 3 weeks previously, and the inner surface of the chest wall had become coated with a layer of granulation tissue about 8 mm thick. The layer facing the cavity and exuding pus is at the right. Overall the cellular population consists mainly of fibroblasts, macrophages (not distinguishable here), and other inflammatory cells. **Arrow:** newly formed capillary. **Bar** = 100 μm.

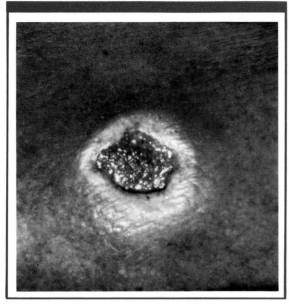

FIGURE 13.7

Example of granulation tissue: "granulating ulcer" after trauma of the leg in a dark-skinned patient. The white dots in the ulcer are highlights and represent granulations. The pale rim represents regenerating epidermis; the melanocytes regenerate poorly and unpredictably. Actual size. (Courtesy of Dr. R.L. Walton, Chicago Medical School, Chicago, IL.)

layer remains richly cellular and vascular, whereas the outer layer produces more collagen and acts as a fibrous capsule.

Granulation tissue is an old surgical term, originally applied to the little red lumps of new tissue that glisten on the raw surface of a healing open wound (Figure 13.7); the term was borrowed later from wound healing and applied to chronic inflammation. In either case we are dealing with new, growing, richly vascular connective tissue.

The lymphatics in chronic inflammation. The development of new blood vessels (*angiogenesis*) is one of the main features of granulation tissue, but what about the lymphatics? Little is known about them, except that they do develop in granulation tissue, with some delay after the blood capillaries (53). Striking photographs were published in 1937 by Pullinger and Florey showing dense networks of new lymphatics appearing after various injuries to the mouse ear (Figure 13.8). This is now known as *lymphangiogenesis* (52). Injury to the cornea induces lymphangiogenesis at the periphery, in the limbus (17). An interesting fact: after one week of sterile peritonitis in the rat, the lymphatic absorp-

tion of oil or particulate matter introduced into the peritoneum is much greater (20).

In essence, more facts are needed, but lymphangiogenesis can definitely occur in granulation tissue.

Granulation tissue develops around many chronic irritants, especially infected tissue; in this case it clearly functions as a natural barrier against bacteria. We will better understand its function after discussing special types of chronic inflammation.

FORMS OF CHRONIC INFLAMMATION

Chronic inflammation takes on different aspects depending on the setting, that is, on the causal agent (e.g., some bacteria emphasize pus formation; silica dust emphasizes fibrosis) and on the location (e.g., a solid organ, a serosal surface). We will now examine some typical settings of chronic inflammation: abscesses, ulcers, inflammation of serosal membranes, organization, granulomas, and fibrosis.

THE ABSCESS

An abscess is a collection of pus in a newly formed cavity. Collections of pus can also develop in preexisting spaces, but they are given special names that have been consecrated by the centuries, such as *empyema* for the pleural cavity and *pyosalpinx* for the fallopian tube (remember that the Greek *py-* is the root for *pus*).

An abscess always begins as a microscopic battle between a parasite—usually a pyogenic bacterium, sometimes amoebae (48)—and an army of neutrophils. The bacteria, which may have arrived by the blood stream or by any other route, produce toxins that kill the local cells; the neutrophils, as they attack the bacteria, secrete enzymes that digest the dead cells, and perhaps some live ones as well. Within a few hours the result is a microscopic cavity filled with cell debris and neutrophils: a *microabscess* (Figure 13.9). Within 2–3 days a layer of granulation tissue develops all around the microabscess (Figure 13.9, bottom); its new blood vessels continue to pour out leukocytes, mainly neutrophils, while fibroblasts build layers of a collagen-rich tissue on the outside. This lifesaving wall of granulation tissue is known as "*pyogenic*" *membrane* because its inner surface (in contact with the offending agent) "produces pus" (Figure 13.6); overall it performs as a highly effective barrier to the spread of infection. What happens next depends on the balance of forces:

- All the bacteria (or amoebae) are killed, the pus becomes sterile, and healing occurs by reabsorption of the sterilized pus. The influx of leukocytes stops because the chemotactic stimulus has disappeared; the content of the abscess becomes essentially a mass of denatured proteins, which macrophages slowly erode. Eventually the pyogenic membrane shrivels concentrically into a scar; its shrinkage is probably helped by an outer layer of fibroblasts that have modulated into contractile cells, *myofibroblasts* (p. 472).

- The battle continues, and the abscess expands (Figure 13.10). It is obvious that abscesses can enlarge, but the precise mechanism has not been studied. Presumably the imprisoned parasites attack and destroy the inner surface of the pyogenic membrane while new layers are added to its outer surface. Pressure within the cavity, both hydrostatic and osmotic, could help enlarge the abscess (remember that pus is hypertonic).

- The abscess empties its contents through a fistula. A *fistula* (Latin for *tube*) is *any pathologic channel from a body cavity to another internal cavity or to the body surface.* A lung abscess can erode its way into a bronchus; an abscess that develops at the tip of the root of a carious tooth can work its way out into the mouth or toward the skin. Fistulae, by the way, can be congenital, traumatic, or inflammatory. In the case of a ruptured abscess, the wall of the fistula gradually becomes lined with granulation tissue: this is an *inflammatory fistula*. Drainage of pus through the fistula continues as long as the infection persists.

Note: An abscess can be sterile from the beginning if it is induced by sterile chemotactic materials.

An established experimental method for producing subcutaneous abscesses in mice is to inject the autoclaved content of mouse cecum (16). In the nineteenth century, a rather barbaric method for treating septicemic patients was to create sterile intramuscular "fixation abscesses" by injecting turpentine. It was hoped that the circulating bacteria would somehow become localized in the abscesses. Some probably did, but we would not recommend the procedure.

The dental abscess is an odd case. An infected root canal is a routine event, but it leads to a

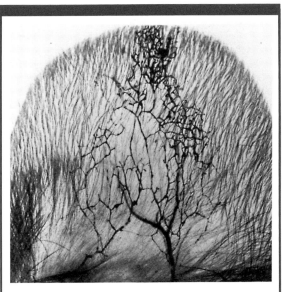

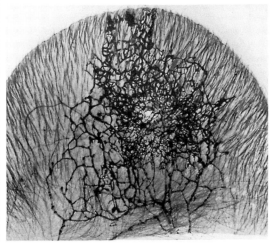

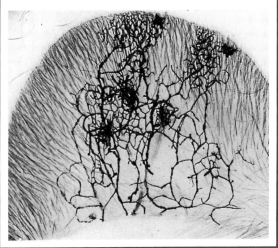

FIGURE 13.8 Proliferation of lymphatics in chronically inflamed skin (mouse ear). A black colloidal suspension of graphite was injected in the margin of the ear. *Top:* Lymphatics of a normal mouse ear. *Center:* Lymphatics, 21 days after induction, with a drop of turpentine, of a small abscess that perforated the ear. *Bottom:* Proliferation of lymphatics at three points where amorphous silica had been injected subcutaneously 3 months previously. (Reproduced with permission from [34].)

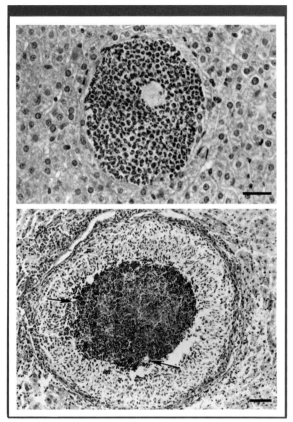

FIGURE 13.9

Microscopic abscesses induced in the liver of hamsters by injecting amoebae (*Entamoeba histolytica*) into the portal vein. *Top:* This animal was sacrificed 6 hours after the inoculation. An amoeba is visible in the lower center of the abscess. **Bar** = 50 μm. *Bottom:* At the 4-day stage, the neutrophils have died (**arrows** point to amoebae), and the necrotic mass is surrounded by a rim of macrophages and fibroblasts. **Bar** = 100 μm. (Reproduced with permission from [48].)

biologically unique situation: granulation tissue mixed with epithelium. Here is what happens. Cavities in teeth are caused by bacteria that may work their way down the dentin canals (Figure 13.11) and eventually reach the pulp, spread along the root, emerge at the tip, and cause a small abscess (Figure 9.3): a collection of pus surrounded by granulation tissue (Figure 13.12). Here is the unique feature: this granulation tissue is often covered by or mixed with layer of squamous stratified epithelium. The mechanism: embryologically the tooth develops inside a cup of epithelium (the *enamel organ*) that determines its shape. The epithelial cup then disappears but leaves behind, on the surface of the tooth's root, little clusters of residual epithelial cells called *rests of Malassez*

(44). When granulation tissue develops at the tip of a root, some of these rests wake up—presumably under the influence of inflammatory growth factors—and grow with the granulation tissue. As far as we know, they never reach the stage of cancerous growth.

Cellulitis or **phlegmon** is essentially the opposite of an abscess: it refers to an acute, overwhelming infection that spreads along the skin and subcutaneous connective tissue before local defenses have a chance to wall it off. Malaise, chills, and fever are usually present; common causes are group A streptococci and *staphylococcus aureus* (22).

> *The name* cellulitis *has nothing to do with cells as we understand them. It is an ancient term meaning inflammation of "cellular tissue"; connective tissue was so called because, when anatomically dissected and stretched, it appears to be formed of thin transparent membranes separating spaces called "cells". (Note: the lay use of the term "cellulitis" refers to the puckered skin of fat thighs. Whatever this condition may be, it is not a recognized pathologic entity).*

ULCERS

An ulcer is a gap in the skin—or a mucosa—that is lined with granulation tissue and has no tendency to heal. The latter feature is the key difference between a wound and an ulcer (Figure 13.13). In ulcers of the skin the little "granules" of the granulation tissue can be very obvious (Figure 13.7).

The lack of healing is not always understood, but a few local causes are clear. For example, ulcers that develop about the ankles in patients with varicose veins can be attributed to poor circulation. The persistence of gastric and duodenal ulcers has long been attributed to the corrosive action of hydrochloric acid, but recent discoveries suggest entirely unpredicted mechanisms: infection with the bacterium *Helicobacter pylori* (9,11) and lack of fibroblast growth factor (FGF), which is degraded by hydrochloric acid (5,46,47). Ulcers in the foot of diabetics are maintained by a lack of sensation (due to diabetic neuropathy), complicated by ischemia and infection (1a). Different mechanisms, of course, lead to different therapies.

The loss of epithelium only, from the skin or from a mucosa, is called an *erosion*. A typical example: corneal erosions due to trauma or infection, which heal quickly by regeneration of the epithelium (p. 20). Recurrent corneal erosions have been attributed to poor adhesion between epithelium and basement membrane (19); in diabetics they are probably due to loss of feeling of the cornea due to nerve damage. Persistent erosions can turn into ulcers.

CHRONIC INFLAMMATION OF SEROSAL SURFACES

A serosal space, such as the pleura or the peritoneum, creates special conditions for inflammation because it offers a large open cavity in which the exudate can accumulate, rather than infiltrating the tight spaces of connective tissue. Accordingly, inflamed serosal spaces can become filled with serous exudate (e.g., *serous pleuritis*) or pus (e.g., *pleural empyema*); or the apposed serosal surfaces may become coated with fibrin (e.g., *fibrinous pericarditis*) (Figures 12.11, 12.12). Histologically there is a thin layer of granulation tissue under the fibrin (Fig. 13.14); plasma exudes from its leaky vessels, coagulates, and produces the fibrin coat.

If the offending agent disappears, this coat can be removed during the healing process, but it may leave a permanent complication called *adhesion*.

Adhesions Adhesions are pathologic connections between two apposed serosal surfaces. Normally the serosal surfaces are prevented from sticking together by the lubricating effect of the mesothelium that coats them. During inflammation the mesothelial lining is partially destroyed, and the apposed surfaces may become glued together, at first, by fibrin: this is a *fibrinous adhesion*, which can be separated (at surgery or during an autopsy) by gentle pulling. The next step is critical: if the fibrin is digested away by macrophages or by the fibrinolytic activity of the serosal fluid, the mesothelium regenerates and healing is complete (38). But if the fibrin is replaced (organized) by granulation tissue, the result is a permanent *fibrous adhesion*. A fibrous adhesion of the entire pleura, pericardium, or peritoneum is called a *symphysis*.

For the function of the lung, a focal adhesion is not critical, but a symphysis is life-threatening. Pericardial symphysis increases the cardiac workload and causes myocardial hypertrophy. In the peritoneum, a single fibrous adhesion can be dangerous by creating a noose through which an intestinal loop can slip and become strangulated. Until the 1940s, an inordinate number of patients who had undergone abdominal surgery developed peritoneal adhesions that contained mysterious microscopic foreign bodies. Finally, it was realized that the talcum powder used to lubricate surgical gloves induced a chronic inflammatory reaction: talcum granulomas (43).

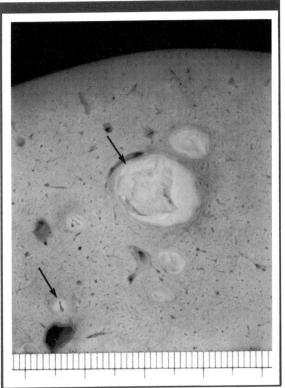

FIGURE 13.10 Multiple abscesses in the liver (**arrows**). From the liver of a 59-year-old man with acute leukemia, who died of sepsis with abscesses in many organs. (Because the liver was fixed before being cut, the pus did not flow out of the abscesses.) Scale in mm.

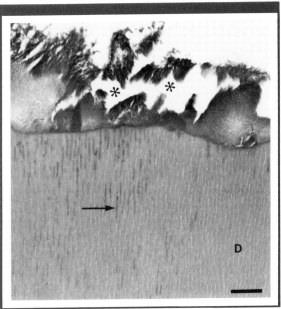

FIGURE 13.11
Surface of a human tooth eroded by cavities. **Asterisks:** Bottom of the cavity, covered by debris of decalcified dentin. The faint white vertical streaks are normal dentinal tubules. **Arrow:** Dentinal tubules that appear basophilic because they are filled with bacteria. The dentin is decalcified by lactic acid produced by the bacteria. **D:** Normal dentin. **Bar** = 50 μm. (Tooth provided by Dr. P.J. Alizzeo, Shrewsbury, MA.)

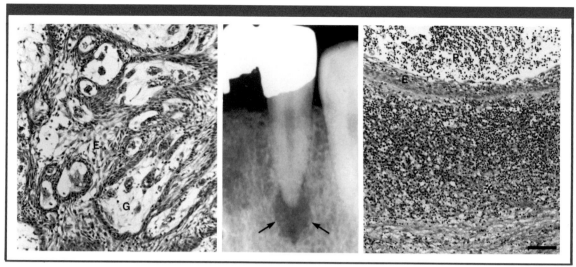

FIGURE 13.12

A mix of granulation tissue and epithelium as observed in dental pathology. *Center:* X-ray of a tooth that has undergone repair for caries (note the metal crown). Some bacteria survived, emerged from the tip of the root, and set up an inflammatory process that caused the bone to be reabsorbed (lucent space between **arrows**). The bone loss could be due to a granuloma, a cyst, or an abscess. Embryologic remains of epithelium (**E**) stimulated by the inflammatory process often proliferate and either mix with the granulation tissue (**G**) (*left*), or line the surface of a pus-filled cavity (*right*). **P** = pus; **E** = epithelium; **asterisk** = granulation tissue overloaded with inflammatory cells. **Bar** = 100 μm. (Left and center reproduced with permission from [34a]. Right: Specimen courtesy of Dr. D. J. Krutchkoff, University of Connecticut, Farmington, CT).

Adhesions can be life-saving, at least in the abdomen. Consider a case of appendicitis: the wall of the appendix is destroyed by bacteria and ready to break open at one point, spilling feces into the peritoneal cavity. This calamity can be averted if the inflammation spreads to the surface of another organ nearby (or even to the abdominal wall); if fibrin glues the two surfaces together, the spot ready to perforate may be covered over. Eventually a fibrous adhesion would be the sole price paid. One organ in the peritoneum is "professionally" prepared to create adhesions: the *omentum.* For this reason surgeons have called it "the policeman of the abdominal cavity."

Inflammation and the Omentum The omentum is a peculiar organ (21). Hanging as it does in front of the intestines, it looks like an afterthought, or maybe a leftover from some embryologic maneuver (which it is, as a large fold of excess peritoneal lining). In fact, the omentum is poised there waiting for trouble. Wherever inflammation may develop in the abdomen, usually by infection (think of appendicitis), it joins the battle; thanks to its many vessels it produces fibrin, becomes attached to the inflamed organ and acts as a barrier to further spread of the bacteria. In essence, it functions as a machine for producing adhesions.

We believe that in this function the omentum is helped by its structure. It is essentially a fibrous membrane perforated by countless holes, making it look like a net (Figure 13.15), in fact its name in German is *Netz* (37). Because of these meshes, it is more easily trapped in a network of inflammatory fibrin (37).

Banjo-String Adhesions The type of adhesions described so far are sometimes called *flat adhesions,* to distinguish them from string-shaped ("banjo-string") adhesions that have a different pathogenesis. These arise in the peritoneum as follows. Imagine that some blood is spilled in the abdominal cavity, that it clots, and that the clot becomes attached to the peritoneal surface at two points 10–15 cm apart. Two organs are thus connected by a soft, rubbery clot. No harm is done, but the end result depends on what happens next. If the clot is dissolved by fibrinolysis or by macrophages, no trouble will develop. But if the clot is colonized by fibroblasts (organized), it will turn into a taut string ready to choke an intestinal loop that may wind around it (37). Needless to say, banjo-string adhesions are always a nuisance.

ORGANIZATION

Organization is the process whereby granulation tissue digests and removes dead tissue, fibrin, or any

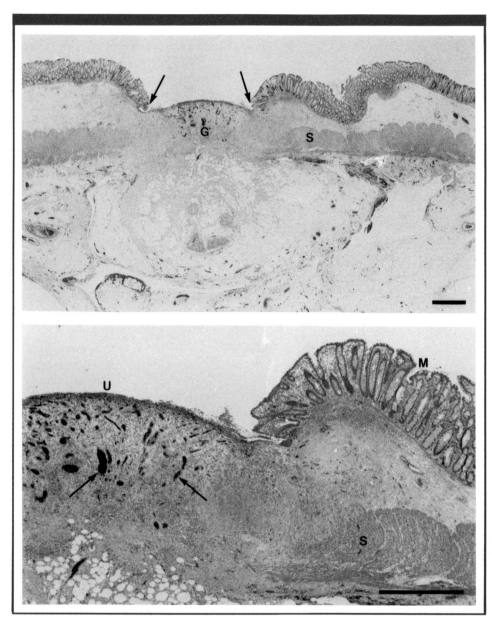

FIGURE 13.13
An ulcer of the colon at a site where a polyp had been excised 12 days earlier. *Top:* The exposed submucosa (between **arrows**) is replaced by granulation tissue (**G**) rich in dilated vessels. The smooth muscle layer (**S**) is interrupted and the inflammatory response expands into the serosa. *Bottom:* Detail. Granulation tissue rich in blood vessels (**arrows**) lines the ulcer (**U**) and has replaced the smooth muscle layer(s). **M** = mucosa **Bars** = 1 mm.

absorbable material such as surgical sponges. The cells that do most of the work are the macrophages.

> The term organization *is not accurate; it derives from an obsolete concept:* "where there was dead tissue there is now live granulation tissue; so, the dead tissue must have been transformed or "organized" into live tissue."

As a large-scale scavenging event, organization is the mechanism that removes infarcts. It can be conveniently studied by implanting pieces of sterile rat liver into another rat's abdominal cavity, the method that we have repeatedly illustrated (p. 191). To recall the key points: the dying liver cells release protein breakdown products; in the meantime the bulk of their proteins coagulates. The omentum becomes attached to the implant within a few hours and begins the process of organization (Figures 8.24–8.29).

Given the notion that infarcts are removed by organization, *how does dead tissue trigger inflammation?* Tissue that is long dead and coagulated actually does not induce inflammation; dying tissue does, by a number of mechanisms. The principal ones are listed here (Figure 13.16).

- *Complement is activated;* the classic membrane attack complex develops in or around necrotic cells (Figure 13.17) (4,39). The activation of C1, the first component of com-

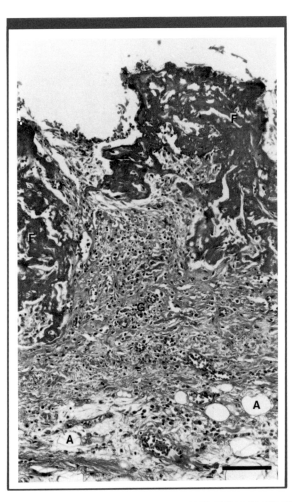

FIGURE 13.14 Fibrinous pericarditis in a case of uremia. The adipose tissue cells at the bottom (**A**) correspond to the epicardium; chronic irritation by an unknown agent (uremia?) has produced a thick layer of granulation tissue (**G**). The plasma oozing from the vessels of the granulation tissue has clotted and produced a ragged fibrin layer (**F**). It is not possible to tell whether fibrin is being produced, reabsorbed, or both. **Bar** = 100 μm.

plement, can be accomplished by components of injured cells (31,36,42,45) and by negatively charged surfaces such as exposed basement membranes. Complement activation means, of course, release of inflammatory anaphylatoxins (C3a, C4a, C5a).

Does this mean that complement is wasted on killing dead cells? Perhaps it gives some dying cells the coup de grâce *(32): experiments on myocardial ischemia showed that an anticomplement treatment reduced the size of the infarct (26,50); it also reduced the influx of leukocytes (18).*

- *Complement-derived anaphylatoxins are released by nonspecific proteolytic enzymes,* even without full-blown activation of complement (13,14,49). In other words, C3, C4, and C5 are cleaved by enzymes unrelated to complement, releasing anaphylatoxins (28,32).
- *Dying tissue releases inflammatory mediators:* histamine and other mediators from dying mast cells, and lysosomal enzymes; among these, the proteases are especially important because they cleave C3, C4, and C5. Products of cell autolysis are probably inflammatory, but they have not been tested.
- *The kinin system is activated* because the exuding plasma contains Hageman factor,

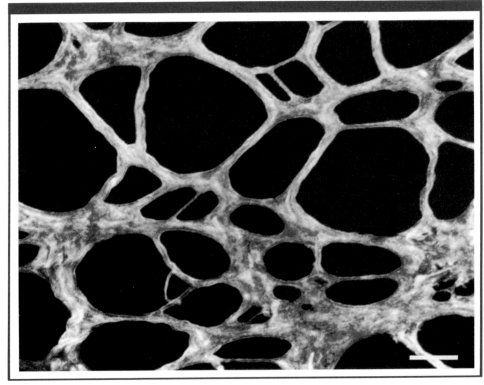

FIGURE 13.15
Dark field micrograph of normal rat omentum, emphasizing its typical net-like structure. Human omentum is similar. (Omentum mounted on a glass slide, unstained. **Bar** = 100 μm.). (Reproduced with permission from [37].)

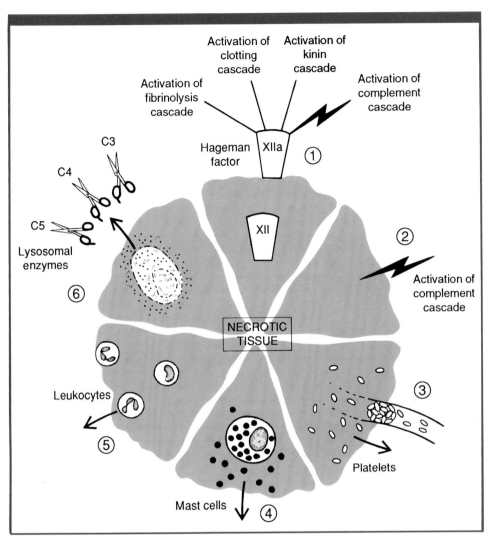

FIGURE 13.16
Why does necrotic tissue cause inflammation? Six likely mechanisms: (1) Plasma in vessels of the dead tissue contains Hageman factor (factor XII of the clotting cascade) which becomes activated by contact with collagen. Activated factor XII activates four cascades, all of which produce inflammatory mediators. (2) Necrotic tissue appears to activate complement directly - mechanism unknown. (3) Vessels of dead tissue contain platelets, which release many inflammatory mediators. (4) Mast cells in the dead tissue release histamine and other inflammatory agents. (5) Leukocytes are attracted into the necrotic tissue, and release inflammatory mediators. (6) Dead cells release lysosomal enzymes, which act on protein substrates, releasing inflammatory mediators (especially anaphylatoxins from complement factors C3, C4, and C5).

and Hageman factor—in contact with collagen—activates kininogen. The resulting bradykinin increases vascular permeability.

- *The clotting cascade is activated,* whereby a permeability-increasing mediator, fibrinopeptide B, is produced. The fibrinolytic cascade is also activated, and products of fibrinolysis are inflammatory; plasmin, the key fibrinolytic enzyme, joins the pool of proteolytic enzymes.
- *Platelet thrombi* develop in surrounding vessels, and the activated platelets release a host of mediators (Figure 9.14).
- *Feedback loops (vicious circles) develop:* the incoming leukocytes release proteolytic enzymes, and these in turn can release mediators as mentioned in the second item of this list (10,49). Leaky vessels supply the

proteolytic enzymes with plasma substrates (C3, C4, C5).

At this point the reader should find it interesting to attempt a two-part quiz, combining cell death and inflammation (note: immunology is not involved):

Question:

(a) If we open the abdomen of a rat 48 hours after implanting a piece of *fresh* liver, what are we likely to see?
(b) If we open the abdomen of a rat 48 hours after implanting a piece of *boiled* liver, what are we likely to see?

Answer:

(a) The fresh liver will be wrapped in inflamed omentum; the two will be glued together by

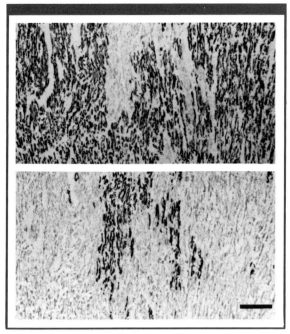

FIGURE 13.17
Presence of complement membrane-attack complex (MAC) in necrotic tissue. *Top:* Myocardium stained for succinic dehydrogenase: the central area devoid of enzyme represents a 6–7 day old infarct. *Bottom:* A consecutive section stained for the C5b-9 complex shows the reverse staining pattern: the complex is present only in the infarct. **Bar** = 250 μm. (Reproduced with permission from [39].)

fibrinous adhesions. Mechanism: the dying liver cells released a variety of peptides, eicosanoids, and other inflammatory mediators that inflamed the omentum, causing it to become attached to the implant. This acute inflammation will slowly merge into chronic inflammation, and eventually the implant will be organized.

(b) The boiled liver can release no mediators: it is essentially an inert mass of denatured protein from which no inflammatory messages arise. It will therefore be ignored by the omentum and will remain free in the abdominal cavity. In other words, it will not be organized. Eventually its surface will be colonized by peritoneal cells, probably macrophages, which will very slowly nibble at it while it slowly calcifies.

Note: After two or three days, an implant of *fresh* liver has released most of its chemical inflammatory messages and has turned into a mass of coagulated protein; therefore, it should no longer be an irritant. Indeed, if it is surgically removed and its core transplanted into another rat, it will remain free, like the boiled liver (24). *This explains why infarcts are removed very slowly:* after a fiery burst of acute inflammation they no longer attract leukocytes and are only nibbled at by the macrophages that happen to be in contact with their surface; sometimes they calcify.

These concepts are illustrated in Figures 13.18 and 13.19.

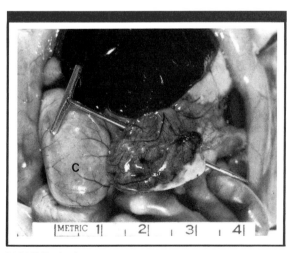

FIGURE 13.18
See color plate 15. Abdominal cavity of a rat 2 days after implantation of a fragment of sterile, fresh liver. The implant has inflamed the omentum, which has wrapped it up. A small area of white, necrotic liver is still visible at lower right (**arrow**). C: cecum. **Bar** = 5 mm.

HOW DOES ACUTE INFLAMMATION RELATE TO CHRONIC INFLAMMATION?

Although the terms *acute* and *chronic* inflammation are used as though they were self-evident, a closer look shows them to be convenient but imprecise. For clarity, let us set aside the clinical use of acute and chronic inflammation, and consider the biological events.

The basic event of inflammation is *the local recruitment of blood components.* If we consider the process from this angle, we find that it includes two types of responses, the first dominated by the neutrophil and the second by the macrophage. We could call the responses by their old names, acute and chronic, but it would be more accurate to call them *stereotyped* and *modulated.*

The acute or stereotyped response takes place almost as fast as a reflex, seconds or minutes after an injury: fluid pours out, closely followed by the neutrophils. We can call this response *stereotyped*

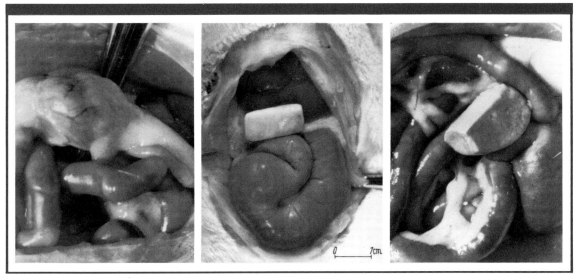

FIGURE 13.19

Long-standing necrotic tissue has lost its ability to trigger acute inflammation. The three panels show the fate of various kinds of liver fragments 1 week after introduction into the peritoneal cavity. *Left:* Fresh liver. Note complete wrapping by the omentum. *Center:* Sterile liver implant that has been transferred daily for 5 days to new recipient animals. It has failed to irritate the peritoneum and is ignored by the omentum. *Right:* A boiled implant that has been similarly ignored. (Reproduced with permission from [24].)

because it is practically immutable: it is the instant reaction to injury, be it an invasion of streptococci, a septic scalpel, or a fall down the stairs. Its purpose is to phagocytize and kill bacteria, with or without the help of plasma proteins, before they can establish a foothold.

The chronic or modulated response takes over if the injurious agent is not immediately removed. Its function is to provide a more sophisticated defense than phagocytosis alone. It is therefore masterminded by the macrophage, which is unequalled as a flexible, multipurpose cell. A macrophage can do almost everything the neutrophil can do, though more slowly. In addition, it can initiate the immune reaction, if required: it can summon lymphocytes, activate fibroblasts, induce new blood vessels, and even cause fever. In a nutshell, it is programmed to organize a powerful second line of defense.

It is important to understand that the stereotyped and modulated inflammatory responses are not phase A and phase B of a single programmed response, but are two overlapping responses, with partially different triggering mechanisms and programs. This explains their various combinations:

- *Acute inflammation followed by chronic,* the most common sequence.
- *Acute and chronic inflammation superimposed.*

A classic example is osteomyelitis due to staphylococcal infection. The first wave of neutrophils is unable to subdue the bacteria, so chronic inflammation sets in (macrophages, lymphocytes, an immune response). However, the staphylococci, being pyogens, attract more neutrophils. Thus, as long as the infection persists, there is continued exudation of neutrophils, *plus* chronic inflammation.

- *Acute inflammation not followed by chronic:* for example, the triple reaction, the sting of the nettle, and the rather similar allergic wheals. Minimal episodes of acute inflammation are also the tiny, unseen, but victorious duels fought every instant between neutrophils and bacteria, especially in the skin, mouth, and gut. We know that they must occur only because, in the absence of neutrophils, the body becomes a breeding ground for microscopic invaders.
- *Chronic inflammation may set in from the start:* such is the case of infection with *Mycobacterium tuberculosis,* against which granulocytes are totally powerless. In these cases a vanishingly brief granulocyte response can be demonstrated (23), but it is practically irrelevant.

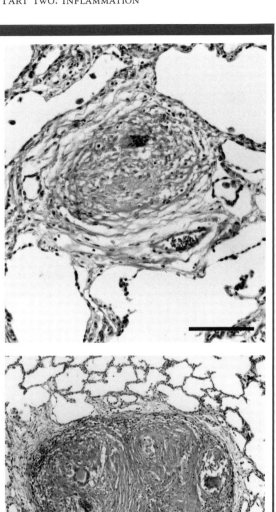

FIGURE 13.20
Tuberculous granulomas in the lung in a case of bacterial dissemination via the blood stream ("miliary" tuberculosis). *Top:* The granuloma consists of macrophages and a few lymphocytes, barely recognizable at this enlargement. Note the giant cell. *Bottom:* Aggregate of tuberculous granulomas. The starting point must have been a single granuloma that then grew by accretion. Note fibrous tissue at the periphery of the granulomas. **Bars** = 100 μm.

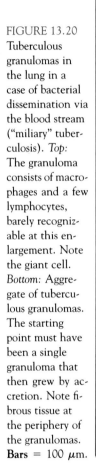

TO SUM UP: It should be obvious that the biological and clinical concepts of acute and chronic inflammation do not match. Biologically, the "chronic", modulated phase begins just hours after the "acute", stereotyped phase. The clinical concept of chronic referring to weeks and months is useful in medical practice, but we should keep in mind that the biological events—fortunately—run faster.

The biologically "chronic" or modulated phase of inflammation provides the sophisticated response required for continuing the fight initiated by the acute (stereotyped) response. It also helps in walling off the injured area: the sterotyped response has no structural borderline, but the wall provided by granulation tissue provides an enclosure that is almost impermeable to bacteria. A special type of walling off is provided by a distinctive modality of chronic inflammation: the *granuloma*, to be examined next.

Granulomatous Inflammation

The cellular infiltrate of a tissue that is chronically inflamed can be arranged according to two patterns: most often it is spread more or less evenly over a large area; other times it is gathered into small, separate, rounded clusters of macrophages that may or may not be joined by a few other cell types, a pattern that can be quite striking. These clusters are *granulomas* (or, for purists, *granulomata*). What do they mean?

The granuloma is Nature's device for dealing with particulate materials that are difficult to eliminate because they are poorly soluble and poorly degradable. These materials include any hard-to-digest microscopic particles that may have found their way into the tissues—thorns, splinters, inhaled asbestos, and so on—or tough bacteria such as *Mycobacterium tuberculosis* and *Mycobacterium leprae* (Figure 13.20). Each granuloma develops around a small quantum of the irritant, which is either free or phagocytized in the center of the granuloma. Sometimes the causal agent can be seen; for example, mycobacteria if they are suitably stained. When the agent is not visible, the observer must run through a mental list of dozens of agents that might be there (67). This is, in fact, the practical interest of the granuloma; it raises a red flag, inscribed: MACROPHAGES AT WORK—TOUGH PROBLEM.

Most granulomas are visible to the naked eye as whitish dots 0.5–1 mm in diameter. They contain no blood vessels, or only a few, which fits with their lack of color as well as their size; oxygen diffuses about 0.5 mm from the capillaries, and thus the macrophages in the center of a granuloma can still function aerobically. Why granulomas contain no vessels is not known; perhaps their macrophages, for reasons known only to them, do not produce angiogenic factor.

Because granulomas are so compact, they can be isolated and analyzed. A classic method is to inject a particulate agent into the portal vein of a mouse; a week or two later the liver is gently homogenized in a blender, and the granulomas can be spun out as tiny grains (Figure 13.21) (89). They can then be incubated, analyzed chemically, or dissociated to study the activity of the various cell components.

TYPES OF GRANULOMAS

The noxious agent buried in the center of the granuloma may be an irritant only in a physical sense, but it may also be antigenic. Accordingly, two kinds of cellular response can develop: a simple foreign-body granuloma or a more complex immune granuloma (55,58,60,61,106) (Figure 13.22).

FOREIGN-BODY GRANULOMAS

Foreign-body granulomas develop around any material perceived by the tissues as extraneous but not antigenic; surgical threads are an example. Foreign-body granulomas are made up primarily of macrophages and their derivatives: giant cells and epithelioid cells. Giant cells can contain dozens and even hundreds of nuclei (Figure 13.23); they arise primarily by fusion of macrophages, although some degree of internal mitosis is possible (72,92). If the foreign body is small enough, it can be entirely contained by a single giant cell; if it is large, the macrophages and giant cells will simply be apposed to its surface. Because giant cells deserve a section of their own, we will deal with them later. Epithelioid cells are sometimes present in foreign body granulomas (98, 101); they were given their peculiar name because they consist of enlarged macrophages so tightly packed as to recall the closeness of epithelial cells. They are much more prevalent in immune granulomas. In hyperlipidemic animals, the macrophages of granulomas turn into foam cells (94).

Fibroblasts form a loose coat around the foreign-body granuloma; as time passes—months, even years—the macrophage component tends to disappear, and the foreign body remains surrounded by a thin fibrous layer, sometimes so thin that the extraneous object appears to lie free in the tissue.

All this sounds straightforward, but how does an inert foreign body attract macrophages? Studies with sterile plastic beads injected into the blood stream suggest that the surface of a foreign body activates the Hageman factor, an important source of inflammatory mediators.

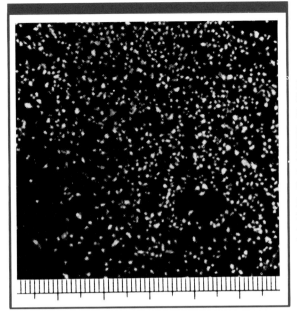

FIGURE 13.21 Suspension of Schistosoma granulomas isolated from mouse liver 8 weeks after infection. Granulomas prepared in this manner can be used for metabolic studies *in vitro*. Scale in mm. (Reproduced with permission from [89].)

It is reasonable to assume that the trauma connected with penetration by a foreign body would spill blood, thus giving the foreign body the opportunity to activate some Hageman factor. Pigeons are deficient in Hageman factor and do not produce granulomas in response to intravenous beads (81,107).

IMMUNE GRANULOMAS

Immune granulomas, also called hypersensitivity granulomas (62), are caused by insoluble particles that are perceived as antigenic and are capable of inducing that particular type of immune response called cell-mediated immunity (CMI) (p. 540). Historically, the prototype for this category of granuloma is that caused by the bacillus of tuberculosis, a disease so prevalent for so long that its granulomas acquired their own name: *tubercle.*

Cell-mediated immunity does not necessarily produce granulomas, but it does so when the antigen is particulate or poorly soluble. The sequence is initiated by the macrophages, which pick up the antigen and present some of it to appropriate T lymphocytes, causing them to respond. The activated T lymphocytes produce IL-2, a T-cell growth factor, which tends to perpetuate the response. Treatment of the animal with cyclosporin A, which blocks cytokine production, also inhibits the formation of granulomas.

The structure of immune granulomas is more varied than just clusters of macrophages (Figure 13.24). Typically, immune granulomas include:

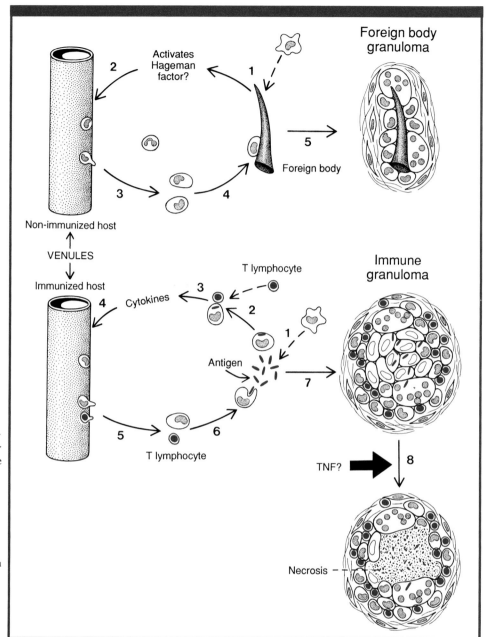

FIGURE 13.22
Two principal types of granulomas. Numbers indicate sequence of events. *Top*: Foreign-body granuloma exemplified by the response to a thorn. The granuloma contains macrophages, macrophage-derived giant cells, and fibroblasts. Lymphocytes are absent. *Bottom*: Immune granuloma. In this case the stimulus is antigenic; in a host previously immunized to this antigen it leads to the formation of a granuloma containing macrophages, fibroblasts, and also lymphocytes (and sometimes granulocytes). This type of granuloma can undergo central necrosis.

- *Macrophages modulated into epithelioid cells*, similar to those of foreign-body granulomas but more numerous (Figure 13.25). The margins of these cells are interdigitated, which fits the name *epithelioid* and can perhaps be interpreted as a useful adaptation for walling off the offending agent (59). Seen by electron microscopy these cells have large nuclei and nucleoli, few organelles, and swollen endoplasmic reticula (88).
- *Lymphocytes*

- Sometimes, *plasma cells*, the antibody secretors, indicating that the immune response to the irritant may occasionally include antibody formation
- A crown of *fibroblasts*

Not always present are macrophages fused into *giant cells*, the purpose of which is not clear (see later); *eosinophils* when the causal agent is a worm or other large parasite; and *mast cells or basophils*. *Granulocytes* are rare in granulomas; of course, if the predominant cells were neutrophils, the

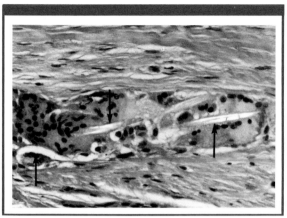

FIGURE 13.23
Foreign-body granuloma in an old surgical scar. Photographed by partially polarized light. The foreign body (**arrows**) is clearly visible; it probably represents the remains of a suture. The granuloma consists almost entirely of multinucleated giant cells.

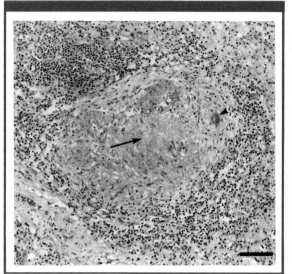

FIGURE 13.24
Tuberculous granuloma in a human lung. The core of the granuloma consists of packed macrophages (epithelioid cells) surrounded by lymphocytes. Note incipient caseous necrosis (**arrow**) and giant cell (**arrowhead**). **Bar** = 100 μm.

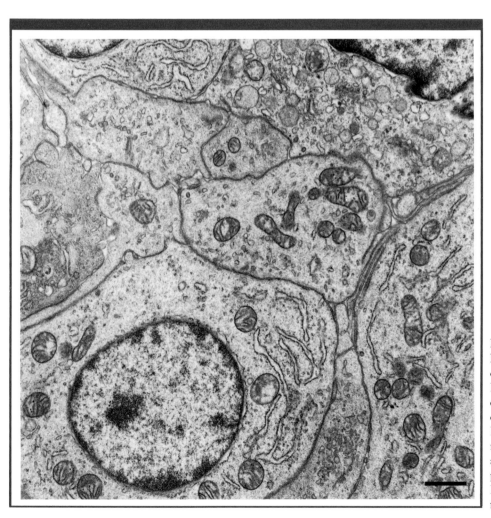

FIGURE 13.25
Electron microscopic aspect of epithelioid cells from a human beryllium granuloma, induced in the skin of a volunteer (chronic berylliosis is caused by industrial exposure to beryllium dust, which induces an immune response). Note the densely packed and interdigitating processes of macrophages. **Bar** = 1 μm. (Courtesy of Dr. W. L. Epstein, University of California, San Francisco, CA).

structure would not be a granuloma but a small abscess.

Responses intermediate between abscess and granuloma do exist: some irritating agents induce cell-mediated immunity and also attract neutrophils. Such is the case with streptococcal wall preparations (74,104,105), which produce—reportedly—large granulomas that are rich in capillaries and filled with neutrophils. There is no official name for these granuloma-abscesses (Figure 13.26). A mixed granuloma–neutrophil response is also produced by a microscopic fungus, *Coccidioides immitis* (Figure 13.27).

The only granulomas containing epithelial (not epithelioid) cells occur at the roots of decaying teeth (dental granulomas); the mechanism is the same as for dental abscesses. The mixture of granulation tissue and epithelial cords can be quite striking (Figure 13.12).

The role of cell-mediated immunity in the pathogenesis of immune granulomas can be demonstrated by injecting intravenously a suspension of nonirritating particles, either blank or loaded with an antigen (64). In a normal animal, plastic beads of either type produces a mild foreign-body

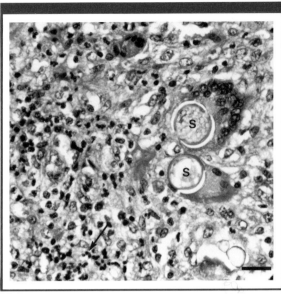

FIGURE 13.27

Focus of infection by a fungus, *Coccidioides immitis*, in a lymph node (not recognizable as such). **S**: Spherules of the fungus, partly surrounded by giant cells. When the spherules break open, they induce an acute inflammatory response, as indicated by the neutrophils seen at the lower left (**arrow**). *This fungus therefore induces both a granulomatous and a purulent response.* There are about 100,000 clinical cases of coccidioidomycosis in the United States each year. **Bar = 25 μm.**

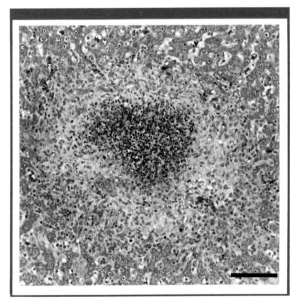

FIGURE 13.26

A sterile "granuloma" produced in the rat by injecting intravenously a preparation of streptococcal cell walls. These so-called granulomas consist of a central mass of neutrophils surrounded by a crown of macrophages: they are actually hybrid lesions, intermediate between granulomas and abscesses. **Bar = 100 μm.** (From a slide kindly provided by Dr. J.D. Geratz of the University of North Carolina, Chapel Hill, NC.).

reaction; in an animal immunized with the specific antigen, the antigen-carrying beads produce a typical immune granuloma (100). Similar results are obtained with Schistosoma eggs injected intravenously (Figure 13.28): the granulomas developing in the lung are much larger if the animal has been previously injected with Schistosoma antigens. Conclusion: the cell-mediated immune response plays a major role in creating this type of granuloma (63,90,102,108). There are many variations to this theme; for example, the role of individual cytokines in the genesis of granulomas can be tested by incorporating a cytokine into plastic beads and then instilling the beads into the trachea to test the effect on the lung (Figure 13.29) (80). Immune granulomas develop very poorly in nude rats, which are incapable of mounting a cell-mediated immune response (60–62,75,104,105): basically, any maneuver to immunosuppress the host—such as X-rays or anti-lymphocyte antibodies—greatly reduces the sizes of immune granulomas, whereas foreign-body granulomas are not affected.

GRANULOMAS AS SECRETORY ORGANS

Using suspensions of granulomas (p. 443), experiments have shown that immune granulomas can secrete many inflammatory mediators (103): cytokines, free radicals, prostaglandins, collagenase (93) and other enzymes, even angiotensin converting enzyme (85), and a variety of other factors (66,69,73,99). The type of secretion depends on the agent (83), the host organ (109), the age of the granuloma, and additional stimuli; but the biological message remains the same: *the granuloma is a device for concentrating activated mononuclear cells against hardy invaders.*

Some of the secretions of granulomas may have general effects, such as increased calcium absorption. Hypercalcemia occurs in several diseases in which myriads of granulomas are produced; such as sarcoidosis, tuberculosis, berylliosis, coccidiomycosis, even silicone injection (76,84,86). It has been found that activated macrophages convert inactive vitamin D3 to the active form (91), which greatly increases calcium absorption in the gut.

CAN GRANULOMAS BE PRODUCED IN VITRO?

Producing granulomas *in vitro* has been attempted by culturing a mixture of "spleen cells," which should include all the cell types required to build a granuloma, together with plastic beads, plain or loaded with cytokines. The result is fairly convincing (Figure 13.30) (95).

NATURAL HISTORY OF GRANULOMAS

Immune granulomas change with time in both structure and function (68,106). It has been suggested that during the life of a granuloma there is a constant flux of macrophages from the periphery to the center (96), but how those in the center disappear is not understood. The growth of the granuloma appears to be autostimulated by TNF secreted by macrophages: antibodies against TNF inhibit the formation of granulomas induced by the attenuated tubercle bacillus BCG (82). The outer fibrous wrapping, which can be striking, is probably accounted for by fibroblast-stimulating factors from macrophages or lymphocytes (104, 105,110). Eventually, *if a granuloma succeeds in eliminating the irritant, it shrinks and disappears,* sometimes leaving a small scar; the same happens if the causal agent is killed by treatment (Figure 13.31). On the other hand, *adjacent granulomas may expand and fuse;* this is especially true of bacterial granulomas such as those of tuberculosis and leprosy.

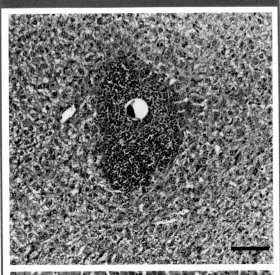

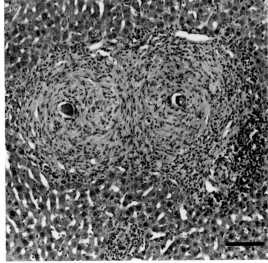

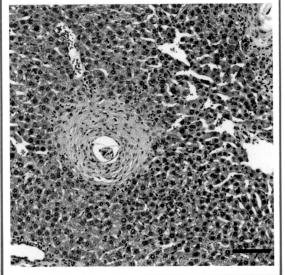

FIGURE 13.28 Life cycle of immune granulomas produced by eggs of *Schistosoma* in mouse liver. *Top:* Early stage. The live egg in the center is surrounded by a dense cellular infiltrate. (At higher power most of these cells are shown to be granulocytes.) *Center:* Two well-developed granulomas consisting mainly of large histiocytes (epithelioid cells) with clusters of lymphocytes at the periphery. *Bottom:* Late stage. A dead Schistosoma egg is surrounded by a dense layer of fibroblasts and collagen. (Some of the cells are surely macrophages, but they cannot be identified in this photograph.) The lymphocytes have disappeared. This stage can be considered a scar. **Bars** = 100 μm. (Specimen kindly provided by Dr. M.J. Stadecker, Department of Pathology, Tufts University School of Medicine, Boston, MA.)

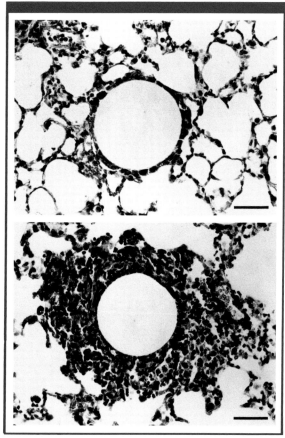

FIGURE 13.29

Role of interleukin-1 in the pathogenesis of granulomas. *Top:* The central white disk represents the cross section of a plain Sepharose (control) bead injected through the trachea into the lung of a mouse. After 3 days it has caused a very mild inflammatory reaction, represented by a single layer of macrophages. *Bottom:* Effect of a bead coupled with interleukin-1. After 3 days it has produced a large granuloma consisting mainly of macrophages. **Bars** = 100 μm. (Reproduced with permission from [80].)

NECROSIS IN IMMUNE GRANULOMAS

Necrosis does not occur in all immune granulomas; it is seen, typically, in those of tuberculosis, syphilis, and rheumatoid arthritis. The necrosis is always of the "coagulation" type (p. 546) and develops in the centers of the granulomas. When adjacent granulomas fuse, the result can be a large mass of necrosis surrounded by a rim of "granuloma" tissue (Figure 13.32); we can call it "tuberculous granulation tissue" because it is richly vascularized (70) (in contrast with individual granulomas, which contain no capillaries). The resulting mass can reach several centimeters in diameter, resembling a tumor, hence the names *tuberculoma* for such lumps that develop in

tuberculosis, *gumma* in syphilis and *rheumatoid nodule* in rheumatoid arthritis. The syphilitic gumma is so-called because the necrosis gives it a rubbery consistency. In tuberculosis the necrosis is rather dry and cheesy, hence the name *caseous necrosis*.

Why does necrosis develop in some immune granulomas? It is natural to blame the bacilli and spirochetes for the granulomas of tuberculosis and syphilis, but a very similar necrosis develops in the sterile granulomas of rheumatoid arthritis, which is a nonbacterial, autoimmune disease (p. 573). So, there must be a nonbacterial explanation for the necrosis of immune granulomas. Nobody knows for sure (71), but it is generally felt that the necrosis in granulomas has something to do with the immunologic phenomenon called hypersensitivity. Prime suspects as chemical indicators are macrophage-derived cytokines such as tumor necrosis factor. We will discuss caseous necrosis in the chapter on immunopathology.

PROS AND CONS OF THE GRANULOMATOUS RESPONSE

Foreign-body granulomas are probably useful; after all, they tend to free the tissues of extraneous material. Immune granulomas have, basically, great survival value. Excellent proof of their value is found in leprosy, which comes in two forms: *tuberculoid,* in which patients produce a hefty granulomatous response, and *lepromatous,* in which the granulomatous response is impaired. Prognosis for the latter form is relatively poor (Figure 13.33). Experimental models confirm this point.

On the other hand, immune granulomas can be harmful. First of all because they occupy space, much of which is not added but is removed from an organ. A tubercle in the lung, for example, is formed at the expense of a small portion of the lung. It is as if macrophages prepared the site for the expanding granuloma by removing local structures. For this reason, granulomas in the retina cause irreversible damage. Furthermore, granulomas exist because they recruit cells by secreting cytokines. These cytokines are presumably washed into the blood and lymph, but any excess might produce unwanted local reactions such as fibrosis, or even general effects ranging from fever to immunosuppression.

Granulomatous diseases number in the hundreds and affect all organs (62,67,79). They can be local to one organ, especially the lung (from

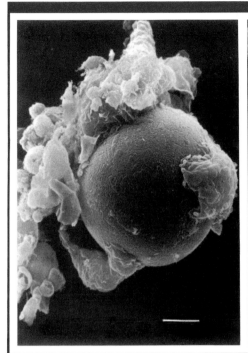
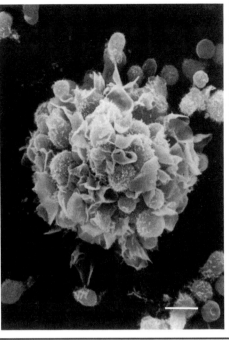

FIGURE 13.30
Granuloma formation *in vitro*. Latex beads were incubated with mouse spleen cells (over 95% macrophages). After incubation for 1 day (**A**) and 3 days (**B**) the beads became progressively covered with macrophages. The effect was enhanced by incubation in the presence of interleukin-1 and tumor necrosis factor α but not in the presence of interleukin-2 or interferon-γ. **Bars** =5μm. (Reproduced with permission from [95].)

inhaling particles) or generalized. The agents of the diseases can be infectious (syphilis, tuberculosis, leprosy, cat-scratch disease), fungal (cryptococcosis), parasitic (schistosomiasis), autoimmune (rheumatic fever), or even inorganic (inhaled beryllium compounds); often the causal agent is unknown. In some granulomatous diseases the granulomas are distinctive enough to suggest the diagnosis; the best example is silicosis, which induces a fibrous response so strong as to be almost unmistakable (p. 456).

Most frustrating of all granulomatous diseases is **sarcoidosis,** in which classic, immune-type, giant-cell granulomas are scattered body-wide, without a hint of their cause. Because the granulomas appear almost anywhere, symptoms are extremely variable and may even be lacking. About two-thirds of the cases recover, either completely or with lung or eye impairment. Inflammatory cells obtained from the lungs of patients with pulmonary sarcoidosis by rinsing the bronchi with saline (bronchoalveolar lavage) show an excess of activated T-helper lymphocytes, precisely those that are essential for recruiting more macrophages and lymphocytes into immune-type granulomas (77,78).

Oddly enough, a depression of cell-mediated immunity has been found in sarcoidosis as well as in regional enteritis (Crohn's disease) and other types of granulomatous diseases, although the granulomas actually represent a cell-mediated immune response. This is a complex problem (62), but a few facts come to the rescue: an excess of circulating T-suppressor over T-helper lymphocytes has been found in several granulomatous diseases, and a circulating immunosuppressor substance has been found not only in humans but also in mice bearing foreign-body granulomas induced by plastic beads (56). That an immune response should produce immunosuppression would not be the first paradox of immunology.

The clinical disease of sarcoidosis is caused by the granulomas themselves; no other lesion seems to occur. In other words, sarcoidosis is the price to pay for an otherwise crucial defensive mechanism, the granuloma.

TO SUM UP: In the big picture of chronic inflammation, granulomas behave like specialized, temporary subcommittees designed for handling tough problems. They may or may not use the mechanisms of the immune response, but they are always programmed by the omnipotent macrophage.

THE GIANT CELL SAGA

Once regarded as a pathologist's curiosity, giant cells—short for multinucleated giant cells—turned out to be the ticket to a Nobel prize and

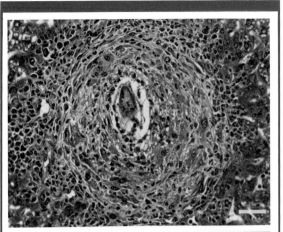

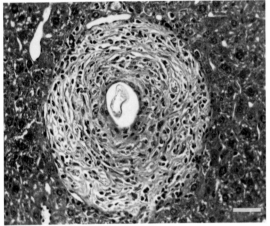

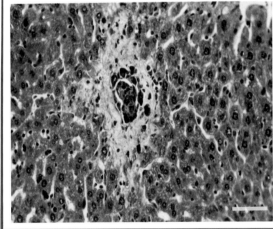

FIGURE 13.31 Regression of schistosomal granulomas in mice treated with a single dose of hycanthone and oxamniquine. *Top:* Granuloma in an untreated mouse. *Center:* After 2 months of treatment the granuloma is sharply defined and contains fewer cells. In the center are an empty and shrunken egg shell. *Bottom:* After 4.5 months, remnants of a Schistosoma egg are surrounded by pigment-laden phagocytic cells and some collagen fibers. **Bars** = 50 μm. (Reproduced with permission from [57].)

then to a commercial boom. They derive from macrophages and are therefore close relatives of the osteoclasts (multinucleated cells associated with bone resorption). The story of the giant cells should be recorded here as a perfect example of how a little seed, in the proper hands, can grow into a forest.

Giant cells were first described by Johannes Müller, Virchow's teacher, in 1838. For a long time they were thought to be "mother cells"; that is, a type of cell that contains many baby cells, perhaps by analogy with the sporocysts of protozoa. Then it was realized that macrophages can give rise to giant cells, either by cell fusion or by nuclear division that is not followed by cell division (124,135).

Structurally, the giant cells of chronic inflammation are essentially macrophages with many nuclei. It is traditional to mention that the nuclei can be arranged in two patterns: either randomly or around the cell periphery (*Langhans type* giant cells, often seen in tuberculosis) (Figure 13.34). The peripheral arrangement is caused by a giant centrosphere in the middle of the cell (129). However, the distinction between the two arrangements has no known significance. Sometimes, especially in sarcoidosis, the giant cells contain beautiful asteroid bodies composed of cytoskeletal fibrils (vimentin) and lipid (Figure 13.35). They may also contain rounded calcified structures called Schaumann bodies. What these inclusions mean is not known (121).

Spontaneous Cell Fusion Giant cells are seen in two pathologic settings:

(a) *Infection with certain bacteria or viruses,* such as the tubercle bacillus or herpes virus (Figure 13.36); under such conditions adjacent macrophages are "zipped" together by a physicochemical effect of lipids or proteins (113) of the infectious particles. Cytokines can also accomplish the fusion (123,130), including interferon gamma (134).

(b) *Giant cells induced by foreign bodies,* either isolated or as part of a granuloma; when they spread over a foreign body they give the impression of trying to swallow it (Figure 13.37).

How do macrophages fuse over a foreign body? Direct studies are lacking, but we can speculate. It is known that the converging edges of two extremely flattened cells creeping over a surface can meet and fuse where they touch, the reason being that the two tightly folded cell membranes no longer repel each other (Figure 13.38) (111). By this mechanism two macrophages could fuse while attempting to engulf the same particle (114).

Mechanisms of Cell Fusion Giant cells have played a major historical role by reviving interest in cell fusion. Cells can fuse spontaneously; they

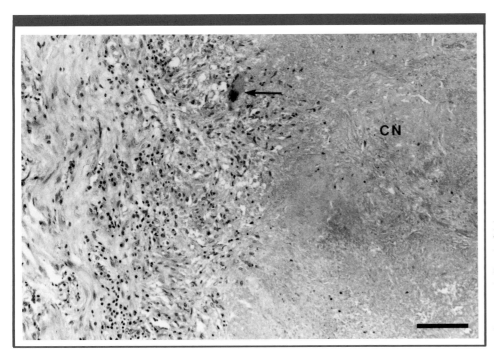

FIGURE 13.32
Transition between tuberculous granulation tissue (left) and caseous necrosis (**CN**). In this field it is obvious that the caseous necrosis is developing by death of the granulation tissue (mostly macrophages = epithelioid cells). **Arrow:** A giant cell. **Bar** = 100 μm.

can also be induced to do so. Both phenomena were well known early in the 1900s by botanists, who even used cell fusion to produce hybrids (115). But somehow the news did not reach the "animal people". Then came, in 1965, Drs. H. Harris and J. F. Watkins of the Sir William Dunn School of Pathology in Oxford (157). Taking the hint from virus-induced giant cells, Harris and Watkins reasoned that if viruses can zip together cells of the same kind, they might also join cells of different species. Sure enough, human cells and mouse cells, in the presence of Sendai virus (convenient because it is not pathogenic for humans), merged into beautiful giant cells; and most important, the giant cells survived (118). These cells were called *heterokarya*. The virus worked even if it was inactivated by UV light, proving that the effect was chemical or physicochemical, unrelated to the infective process.

Just 48 hours after this study appeared in Nature, *a cartoon in the* London Daily Mirror *(Figure 13.39) (117) showed that the press was quick to grasp the importance of the experiment.*

Not all experimental fusions are successful, although some mind-boggling combinations have survived for a time, such as between human and carrot, or human and tobacco leaf (120). A

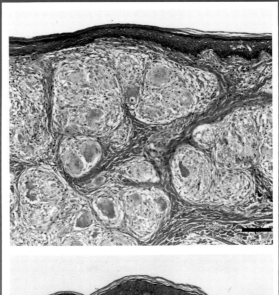

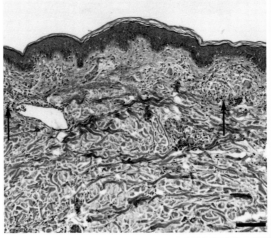

FIGURE 13.33
Two forms of leprosy. *Top:* Tuberculoid leprosy of the skin. The dermis is packed with granulomas; almost every one contains one or more giant cells. This pattern corresponds to a vigorous response of the immune system. *Bottom:* Lepromatous leprosy. There is a diffuse, although not very obvious, inflammatory infiltrate (**arrows**) of the dermis, with no tendency to form granulomas. This pattern corresponds to a partially suppressed immune system. **Bars** = 100 μm.

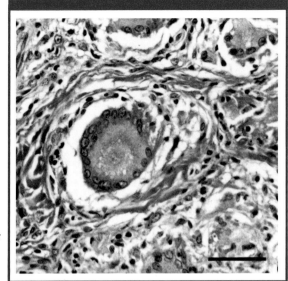

FIGURE 13.34 Typical multi-nucleated giant cell in a case of leprosy of the skin. It occupies much of the granuloma; the surrounding clear halo is an arte-fact. **Bar** = 50 μm.

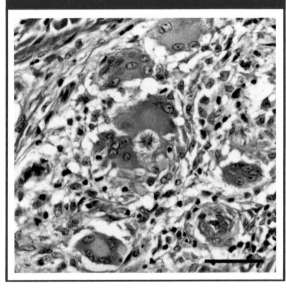

FIGURE 13.35 Giant cells in a case of leprosy of the skin, one of them containing a typical "aster-oid body." The field includes sev-eral coalescent, ill-defined granu-lomas. **Bar** = 50 μm.

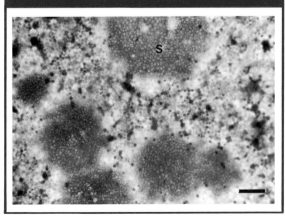

FIGURE 13.36 An example of cell fusion by a herpes virus. Cul-ture of human ma-lignant epithelial cells (HEp-2) 24 hours after infec-tion with a her-pes virus. Many cells have been induced to fuse, producing large syncytia (S). **Bar** = 500 μm.

typical result of such disparate fusions is the following: the two nuclei of the heterokaryon enter mitosis together; then a single spindle is formed, and the two mononuclear daughter cells contain, *in a single nucleus*, the chromosomes of both parent cells (117). In successive mitoses, some chromosomes can be eliminated, a fact that can be used for mapping single human chromo-somes. This approach has opened up a new branch of genetics.

Of course, fusions between normal and tumor cells came early in the experimental agenda. At first they seemed to show that malignancy (as a pessimist might have guessed) tends to be domi-nant in such fusions, but more work reversed this conclusion (p. 904). This is where the commer-cial boom occurred: two imaginative scientists (122) had the idea of fusing a malignant, and therefore immortal, plasma cell with a normal, mortal cell that secretes a certain protein: *this fusion produces a protein-secreting cell that is also immortal.* From this single fused cell one can then grow an artificial tumor or *hybridoma* that will continue to secrete that protein *in vitro* in potentially unlimited amounts: at long last a contribution to human welfare by tumors. This was the key to monoclonal antibodies. Cell fusion can now be induced by a host of reagents such as polyethylene glycol, with cytokines (132,133), and even with electricity (112,131). In 1984 the Nobel prize committee chose to reward the application of cell fusion to the production monoclonal antibodies rather than to the original idea.

One hope raised by the heterokarya did not material-ize: the possibility of alleviating world famine by creating a new generation of plant hybrids. The advent of genetic engineering in 1977 provided a more effective method (116).

Biological Significance of Giant Cells Apart from the inspiration that they provided to researchers, to this day we know of no specific function of giant cells, beyond the status of glorified macrophages. For some time they were maligned: it was said that they were less phagocytic (126) and slower moving (125) than their parent cells, and even that they represented a way to get rid of obsolete macro-phages. Their half-life, estimated from transplanta-tion experiments, was said to be only a few days (127), a figure that we find unlikely. More recent work finds the giant cell to be metabolically at least as active as a regular macrophage (128); one study found its oxygen burst to be 20–30 times greater (123).

It has been suggested that giant cells may have a survival value for viruses, by allowing them to jump from one cell to the next without being exposed to the intercellular fluid, which might contain dangerous antibodies. They are certainly useful to the pathologist: they provide a diagnostic hint that something abnormal is lurking in the tissue, perhaps a foreign body, perhaps an infectious agent.

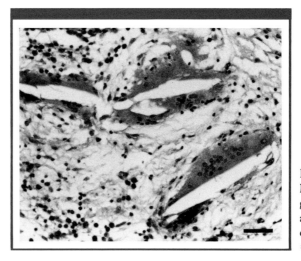

FIGURE 13.37
Multinucleated giant cells around crystals of cholesterol. **Bar** = 50 μm.

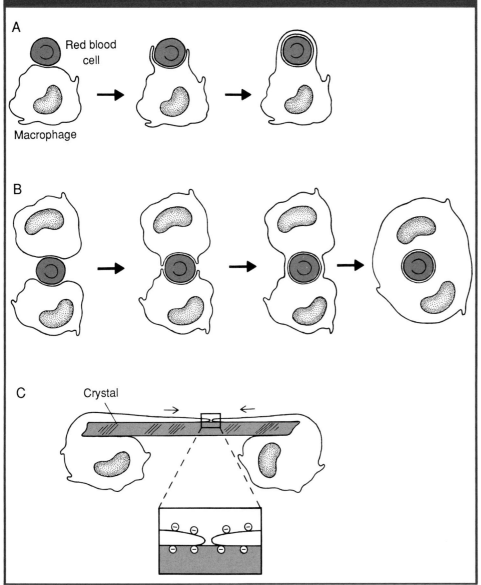

FIGURE 13.38
Showing how phagocytosis may lead to the fusion of macrophages. **A:** phagocytosis of a red blood cell by a macrophage. The red blood cell is engulfed by a "crater" arising from the cell membrane; the rim of the crater then fuses with itself and closes over the red blood cell. **B:** two macrophages attempting to engulf the same red blood cell. The two apposed craters may fuse along their rims. **C:** fusion of two macrophages over the surface of a crystal. The two thin lamellipodia may fuse because the radius of curvature of the cell membranes at their advancing edge (*inset*) is so small that the negative charges are spread apart, whereby the apposed folds do not repel each other. (Adapted from [114].)

FIGURE 13.39
Cartoon from
*The London Daily
Mirror* of February 15, 1965. Response to the
news that cells
"from man and
mouse" had been
fused into viable
hybrids. (Reproduced with permission from
[117].)

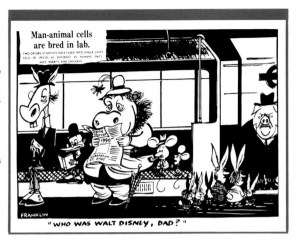

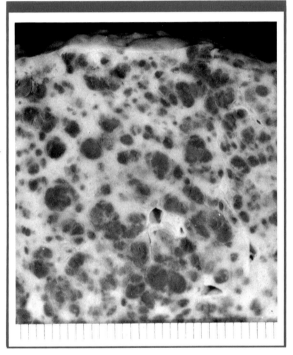

FIGURE 13.40
Example of fibrosis: cut surface of
a cirrhotic liver
from a chronic alcoholic. The
dark nodules represent normal or
regenerating
liver tissue; the
whitish background is the
newly formed fibrous tissue typical of cirrhosis.
Scale in mm.

Fibrosis

Fibrosis is any excess of fibrous tissue. As we
understand it, it is a response of fibroblasts to
stimulation by cytokines, typically produced in
chronic inflammation. Fibrosis is therefore, in the
first place, an aspect of defense processes. In
chronic inflammation it can be helpful by contributing to the walling off of infected areas; the outer
wall of an abscess is a layer of fibrous tissue.
Fibrosis is also the end-point of wound healing: the
scar that restores the continuity of severed tissues.

However, fibrosis can also contribute to disease:
an excessive or inappropriate stimulus can induce
fibrosis throughout an organ (interstitial fibrosis),
typically the lung, and impair its function.

> Cirrhosis *is now applied rather loosely to mean a
> severe, progressive fibrosis of the liver and occasionally of the pancreas, although the term was
> originally coined to mean* yellowness *(p. 78).*

Fibrotic tissue is whitish to the naked eye because of its high collagen content (Figure 13.40).
For the same reason it is also firm, or even hard:
hence the terms *sclerosis* and *sclerotic* (from the
Greek *sklerós*, hard). A classic example are the
thick white plaques sometimes found on the
parietal pleura or diaphragm, which consist almost
entirely of collagen and are most likely related to
the inhalation of asbestos particles (Figure 13.41)
(169).

BIOLOGY OF FIBROSIS
The cells of fibrotic tissue are mainly fibroblasts,
sometimes mixed with myofibroblasts (157).

> *An exception: in the liver, the cells responsible for
> producing most of the fibrosis are thought to be the
> star-shaped, fat-storing "lipocytes" or Ito cells
> (145,146).*

The collagen of fibrotic tissues consists of the
ordinary types I and III (143), and its chemical
composition is normal. But there is evidence, at
least in the lung, for a "fibrotic" collagen characterized by an excess of hydroxylation and crosslinking (168). Another exception occurs in the
fibrosis of diabetes, in which glycation is thought
to make the fibers more resistant to enzymatic
attack (p. 267). As fibrotic lesions age, collagen
becomes more and more cross-linked and reabsorption becomes virtually impossible (168).

If fibrotic tissue contains enough cells (myofibroblasts, fibroblasts), it may slowly contract,
creating mechanical problems. Myofibroblasts
have been found in all such cases. For example: the
contraction of the heart's *chordae tendineae* as a
consequence of rheumatic endocarditis (usually on
the mitral valve) leads to deformation and malfunction of the valve; the contracting tissue contains
myofibroblasts (23a). The fibrotic lung contains a
large number of myofibroblasts (138). Cirrhotic
livers contract strongly enough to impair the flow of
portal blood and to produce ascites (p. 607).

Fibrosis with shrinkage, as seen in cirrhotic livers, can also occur in the kidney. The so-called contracted kidney can be shriveled to a fraction of normal size as the end result of several conditions (especially chronic inflammation and ischemia). Myofibroblasts may be blamed for some of the shrinkage of the kidney (164) and of the liver (154), but the small size of the contracted kidney and of shrunken cirrhotic livers is also due to loss of parenchyma.

Contraction of the fibrotic tissue does not occur when the stiff collagen component is overwhelming, as in keloids or in asbestosis plaques (Figure 13.41) (139).

STIMULI THAT INDUCE FIBROSIS

Cytokines Powerful inducers of fibrosis are to be found among the cytokines (144,176). These products of macrophages and lymphocytes affect fibroblasts in many ways: they induce them to move by chemotaxis, to divide, to secrete collagen or collagenase; they can also inhibit any of these functions (156) (Figure 13.42).

The most important monocyte products affecting fibroblasts are interleukin-1 (IL-1), tumor necrosis factor alpha (TNF-alpha), platelet-derived growth factor (PDGF), transforming growth factor beta

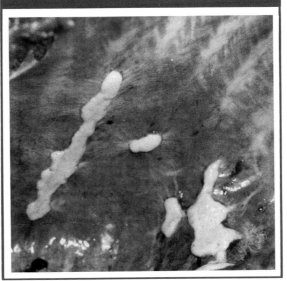

FIGURE 13.41
Thick, whitish fibrous plaques typical of exposure to asbestos. Photograph taken at autopsy, showing the inner surface of the chest; natural size.

(TGF-beta), which is also a lymphokine, and the two fibroblast growth factors (FGF), acidic and basic. Other factors are secreted by lymphocytes (175).

Proof that these cytokines really induce fibrosis has been obtained in many ways: by infusion into the tissues, by demonstrating that tissue cells are actively synthesizing a given cytokine, and by preventing fibrosis by means of anticytokine-antibody (Figure 13.43) (167).

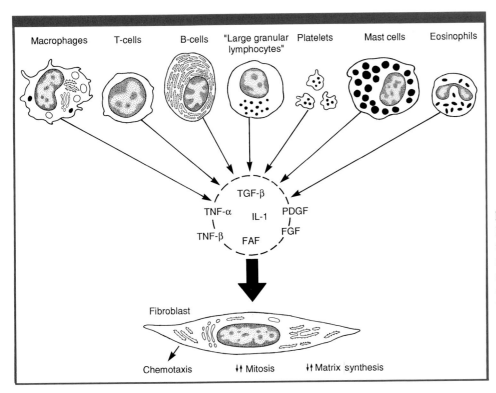

FIGURE 13.42
Many cell types can stimulate the fibroblasts, by means of the chemical messengers shown in the box. Conspicuously absent from the group of stimulating cells are the neutrophils; the eosinophils are almost certainly involved. The stimulated fibroblasts may respond by chemotaxis, by proliferation, or by secretion of collagen and other macromolecules. (Adapted from [62].)

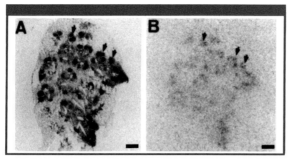

FIGURE 13.43
Tumor necrosis factor is involved in fibrosis. **A:** Histologic section of mouse lung. Instilled silica particles produced densely fibrous silicotic nodules (**arrowheads**). **B:** Autoradiograph of the same section after it was hybridized with a probe for TNF messenger RNA. The silver grains of the autoradiograph are deposited over the silicotic nodules (**arrows**) but not over the rest of the lung. **Bars** = 1000 μm. (Reproduced with permission from [167].)

Serotonin Serotonin is the only mediator of acute inflammation to produce fibrosis, at least under pathologic conditions.

The first hint that serotonin produces fibrosis came in the 1930s, from the autopsy of patients with liver metastases of carcinoids, which are endocrine tumors that secrete, among other molecules, serotonin. There was a fibrous thickening of the valves and of the endocardium on the right side of the heart, an unusual location in that most cardiac pathology is on the left side (Figure 9.21). The explanation: serotonin liberated by liver metastases reaches the right heart, causes the changes, and is then inactivated by the endothelial angiotensin-converting enzyme as it passes through the lung (170). Indeed, serotonin is now

recognized as a mitogen for fibroblasts (172). Accordingly, endocardial fibrosis is fairly rich in cells.

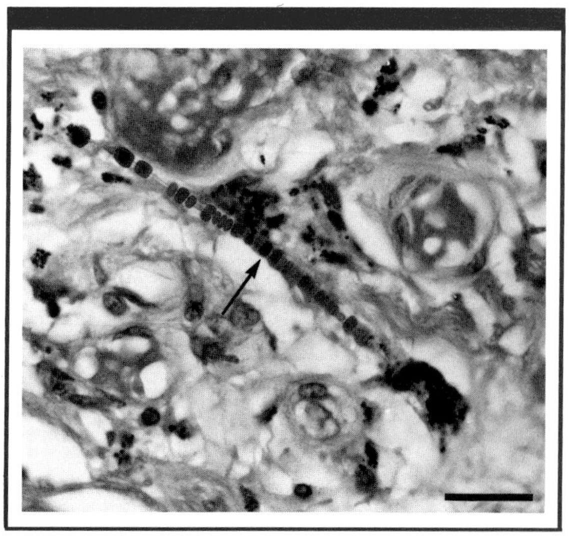

Drugs Several forms of sclerosis are iatrogenic: a worrisome development because some of the incriminated drugs are invaluable. A few patients treated for migraine develop ureteral constriction caused by retroperitoneal fibrosis (160), whereby a tough, glistening, wood-hard mass of fibrous tissue 2–6 cm thick (160,165) encases the ureters, the large vessels, and other retroperitoneal structures. The main drug involved is methysergide, a vasoconstricting ergot derivative. An intriguing fact is that methysergide is a serotonin antagonist, as is lysergic acid diethylamide (LSD), which can cause the same complication. Several other drug families have been incriminated, including beta blockers. Beta blockers include in their list of possible side effect: Peyronies's disease, a slow retraction of the penile shaft.

Totally unexplained are the bizarre localizations of fibrosis: why should a drug taken orally affect just the retroperitoneal tissues or the penis? All we can say is that fibroblasts can be capricious in their responses to drugs. For example, depending on their anatomic location fibroblasts may have different life spans (161), different surface markers or patterns of synthesis (173), or varying propensities to modulate into myofibroblasts (147); even two cells arising from the same mitosis may grow at very different rates (161).

Silica and Asbestos Particles These powerful agents of fibrosis (Figure 13.44) elicit an almost pure mass of collagen, which can feel quite as hard as wood (Figure 13.45). Both silica and asbestos are said to stimulate the fibroblasts in more than one way (136,140,151,159) and to involve other cells, especially macrophages (Mϕ). For example:

- silica → fibroblasts
- silica → Mϕ death → fibroblasts
- silica → Mϕ (monokines) → fibroblasts
- silica →Mϕ (monokines) → T-lymphocytes (lymphokines) → fibroblasts

There is a hidden message in the last mechanism on this list: could it be that macrophages "put lymphocytes to work" and get them to secrete lymphokines without involving the immune response (141)? To use current lingo, a nonimmune task should not be in the job description of T-lymphocytes; but it does not seem impossible to us that some lymphocytes could be induced to participate in run-of-the-mill, nonimmune inflam-

FIGURE 13.44
Rod-shaped, beaded structure typical of an asbestos body (**arrow**). It was found in the lung of a patient who had been chronically exposed to asbestos and developed fibrosis of the lung (asbestosis). **Bar** = 25 μm.

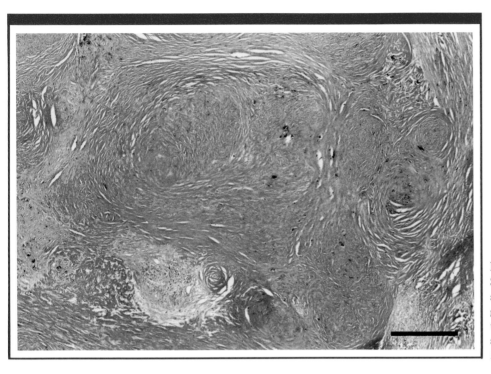

FIGURE 13.45
Silicotic nodules in the hilar node of a miner's lung: dense whorls of collagen fibers with few cells. A view of this field in polarized light would show scattered grains of silica. **Bar** = 500 μm.

mation. For some reason the literature is virtually silent on this important topic, perhaps because it implies immunologic heresy.

Ischemia That ischemia is well-established as a cause of fibrosis may strike the reader as peculiar because lack of blood supply should tend to inhibit all cellular activities, including collagen synthesis. Yet hypoxia favors collagen synthesis *in vitro* (162). The explanation may lie in the discovery that lactate, a product of anaerobic metabolism, favors collagen synthesis (153,171).

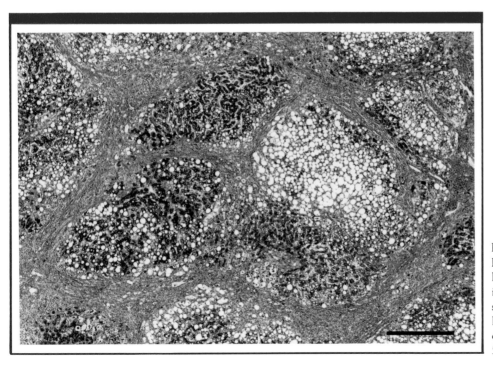

FIGURE 13.46
Example of scarring: cirrhosis of the liver in an alcoholic. The liver tissue is criss-crossed by bands of fibrous tissues. Many hepatocytes contain droplets of fat. (Masson trichrome, a special blue stain for collagen.) **Bar** = 500 μm.

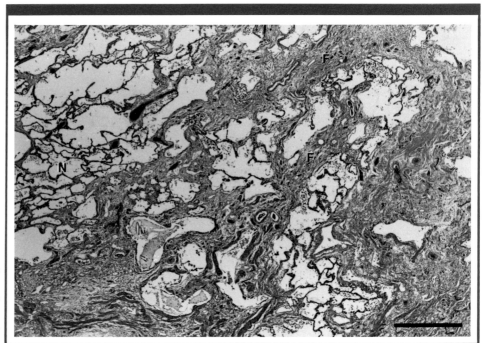

FIGURE 13.47
Idiopathic fibrosis of the lung. Strands of fibrous tissue (**F**) infiltrate the parenchyma; small patches of lung tissue are spared and nearly normal (**N**). The paucity of inflammatory cells indicates that this is a long-standing lesion. **Bar** = 1 μm.

SUNDRY CAUSES OF FIBROSIS

Alcohol abuse causes fibrosis (cirrhosis) of the liver (Figure 13.46), but the mechanism that stimulates collagen synthesis by the lipocytes appears to be indirect, via acetaldehyde (152); in the cirrhotic liver it is possible that the lipocytes are further activated by growth factors provided by surrounding cells (145). Alcoholics are especially prone to develop a bizarre condition, *Dupuytren's disease:* a fibrosis and contraction of the palmar fascia, which deforms the hand.

In some diseases fibrosis is secondary and related to scarring. For example, in **cystic fibrosis** *(or mucoviscidosis), the most common lethal genetic disease in Caucasians (141) fibrosis of the pancreas, lungs, liver, salivary glands, and other organs is secondary to obstruction of excretory canals by plugs of abnormally viscid mucus. The basic defect is a molecular cell-membrane disorder leading to failed chloride export and excessive sodium absorption; how this relates to abnormally viscid mucus is not certain. In* **retrolental fibroplasia** *(or retinopathy of prematurity) the mechanism is thought to be spasm of the immature retinal ar-*

terioles in response to oxygen therapy, followed by retinal damage and a proliferative fibrovascular response.

Sometimes the cause of fibrosis is unknown. Such is the case for idiopathic pulmonary fibrosis (Figure 13.47). Another peculiar disease in this category is **idiopathic retractile mesenteritis,** *in which the mesentery becomes fibrous and contracts into a palpable mass, sometimes leading to intestinal obstruction (155).*

TO SUM UP: The many diseases involving fibrosis, either generalized as scleroderma (p. 575) or localized as silicosis of the lungs, are incapacitating because the fibrous tissue is stiff and interferes with function; and when it contracts, it makes matters worse. All sclerosing conditions are difficult to treat or untreatable (174). *However, there is nothing intrinsically irreversible even in the toughest fibrotic plaques.* Experimentally, even cirrhosis of the liver can be reversed, up to a point (137,166). Several cell types, including fibroblasts, produce collagenase. When chronic inflammation is resolved, much of its fibrotic component may shrivel away. The problem is that we do not know how to program the fibroblasts to demolish their constructions.

References

Chronic Inflammation

1. Cavender DE. Lymphocyte adhesion to endothelial cells in vitro: models for the study of normal lymphocyte recircu-lation and lymphocyte emigration into chronic inflammatory lesions. J Invest Dermatol 1989;93(suppl.):88S-95S.

2. Davis PB. Cystic fibrosis: new perceptions, new strategies. Hosp Pract 1992;27:79–118.

3. Duijvestijn AM, Horst E, Pals ST, et al. High endothelial differentiation in human lymphoid and inflammatory tissues defined by monoclonal antibody HECA-452. Am J Pathol 1988;130:147–155.

4. Engel AG, Biesecker G. Complement activation in muscle fiber necrosis: demonstration of the membrane attack complex of complement in necrotic fibers. Ann Neurol 1982;12:289–296.

5. Folkman J, Szabo S, Stovroff M, McNeil P, Li W, Shing Y. Duodenal ulcer. Ann Surg 1991;214:414–427.

6. Freemont AJ, Ford WL. Functional and morphological changes in post-capillary venules in relation to lymphocytic infiltration into BCG-induced granulomata in rat skin. J Pathol 1985;147:1–12.

7. Freemont AJ, Jones CJP. Endothelial specialization of salivary gland vessels for accelerated lymphocyte transfer in Sjögren's syndrome. J Rheumatol 1983;10:801–804.

8. Freemont AJ, Jones CJP, Bromley M, Andrews P. Changes in vascular endothelium related to lymphocyte collections in diseased synovia. Arthritis Rheum 1983;26: 1427–1433.

9. Genta RM, Lew GM, Graham DY. Changes in the gastric mucosa following eradication of Helicobacter pylori. Mod Pathol 1993;6:281–289.

10. Goldstein IM, Weissmann G. Generation of C5-derived lysosomal enzyme-releasing activity (C5a) by lysates of leukocyte lysosomes. J Immunol 1974;113:1583–1588.

11. Hentschel E, Brandstätter G, Dragosics B, et al. Effect of ranitidine and amoxicillin plus metronidazole on the eradication of Helicobacter pylori and the recurrence of duodenal ulcer. N Engl J Med 1993;328:308–312.

12. Hill JH, Ward PA. C3 leukotactic factors produced by a tissue protease. J Exp Med 1969;130:505–518.

13. Hill JH, Ward PA. The phlogistic role of C3 leukotactic fragments in myocardial infarcts of rats. J Exp Med 1971;133:885–900.

14. Iguchi T, Ziff M. Electron microscopic study of rheumatoid synovial vasculature. J Clin Invest 1986;77:355–361.

15. Jalkanen S, Steere AC, Fox RI, Butcher EC. A distinct endothelial cell recognition system that controls lymphocyte traffic into inflamed synovium. Science 1986;233: 556–558.

16. Joiner KA, Onderdonk AB, Gelfand JA, Bartlett JG, Gorbach SL. A quantitative model for subcutaneous abscess formation in mice. Br J Exp Pathol 1980;61:97–107.

17. Junghans BM, Collin HB. Limbal lymphangiogenesis after corneal injury: an autoradiographic study. Curr Eye Res 1989;8:91–100.

18. Katori M, Kanayama T, Sasaki K, Ueno A, Takagi M, Yamashina S. Biphasic accumulation of leukocytes in rat cardiac infarct tissue caused by leukotriene B4 and complement. Jpn J Pharmacol 1989;50:234–238.

19. Kaufman HE, McDonald MB, Barron BA, Waltman SR. The cornea. New York: Churchill Livingstone, 1988.

20. Levine S. Postinflammatory increase of absorption from peritoneal cavity into lymph nodes: particulate and oily inocula. Exp Mol Pathol 1985;43:124–134.

21. Liebermann-Meffert D, White H. The greater omentum. Berlin: Springer-Verlag, 1983.

22. Lindbeck G, Powers R. Cellulitis. Hosp Pract 1993;28 (suppl. 2):10–14.

23. Lurie MB. Resistance to tuberculosis: experimental studies in native and acquired defensive mechanisms. Cambridge, MA: Harvard University Press, 1964.

23a. Majno and Joris (unpublished results)

24. Majno G, LaGattuta M, Thompson TE. Cellular death and necrosis: chemical, physical and morphologic changes in rat liver. Virchows Arch Pathol Anat 1960;333:421–465.

25. Majno G. The healing hand: man and wound in the ancient world. Cambridge, MA: Harvard University Press, 1975.

26. Maroko PR, Carpenter CB, Chiariello M, et al. Reduction by cobra venom factor of myocardial necrosis after coronary artery occlusion. J Clin Invest 1978; 61:661–670.

27. Matsuki Y, Yamamoto T, Hara K. Interleukin-1 MRNA-expressing macrophages in human chronically inflamed gingival tissues. Am J Pathol 1991;138:1299–1305.

28. McManus LM, Kolb WP, Crawford MH, O'Rourke RA, Grover FL, Pinckard RN. Complement localization in ischemic baboon myocardium. Lab Invest 1983;48:436–447.

29. Nightingale G, Hurley JV. Relationship between lymphocyte emigration and vascular endothelium in chronic inflammation. Pathology 1978;10:27–44.

30. Oppenheimer-Marks N, Ziff M. Binding of normal human mononuclear cells to blood vessels in rheumatoid arthritis synovial membrane. Arthritis Rheum 1986;29: 789–792.

31. Pinckard RN, Olson MS, Giclas PC, Terry R, Boyer JT, O'Rourke RA. Consumption of classical complement components by heart subcellular membranes in vitro and in patients after acute myocardial infarction. J Clin Invest 1975;56:740–750.

32. Pinckard RN, O'Rourke RA, Crawford MH, et al. Complement localization and mediation of ischemic injury in baboon myocardium. J Clin Invest 1980;66: 1050–1056.

33. Pitzalis C, Kingsley G, Haskard D, Panayi G. The preferential accumulation of helper-induced T lymphocytes in inflammatory lesions: evidence for regulation by selective endothelial and homotypic adhesion. Eur J Immunol 1988;18:1397–1404.

34. Pullinger BD, Florey HW. Proliferation of lymphatics in inflammation. J Pathol Bacteriol 1937;45:157–170.

34a. Regezi, JA, Sciubba, JJ Oral Pathology. Clinical-Pathologic Correlations. Philadelphia, PA: WB Saunders, 1989.

35. Rossen RD, Michael LH, Kagiyama A, et al. Mechanism of complement activation after coronary artery occlusion: evidence that myocardial ischemia in dogs causes release of constituents of myocardial subcellular origin that complex with human C1q in vivo. Circ Res 1988;62:572–584.

36. Rossen RD, Swain JL, Michael LH, Weakley S, Giannini E, Entman ML. Selective accumulation of the first component of complement and leukocytes in ischemic canine heart muscle. A possible initiator of an extra myocardial mechanism of ischemic injury. Circ Res 1985;57:119–130.

37. Ryan GB, Grobéty J, Majno G. Postoperative peritoneal adhesions. A study of the mechanisms. Am J Pathol 1971;65:117–148.

38. Ryan GB, Grobéty J, Majno G. Mesothelial injury and recovery. Am J Pathol 1973;71:93–112.

39. Schäfer H, Mathey D, Hugo F, Bhakdi, S. Deposition of the terminal C5b-9 complement complex in infarcted areas of human myocardium. J Immunol 1986; 137:1945–1949.

40. Schoefl GI. Studies on inflammation. III. Growing capillaries: their structure and permeability. Virchows Arch Pathol Anat 1963;337:97–141.

41. Schoefl GI, Majno G. Regeneration of blood vessels in wound healing. Adv Biol Skin 1964;5:173–193.

42. Seifert PS, Catalfamo JL, Dodds WJ. Complement C5a

(desArg) generation in serum exposed to damaged aortic endothelium. Exp Mol Pathol 1988;48:216-225.

43. Sheikh KMA, Duggal K, Relfson M, Gignac S, Rowden G. An experimental histopathologic study of surgical glove powders. Arch Surg 1984;119:215–219.

44. Spouge JD. A new look at the rests of Malassez. A review of their embryological origin, anatomy, and possible role in periodontal health and disease. J Periodontol 1980; 51:437–444.

45. Storrs SB, Kolb WP, Pinckard RN, Olson MS. Characterization of the binding of purified human C1q to heart mitochondrial membranes. J Biol Chem 1981;256: 10924–10929.

46. Szabo S, Folkman J, Vattay P, Morales RE, Kato K. Duodenal ulcerogens: effect of FGF on cysteamine-induced duodenal ulcer. In: Halter F, Garner A, Tytgat GNJ, eds. Mechanisms of peptic ulcer healing. (Falk Symposium 59). Dordrecht: Kluwer Academic Publishers, 1990:139–150.

47. Szabo S, Vattay P, Scarbrough E, Folkman J. Role of vascular factors, including angiogenesis, in the mechanisms of action of sucralfate. Am J Med 1991;91(suppl 2A):158S-160S.

48. Tsutsumi V, Mena-Lopez R, Anaya-Velazquez F, Martinez-Palomo A. Cellular bases of experimental amebic liver abscess formation. Am J Pathol 1984;117: 81–91.

49. Ward PA, Hill JH. C5 chemotactic fragments produced by an enzyme in lysosomal granules of neutrophils. J Immunol 1970;104:535–543.

50. Weisman HF, Bartow T, Leppo MK, et al. Soluble human complement receptor type 1: in vivo inhibitor of complement suppressing post-ischemic myocardial inflammation and necrosis. Science 1990;249:146–151.

51. Weissman IL, Butcher EC, Rouse RV, Scollay RG. Cell-cell interactions in the establishment and maintenance of lymphoid tissue architecture. In: Sercarz E, Cunningham AJ, eds. Strategies of immune regulation. New York: Academic Press, 1980:77–94.

52. Witte MH, Witte CL. Lymphatics and blood vessels, lymphangiogenesis and hemangiogenesis: from cell biology to clinical medicine. Lymphology 1987;20:257–266.

53. Yoffey JM, Courtice FC. Lympathics, lymph and the lymphomyeloid complex. London: Academic Press, 1970.

54. Ziff M, Cavender D, Haskard D. Pathogenetic factors in rheumatoid synovitis. Br J Rheumatol 1988;27(suppl II):153–156.

Granulomatous Inflammation

55. Adams DO. The biology of the granuloma. In: Ioachim HL, ed. Pathology of granulomas. New York: Raven Press, 1983:1–20.

56. Allred DC, Kobayashi K, Yoshida T. Anergy-like immuno-suppression in mice bearing pulmonary foreign-body granulomatous inflammation. Am J Pathol 1985;121: 466–473.

57. Andrade ZA, Grimaud J-A. Morphology of chronic collagen resorption. A study on the late stages of schistosomal granuloma involution. Am J Pathol 1988; 132:389–399.

58. Boros DL. The granulomatous inflammatory response: an overview. In: Boros DL, Yoshida T, eds. Basic and clinical aspects of granulomatous diseases. New York: Elsevier-North Holland, 1980:1–14.

59. Boros DL. Experimental granulomatous disease. In: Fanburg BL, ed. Sarcoidosis and other granulomatous diseases of the lung. New York: Marcel Dekker, 1983: 403–449.

60. Boros DL. Experimental granulomatosis. Clin Dermatol 1986;4:10–21.

61. Boros DL. Immunoregulation of granuloma formation in murine Schistosomiasis mansoni. Ann NY Acad Sci 1986;465:313–323.

62. Boros DL. Hypersensitivity granulomas. In: Middleton E Jr, Reed CE, Ellis EF, Adkinson NF Jr, Yunginger JW, eds. Allergy: principles and practice, 3rd ed, vol 1. St. Louis: CV Mosby, 1988:275–294.

63. Boros DL, Warren KS. Delayed hypersensitivity-type granuloma formation and dermal reaction induced and elicited by a soluble factor isolated from Schistosoma mansoni eggs. J Exp Med 1970;132:488–507.

64. Boros DL, Warren KS. Specific granulomatous hypersensitivity elicited by bentonite particles coated with soluble antigens from schistosome eggs and tubercle bacilli. Nature 1971;229:200–201.

65. Boros DL, Warren KS. Effect of antimacrophage serum on hypersensitivity (Schistosoma mansoni egg) and foreign body (divinyl-benzene copolymer bead) granulomas. J Immunol 1971;107:534–539.

66. Boros DL, Warren KS, Pelley RP. The secretion of migration inhibitory factor by intact schistosome egg granulomas maintained in vitro. Nature 1973;246:224–226.

67. Boris DL, Yoshida T, eds. Basic and clinical aspects of granulomatous diseases. New York: Elsevier-North Holland, 1980.

68. Chensue SW, Boros DL. Modulation of granulomatous hypersensitivity. I. Characterization of T lymphocytes involved in the adoptive suppression of granuloma formation in Schistosoma mansoni-infected mice. J Immunol 1979;123:1409–1414.

69. Chensue SW, Kunkel SL, Higashi GI, Ward PA, Boros DL. Production of superoxide anion, prostaglandins, and hydroxyeicosatetraenoic acids by macrophages from hypersensitivity-type (Schistosoma mansoni egg) and foreign body-type granulomas. Infect Immun 1983;42: 1116–1125.

70. Courtade ET, Tsuda T, Thomas CR, Dannenberg AM Jr. Capillary density in developing and healing tuberculous lesions produced by BCG in rabbits. Am J Pathol 1975;78:243–260.

71. Dannenberg AM Jr, Tomashefski JF Jr. Pathogenesis of pulmonary tuberculosis. In: Fishman AP, ed. Pulmonary diseases and disorders, 2nd ed, vol 3. New York: McGraw-Hill, 1988:1821–1842.

72. Dreher R, Keller HU, Hess MW, Roos B, Cottier H. Early appearance and mitotic activity of multinucleated giant cells in mice after combined injection of talc and prednisolone acetate. A model for studying rapid histiocytic polykarion formation in vivo. Lab Invest 1978;38:149–156.

73. Elliott DE, Righthand VF, Boros DL. Characterization of regulatory (interferon-α/β) and accessory (LAF/IL 1) monokine activities from liver granuloma macrophages of Schistosoma mansoni-infected mice. J Immunol 1987;138: 2653–2662.

74. Geratz JD, Tidwell RR, Schwab JH, Anderle SK, Pryzwansky KB. Sequential events in the pathogenesis of streptococcal cell wall-induced arthritis and their modulation by bis(5-amidino-2-benzimidazolyl)methane (BABIM). Am J Pathol 1990;136:909–921.

75. Ginsburg CH, McCluskey RT, Nepom JT, et al. Antigen- and receptor-driven regulatory mechanisms. X. The induction and suppression of hapten-specific granulomas. Am J Pathol 1982;106:421–431.

76. Greenaway TM, Caterson ID. Hypercalcemia and lipoid pneumonia. Aust N Z J Med 1989;19:713–715.

77. Hunninghake GW, Crystal RG. Pulmonary sarcoidosis. A disorder mediated by excess helper T-lymphocyte

activity at sites of disease activity. N Engl J Med 1981;305:429–434.

78. Hunninghake GW, Crystal RG. Mechanisms of hyper-gammaglobulinemia in pulmonary sarcoidosis. Site of increased antibody production and role of T lymphocytes. J Clin Invest 1981;67:86–92.

79. Ioachim HL, ed. Pathology of granulomas. New York: Raven Press, 1983.

80. Kasahara K, Kobayashi K, Shikama Y, et al. Direct evidence for granuloma-inducing activity of interleukin-1. Am J Pathol 1988;130:629–638.

81. Kellermeyer RW, Warren KS. The role of chemical mediators in the inflammatory response induced by foreign bodies: comparison with the schistosome egg granuloma. J Exp Med 1970;131:21–39.

82. Kindler V, Sappino A-P, Grau GE, Piguet P-F, Vassalli P. The inducing role of tumor necrosis factor in the development of bactericidal granulomas during BCG infection. Cell 1989;56:731–740.

83. Kobayashi K, Allred C, Castriotta R, Yoshida, T. Strain variation of bacillus Calmette-Guerin-induced pulmonary granuloma formation is correlated with anergy and the local production of migration inhibition factor and interleukin 1. Am J Pathol 1985;119:223–235.

84. Kozeny GA, Barbato AL, Bansal VK, Vertuno LL, Hano JE. Hypercalcemia associated with silicone-induced granulomas. N Engl J Med 1984;311:1103–1105.

85. Krulewitz AH, Stadecker MJ, Wright JA, Fanburg BL. Angiotensin-1-converting enzyme activity of murine macrophages isolated from granulomas elicited by eggs of Schistosoma mansoni. Infect Immun 1983;41:39–43.

86. Lemann J Jr, Gray RW. Calcitriol, calcium, and granulomatous disease. N Engl J Med 1984;311:1115–1117.

87. Lurie MB. Resistance to tuberculosis: experimental studies in native and acquired defensive mechanisms. Cambridge, MA: Harvard University Press, 1964.

88. Narayanan RB, Badenoch-Jones P, Turk JL. Experimental mycobacterial granulomas in guinea pig lymph nodes: ultrastructural observations. J Pathol 1981;134:253–265.

89. Pellegrino J, Brener Z. Method for isolating schistosome granulomas from mouse liver. J Parasitol 1956;42:564.

90. Perrotto JL, Warren KS. Inhibition of granuloma formation around Schistosoma mansoni eggs. IV. X-irradiation. Am J Pathol 1969;56:279–291.

91. Rook GAW, Taverne J, Leveton C, Steele J. The role of gamma-interferon, vitamin D₃ metabolites and tumour necrosis factor in the pathogenesis of tuberculosis. Immunology 1987;62:229–234.

92. Ryan GB, Majno G. Inflammation. Kalamazoo, MI: The Upjohn Company, 1977.

93. Salthouse TN, Matlaga BF. Collagenase associated with macrophage and giant cell activity. Experientia 1972; 28:326.

94. Schwartz CJ, Ghidoni JJ, Kelley JL, Sprague EA, Valente AJ, Suenram CA. Evolution of foam cells in subcutaneous rabbit carrageenan granulomas. I. Light-microscopic and ultrastructural study. Am J Pathol 1985;118:134–150.

95. Shikama Y, Kobayashi K, Kasahara K, et al. Granuloma formation by artificial microparticles in vitro. Am J Pathol 1989;134:1189–1199.

96. Stadecker MJ, Wright JA. Distribution and kinetics of mononuclear phagocytes in granulomas elicited by eggs of Schistosoma mansoni. Am J Pathol 1984;116:245–252.

97. Tanaka A, Emori K. Epithelioid granuloma formation by a synthetic bacterial cell wall component, muramyl dipeptide (MDP). Am J Pathol 1980;98:733–748.

98. Tanaka A, Emori K, Nagao S, et al. Epitheloid granuloma formation requiring no T-cell function. Am J Pathol 1982;106:165–170.

99. Truden JL, Boros DL. Collagenase, elastase, and nonspecific protease production by vigorous or immunomodulated liver granulomas and granuloma macrophages/eosinophils of S. mansoni-infected mice. Am J Pathol 1985;121:166–175.

100. Unanue ER, Benacerraf B. Immunologic events in experimental hypersensitivity granulomas. Am J Pathol 1973;71:349–364.

101. van der Rhee HJ, van der Burgh-de Winter CPM, Daems WT. The differentiation of monocytes into macrophages, epitheloid cells, and multinucleated giant cells in subcutaneous granulomas. I. Fine structure. Cell Tissue Res 1979;197:355–378.

102. von Lichtenberg F. Studies on granuloma formation. III. Antigen sequestration and destruction in the schistosome pseudotubercle. Am J Pathol 1964;45:75–93.

103. Wahl SM. Fibrosis: bacterial-cell-wall-induced hepatic granulomas. In: Gallin JI, Goldstein IM, Snyderman R, eds. Inflammation. Basic principles and clinical correlates. New York: Raven Press, 1988:841–860.

104. Wahl SM, Allen JB, Dougherty S, et al. T lymphocyte-dependent evolution of bacterial cell wall-induced hepatic granulomas. J Immunol 1986;137:2199–2209.

105. Wahl SM, Hunt DA, Allen JB, Wilder RL, Paglia L, Hand AR. Bacterial cell wall-incuded hepatic granulomas. An in vivo model of T cell-dependent fibrosis. J Exp Med 1986;163:884–902.

106. Warren KS. A functional classification of granulomatous inflammation. Ann NY Acad Sci 1976;278:7–18.

107. Warren KS. The cell biology of granulomas (aggregates of inflammatory cells) with a note on giant cells. In: Weissmann G, ed. The cell biology of inflammation. Amsterdam: Elsevier-North Holland Biomedical Press, 1980:543–557.

108. Warren KS, Domingo EO, Cowan RBT. Granuloma formation around schistosome eggs as a manifestation of delayed hypersensitivity. Am J Pathol 1967;51:735–756.

109. Weinstock JV, Boros DL. Organ-dependent differences in composition and function observed in hepatic and intestinal granulomas isolated from mice with schistosomiasis mansoni. J Immunol 1983;130:418–422.

110. Wyler DJ, Stadecker MJ, Dinarello CA, O'Dea JF. Fibroblast stimulation in schistosomiasis. V. Egg granuloma macrophages spontaneously secrete a fibroblast-stimulating factor. J Immunol 1984;132:3142–3148.

The Giant Cell Saga

111. Bangham AD. The adhesiveness of leukocytes with special reference to zeta potential. Ann NY Acad Sci 1964;116:945–949.

112. Beers RF Jr, Bassett EG, eds. Cell fusion: gene transfer and transformation (Miles International Symposium Series, No. 14). New York: Raven Press, 1984.

113. Blobel CP, Wolfsberg TG, Turck CW, Myles DG, Primakoff P, White JM. A potential fusion peptide and an integrin ligand domain in a protein active in sperm-egg fusion. Nature 1992;356:248–252.

114. Chambers TJ. Fusion of macrophages following simultaneous attempted phagocytosis of glutaraldehyde-fixed red cells. J Pathol 1977;122:71–80.

115. Constabel F, Cutler AJ. Protoplast fusion. In: Fowke LC, Constabel F, eds. Plant protoplasts. Boca Raton, FL: CRC Press, 1985:53–65.

116. Gasser CS, Fraley RT. Genetically engineering plants for crop improvement. Science 1989;244:1293–1299.

117. Harris H. Cell fusion. The Dunham Lectures. Oxford: Clarendon Press, 1970.

118. Harris H, Watkins JF. Hybrid cells derived from mouse

and man: artificial heterokaryons of mammalian cells from different species. Nature 1965;205:640–646.

119. Harris H, Watkins JF, Ford CE, Schoefl GI. Artificial heterokaryons of animal cells from different species. J Cell Sci 1966;1:1–30.

120. Jones CW, Mastrangelo IA, Smith HH, Liu HZ, Meck RA. Interkingdom fusion between human (HeLa) cells and tobacco hybrid (GGLL) protoplasts. Science 1976; 193:401–403.

121. Kirkpatrick CJ, Curry A, Bisset DL. Light- and electron-microscopic studies on multinucleated giant cells in sarcoid granuloma: new aspects of asteroid and Schaumann bodies. Ultrastruct Pathol 1988;12: 581–597.

122. Köhler G, Milstein C. Continuous cultures of fused cells secreting antibody of predefined specificity. Nature 1975;256:495–497.

123. Kreipe H, Radzun HJ, Rudolph P, et al. Multinucleated giant cells generated in vitro. Terminally differentiated macrophages with down-regulated c-fms expression. Am J Pathol 1988;130:232–243.

124. Mariano M, Spector WG. The formation and properties of macrophage polykaryons (inflammatory giant cells). J Pathol 1974;113:1–19.

125. Papadimitriou JM, Kingston KJ. The locomotory behaviour of the multinucleate giant cells of foreign body reactions. J Pathol 1976;121:27–36.

126. Papadimitriou JM, Robertson TA, Walters MN-I. An analysis of the phagocytic potential of multinucleate foreign body giant cells. Am J Pathol 1975;78:343–358.

127. Papadimitriou JM, Sforsina D, Papaelias L. Kinetics of multinucleate giant cell formation and their modification by various agents in foreign body reactions. Am J Pathol 1973;73:349–364.

128. Papadimitriou JM, Van Bruggen I. Evidence that multinucleate giant cells are examples of mononuclear phagocytic differentiation. J Pathol 1986;148:149–157.

129. Sapp JP. An ultrastructural study of nuclear and centriolar configurations in multinucleated giant cells. Lab Invest 1976;34:109–112.

130. Sone S. Functions of multinucleated giant cells formed by fusing rat alveolar macrophages with lymphokines containing macrophage fusion factor. Lymphokine Res 1984;3:163–173.

131. Sowers AE, ed. Cell fusion. New York: Plenum Press, 1987.

132. Tominaga S-I. Interferon induces cell fusion and the formation of multinuclear cells in a culture of Ehrlich ascites tumor cells. J Cell Physiol 1988;135:350–354.

133. Weinberg JB, Hobbs MM, Misukonis MA. Recombinant human α-interferon induces human monocyte polykaryon formation. Proc Natl Acad Sci USA 1984; 81:4554–4557.

134. Weinberg JB, Hobbs MM, Misukonis MA. Phenotypic characterization of gamma interferon-induced human monocyte polykaryons. Blood 1985;66:1241-1246.

135. Weiss LP, Fawcett DW. Cytochemical observations on chicken monocytes macrophages and giant cells in tissue culture. J Histochem Cytochem 1953;1:47-65.

Fibrosis

136. Aalto M, Potila M, Kulonen E. The effect of silica-treated macrophages on the synthesis of collagen and other proteins in vitro. Exp Cell Res 1976;97:193–202.

137. Abdel-Aziz G, Lebeau G, Rescan P-Y, et al. Reversibility of hepatic fibrosis in experimentally induced cholestasis in rat. Am J Pathol 1990;137:1333-1342.

138. Adler KB, Low RB, Leslie KO, Mitchell J, Evans JN.

139. Beattie J. The asbestosis body. In: Davies CN, ed. Inhaled particles and vapours. Oxford: Pergamon Press, 1961:434–442.

140. Craighead JE, Mossman BT. The pathogenesis of asbestos-associated diseases. N Engl J Med 1982;306: 1446–1455.

141. Davis PB. Cystic fibrosis: new perceptions, new strategies. Hosp Pract 1992;11:79–118.

142. Davis GS. Pathogenesis of silicosis: current concepts and hypotheses. Lung 1986;164:139–154.

143. De Crombrugghe B, Liau G, Setoyama C, Schmidt A, McKeon C, Mudryj M. Structural and functional studies on the interstitial collagen genes. Ciba Found Symp 1985;114:20–33.

144. Elias JA, Jimenez SA, Freundlich B. Recombinant gamma, alpha, and beta interferon regulation of human lung fibroblast proliferation. Am Rev Respir Dis 1987; 135:62–65.

145. Friedman SL, Bissell DM. Hepatic fibrosis: new insights into pathogenesis. Hosp Pract 1990;25:43–50.

146. Friedman SL, Roll FJ, Boyles J, Bissell DM. Hepatic lipocytes: the principal collagen-producing cells of normal rat liver. Proc Natl Acad Sci USA 1985;82: 8681–8685.

147. Gabbiani G, Hirschel BJ, Ryan GB, Statkov PR, Majno G. Granulation tissue as a contractile organ. A study of structure and function. J Exp Med 1972;135: 719–734.

148. Goldstein RH, Fine A. Fibrotic reactions in the lung: the activation of the lung fibroblast. Exp Lung Res 1986;11:245–261.

149. Graham JR, Suby HI, LeCompte PR, Sadowsky NL. Fibrotic disorders associated with methysergide therapy for headache. N Engl J Med 1966;274:359-368.

150. Green MC, Sweet HO, Bunker LE. Tight-skin, a new mutation of the mouse causing excessive growth of connective tissue and skeleton. Am J Pathol 1976; 82:493–512.

151. Heppleston AG. Cellular reactions with silica. In: Bendz G, Lindqvist I, eds. Biochemistry of silicon and related problems. New York: Plenum Press, 1977:357–379.

152. Holt K, Bennett M, Chojkier M. Acetaldehyde stimulates collagen and noncollagen protein production by human myofibroblasts. Hepatology 1984;4:843–848.

153. Hunt TK, Conolly WB, Aronson SB, Goldstein P. Anaerobic metabolism and wound healing: an hypothesis for the initiation and cessation of collagen synthesis in wounds. Am J Surg 1978;135:328–332.

154. Irlé C, Kocher O, Gabbiani G. Contractility of myofibroblasts during experimental liver cirrhosis. J Submicrosc Cytol 1980;12:209–217.

155. Kelly JK, Hwang W-S. Idiopathic retractile (sclerosing) mesenteritis and its differential diagnosis. Am J Surg Pathol 1989;13:513–521.

156. Kovacs EJ. Fibrogenic cytokines: the role of immune mediators in the development of scar tissue. Immunol Today 1991;12:17–23.

157. Kuhn C, McDonald JA. The roles of the myofibroblast in idiopathic pulmonary fibrosis. Ultrastructural and immunohistochemical features of sites of active extracellular matrix synthesis. Am J Pathol 1991;138: 1257–1265.

158. Last JA, Reiser KM. Effects of silica on lung collagen. Ciba Found Symp 1986;121:180–193.

159. Lemaire I, Beaudoin H, Massé S, Grondin, C. Alveolar macrophage stimulation of lung fibroblast growth in

Contractile cells in normal and fibrotic lung. Lab Invest 1989;60:473–485.

asbestos-induced pulmonary fibrosis. Am J Pathol 1986; 122:205–211.

160. Lepor H, Walsh PC. Idiopathic retroperitoneal fibrosis. J Urol 1979;122:1-6.

161. Leroy EC. Collagen deposition in autoimmune diseases: the expanding role of the fibroblast in human fibrotic disease. Ciba Found Symp 1985;114:196-207.

162. Levene CI, Bates CJ. The effect of hypoxia on collagen synthesis in cultured 3T6 fibroblasts and its relationship to the mode of action of ascorbate. Biochim Biophys Acta 1976;444:446–452.

163. Martinet Y, Rom WN, Grotendorst GR, Martin GR, Crystal RG. Exaggerated spontaneous release of platelet-derived growth factor by alveolar macrophages from patients with idiopathic pulmonary fibrosis. N Engl J Med 1987;317:202-209.

164. Nagle RB, Kneiser MR, Bulger RE, Benditt EP. Induction of smooth muscle characteristics in renal interstitial fibroblasts during obstructive nephropathy. Lab Invest 1973;29:422–427.

165. Ormond JK. Idiopathic retroperitoneal fibrosis: a discussion of the etiology. J Urol 1965;94:385–390.

166. Pérez Tamayo R. Cirrhosis of the liver: a reversible disease? Pathol Annu 1979;14:183–213.

167. Piguet PF, Collart MA, Grau GE, Sappino A-P, Vassalli P. Requirement of tumour necrosis factor for development of silica-induced pulmonary fibrosis. Nature 1990; 344:245–247.

168. Reiser KM, Last JA. A molecular marker for fibrotic collagen in lungs of infants with respiratory distress syndrome. Biochem Med Metab Biol 1987;37:16-21.

169. Roberts WC, Ferrans VJ. Pure collagen plaques on the diaphragm and pleura. Gross, histologic and electron microscopic observations. Chest 1972;61: 357–360.

170. Roberts WC, Sjoerdsma A. The cardiac disease associated with the carcinoid syndrome (carcinoid heart disease). Am J Med 1964;36:5–34.

171. Savolainen E-R, Leo MA, Timpl R, Lieber CS. Acetaldehyde and lactate stimulate collagen synthesis of cultured baboon liver myofibroblasts. Gastroenterology 1984;87:777–787.

172. Seuwen K, Magnaldo I, Pouysségur J. Serotonin stimulates DNA synthesis in fibroblasts acting through 5-HT_{1B} receptors coupled to a G_i-protein. Nature 1988; 35:254–256.

173. Trelstad RL, Birk DE. The fibroblast in morphogenesis and fibrosis: cell topography and surface-related functions. Ciba Found Symp 1985;114:4–19.

174. Uitto J, Ryhänen L, Tan EML, Oikarinen AI, Zaragoza EJ. Pharmacological inhibition of excessive collagen deposition in fibrotic diseases. Fed Proc 1984;43:2815–2820.

175. Wahl SM, Allen JB. T lymphocyte-dependent mechanisms of fibrosis. Prog Clin Biol Res 1988;266:147–160.

176. Wahl SM, Wong H, McCartney-Francis N. Role of growth factors in inflammation and repair. J Cell Biochem 1989;40:193–199.

Wound Healing

CHAPTER 14

Healing by First
Intention: Closed
Aseptic Wounds

Healing by
Second Intention

Experimental Models of
Wound Healing

The Pace of
Wound Healing

Disorders of
Wound Healing

The grand scenario of wound healing combines three processes: *hemostasis*, because vessels are open; *inflammation*, because there has been injury; and *regeneration*, because structures have been severed or destroyed (Figure 8.1). The basic plan of the repair process, overall, is always the same: to close the gap and seal it with a scar. The details, however, vary, depending on the presence or absence of bacteria, the nature of the wound (open or closed), the blood supply, the amount of dead tissue to be eliminated (as in bruised wounds), the type of wounded tissue, and many other factors.

The most favorable situation for healing is a closed, noninfected sutured wound; this is known as an *incisional* wound, as opposed to an *excisional* wound whereby a piece of skin is cut out. Here healing can start immediately because there is no significant bacterial population and virtually no dead tissue to eliminate. The ancient surgical term for this situation is *healing by first intention.* In contrast, healing is delayed if there is infection or if the wound remains open due to loss of tissue. These two conditions are hurdles that must be overcome before the wound can close; thus healing is said to occur *by second intention* (Figure 14.1).

There is something rather quaint about this ancient notion of "intention." For one thing, who is supposed to have the intention, the wound or the surgeon? Almost 1000 years ago, in the Canon of Avicenna— one of the pillars of Arabic medicine—it was clearly the surgeon who displayed therapeutic "intentions" appropriate to the type of injury (2a). In the surgical writings of the later Middle Ages, e.g. by Guy de Chauliac (1300–1368), healing intentions are sometimes attributed to the surgeon, sometimes to the wound or to Nature (26). In today's medical jargon it is assumed that the intention is expressed by the wound itself.

Healing by First Intention: Closed Aseptic Wounds

We will now describe the healing of a noninfected, sutured incisional wound. Technically all wounds are infected to some degree, but in aseptic surgery the number of bacteria is so small that healing is not disturbed. The sequence of events (Figure 14.2) is fairly constant, but the timing indicated below is merely indicative: depending on the conditions it may be cut by half or doubled.

HEMOSTASIS: WITHIN SECONDS TO MINUTES

The first priority is to stop the bleeding (hemostasis); and as usual the programming is

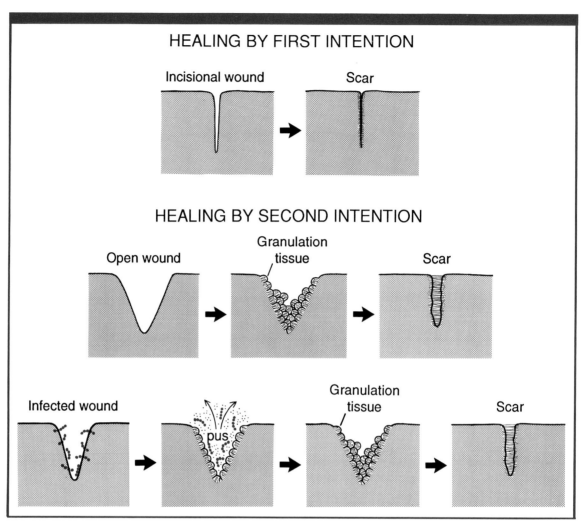

FIGURE 14.1

Wound healing by first and second intention. *Top:* Healing by first intention in a closed, noninfected wound, such as a surgical incision. The margins are apposed, and healing proceeds directly to produce a scar. *Center:* Healing by second intention in an open wound (not infected). The gaping wound is first filled by granulation tissue, which then contracts and turns into a scar. *Bottom:* Healing by second intention in an infected wound (red dots represent bacteria). The wound becomes lined with granulation tissue, which produces pus until the bacteria are eliminated. Thereafter the granulation tissue contracts and produces a scar.

admirable. The severed arterioles contract and the spilled blood clots. Generally speaking, blood can be induced to clot by either one of two mechanisms, called "instrinic" and "extrinsic" (p. 617): (a) by coming in contact with collagen, and (b) by mixing with a "tissue factor" released by injured cells. Both mechanisms are triggered in a wound, and so the blood clots without delay. This helps to stop the bleeding. In the meantime, platelets pile up on the mouths of the bleeding vessels and create plugs called *thrombi*, another essential mechanism of hemostasis. The details will be discussed later (p. 612).

The clotted blood also forms a tenuous network (not quite a glue) that connects the two faces of the wound in the so-called "wound space". Here is another example of Nature's economy: products of the clotting mechanism help initiate the healing processes. Thrombin, the enzyme that generates fibrin, attracts macrophages and causes fibroblasts to replicate; and platelet-derived growth-factor (PDGF), released by degranulating platelets, is also a mitogen and a chemotaxin for fibroblasts (19).

INFLAMMATION: WITHIN MINUTES TO HOURS

The next priority is to ward off bacteria. Here is another example of masterful design. The wound

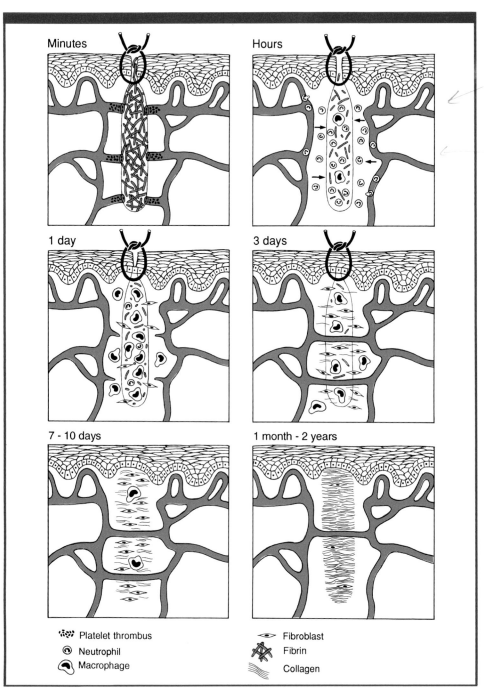

Minutes

Hours

1 day

3 days

7 - 10 days

1 month - 2 years

thrombin (makes fibrin) calls MΦs + come + scavenge; also fbs replicate

neutrs automatically called in - prophylaxis!

Legend:
- ░ Platelet thrombus
- ⓝ Neutrophil
- ⬤ Macrophage
- ⬥ Fibroblast
- ✳ Fibrin
- 〰 Collagen

FIGURE 14.2

Wound healing by first intention: diagram of the principal steps.

has no way to "know" whether it is infected or not; therefore, to avoid a potentially dangerous loss of time, inflammation is triggered automatically without waiting for the bacteria to do so. So, as we saw in earlier chapters, a host of inflammatory mediators are generated, an exudate of cells and fluid begins to pour out of the venules, the arterioles dilate to increase the supply, and leukocytes crawl around looking for prey. (If they find any, the battle is on, and more leukocytes are called in.) However, in a sterile wound the number of leukocytes in the exudate is never enough to qualify as pus. Scavenging of debris, including the remains of spent neutrophils, begins immediately. The tissues next to the wound swell up a little because of the inflammatory edema. In the expanded connective tissue spaces, the exudate clots and forms a fine network of fibrin; this may offer the leukocytes an extra surface against which they can trap bacteria (*surface phagocytosis*).

SCAB FORMATION

A scab begins to form as exudate seeps out of the sutured wound and appears on the surface of the skin; it clots and eventually dries up. This process continues and builds up a scab, which has an important function: it seals off the wound from the environment and prevents bacteria from penetrating. *The scab is a natural dressing* (40).

MIGRATION OF FIXED CELLS: WITHIN 24 HOURS

By 24 hours even some stationary cells begin to move: the fibroblasts, the epidermal cells and even the endothelium (47).

The leukocytes attracted to the wound now include more monocytes (108), which settle in the wound space and around it; they phagocytize the remains of the neutrophils, which continue to arrive and die within hours of their arrival. As the macrophages scavenge, they become activated; they secrete cytokines that direct the activities of all other cells.

The network of fibrin continues to grow from the fibrinogen supplied by the inflammatory exudate. Mechanically it is not very tough, but it plays another important role: fibrin filaments coated with the plasma protein fibronectin (Figure 14.3) are suitable as footholds for the epidermal cells and migrating fibroblasts (44). By 24 hours, the fibroblasts come out of their torpor, enlarge and begin to migrate into the wound space, hauling themselves along the coated filaments of fibrin (66). One of their chemotactic calls may be platelet-derived growth factor released by platelets that have been spent in the process of hemostasis.

The epidermal cells are mobilized within hours (86). Basal cells on the edge of the cut, triggered perhaps by the sudden absence of a neighbor—the "free-edge effect" (80)—flatten out and creep over the denuded area (Figure 2.9); the cells at the leading edge are phagocytic, which may help them to eat their way along *under the forming scab* (80). They advance by a leapfrog or a caterpillar motion, as discussed earlier (p. 20). This migration is an apparent exception to the rule that basement membranes guide epithelia because, in this case, there is no basement membrane. Histochemical studies have shown that the substrate over which the epithelial cells accept to glide is a mixture of fibrin and fibronectin (113); the latter is supplied by plasma and by the activated fibroblasts (15). Normal basal cells of the epidermis have no receptors for fibronectin, but regenerating ones do (42, 45). The gliding cells advance at a rate of 2–3 cell diameters per hour or roughly 0.5 mm/day; the speed record is held by amphibian epidermis, which migrates 10 times faster (122).

> *It may seem strange that the epithelium should advance faster in a cold-blooded animal, but we can theorize as follows. Imagine an open wound in the skin of a frog that is out in the air; the surface will be covered by a clot, which becomes a scab. Now, if the frog goes swimming, precious electrolytes may be lost to the hypotonic water of the pond. Therefore it is urgent to cover the wound with a watertight layer: the fastest way is for the regenerating epithelium to creep over the scab (96) instead of having to burrow beneath it.*

Capillary sprouts are not easy to see at 24 hours by light microscopy (the earliest are simply endothelial pseudopodia reaching out through the basement membrane) but they are already developing in both faces of the wound in response to

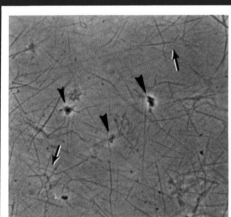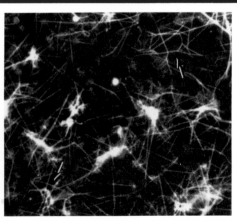

FIGURE 14.3
Clot of human blood. *Left:* Phase contrast photograph shows fibrin strands (**arrows**) and platelets (**arrowheads**). *Right:* Photograph in ultraviolet light after immunofluorescent staining of fibronectin with specific antibody, showing that fibronectin is present in the fibrin strands. (Reproduced with permission from [41].)

angiogenic factors, and grow toward the wound space. Anoxia is a major factor in stimulating vascular ingrowth. In the wound space, oxygen tension is close to zero; if it is artificially raised, angiogenesis stops (65). This phase of angiogenesis is another feat of the macrophages. Those that have migrated into the wound space become anoxic, and *anoxia causes them to secrete a factor that stimulates capillary outgrowth* (64), probably TNF alpha (69). High concentrations of lactate, such as occur in wounds, have the same effect (59). What a beautiful mechanism.

REGENERATION: 3 DAYS

As regards inflammatory cells, by 2–3 days the monocytes begin to outnumber the neutrophils (108). Regeneration, which had started by day one, now dominates the picture. The advancing epidermal cells undermine the scab, which eventually falls off; the timing depends a great deal on the size of the scab. Where the epidermis is perforated by a suture thread, a strange thing happens: epidermal cells grow down into the suture track like a tube surrounding the thread (Figure 14.4). After all, this should be expected because epithelia tend to grow over raw tissue surfaces. (This is the principle exploited when earlobes are perforated and a wire is left in place until healing occurs.)

The activated fibroblasts are in full swing. Responding to growth factors they multiply and produce collagen fibrils: type III as a start (81). They also

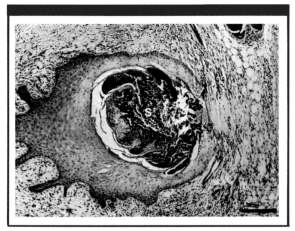

FIGURE 14.4
Cross section of a suture thread (**S**) in the depth of a wound in the skin of a pig. The thread is almost completely surrounded by epidermis. The mechanism: on the surface of the skin, where the suture thread penetrates into the tissue, the regenerating epidermis tends to plunge into the tunnel created by the suture. **Bar** = 200 μm. (Reproduced with permission from [86].)

secrete proteoglycans—but (for reasons unknown) few elastic fibers.

Angiogenesis (the regeneration of blood vessels) (p. 755) has progressed enough after 2–3 days for some sprouts to join up tip to tip (56). This marvellous encounter is called *inosculation* (*osculare* is Latin for kissing) (20, 101). The crowd of new fibroblasts mingles with the new capillaries to form the beginning of granulation tissue.

EARLY SCARRING: 7–10 DAYS

Within a week the wound space has had the time to fill with granulation tissue: very little is needed, because the two faces of the wound are so close. A network of capillaries has bridged the wound space. The lymphatics begin to regenerate with some delay after the blood capillaries; their advancing tips never seem to link up with tips of blood vessels (122), perhaps because they carry different "recognition" molecules. Slowly the granulation tissue acquires more and more collagen fibers and begins to look more and more like the fibrous mass called a scar.

Throughout the wound, scavenging by the macrophages continues and eventually the fibrin is also removed. Collagen type I begins to appear (17, 35, 81).

Although the epidermis has regenerated, skin appendages such as hair and sweat glands do not develop; this lack is an everyday observation in surgical wards. (The rabbit stands out as a glaring exception [7].) Human scars not only are hairless but also are usually pale, especially on black skin, because melanocytes regenerate poorly (p. 22). Yet hyperpigmented scars do occur, in white as well as in black skin; the reason is not understood.

SCAR MATURATION: 1 MONTH–2 YEARS

Ultimately, the scar will be a mass of fibrous tissue with many collagen fibers, few cells and few vessels (Figure 14.5), but the process of maturation is slow. As time passes, most cells vanish; apoptosis has been observed in fibroblasts and endothelial cells (25). Eosinophils sometimes appear in the late phases of wound healing; perhaps they contribute helpful growth factors (116). The collagen becomes more and more cross-linked; elastic fibers remain few, so that scars have little recoil, and eventually tend to stretch. Many capillaries disappear so that old scars appear white (2).

However, it takes many months, even a year or two, for a surgical scar to change from pink to white. The local turnover of collagen remains high

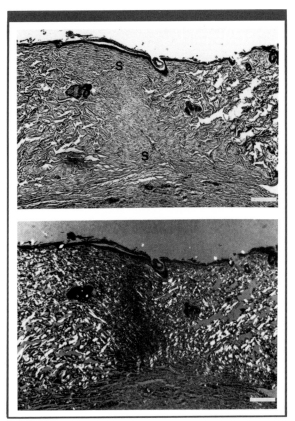

FIGURE 14.5
The arrangement of scar collagen is not "normal." Dermal scar from a 100-day old (tape-closed) skin wound in the rat. *Top:* Viewed in ordinary light. The scar (S-S) can be recognized because it is made of collagen bundles thinner than those of the surrounding dermis. *Bottom:* viewed in polarized light, normal collagen appears bright (birefringent) because it consists of thick bundles of parallel fibrils; scar collagen is dark (not birefringent) because it is made of thin fibrils arranged in a disorderly fashion. **Bars** = 250 μm. (Reproduced with permission from [32].)

for years; this is why, in the days of scurvy, old scars would break down during a long trip at sea (p. 252).

Even a mature scar is never as strong as normal skin. The tensile strength remains below normal (Figure 14.6) (70, 89). Boxers are aware of this problem: scars break open more easily than normal skin.

The term *scar* is applied also to the end result of injuries other than wounds. An infarct, for example, heals with a scar (Figure 14.7).

THE CHEMICAL MEDIATORS OF WOUND HEALING

In the early hours of a wound, the mediators are those of acute inflammation. For example: injured mast cells release the histamine that causes hyperemia, and a variety of stimulated cells release

prostaglandins. Platelets from hemostatic plugs promptly die and release serotonin (a vasoconstrictor) and a host of other mediators (p. 328). Venular leakage can result from histamine, leukotrienes, and serotonin released by platelets. Chain reactions occur: clotting is accompanied by the activation of kallikrein, which produces bradykinin; bradykinin induces prostaglandins (120). Leukocytes are attracted by leukotriene B_4 and by many products of proteolysis. Proteolytic enzymes spring from many sources (lysosomes of broken cells and platelets, mast cell granules, plasmin from the activated fibrinolytic system), and they act on a variety of proteins to produce mediators (substrates include complement molecules C3, C4, C5, kininogen, and fibrin). The reader is referred to the synoposis of Figure 14.2. Complement, by the way, helps attract neutrophils but it is not essential to wound healing (119). Within hours, the mediators of acute inflammation fade away and the principal role goes to a variety of cytokines and growth factors, especially platelet-derived growth factor (PDGF) and the angiogenic tumor necrosis factor alpha (TNF alpha) (63). Some of these factors are certainly released by platelets, especially in the early hours, but the macrophages provide sustained release. Within 2–3 days the macrophages take over as the "overseers" of the healing process, as proven by the following experiments: in animals depleted of neutrophils, wound healing proceeds on schedule (108), but in the absence of monocytes and macrophages the wound becomes filled with fibrin and all manner of debris, including dead neutrophils; fibroblasts do not appear until day 5, and fibrosis is significantly reduced, so that by 10 days the wound appears "extremely immature" (68): fibroblasts are among the cells that take orders from macrophages.

Healing by Second Intention

Wound healing can be delayed under two circumstances: if the wound is infected, or if it is gaping (Figure 14.1).

HEALING OF INFECTED WOUNDS

If the raw surface of a wound is infected, waves of neutrophils flood it. Even if the wound is sutured, the apposed surfaces cannot attach to each other, because they are separated by pus (Figure 14.1).

Eventually, the two surfaces are covered by a layer of granulation tissue producing pus, similar to the pyogenic membrane of an abscess (p. 434). In fact, it could be said that an infected wound behaves very much like a cup-shaped abscess. Healing cannot begin until the infection has been overcome; at that point the wound, filled with granulation tissue, becomes an *open wound*. It then heals in a special manner, as we will now explain.

HEALING OF OPEN WOUNDS

The healing of an open wound, surgical (excisional) or accidental, presents a special problem because the gap must somehow be filled. Trees solve this problem simply by a slow ingrowth from the margins. We vertebrates, too, produce some filling (granulation tissue); but we also have a faster mechanism. Consider the large open wound shown in Figure 14.8. After a lag period of 5–9 days, the wound margins move toward each other as if pulled by an invisible force (89). This phenomenon, *wound contraction*, can be demonstrated in experimental animals by placing tattoo marks on the margins of an open wound and watching their displacement. What is the nature of the pulling force?

Open wounds contract by at least two mechanisms. During the first few days, *it is the scab that contracts.* In an open wound not covered with a moist dressing, the scab consists mainly of dried-up fibrin. As it dries it shrinks; and being firmly anchored to the tissues beneath, it can reduce the surface of a small open wound by about half.

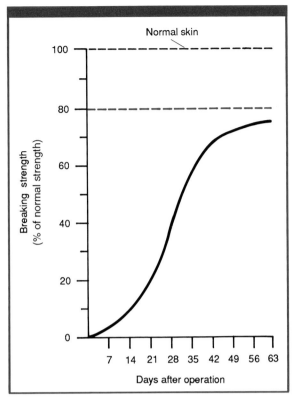

FIGURE 14.6 Breaking strength of a healing wound in rat skin. The strength of the final scar is about 80% of that of normal skin. (Reproduced with permission from [70].)

Another contraction mechanism begins to operate after about a week; its physical pull is quite strong (58). In the past this seemed mysterious, because wounds—open or not—were not known to contain cells capable of contracting. Eventually it was the good fortune of our laboratory to show that open wounds acquire a special set of contractile cells, the myofibroblasts.

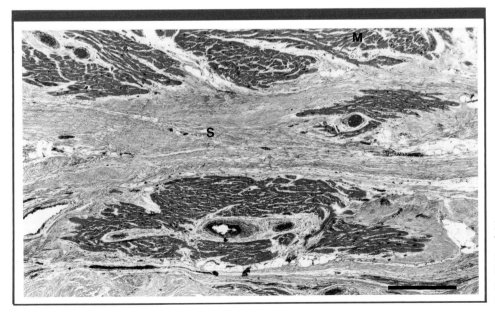

FIGURE 14.7 Typical scars (**S**) criss-crossing the myocardium (**M**): the end result of a healed infarct. The scar tissue consists mainly of collagen with few cells. **Bar** = 500 μm.

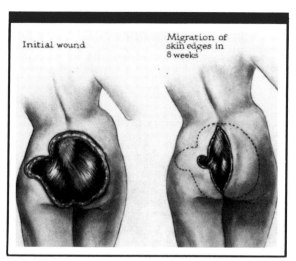

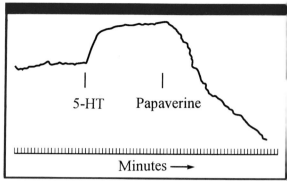

FIGURE 14.9
Proof that granulation tissue is a contractile organ. Responses of a strip of granulation tissue obtained from a 25-
day-old granuloma pouch. The strip was connected to a
recording needle and then stimulated with a contractant
(5-hydroxytryptamine = serotonin), followed by a relaxant,
papaverin. (Adapted from [103].)

ENTER THE MYOFIBROBLASTS

The adventurous quest for the myofibroblasts has
been told elsewhere (77). It led us as far as
investigating the method used for head-shrinking,
Amazonian style. Eventually we became convinced that the secret was in the fibroblasts, and
after moving to Geneva we joined forces with G.
Gabbiani and G.B. Ryan. Using the electron
microscope, we looked at several kinds of granulation tissue (including that of open wounds) and
found that many fibroblasts contained more fibrils
than usual. But did these fibrils have anything to
do with contraction? In a previous study on
endothelial cells, Majno and Leventhal (79) had
used the "accordeon" deformation of the nucleus
as an indicator of cellular contraction, and we
found to our delight that many of the fibroblast
nuclei did show the typical accordeon folds (33).
However, when these findings were reported at an
international meeting, the reception was cool:
morphologic evidence could only suggest contraction, it could not prove it. We had submitted a
hypothesis, not a fact. The challenge, at this
point, was to provide *functional* evidence that
wound fibroblasts contract.

We offer this challenge, year after year, to the
students in our Pathology course, adding that the
solution has to be simple and inexpensive. The
solution actually devised by one of us (GM) was to
take a strip of granulation tissue (for example,
from an open wound 10 days old), suspend it in a
bath as physiologists do with muscle, and stimulate
it with a smooth muscle contractant, such as
bradykinin. It worked (Figure 14.9) (78). To
behold that strip of supposedly inert connective
tissue shorten under our eyes was a rare experi-

ence. The first granulation tissue that we tested we
obtained from a "rat granuloma pouch" (p. 472); it
responded to contractants and relaxants much like
smooth muscle, only not as intensely. It was
fortunate that we began with that preparation: our
first experiment with wound tissue (from a 10-day
open wound of a rat) was negative. The wound
had already contracted *in vivo* and understandably
the granulation tissue refused to contract any
further. Minutes later we realized our conceptual
error and dowsed the strip with a smooth muscle
relaxant: it relaxed.

We concluded from these and other experiments that under certain conditions, such as in
open wounds, fibroblasts modulate into a contractile phenotype (33, 34) for which one of us
(GM) proposed the name **myofibroblast** (78).
The reason for introducing a new name was largely
the notion, well known to anthropologists, that in
the human world things truly exist only when they
have a name. The rapid career of the myofibroblast confirmed this notion. In essence, we had
shown that *the granulation tissue that fills an open
wound is a temporary contractile organ.*

Structure and Function of the Myofibroblasts

Obviously, if isolated fibroblasts became shorter,
the surrounding tissue would not contract at all.
So, in modulating to myofibroblasts, they develop
structural features that would be expected from
cells designed to pull (33, 34): (a) *intercellular
fibrils* with dense bodies resembling those of
smooth muscle (Figure 14.10); (b) *microtendons*, a
name that we like to use for fibrous bundles that

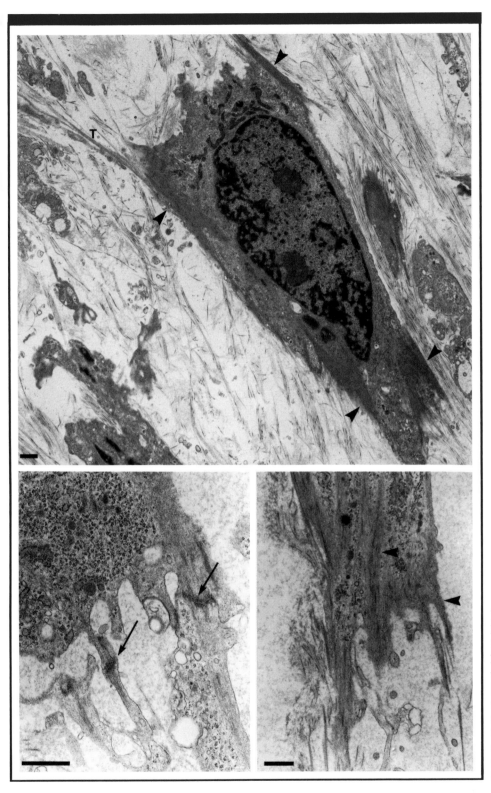

FIGURE 14.10
Myofibroblasts. *Top:* Overall view. Bundles of intracellular fibrils (**arrowheads**), some of which are continuous with extracellular "microtendons" (**T**). (From a human stenotic mitral valve). *Bottom left:* Junctions (**arrows**) between adjacent myofibroblasts. *Bottom right:* Bundles of fibrils (**arrowheads**) extending into cell processes. (From an 11-day open wound in a rat). **Bars** = 1 μm.

emerge from the cell, continuing the direction of intracellular fibrils (102) ("fibronexus" is the official name for this arrangement); (c) *intercellular junctions* of various kinds, especially gap junctions (Figure 14.10), such as are never seen among ordinary fibroblasts. In fact, normal fibroblasts avoid contact between each other by "contact inhibition". Overall these changes cause the myofibroblast to resemble, but not to become, a smooth muscle cell (25, 38)

The fibrillar equipment of the myofibroblasts has been extensively studied by G. Gabbiani's group (105); the distinctive feature is the transient expression of alpha-smooth muscle actin (25) which can be induced by heparin (27). The same group described various phenotypes of myofibroblasts, depending on the filaments present (61, 109) and found that myofibroblasts secrete collagen type III, typical of early repair (105).

While it is generally agreed that myofibroblasts are cells intermediate between fibroblasts and smooth muscle cells, exactly how they use their contractile machinery is not entirely clear. They seem to exert their pull in two very different ways:

- By shortening, in the manner of smooth muscle cells. Since the myofibroblasts are connected to each other as well as to the stroma, if each one becomes shorter the overall result is similar to that of a contracting muscle.
- By a stationary hand-over-hand mechanism (48). This mechanism—still hypothetical—can be understood by imagining a sailor hauling in an anchor; the sailor produces traction but does not have to become shorter in the process. This concept was suggested by the fact that cultured fibroblasts (myofibroblasts) seeded in a gel of collagen are able to contract the gel, as we will explain shortly.

Little is known about the message, or messages, that induce fibroblasts to modulate into myofibroblasts. Clearly there is something about an open wound that induces the modulation; *myofibroblasts develop in open wounds, where contraction is necessary, but not in closed wounds, where it is not.* In fact this is why the myofibroblasts were not discovered earlier: all experimenters who had studied healing

by electron microscopy had used incisional wounds. But how do the fibroblasts perceive that a wound is open? This is the next challenge. We suspect that chemical as well as physical factors are involved. *Traction* alone can induce fibroblasts to modulate into myofibroblasts; this was shown by stretching the skin of a mouse for 4–6 days, by means of a spring-loaded device (112). Cultured fibroblasts promptly modulate into myofibroblasts (16, 103, 105), presumably because they receive the message "this is an open wound."

It would be important to understand the molecular mechanisms of this modulation, because it often leads to trouble.

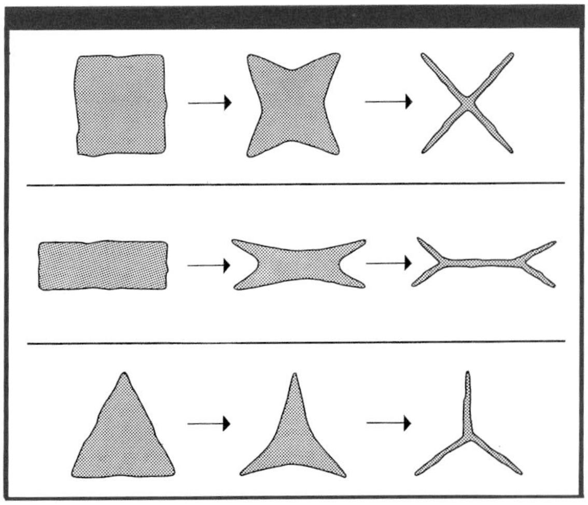

Misdeeds of the Myofibroblast The contraction of open wounds is not always wanted. Burns are the best example: a burn encircling an arm is an open wound; accordingly, myofibroblasts appear and produce enough traction to lock the elbow into a permanent fixture or even to hamper the circulation. By the same mechanism, burns of the face or neck can produce disfiguring scars. Besides wounds, myofibroblasts have been found in cirrhosis of the liver, in the so-called *contracted kidney*, and in many diseases in which fibrosis and contraction of connective tissue are central features (105).

To this day the only method for preventing the contraction of an open wound in humans is to cover it with a graft. Drugs have been tried but without much success.

Myofibroblasts: loose ends. The story of myofibroblasts is far from complete. Myofibroblasts have been found in many normal tissues, such as the lung (105), and it may be that cells other than fibroblasts, even macrophages, can modulate into a contractile phenotype (6, 9, 105). The mechanism of the modulation remains an open issue; it has been reported that platelet-derived growth factor BB (PDGF-BB) and transforming growth factor beta 1 (TGF-beta 1) inhibit the fibroblast-to-myofibroblast modulation in rabbit wounds (93), yet TGF-beta accelerated the contraction of a collagen gel (83), presumably because the effect of cytokines depends a great deal on their environment. In pigs, the contraction of open wounds can be reduced by covering the area with an artificial collagen/elastin dermal substitute seeded with "stromal cells" (lipoblasts?) obtained from subcutaneous fat (28).

SHAPES OF OPEN WOUNDS AND SHAPES OF SCARS

An open wound contracts as if its margins were being drawn toward the center; this means that

FIGURE 14.11 Open wounds of the three shapes shown (*left*) will contract and produce scars of predictable geometric patterns (*right*). (Reproduced with permission from [76].)

the final shape of the scar depends on the original shape of the wound. For example, as is well known to plastic surgeons, a square wound will lead to a star-shaped scar and a triangular wound to a Y-shaped scar (Figure 14.11). One way to understand these geometric results is to imagine 40 turtles standing in a square and facing inward at right angles to the sides of the square; if they all walk straight forward, they must come to a halt in the formation of a star (Figure 14.12) (76). Using the same example, we can predict that there must be a problem in the healing of round wounds; as matter of fact, it was known in Hippocratic times that a round wound heals more quickly if it is cut into a different shape (76). Experimental round wounds in rabbits do heal more slowly than square wounds of the same surface area: eventually they do heal because the circular shape slowly turns into an oval, then the oval becomes narrower, and finally it heals like a linear wound. This is intuitive. If a round wound were to heal by contraction, its margins would have to condense to a point, which is patently impossible.

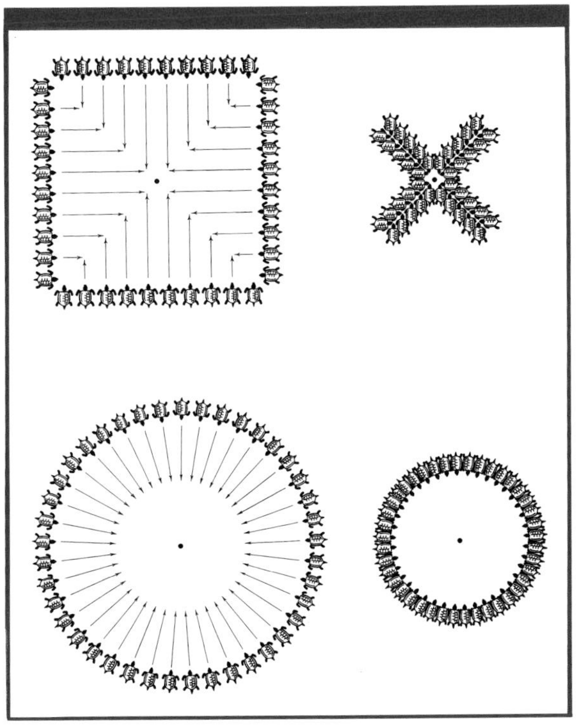

Experimental Models of Wound Healing

Because wounds are such a basic medical problem, a great deal of effort has gone into developing experimental models: not a simple task, because laboratory animals naturally tend to "work" on their wounds and interfere with the experiment.

THE RABBIT EAR CHAMBER

A classic device is the rabbit ear chamber (Figure 14.13): in essence, a small hole is punched in a rabbit ear, which is then sandwiched between two coverslips; the hole fills up with blood, and over the next few weeks one can observe, under the microscope, the ingrowth of blood vessels that organize the clot, i.e., replace it with living tissue (Figure 14.14). Careful drawings made by Sandison and by the Clarks in the 1920s and 1930s show very nicely how the vascular network develops (Figure 14.15) (13, 104). A recent improvement to the ear chamber has been the introduction of oxygen electrodes, which have confirmed that oxygen pressure in the center of the wound, where the macrophages are at work, is close to zero (Figure 14.16) (53).

SPONGES AND CYLINDERS

To examine the chemistry of granulation tissue, one can implant a small absorbable sponge, let it be infiltrated by granulation tissue, and then recover it for study at various times (50). To analyze the nature and properties of "wound fluid," one can slip a hollow object such as a cylinder of

FIGURE 14.12
The "turtle experiment" illustrating how open wounds heal. The rows of turtles represent the margins of skin wounds. *Top:* In a square wound, an inward motion of the margins leads to a star-shaped scar. *Bottom:* If the wound is perfectly circular, it cannot heal solely by contraction because its margins cannot condense into a point. Large circular wounds heal by becoming oblong; later they close with a linear scar. (Reproduced with permission from [76].)

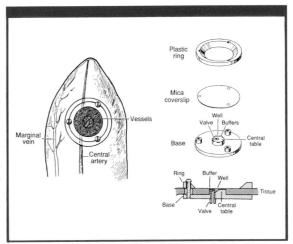

FIGURE 14.13
Rabbit ear chamber, a tool for the study of wound healing *in vivo. Left:* The chamber as installed in the ear. *Right:* Exploded view of the chamber and cross section of the chamber installed *in vivo.* (Adapted from [84].)

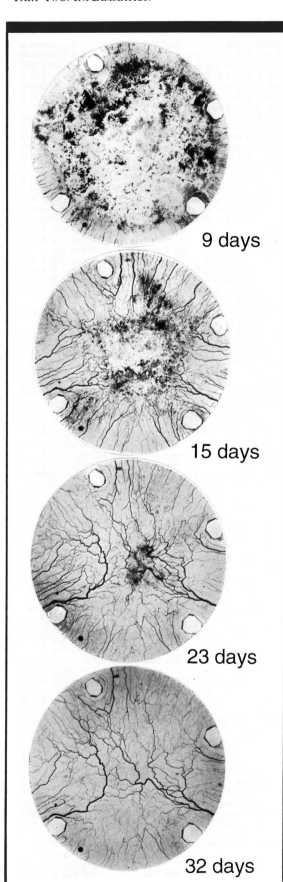

FIGURE 14.14 Serial photographs through a rabbit ear chamber, showing the progressive ingrowth of blood vessels and the organization of the central blood clot at various times after chamber was installed. (Reproduced with permission from [14].)

9 days

15 days

23 days

32 days

wire mesh under the skin of an experimental animal (53, 125); after a few days the space is filled with wound fluid, which is not quite the same as inflammatory exudate.

EYE INJURIES

Studies on eye injuries have illustrated many points, such as the angiogenic power of macrophages (Figure 14.17); they also have provided spectacular three-dimensional views of angiogenesis (Figure 14.18).

THE AIR POUCH (SELYE POUCH)

Besides open wounds, a highly standardized method for producing sheets of granulation tissue is the "granuloma pouch" or "Selye pouch" (Figure 14.19) (34). On the back of a rat, using a syringe, 20 ml of air are injected subcutaneously, followed by 1 ml of 1 percent croton oil, a powerful irritant. Within a few days the wall of the air pouch is filled with exudate and lined by granulation tissue. It can be excised as an egg-shaped organ, and the granulation tissue (which, unlike that of an open wound, is aseptic) can be studied microscopically or measured in various ways. If left alone, the pouch shrinks—it is loaded with myofibroblasts (34)—and disappears in about 3 months.

COLLAGEN LATTICE

This model is an *in vitro* system that addresses the mechanism of connective tissue contraction; it has produced some intriguing facts (5). The principle is to pour into a round dish a solution of collagen mixed with cultured fibroblasts (which are therefore modulated to myofibroblasts). The solution gels into a fibrillar matrix that imprisons the cells. Within 24 hours the gel shrinks to 1/28th of the original area, extruding water; TGF-beta accelerates the contraction (83) (Figure 14.20). Why does the lattice shrink? Seen by electron microscopy, the cells appear to be largely isolated, but they do have attachments to the collagen fibrils (1, 43, 82).

The Pace of Wound Healing

Mankind has been trying for millenia to accelerate wound healing, be it with spider webs, manure, or more orthodox drugs (95). However, by the early twentieth century, pessimism began to prevail: the view was widely adopted that *wounds heal at maximal rate*, meaning that no drug could possibly speed up the process. This dogma is now somewhat threatened as growth factors are tested on wounds (90); some growth factors do stimulate wound healing in experimental models (Figure 14.21) (39, 72) and in humans (8), but the cost is prohibitive. At the time of this writing there is no routine use of such factors in surgery.

> *Mammals lick their wounds. Mouse salivary glands secrete large amounts of nerve growth factor and epidermal growth factor. In mice deprived of sublingual and submaxillary glands, open wounds contract more slowly (57) and corneal ulcers heal poorly (117). Even in humans, wounds in the mouth heal quickly and without infectious complications, despite a teeming bacterial flora. The mechanism is not clear.*

Mucosal wounds in general heal faster than skin wounds (106). When a *muscularis mucosae* exists, it contracts and reduces the area of the wound. This is why mucosal biopsies can be taken routinely, even from the rectum.

Age is a factor in the rate of healing. Although armies are not known for basic research, an exception should be made for the wound healing laboratory of the French army during World War I: Alexis Carrel and his group discovered that open wounds in older persons close more slowly (36). Wound healing in the fetus will be discussed next.

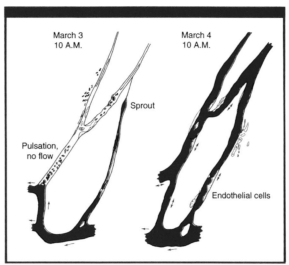

FIGURE 14.15
Advancing edge of a capillary network as seen in the rabbit ear chamber. The two drawings are of the same field and were made 24 hours apart. (Reproduced with permission from [14].)

bacteria beyond which clinical infection results: this is currently set at 10^5 bacteria per gram of tissue or per milliliter of biologic fluid. This figure varies surprisingly little with different organisms (49).

Infection and Oxygen It is an axiom of surgery that *the resistance of wounds to infection is proportional to their blood supply* (54). As we have seen, blood protects against infection in many ways. A key factor is the oxygen supply. Leukocytes can move about and phagocytize anaerobically, but

Disorders of Wound Healing

The process of healing is powerfully programmed and very difficult to obstruct, but it has its enemies. Some are iatrogenic: glucocorticoids, given during the first 3 days after injury, retard wound healing. Delays are caused also by the cachexia induced by malignant tumors, X-ray therapy, and many antineoplastic agents; this can create a problem when surgery is needed during the treatment of tumors (10, 107). Diabetics have a fivefold greater risk than nondiabetics of wound infection (10); not only is their inflammatory response defective (p. 503) but also there are subtle defects of the microcirculation and of the granulation tissue (37, 121). Malnutrition, including lack of vitamin C (scurvy), can also impair wound healing.

The two main complications of wound healing are infection, which is the most common (51), and keloids.

WOUND INFECTION

No skin wound can be totally free from bacterial contamination, but there is a critical number of

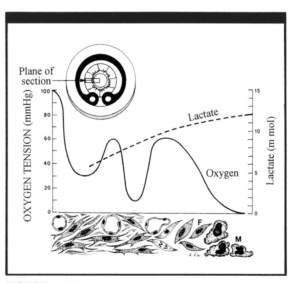

FIGURE 14.16
Oxygen and lactate levels in the rabbit ear chamber. Tissue sample oriented as shown in the inset at top. The peaks of oxygen concentration correspond to vessels. The cells at the advancing front, shown at bottom, are macrophages (**M**) and fibroblasts (**F**); they live in a low-oxygen, high-lactate environment. (Reproduced with permission from [52].)

FIGURE 14.17 Dense growth of vascular sprouts in guinea pig cornea. To illustrate the angiogenic property of macrophages, the cornea was injected with activated peritoneal macrophages, and 7 days later all vessels were perfused with carbon black. **Arrows:** Injection site. (Reproduced with permission from [94].)

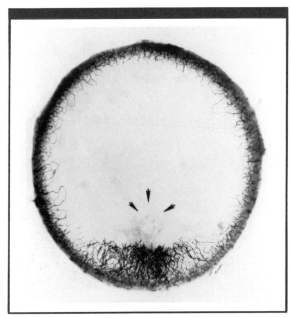

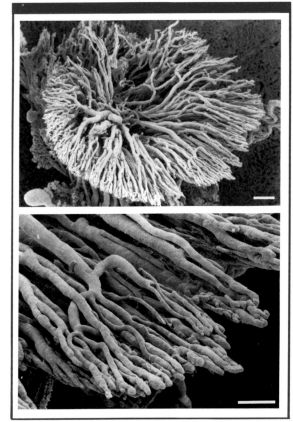

FIGURE 14.18
Burst of angiogenesis in the eye of a rabbit. These vessels grew into the vitreous body (normally avascular) in response to an injection of cultured skin fibroblasts 3 months earlier. The vessels were then injected with plastic, and all tissues were removed by corrosion. *Top:* Normal view of the vascular fan. **Bar = 200 μm.** *Bottom:* Higher power showing advancing vascular loops. **Bar = 100 μm.** (Reproduced with permission from [115].)

they depend on oxygen for killing some bacteria; for example, *Staphylococcus aureus* and *E. coli* are killed at rates proportional to oxygen tension, whereas pneumococci are killed independently of oxygen tension. In essence, *leukocytes deprived of oxygen behave like leukocytes in chronic granulomatous disease: the oxygen burst is impaired* (54).

If wounded rabbits are kept in various concentrations of oxygen, and *Pseudomonas aeruginosa* are injected into the wounds, the bacteria are cleared much faster from the rabbits breathing the highest oxygen concentrations (54, 55). In this context, it has been said that oxygen acts as an antibiotic (62).

Infection and Foreign Bodies Foreign bodies such as dirt or splinters can create serious complications even if they are chemically inert because they have the odd property of favoring infection. This is why surgeons submit accidental wounds to careful cleaning and do not immediately suture dirty wounds. Foreign bodies favor infection in three ways:

- They can be a source of bacteria.
- They lower the infectious dose of bacteria.
- They make the infection harder to treat.

The first way is self-evident. The second has been more difficult to understand, but the facts are impressive: in experiments on courageous volunteers in the 1950s, virulent staphylococci were introduced into the skin, with or without a surgical suture. The suture lowered the infectious dose of bacteria to 100 staphylococci, enhancing their virulence at least 10,000 times (30, 85).

There are at least two mechanisms for this enhanced virulence: First, the foreign body acts as a decoy and distracts the phagocytes, which waste their precious granules in attempts to phagocytize it.

If a small, sterile plastic cage is implanted under the skin of a guinea pig, as few as 100 Staph aureus suffice to infect, whereas even 10^8 bacteria fail to produce an abscess in normal guinea-pig skin (125). If the neutrophils in the cage are tested later, they are found to have developed a phagocytic defect (124): loss of ammunition as a result of "frustrated phagocytosis" (p. 404).

As for the second mechanism: some bacteria that stick to surfaces bury themselves under a thick layer of slime, more politely referred to as an exopolymer (Figure 14.22). The reader may wonder why this does not happen in ordinary bacterial cultures. The answer: in the competitive situation of a natural environment, where many types of bacteria coexist, selection favors those bacteria that are protected; the protection is achieved by sticking to a suitable surface under the cover of a slime, actually a tangle of branching macromolecules. In a pure culture the advantage is lost, and no slime is produced (23). This is true for any aquatic ecosystem in nature: for every free-floating organism there are 1–10 thousand growing in biofilms on submerged surfaces (22). The urinary pathways, or any canal in the body's plumbing, are potential targets for such ecosystems; urinary catheters can become coated with slimy layers of bacteria dozens of cells and hundreds of micrometers thick (22). In essence, *staphylococci growing on a urinary catheter are simply doing what they would do in their natural environment* (11). Dentists have been aware of these facts for a long time because the crevices around a tooth, where dental plaque flourishes, is one of these natural ecosystems (114). Bacteria buried in the slime are at least partially shielded not only from phagocytes (60, 118) and lymphocytes (91) but also from antibodies, opsonins, and antibiotics (21).

In these days of catheters, invasive procedures, and plastic prostheses, infection related to foreign bodies is becoming increasingly common. As for sutures, the Centers for Disease Control now recommend monofilament threads to reduce the surface area and thereby the risk of infection (31).

HYPERTROPHIC SCARS AND KELOIDS

Aberrations of scar formation are the nightmare of plastic surgeons and of their patients. In some individuals the smallest wound, even that left by piercing an ear, can lead to an overgrowth of the scar. If the scar develops into a raised, firm ridge, it is called a *hypertrophic scar*, which can regress. If the overgrowth exceeds the borders of the scar, it is called a *keloid*, which does not regress. Keloid is Greek for claw-like, and therefore cancer-like. This connection has yet to be proven, although some keloids truly suggest tumor growth (Figure 14.23). Histologically, all one sees is a tremendous overproduction of collagen (Figure 14.24); biochemically, collagen metabolism is abnormally high in keloids even after 10 years (3). Excision of a keloid simply creates another one. However, keloids are capricious: a wound in one part of the body may produce a keloid, but in another it may not. Blacks are especially prone to keloid development. Theories abound (18), but there is no explanation for this distressing condition.

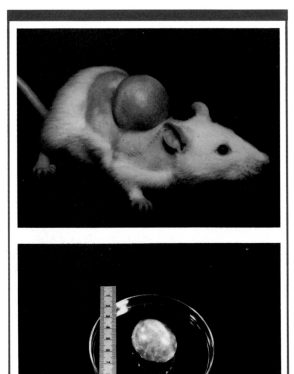

FIGURE 14.19
Top: The "granuloma pouch" method for the study of inflammation. Air (20 ml) is injected under the rat's skin, followed by a small volume of irritant; the skin remains intact. *Bottom:* 2–3 weeks later a pouch of granulation tissue can be excised and studied. It contains air and exudate. Scale in cm. (Courtesy of Dr. G.B. Ryan, University of Melbourne, Melbourne, Australia.)

"Proud Flesh" Hypertrophy of granulation tissue sometimes occurs during wound healing. An overenthusiastic granulation tissue grows above the surface of the surrounding skin (Figure 14.25), but it can be brought under control by cauterization with silver nitrate. This condition was once known by the medieval name of *proud flesh* (a

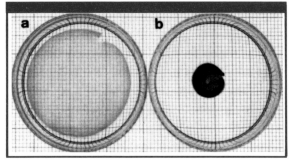

FIGURE 14.20
Stimulation of "cultured fibroblasts" to contract their substrate. Two dishes were coated with a layer of collagen, seeded with 1 million fibroblasts, and stained after 5 days. **a:** Control. **b:** Stimulation with transforming growth factor beta (TGF-β). Scale in mm. (Reproduced with permission from [83].)

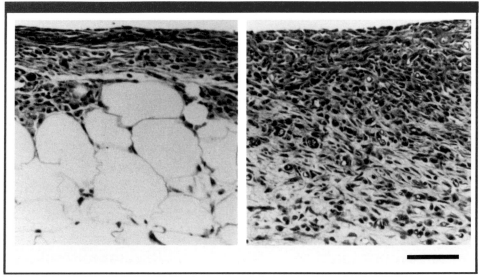

FIGURE 14.21
Stimulation of wound healing with recombinant PDGF in square open wounds on the backs of genetically diabetic mice. *Left:* Control wound in a diabetic mouse treated with control solution for 5 days shows minimal cellular invasion and granulation tissue formation. *Right:* 5-day diabetic wound treated with recombinant PDGF shows marked increase in the thickness, cellularity, and vascularity of the granulation tissue. **Bar** = 500 μm. (Reproduced with permission from [39].)

similar expression is still current in carpentry: in covering a wall with plaster the surface above a hole must be slightly "prouded"). In children, an overgrowth of granulation tissue can obstruct the opening of a long-term tracheostomy tube (98); occasionally an overgrowth occurs at the navel after shedding of the umbilical cord ("umbilical granuloma").

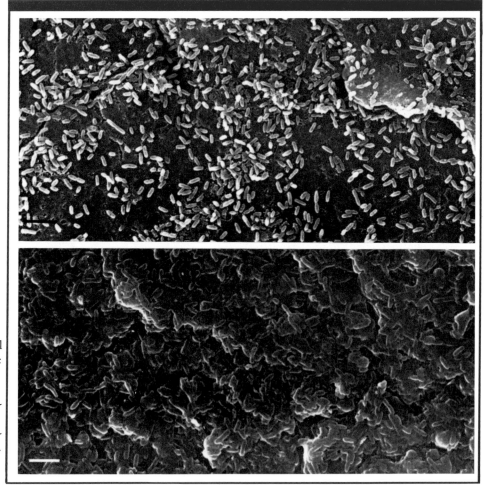

FIGURE 14.22
Behavior of *Pseudomonas aeruginosa* on the surface of a catheter material that is bathed in artificial urine. *Top:* Colonization of the surface after 2 hours of exposure to the bacteria-laden medium. *Bottom:* The same after 8 hours; the surface is now covered by a thick film in which the bacterial cells are buried. **Bars** = 5 μm. (Reproduced with permission from [24].)

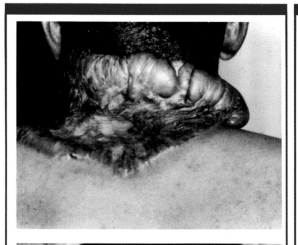

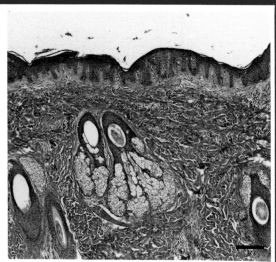

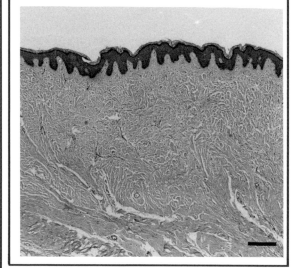

FIGURE 14.24
Comparison of normal skin and keloid tissue. *Top:* Control skin. *Bottom:* Keloid. The dermis is replaced by a meshwork of thick collagen fibers without many cells. Note lack of glands and hair. **Bars =** 250 μm.

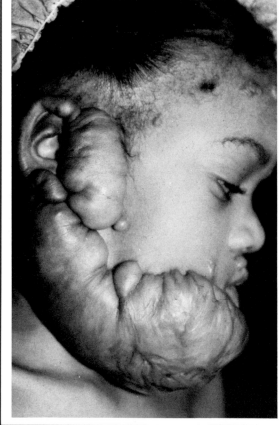

FIGURE 14.23
Top: Keloid of the neck, following an infection. *Bottom:* Extensive keloid of the face, following a burn of the ear and two grafting operations. (Reproduced with permission from [87, 88].)

SUNDRY DISTURBANCES

Diabetes entails defective wound healing and decreased resistance to infection; the mechanisms are many and not well understood. Hyperglycemia alone impairs leukocyte chemotaxis (71). **Paralysis**

from different causes is often accompanied by poor healing; denervation was shown to reduce the tensile strength of scars in rabbits (75). In **germ-free animals** incisional wounds heal normally (4) but it would be more interesting to know what happens with open wounds. A special variety of germ-free healing occurs also in the **fetus.** Experimentally, incisional wounds in the fetus heal perfectly, without a scar; open wounds may heal by contraction, but in some species they do not heal at all (73, 74, 111). In a 20-week human fetus that suffered amputations due to amniotic bands, there was no acute inflammatory response, no granulation tissue, and no removal of necrotic tissue (amniotic bands are abnormal, tough cords derived from the amniotic membrane; they can strangle and even sever parts of the fetus) (99). We tend to think of embryonic

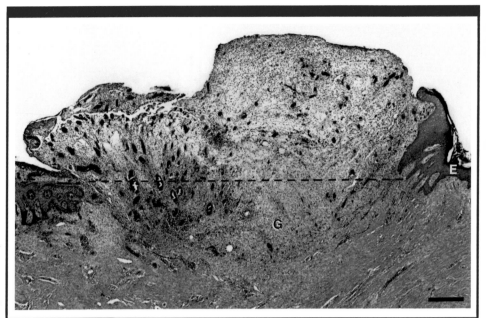

FIGURE 14.25
Excessive granulation tissue (proud flesh), in an ulcer of the skin. The granulation tissue (**G**) rises higher than the epidermis (**E**). Cauterization with silver nitrate controls the hypertrophy, but the biological question (why this overgrowth happens) remains unanswered. Perhaps an excess of growth factors? **Bar** = 500 μm.

tissue as omnipotent, but we should also remember that the fetus is neutropenic, lacks an immune response, and has less oxygen available than a mountaineer at the top of Mount Everest (74).

TO SUM UP: Wound healing is one of the marvels of Nature. Its mechanisms evolved in a world saturated with bacteria, which may explain its effectiveness in dealing with infection. Indeed, some surgeons maintain (privately) that "a little bit of infection" accelerates the healing.

The efficiency of wound healing has been well tested in the course of medical history: the most unsavory materials were used as surgical dressings (Galen favored dove dung), yet healing occured anyway. Today we are still looking for ways to speed up the process. Recombinant growth factors are not yet used clinically, but they have already undermined the ancient dogma that normal wound healing occurs at its maximal rate. Among the major challenges that lie ahead: find a way to prevent wound contraction when it is not wanted.

References

1. Allen TD, Schor SL. The contraction of collagen matrices by dermal fibroblasts. J Ultrastruct Res 1983;83:205–219.
2. Ausprunk DH, Falterman K, Folkman J. The sequence of events in the regression of corneal capillaries. Lab Invest 1978;38:284–294.
2a. Avicenna. *Liber Canonis.* Translated from Arabic to Latin by Gerard of Cremona. Printed in Venice, 1507; photographically reproduced by G. Olms Verlag, Hildesheim, 1964; pp. 79/r col.2, 446 r/col.2.
3. Bailey AJ, Bazin S, Sims TJ, Le Lous M, Nicoletis C, Delaunay A. Characterization of the collagen of human hypertrophic and normal scars. Biochim Biophys Acta 1975;405:412–421.
4. Bauer H. Cellular defence mechanisms. In: Coates ME, Gordon HA, Wostmann BS, eds. The germ-free animal in research. London and New York: Academic Press, 1968:210–226.
5. Bell E, Ivarsson B, Merrill C. Production of a tissue-like structure by contraction of collagen lattices by human fibroblasts of different proliferative potential in vitro. Proc Natl Acad Sci USA 1979;76:1274–1278.
6. Bhawan J, Majno G. The myofibroblast. Possible derivation from macrophages in xanthogranuloma. Am J Dermatopathol 1989;11:255–258.
7. Breedis C. Regeneration of hair follicles and sebaceous glands from the epithelium of scars in the rabbit. Cancer Res 1954;14:575–579.
8. Brown GL, Nanney LB, Griffen J, et al. Enhancement of wound healing by topical treatment with epidermal growth factor. N Engl J Med 1989;321:76–79.
9. Campbell GR, Ryan GB. Origin of myofibroblasts in the avascular capsule around free-floating intraperitoneal blood clots. Pathology 1983;15:253–264.
10. Carrico TJ, Mehrhof AI Jr, Cohen IK. Biology of wound healing. Surg Clin North Am 1984;64:721–733.
11. Christensen GD, Baddour LM, Hasty DL, Lowrance JH, Simpson WA. Microbial and foreign body factors in the pathogenesis of medical device infections. In: Bisno AL, Waldvogel FA, eds. Infections associated with indwelling

medical devices. Washington, DC: American Society for Microbiology, 1989:27–59.

12. Chvapil M, Koopmann CF Jr. Scar formation: physiology and pathlogical states. Otolaryngol Clin North Am 1984;17:265–272.

13. Clark ER, Clark EL. Observations on living preformed blood vessels as seen in a transparent chamber inserted into the rabbit's ear. Am J Anat 1931;49:441–477.

14. Clark ER, Hitschler WJ, Kirby-Smith HT, Rex RO, Smith JH. General observations on the ingrowth of new blood vessels into standardized chambers in the rabbit's ear, and the subsequent changes in the newly grown vessels over a period of months. Anat Rec 1931;50:129–160.

15. Clark RAF, Winn HJ, Dvorak HF, Colvin RB. Fibronectin beneath reepithelializing epidermis in vivo: sources and significance. J Invest Dermatol 1983;80:026s-030s.

16. Clark RAF. Overview and general considerations of wound repair. In: Clark RAF, Henson PM, eds. The molecular and cellular biology of wound repair. New York: Plenum Press, 1988:3–33.

17. Clark RAF, Henson PM, eds. The molecular and cellular biology of wound repair. New York: Plenum Press, 1988.

18. Cohen IK, McCoy BJ. Keloid: biology and treatment. In: Dineen P, Hildick-Smith G, eds. The surgical wound. Philadelphia: Lea & Febiger, 1981:123–131.

19. Colvin RB. Wound healing processes in hemostasis and thrombosis. In: Gimbrone MA Jr, ed. Vascular endothelium in hemostasis and thrombosis. Edinburgh: Churchill Livingstone, 1986:220–241.

20. Converse JM, Smahel J, Ballantyne DL Jr, Harper AD. Inosculation of vessels of skin graft and host bed: a fortuitous encounter. Br J Plast Surg 1975;28:274–282.

21. Costerton JW. Effects of antibiotics on adherent bacteria. In: Sabath LD, ed. Action of antibiotics in patients. Bern: Hans Huber Publishers, 1982:160–176.

22. Costerton JW. The etiology and persistence of cryptic bacterial infections: a hypothesis. Rev Infect Dis 1984; 6(suppl 3):S608-S616.

23. Costerton JW, Geesey GG, Chen, K-J. How bacteria stick. Sci Am 1978;238:86–95.

24. Costerton JW, Watkins L. Adherence of bacteria to foreign bodies: the role of the biofilm. In: Root RK, Trunkey DD, Sande MA. New surgical and medical approaches in infectious diseases. New York: Churchill Livingstone, 1987:17–30.

25. Darby I, Skalli O, Gabbiani G. α-Smooth muscle actin is transiently expressed by myofibroblasts during experimental wound healing. Lab Invest 1990;63:21–29.

26. de Chauliac G. On wounds and fractures. (Translated by WA Brennan). Chicago: Translator, 1923.

27. Desmoulière A, Rubbia-Brandt L, Crau G, Gabbiani G. Heparin induces α-smooth muscle actin expression in cultured fibroblasts and in granulation tissue myofibroblasts. Lab Invest 1992;67:716–726.

28. de Vries HJC, Middelkeep E, van Heemstra-Hoen M, Wildevuur CHR, Westerhof W. Stromal cells from subcutaneous adipose tissue seeded in a native collagen/elastin dermal substitute reduce wound contraction in full thickness skin defects. Lab Invest 1995;73:532–540.

29. Dunphy JE. Practical accomplishments and future prospects. In: Dunphy JE, Van Winkle W Jr, eds. Repair and regeneration. New York: McGraw-Hill, 1969:349–358.

30. Elek SD, Conen PE. The virulence of Staphylococcus pyogenes for man. A study of the problems of wound infection. Br J Exp Pathol 1957;38:573-586.

31. Fishman M. Microbial adherence and infection—clinical relevance. Infect Control 1986;7:181–184.

32. Forrester JC, Zederfeldt BH, Hayes TL, Hunt TK. Mechanical, biochemical and architectural features of repair. In: Dunphy JE, Van Winkle W Jr, eds. Repair and regeneration. New York: McGraw-Hill, 1969:71–85.

33. Gabbiani G, Ryan GB, Majno G. Presence of modified fibroblasts in granulation tissue and their possible role in wound contraction. Experientia 1971;27:449–550.

34. Gabbiani G, Hirschel BJ, Ryan GB, Statkov PR, Majno G. Granulation tissue as a contractile organ. A study of structure and function. J Exp Med 1972;135:719–734.

35. Gay S, Viljanto J, Raekallio J, Pentinnen R. Collagen types in early phases of wound healing in children. Acta Chir Scand 1978;144:205–211.

36. Goodson WH III, Hunt TK. Wound healing and aging. J Invest Dermatol 1979;73:88–91.

37. Goodson WH III, Radolf J, Hunt TK. Wound healing and diabetes. In: Hunt TK, ed. Wound healing and wound infection. New York: Appleton-Century-Crofts, 1980:106–117.

38. Gown AM. The mysteries of the myofibroblast (partially) unmasked. Lab Invest 1990;63:1–3.

39. Greenhalgh DG, Sprugel KH, Murray MJ, Ross R. PDGF and FGF stimulate wound healing in the genetically diabetic mouse. Am J Pathol 1990;136:1235-1246.

40. Grillo HC. Research in wound healing. In: Ballinger F, ed. Research metholds in surgery. The National Cancer Institute, 1964:235–254.

41. Grinnell F. Fibronectin and wound healing. J Cell Biochem 1984;26:107-116.

42. Grinnell F. The activated keratinocyte: up regulation of cell adhesion and migration during wound healing. J Trauma 1990;30(suppl 12):S144-S149.

43. Grinnell F. Fibroblast reorganization of three-dimensional collagen gels and regulation of cell biosynthetic function. In: Okamura S, Tsuruta S, Imanishi Y, Sunamoto J, eds. Fundamental investigations on the creation of biofunctional materials. Kyoto, Japan: Kagaku-Dojin, 1991: 33–43.

44. Grinnell F, Billingham RE, Burgess L. Distribution of fibronectin during wound healing in vivo. J Invest Dermatol 1981;76:181–189.

45. Grinnell F, Toda, K-I, Takashima A. Activation of keratinocyte fibronectin receptor function during cutaneous wound healing. J Cell Sci Suppl 1987;8:199-209.

46. Gristina AG, Oga M, Webb LK, Hobgood CD. Adherent bacterial colonization in the pathogenesis of osteomyelitis. Science 1985;228:990–993.

47. Grotendorst GR, Martin GR. Cell movements in wound-healing and fibrosis. Rheumatology 1986;10:385–403.

48. Harris AK, Wild P, Stopak D. Silicone rubber substrata: a new wrinkle in the study of cell locomotion. Science 1980;208:177–179.

49. Heggers JP. Variations on a theme. In: Heggers JP, Robson MC, eds. Quantitative bacteriology: its role in the armamentarium of the surgeon. Boca Raton, FL: CRC Press, 1991:15–23.

50. Holund B, Junker P, Garbarsch C, Christoffersen P, Lorenzen I. Formation of granulation tissue in subcutaneously implanted sponses in rats. Acta Pathol Microbiol Scand Sect A 1979;87:367–374.

51. Hunt TK, ed. Wound healing and wound infection. New York: Appleton-Century-Crofts, 1980.

52. Hunt TK. Prospective: a retrospective perspective on the nature of wounds. Prog Clin Biol Res 1988;266:xiii–xx.

53. Hunt TK, Andrews WS, Halliday B, et al. Coagulation and macrophage stimulation of angiogenesis and wound healing. In: Dineen P, Hildick-Smith G, eds. The surgical wound. Philadelphia: Lea & Febiger, 1981:1–18.

54. Hunt TK, Knighton DR, Price DC, et al. Oxygen in the prevention and treatment of infection. In: Root RK,

Trunkey DD, Sande MA, eds. New surgical and medical approaches in infectious diseases. New York: Churchill Livingstone, 1987:1–16.

55. Hunt TK, Linsey M, Grislis G, Sonne M, Jawetz E. The effect of differing ambient oxygen tensions on wound infection. Ann Surg 1975;181:35–39.

56. Hunt TK, Van Winkle W Jr. Normal repair. In: Hunt TK, Dunphy JE, eds. Fundamentals of wound management. New York: Appleton-Century-Crofts, 1979:2–67.

57. Hutson JM, Niall M, Evans D, Fowler R. Effect of salivary glands on wound contraction in mice. Nature 1979;279:793–795.

58. James DW. Wound contraction—a synthesis. Adv Biol Skin 1964;5:216-230.

59. Jensen JA, Hunt TK, Scheuenstuhl H, Banda MJ. Effect of lactate, pyruvate, and pH on secretion of angiogenesis and mitogenesis factors by macrophages. Lab Invest 1986;54:574–578.

60. Johnson GM, Lee DA, Regelmann WE, Gray ED, Peters G, Quie PG. Interference with granulocyte function by Staphylococcus epidermis slime. Infect Immun 1986;54:13–20.

61. Kapanci Y, Burgan S, Pietra GG, Conne B, Gabbiani G. Modulation of actin isoform expression in alveolar myofibroblasts (contractile interstitial cells) during pulmonary hypertension. Am J Pathol 1990;136:881–889.

62. Knighton DR, Halliday B, Hunt TK. Oxygen as an antibiotic. A comparison of the effects of inspired oxygen concentration and antibiotic administration on in vivo bacterial clearance. Arch Surg 1986;121:191–195.

63. Knighton DR, Fiegel VD. The macrophages: effector cell wound repair. Prog Clin Biol Res 1989;299:217–226.

64. Knighton DR, Hunt TK, Scheuenstuhl H, Halliday BJ, Werb Z, Banda MJ. Oxygen tension regulates the expression of angiogenesis factor by macrophages. Science 1983;221:1283–1285.

65. Knighton DR, Silver IA, Hunt TK. Regulation of wound-healing angiogenesis—effect of oxygen gradients and inspired oxygen concentration. Surgery 1981;90:262–270.

66. Knox P, Crooks S, Rimmer CS. Role of fibronectin in the migration of fibroblasts into plasma clots. J Cell Biol 1986;102:2318–2323.

67. Kuwabara T, Perkins DG, Cogan DG. Sliding of the epithelium in experimental corneal wounds. Invest Ophthalmol 1976;15:4–14.

68. Leibovich SJ, Ross R. The role of the macrophage in wound repair. A study with hydrocortisone and antimacrophage serum. Am J Pathol 1975;78:71-100.

69. Leibovich SJ, Wiseman DM. Macrophages, wound repair and angiogenesis. Prog Clin Biol Res 1988;266:131–145.

70. Levenson SM, Geever EF, Crowley LV, Oates JF III, Berard CW, Rosen H. The healing of rat skin wounds. Ann Surg 1965;161:293–308.

71. Levenson SM, Demetriou AA. Metabolic factors. In: Cohen IK, Diegelmann RF, Lindblad WJ, eds. Wound healing: biochemical and clinical aspects. Philadelphia: WB Saunders 1992:248–273.

72. Li AKC, Koroly MJ, Schattenkerk ME, Malt RA, Young M. Nerve growth factor: acceleration of the rate of wound healing in mice. Proc Natl Acad Sci USA 1980;77:4379–4381.

73. Longaker MT, Whitby DJ, Adzick NS, et al. Studies in fetal wound healing. VI. Second and early third trimester fetal wounds demonstrate rapid collagen deposition without scar formation. J Pediatr Surg 1990;25:63–69.

74. Longaker MT, Adzick NS. The biology of fetal wound healing: a review. Plast Reconstr Surg 1991;87:788–798.

75. Lusthaus S, Shoshan S, Benmeir P, Livoff A, Ashur H, Vardy D. Effect of denervation on incision wound scars in rabbits. J Geriat Dermatol 1993;1:11-14.

76. Majno G. The healing hand. Man and wound in the ancient world. Cambridge, MA: Harvard University Press, 1975.

77. Majno G. The story of the myofibroblasts. Am J Surg Pathol 1979;3:535-542.

78. Majno G, Gabbiani G, Hirschel BJ, Ryan GB, Statkov PR. Contraction of granulation tissue in vitro: similarity to smooth muscle. Science 1971;173:548-550.

79. Majno G, Leventhal M. Pathogenesis of histamine-type vascular leakage. Lancet 1967;2:99–100.

80. McCarthy JB, Sas DF, Furcht LT. Mechanisms of parenchymal cell migration into wounds. In: Clark RAF, Henson PM, eds. The molecular and cellular biology of wound repair. New York: Plenum Press, 1988:281–319.

81. McPherson JM, Piez KA. Collagen in dermal wound repair. In: Clark RAF, Henson PM, eds. The molecular and cellular biology of wound repair. New York: Plenum Press, 1988:471–496.

82. Mochitate K, Pawelek P, Grinnell F. Stress relaxation of contracted collagen gels: disruption of actin filament bundles, release of cell surface fibronectin, and downregulation of DNA and protein synthesis. Exp Cell Res 1991;193:198–207.

83. Montesano R, Orci L. Transforming growth factor β stimulates collagen-matrix contraction by fibroblasts: implications for wound healing. Proc Natl Acad Sci USA 1988;85:4894–4897.

84. Moses JM, Ebert RH, Graham RC, Brine KL. Pathogenesis of inflammation. I. The production of an inflammatory substance from rabbit granulocytes in vitro and its relationship to leucocyte pyrogen. J Exp Med 1964;120:57–82.

85. Noble WC. The production of subcutaneous staphylococcal skin lesions in mice. Br J Exp Pathol 1965;46:254–262.

86. Ordman LJ, Gillman T. Studies in the healing of cutaneous wounds. I. The healing of incisions through the skin of pigs. Arch Surg 1966;93:857–882.

87. Peacock EE Jr. Pharmacologic control of surface scarring in human beings. Ann Surg 1981;193:592:597.

88. Peacock EE Jr. The wound repair. Philadelphia: WB Saunders, 1984.

89. Peacock EE Jr, Van Winkle W Jr. Surgery and biology of wound repair. Philadelphia: WB Saunders, 1970.

90. Pessa ME, Bland KI, Copeland EM III. Growth factors and determinants of wound repair. J Surg Res 1987;42:207–217.

91. Peters G, Gray ED, Johnson GM. Immunomodulating properties of extracellular slime substance. In: Bisno AL, Waldvogel FA, eds. Infections associated with indwelling medical devices. Washington, DC: American Society for Microbiology, 1989:61–74.

92. Pierce GF, Tarpley JE, Yanagihara D, Mustoe TA, Fox GM, Thomason A. Platelet-derived growth factor (BB Homodimer), transforming growth factor-β1, and basic fibroblast growth factor in dermal wound healing. Am J Pathol 1992;140:1375–1388.

93. Pierce GF, Vande Berg J, Rudolph R, Tarpley J, Mustoe TA. Platelet-derived growth factor-BB and transforming growth factor beta-1 selectively modulate glycosaminoglycans, collagen, and myofibroblasts in excisional wounds. Am J Pathol 1991;138:629–646.

94. Polverini PJ, Cotran RS, Gimbrone MA Jr, Unanue ER. Activated macrophages induce vascular proliferation. Nature 1977;269:804–806.

95. Prudden JF, Wolarsky ER, Balassa L. The acceleration of healing. Surg Gynecol Obstet 1969;128:1321–1326.

96. Repesh LA, Oberpiller JC. Ultrastructural studies on migrating epidermal cells during the wound healing stage of regeneration in the adult newt, *Notophthalmus viridescens*. Am J Anat 1980;159:187–208.

97. Root RK, Trunkey DD, Sande MA. New surgical and medical approaches in infectious diseases. Contemporary issues in infectious diseases, vol 6. New York: Churchill Livingstone, 1987.

98. Rosenfeld RM, Stool SE. Should granulomas be excised in children with long-term tracheotomy? Arch Otolaryngol Head Neck Surg 1992;118:1323–1327.

99. Rowlatt U. Intrauterine wound healing in a 20 week human fetus. Virchows Arch A Path Anat Histol 1979;381:353–361.

100. Rudolph R. Inhibition of myofibroblasts by skin grafts. Plast Reconstr Surg 1979;63:473–480.

101. Rudolph R, Ballantyne DL Jr. Skin grafts. In: McCarthy JG, May JW Jr, Littler JW. Plastic surgery, vol 1. Philadelphia: WB Saunders, 1990.

102. Ryan GB, Cliff WJ, Gabbiani G, et al. Myofibroblasts in human granulation tissue. Hum Pathol 1974;5:55–67.

103. Ryan GB, Majno G. Inflammation. (A Scope Publication.) Kalamazoo, MI: The Upjohn Company, 1977.

104. Sandison JC. Observations on the growth of blood vessels as seen in the transparent chamber introduced into the rabbit's ear. Am J Anat 1928;41:475–496.

105. Schürch W, Seemayer TA, Gabbiani G. Myofibroblast. In: Sternberg SS, ed. Histology for pathologists. New York: Raven Press, 1992.

106. Sciubba JJ, Waterhouse JP, Meyer J. A fine structural comparison of the healing of incisional wounds of mucosa and skin. J Oral Pathol 1978;7:214-227.

107. Shamberger R. Effect of chemotherapy and radiotherapy on wound healing: experimental studies. Recent Results Cancer Res 1985;98:17–34.

108. Simpson DM, Ross R. The neutrophilic leukocyte in wound repair. A study with antineutrophil serum. J Clin Invest 1972;51:2009–2023.

109. Skalli O, Schürch W, Seemayer T, et al. Myofibroblasts from diverse pathologic settings are heterogeneous in their content of actin isoforms and intermediate filament proteins. Lab Invest 1989;60:275–285.

110. Somasundaram K, Prathap K. Intra-uterine healing of skin wounds in rabbit foetuses. J Pathol 1970;100:81–86.

111. Somasundaram K, Prathap K. The effect of exclusion of anmiotic fluid on intra-uterine healing of skin wounds in rabbit foetuses. J Pathol 1972;107:127-130.

112. Squier CA. The effect of stretching on formation of myofibroblasts in mouse skin. Cell Tissue Res 1981;220:325–335.

113. Stenn KS, DePalma L. Re-epithelialization. In: Clark RAF, Henson PM, eds. The molecular and cellular biology of wound repair. New York: Plenum Press, 1988:321–335.

114. Taichman NS, Tsai C-C, Shenker BJ, Boehringer H. Neutrophil interactions with oral bacteria as a pathogenic mechanism in periodontal diseases. Adv Inflam Res 1984;8:113–142.

115. Tano Y, Chandler DB, Machemer R. Vascular casts of experimental retinal neovascularization. Am J Ophthalmol 1981;92:110–120.

116. Todd R, Donoff BR, Chiang T, et al. The eosinophil as a cellular source of transforming growth factor alpha in healing cutaneous wounds. Am J Pathol 1991;138:1307–1313.

117. Tsutsumi O, Tsutsumi A, Oka T. Epidermal growth factor-like, corneal wound healing substance in mouse tears. J Clin Invest 1988;81:1067–1071.

118. Vaudaux PE, Zulian G, Huggler E, Waldvogel FA. Attachment of *Staphylococcus aureus* to polymethylmethacrylate increases its resistance to phagocytosis in foreign body infection. Infect Immun 1985;50:472–477.

119. Wahl SM, Arend WP, Ross R. The effect of complement depletion on wound healing. Am J Pathol 1974;74:73–90.

120. Williams TJ. Factors that affect vessel reactivity and leukocyte emigration. In: Clark RAF, Henson PM, eds. The molecular and cellular biology of wound repair. New York: Plenum Press, 1988:115–147.

121. Williamson JR, Chang K, Rowold E, et al. Diabetes-induced increases in vascular permeability and changes in granulation tissue levels of sorbitol, *myo*-inositol, *chiro*-inositol, and *scyllo*-inositol are prevented by sorbinil. Metabolism 1986;35(suppl 1):41–45.

122. Winter GD. Movement of epidermal cells over the wound surface. Adv Biol Skin 1964;5:113–127.

123. Yoffey JM, Courtice FC. Lymphatics, lymph and the lymphomyeloid complex. London: Academic Press, 1970.

124. Zimmerli W, Lew PD, Waldvogel FA. Pathogenesis of foreign body infection. Evidence for a local granulocyte defect. J Clin Invest 1984;73:1191–1200.

125. Zimmerli W, Waldvogel FA, Vaudaux P, Nydegger UE. Pathogenesis of foreign body infection: description and characteristics of an animal model. J Infect Dis 1982;146:487–497.

General Effects of
Local Injury and
Inflammation

CHAPTER 15

Fever

Leukocytosis

The Acute Phase
Response

Increased Erythrocyte
Sedimentation Rate

Other General Effects
of Local Injury

In the economy of the body, injury (even if local) tends to affect the body as a whole. The chemical messages that escape from a focus of injury are of two kinds: (a) molecules from ruptured cells (such as lysosomal enzymes) that may be important in triggering inflammation but have few known general effects (p. 217), and (b) inflammatory mediators, primarily polypeptides (cytokines), that have a local function but may enter the blood stream in sufficient amounts to have biological effects. Bacterial products may also follow that route. On the whole, *the general effects are standard, that is, nonspecific.* Four such effects stand out; they can develop within one day of any significant injury:

• Fever: the body temperature rises
• Leukocytosis: the number of circulating leukocytes usually increases
• Acceleration of the erythrocyte sedimentation rate: simply stated, something peculiar happens to the red cells. If a sample of blood is withdrawn from an injured person, prevented from clotting, and allowed to stand, the red cells settle more quickly than normal. This phenomenon depends in turn on the next item in this list.

• The acute phase response: this response is a set of changes in the plasma proteins that is due to the fact that the liver undergoes a shift in its pattern of protein synthesis.

Disparate as they may seem, all these general effects of local injury can be reproduced by injecting macrophage products, such as *tumor necrosis factor (TNF), interleukin-1 (IL-1), or IL-6* (12). These cytokines are generated in almost any focus of inflammation, and they are extremely potent: TNF, as we will see, is the main agent of cachexia in individuals with malignant tumors. It is no wonder that one does not feel too well after a fracture or any other supposedly local mishap. Some of the general effects are obviously beneficial; others are not well understood.

Fever

Fever can be recognized by doctors, and mothers, without the benefit of a thermometer. It is often mentioned in the oldest Akkadian tablets and in the Hippocratic books (2,3,40). The Romans, perhaps because they were harassed by malaria, saw fit to give it a heavenly patron, the goddess *Febris* (41).

The first thermometer for measuring body temperature was designed around 1611 by Santorio Santorio, who probably borrowed the basic idea from his colleague in Padua, Galileo. However, the principle of thermometry was not adopted in routine medical practice until the mid-1800s (30).

THE GENESIS OF FEVER

Body temperature is regulated by a nucleus in the anterior hypothalamus, which functions as a thermostat, controlling the balance between heat production and heat loss. Stated in the simplest terms: fever develops when the thermostat is switched to a higher setting. For the body to reach a higher temperature, heat loss by the skin is reduced by vasoconstriction, so for a short time during a rising fever the skin, paradoxically, becomes cool. The moment of switching is clinically apparent as a chill, which means that the environmental temperature is suddenly perceived as too cool.

What resets the thermostat? The hunt for a chemical cause goes back to the 1800s.

In 1866 a German medical student, inspired by Billroth, the eminent surgeon–musician friend of Brahms, injected filtered autogenous pus into a cat and found that it produced fever (3,58). The cat escaped, but the experiment proved that pus contained "pyrogens." However, it remained to be decided whether these pyrogens were bacterial, leukocytic, or both. After nearly a century, in 1953, in a series of experiments that were hailed as classic, Bennett and Beeson proved that a preparation of "granulocytes" produced fever (6,58); many years later it turned out that the effect of Bennett's and Beeson's preparation was due primarily to a small fraction of contaminating monocytes (25).

Even after these early experiments suggested that leukocytes were the source of endogenous pyrogens, the next step was difficult to accomplish because fresh leukocytes contain no fever-inducing material. Monocytes *produce* endogenous pyrogenic cytokines (including TNF, IL-1, IL-6, and MPI-1) (11) only when they are exposed to certain phagocytizable exogenous (bacterial) pyrogens, especially endotoxin. These cytokine pyrogens affect the anterior hypothalamus by increasing the local synthesis of prostaglandin E_2 (PGE_2). *Aspirin opposes fever precisely by inhibiting cyclooxygenase in the hypothalamus.* TNF can also stimulate the hypothalamic center directly (37). With these facts at hand, it was easy to understand why endogenous pyrogens, injected intravenously, act almost immediately, whereas exogenous (bacterial) pyrogens act only after a delay of at least 30 minutes.

Exogenous pyrogens are many. The prototype is endotoxin, a lipopolysaccharide of the wall of gram-negative bacteria. Endotoxin lurks almost everywhere and causes much trouble to manufacturers of medical supplies, whose products must be pyrogen-free. Other exogenous pyrogens are found in gram-positive bacteria, viruses, and fungi.

IS FEVER USEFUL?

Sir William Osler, the "modern Hippocrates," once wrote that "Humanity has but three great enemies: fever, famine and war. Of these by far the greatest, by far the most terrible, is fever" (48). A century later it appears that Osler was equating fever with infection, and infections are indeed a great scourge. And they cause fever. But blaming fever for the misdeeds of infection is assuming guilt by association. In 1927, just eight years after the death of Osler, the Nobel prize for medicine was given to Wagner-Jauregg for his method of treating neurosyphilis with fever by actually giving malaria to the patients (30); the basic idea was to cook the spirochetes, which are known to die at temperatures above 41°C (30). There are strains of pneumococci that die at temperatures as low as 40°C, easily within reach of fever in rabbits; pneumococcal virulence in this animal can actually be correlated with the ability of the cocci to survive at 41°C (30). These facts and many others (30,32,39) argue for a useful effect of fever in infections.

In mammals, however, it has been difficult to prove beyond doubt that fever has a general survival value. The experimental procedure is to compare the survival of two groups, one treated and one not treated with antipyretics; thus one can always argue that antipyretics might have effects other than decreasing body temperature. The problem was solved ingeniously by a physiologist who chose to study animals in which body temperature can be raised or lowered without drugs: lizards (Figure 15.1) (30).

Like snakes and other poikilotherms, lizards set their own temperature either by exposing part of their body to the sun, just enough to produce the desired overall temperature, or by moving back and forth between sun and shade. Kluger placed his small iguanas in a sand box, part of which was warmed by heat lamps; the lizards were free to shuttle back and forth between the warm and the cool parts, and thereby to choose their own temperature anywhere between that of the room and 50°C. They chose about 38°C; but if they had been injected with appropriate gram-negative

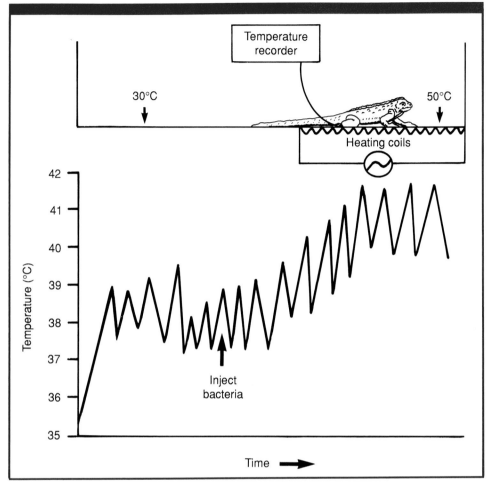

FIGURE 15.1

Top: Self-regulation of body temperature in the lizard *Dipsosaurus dorsalis*, kept in a sand box. Left side of sand box is set at 30°C. Lizard moves back and forth between the two sides, thereby selecting its appropriate body temperature, 38°C (measured by a thermocouple inserted into the cloaca and taped to the tail). *Bottom:* Self-induced fever in a lizard injected with pathogenic bacteria. Before the injection: The lizard migrates back and forth, maintaining an average temperature of about 38°C.) A few hours after being inoculated with pathogenic bacteria (**arrow**), the lizard begins to adjust its body to higher temperatures, eventually reaching 43°C. (Reproduced with permission from [30].)

bacteria (reptilian pathogens) they gave themselves fever by choosing 42°C. If they were prevented from doing so and kept at 38°C, within 24 hours half of them were dead. A similar experiment can be done with fish swimming in communicating tanks at different temperatures (30).

Kluger's experiments prove beyond doubt that fever *can* have survival value. In retrospect, this is logical. The capacity to react to infection with fever has been found in all vertebrates that have been tested (30). If evolution has preserved this energy-consuming reaction for so long, it is not likely to be worthless. An exception should be made for high fevers, beyond the 40–41°C range, which are generally considered dangerous. The truth therefore seems to be in the camp of Thomas Sydenham, the "English Hippocrates" (1624–1689), who wrote some 300 years ago that "fever is Nature's engine which she brings into the field to remove her enemy" (30).

How can fever be useful? The bacteria-killing effect may not be the only answer. It is proven that

leukocytes move faster as temperature rises (Figure 15.2), and many other cellular functions may be involved (14,30). Recent studies show, for example, that both IL-1 and TNF are more effective at higher temperatures (TNF kills more tumor cells [37]).

To conclude, it may seem that the time should have come to reexamine the reflex habit of "curing fevers" with aspirin and the like (30,31). Yet, in practice, fevers continue to be "cured". We can see several reasons. One is that the experimental evidence is marred by a few exceptions: in a recent review, 13 experimental models showed that fever helped against infection, 3 that it made matters worse (39). However, exceptions should not negate the rule. Similarly, it was reported in the 1960s that in humans there was no correlation between fever and survival, but more recent data show a positive correlation (39). Last, antipyretics are also analgesics, and make patients feel more comfortable; thus there is no good reason to withdraw aspirin in self-limited infections. In essence, the data show that "the best approach to

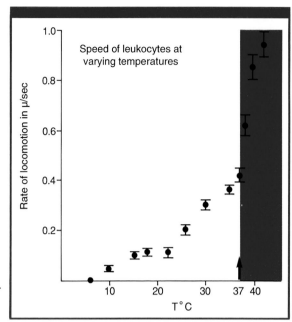

FIGURE 15.2
Rate of locomotion of human neutrophils as a function of temperature. **Red bar:** Range of fever. (Adapted from [46].)

fever would apparently be to let it run its course" (39)—at least in severe infections.

COMPARISON WITH HYPERTHERMIA

Hyperthermia refers to an increase in body temperature *above* the thermostat setting which remains normal; it is therefore improper to use this term interchangeably with fever (52,53). The body becomes hyperthemic *when heat dissipation cannot keep up with the amount of heat produced or absorbed.* Classic examples are heat stroke, a hazard of hot environments, and exertion heat stroke, typically seen in untrained joggers; in this latter case rectal temperatures can exceed 41.5°C (26).

Hyperthermia has attracted much interest since it became a therapeutic modality in cancer (p. 937). Using focal hyperthermia produced with radio waves, minimal necrosis of muscle begins to occur after 30 minutes at 40–43°C (44). Cell membranes are irreversibly damaged at temperatures between 41 and 45°C; both proteins and lipids are probably affected (38). It is no wonder that body temperatures exceeding 41°C (106°F) should be regarded as medical emergencies (13).

Malignant hyperthermia syndrome *(fulminant hyperthermia) is a genetic disease of humans, swine, cats, dogs, and horses; it is a sudden hypermetabolic state of striated muscle that is unleashed accidentally in 1 in 10,000–15,000 general anesthesias. The cause appears to be an excessive release of calcium by the sarcoplasmic reticulum in response to neuronal stimulation (49a). The syndrome can be triggered in* swine and horses by sudden stress (47). In the 1950s, 30 members of one family died of anesthesia before the disease was recognized (24). The temperature can rise at the rate of 1°C every 5 minutes, reaching 44.4°C in humans and 48.2°C in a strain of predisposed swine. Aspirin is quite useless in such cases because the target of aspirin is the thermostat, which is not involved.

Leukocytosis

Human blood contains 4,000–10,000 leukocytes per mm^3; numbers above and below these limits denote *leukocytosis* and *leukopenia*. The predominant leukocyte in human blood is the neutrophil; in rats and mice, the predominant cell is the lymphocyte (Table 15.1).

Neutrophilia (neutrophil leukocytosis) is a common effect of injury and especially of infections with pyogenic (pus-generating) bacteria (Table 15.2). It has survival value by helping to recruit more leukocytes to the battlefield. Normally more than half of all neutrophils are not circulating but are held in a "loosely marginating" pool (1); *loosely* means that wherever these neutrophils may be, margination is not followed by diapedesis. These neutrophils are immediately available and can be released by stress and exercise, and artifically by an injection of epinephrine.

Leukocytosis induced by trauma or infection is sustained by the colony-stimulating factors (CSFs) (45), small glycoproteins that promote bone-marrow hyperplasia; in and around injured tissues they can be produced by many cell types, including monocytes and endothelial cells (51). After trauma, greatly increased levels of CSFs appear in

Table 15.1
White Blood Cells: Normal Counts

	HUMAN ADULTS	RATS
Total (per-μl)	4,000–11,000	6,000–18,000
Neutrophils	60%	15–20%
Eosinophils	3%	1–4%
Basophils	0.6%	Rare
Monocytes	4%	6%
Lymphocytes	33%	86%

Table 15.2
Neutrophil Leukocytosis:
Major Causes

Physiologic	Exercise
	Stress
	Epinephrine
	Steriod therapy
Infections	Bacterial, especially pyogenic bacteria; some fungal, parasitic, and viral diseases
Inflammation	Burns
	Necrosis (e.g. myocardial and pulmonary infarction, trauma)
	Connective tissue ("collagen") diseases: myositis, vasculitis
Metabolic disorders	Ketoacidosis
	Uremia
	Eclampsia
	Gout
Other:	Tumors of many types
	Acute hemorrhage or hemolysis
	Idiopathic

Adapted from (10)

the serum and in the urine, where they were first detected (57).

Few drugs cause leukocytosis, in contrast with the many that cause leukopenia. Corticosteroids lead to leukocytosis by several mechanisms: they impair the diapedesis of leukocytes, prolong their life span, and enhance their release from the bone marrow.

The Acute Phase Response

The acute phase response is a prominent but still poorly understood phenomenon (21,35,36). Within hours of injury (such as trauma, surgery, infection) the pattern of protein synthesis by the liver is drastically altered, as shown by the composition of the plasma: for some proteins, such as albumin, liver synthesis is decreased (these have been called "negative" acute phase reaction proteins); for others, such as fibrinogen, it is increased (these are the "positive" acute phase proteins, shown in Table 15.3). Despite its name, the acute phase reaction can become chronic. It is triggered by cytokines (TNF, IL-1, IL-6) released by cells of an inflammatory focus (macrophages, endothelium, fibroblasts). Of course, the liver cells can only respond if the focus of inflammation can produce enough cytokines (a pimple will not do); in practice, if the inflammatory focus is large enough to alert the liver cells, it is large enough to cause clinical concern.

Table 15.3
Positive Acute Phase Proteins in Humans

PROTEIN	NORMAL PLASMA CONCENTRATION (MG/DL)	OBSERVED INCREASE	SELECTED BIOLOGIC FUNCTIONS
Ceruloplasmin	15–60	50%	Cu transport; free radical scavenger
C3 (complement component)	80–170	50%	Modification of inflammation; host defense
α_1-Acid glycoprotein	55–140	2–3×	Modification of inflammation
α_1-Antitrypsin	200–400	2–3×	Protease inhibition
Haptoglobin	40–180	2–3×	Hemoglobin transport
Fibrinogen	200–450	2–3×	Coagulation
C-reactive protein	<0.5	100–1000×	Inflammation, host defense
Protein SAA	<10	100–1000×	Unknown

Adapted from (21)

Some features of the acute phase response have been noticed after infarcts, and in patients with malignant tumors, as well as in pregnancy and in the early neonatal state. This suggests that the changes can be helpful; and for some of the "positive" proteins a helpful role can indeed be rationalized (Table 15.3). For example:

- *Decrease in plasma iron* (hypoferremia or hyposideremia): this can be understood as an antibacterial measure, because iron is a growth factor for many bacteria (8,56).

This change has a complicated 3-step mechanism: the activated neutrophils release lactoferrin, an iron-binding protein; lactoferrin snatches away the iron from serum transferrin, another iron-binding protein; and finally, the iron-laden lactoferrin is phagocytized by the monocyte-macrophage system and stored away as ferritin (55). A hyposideremia after infection was found even in lizards (23).

- *Increase in C3:* this molecule is the key component of complement; as such it is an essential antibacterial weapon.
- *Increase in ceruloplasmin:* this blue, copper-containing protein, can act as a scavenger of free radicals, clearly a defensive function (22).
- *Increase in C-reactive protein* (CRP): CRP appears to be part of a beautiful system: IL-1 stimulates the secretion of CRP; CRP binds to damaged tissue components, and makes them better suited for phagocytosis (i.e. it is an opsonin); the macrophages take up the complex, and become activated, thereby secreting more IL-1.
- *Increase in alpha-1-antitrypsin:* this protein inactivates dangerous proteases that might be released by damaged cells.
- *Increase in fibrinogen:* this molecule is essential for coagulation, which is be needed for stopping hemorrhages resulting from injury.

By contrast, it is very difficult to rationalize the enormous increase in SAA (serum amyloid A). If the concentration of a plasma protein rises one-thousandfold, as can occur with SAA, it would seem that this protein plays some important role; but all we know for the time being about this particular change is that, in the long run, the price of high SAA can be amyloidosis, a lethal disease (p. 268). Another baffling fact about SAA is its molecular structure, which is similar to that of CRP: it has been likened to a cluster of five berries (hence the name *pentraxins* for this class of pro-

teins) (p. 270, 277) (4,21). SAA is associated with high-density lipoproteins (HDL) and appears to depress the type of immune response called delayed hypersensitivity; we have already mentioned its hazard as an amyloid precursor. CRP is quite harmless and has an interesting history (43,49).

The C-reactive protein was discovered in 1930 at the Hospital of the Rockefeller Institute in the days when pneumococcal pneumonia was deadly. The study of type-specific antibodies against pneumococci was a top priority because they were the only known way to treat the disease. Something very strange turned up in the serum of febrile patients admitted with pneumonia: it invariably contained a protein that reacted specifically with a crude pneumococcal antigen named "fraction C"; however, it was not likely to be an antibody because it appeared too soon. In fact, it behaved in a way that was opposite to that of antibodies: it began to drop while type-specific agglutinating antibodies rose. Even more baffling was the subsequent finding that this C-reactive protein also appeared in the serum of patients with other acute diseases (43). The logical conclusion was that CRP could not be a specific effect of pneumonia; it was somehow related to the acute phase of disease in general. Soon, other proteins were found to behave in a similar fashion. Thus were born two rather unwieldy names, the C-reactive protein and the acute phase response.

Intensive studies of CRP (21,36) suggest that it can bind to a number of surfaces and influence several functions of the blood (e.g., platelet aggregation).

CRP responds so fast to acute disease that it has been proposed as a clinical barometer to assess the severity of a patient's condition (21). In practice, however, few hospitals use this test (54); it is much simpler to measure the erythrocyte sedimentation rate, which reflects the rise of another acute phase protein, fibrinogen.

Increased Erythrocyte Sedimentation Rate

Although some authors (29) consider it quaint, the simple test of measuring the erythrocyte sedimentation rate (ESR) continues to be a reliable screening test for the medical practitioner. In about 1 hour it can answer two basic questions: Is there tissue damage somewhere in this patient? If so, how severe is the damage? For this reason, this test was widely used for the prognosis of tuberculosis and syphilis in patients before the advent of antibiotics.

The principle was discovered in 1894 and forgotten (34), and then rediscovered in a classic paper by Fårhaeus in 1929 (16).

The principle of the ESR test is the following. Normally, the blood forms a stable suspension because the density of the red blood cells (1.09) is close to that of the plasma (1.03). Therefore, if blood (2 ml) is anticoagulated and poured into a vertical tube, the red blood cells settle very slowly; after 1 hour, they have settled only 0–10 mm in men and 1–15 mm in women as measured by the commonly used Westergren method.

The driving force that causes the red blood cells to fall is their weight (generally speaking, the weight of spherical particles increases by the cube of the radius). This driving force is opposed by the resistance offered by the plasma, which increases only with the radius of the falling particles (17). This means that the larger the particles, the faster they fall: stones sink faster than sand. Now, the red blood cells in blood taken during an acute phase reaction tend to aggregate into **rouleaux** (rolls) resembling piles of coins (Figure 15.3). The rouleaux are the equivalent of stones: they sink faster.

What produces rouleaux? Under normal conditions the red blood cells repel each other by their similar charges; but if the plasma contains a large number of elongated molecules such as fibrinogen, these molecules tend to become attracted by the surfaces of the red blood cells (reason unknown), and this coating reduces the repelling effect of the surface charges (21). Because fibrinogen is one of the positive acute phase proteins, the ESR reflects the acute phase response (Figure 15.4). Rouleaux can also be seen on blood smears (Figure 15.5), but this fact is not used as a test.

It must be understood that the ESR test is very nonspecific; after all, it reflects the nonspecific acute phase response. It should be used only as a quick way to find out if "something is really wrong" while remembering that a normal value may not exclude diseases that are unrelated to tissue damage, including many malignancies. It can even reflect pregnancy. As a matter of fact, it was discovered in the course of a study of blood changes in pregnancy.

The phenomenon of increased sedimentation rate was observed in antiquity and had an enormous impact on medical practice well into the 1800s. It was customary in bloodletting, from the time of Hippocrates and for 2200 years afterward, to collect the blood in a basin, where it eventually clotted. If a patient's ESR was high, the red blood cells might be

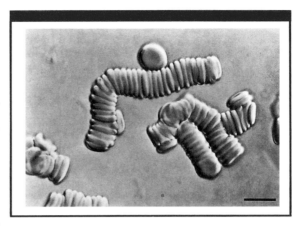

FIGURE 15.3
Red blood cells forming typical rouleaux, by interference microscopy. **Bar** = 10 μm. (Reproduced with permission from [7].)

able to settle a few millimeters before clotting; then, when clotting did occur, the blood would be divided into two layers as in Figure 15.6: a bottom red layer and a superficial whitish jelly (actually a fibrin clot) called the buffy coat. To ancient observers this meant that the blood in that patient contained an abnormal whitish material, supposedly the pernicious "phlegm"; such blood was referred to as "sizy" and the fibrin layer became known as the phlogistic crust (crusta phlogistica). The logical therapy was to draw more blood so as to remove more of that pernicious phlegm. As more and more blood was drawn, the patient became anemic; and because anemia accelerates the sedimentation rate, the cycle was self-perpetuating (16). Worse yet, pregnant women were systematically bled well into the past century, because, as we mentioned, their ESR is always accelerated (16). Nobody knows how many patients died of this therapy. Such is the power of theory.

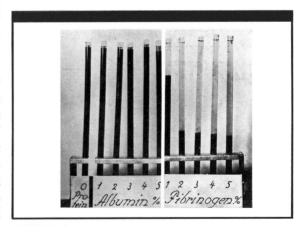

FIGURE 15.4
Mechanism of accelerated sedimentation rate, demonstrated by suspending red blood cells in solutions of plasma proteins. Albumin solutions of increasing concentrations (1.3–6.3%) do not increase the sedimentation rate of red blood cells after 3 hours. Fibrinogen solutions of 1–5% do increase the sedimentation rate (normal concentration of fibrinogen in plasma: 0.15–0.35 g/100 ml). (Reproduced with permission form [15].)

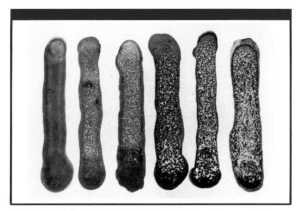

FIGURE 15.5
Blood smears prepared from six drops of blood with sedimentation rates of 2, 7, 28, 40, 68, and 102 mm/h (from left to right). The subjects were, respectively, a healthy man, a healthy woman, a pregnant woman, a man with appendicitis, a man with pneumonia, and a man with sepsis. The increasingly granular aspect of the smears is due to the formation of rouleaux. (Reproduced with permission from [15].)

FIGURE 15.6
Buffy coat produced by blood with a high sedimentation rate: a phenomenon that had a tremendous impact on the history of medicine. (Reproduced with permission from [15].)

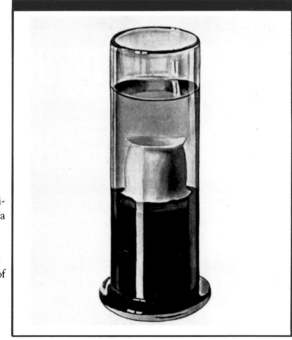

Other General Effects of Local Injury

The *sleepiness* and *lack of appetite* (anorexia) that appear after serious injury are best considered as part of the acute phase response, and therefore as cytokine-induced (35). The same is true for the typical anemia of chronic inflammation, due in part to de*pressed production of erythropoietin. The mechanism of muscular pain* (myalgia) so common in fever is not well understood; however, it is a fact that striated muscle during the acute phase response shows accelerated proteolysis; the effect can be duplicated by IL-1, and it is reversed by aspirin, which indicates that it is mediated by prostaglandins (5).

Severe injury also elicits what is known to the public as *stress*, scientifically the *hypothalamic-pituitary-adrenal stress response*. This is a complex, non-specific endocrine response that has been the topic of many volumes (50). It may occur also after psychological challenges, in the absence of physical damage (20,42). Among its many effects we will cite two: it depresses some cellular inflammatory functions (27) and increases the susceptibility to the common cold in humans (9).

This endocrine stress response intersects with the acute phase response in that it can be initiated by IL-1 and IL-6 (35); indeed, corticosteroids can be considered as cofactors of the acute phase response (35). It is no wonder that the metabolic consequences of injury are so complex.

Last but not least, *a generalized protective effect of inflammation* has been described at the Pasteur Institute in Paris (18), using an experimental model based on granulomas in mice. We have already mentioned that granulomas can be construed as organs of internal secretion (p. 447). Talcum-induced granulomas generate a protein that protects mice against an otherwise lethal infection (19) and exerts a cytostatic effect against a highly malignant mouse tumor (18). This amounts to a general increase in resistance, which is a sort of bonus in addition to the local protective effect of inflammation.

TO SUM UP: there is no such thing as a purely local injury. Almost immediately after the local alarm is sounded, cytokines deliver messages to the white blood cells, to the red blood cells, to the liver, and to the thermostat in the brain; at the same time an endocrine response is unleashed, hormones step in, and the entire body becomes involved. We will recall once again the similarity between the microcosm of the cell (remember the heat-shock proteins, p. 175) and the macrocosm of the liver: both respond to injury by altering their pattern of protein synthesis, and for the same basic reason—adjusting priorities.

References

1. Athens JW, Haab OP, Raab SO, et al. Leukokinetic studies. IV. The total blood, circulating and marginal granulocyte pools and the granulocyte turnover rate in normal subjects. J Clin Invest 1961;40:989–995.

2. Atkins E. Fever: its history, cause, and function. Yale J Biol Med 1982;55:283–289.

3. Atkins E. Fever: the old and the new. J Infect Dis 1984;149:339–348.

4. Baltz ML, de Beer FC, Feinstein A, et al. Phylogenetic aspects of C-reactive protein and related proteins. Ann NY Acad Sci 1982;389:49–75.

5. Baracos V, Rodemann HP, Dinarello CA, Goldberg AL. Stimulation of muscle protein degradation and prostaglandin E_2 release by leukocytic pyrogen (interleukin-1). N Engl J Med 1983;308:553–558.

6. Bennett IL Jr, Beeson PB. Studies on the pathogenesis of fever. I. The effect of injection of extracts and suspensions of uninfected rabbit tissues upon the body temperature of normal rabbits. J Exp Med 1953;98:477–492.

7. Bessis M. Living blood cells and their ultrastructure. New York: Springer-Verlag, 1973.

8. Bullen JJ. The significance of iron in infection. Rev Infect Dis 1981;3:1127–1138.

9. Cohen S, Tyrrell DAJ, Smith AP. Psychological stress and susceptibility to the common cold. N Engl J Med 1991;325:606–612.

10. Dale DC. Leukocytosis, leukopenia, and eosinophilia. In: Wilson JD, Braunwald E, Isselbacher KJ, et al., eds. Harrison's principles of internal medicine, 12th ed. New York: McGraw-HIll, 1991.

11. Davatelis G, Wolpe SD, Sherry B, Dayer J-M, Chicheportiche R, Cerami A. Macrophage inflammatory protein-1: a prostaglandin-independent endogenous pyrogen. Science 1989;243:1066–1068.

12. Dinarello CA. The endogenous pyrogens in host-defense interactions. Hosp Pract 1989;24:111–128.

13. Donaldson JF. Therapy of acute fever: a comparative approach. Hosp Pract 1981;16:125–138.

14. Duff GW, Durum SK. Fever and immunoregulation: hyperthermia, interleukins 1 and 2, and T-cell proliferation. Yale J Biol Med 1982;55:437–442.

15. Fåhraeus R. The suspension-stability of the blood. Acta Med Scand 1921;55:1–228.

16. Fåhraeus R. The suspension stability of the blood. Physiol Rev 1929;9:241–274.

17. Florey HW. General pathology, 4th ed. Philadelphia: WB Saunders, 1970.

18. Fontan E, Fauve RM. Inflammation and anti-tumor resistance. IV. Induction of cytostatic activity of murine peritoneal cells by a mouse granuloma protein. Int J Cancer 1988;42:267–272.

19. Fontan E, Fauve RM, Hevin B, Jusforgues H. Immunostimulatory mouse granuloma protein. Proc Natl Acad Sci USA 1983;80:6395–6398.

20. Ganong WF. The stress response—a dynamic overview. Hosp Pract 1988;23:155–171.

21. Gewurz H. Biology of C-reactive protein and the acute phase response. Hosp Pract 1982;17:67–81.

22. Goldstein IM, Kaplan HB, Edelson HS, Weissmann G. Ceruloplasmin. A scavenger of superoxide anion radicals. J Biol Chem 1979;254:4040–4045.

23. Grieger TA, Kluger MJ. Fever and survival: the role of serum iron. J Physiol 1978;279:187–196.

24. Gronert GA. Malignant hyperthermia. Anesthesiology 1980;53:395–423.

25. Hanson DF, Murphy PA, Windle BE. Failure of rabbit neutrophils to secrete endogenous pyrogen when stimulated with staphylococci. J Exp Med 1980;151:1360–1371.

26. Hanson PG, Zimmerman SW. Heatstroke in road races. N Engl J Med 1979;300:96–97.

27. Henricks PAJ, Binkhorst GJ, Nijkamp FP. Stress diminishes infiltration and oxygen metabolism of phagocytic cells in calves. Inflammation 1987;11:427-437.

28. Isselbacher KJ, Adams RD, Braunwald E, Petersdorf RG, Wilson JD, eds. Harrison's principles of internal medicine, 9th ed. New York: McGraw-Hill, 1980.

29. Jandl JH. Blood. Boston: Little, Brown, 1987.

30. Kluger MJ. Fever. Its biology, evolution, and function. Princeton, NJ: Princeton University Press, 1979.

31. Kluger MJ. Phylogeny of fever. Fed Proc 1979;38:30–34.

32. Kluger MJ. Fever revisited. Pediatrics 1992; 90:846–850.

33. Konijn AM, Hershko C. Ferritin synthesis in inflammation. I. Pathogenesis of impaired iron release. Br J Haematol 1977;37:7–16.

34. Kucharz E. 80th anniversary of the discovery of erythrocyte sedimentation rate. Mater Med Pol 1975;7:344–346.

35. Kushner I. Regulation of the acute phase response by cytokines. Perspect Biol Med 1993;34:611–622.

36. Kushner I, Volanakis JE, Gewurz H, eds. C-reactive protein and the plasma protein response to tissue injury. Ann NY Acad Sci 1982;389.

37. Le J, Vilcek J. Tumor necrosis factor and interleukin 1: cytokines with multiple overlapping biological activities. Lab Invest 19872;56:234–248.

38. Lepock JR. Involvement of membranes in cellular responses to hyperthermia. Radiat Res 1982;92:433–438.

39. Mackowiak P. Fever: modern insights into an ancient clinical sign. Contemp Intern Med 1992;4:17–28.

40. Majno G. The healing hand: man and wound in the ancient world. Cambridge, MA: Harvard University Press, 1975.

41. Majno G. The ancient riddle of sepsis. J Infect Dis 1991;163:937–945.

42. Makara GB. Mechanisms by which stressful stimuli activate the pituitary-adrenal system. Fed Proc 1985;44:149–153.

43. McCarty M. Historical perspective on C-reactive protein. Ann NY Acad Sci 1982;389:1–10.

44. Meshorer A, Prionas SD, Fajardo LF, Meyer JL, Hahn GM, Martinez AA. The effects of hyperthermia on normal mesenchymal tissues. Arch Pathol Lab Med 1983;107:328–334.

45. Metcalf D. The molecular control of normal and leukaemic granulocytes and macrophages. Proc R Soc Lond [Biol] 1987;230:389–423.

46. Nahas GG, Tannieres ML, Lennon JF. Direct measurement of leukocyte motility: effects of pH and temperature. Proc Soc Exp Biol Med 1971;138:350-352.

47. Olgin J, Argov Z, Rosenberg H, Tuchler M, Chance B. Non-invasive evaluation of malignant hyperthermia susceptibility with phosphorus nuclear magnetic resonance spectroscopy. Anesthesiology 1988;68:507–513.

48. Osler W. The study of the fevers of the South. JAMA 1896;26:999–1004.

49. Pepys MB, Baltz ML. Acute phase proteins with special reference to C-reactive protein and related proteins (pentaxins) and serum amyloid A protein. Adv Immunol 1983;34:141–212.

49a. Rubenstein E. Malignant hyperthermia. In: Rubenstein E, Federman DD (eds). *Scientific American Medicine*. New York: Scientific American, Inc., 1993; Sect. 8V, pp. 1–2.

50. Selye H. Stress without distress. Philadelphia: JB Lippincott, 1974.

51. Sieff CA, Tsai S, Faller DV. Interleukin 1 induces cultured human endothelial cell production of granulocyte-macrophage colony-stimulating factor. J Clin Invest 1987;79:48–51.

52. Simon HB. Hyperthemia. In: Desforges JF, ed. Current concepts. N Engl J Med 1993;329:483–488.

53. Stitt JT. Fever versus hyperthermia. Fed Proc 1979; 38:39–43.

54. Van Lente F. The diagnostic utility of C-reactive protein. Hum Pathol 1982;13:1061–1063.

55. Van Snick JL, Masson PL, Heremans JF. The involvement of lactoferrin in the hyposideremia of acute inflammation. J Exp Med 1974;140:1068–1084.

56. Ward CG, Hammond JS, Bullen JJ. Effect of iron compounds on antibacterial function of human polymorphs and plasma. Infect Immun 1986;51:723–730.

57. Weiner HL, Robinson WA. Leukopoietic activity in human urine following operative procedures. Proc Soc Exp Biol Med 1971;136:29–33.

58. Wood WB Jr. Studies on the cause of fever. N Engl J Med 1958;258:1023-1031.

Variations and Aberrations of the Inflammatory Response

Inflammation in Tissues Devoid of Blood Vessels

Inflammation in Different Organs

Inflammation in Organs with a Blood-Tissue Barrier

Inflammation in the Newborn

Inflammation in Invertebrates

Life Without Inflammation: The Case of Plants

Inflammation as a Cause of Damage

Failures of the Inflammatory Response

The inflammatory response always obeys its own basic rule—to create an exudate—but the intensity of the process, its side effects and the final result vary a great deal according to the tissue, the age and state of health of the subject, as well as many other factors. The inflammatory response can also be defective for congenital or acquired reasons.

Inflammation in Tissues Devoid of Blood Vessels

By definition, inflammation is a response to injury of vascularized tissues. What happens if there are no vessels are present? The lost cells will simply regenerate if they can, and an inflammatory response may develop in the nearest vascularized tissue.

THE CASE OF THE CORNEA

The cornea has no vessels. If it is scratched, surprisingly, some neutrophils appear in the scratch, but they do not crawl in from the rim (the *limbus*)—they "jump over" from the covering eyelid. Historically these leukocytes caused much trouble: because they were not seen wandering in from the rim, they were taken as proof that corneal fibroblasts could turn into leukocytes. The scratch itself will heal by epithelial regeneration, without becoming truly inflamed, unless bacteria take over. If the injury is severe or persistent, blood vessels grow toward it from the limbus; they advance within the thickness of the cornea like a whitish, opaque sheet called **pannus** (Latin for sheet). The pannus reaches its target, becomes granulation tissue, and the cornea then can develop inflammation as any other vascularized tissue. Eventually the pannus may regress.

ARTICULAR CARTILAGE

In arthritis the inflammatory process rages in the synovial membrane; the cartilage itself is involved only passively, being bathed in the inflammatory exudate. This kind of bath is not a treat, because leukocytes can damage the cartilage matrix. In the long run the entire layer of cartilage may be destroyed and replaced by a vascular *pannus* arising from the rim of the articular surface. The lack of articular cartilage leads to arthritis.

Inflammation in Different Organs

This topic has not been studied in detail, but the following are two clear cut cases.

INFLAMMATION IN THE CENTRAL NERVOUS SYSTEM

For most organs it is almost automatic to consider the sequence *injury* → *inflammation,* but in the central nervous system the sequence is rather *injury* → [*inflammation + ischemia + free radical damage*]. Ischemia tends to develop as a secondary effect because nervous tissue is tightly packed (it has almost no extracellular spaces), it has no lymphatic drainage, and being locked inside a box of bone, it cannot swell or expand to accommodate the exudate. If it does become acutely inflamed, the sorry sequence of events is:

- leaky vessels produce exudate and increase tissue pressure;
- a rise in tissue pressure causes ischemia (13,21);
- should this ischemia abate, reperfusion and reoxygenation of ischemic tissues generate free radicals (p. 687);
- nervous tissue is especially sensitive to free radical damage because myelin is rich in lipids, which are favorite targets of free radicals;
- any red blood cells spilled out by injury or by the inflammatory response release hemo-

globin and thereby create the conditions for iron-dependent generation of free radicals (45);
- any parenchymal damage due to inflammation will not be followed by significant regeneration.

INFLAMMATION IN THE KIDNEY

As few as ten *Escherichia coli* or staphylococci injected into the renal medulla of some experimental animals can start an infection, whereas over 10,000 are needed to infect the cortex (27). The inflammatory response in the medulla is thought to be poor for several reasons, including a lower blood supply and a hypertonic extracellular fluid that depresses phagocytosis by the polymorphs.

Inflammation in Organs with a Blood-Tissue Barrier

These include the brain and cord, the nerves, the testes and apparently also the superficial layer of the dermis (p. 303). The organ most studied is the brain (39,57). We have posed the key question to several experts, namely, what happens when the blood–brain barrier is broken down? The answers provided only one hard fact: *in the short run (hours) a breakdown of the barrier is not critical.* This can be shown experimentally; a standard way to break down the barrier is to inject hypertonic solutions (Figure 16.1). As a matter of fact, much effort is being spent on producing temporary breakdown of the blood–brain barrier in order to increase the local delivery of drugs, such as antibiotics. Around brain abscesses the barrier is broken (39).

Inflammation in the Newborn

The inflammatory response in the newborn is defective in almost all respects, and the immune response is also defective. In fact, *the human neonate can be considered an immunocompromised host* (Table 16.1). (15,55). The diminished responsiveness of the newborn extends to the blood vessels (32), as has been demonstrated quite dramatically in rodents (28). Correspondingly, and disappointingly, neonatal sepsis is still a major problem in the United States; its incidence is still 1–10 cases for every 1000 live births, accounting

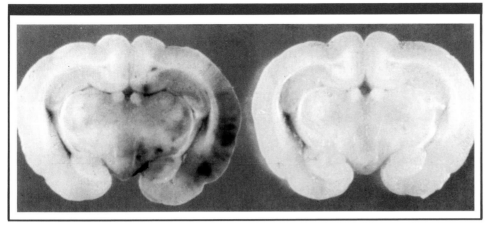

FIGURE 16.1
Coronal sections of two rabbit brains. In both rabbits the blood–brain barrier was broken with a hypertonic solution of urea (2 Osm) injected into the right carotid artery. Evans blue was injected intravenously before the dose of urea in the first animal (*left*) and 30 minutes after the dose of urea in the second animal (*right*). A broken barrier is indicated by the dark staining; the damage is repaired within 30 minutes. (Reproduced with permission from [42].)

for 30 percent of all neonatal deaths (59). It is clear that newborns are not well prepared to fight infections.

Inflammation in Invertebrates

If we attempt to reconstruct the evolution of the inflammatory response by studying it in animals simpler than warm-blooded vertebrates, we find that its simplest expression is phagocytosis, which is already present in single-cell creatures (p. 296), together with the heat-shock response. When blood vessels appear, with them comes diapedesis.

TABLE 16.1
Defects of Inflammation in the Newborn

Increased neutrophil rigidity
Reduced neutrophil and monocyte chemotaxis
Reduced neutrophil and monocyte locomotion
Reduced neutrophil and monocyte adherence
Reduced neutrophil anaerobic glycolysis
Reduced neutrophil bactericidal ability
Reduced serum opsonic ability
Reduced complement components (one-third to one-half)
Reduced antibody response
Reduced cell-mediated immune response

Adapted from (43)

Thus, despite the lack of *rubor* and *calor*, a simplified version of inflammation exists also in invertebrates (8). Remember that Metchnikoff's pioneer work on inflammation was done on starfish larvae and water fleas. His book, incidentally, *Lectures on the Comparative Pathology of Inflammation*, is still unsurpassed, still in print (34), and still great reading. Much is known about inflammation in mollusks and especially oysters, presumably because they make good food and beautiful pearls. Foreign bodies that penetrate into the body of mollusks are submitted to *encapsulation* (16): they are surrounded by all-purpose blood cells called *hemocytes*, which form a sort of granuloma, with an outer fibrous layer as one might also expect in vertebrates. Any parasite or foreign body that is trapped between the body of an oyster and its shell will irritate the covering epithelium of the body, called *mantle*; eventually it will be coated—on the mantle side—with the normal secretion of the mantle, which is *nacre* or mother-of-pearl. This accident, called *nacrezation*, produces half a pearl; the trick of producing a whole pearl is accomplished by grafting into the body of an oyster a piece of mantle, next to a spherical object; the epithelium of the mantle then will grow over the sphere and continue to produce mother-of-pearl. In 2–3 years the coat will be thick enough to produce the effect of a natural pearl (Figure 16.2).

There are analogous processes in human pathology. In certain malignant tumors of the epidermis (squamous cell carcinomas), pegs of epidermis invade the dermis. The basal cells are on the outside, and they tend to differentiate into mature squamous cells toward the core of the peg. Under these conditions the center of the peg, seen in

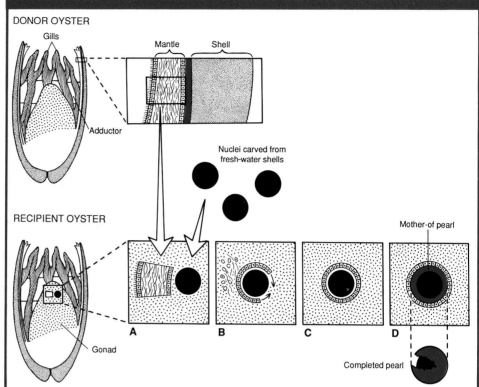

FIGURE 16.2
The method used in Japan for producing cultured pearls exploits mechanisms typical of wound healing. **A:** A square piece of mantle from a donor oyster is implanted into the gonad of a recipient oyster, next to a sphere carved from a freshwater shell; the size of sphere determines the size of future pearl. **B:** Epithelium of the mantle, which normally produces mother-of-pearl, grows over the surface of the sphere. **C:** Epithelial cells continue to produce mother-of-pearl. **D:** After about 2 years, the process is complete. (Drawn with the aid of Prof. Koji Wada, Faculty of Bioresources, Mie University, Japan.)

cross section, appears to contain a lump of shed keratinocytes, actually called a "pearl" (p. 751). The same process occurs on a larger scale when a sphere of epidermal cells grows beneath the skin, as an *epidermoid* cyst filled with shed cells. Such cysts are sometimes formed by traumatic displacement of epidermis into the subcutaneous tissue; more often they develop from hair follicles (Figure 16.3).

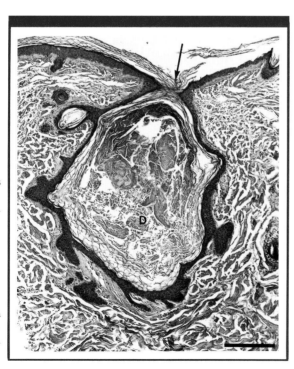

FIGURE 16.3
Epidermoid cyst filled with desquamated cells (**D**). In this case a connection with the epidermis is present (**arrow**). **Bar** = 250 μm. (Specimen kindly provided by Dr. A.B. Ackerman, Thomas Jefferson University Medical Center Philadelphia, PA.)

Life Without Inflammation: The Case of Plants

Plants have no migrating cells and no phagocytes; to defend themselves against invading organisms, plant tissues depend on a variety of mechanisms. One is to *sacrifice the injured part* by walling it off so that it will die, and with it dies the pathogen (Figure 16.4) (1). In animal tissues a similar process is called *sequestration:* a piece of infected tissue is isolated in a cavity (i.e., in an abscess) and contained there for long periods; bone sequestra in osteomyelitis can be retained for years. Plants also respond with general adaptations such as the production of protease inhibitors, which happen to be toxic to pathogens and pests (4). It certainly is amazing that phagocytosis plays no role in defense. However, chemotaxis does

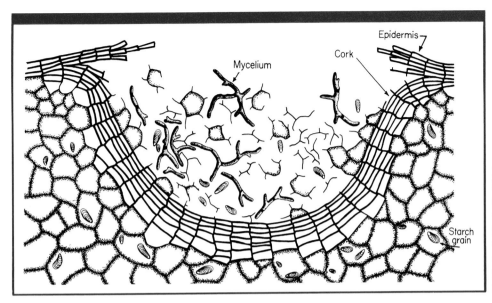

FIGURE 16.4
Surface of a potato invaded by a fungus. The potato responds by forming a dense layer of cork cells beyond the point of infection; this inhibits further invasion, blocks the spread of toxic substances, and deprives the pathogen of nourishment. (Adapted from [41a].)

exist in plants; it was actually discovered in fern gametes (p. 386).

Inflammation as a Cause of Damage

Inflammation can go wrong—by excess or by default. The first aberration damages the body, the second fails to protect it. It is not surprising that inflammation should cause damage. After all, a major purpose of inflammation is to inflict damage to live cells (parasites), and it is to be expected that innocent bystander cells may also be hurt. As a matter of fact, it is still not clear how the aggressive cells, especially the killer cells, escape being hurt by their own weapons, be they enzymes, oxygen metabolites, or perforin-type molecules.

Inflammation is a nuisance in all diseases caused by the immune response. The reason is that the immune response "borrows" inflammation as one of its effector mechanisms for destroying its targets. The targets, however, are not necessarily dangerous. A prime example is hay fever. Pollen is harmless, but it becomes a problem when the immune system creates an allergic response against it (p. 522). A vast number of such diseases exist, including all the autoimmune conditions (one of the most distressing is rheumatoid arthritis). In none of these situations does inflammation have

any survival value. To the contrary, it is a fair target for anti-inflammatory therapy.

The "Crystal Diseases" Several diseases are based on the deposition of microscopic endogenous crystals in the tissues, especially in the joints (pp. 141, 417). The crystals themselves are not greatly irritating to the tissues; but when they are deposited in a joint, an acute inflammatory response ensues. Why? One theory is that the crystal surface binds IgG and thereby activates complement (22). The resulting influx of activated leukocytes is deleterious to the articular cartilage. As in hay fever, damage is caused by inflammation that is triggered by conditions that seem to us, as observers or victims, inappropriate.

The Adult Respiratory Distress Syndrome The adult respiratory distress syndrome (ARDS) is a lung disorder that stands in a category by itself. It occurs typically in shock (p. 703), and especially in septic shock. It leads to diffuse alveolar damage and respiratory failure, with a mortality rate over 50 percent. It is in part the result of inflammatory mechanisms gone awry. The pathogenesis varies, but the following steps seem clear: leukocytes are activated in the circulation (this may be due to endotoxin or to intravascular activation of complement, which produces C5a, which activates the leukocytes); activation then causes the leukocytes to aggregate and to become trapped in the lungs, where they cause damage by releasing oxygen metabolites and enzymes (31, 52).

Failures of the Inflammatory Response

Inflammation may be inadequate for accidental or congenital reasons. In either case, the result is a greater risk of infection.

Acquired Defects of Inflammation

Leukocytes fail because they cannot be properly delivered to an injury site by the microcirculation, because they are too few, or because they are defective; plasma components can be insufficient or exhausted. Here are some examples of leukocyte failure:

- **Inadequate delivery of blood** Every surgeon knows that poor blood supply is a major cause of inadequate inflammation and therefore of infection, especially in skin

---

TABLE 16.2
Neutropenia: Major Causes

BY DECREASED PRODUCTION
- X-rays
- A large variety of drugs (antineoplastic agents, some antihistamines, antibiotics, analgesics, tranquilizers, anti-inflammatory agents, many others)
- Some infections (tuberculosis, malaria, hepatitis, typhoid, overwhelming sepsis)
- Starvation, anorexia nervosa
- Folate deficiency, especially in alcoholics
- Vitamin B12 deficiency

BY PERIPHERAL TRAPPING OR DESTRUCTION
- Diseases with splenectomy (e.g., congestive splenomegaly, Gaucher's disease, sarcoidosis)
- Anaphylaxis, cardiopulmonary bypass (due to clumping followed by trapping)
- Some autoimmune disorders (e.g., systemic lupus erythematosus)
- Autoimmune neutropenia (antineutrophil antibodies)
- Some drugs (e.g., mercurial diuretics)

Adapted from (9)

---

flaps. Remember that hypoxic leukocytes are ineffective against many bacteria. It follows that hypoxic tissues are much more susceptible to infection than normal tissues, as can be shown most dramatically with experimental skin flaps (24). Hypoxia and ischemia are multiplied in *circulatory shock,* which is generalized inadequate flow: in shock, bacteria can multiply out of control almost anywhere, but especially in the gut. In essence, ischemia frustrates inflammation: it allows bacteria to multiply unhindered, by leukocytes and complement, and by antibiotics injected intravenously.

- **Inadequate numbers of leukocytes** Neutropenia can be due to a variety of conditions (Table 16.2). In general, the risk of infection increases as the number of neutrophils per cubic millimeter drops below 1000–500. Monocytopenia appears to be less dangerous than neutropenia; it is seen after stress or glucocorticosteroid therapy and during many acute infections.

- **Lack of spleen** Splenectomy exposes a patient to the risk of sepsis, especially by pneumococci. There is a heightened risk of infection immediately after splenectomy (49) as well as a long range risk due to several factors. One is, obviously, the loss of macrophages (those of the spleen are especially able to phagocytize bacteria that are not well opsonized, hence they play a critical role in the nonimmune host [3]). Add to this a loss of antibody production; a defect in monocyte chemotaxis; and an impairment of phagocytosis due to reduced production of two opsonins, tuftsin and properdin (50,51,56).

- **Overworked littoral macrophages** Whenever the RES/MPS system (p. 297) is flooded with excess material to phagocytize, a so-called blockade develops. This event has been measured: in rats, if the system is challenged twice in a sequence with intravenous injections of carbon black, the second time it will respond less effectively (p. 300) (2). Clinical settings of blockade can be induced by intravascular hemolysis, which amounts to blockade by hemoglobin and red cell ghosts (29). Circulating antigen–antibody complexes have a similar effect.

- **Impairment of leukocytes by severe burns**

Extensive burns imply a greatly increased risk of infection, due at least in part to leukocyte "exhaustion": thermal injury generates large amounts of chemotaxins, especially C5a, resulting in generalized activation of neutrophils. The neutrophils respond by secreting their specific granules and become ineffective (10,36). When the leukocyte population has lost most of its granules (5–15 days), septic complications reach their peak (11).

- **Impairment of leukocytes by alcoholic intoxication** Alcohol abuse carries a risk of infection, especially of the lungs (25). In the preantibiotic era, lobar pneumonia of drunkards was an everyday occurrence in city hospitals. In alcohol intoxication, leukocytes adhere abnormally and migrate poorly. This was shown by adherence tests *in vitro* using nylon wool and by skin-window tests on volunteers (20).
- **Drugs** Many drugs depress leukocyte function or production. Leukocyte adherence *in vitro* is decreased by steroids, salicylates, colchicine, and local anesthetics; and because adherence is the first step to leukocyte emigration, these same drugs decrease chemotaxis *in vivo* (44). Other drugs with antiinflammatory side-effects are tetracycline, chloroquine, chloramphenicol, and halothane (44,58). Anti-inflammatory drugs are the basis of treatment for autoimmune diseases, and of course they are a two-edged sword (46).
- **Diabetes** A variety of defects in inflammation and wound healing accompany diabetes (40): impaired chemotaxis and phagocytosis (17,37), delayed wound closure and contraction, defective granulation tissue (61), inhibition of collagen synthesis (54), and microcirculatory disturbances, including increased vascular permeability (60).
- **Cancer** Defects of leukocyte function are often associated with cancer, and at least two types of chemotaxis inhibitors have been found in the serum of cancer patients (30). However, the principal mechanism of inflammatory failure in cancer is chemotherapy, which affects the bone marrow as well as the cancer.

Interestingly, the same French laboratory that described an antiinflammatory effect of cancer

cells (14) later found an antitumor effect of inflammatory cells (23).

- **Viral and bacterial infections** Certain infectious agents interfere with leukocyte function. The dangerous *Entamoeba histolytica* evades the only cell that can engulf it, the monocyte/macrophage, by means of a specific chemotaxis inhibitor; neutrophils are not affected by it (19).
- **Malnutrition** Though it is known that malnutrition impairs the leukocytes (47,48), this topic has been poorly explored (38).

CONGENITAL DEFECTS OF INFLAMMATION

The most common congenital defect of inflammation in humans is just being a newborn, as mentioned above. In addition, there are about 20 congenital diseases of the inflammatory response. Although generally rare, as experiments of nature they have been very useful for deciphering normal mechanisms of inflammation (18a).

Congenital Defects of Leukocytes When a malfunction of leukocytes is suspected, a battery of tests is available (33,58). Defects include anomalies of leukocyte adherence, chemotaxis, phagocytosis, and bacterial killing—alone or combined. The lack of one function may affect several others; for instance, the lack of adhesion also affects motility over a substrate (17,41,58). Leukocyte adhesion deficiency (LAD) has already been mentioned (p. 398) (Figure 16.5); a few other examples are listed:

- **Chronic granulomatous disease (CGD)** In this miserable condition, neutrophils, macrophages and eosinophils are unable to produce an oxygen burst in response to stimulation (Figure 16.5). Chronic infections usually develop during the first year of life; inflammation, both suppurative and granulomatous, is excessive but ineffective. This syndrome can be produced by several molecular defects; although rare, it has attracted great interest because it is an experiment of nature that demonstrates the role of the oxygen burst (18a).
- **Myeloperoxidase (MPO) deficiency** This deficiency is quite common: the use of peroxidase stain for routine leukocyte differential counts has revealed it in one of every 1,200 individuals. It affects neutrophils and monocytes but not eosinophils. Oddly

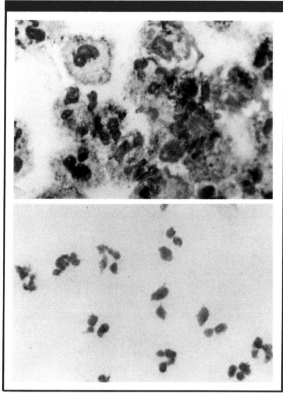

FIGURE 16.5

Oxidative defect of neutrophils, from a child with chronic granulomatous disease. *Top:* Normal human neutrophils stimulated for 40 minutes with phorbol myristate acetate and tested for their ability to reduce the dye nitroblue tetrazolium (NBT). Note the abundance of dark granules, blue in the original specimen. *Bottom:* Defective leukocytes can be demonstrated by a nuclear stain, but they contain no reaction product. (Courtesy of Ms. Julia Metcalf and Dr. John I. Gallin, National Institute of Allergy and Infectious Diseases.)

enough, few of these patients have problems with bacterial infections, probably because the defective cells show increased activity of the NADPH-oxidase system producing superoxide anion. MPO deficiency can also be acquired: for instance, in pregnancy, anemia, and leukemia.

- **Congenital lack of specific granules** Discovered in children with recurrent infections, this lack was "useful" in showing that these granules are a source not only of the anti-bacterial lactoferrin but also of receptors for chemotaxins. As the granules fuse with the plasma membrane, the receptors on the inner surfaces of the granules are transferred to the outer surface of the plasma membrane (Figure 11.6) (18).

- **Job's syndrome** This skin disease was named, somewhat inaccurately, from the Bible: *So went Satan forth from the presence of the Lord, and smote Job with sore boils from the sole of his foot unto his crown* (Job 2:7). The biblical Job was an adult, whereas most of Job's syndrome patients begin to suffer from infections during the first weeks of life (multiple, torpid, skin abscesses) (41). Strangely enough, these patients turn out to have very high IgE levels (hyper IgE syndrome). How this syndrome relates to the disease is not clear. Chemotaxis is depressed, especially for monocytes, but not always.

- **Other congenital defects of inflammation are attributed to dysfunction of the microtubules,** which are important for locomotion as well as for phagocytosis. Instances are the *Chediak–Higashi syndrome,* characterized by multiple phagocytosis defects and large granules in all granulocytes; and the *immotile cilia syndrome,* which mainly concerns a dysfunction of the ciliary microtubules (p. 156).

- **Congenital defects of the complement system** are discussed on p. 344.

TO SUM UP: We take inflammation for granted because (speaking for all vertebrates) it rarely lets us down; but when it does, we realize how essential it is for survival. It works even behind the scenes, in everyday life, even in the absence of overt disease. Individuals with leukocyte adhesion deficiency develop overwhelming gum infections: this tells us that anonymous leukocytes are constantly fighting duels around our teeth, keeping the bacteria under control. Among the congenital failures of inflammation, it is interesting to see that the most common is represented by the neonatal state. Among the acquired failures, many are iatrogenic and accompany immunosuppression, the ultimate failure of our defense systems (p. 585). We should not complain that the mechanisms of inflammation are so redundant.

References

1. Agrios GN. Plant Pathology. San Diego: Academic Press, 1988.

2. Biozzi G, Benacerraf B, Halpern BN. Quantitative study of the granulopectic activity of the reticulo-

endothelial system. II. A study of the kinetics of the granulopectic activity of the R.E.S. in relation to the dose of carbon injected. Relationship between the weight of the organs and their activity. Br J Exp Pathol 1953;34:441–457.

3. Bohnsack JF, Brown EJ. The role of the spleen in resistance to infection. Annu Rev Med 1986;37:49–59.

4. Bowles D. Signals in the wounded plant. Nature 1990;343:314–315.

5. Bryant RE. Pus: friend or foe? In: Root RK, Trunkey DD, Sande MA, eds. New surgical and medical approaches in infectious diseases. Contemporary issues in infectious diseases, vol 6. New York: Churchill Livingstone, 1987:31-48.

6. Burke JF. The effective period of preventive antibiotic action in experimental incisions and dermal lesions. Surgery 1961;50:161–168.

7. Burke JF. Wound infection and early inflammation. Monogr Surg Sci 1964;1:301–345.

8. Cohen N, Sigel MM, eds. The reticuloendothelial system. A comprehensive treatise, vol 3, phylogeny and ontogeny. New York: Plenum Press, 1982.

9. Dale DC. Leukocytosis, leukopenia, and eosinophilia. In: Wilson JD, Braunwald E, Isselbacher KJ, et al., eds. Harrison's principles of internal medicine, 12th ed. New York: McGraw-Hill, 1991.

10. Davis JM, Dineen P, Gallin JI. Neutrophil degranulation and abnormal chemotaxis after thermal injury. J Immunol 1980;124:1467–1471.

11. Duque RE, Phan SH, Hudson JL, Till GO, Ward PA. Functional defects in phagocytic cells following thermal injury. Am J Pathol 1985;118:116–127.

12. Erickson CA, Nuccitelli R. Embryonic fibroblast motility and orientation can be influenced by physiological electric fields. J Cell Biol 1984;98:296–307.

13. Faden AI. Pharmacotherapy in spinal cord injury: a critical review of recent developments. Clin Neuropharmacol 1987;10:193–204.

14. Fauve RM, Hevin B, Jacob H, Gaillard JA, Jacob F. Antiinflammatory effects of murine malignant cells. Proc Natl Acad Sci USA 1974;71:4052–4056.

15. Fleer A, Gerards LJ, Verhoef J. Host defence to bacterial infection in the neonate. J Hosp Infect 1988;11 (suppl A):320–327.

16. Fletcher TC, Cooper-Willis CA. Cellular defense systems of the mollusca. In: Cohen N, Sigel MM, eds. The reticuloendothelial system. A comprehensive treatise, vol 3, phylogeny and ontogeny. New York: Plenum Press, 1982:141–166.

17. Forehand JR, Johnston RB. Phagocytic defects. Clin Immunol Allergy 1985;5:351–369.

18. Gallin JI, Fletcher MP, Seligmann BE, Hoffstein S, Cehrs K, Mounessa N. Human neutrophil-specific granule deficiency: a model to assess the role of neutrophil-specific granules in the evolution of the inflammatory response. Blood 1982;59:1317–1329.

18a. Gallin, JI. Disorders of Phagocytic Cells. In: Gallin, JI, Goldstein, IM, and Snyderman, R (eds). Inflammation: Basic Principles and Clinical Correlates, 2nd ed. New York: Raven Press, 1992.

19. Giménez-Scherer JA, Pacheco-Cano MG, de Lavín EC, Hernández-Jáuregui P, Merchant MT, Kretschmer RR. Ultrastructural changes associated with the inhibition of monocyte chemotaxis caused by products of axenically grown Entamoeba histolytica. Lab Invest 1987;57:45–51.

20. Gluckman SJ, MacGregor RR. Effect of acute alcohol intoxication on granulocyte mobilization and kinetics. Blood 1978;52:551–559.

21. Hall ED. Free radicals and CNS injury. Crit Care Clin 1989;5:793–805.

22. Hasselbacher P. Crystal-protein interactions in crystal-induced arthritis. In: Weissmann G, ed. Advances in inflammation research. New York: Raven Press, 1982: 25–44.

23. Hevin M-B, Friguet B, Fauve RM. Inflammation and anti-tumor resistance. V. Production of a cytostatic factor following cooperation of elicited polymorphonuclear leukocytes and macrophages. Int J Cancer 1990;46:533–538.

24. Hunt TK, Knighton DR, Price DC, et al. Oxygen in the prevention and treatment of infection. In: Root RK, Trunkey DD, Sande MA, eds. New surgical and medical approaches in infectious diseases. New York: Churchill Livingstone, 1987:1–16.

25. Kass EH. Changing ecology of bacterial infections. Arch Environ Health 1963;6:19–25.

26. Kucharz E. 80th anniversary of the discovery of erythrocyte sedimentation rate. Mater Med Pol 1975;7:344–346.

27. Leaf A, Cotran RS. Renal pathophysiology. New York: Oxford University Press, 1976.

28. Little RA. Changes in the reactivity of the skin blood vessels of the rabbit with age. J Pathol 1969;99:131–138.

29. Loegering DJ, Grover GJ, Schneidkraut MJ. Effect of red blood cells and red blood cell ghosts on reticuloendothelial system function. Exp Mol Pathol 1984;41: 67–73.

30. Maderazo EG, Anton TF, Ward PA. Serum-associated inhibition of leukotaxis in humans with cancer. Clin Immunol Immunopathol 1978;9:166–176.

31. Malech HL, Gallin JI. Neutrophils in human diseases. N Engl J Med 1987;317:687–694.

32. Matheson A, Nierenberg M, Greengard J. Reactivity of the skin of the newborn infant. Pediatrics 1962; 10:181–197.

33. Metcalf JA, Gallin JI, Nauseef WM, Root RK. Laboratory manual of neutrophil function. New York: Raven Press, 1986.

34. Metchnikoff E. Lectures on the comparative pathology of inflammation, 1892. (Translated from the French by Starling FA, Starling EH). New York: Dover Publications, 1968.

35. Mims CA. The pathogenesis of infectious disease. London: Academic Press, 1976.

36. Moore FD Jr, Davis C, Rodrick M, Mannick JA, Fearon DT. Neutrophil activation in thermal injury as assessed by increased expression of complement receptors. N Engl J Med 1986;314:948–953.

37. Naghibi M, Smith RP, Baltch AL, et al. The effect of diabetes mellitus on chemotactic and bactericidal activity of human polymorphonuclear leukocytes. Diabetes Res Clin Pract 1987;4:27–35.

38. Neumann CG. Nonspecific host factors and infection in malnutrition—a review. In: Suskind RM, ed. Kroc Foundation series vol 7. Malnutrition and the immune response. New York: Raven Press, 1977:355–374.

39. Neuwelt EA, ed. Implications of the blood-brain barrier and its manipulation, vol 2. New York: Plenum Medical Book Company, 1989.

40. Pickup JD, Williams G. Textbook of diabetes, vol 2. Oxford: Blackwell Scientific Publications, 1991.

41. Quie PG. Phagocytic cell dysfunction. J Allergy Clin Immunol 1986;77:387-398.

41a. Ramsey, GB. A form of potato disease produced by Rhizoctonia. J Agric Res 1917;9:421–426.

42. Rapoport SI, Hori M, Klatzo I. Testing of a hypothesis for osmotic opening of the blood-brain barrier. Am J Physiol 1972;223:323–327.

43. Regelmann WE, Mills EL, Quie PG. Immunology of the newborn. In: Feigin RD, Cherry JD, eds. Textbook of pediatric infectious diseases, vol 1, 2nd ed. Philadelphia: WB Saunders, 1987:921–939.

44. Roberts R, Gallin JI. The phagocytic cell and its disorders. Ann Allergy 1983;50:330–343.

45. Sadrzadeh SMH, Anderson DK, Panter SS, Hallaway PE, Eaton JW. Hemoglobin potentiates central nervous system damage. J Clin Invest 1987;79:662–664.

46. Seldin MF, Steinberg AD. Immunoregulatory agents. In: Gallin JI, Goldstein IM, Snyderman R, eds. Inflammation: basic principles and clinical correlates. New York: Raven Press, 1988:911–934.

47. Selvaraj RJ, Bhat KS. Phagocytosis and leucocyte enzymes in protein-calorie malnutrition. Biochem J 1972;127:255–259.

48. Seth V, Chandra RK. Opsonic activity, phagocytosis, and bactericidal capacity of polymorphs in undernutrition. Arch Dis Child 1972;47:282–284.

49. Shatney CIH. Complications of splenectomy. Acta Anaesth Belg 1987;38:333–339.

50. Shaw JHF, Print CG. Postsplenectomy sepsis. Br J Surg 1989;76:1074-1081.

51. Simon M Jr, Djawari D, Hohenberger W. Impairment of polymorphonuclear leukocyte and macrophage functions in splenectomized patients. N Engl J Med 1985;313:1092.

52. Smedley LA, Tonnesen MG, Sandhaus RA, et al. Neutrophil-mediated injury to endothelial cells. Enhancement by endotoxin and essential role of neutrophil elastase. J Clin Invest 1986;77:1233–1243.

53. Smith RM, Curnutte JT. Molecular basis of chronic granulomatous disease. Blood 1991;77:673–686.

54. Spanheimer RG. Direct inhibition of collagen production in vitro by diabetic rat serum. Metabolism 1988;37:479–485.

55. Stiehm ER. The human neonate as an immunocompromised host. In: Verhoef J, Peterson PK, Quie PG, eds. Infections in the immunocompromised host—pathogenesis, prevention and therapy. Amsterdam: Elsevier-North Holland Biomedical Press, 1980:77–94.

56. Styrt B. Infection associated with asplenia: risks, mechanisms, and prevention. Am J Med 1990;88(suppl 5N):33N-42N.

57. Suckling AJ, Rumsby MG, Bradbury MWB, eds. The blood-brain barrier in health and disease. Chichester, England: Ellis Horwood Ltd., 1986.

58. van der Valk P, Herman CJ. Leukocyte functions. Lab Invest 1987;57:127-137.

59. Wasserman RL. Neonatal sepsis: the potential of granulocyte transfusion. Hosp Pract 1982;17:95–104.

60. Williamson JR, Chang K, Tilton RG, et al. Increased vascular permeability in spontaneously diabetic BB/W rats and in rats with mild versus severe streptozocin-induced diabetes. Diabetes 1987;36:813–821.

61. Yue DK, Swanson B, McLennan S, et al. Abnormalities of granulation tissue and collagen formation in experimental diabetes, uraemia and malnutrition. Diab Med 1986;3:221–225.

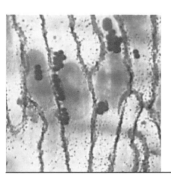

PART # THREE

IMMUNOPATHOLOGY

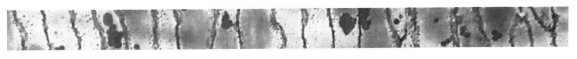

Hypersensitivity Reactions

CHAPTER **17**

Introduction

Both the inflammatory and the immune responses are essential to survival; however, both processes—like all things biological—can go wrong. We have already talked about the failures of inflammation. In the next few chapters we will deal with failures of the immune response:

it can do too much (*hypersensitivity*), it can do too little (*immunodeficiency*), or it can attack the wrong target (*autoimmunity*).

We assume that the reader is familiar with the basic concepts of immunology, which is, essentially, the saga of antigen. Readers seeking background in immunology have a choice of excellent texts (1, 70).

Since we are about to describe the *bad* deeds of the *immune* response, we should comment on the schizophrenic use of the word "immune," which is confusing for the novice. Immunity sounds like a good thing; according to the *Dictionary of Immunology* (71), it means "having a high degree of natural or acquired resistance to a disease." However, by extension, it also includes any altered state that results from exposure to an antigen—*whether the altered state is good, bad, or indifferent.* Hay fever is therefore an immune phenomenon even though it makes life miserable. We have no choice but to follow this ambivalent usage and to speak of "vaccines that render a person immune to infection" as well as of "immune reactions that cause disease."

The word immune *really means tax exempt (from in-, not, and* munus, *tax or money) just as* municipal *means tax-taking. These were fiscal terms in ancient Rome; eventually the word* immune *crossed over from politics into medicine and came to mean disease-exempt. The jump may not be so great; a noted historian, W.H. McNeill, equated taxes with disease, proposing that people are caught between* microparasites *(such as bacteria and viruses) and* macroparasites *(other people, singly or assembled in governments) (46). The pathology caused by macroparasites would probably fill a book much larger than the present one.*

A note on terminology: textbooks of immunology are apt to mention the various cells of the immune family by means at "adjuncts" that refer to the surface CD antigens that characterize them. CD stands for clusters of differentiation; over 100 such antigens are presently known (1). To complicate matters, the CD terminology is riddled with synonyms. T-helper cells, for example, are ritually called CD4+ CD8− T-helper cells, and suppressor/cytotoxic T cells carry the prefix CD4− CD8+. For our purpose we consider these adjuncts unnecessary.

The Weapons of the Immune Response

To understand the damage that can be wrought by the immune response when its weapons are misused, we should briefly review those weapons. The most important are two: inflammation and cell killing.

INFLAMMATION AND THE IMMUNE RESPONSE

Inflammation and the immune response are both defensive mechanisms, which may function separately or jointly. They differ in one basic aspect. *Inflammation is nonspecific:* it is triggered by virtually any type of injury and varies little with different causal agents. In contrast, *the immune response is specifically aimed at certain molecular structures* (anti-

gens) recognized as foreign; however, *it often uses inflammation as one of its effector arms.* Why?

Consider how the immune response is organized. It generates two main types of specific weapons: *antibodies* and *killer cells.* For several reasons, both become vastly more powerful with the help of nonspecific inflammation. For example:

- Antibodies are obviously useful, but they are large molecules that are mostly confined to the bloodstream. How can they escape and reach their targets? The solution is to increase the permeability of blood vessels. Inflammation is programmed to do just that.
- Antibodies are relatively harmless by themselves. They are molecular labels that identify targets that should be destroyed. But what will destroy these targets? The deed is done by various inflammatory cells, which are programmed to destroy any target labeled with antibody. It is therefore obvious that inflammation is a major ally of the antibody response.
- Antibodies can combine with toxins and other soluble antigens, forming complexes; but who will eliminate those complexes? The best candidates are the macrophages—another reason to invoke the inflammatory response—which will summon more macrophages.
- Killer cells are a magnificent invention, but they too are confined to the bloodstream and need help to reach their targets. Inflammation has all the necessary mechanisms for helping these cells migrate out of the vessels.

All this explains why the immune response can benefit from the inflammatory response. It triggers inflammation by inciting the release of inflammatory mediators; T-helper cells are largely in charge of this function. Although inflammation and the immune response can be triggered separately, as shown in Figure 17.1, whenever the immune response is triggered, inflammation follows sooner or later.

CELL KILLING: A SPECIALTY OF THE IMMUNE SYSTEM

When killer cells were first described, we greeted the news with skepticism: it sounded so human. Could such violence really extend to cells? Today we have no doubt: even paramecia kill each other (21). The main function of the immune system is to find target cells and kill them. The targets are mostly bacteria, virus-infected cells and tumors—but unfortunately, they can also be surgically

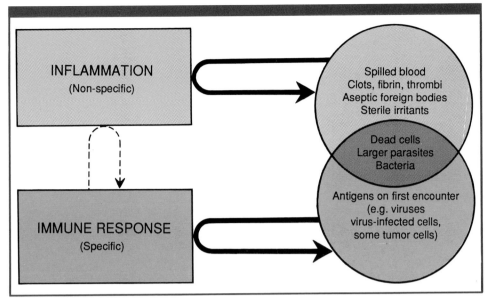

FIGURE 17.1
Interrelations between inflammation and the immune response. Some agents (*top right*) elicit only inflammation; other agents, namely antigens not previously encountered (*bottom right*), elicit only an immune response; other agents (*overlapping areas*) can elicit both at the same time. Eventually the immune response "borrows" the inflammatory response (*dashed arrow*): this occurs when an antigen is introduced into a specifically sensitized host.

transplanted cells (grafts). Several cell types are now known to have the propensity to be cytotoxic: natural killer (NK) cells, cytotoxic T and B lymphocytes, macrophages, and some lymphoma cell lines (38). These cells kill in different ways.

> *Cytotoxic is a rather confusing term in a medical environment. A patient is called "toxic" if passively suffering from symptoms of intoxication, whereas a cytotoxic cell is actively engaged in killing other cells. It may help to remember that in ancient Greek tóxon meant bow (and arrow) (42); eventually, toxic material came to mean poison for the arrow and then poison in general. Cytotoxic cells are best remembered by thinking of them as holding bows and arrows.*

Seen in action, killer cells are impressive. Minutes after they have fastened upon their target (72), the victim undergoes violent "blebbing"; and within a few minutes or hours it dies (77, 92). Then the killer cell can wander off to repeat its performance on two or three other targets (6) (Figures 17.2, 17.3).

Why do target cells die? After heated debates some of the dust is settling (6). The type of cell death is apoptosis; and if all means of cell-to-cell killing are included, no less than four lethal mechanisms have emerged: (a) inserting plugs into the cell membrane; (b) producing "burns" with oxygen-derived free radicals; (c) producing toxic damage with cytokines such as TNF; and (d) inducing suicide, associated with (a) and (c). These mechanisms are not mutually exclusive.

Inserting Plugs This was the first mechanism to be worked out. A killer cell, such as a cytotoxic

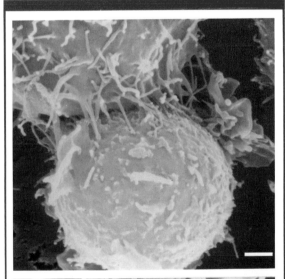

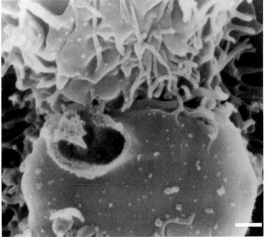

FIGURE 17.2
Top: Killer cell makes contact with the smaller target cell (a tumor cell). *Bottom:* Tumor cell is swollen; a large hole has developed. **Bars** = 2 μm. (Reproduced with permission from [92]. Electron micrograph by Gilla Kaplan, Ph.D., Laboratory of Cellular Physiology and Immunology, The Rockefeller University, New York.)

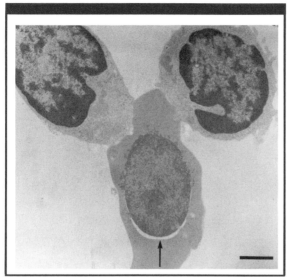

FIGURE 17.3

Two B lymphocytes attacking and lysing an antibody-coated, red blood cell of a chicken. Nucleus of the target cell appears to be disintegrating; the dilatation of the perinuclear cisterna (**arrow**) is a sign of cell injury. Note: Not all lymphocytes are capable of this performance; these B lymphocytes were obtained from tumor-bearing mice. **Bar** = 1 μm. (Reproduced with permission from [38].)

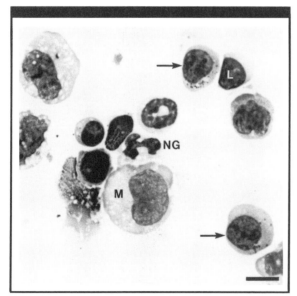

FIGURE 17.4

Cells obtained from mouse liver. *Arrows:* natural killer cells, also called large granular leukocytes; **M** = monocyte/macrophage, **NG** = nucleus of granulocyte; **L** = lymphocyte. Stain: Wright-Giemsa. **Bar** = 10 μm. (Preparation courtesy of K.W. McIntyre, University of Massachusetts Medical Center, Worcester, MA.)

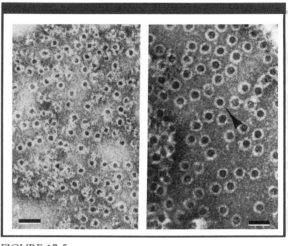

FIGURE 17.5

Comparing membrane lesions formed by complement and by cytotoxic lymphocytes. *Left:* Human complement lesions; internal diameter 100 Å. *Right:* Lesions due to polymerized mouse perforin 1 (*arrowhead*), internal diameter 160 Å. **Bars** = 0.05 μm. (Reproduced with permission from [60].)

lymphocyte or an NK cell (Figure 17.4), begins by identifying their specific target; NK cells, most distinctively, do so by means of receptors that tell them "this is NOT a target" (9a). Attachment is followed by internal rearrangements that bring a wave of calcium and the secretory granules to the contact zone. Then, within 5–15 minutes, the granules are extruded into the intercellular space, and the target cell is perforated and dies (58). The granules contain a protein called *perforin* (or *cytolysin*) that assembles within the victim's membrane and creates stable holes (Figure 17.5), very similar to those produced by the lethal membrane attack complex of complement (p. 339) (59).

> *Perforin has 30 percent homology with the C9 component of complement. The perforin plug is produced by many molecules of perforin stacked side by side whereas the complement plug contains C5, C6, C7, C8, and up to 18 molecules of C9 (16). The internal diameter of the perforin plug is slightly larger (100–200 Å).*

At first the discovery of the perforin plug appeared to be the perfect solution to cell killing. The similarity with complex-mediated killing seemed inescapable. But then some surprising facts came to light: target cells may die even if the killer cell is prevented from secreting its supposedly lethal granules (86). Antibodies against perforin prevent killing by NK cells but not by T cells (6, 25). On the other hand, the DNA of a target cell begins to break down within minutes of the attack (19,73), as occurs in apoptosis (Figure 5.32). Thus, another scenario came to light: the killer cell induces its victim to commit suicide (87).

Behold: a form of violence that has few parallels in the human model. It has been called *enforced suicide* (91).

The last word is not yet in, but it seems that cytotoxic lymphocytes and NK cells kill by two mechanisms: a fast mechanism based on perforin and a slower one based on an NK cytotoxic factor or leukalexin (7).

Producing Burns Damage to the plasma membrane of target cells by oxygen-derived free radicals is typical of granulocytes and macrophages (51).

Inflicting Toxic Damage Such damage is typical of activated macrophages, which can kill by means of tumor necrosis factor in the immunologic process known as ADCC (p. 527) (20, 44, 94); similarly, activated T lymphocytes can kill by means of lymphotoxin. *Both these cytokines induce apoptosis* (7).

Combinations of Weapons Plugs, burns, and poisons are used by various cells in differing combinations (6, 33):

- Eosinophils use plugs and burns.
- Lymphocytes use plugs and poisons.
- Macrophages use burns and poisons.

We know of no cell that uses all three.

Killer cells have become a hot topic in immunology. However, remember that cell killing is not a prerogative of the immune response: NK cells are ready to perform on first encounter.

Hypersensitivity Reactions

The term *hypersensitivity reaction* applies to an immune response that is unnecessary or exaggerated so that *the response becomes a greater hazard than the antigen that triggers it.*

What response can be excessive? To understand this, recall that the immune system exerts its function—basically—by means of two effector arms: *producing antibodies*, which are manufactured by modified B lymphocytes (plasma cells) and *producing cells* (mainly T lymphocytes), which destroy target cells and elicit inflammation. Trou-

ble in terms of excessive response can develop along the pathway of either arm. This concept is laid out in Table 17.1, an overview of hypersensitivity mechanisms, based on the classification proposed by Coombs and Gell in 1975 (12). In essence, this table shows that, just as there are two ways to deal with antigens (the B-cell and the T-cell pathways), there are two main categories of hypersensitivity responses. One depends on B cells and thus on antibody production, and includes three subgroups labeled Types I, II, and III. The other (Type IV) depends on T cells and has nothing to do with antibody production. Because antibodies are molecules in solution, instantly available for reactions, Type I, II, and III responses develop very rapidly (seconds to hours) and are therefore also known as immediate-type hypersensitivity reactions; because cells are mobilized slowly and need time to kill or to synthesize their chemical messengers, the Type IV response is also known as *delayed-type hypersensitivity* (DTH; the delay is of the order of 12–18 hours), or cell-mediated hypersenstivity.

The key feature of Table 17.1 is the right-hand column: note the various arrangements of the antibody molecules. Once these are understood, the three antibody-mediated types of hypersensitivity are not difficult to remember. Besides, Type I is unforgettable.

Hypersensitivity Type I: Anaphylactic

Many of us have heard of an outdoor party that turned to tragedy when someone was stung by a bee, collapsed, and died. An episode of this kind happens about 40 times a year in the United States. This is anaphylaxis (anaphylactic shock). The basic mechanism of this catastrophic event was discovered because of a cruise on a royal yacht. Later it turned out that the acute episode called anaphylaxis was just the tip of an iceberg: today we know of a whole gamut of anaphylactic reactions, all based on the same mast-cell mechanism. Besides anaphylaxis, this group includes a variety of less-threatening conditions that are also called *allergies*, at least in the United States: hay fever (allergic rhinitis), food allergies, some skin rashes, and allergic asthma. All anaphylactic reactions involve acute degranulation of mast cells. Degranulation is induced by exposure to an antigen in individuals

TABLE 17.1

The Four Principal Types of Hypersensitivity

TYPE I: ANAPHYLACTIC

Key is the mast cell

Antibody (IgE) is bound to mast cells "by the tail" (Fc segment cytophilic binding)

Degranulation occurs when antigen hits the mast cell

No cells die

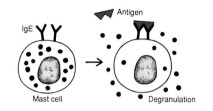

TYPE II: CYTOTOXIC

Antibody (non-IgE) binds to an antigenic surface, cell or basement membrane, by the Fab segments (cytotoxic binding)

The carpet of fixed antibody fixes leukocytes and activates complement, thereby attracting more leukocytes

Damage to the antigenic surface is done by complement and by leukocytes

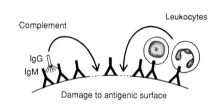

TYPE III: COMPLEX-MEDIATED

Complexes are formed by antigen + antibody

Complexes fix leukocytes and activate complement, thereby attracting more leukocytes

Damage to any tissue nearby is done mainly by neutrophils

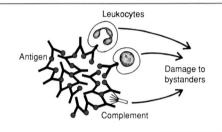

TYPE IV: CELL-MEDIATED

No antibody is involved

Only cells participate

Target antigenic cells are killed by killer cells and lymphokines

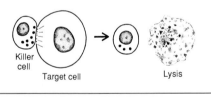

(Left margin labels: IMMEDIATE for Types I–III, DELAYED for Type IV)

---

whose mast cells are coated with the specific antibody to that antigen. The degranulation can be general, in which case it may kill, or local, in which case it causes disease but rarely death. In essence, we are dealing with endogenous overdoses of mast-cell products (80).

The villains, to be precise, are not only the mast cells but also their circulating relatives, the basophils (other cells play lesser roles). When it was realized that mast cells are programmed to coat themselves with antibody and to act in that uniform as agents of the immune reaction, something like a mast-cell cult developed. And rightly so: no other group of cells is equipped to kill the whole body in a few minutes.

But let us begin from the beginning, aboard a royal yacht (Figure 17.6).

In 1901 Prince Albert of Monaco, who was interested in marine biology, set to sea on the Princess Alice II to work out the mechanism of poisoning by the Portuguese man-of-war, a stinging jellyfish that can be a nuisance on Mediterranean beaches (Figure 17.7). The ship was equipped with labs for animal experiments; Paul Portier was the resident scientist. To supervise the experiments, Prince Albert invited a senior scholar, Charles Richet (1850–1935), who was also a writer and an eminent physiologist; it was he who found that dog panting is a cooling device (29). As the ship cruised along, a number of dogs, ducks, pigeons, and frogs were injected with jellyfish extracts; the only finding worthy of note was that the animals tended to "fall asleep," perhaps by a neurotoxic effect. After the voyage, Richet continued the experiments on dogs using sea anemones, which cost less. Would their poison have the same narcotic effect as that of the Portuguese man-of-war? He tried several doses, and, again for economic reasons, he used the same dog for more than one injection. So, Dog Neptune, for example, received three nonlethal doses on days 1, 3, and 27 (68); the first two had no apparent harmful effect, but after the third one, he suddenly keeled over, convulsed, vomited, and died after 25 minutes (62). Portier and Richet were utterly amazed, having anticipated, if anything, an immunizing (prophylactic) effect of repeated doses. Dog Neptune—and others after him—seemed to show the reverse effect. Groping for a Greek word to mean "reversed protection" they settled on anaphylaxis (61, 78). As Greek goes it was a poor choice, but 12 years later Richet was awarded the Nobel prize for having opened a new field of immunology. Actually, anaphylaxis had been seen by others before him, but nobody had generalized from it. Neither Richet nor Portier lived long enough to learn its basic mechanism.

MECHANISMS OF ANAPHYLACTIC HYPERSENSITIVITY

We are now able to explain in some detail what happened to those unfortunate dogs. Portier and Richet had come upon the phenomenon of *generalized* anaphylactic hypersensitivity: massive, allergic mast-cell degranulation (Figure 17.8). For an anaphylactic response to occur—whether it be local (as in hay fever) or generalized—the antigenic material must have the property of inducing antibodies of the IgE class. In most mammals, IgE antibodies bind to the surfaces of mast cells, but note this key fact: if we liken the shapes of immunoglobulin molecules to lobsters, an IgE molecule binds to a mast cell by its "tail" (i.e., by the Fc portion), and the "claws" float free, ready to bind antigen. This type of binding is called *cytophilic* (cell-friendly), and in fact, the mast cell is not at all troubled by its antigenic coat: it has receptors for the very purpose of acquiring it as part of its normal life (later we will see why). When the specific antigen to these antibodies comes along and binds to their outstretched claws, it triggers degranulation; to do so it must be at least divalent so that it can bind two adjacent molecules of IgE together (Figure 17.9).

But beware: mast cells can be induced to degranulate by any of hundreds of molecules that

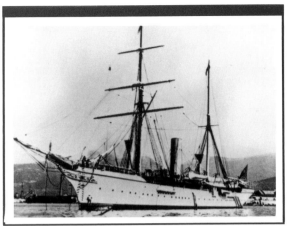

are wholly unrelated to IgE and to anaphylactic hypersensitivity, the so-called histamine liberators (p. 525). Mast cells also degranulate in response to two purely experimental tricks: one is to use antibodies against the bound IgE antibody, the other is to use antibodies against the surface IgE receptor.

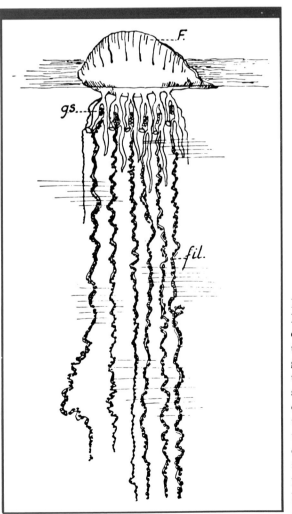

FIGURE 17.7
Portuguese man-of-war floating in the sea. The dangerous sting of this mollusk inspired the Prince of Monaco to initiate research that led to the discovery of anaphylaxis. (Reproduced with permission from [61].)

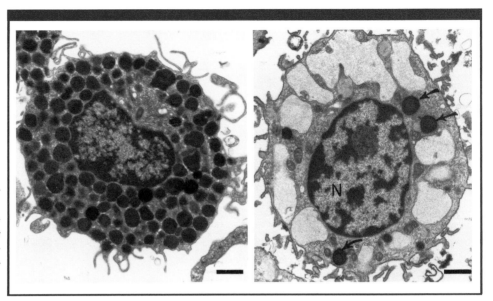

FIGURE 17.8
Mast cells isolated from the human lung. *Left:* Normal cell. *Right:* Degranulating cell, fixed 10 minutes after the degranulation stimulus (challenge with anti-IgE); clear spaces represent swollen granules; there are few residual granules. **Arrows:** Lipid bodies. **N:** Nucleus. **Bars** = 1 μm. (Reproduced with permission from [17, 18].)

DEGRANULATION: TWO WAVES OF MAST-CELL PRODUCTS

What mast cells do for a living is not entirely clear (p. 329); but when they become troublemakers, their enormous secretory resources come to light.

The response is immediate, but the effects become clinically apparent in two waves.

The Immediate Response Within seconds after the stimulus to degranulate, histamine is released

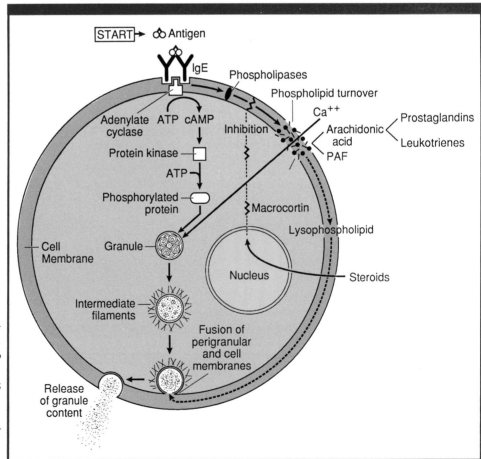

FIGURE 17.9
Proposed sequence of metabolic events in a mast cell activated by antigen bridging a pair of IgE molecules. Transduction of the stimulus leads to degranulation as well as to perturbation of cell-membrane phospholipids; this leads to the production of arachidonic acid metabolites and of platelet activating factor. Note the inhibitory pathway mediated by macrocortin. (Adapted from [4].)

from storage in the granules; in rats, serotonin comes with it. The result is vascular leakage, which causes local swelling in many places, including the skin and (more ominously) the larynx. Circulating histamine contributes to a drop in blood pressure, to constriction of the bronchi, and to other smooth muscle effects. At the same time the mast cell puts the phospholipids in its membranes to work, producing three sets of mediators (p. 345): leukotrienes, prostaglandins, and platelet activating factor (PAF) (64–66, 89). Prostaglandin D2 and leukotriene C4 are powerful bronchoconstrictors, and the latter makes the spasm worse by stimulating the secretion of mucus: thus the victim has plenty of reasons for suffering from air hunger, although the greatest threat of suffocation (in anaphylaxis) comes from edema of the larynx. Other factors released during this phase are chemotactic for neutrophils and eosinophils, but it takes some time (hours) for these cells to respond in significant numbers.

At this point the mast cells have fired their first, double-barreled shot, but there is more to come.

The Late-Phase Reaction After 2–4 hours, the late-phase reaction begins; it peaks at 6–12 hours and can last 1–2 days or longer. It has been observed not only in the skin but also in the nose (in hay fever) and in the bronchi (37). *Biopsies have shown an inflammatory exudate* (whereas during the early reaction there is almost pure edema) with eosinophils, basophils, neutrophils, and some macrophages; many granules are spilled around, from degranulated mast cells, basophils, and eosinophils (Figure 17.10). One hypothesis is that the granules spilled from the mast cells slowly release their bound proteases (tryptase and chymase, p. 330), which act on plasma proteins of the edema to produce inflammatory mediators; the eosinophils participate with their own toxic products (10, 36). In other words, at this stage the initiating antigen is not necessarily involved (35). *Intradermal injections of mast-cell granules produce late-phase reactions* (31). It has also been suggested that late-phase reactions involve activated eosinophils, which secrete their cytolytic *major basic protein* (75).

WHY DO SOME ANTIGENS INDUCE AN IgE RESPONSE?

The crucial feature that makes some antigens capable of inducing anaphylactic reactions is their ability to induce the synthesis of antibodies of the IgE type. Why do they "choose" that type? If they induced IgG or IgM antibodies, allergic patients

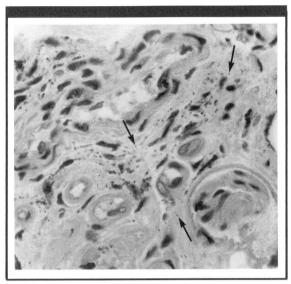

FIGURE 17.10
Pathogenesis of the late-phase allergic reaction. Biopsy of the skin 5 hours after the intradermal injection of antigen in a sensitized patient. Note the degranulating mast cells and the free mast-cell granules (**arrows**) which are thought to be responsible for the late-phase reaction. (Reproduced with permission from [31].)

would presumably be trouble-free. The answer is not wholly satisfactory, but it includes at least five factors:

- The type of antigen
- The route of antigen administration
- Genetic factors
- Environmental factors
- In laboratory experiments, the type of "adjuvant" (see further) injected with the antigen.

In children, the cumulative risk of developing some allergic condition was found to be 10 percent if neither parent had a history of allergy; if one or both parents were allergic, it rose to about 25 percent and 50 percent, respectively (Figure 17.11) (87). Many allergens are obviously environmental, and they *penetrate through mucosae:* pollens, house dust, animal dandruff, insect stings, and foods. Diesel exhaust particles have an adjuvant effect on IgE production, at least in mice, and this may have something to do with the rapid increase of allergies in industrialized countries (83).

THE PHARMACOLOGY OF ALLERGY: LINKS BETWEEN PATHOGENESIS AND THERAPY

Pharmacology helps us understand the mechanisms of allergic lesions (Figure 17.12). For example (56):

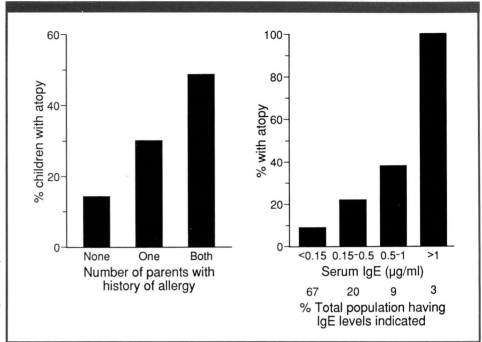

FIGURE 17.11
Risk factors in allergy. *Left:* A family history of allergy increases the risk of developing allergies. *Right:* The higher the concentration of IgE in the serum, the greater the chance of developing allergies. (Adapted from [70].)

- *Inhibitors of degranulation* prevent but do not treat anaphylactic manifestations; it is patently useless to give cromolyn sodium, the best known inhibitor of degranulation, to someone who has already degranulated.
- *Epinephrine and other adrenergic agonists* can be lifesaving. They act by stimulating adrenergic alpha and beta receptors, which raise the cell's level of cAMP and stops degranulation. Epinephrine also dilates the bronchi and constricts arteries; hence it has long been the drug of choice in anaphylactic shock and other allergies. Even the Romans knew that a decoction of *ephedra* is helpful for asthma (42).
- *Antihistamines* are effective in many conditions (such as urticaria, but not in others such as asthma, because *histamine is only one of the mediators released by mast cells.* It is well to remember that mast cells differ from one body site to another (p. 330).
- *Antiinflammatory agents:* aspirin is generally

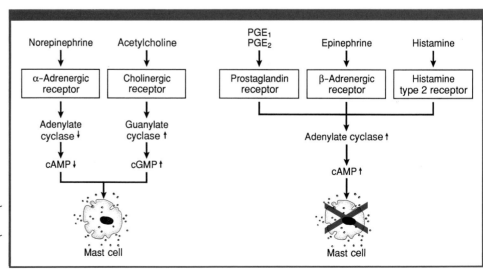

FIGURE 17.12
Modulation of mast-cell degranulation by drugs. *Left:* Release is stimulated by decreased cAMP or increased gGMP. *Right:* Release is inhibited by increased cAMP. (Adapted from [69].)

avoided in treating asthma because it makes things worse. The mechanism is thought to be the following: aspirin inhibits the cyclo-oxygenase pathway of arachidonic acid metabolism, which releases prostaglandins; this inhibition makes more substrate available for the lipoxygenase pathway, which produces leukotrienes (some of which are bronchoconstrictors, and make asthma worse). Corticoids take effect only after several hours, so they are useful for preventing and treating late reactions.

- Desensitization therapy by injecting the offending antigen might sound contradictory and dangerous to the novice, but there is of course a theory behind it. The allergen is *injected,* which is not its natural route of entry; most allergens are inhaled or swallowed and therefore penetrate the mucosal membranes. The idea is that the different route of entry will elicit a non-IgE antibody, such as IgG. Purpose: circulating IgG might be able to "grab" any antigen that penetrates the body barriers, before it can reach the IgE antibody on the mast cells (this grabbing is what is meant by "*blocking* antibodies"). There is evidence that this mechanism does work, although anaphylactic accidents (rarely) do occur during the therapy.

A loose end for readers with strong nerves. The authors of this book were profoundly shocked one day by reading that anaphylaxis can be produced in mice that are congenitally deficient in mast cells (26, 30). A reflex telephone call produced the following data. (a) These mice have some mast cells (less than 1 percent of normal) plus a normal amount of basophils (83): perhaps this is enough. (b) Perhaps other cells contribute to the anaphylactic response (platelets, macrophages?). (c) The central dogma of anaphylaxis "has not been demolished." So we trust.

Psychology and the Mast Cells The lore on this subject includes the story of the asthmatic patient hypersensitive to the perfume of roses, who visited an art museum and developed an asthmatic attack before a painting of roses. This sequence has been confirmed experimentally. If guinea pigs hypersensitive to an antigen are submitted to a Pavlovian conditioning procedure whereby the nose is repeatedly swabbed with the antigen coupled with a smell, after some time the guinea pigs begin to release histamine into the bloodstream when presented with the smell alone (74). Similar results were obtained with rats, this time by combining the antigen with an audiovisual cue (39). These and other experiments suggest that the central nervous system may be involved in modulating mast-cell degranulation as well as in other mechanisms of mediator release: hypnotic suggestion can decrease the flare (though not the wheal) of the triple response (p. 366) (93). We will return to the role of the nervous system (p. 587).

Diseases Related to Anaphylactic Hypersensitivity

Anaphylactic shock (a whole-body response) is the most spectacular manifestation of anaphylactic hypersensitivity, but the same mast-cell IgE mechanism is shared by a number of local conditions called "allergies," such as hay fever. We will now review both the generalized and the local responses.

ANAPHYLACTIC SHOCK

As we have seen, this is a fearful acute clinical syndrome. It is always the result of generalized degranulation, but its manifestations vary from one species to another because the pharmacologic effects of the mediators involved are species-related.

In humans, anaphylactic shock is well known as a result of insect stings. Note, incidentally, the pharmacologic wizardry displayed in yellow-jacket venom, which can do much worse than simply induce allergy (Table 17.2; Figure 17.13). Drugs can also induce anaphylactic sensitization and shock; anaphylaxis by penicillin kills 500 people every year (13). Tiny amounts of antigen may suffice, even a vaccination. As to the clinical picture, the patient typically begins to feel faint; common symptoms are itching of the palms and soles or the genital area, and skin rashes that resemble the sting of the nettle (urticaria); nausea, vomiting, and diarrhea may develop within minutes. Some individuals plunge into cardiovascular collapse: histamine causes leakage from the venules throughout the body, and the resulting loss of plasma volume causes the blood pressure to drop, while the heart rate speeds up (Figure 17.14) (81). Other victims develop air hunger from bronchial spasm or hoarseness from laryngeal edema (there are many mast cells in the

TABLE 17.2

Some Ingredients of Yellow-Jacket Venom

Ingredients	Effects
Histamine, serotonin, bradykinin	Major inflammatory mediators; kinins produce pain
Histidine decarboxylase	Produces histamine
Phospholipase A and B	May initiate cascade of prostaglandin and leukotriene inflammatory mediators
Protease	May produce more inflammatory mediators by acting (e.g., on complement components)
Hyaluronidase	Favors spread of other molecules in connective tissue
Norepinephrine, epinephrine (vasoconstrictors)[a]	May slow the removal of other agents

[a]The pharmacologic wisdom of yellow-jacket venom is truly diabolical, the essence of textbook inflammatory knowledge. These two ingredients are currently used in local anesthetics to hold the injected drug in place as long as possible; perhaps their purpose in yellow-jacket venom is similar. For other ingredients (e.g., cholinesterase) a rationale is not obvious.

Adapted from (67).

larynx, and they account for some deaths). There may be a relapse after an initial improvement, surely by the mechanism of the late-phase reaction. The mortality of anaphylactic shock is about 10 percent.

In the guinea pig, the effect is essentiall asphyxia. If a guinea pig is sensitized intradermally with bovine albumin and challenged intravenously 3 weeks later, it will begin to scratch its nose within seconds (itching from local degranulation);

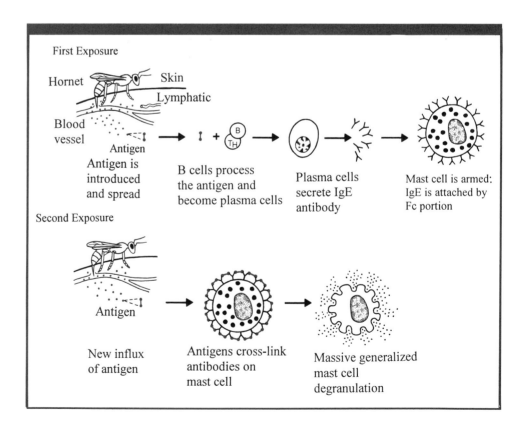

FIGURE 17.13
Mechanism of anaphylaxis after a sting (e.g., by a hornet).

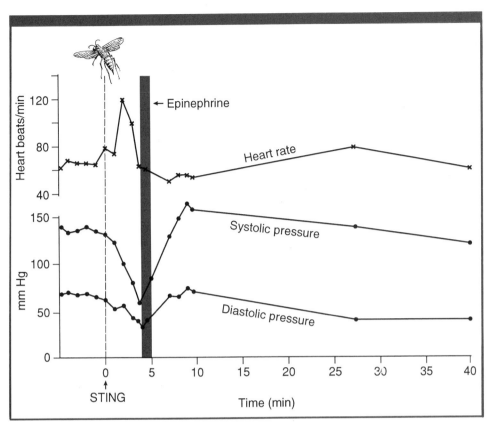

FIGURE 17.14
Effects of anaphylactic shock on human heart rate and blood pressure. This experiment was carried out in a critical care setting, with the purpose of selecting the best possible treatment. Note the very short interval between the sting by a real insect and the general effects. (Reproduced with permission from [81].)

it gasps for air, collapses, and dies within minutes. Autopsy shows *overinflated* lungs—because the constricted bronchi let air in but not out—even after the lungs are removed from the body (Figure 17.15). The blood shows a *prolonged clotting time*, probably due to release of heparin into the blood, and *leukopenia*, which is attributed to leukocyte clumping and retention of the clumps in the lung, an effect of platelet activating factor released by mast cells (p. 347). Thus, in the guinea pig, the effects are dominated by spasm of the bronchial musculature. Curiously, anaphylaxis in the guinea pig depends on IgG; otherwise, the mechanism is the same as in other animals.

In the dog, the main effect is a constriction of the hepatic veins, resulting in diarrhea and vomiting. In the rabbit, the critical event seems to be pulmonary hypertension and right heart failure, perhaps because too many pulmonary capillaries are blocked by leukocyte emboli (remember the platelet–leukocyte aggregates induced by PAF).

LOCAL MANIFESTATIONS OF ANAPHYLACTIC HYPERSENSITIVITY

Portier and Richet could never have guessed that hay fever, food allergies, urticaria (hives), and

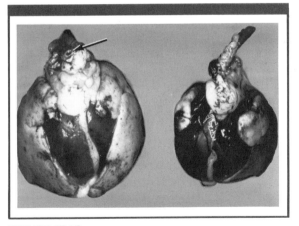

FIGURE 17.15
Heart and lungs of two guinea pigs. *Left:* This guinea pig had been sensitized with albumin and was challenged 21 days later with an intravenous dose of albumin; death from anaphylactic shock followed within 10 minutes. The lungs after dissection remained expanded due to bronchial spasm trapping air in the lungs; yet the trachea was open (**arrow**). *Right:* Normal guinea pig: the lungs (barely visible behind the heart) have collapsed due to their natural elasticity. Conclusion: anaphylactic shock causes spasm in the bronchi. Slightly enlarged.

asthma all belong to the same family as anaphylactic shock. In fact, for many years they were lumped into a mysterious category of disorders called **atopic** (a Greek term for bizarre or out of place), the reason being that—although they had the hallmarks of antigen–antibody reactions—no circulating antibody was demonstrable. The reason was the very low level of IgE antibody in the blood. All these local forms of anaphylactic response follow local applications of antigen, such as pollen on the nasal mucosa.

Hay Fever Allergic rhinitis, also called hay fever, is more prevalent in developed countries, where it affects 10–15 percent of the population (87). It offers a classic example of hypersensitivity because the inhalation of harmless pollen sets up an intense and wholly unnecessary inflammatory response, creating a considerable nuisance to the patient. The mechanism of allergic rhinitis is summarized in Figure 17.16.

Why does the sneeze come so soon after a sniff of hay? It should take time for the antigen to reach the mast cells lying under the epithelium. We have consulted some eminent immunologists, both normal and allergic, but elicited no good answer. We were told that the antigens of some allergenic particles, such as the feces of house mites, are very soluble in water and therefore quickly extracted (84); we were also reminded that some mast cells sit on the mucosa, out in the breeze (55), and may "somehow" accelerate the passage of the antigen. However, we found no electron microscopic proof of the statement (52) that they can increase the permeability of epithelia, as they can with venular endothelium. Someone should try to work this out.

A curious aspect of hay fever is that the nasal mucosa, constantly inflamed, eventually becomes hypertrophic and "grows out" in the form of polyps that may even appear at the nostrils (Figures 17.17, 17.18): soft, oblong masses that interfere with breathing and must be surgically removed, but may recur. We suspect that these polyps are a response to growth factors secreted by the inflammatory cells, but they carry no threat of malignant transformation. We know of only one comparable phenomenon in pathology: the outgrowth of

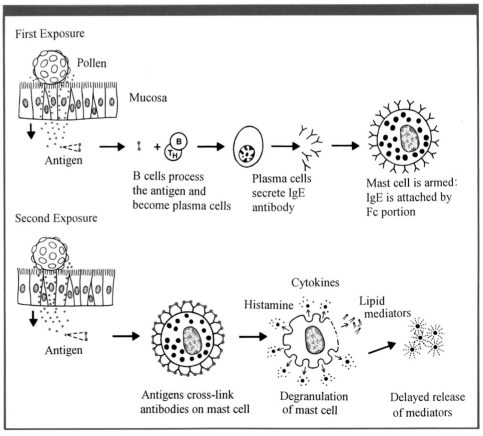

FIGURE 17.16
The mechanism of a mucosal allergy: hay fever (allergic rhinitis).

finger-shaped "villi" from synovial membranes when they are chronically inflamed, such as in rheumatoid arthritis.

Food Allergies Allergies to various foods are due to antigens that manage to cross the barrier of the intestinal epithelium, probably transcytosed by absorptive cells and by the specialized M-cells that lie over Peyer's patches and solitary lymphoid follicles (Figure 17.19) (47, 53, 54). If the patient has been sensitized, the effect can remain localized to the gut: the mucosal mast cells degranulate, leading indirectly to diarrhea. However, the amount of antigen absorbed is often large enough to reach (by the bloodstream) other target organs such as the skin, causing urticaria, or the lungs, causing asthma. Nuts, strawberries, and shellfish are among the common culprits.

It was a food allergy that began to clarify the basic mechanism of all atopic lesions. The breakthrough came in 1921, in Breslau. Dr. Heinz Küstner wondered why he became ill every time he ate cooked fish or shellfish. So he worked out a scientific deal with Dr. Prausnitz who, acting as guinea pig, received 0.1 ml of Küstner's serum in his skin, followed 1 day later by 0.1 ml of fish extract. Thus was born the classic Prausnitz–Küstner reaction. Interestingly, when the result was published, the gentleman who acted as the guinea pig became the senior author: the P of the PK reaction (63).

The principle of the PK reaction is to inject a minute amount of serum from the allergic subject into the skin of a normal volunteer; 24–48 hours later the suspected antigen is injected into the same site. If a wheal develops within 90 minutes, the reaction is positive. This waiting period after the serum injection allows time for the IgE antibody to combine with the mast cells; in some cases the time can be shortened to 45 minutes. The site remains reactive for 4–6 weeks; it can also be challenged by taking the antigen by mouth. The PK reaction is now dropping out of fashion because it involves the injection of human serum.

Allergic Asthma In developed countries, allergic asthma occurs in about 5 percent of adults and almost twice as many children (45); the percentage is lower in developing countries (87).

The sequence of events leading to an allergic asthma attack is similar to that of hay fever: the bronchial mucosa contains mast cells coated with IgE antibody against a specific antigen such as horse hair; inhalation of that antigen leads to mast-cell degranulation and bronchospasm.

Recent evidence indicates that macrophages in

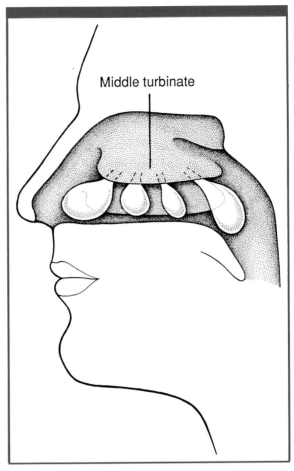

Middle turbinate

FIGURE 17.17
Nasal polyps, as seen in patients with allergic rhinitis (hay fever). Such polyps, which can completely occlude the nose, are soft structures arising from the nasal mucosa, usually beneath the middle turbinate, a shell-like bone. They are easily removed surgically but tend to recur. (Modified from [15].)

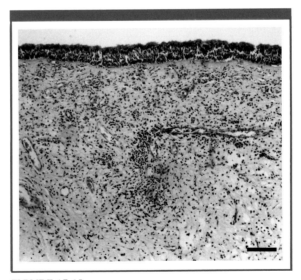

FIGURE 17.18
Histology of a nasal polyp. The surface epithelium is of the upper respiratory type; beneath it is edematous connective tissue with many vessels and a diffuse infiltrate of macrophages, lymphocytes, plasma cells, and eosinophils (not distinguishable at this enlargement). **Bar** = 100 μm.

FIGURE 17.19
Macromolecular
transport across
the epithelium of
the gut by an M
cell (**M**) over a
Peyer's patch in
the mouse. Horse-
radish peroxidase
injected into the
lumen of the gut
is being trans-
ported by vesicles
(**arrows**) into the
subepithelial
space. Note a
macrophage
(**Mφ**) surrounded
by lymphocytes
(**L**). **Bar** = 2
μm. (Repro-
duced with per-
mission from
[53].)

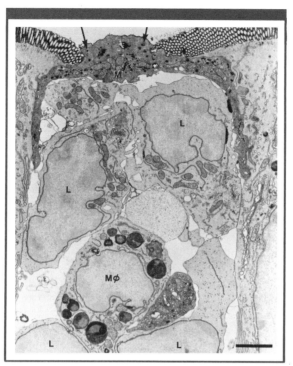

Urticaria This itchy rash (also called hives) is caused by local mast-cell degranulation of any kind, not just by the IgE mechanism (Figure 17.20). We mentioned hives in relation to anaphylactic shock. The name *urticaria* comes from the latin *urtica* for nettle. The rash appears very rapidly and can disappear in less than an hour, much like the sting of the nettle. As a matter of fact, the similarity goes much deeper. The weapon of the nettle is similar to a tiny glass syringe (Figure 17.21) which pierces the skin and injects—believe it or not—histamine and serotonin plus acetylcholine, which degranulates mast cells (40). Think how many millions of years it must have taken for the nettle to work out this mix of inflammatory mediators, including the refinement of adding to the histamine an agent that degranulates mast cells (as if saying "if my histamine doesn't bother you, maybe yours will").

Atopic dermatitis (or atopic eczema). This dermatitis is a weepy sort of rash that occurs in about 3 percent of children under 5 years old, as well as in adults; it does have an allergic, IgE–mast cell component, but its pathogenesis is much more complex and includes a cell-mediated response (27).

WHY ANAPHYLACTIC RESPONSES HAPPEN—MAYBE

Anaphylactic responses are a nuisance at best, so why do they happen? Students never fail to ask

the bronchial mucosa or free in the bronchial lumen are activated and contribute a large share of inflammatory mediators (22). The key point to remember is that the bronchi come under multiple attack by mast-cell and macrophage mediators: histamine, leukotrienes, prostaglandin E$_2$, and platelet activating factor cooperate in causing bronchospasm, vascular leakage (which means mucosal edema), hypersecretion of mucus, and an infiltrate of eosinophils and other inflammatory cells. To make matters worse, some mediators such as PAF increase the responsiveness of the bronchi to other mediators (9, 64–66).

Allergic asthma tends to become chronic; when this occurs, the bronchial mucosa shows changes of chronic inflammation, which require anti-inflammatory treatment (5).

The term asthma *was used in Hippocratic days to mean air hunger. Today it refers to an increased responsiveness of the bronchi, which become constricted in response to stimuli that would not affect normal lungs. The stimuli are sometimes clearly antigenic, but some are nonspecific, such as cold, exercise, or stress. The lungs are abnormally distended; the combination of constricted bronchi and distended lungs recalls the findings in guinea pig anaphylaxis (p. 520). The bronchi are partially plugged by an excess of mucus secretion. They also show an eosinophilic infiltration of the mucosa, and hypertrophy of the musculature (Figure 7.30).*

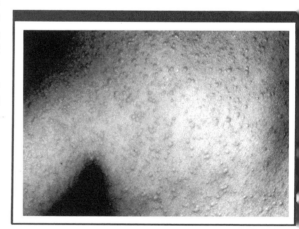

FIGURE 17.20
Close-up view of the skin in a case of severe urticaria (hives), characteristic of sudden, generalized mast-cell degranulation. In this case the degranulation was produced by an unusual mechanism: running in place for 10 minutes by a patient suffering from cholinergic urticaria. These patients are hypersensitive to cholinergic mediators; the mechanism is poorly understood. (Reproduced with permission from [32].)

this question, and neither do their teachers. Anaphylaxis kills and serves no purpose; asthma is crippling and sometimes fatal. Do these responses imply a wrong turn in the evolution of the immune system?

Nobody knows for sure, but here is a possible explanation: we may be dealing with an adaptation leftover from primal days when infestations with worms were prevalent. Consider the following facts: Worms tend to induce an IgE antibody response; all modern populations with a high "worm burden" also have a high plasma IgE titer and a high eosinophil count; local lesions caused by worms are rich in eosinophils, as are all anaphylactic responses (because degranulating mast cells produce chemotaxins for eosinophils); and finally, eosinophils appear to be specialized for killing worms (p. 322). Putting all this together, we can speculate that our distant, worm-ridden ancestors, having developed a high IgE titer, put it to use by evolving an IgE-mast–cell mechanism for attracting eosinophils—the best qualified cells for the job of killing such parasites. Although the worm burden has abated (at least in some places), we still respond to some environmental antigens, such as pollen instead of worms, by the same IgE-mast–cell mechanism—which has now become inappropriate.

Skeptic? Hear this. Guinea pigs attacked by ticks for the second time reject them by a basophil-related mechanism (83); whereas mice that are congenitally deficient in mast cells are unable to reject ticks, at least in one model (43).

ANAPHYLACTOID REACTIONS

Red flag: this is a simple concept but a source of confusion. The key to avoiding confusion is to realize that we are momentarily stepping out of immunology: *mast cells can degranulate massively for a variety of reasons that have nothing to do with IgE or immunology.* The result is a generalized effect that *looks* anaphylactic (hypersensitivity Type I) but is not; hence the name **anaphylactoid.** The agents capable of inducing this nonimmunologic effect are called **histamine liberators;** several hundred have been identified (34, 57).

This type of degranulation can occur in response to drugs, endogenous agents, cold, and even exercise and psychological mechanisms (2, 50). For reasons not understood, the degranulation response does not occur in all individuals. A small selection of histamine liberators is shown in Table 17.3; note that it includes complement

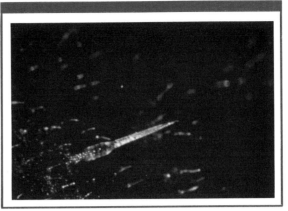

FIGURE 17.21
See color plate 16. Stinging hair on the leaf of a nettle, a plant of the genus *Urtica*, ready to inflict *urticaria* by injecting a sophisticated mix of inflammatory mediators. (About 25×).

products (anaphylatoxins). Among the drugs, note morphine; that called 48/80 is commonly used experimentally when it is necessary to deprive a rat of its mast cells. Remember that there are major species differences as well as local differences in the reactivity of mast cells (p. 329): no single agent is known to degranulate them in all tissues.

The name *anaphylactoid,* proposed by Selye in 1968 (79), means that the overall effect is virtually identical to that of anaphylaxis; in fact

---

TABLE 17.3
Nonimmunologic Mast-Cell Degranulating Agents[a] (Histamine Liberators)

Morphine, opiates
Curare and other muscle relaxants
Radiocontrast media (intravenous)
Dextrans, iron-dextran; plasma expanders
Mannitol
Polymyxin B and other highly charged
    antibiotics
Many chemotherapeutic agents
Components of bee venom (MCD peptide,
    melittin)
Some foods (perhaps strawberries) (3)
Compound 48/80 (in experimental animals)
Eggwhite (intraperitoneal, in rats)

[a]These are just a few examples. Some agents (e.g., the first three items) affect only certain individuals; the reason is unknown.

From (3, 79, 89).

degranulation can be even faster (14). A classic setting is the intravenous administration of iodinated contrast media in preparation for X-ray workup (e.g., pyelography). Most patients develop acute symptoms within 1–3 minutes. Another classic setting, oddly enough, is an insect sting, which is usually cited as the classic example of the anaphylactic mechanism: bee venom contains at least three histamine liberators, melittin, phospholipase, and a "mast-cell degranulating peptide" (67). Treatment is the same as for anaphylaxis, which may explain why clinically oriented textbooks tend to ignore the anaphylactoid mechanism.

Note: Two mechanisms can lead to an anaphylactoid response (8): (a) a direct effect on mast cells and (b) the intravascular activation of complement, most often due to intravenous injection of iodinated radiologic contrast media (28). Complement degranulates mast cells by means of C3a, C4a, and C5a, the so-called anaphylatoxins.

The main reason for our insistence on discussing the anaphylactoid response is that some drugs can unleash a catastrophic reaction that requires an instant response.

> *Pure histamine intoxication—unrelated to mast cells—can occur during dinner at a restaurant, as* scombroid poisoning. *It usually occurs with fish of the scombroid families, which include tuna. The probable mechanism: improper cleaning of the fish that is followed by spoiling. After bacterial enzymes release histamine from histidine, a few mouthfuls of fish provide a toxic dose of histamine. Symptoms are flushing, headache, vomiting, diarrhea, swelling of the face and tongue, and sometimes respiratory distress (49). Allergy is not involved: this is straight histamine poisoning. No deaths have occurred.*

Hypersensitivity Type II: Cytotoxic

Take another look at Table 17.1. *Type I* hypersensitivity is based on antibody that has become attached—by the tail according to the lobster model—and only to mast cells. The host runs into trouble as soon as the antigen comes along because the mast cells were previously primed to degranulate when it arrives. However, the trouble goes no farther than degranulation; no cells are destroyed, and the mast cells regenerate their granules. In TYPE II hypersensitivity, mast cells are not involved; antibody binds to an antigenic surface, "claws down" as it ordinarily does when it labels a target for destruction, but there is a hitch: *the target is harmless.* The host runs into trouble because specific structures are targeted and destroyed for no good reason, either by complement or by leukocytes.

Let us quickly review what an antibody is supposed to do when it works properly as a protector. *The key feature of an antibody is that it does not destroy; it has no means to do so. Antibody is essentially a label that marks a target for destruction by some other mechanism.* As antibody molecules attach themselves to and carpet a surface that they recognize as foreign, their tails stick out; and that carpet of bristling Fc segments is the label.

> *There are some exceptions to the rule that antibody has no direct effect on its target. When it binds to a cell receptor, it may inactivate it; it may also activate it by mimicking the normal ligand. When antibody binds to a free-floating toxic molecule, it inactivates the molecule; hence the clinical use of antibodies as antitoxins.*

Now, envision an antigenic surface coated with antibody molecules; usually it is the surface of a bacterium or virus. To defend ourselves against the invader, we need some watchful agent floating around in our body fluids that can recognize the carpet-of-antibody signal and attack the surface under it. There are two such roving guardians (Figure 17.22).

ANTIBODY-DEPENDENT COMPLEMENT-MEDIATED CYTOTOXICITY

One type of roving guardian is the first component of complement, C1, that beautiful flower-shaped molecule that responds to antibody tails by activating complement. A molecule of C1 recognizes two properly spaced Fc segments, becomes activated, and brings down a shower of membrane attack complexes (MACs). These MACs mercilessly perforate the labeled surface if it is a cell membrane. In the process of complement activation a split product of C3 is also produced (C3b, an opsonin) that attaches to the foreign surface and makes it more appetizing to phagocytes. So far, the carpet-of-antibody signal has brought down two curses on the labeled surface: perforation and phagocytosis. But this is not all.

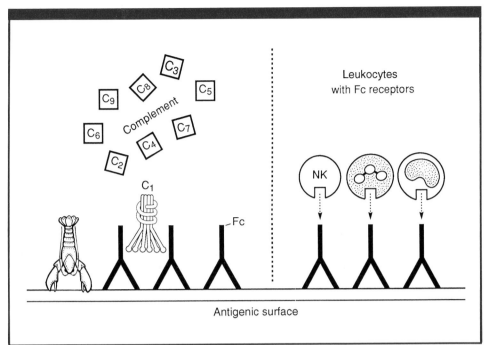

FIGURE 17.22
Surfaces coated with antibody can be attacked by two mechanisms: by complement (*left*) and by various types of leukocytes bearing receptors for the Fc portion of the globulin molecule (*right*). The result is known as antibody-dependent cytotoxicity, either complement-mediated or cell-mediated (ADCC). For these mechanisms to work, the immunoglobulin molecules must be bound "tails up."

ANTIBODY-DEPENDENT CELL-MEDIATED CYTOTOXICITY

The second type of roving guardian includes all leukocytes endowed with Fc receptors. If the invader is too large to be phagocytized in one gulp, the antibody label can take care of the matter by bringing onto the invader yet other curses: NK cells, monocytes, neutrophils, and eosinophils (Figure 4.4). All these cell types bind to the carpet of Fc segments, become activated, blast it with granules and free radicals, and then crawl away to meet the next invader. This modality of attack is called ADCC (antibody-dependent cell-mediated cytotoxicity), another poor acronym. ADCC, a stab-and-run mechanism, appears well suited for killing parasites too large to be phagocytized; eosinophils probably use it in their attack on worms (Figures 17.23, 17.24) (98; 99). This is the same phenomenon that we described earlier as *frustrated phagocytosis* (p. 404), which occurs when a phagocyte flattens itself against an object too large to engulf. However, it looks (to us) much more like a purposeful kiss of death than an act of frustration. The problem with ADCC is the difficulty of proving that it actually occurs *in vivo*.

Note a cunning feature of the leukocyte Fc receptors: they bind tightly to Fc segments presented by antibodies fixed on a surface, but they bind very *loosely to free antibody molecules. This is advantageous. If the surface of the leukocytes had a high affinity for Fc fragments, the leukocyte would always be coated and would lose the freedom to bind where necessary.*

DISEASES PRODUCED BY THE "TYPE II" MECHANISM

The binding of antibody to a surface causes disease when the surface thus marked for destruction is a normal part of the body. Examples:

ABO Mismatch In an ABO-mismatched blood transfusion, the foreign surfaces are those of the

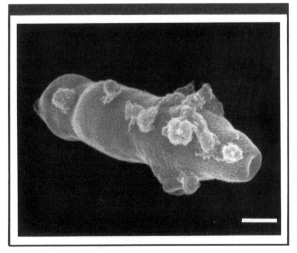

FIGURE 17.23
Scanning electron micrograph: leukocytes adhering to a schistosomulum that was preincubated in antibody and complement. **Bar** = 10 μm. (Reproduced with permission from [99].)

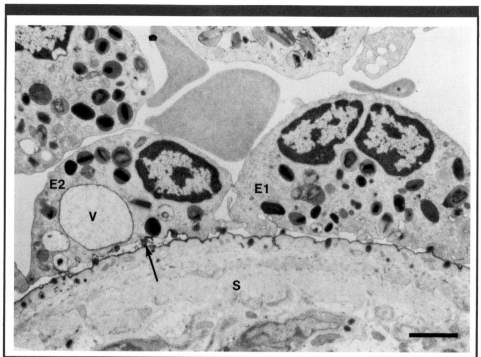

FIGURE 17.24

After 2 minutes of incubation with schistosome larvae, two eosinophils (**E1, E2**) attacking a larva (**S**). **E1** is simply attached; **E2** has begun to degranulate against the larval surface (**arrow** points to dense material probably discharged by the eosinophil). This type of attack may lead to death of the parasite. Vacuoles such as **V** are formed by the membranes of discharged granules. **Bar** = 1 μm. (Reproduced with permission from [100].)

injected, mismatched red blood cells; they are recognized by a natural antibody in the plasma of the ill-matched recipient, coated, and instantly attacked by complement (Table 17.4).

The ABO system works as follows. Human red blood cells carry a number of antigens including two major ones called A and B. The red blood cells of an individual may be A, B, AB, or O (with neither antigen). Now a peculiar fact complicates the situation: individuals with type A blood also carry ready-made anti-B antibodies in their blood, type B individuals carry anti-A, type O individuals carry both anti-A and anti-B, and type AB

individuals carry neither antibody. You may wonder how anyone who has never been exposed to foreign red blood cells could have antibodies against them. Though nobody knows for sure, these antibodies are probably against antigens of the flora of the gut, which happen to be very similar to antigens on red blood cells.

With this premise, imagine an A individual receiving B blood. Because type A blood carries anti-B antibodies, the transfused B cells are greeted by instant antibody coating followed by complement activation, massive hemolysis, and generalized capillary obstruction by red blood cell aggregates. The symptoms of this major emergency resemble those of anaphylaxis because of the release of complement anaphylatoxins C5a and C3a, which cause mast-cell and basophil degranulation.

Mother—Fetus Mismatch This mismatch occurs when mother and fetus are Rhesus incompatible. This incompatibility is due to the antigen called RhD. The setting, somewhat simplified: an RhD-negative mother (i.e., a mother with no RhD antigen on her red blood cells) gives birth to an RhD-positive baby. Due to the trauma of birth, some of the baby's red blood cells find their way into the bloodstream of the mother, causing the mother to make anti-RhD antibody of the IgG type, which happens to be able to cross the placental barrier. So *the next baby* with an RhD-

TABLE 17.4
Blood Groups of the ABO Series[a]

Blood Group	Contains Antigen	Contains Antibody	Will Hemolyse
A	A	Anti-B	B
B	B	Anti-A	A
AB	A & B	—	—
O	H	Anti-A & anti-B	A & B

[a]The series responsible for the most severe transfusion reactions.

positive father will receive a constant infusion of antibodies against its RhD-positive red blood cells; the antibody opsonizes the red blood cells, exposing them to phagocytosis by macrophages (Figure 17.25). The fetus becomes anemic; it will desperately try to compensate by making new red blood cells, including immature forms (erythroblasts, hence the ancient name of *erythroblastosis foetalis* for Rhesus incompatibility). The preventive treatment is not only effective but also conceptually satisfying: during the birth of the first baby the mother is given anti-RhD antibody, which rids her of the intruding fetal red blood cells.

Normal Surfaces Become Antigenic A normal surface is sometimes made foreign by a pathologic mechanism. The most common offenders are drugs, which can combine with surface molecules of any kind of blood cells and make them antigenic; the resulting antibodies—depending on the target cell—will then deplete the patient's erythrocytes, granulocytes, or platelets (anemia, agranulocytosis, and thrombocytopenia). Why this happens in some individuals is not known. Normal basement membranes somehow become antigenic in Goodpasture's disease, a hemorrhagic condition of the lungs and kidneys (p. 574).

Targeting Allografts Vascular endothelium of an allograft is recognized by the recipient's immune system as foreign. Coating of the graft's blood vessels by antibody is one of the mechanisms of rejection (p. 562).

Targeting Receptors *This is a form of autoimmunity.* It stands to reason that antibodies attached to a receptor will interfere with its function, either suppressing or stimulating it. Nature has provided several experiments of this kind, notably myasthenia gravis and two diseases of the thyroid, thyrotoxicosis (Graves' disease) and Hashimoto's disease (p. 571).

Hypersensitivity Type III: Complex-Mediated

Type III hypersensitivity (Table 17.1) is based on the fact that antibodies combine with soluble antigens to form antigen–antibody *complexes* (also called immune complexes). The complexes activate complement, which attracts leukocytes, and damage occurs. Here is a paradox: complex

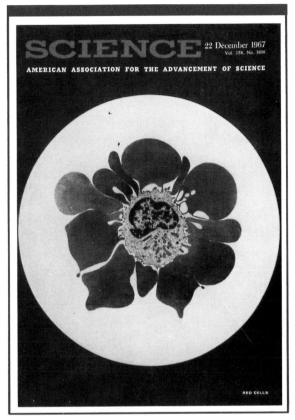

FIGURE 17.25
Classic "rosette" of red blood cells attached to a human monocyte. The mechanism: some anti-red blood cell antibodies, including autoantibodies, fix little or no complement but cause the red blood cells to become very sticky for monocytes. This sticking is followed in due time, by phagocytosis. Such is the sequence of events in *erythroblastosis foetalis*, caused by Rh incompatibility. (Reproduced with permission from [118].)

formation is precisely what antibodies are supposed to do when they encounter bacterial products, viruses, and other antigens in solution. How does this defensive mechanism become dangerous? Very simple: when large amounts of complex are formed, large amounts of complement are activated, and large numbers of activated leukocytes appear on the scene. Activated leukocytes are, as we have seen many times, dangerous cells. Type III hypersensitivity occurs when the body is flooded with antigen; in some cases the masses of complexes are large enough to plug capillaries. Too much is too much, especially when complement and leukocytes are involved. *Note: What we call "complexes" in vivo correspond to precipitates in vitro.* It follows that complex disease occurs only with those antigens that induce precipitating antibodies in the laboratory.

> We may be belaboring the obvious, but let it be clear that by complexes we mean antigen–antibody complexes, not lumps of antigen.

Let us try to visualize the role of antigen–antibody complexes in a hypersensitive reaction. When large amounts of polyvalent antigens react with antibodies that are floating free in the extracellular spaces (rather than fixed to surfaces), the complexes aggregate and form fluffy masses, just like a precipitate *in vitro*. The outer surface of these masses bristles with Fc tails (i.e., lobster tails, with the claws pointing inward, clinging to antigen). Now, as we just explained for hypersensitivity Type II, body fluids (and especially the blood) contain two kinds of roving guardians on the lookout for carpets of antibodies: complement (C1,) and cells with Fc receptors. In Type II hypersensitivity, the carpets are formed on fixed substrates, mostly cell membranes, and the roving guardians focus their attacks on those cells. In Type III, it is the outer surfaces of the antigen–antibody complexes that is attacked. Of course, attack on the complexes does no harm, but damage is caused to any cells that happen to be lying around. The main culprits are granulocytes, which in their "feeding frenzy" release their arsenal of granules and free radicals (p. 322).

To clarify these mechanisms, we will describe two classic models in which complexes are formed experimentally *in vivo*. To do so we must choose antigens capable of inducing precipitating antibodies (otherwise there will be no complexes); and the antibodies must activate complement (IgG and IgM fill the bill; IgA can activate complement by the alternative pathway).

- In the first model of complex-mediated hypersensitivity, antigen is injected *into the skin* of an animal previously immunized against that antigen; in this case the complexes form mainly *in the tissues* at the site of reinjection. This is therefore a model of *local* complex-mediated hypersensitivity.
- In the second model, antigen and antibody are caused to meet in the bloodstream;

complexes therefore cause injury primarily in the *vascular system*. This is therefore a model of *general* complex-mediated hypersensitivity.

A MODEL OF LOCAL COMPLEX-MEDIATED HYPERSENSITIVITY: THE ARTHUS PHENOMENON

The **Arthus phenomenon** consists of the development of a hemorrhagic, necrotic skin lesion where antigen has been injected into an animal previously immunized against that antigen (Figure 17.26).

We should first introduce Dr. Maurice Arthus (you may pronounce *Arthus* the English way, as long as you realize that it should be French). In the late 1800's lives were being saved by treating cases of diphtheria, tetanus, and scarlet fever with a new method discovered in 1890 by von Behring: subcutaneous injections of "antitoxins" (i.e., serum from immunized horses). When two such injections were given a few weeks apart, a local swelling sometimes appeared after the second injection. Why? In 1903 Dr. Arthus (95) tried to answer this question. Working at the Pasteur Institute in Lille, France, he injected horse serum subcutaneously and aseptically to some rabbits, 5 ml every 6 days in different places. A few hours after the fourth injection, a soft edema appeared at the injection site; the fifth and sixth injections produced a firmer swelling; the seventh and eighth infection caused a hemorrhagic patch (Figure 17.26) that became necrotic and eventually healed. Dr. Arthus did not study the mechanism but warned clinicians that horse serum, if injected repeatedly, could cause local necrosis. We should add that *when local changes develop, they begin to appear 4–6 hours after the injection* (we will soon see why).

Eventually, the mechanism was worked out (Figure 17.27) (100, 102, 113). The injections of horse serum are absorbed, and the rabbit becomes increasingly hyperimmunized. By the seventh injection there is so much precipitating antibody in the circulation and interstitial spaces that a large subcutaneous injection of antigen can react with it and create a massive amount of antigen–antibody complex. Exactly where the initial meeting of antigen and antibody occurs has not been determined, but we believe there is enough antibody in the extracellular fluid to initiate the reaction; also, the trauma of the needle might cause some mixing of blood and injected serum. Anyway, as soon as some complex forms, the first

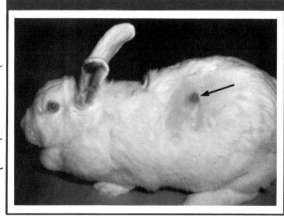

FIGURE 17.26 Typical Arthus reaction. The rabbit was sensitized to bovine gamma globulin with six subcutaneous injections (one every 3 days). The seventh injection produced this hemorrhagic necrosis (**arrow**); it was photographed 24 hours later.

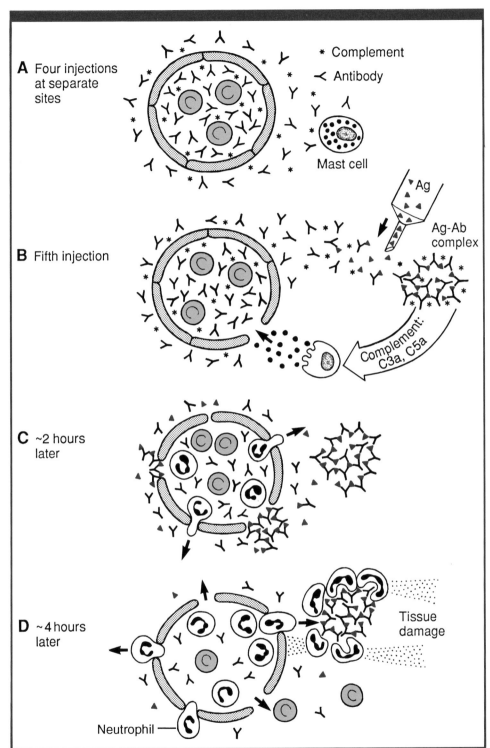

FIGURE 17.27

Mechanism of vascular injury by the Arthus reaction. **A:** Conditions that predispose to an Arthus reaction: precipitating antibodies are present in the plasma and also in the interstitium, where mast cells lie waiting. **B:** Injection of antigen at this stage creates antigen–antibody complexes, which activate complement; anaphylatoxins of complement (C3a, C4a, C5a) degranulate the mast cells, releasing histamine, which creates gaps in the venules. **C:** Antibody escapes through the venular gaps and creates massive antigen–antibody complexes. Complement activation produces chemotactic molecules, by which neutrophil emigration is initiated. **D:** Activated neutrophils phagocytize the complexes; in the process they release enzymes that cause further damage to the vascular wall and surrounding tissues. The venular basement membrane is also digested, which explains the escape of red blood cells into the tissues (hemorrhage).

component of complement, C1, settles on it and activates the complement cascade; anaphylatoxins are released (C3a, C4a, and C5a), the mast cells degranulate and release histamine, endothelial gaps develop in the venules, and large amounts of intravascular antibody combine with the antigen. Electron micrographs actually show fluffy masses of complex in the lumen; leukocytes are also attracted (Figure 17.28) (95, 121).

The crowd of granulocytes attracted by complement chemotaxins is remarkable; in principle the granulocytes are summoned to remove the com-

FIGURE 17.28 Electron micrograph of ongoing Arthus reaction in the wall of a rabbit venule (3 minutes after injection of antigen). Note the gap in the endothelium filled with an amorphous mass of antigen–antibody complex. **E:** Endothelium. **G:** Emigrating granulocyte. **AA:** Antigen–antibody complex. **Arrowheads:** Basement membrane. **Bar** = 1 μm. (Reproduced with permission from [162].)

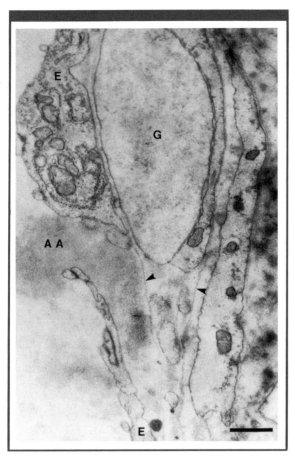

plex, but in their fury of activation they spill enough enzymes and free radicals to destroy the venular wall as they cross it (Figure 17.29). The Arthus phenomenon was one of the first lesions to

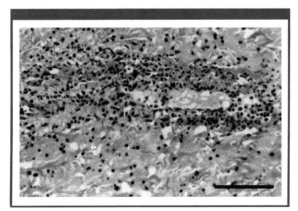

FIGURE 17.29
Typical venule in an Arthus lesion. Emigrating neutrophils are crowded in and around the wall of the venule, which is injured in the process. From the skin of a rabbit hyperimmunized against bovine albumin, 4 hours after the seventh local injection of albumin. **Bar** = 100 μm.

reveal the destructive power of the otherwise friendly neutrophils. *No Arthus lesion can be produced in an animal depleted of leukocytes or of complement* (102, 113, 127). As for the hemorrhage and necrosis observable with the naked eye, they are explained by the venular lesions just described; the delay of 4–6 hours is the time required for all these events to unfold.

> The Arthus phenomenon lends itself to classic immunologic games: it can be obtained as a passive Arthus (serum from a prepared rabbit is given intravenously to a second rabbit, which becomes immediately able to produce an Arthus reaction upon injection with antigen); or a reversed passive Arthus (antigen is injected intravenously, and antibody is injected locally: an Arthus lesion develops promptly if the doses are right) (113).

In a modern clinical setting, a skin reaction as Arthus described it should never be seen because proteins should not be injected locally in large amounts as they were 100 years ago. However, the basic mechanism is at work in a variety of lesions thought to be caused by complex—for example, in the *vasculitis* produced in the "serum sickness" model of complex-induced disease, as we will now explain.

GENERAL MODEL OF COMPLEX-MEDIATED HYPERSENSITIVITY: SERUM SICKNESS

As often happens in immunology, this mechanism of disease was first observed clinically, then worked out in the laboratory.

Clinical Serum Sickness This condition used to be called "serum fever" or "serum rash" because of the clinical symptoms that appear after a *single* large subcutaneous injection of horse serum. The condition has almost vanished in its original form, because injections of horse serum are rarely indicated (116). However, serum sickness is still with us because it can be produced by a different mechanism: *a number of drugs—as a side effect—combine with plasma proteins and turn them into antigens.* The result is the same as with serum sickness: *a lot of foreign protein circulating in the blood* (112).

We hope the reader was intrigued by the "catch" planted in the previous paragraph: serum sickness was caused by a *single* injection of serum, whereas immune responses are typically induced by a second challenge. Strange but true. There is no breaking of immunologic rules. *In reading what follows, keep in mind that a single large injection of antigen is absorbed by the lymphatics over many days, and basically works like a series of daily injections.*

The natural history of serum sickness was worked out in 1905 by von Pirquet and Schick in the Department of Scarlet Fever and Diphtheria at the St. Anna pediatric hospital in Vienna. The work was reported in a small book called *Serumkrankheit*.

When Dr. Schick was asked to revise the book 45 years later, he found nothing to change and so republished it as it was (126). We know of very few books that could stand that test; another is Metchnikoff's Lectures on the Comparative Pathology of Inflammation, *which was reprinted in a paperback edition after 77 years (118).*

The children in that Viennese hospital ward were treated for diphtheria or scarlet fever with antibodies from immunized horses; in practice this required huge subcutaneous doses (up to 200 ml) of horse serum. Eight to 12 days later the "Serumkrankheit" was expected; its incidence increased with the dose of serum (85% after 100–200 ml, 22% after 10–30 ml). The signs and symptoms were very much the same as those seen today in cases of drug hypersensitivity:

- A slight but painful swelling of the regional lymph nodes draining the injection site (the nodes were beginning to make antihorse-serum antibody).

- Fever and an uncomfortable itchy rash.
- Some edema, or rather fluid retention, not always visible (it was von Pirquet who first had the idea of judging the extent of edema by weighing the patient) (Figure 17.30).
- Joint pains, which were common and significant though the objective signs were minimal.
- A precipitous drop in the number of leukocytes in the peripheral blood when the symptoms appeared (presumably because the leukocytes, activated by mast-cell PAF, tend to clump, and the clumps are filtered out by the lungs).
- A mild albuminuria, but no renal disease ever developed.

Overall, *serum sickness was a nuisance but not a life-threatening event*; no patient ever died of it though two came close (125). For the Viennese team, the nuisance was acceptable because there was no alternative treatment. Antitoxic serum was the only rational therapy available. What had been tried previously was hopelessly empirical: intravenous injections of lamb blood or of milk with sugar (126). Anyway, the antisera really helped (123), and mortality by diphtheria dropped dramatically (Figure 17.31). Von Behring, the pioneer of this treatment, was rewarded with the Nobel prize.

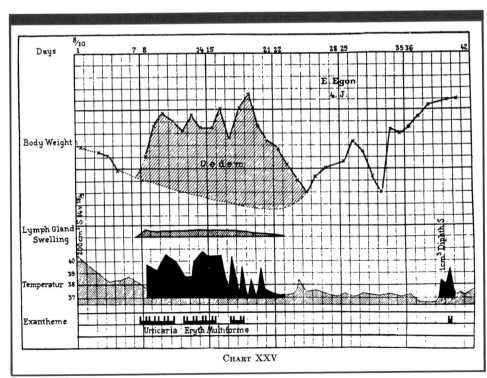

CHART XXV

FIGURE 17.30
Manifestations of serum sickness in a 4-year-old child hospitalized for diphtheria around the year 1900. Upon admission he received 200 ml of antidiphtheric serum subcutaneously. Typically, on day 8, urticaria and swelling of the lymph nodes developed. Fever appeared shortly thereafter. The skin eruption changed aspect after a few days; this also is typical. The generalized edema was assessed by changes in body weight. On the day 39, note the effect of a subcutaneous injection of 1.0 ml of "diphtheria serum for immunization." This time the response is immediate: fever and rash. See text for explanation. (Original diagram from [126].)

FIGURE 17.31
Drop in mortal-
ity from diphthe-
ria coincident
with the avail-
ability of anti-
diphtheric serum
(Prussia, about
1895; children
under 15). The
morbidity re-
mained un-
changed. (Re-
drawn from
[123].)

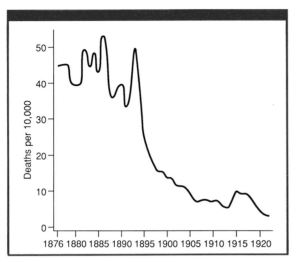

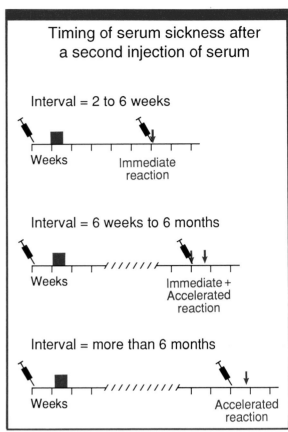

FIGURE 17.32
This diagram answers the question, "Can one have serum
sickness twice in a row?" using data reported by von Pirquet
and Schick in 1905. Syringes indicate injection of horse
serum; arrows indicate recurrence of serum sickness. The
left part of the diagram shows that after the first injection
of horse serum, serum sickness (**red square**) developed
between 8 and 12 days. *Top:* If a second injection was given
within 6 weeks, serum sickness reappeared immediately
because the patient still had circulating antibodies. *Center:*
If the second injection was given between 6 weeks and 6
months after the first, serum sickness again reappeared
immediately because of some circulating antibody, and
memory cells produced a third episode of serum sickness (an
accelerated reaction) about a week later. *Bottom:* if the
second injection was given more than 6 months after the
first, no circulating antibody was left; so there was no
immediate reaction, but the memory cells produced an
accelerated reaction after less than a week.

*Test your grasp of the antibody response. Von Pirquet
and Schick reported that some children had to receive
two injections of horse serum: for example, the first
to treat diphtheria, the second to treat scarlet fever. In
these cases the timing of the second attack of serum
sickness differed according to the interval between the
first and second injection of serum. The pattern
observed depended on whether the two treatments
were separated by 2 to 6 weeks, 6 weeks to 6
months, or more than 6 months. Why? The answer
is in Figure 17.32 (126, p. 79).*

PATHOGENESIS OF SERUM SICKNESS: ENTER THE RABBIT

Serum sickness remained somewhat obscure until
the late 1960s. One of its puzzling features was that
it broke the two-shot rule of immunology: the
immune response appeared after a single injection
of foreign protein. The mechanism was finally
worked out by Dixon, Cochrane, and others using
rabbits injected with bovine serum albumin
(101, 107). The basic method of this study was to
maintain, to begin with, the one-shot injection
but to give the dose intravenously, a more
controllable route.

The main findings are summarized in Figure
17.33, which has become a classic. In essence: the
amount of circulating antigen drops, slowly at first
as it is phagocytized or escapes from the blood, and
then faster as it is bound by increasing amounts of
newly formed antibody. For 12 days no free antibody can be found because as long as antigen circulates, all the antibody is complexed. At about day
13 all the injected antigen has been used up (either
phagocytized or complexed) and now free antibody
appears. Morphologic injury develops (reversibly)
between days 8 and 15, mainly in the "blood container" in which the complexes circulate (heart and
arteries), in the blood filters (the renal glomeruli),
and in the joints (reminiscent of clinical serum
sickness). *The lesions are mild and reversible because
the supply of antigen is limited by the one-shot approach.*

*That lesions develop in the blood container seems to
make sense, but then why do lesions spare the venous*

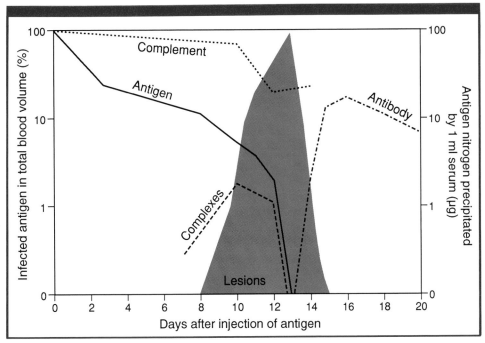

FIGURE 17.33
Sequence of events in classic "one-shot" serum sickness in the rabbit. No antibody is detected in the blood before day 13 because it combines with antigen and forms complexes. After all the antigen has been complexed, antibody can be detected. Note the behavior of complement, which correlates with complex formation. The colored area indicates the time and intensity of lesions. (Reproduced with permission from [106].)

side? And why are the joints affected? We found no satisfactory answers.

Human diseases caused by the serum-sickness mechanism are usually chronic, which means that the supply of complexes is also chronic. Therefore, a *chronic model* of experimental serum sickness was developed, by giving rabbits daily injections of antigen (108). These experiments became especially important because they showed that *the size of the complexes is critical;* and their size, as you may recall, depends on the relative concentrations of antigen and circulating antibody (Figure 17.34). This means that the size of the complexes depends on the antibody response of the rabbit:

• *Some rabbits produce huge amounts of anti-body.* Complexes formed under such conditions—antibody excess—are very large, easily removed by the littoral phagocytes of the RES/MPS (p. 297), and little or no disease ensues.

• *Other rabbits are "minimal responders,"* which leads to very small complexes as expected from the condition of antigen excess. Such complexes are too small to activate complement and to be pathogenic.

• *Medium responders are most at risk.* Their complexes are just large enough to be pathogenic but small enough to circulate for a long time; they become trapped in filtering organs, activate complement, and cause disease.

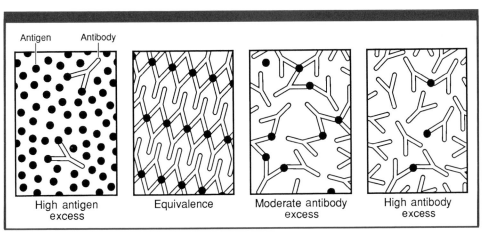

FIGURE 17.34
Antigen–antibody complexes vary in size depending on the concentration of the reactants. When complexes develop in the bloodstream, the larger complexes (formed at the equivalence point) are easily removed by the RES/MPS and cause no harm; the complexes more apt to cause damage are those of medium size, which develop in moderate antibody excess. (Adapted from [69].)

Question: why do the various rabbits respond differently? Is it not a fact that the immune response is programmed, and thus should proceed in a standard fashion? The unsatisfactory answer is that even though the immune response is certainly programmed, individuals have different responses, quantitatively and sometimes even qualitatively. The individual's genetic makeup is important; just consider that not everybody becomes allergic to pollen.

The lesions in experimental serum sickness are important as a model for human diseases. Because complexes are developing in the blood, lesions develop in the blood container and its main filter: the arteries, the heart, and the glomeruli. Not every detail is understood (108).

Arteritis Surprisingly, inflammation of the arteries is focal and hits only the small branches, especially those of the coronaries (Figure 17.35). Visualize the lesion of arteritis as a small sphere of acute inflammation encasing a short segment of an artery; typically, the wall is necrotic and infiltrated with fibrin (a combination empirically described as **fibrinoid necrosis**). Immunofluorescence shows antigen, antibody, and complement in the lesion.

There is no doubt that the medial necrosis is caused by the activated polymorphs, attracted by activated

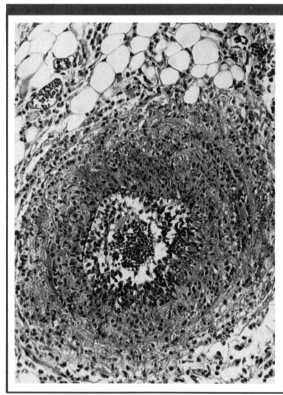

FIGURE 17.35 Arteritis in experimental serum sickness (rabbit). The intima is attacked and destroyed by leukocytes; in a more advanced stage the media is also destroyed. The main inflammatory cell is the neutrophil (not recognizable here). (Courtesy of Dr. C.G. Cochrane, Department of Immunology, Research Institute of Scripps Clinic, La Jolla, CA.)

complement; but beyond this, the pathogenesis of complex-induced arteritis is not clear. Complexes are too large to cross the endothelium. To overcome this difficulty the following theoretical sequence has been proposed (96, 114): the circulating antigen induces some IgE (as well as IgG and IgM) → the IgE sensitizes mast cells and circulating basophils → some basophils settle on the arterial intima and release histamine → endothelial gaps are formed → the door opens for the complexes. As far as we know, the basophil mechanism is purely theoretical. It has never been verified. We prefer to believe that all the proteins involved cross the endothelium by transcytosis and then react within the arterial wall.

Cardiac Lesions Lesions are especially obvious on the valves. Small platelet masses (thrombi) attach to the luminal surfaces of the valve flaps where they come into contact when the valves snap shut: this area is thought to be prone to microtrauma, especially if the valves are misshaped. It is conceivable that small patches of endothelium are removed by this mechanism; complexes could then penetrate into the underlying connective tissue, activate complement, attract leukocytes, and induce platelet deposition—but this is largely speculative. There are also diffuse mononuclear cell inflammatory infiltrates throughout the heart.

Glomerular Lesions These lesions are partially accounted for by the filtering mechanism: lumps of protein precipitate appear along the capillary basement membrane (Figure 17.36) (p. 573). Oddly enough, electron microscopy sometimes shows them on the outer surface of the basement membrane, which would seem analogous to finding coffee grounds on the brew side of a coffee filter. One explanation is that antigens seep through the basement membrane filter and form complexes with antibodies where they are stopped—against the surfaces of the podocytes. However, a number of factors, such as molecular charge, affect the deposition of the complexes. Ultimately, this buildup of foreign material leads to hyperplasia of the mesangial cells (which lie outside the capillaries and phagocytize the complexes) and of the Bowman's capsule (Figure 17.37).

Here is a challenge. Neutrophils are always attracted by complexes, yet the glomerular lesions of serum sickness are notoriously poor in neutrophils. Depletion of leukocytes abolishes arteritis but not glomerular lesions. This remains a mystery. We propose our own explanation, which has not yet been tested: the lumps of complex do activate

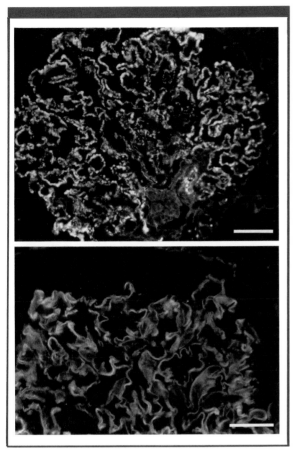

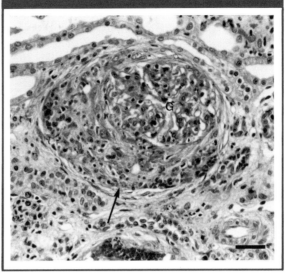

FIGURE 17.37
Glomerulus from the kidney of a rabbit in which chronic serum sickness was induced. The glomerular tuft (**G**) has been squeezed to about half its normal size by hyperplasia of the cells lining Bowman's capsule (**arrow**). This is but one of several misfortunes that can befall the glomerulus in chronic serum sickness. **Bar** = 25 μm. (Specimen kindly supplied by Dr. C.G. Cochrane, Scrips Clinic, La Jolla, CA.)

HOW DO COMPLEXES CAUSE INJURY?

The most convincing experiment showing that leukocytes cause damage in complex-induced lesions is to test animals that have been depleted of leukocytes with nitrogen mustard or antileukocyte serum (108). In such animals Arthus lesions, arteritis, and synovitis are suppressed even though the masses of complexes are present; the suppression occurs also if complement is depleted (100).

The mediation of glomerular injury is more complicated; it depends in part on the type of antibody involved. If rabbits are injected with IgG1 anti-glomerular–basement membrane antibodies, the resulting glomerular injury is neutrophil-dependent; with IgG2 antibodies it is not. In the latter case, the mediation of the injury is not yet known (107). *Note:* we should warn our readers that the mechanisms whereby complexes are deposited in the glomeruli are many and complicated (p. 539).

A basic question: how do the lesions of serum sickness relate to the Arthus lesion? Answer: they are very similar. *The neutrophil-rich lesions of serum sickness are essentially small Arthus lesions;* both types of lesion are caused by a local deposit of complex that summons a swarm of leukocytes. Remember that in both local and general models

FIGURE 17.36
Immunofluorescence staining of the glomerular basement membrane using antihuman IgG antibody. *Top:* Typical "lumpy-bumpy" pattern of fluorescence is due to clumps of antigen–antibody complexes deposited along the capillary basement membrane; from a patient with membranous glomerulonephritis (of unknown cause). *Bottom:* this linear (continuous) pattern of fluorescence occurs when the basement membrane is evenly coated with IgG antibody; from a patient with Goodpasture's disease, caused by an antibody against the glomerular basement membrane. **Bars** = 25 μm. (Courtesy of Dr. G. Andres, University of Buffalo, Buffalo, NY.)

complement, but the chemotactic by-products are washed out with the filtrate before they can diffuse back into the lumen of the capillary. Glomerular capillaries are unique with regard to their perfusion physiology: they filter under high pressure (60 mm Hg, almost four times the pressure in skin capillaries) and do not reabsorb.

Injury of the Joints Joints are not always affected in serum sickness, but when they are, injury consists of synovial edema with fibrin deposits and mononuclear infiltrates.

of disease, we are dealing with the same basic principle: complex-induced injury. The glomerular lesions of serum sickness are special because they depend largely on the function of filtration, but they also depend on complexes that activate complement and attract leukocytes.

> *Von Pirquet and Schick sometimes injected their children with a second dose of serum: did this produce Arthus lesions? In fact, they did notice local redness and swelling, although not an all-out, necrotic, and hemorrhagic Arthus lesion. These local changes were noticed even a week or so after the first injection. Presumably enough antigen was left over at the injection site to react with the newly formed antibody.*

HUMAN DISEASES MEDIATED BY ANTIGEN–ANTIBODY COMPLEXES

Antigen–antibody complexes are thought to participate in many human diseases. How are these diseases recognized? Microscopy is helpful: any focal arteritis or vasculitis is suspect. The next step is to analyze the lesions by immunohistochemistry: if complexes are present, they should be demonstrable with antibodies against complement and against immunoglobulin (representing antibody). The search for antigen is far more difficult because in most cases there is no clue as to what it may be. There are also methods for identifying complexes in the blood, even if the antigen is unknown (107).

The best examples of complex-mediated diseases in humans are *polyarteritis nodosa* and *glomerulonephritis;* two others, *systemic lupus erythematosus* and *rheumatoid arthritis* will be described in relation to autoimmune disease (p. 569).

Polyarteritis Nodosa Polyarteritis nodosa (PAN) looks like an exaggerated version of serum sickness arteritis except that it tends to be deadly. It affects small and medium-sized arteries, and it is strictly segmental: *nodosa* means knotty, and the knots are spherical inflammatory foci encasing a short segment of artery, as also seen in experimental models of complex-mediated arteritis (p. 000) (Figures 17.38, 17.39). The inflammatory foci tend to be located at bifurcations and can progress to several complications: the inflamed arterial segments may literally blow out and bleed or simply expand into small aneurysms that can be seen on arteriograms; they can also become thrombosed and cause infarcts in the tissues downstream. Clinically, PAN prefers young adult males; it usually presents as a fever of unknown origin, accompanied by malaise and a variety of symptoms depending on the prevailing localization (often the kidney). Diagnosis depends on a biopsy taken from an organ that appears to be especially affected, such as kidney, muscle, or skin. The pathogenesis is not well understood and may be autoimmune. Antibodies against leukocytes are present, and their titer correlates with severity; 30 percent of the patients have hepatitis B antigen in the serum. Globulin and complement can be found in the lesions. Left untreated, PAN is usually fatal; corticosteroids improve the 5-year survival to 48 percent.

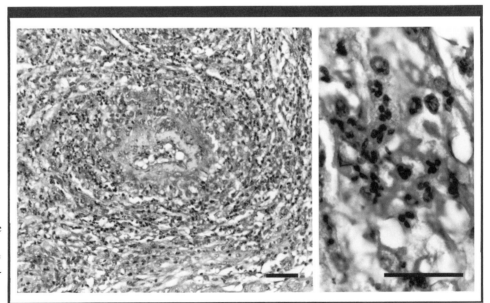

FIGURE 17.38

Left: Believe it or not, this was once an artery. It has been largely destroyed by periarteritis nodosa. **Bar** = 50 μm. *Right:* Cells infiltrating the artery wall are mostly neutrophils and macrophages. **Bar** = 25 μm.

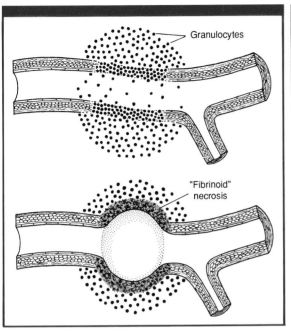

FIGURE 17.39
Structural changes in polyarteritis nodosa. *Top*: Inflammatory cells, mainly granulocytes (neutrophils and eosinophils), are attracted to a segment of the arterial media (presumably by products of complement activation caused by antigen–antibody complexes). *Bottom*: Necrosis of that segment, which becomes soaked with fibrin (fibrinoid necrosis), followed by aneurysmal dilatation.

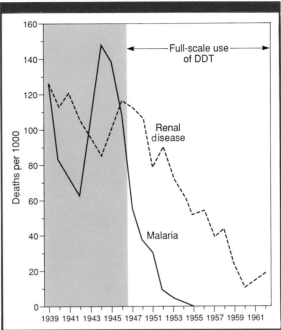

FIGURE 17.40
Evidence that malaria showers the kidney with antigen–antibody complexes, causing renal disease. In a part of British Guiana, between 1939 and 1959, the full-scale use of DDT decreased not only the number of deaths from malaria, but also the deaths from chronic renal disease due to antigen–antibody complex deposition in the glomeruli. (Reproduced with permission from [110].)

PAN is but one of many forms of vasculitis, which may affect any artery from the aorta to the microcirculation. An immune (and autoimmune) pathogenesis is often likely but not always demonstrable. The vasculitides are a vast family of lesions that are, on the whole, poorly understood (103). Note: A form of mononuclear-cell vasculitis in mice depends on Type IV (cell-mediated) hypersensitivity (119).

Glomerulonephritis Glomerular inflammation due to showers of complexes occurs as a complication of many human diseases. All that is needed is some mechanism that injects antigens into the blood; tumors can do it, and so can many chronic infections such as syphilis (115) and malaria. In fact, it was noticed in a field study in Africa that when malaria was eradicated from a region, the associated glomerular disease tended to disappear with it (Figure 17.40) (110).

The best-known example of glomerular complex disease in man is *poststreptococcal glomerulonephritis*. The sequence begins with a throat infection with certain strains of streptococcus;

streptococcal antigens are released into the blood, antibodies are formed, and the resulting complexes are retained by the glomeruli.

The statement that "complexes are retained" may not be entirely accurate. It has been suggested that a bacterial antigen first seeps across the glomerular capillary wall and becomes deposited in the mesangium; later it is joined by the antibody. This complex then stimulates mesangial cell proliferation (Figure 17.41) (129).

Note: The most common form of complex-mediated renal disease is caused, oddly enough, by complexes of IgA, the immunoglobulin that is normally secreted by mucosal surfaces (109).

The clinical effect of glomerular complexes is the so-called nephrotic syndrome; protein is lost into the urine by excessive permeability of the glomerular capillary, probably caused by the membrane-attack complex of activated complement.

Hypersensitivity Pneumonia This is another group of diseases in which antigen–antibody complexes are thought to intervene: namely

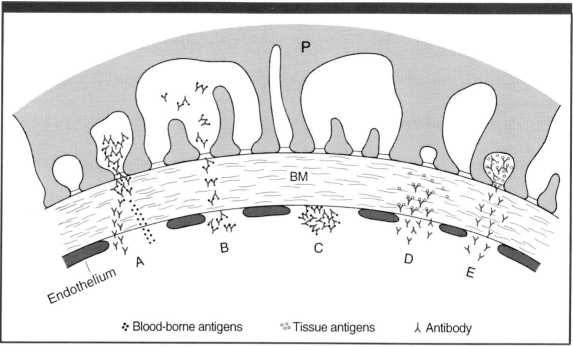

FIGURE 17.41

Various mechanisms leading to the deposition of antigen-antibody complexes against, within or beyond the glomerular basement membrane (**BM**). **A:** Antigen and antibody penetrate separately, and complexes develop within or beyond the basement membrane. **B:** Small complexes penetrate and cross the basement membrane. **C:** Large complexes are retained against the luminal (subendothelial) surface of the basement membrane. **D:** A component of the basement membrane becomes antigenic, elicits antibodies, and complexes are formed within the basement membrane. **E:** Antigens appear on the surface of the podocyte (**P**), and antibodies are trapped in that location. (Adapted from [104].)

chronic lung diseases caused by organic dusts, most of them job-related. Examples are pigeon breeder's disease (inhalation of dust of dried pigeon feces), farmer's lung (inhalation of an *actinomyces*), humidifier lung, as well as mushroom picker's, cheese washer's, paprika slicer's, maple-bark stripper's, wood trimmer's, chicken plucker's, and even sauna-bather's disease, plus sequoiosis in the lumber industry and many others (124). The plasma of these patients contains precipitating antibodies to the various antigens as required to produce complexes and Arthus- or serum sickness-type lesions. Inhalation of the antigen causes symptoms (coughing, chills, fever, and dyspnea) with a delay of 4–12 hours, which falls between the delay typical of the Arthus mechanism and that of delayed-type (cell-mediated, Type IV) hypersensitivity. The pathogenesis is not yet clear; it may include components of Type I hypersensitivity (allergic asthma) as well as of Type III (complex-mediated) and Type IV (cell-mediated) hypersensitivity. A reminder that human classifications do not always fit with those of Nature.

Hypersensitivity Type IV: Delayed Type or Cell-Mediated

Unlike the three types of hypersensitivity described so far, this fourth type does not depend on circulating antibodies. To understand this rather intricate topic, we can reason as follows. It so happens that some infectious agents, such as the tubercle bacillus, do not induce a significant antibody response, or induce antibodies that have no protective effect. This deprives the host of a major mechanism of defense. Fortunately, the immune system has another effector arm: sensitized lymphocytes, and these do become responsible for the host's defense. This type of lymphocyte-dependent defense is called *cell-mediated immunity* or CMI. We find it at work in many infectious diseases, such as tuberculosis: specifically sensitized lymphocytes secrete cytokines that recruit and activate other lymphocytes as well as macrophages, and together they fight the parasite. The typical result is the *immune granuloma* (a lump of macrophages and lymphocytes in which the invader is buried) such as we described it in an earlier chapter.

If the story of cell-mediated immunity (CMI) ended here, it would not belong in a chapter on hypersensitivity; yet we must deal with it because—as all biological mechanisms—it can go wrong. It becomes a nuisance when it is unleashed against antigens that are by themselves quite harmless, such as urushiol, the "irritant" of poison ivy. There is nothing to be gained by mounting a violent inflammatory response against the leaves of poison ivy, against metal earrings, or against the countless chemicals that produce this so-called *contact dermatitis*. A basic feature of this response is that it is much slower than the anaphylactic reactions, because lymphocytes take 12–24 hours to gather on the spot in sufficient numbers and to produce large amounts of cytokines; for this reason this response is called *delayed-type hypersensitivity* or DTH. So far, then, we can conclude that DTH is the "nuisance version" of CMI.

Nobody could doubt that the DTH of poison ivy is pure nuisance; but the distinction between CMI and DTH becomes blurred when the two coexist, as happens in many chronic infections. For example, in a patient suffering from pulmonary tuberculosis, CMI is presumably at work fighting the bacteria in the lungs; but if the patient's skin is tested by injecting suitable, *harmless* antigens of *Mycobacterium tuberculosis*, such as tuberculin or PPD, a local DTH response is obtained—as some readers will know, if they have been tested for tuberculosis. A similar skin reaction, using the appropriate bacterial antigens, can be demonstrated in the other diseases in which CMI is induced. Tuberculin and PPD, injected into the skin of normal, noninfected individuals, have no effect. *So here we have a combination of helpful CMI and nuisance DTH.* This DTH tells us that the person is hypersensitive to some bacterial protein, but does it also tell us that the individual is protected from the corresponding infection? Experience shows that it does not. Most importantly: are CMI and DTH due to different subsets of lymphocytes? This too has been debated for decades. Until the experts have settled this issue, *we choose to assume that CMI is caused a subset of "well informed" lymphocytes, and DTH by a subset of their misguided colleagues.*

We shall return to this thorny issue; in the meantime, the following pages will become easier to absorb if the reader will keep in mind that we are trying to explain the two typical examples of

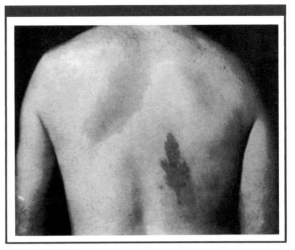

FIGURE 17.42

Contact dermatitis, a classic example of cell-mediated hypersensitivity. This gardener complained of rashes on the hands and forearms during the chrysanthemum season. A chrysanthemum leaf was strapped to his skin for 24 hours, and this is the result. There were pinhead vesicles all over the reddened area, much as with poison ivy. (Reproduced with permission from [154a].)

DTH: poison ivy (or any contact dermatitis) and the tuberculin reaction.

EXPERIMENTAL MODELS OF DELAYED-TYPE HYPERSENSITIVITY

As seen under the microscope, DTH begins in the same way as CMI: *a focus of inflammation consisting mainly of lymphocytes and macrophages*—a deceptively simple image, not yet fully explained.

Contact Dermatitis This skin lesion is excellent for illustrating the nuisance value of DTH (Figures 17.42, 17.43). Somehow, *sensitization through the intact skin favors the development of DTH*, perhaps

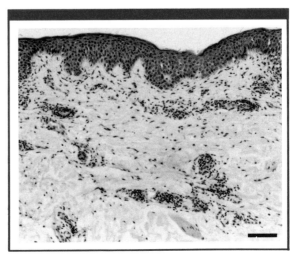

FIGURE 17.43
Contact dermatitis in human skin. Despite the very obvious and itchy clinical picture, histology is limited to a not-very-impressive infiltrate of mononuclear cells, mainly in perivascular cuffs. **Bar** = 100 μm.

because the antigen combines with a component of the epidermis (the antigen can be rubbed in with an ointment, but in some individuals just the contact with a metal surface may suffice). The resulting compound is taken up by Langerhans' cells that are lurking in the epidermis; then these cells migrate to the lymph nodes where they present their catch to T-lymphocytes. Specifically sensitized T-lymphocytes are then produced and released into the circulation (the sequence requires 2–3 weeks). From this time on, if the skin of this individual is challenged again with the same antigen, a local DTH response will occur. Its pathogenesis has been studied a great deal using the sensitizer DNCB (dinitrochlorobenzene) (Figure 17.44). The main problem is to explain how the cells get there: the final word is not yet in (Figure 17.45). Once sensitized T-lymphocytes are circulating, they must be recruited at the challenged site. Much evidence suggests that the endothelium of the local venules is able to pick up antigen from the perivascular spaces and present it to the circulating cells; the specific memory T-cells would then stop, exit, and become activated (163, 164). this group of activated T-cells might provide enough lymphokines to recruit nonspecific T-cells and macrophages. Another wave of emigrant lymphocytes and monocytes will follow if the microvascular endothelium, activated by cytokines, were to express the adhesion proteins ICAM-1 and VCAM-1 (163, 164).

Although the DTH lesion is typically composed of mononuclear cells, a few neutrophils are usually present during the early phases, much to the disappointment of students, who would prefer clear-cut situations (150, 156). There are also scattered filaments of fibrin, which explain the firmness noticed on palpation (138). The presence of fibrin implies that some vessels must be leaky, and so they are. Leakage begins 3–6 hours after skin testing and peaks at 24 hours (131, 182); some of the leaky vessels are capillaries (182).

Adjuvants An *adjuvant* is "a substance that enhances, nonspecifically, the immune response to an antigen" (168). Because adjuvants favor the induction of a cell-mediated response (sensitized T-lymphocytes) as well as the production of antibodies (via the B-cell pathway), they are often used, experimentally, for the study of the cell-mediated response: an antigen, which alone will induce mainly antibodies, is injected together with an appropriate adjuvant, and both types of responses will be obtained.

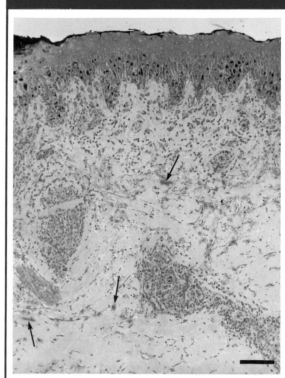

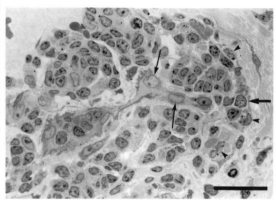

FIGURE 17.44

Focus of inflammation produced by delayed-type hypersensitivity. *Top:* Histology of a 72-hour contact dermatitis produced in a human volunteer with dinitrochlorobenzene. Mononuclear cells are scattered throughout and collected in cuffs about venules. Note the strands of fibrin (**arrows**), which confer the typical firmness to this lesion. **Bar** = 100 μm. *Bottom:* Higher magnification shows the perivascular mononuclear cell infiltrate typical of delayed hypersensitivity. **Arrowheads:** Three basophils, partially degranulated, another typical feature of delayed hypersensitivity reactions in humans. **Thin arrows:** Hypertrophic endothelial cells. **Thick arrow:** Mast cell. **Bar** = 25 μm. (*Top* reproduced with permission from [148]. *Bottom* courtesy of Dr. H.F. Dvorak, Beth Israel Hospital, Harvard Medical School, Boston, MA.)

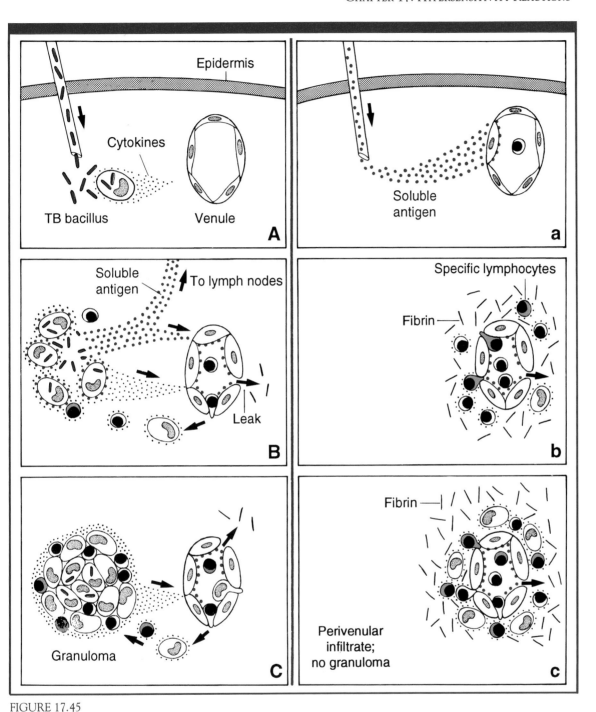

FIGURE 17.45
Comparing the tissue reactions to tubercle bacilli and to tuberculin (or PPD). *Left:* **A:** Tubercle bacilli are phagocytized by macrophages, which become activated and produce cytokines. **B:** The cytokines activate the endothelium of a venule, and cause it to leak; this endothelium is also reached by antigen from the tubercle bacilli, and presents it toward the lumen. (Some of this antigen, carried by the lymph, reaches the regional lymph nodes where an immune response is elicited). Macrophages and lymphocytes (by now some are specifically sensitized) are trapped and emigrate toward the focus of infection. **C:** *End result: a granuloma is formed,* consisting mainly of macrophages and lymphocytes, some of which are specifically sensitized. The granuloma produces cytokines which activate macrophages and vascular endothelia in the neighborhood. Venular leakage leads to fibrin deposition. *Right:* **a:** Tuberculin (or PPD) injected into the tissue diffuses toward a venule; endothelial cells pick up this antigenic material and present it toward the lumen. **b:** The activated venular endothelium becomes leaky, it also traps circulating lymphocytes (specific and non-specific) and monocytes, which emigrate. **c:** *End result:* an activated venule surrounded by a cuff of mononuclear cells and some fibrin. *No granuloma is formed.*

Therefore, given an antigen, the classic procedure for obtaining a cell-mediated response is to inject that antigen into the skin, mixed with a messy substance called *Freund's complete adjuvant*, which consists of heat-killed tubercle bacilli suspended in mineral oil. So effective is this method that it will even twist the arm of the immune system to react against the body's own tissue when this tissue is minced, mixed with Freund's adjuvant, and injected.

This peculiar oily ritual calls for some explanation. How could anyone dream up such a nasty mixture as Freund's adjuvant?

It all began when Louis Dienes asked himself—in North Carolina in the late 1920s—why tuberculous guinea pigs developed a delayed-type skin hypersensitivity to tuberculin (146). Perhaps it had something to do with the peculiar tuberculous "granulation tissue"? He injected some egg white into the granulation tissue of his tuberculous guinea pigs; and sure enough, the guinea pigs developed a delayed tuberculin-type response also to the egg white. Did this depend on some action of the live tubercle bacilli? Dr. Dienes injected some normal guinea pigs with heat-killed Mycobacterium tuberculosis, which produced a strong inflammatory response. When he injected egg white into this mass, he again obtained a delayed-type hypersensitivity against egg white. So the mycobacteria somehow had the property of enhancing delayed-type hypersensitivity toward an antigen injected with them. At that time Jules Freund, a fellow Hungarian, was working with Dienes (177). In 1942 Freund and McDermott introduced the mineral oil, plus a lanolin-type solvent, which made it easier to suspend the bacilli (151). The trend to adjuvants was on. By the way, Freund and McDermott also found that their mixture, injected with horse serum, enhanced the DTH as well as antibody formation.

Note: *Freund's adjuvant is generally used to push the immune response in the direction of DTH, and it works; but the antibody response is also increased* (156).

Today the list of adjuvants is long (154). It includes aluminum hydroxide (alum, the only adjuvant licensed for use in humans) and bacterial products such as lipopolysaccharide (LPS) and muramyl dipeptide (MDP); MDP is thought to be the minimal sequence capable of replacing the whole tubercle bacillus (137). Some adjuvants favor cell-mediated immunity, others the antibody response (129). Recently added are the versatile *liposomes* (p. 213), which have the advantage of being nontoxic.

How do adjuvants work? Probably by two mechanisms: they form a depot that prolongs the contact between antigen and antigen-presenting cells, and they activate macrophages (130, 154).

Delayed-Type Hypersensitivity and Tuberculosis

Delayed hypersensitivity is so closely associated with tuberculosis, biologically as well as historically, that a brief review of this disease is essential. The very word *allergy* was coined in relation to skin tests in tuberculous patients. Tuberculosis as a social problem had begun to disappear from the level of consciousness in the Western world (until AIDS brought it back), but on a global level it still remains the most prevalent infection: half of the world's population is infected (152), active cases amount to 2 billion and cause 3 million deaths per year (175). The decline of tuberculosis in Western cultures teaches a humbling lesson, at least for medical scientists: it began long before the advent of effective therapy and was probably related to changing social, nutritional, and hygienic conditions (Figure 17.46) (147).

Tuberculosis as a disease suggests two main thoughts. First, it is predominantly a lung infection: *Mycobacterium tuberculosis* is an obligate aerobe, and the lung offers the best oxygen supply. Second, the tubercle bacillus has worked out a way to be a nearly perfect parasite: it tends to produce slow, indolent tissue responses, whereby the host becomes chronically ill and transmits bacteria to

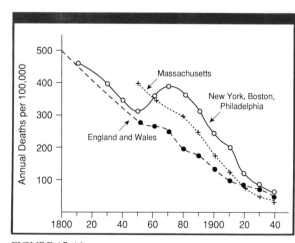

FIGURE 17.46

Mortality from pulmonary tuberculosis 1800–1940. Deaths began to decline long before specific therapy became available (streptomycin, in the 1940s). The transient increase in mortality that began around 1850 in the large cities of the United States may reflect a sudden influx of Irish immigrants. (Reproduced with permission from [147].)

others but does not die of the infection, at least not for many years. The body mounts an immune response that teeters on the adequate. The infected tissues tend to heal by scarring and to contain the infection, but they also tend to melt into a semifluid necrotic mass that spreads the infection. The two tendencies can coexist in the same lung (145). The balance between healing and progression depends on factors that are poorly understood. Hypersensitivity is probably involved, and that is why we discuss tuberculosis here; but be prepared for disappointment: the role of hypersensitivity in tuberculosis is still not clear.

This discussion concerns tuberculosis caused by Mycobacterium tuberculosis hominis, *the human strain. In AIDS the infection is mostly due to M.* tuberculosis avium, *once typical of birds, which produces a different type of disease, less centered on the lungs; the skin test with PPD is positive, although not as strongly as in infections with the human strain.*

Tuberculosis: The Clinical Footsteps Unpasteurized milk may contain the bovine strain *Mycobacterium tuberculosis bovis,* which can cause infection by penetrating through the tonsils. The ensuing disease is tuberculosis of the cervical lymph nodes (183). However, most human cases of tuberculosis not related to AIDS are caused by *Mycobacterium tuberculosis hominis* spread by airborne particles from infectious patients, perpetuating the cycle of pulmonary tuberculosis. The events we now describe as *primary tuberculosis* were once typical of childhood, but improved preventive measures have raised the age of first exposure to early adulthood, or even later.

Inhaled clusters of bacteria reach the alveoli if they are small enough (1–3 bacteria; one bacillus is 5 μm long). Larger particles hit the bronchial mucosa and are transported back up by the so-called mucociliary elevator and eventually are coughed out or swallowed. The mucosae of the bronchi and the digestive tract are fairly resistant to infection (145).

The alveolar macrophages phagocytize the bacilli, and the battle is on (Figure 17.47) (130, 141, 143, 172). You may recall the cunning survival strategy of phagocytized tubercle bacilli, which prevent the fusion of the phagosome with lysosomes (p. 141). So the bacilli continue to grow within the macrophages and eventually kill many of them (the mechanism is not clear). New macrophages replace the dead ones, and within a few weeks the *primary lesion* has developed; this is a

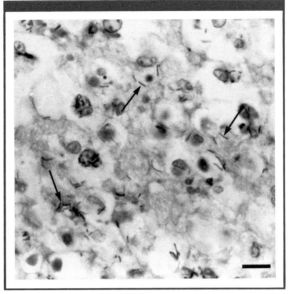

FIGURE 17.47 Phagocytosis of *Mycobacterium tuberculosis* by alveolar macrophages (**arrows**). in a case of tuberculous pneumonia. Acid-fast stain. **Bar** = 10 μm.

firm nodule 4–16 mm in diameter, often visible in X-rays, consisting of a necrotic "caseous" (cheesy) center surrounded by live macrophages, lymphocytes, and a fibrous layer (Figure 17.48). Some bacilli escape along the lymphatics and establish one or more infections in the hilar lymph nodes. The combination of the primary nodule with the infected hilar nodes constitute the *primary complex* or *Ghon complex.* After 1–2 months the bacilli have released enough antigenic material to give a positive skin test (to be discussed later); other

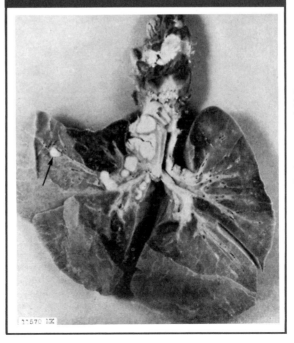

FIGURE 17.48 Rapidly progressing tuberculosis in the lungs of a 19-month-old infant. The small primary lesion in the middle lobe of the right lung (**arrow**) gave rise to greatly enlarged, caseous hilar peritracheal lymph nodes. (Reproduced with permission from [166].)

clinical evidence of infection may be lacking, except for a mild fever.

The primary complex in most cases stops growing and "heals" with partial calcification. It does not truly heal because some live bacilli probably survive in a dormant state, ready to reactivate the lesion, perhaps throughout the patient's lifetime. An individual with healed primary infection may never hear from it again, or may proceed to what is called *post-primary tuberculosis*. Bacteria spreading by the bloodstream may set up a new focus elsewhere in the lung or in any other part of the body. By now the immune system is prepared, and any charge of tubercle bacteria is met by a swift response: they are enclosed in a granuloma called *tubercle* (p. 443). Sometimes a large number of bacteria penetrate into the bloodstream at the same time and seed tubercles throughout the lung or the whole body: this is *miliary tuberculosis*, so called because the countless tiny, whitish granulomas, all of the same age— seen at autopsy—suggest comparison with millet seeds (Figure 17.49).

Wherever the post-primary tuberculous infection may start, it tends to follow the same natural history. The first lesion is a granuloma; the granuloma grows by accretion, several granulomas fuse into a larger mass that is interspersed with fibrous tissue; and this mass of newly formed tissue develops foci of coagulation necrosis of a special type called *caseous necrosis* (Figure 17.50). The tissue around the necrosis has the same cellular constituents as the tuberculous granuloma (p. 443); the entire necrotic mass with its wrapping may in fact be considered a giant granuloma.

Caseous Necrosis and Hypersensitivity Caseous necrosis deserves special attention (145). With apologies to cheese lovers, it really does look like semidried cream cheese. *It is biologically different from the necrosis of an infarct,* because it is saturated with mycobacterial products, which may explain why the macrophages around it do not appear eager to nibble at it. Small amounts of caseous necrosis can probably be cleared (140), but a large focus is never surrounded by a healthy scavenging layer of granulation tissue such as that around an infarct.

Caseous necrosis differs from the coagulation necrosis of an infarct also because it can expand. The cells gathered around it (mainly macrophages) die and join the necrotic mass; then a new barrier of macrophages develops just outside, and so the cycle continues. By this mechanism a tuberculous lymph node can enlarge like a tumor; indeed the term *tuberculoma* is used for such expanding masses, to which the brain is especially prone.

Another peculiar feature of caseous necrosis is that it can undergo liquefaction, that is, it becomes semifluid (140, 144, 145). This is a serious complication for a number of reasons: (a) the resulting creamy fluid is an excellent culture medium for mycobacteria, which can grow in it profusely; (b) accelerated growth favors the appearance of mutants, which complicates therapy; (c) when liquefaction occurs in the lung, the fluid mix is easily aspirated and spread throughout the bronchi; and (d) the high concentration of bacteria and bacterial products tends to cause a necrotic response, much like a large dose of intradermal tuberculin may cause

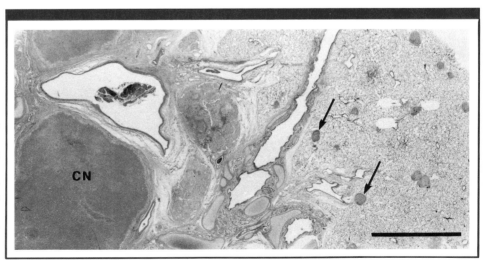

FIGURE 17.49
Progression of a tuberculous infection that killed a malnourished infant. **CN:** Caseous necrosis in hilar lymph node draining a primary complex (not shown). **Arrows:** Miliary tubercles due to hematogenous dissemination of tubercle bacilli. The miliary granulomas are all equal in size, indicating a single episode of dissemination. **Bar** = 5 mm.

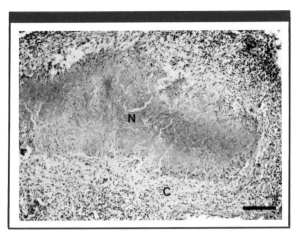

FIGURE 17.50
Tuberculous granuloma of the lung with extensive central necrosis (**N**). The live part of the granuloma is represented by a rim of cells (**C**): macrophages, lymphocytes, and fibroblasts, not recognizable at this enlargement. Whether the necrosis is encroaching further upon the surrounding cells, or whether the macrophages are invading the necrosis, cannot be decided on this section. **Bar** = 100 μm.

necrosis in the skin of a patient with active tuberculosis.

Is caseous necrosis helpful, harmful, or indifferent? After a century of speculation we seem finally to have an answer rather than a guess (142). By comparing the tuberculous lungs of two strains of rabbits, one resistant and one susceptible, A. Dannenberg concluded that caseous necrosis is helpful because it stops the growth of bacilli: its anoxic environment chokes them. They can survive but not multiply. If liquefaction develops, of course, it is quite another matter.

What is the mechanism of caseous necrosis? As we mentioned earlier, mycobacteria produce no toxins and no enzymes; therefore it is generally thought that caseous necrosis is a manifestation of delayed-type hypersensitivity: a "mass burial" of inflammatory and parenchymal cells that are destroyed by mechanisms of immunity designed to eliminate bacteria. Several factors could contribute to the massive cell death; we will list three, but more have been suggested (168):

- Conscientious but blind cytotoxic T-cells that destroy antigen-presenting macrophages because—for the T-cells—any surface coated with specific antigen is a legitimate target.
- Macrophages and, perhaps, NK cells that become nonspecifically cytotoxic by lymphokine activation.

- Cytokines, especially tumor necrosis factor (TNF). It has been shown that *Mycobacterium tuberculosis* not only triggers the release of TNF, but also makes the cells of the host more sensitive to the toxicity of TNF (168).

Other mechanisms have been proposed that may contribute to caseous necrosis (140): ischemia due to thrombosed vessels (activated macrophages do produce procoagulant factors), activation of complement with injury of bystander cells, hydrolytic enzymes, and reactive oxygen intermediates released by macrophages and neutrophils.

A strong argument in favor of hypersensitivity as a cause of caseous necrosis is provided by other diseases characterized by granulomas with a necrotic center. A classic example is *tertiary syphilis*. At this late stage of the disease the syphilitic granulomas contain very few spirochetes, and their necrotic center is best explained as a hypersensitivity reaction. As the caseous necrosis of tuberculosis, it tends to enlarge in tumor-like fashion.

In the past it was customary to insist on the difference between syphilitic and tuberculous necrosis. Grossly, in syphilis, the necrotic mass is firm and rubbery rather than cheesy (hence the name gumma); histologically, the outlines of the tissue are partially preserved. But biologically these are not very significant features. What counts is that in both diseases there is extensive focal necrosis explainable only in terms of an immune response.

Even more compelling is the comparison of tuberculous necrosis with the so-called *rheumatoid nodules*, which contain no infectious agent at all. They are found in two diseases with a strong hypersensitivity component: rheumatoid arthritis and acute rheumatic fever. Rheumatoid nodules, like tuberculous lymph nodes, can grow to tumor size (p. 574). There is no way at all to explain them—and their central necrosis—except by a hypersensitivity mechanism.

With these facts in mind, we can now return to DTH in tuberculosis.

EVENTS AT THE IMMUNOLOGICAL LEVEL: THE TUBERCULIN STORY

Robert Koch, who discovered the tubercle bacillus in 1882, announced 8 years later that he had discovered a cure for tuberculosis. The magic drug was **tuberculin,** actually a highly impure solution obtained by filtering mycobacterial cultures (157,

158). The result was enormous acclaim, promptly followed by enormous disappointment: tuberculin simply did not work. Nobody was cured (171).

Koch had to swallow his pride, but two events provided him with some consolation. He received the Nobel prize in 1905 for his overall research on tuberculosis, and in the meantime an eminent clinician, the Baron von Pirquet of serum-sickness fame (p. 533) (134), discovered that tuberculin was very useful, if not for the therapy—at least for the diagnosis of tuberculosis. Applied over a scratch in the skin of infected individuals, it produced a striking, delayed inflammatory response. This was the birth of the tuberculin test (Figure 17.51). Then, in 1906, von Pirquet (who had long experience with both serum sickness and tuberculosis) proposed the term *allergy* to mean any altered state of reactivity, be it to tuberculin or to any other "organic, living or non-living poison" (181). The term was promptly adopted. In Europe it is generally used in the original sense of any increased state of reactivity, whatever the type of hypersensitivity, whereas in the United States its use is often restricted to Type I hypersensitivity, that is, to allergies of the hay-fever type. Incidentally, the tuberculin test became crucial early in the nineteenth century for identifying and eliminating all cattle infected with bovine tuberculosis.

The existence of an allergy to tuberculin raised a burning question that has not been wholly answered to this day: tuberculin allergy is obvious, but how does it relate to resistance? In other words, is the individual better off because of this allergy?

To approach this question we will begin by presenting a fact observed by Koch, the *Koch phenomenon* (158, 166):

> *If a normal guinea pig is inoculated with a pure culture of tubercle bacilli, the wound, as a rule, closes and in the first few days seemingly heals. After ten to fourteen days, however, there appears a firm nodule which soon opens, forming an ulcer that persists until the animal dies. Quite different is the result if a tuberculous guinea pig is inoculated with tubercle bacilli. For this purpose it is best to use animals that have been infected four to six weeks previously. In such an animal, also, the little inoculation wound closes at first, but in this case no nodule is formed. On the next or second day, however, a peculiar change occurs at the inoculation site. The area becomes indurated and assumes a dark color, and these changes do not remain limited to the inoculation point, but spread to involve an area 0.5– 1.0 cm in diameter. In the succeeding days it becomes evident that the altered skin is necrotic. It finally sloughs, leaving a shallow ulcer which usually heals quickly and permanently, and the regional lymph nodes do not become infected. The action of tubercle bacilli upon the skin of a normal guinea pig is thus entirely different from their action upon the skin of a tuberculous one. This striking effect is produced not only by living tubercle bacilli, but also by dead bacilli, whether killed by prolonged low temperature, by boiling, or by certain chemicals.*

We must agree with Koch that the second exposure to mycobacteria (or even to mycobacterial extracts) elicits a different and more violent response than the first exposure. The tuberculin test gives us the same information: if a patient with active tuberculosis is given a tuberculin test (not a recommended procedure) the result may be a patch of hemorrhagic necrosis; in other words, a Koch phenomenon. *But is this exaggerated response an advantage?* In the original model of Koch, the guinea pig dies anyway, so there is no effective vaccination.

In Koch's time, von Pirquet noticed that in patients with advanced, terminal tuberculosis the tuberculin test became weaker (the poorly understood phenomenon of *anergy*); this led him to conclude that the skin test measured the strength of the body's response to the infection. But later it was found that animals highly resistant to tuberculosis, such as rats, develop a weak tuberculin test when infected; whereas guinea pigs, which are highly susceptible to tuberculosis, develop a strong test (166, 183).

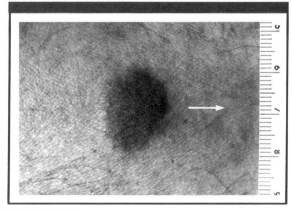

FIGURE 17.51

Strongly positive tuberculin test (photographed at 48 hours) on the forearm of a 60-year-old man in good health. At age 10 he had suffered a primary tuberculous infection, which clinically healed. Despite the 50-year interval between the infection and this tuberculin test, the local reaction was so intense that at 24 hours a lymphangitic streak appeared on the proximal side of the lesion, in the direction of lymph flow (*arrow*). Scale in centimeters.

So, how does the tuberculin test relate to the body's actual defenses against the infection? This topic is still riddled with controversy, but we can conclude with a few defensible statements:

- The chronic inflammatory reaction against tuberculosis is caused by living bacteria; the tuberculin reaction is obtained with a solution of selected antigens; therefore the two responses may overlap biologically, but they are not entirely comparable. The difference corresponds to CMI versus DTH, as illustrated in Figure 17.45.
- The skin test in tuberculosis or other infections that induce cell-mediated response tell us that the individual has been *exposed* to a given infectious agent, but clinical experience shows that they do not measure the *effectiveness* of the body's defenses (140).
- Perhaps a measure of the body's defenses could be obtained if the skin test were done with another bacterial antigen, selected to represent CMI rather than DTH (136).

This brings us to discuss vaccination against tuberculosis.

Vaccination Against Tuberculosis: The BCG Controversy We have lived through the disappointment of tuberculin as a cure; what about vaccination? The scene now moves to the Pasteur Institute in Lille, where the birth of the Arthus phenomenon took place in the early 1900s. By treating tubercle bacilli with ox bile, Albert Calmette and Camille Guérin managed to obtain an attenuated strain; in 1921 they proposed it as a vaccine for human use, by mouth, under the name BCG (for bacillus Calmette–Guérin) (133, 169). It was soon found that BCG causes the tuberculin test to be positive. Since then, the world is divided into two camps (165). In the United States, BCG is not used because the reported effectiveness is not obvious and because it has the built-in drawback just mentioned: vaccinated individuals become tuberculin-positive, which makes the tuberculin test useless for diagnosing a tuberculous infection. The vaccine does not *prevent* infection; it is said to provide better protection against the disease (159), but the extent of this protection is unclear. Epidemiologic studies yielded answers ranging from 80 percent to zero (152, 179, 180). The BCG vaccine is still one of the most widely used vaccines on a global scale; the Pasteur Institute in Paris is searching for ways to improve its effectiveness. The question is still open.

Meaning of a Positive Tuberculin Test Let it be clear that Koch's "old tuberculin" (actually called OT) is now replaced by a more standardized mixture called purified protein derivative (PPD); the scratch test, still used for other diseases, is replaced by an intradermal injection, as proposed by Charles Mantoux in 1910. This "Mantoux test" is considered positive if the reaction reaches at least 10 mm in diameter in 24 hours (165) *and* is accompanied by stiffening of the skin, as tested by lifting a fold between thumb and forefinger. This feature (which is rarely absent (132)) is especially useful when the tuberculin test is done on pigmented skin.

A positive test means that the patient has been infected with tubercle bacilli or has been vaccinated with BCG. It does not mean that there is active disease, although this is a possibility. In the United States, a positive PPD test in an individual who has not been vaccinated means that treatment for tuberculosis is recommended. Because hepatitis is a possible side-effect of that treatment and because this risk increases with age, the two risks must be weighed. *The treatment usually causes the PPD test to become negative within months or years* (183): this is the best proof available that mycobacteria do survive in the lesion.

Note: Repeated injections of tuberculin in a "negative" individual can induce a positive response, but this response is transient.

Four Types of Hypersensitivity: Some Closing Questions

We have reviewed and explained four basic mechanisms whereby the immune system reacts with vigor against harmless antigens—much like Don Quijote attacking windmills. Now we can step back and ask some broader questions.

COULD THERE BE MORE THAN FOUR TYPES OF HYPERSENSITIVITY?

There probably are more types, if we turn to subgroups. *Stimulatory hypersensitivity,* which has been called Type V, includes those situations in which antibodies bound to a cell receptor activate it; a human example is provided by some hyperthyroid patients who have antibodies against thyroid cell receptors for the pituitary thyroid-stimulating hormone (Graves' or Basedow's disease, p. 571).

There are several experimental examples of similar mechanisms. **Jones–Mote** or **cutaneous basophil hypersensitivity is** a skin response very rich in basophils obtained by sensitizing animals with antigen alone (without adjuvant) (148). The response develops faster than the tuberculin response and disappears faster. The biological significance of the basophil's presence is not clear.

IS THERE ANY "HYPERSENSITIVITY" UNRELATED TO THE IMMUNE RESPONSE?

We know two; both are based on injecting something into a prepared animal, and both are somewhat mysterious. One is calciphylaxis (p. 242), the other is the Shwartzman phenomenon.

The Shwartzman Phenomenon This experimental phenomenon, also called the *Shwartzman reaction*) is a puzzling observation dating from 1928 that is still incompletely understood but may hold the key to some human lesions in endotoxemia. It deserves mention here because it implies that a patch of skin becomes hemorrhagic only after a second insult. It comes in two varieties, local and generalized, and it works almost exclusively in rabbits.

To elicit the *local Shwartzman reaction,* a small dose of endotoxin is injected intradermally into a rabbit; no visible changes appear, although microscopically the dermis shows a leukocytic infiltrate with a predominance of neutrophils (162, 172, 178). Then, 24 hours later, a second injection of endotoxin is given intravenously, and a necrotic–hemorrhagic lesion develops at the first injection site (Figure 17.52). The interval between the two injections can be shorter, but not as short as 2 hours; 48 hours after the first injection the local predisposition disappears (174). What brings about the reaction is not yet clear, but a recent overview by Cotran and Pober (1990) suggests that several "new" players are involved: activation and/ or sensitization of the endothelium by the first injection, increased leukocyte aggregation induced by the second endotoxin injection, and possible roles for TNF and IL-1 and for the complement system. If the rabbit is depleted of leukocytes, the effect is abolished (176) as is the Arthus skin lesion (p. 532). The topic may sound complicated, but we have actually oversimplified it. It is currently of interest because it may overlap with TNF-induced tumor necrosis. Indeed, the local Shwartzman phenomenon and the Koch phenomenon have similarities: both seem to

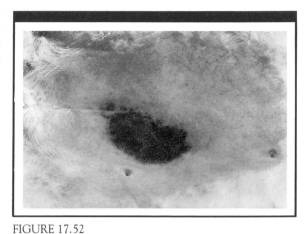

FIGURE 17.52
The local Shwartzman phenomenon. Abdominal skin of a living rabbit that received first an intradermal injection of endotoxin (meningococcus culture filtrate); then the same endotoxin was injected intravenously 24 hours later. Four hours after the second injection, this hemorrhagic lesion appeared. (Reproduced with permission from [174].)

depend on TNF release in skin primed by bacterial toxins (167).

The generalized Shwartzman reaction, which should really be called the Sanarelli–Shwartzman reaction (153, 162), is produced by injecting both doses of endotoxin intravenously (in rabbits) 24 hours apart; a disseminated intravascular coagulation follows, which may produce bilateral cortical necrosis of the kidney (Figure 17.53) and death. There is no final explanation at this time. One theory runs as follows (170). The first injection of endotoxin produces widespread platelet destruction and release of thromboplastin, but the RES/ MPS (p. 297) manages to remove the microscopic fibrin clots. The second injection has the same effect, but this time the RES/MPS is overwhelmed ("blockaded," p. 300), and microvascular occlusion follows. An interesting variant: *in pregnant rabbits a single intravenous injection suffices,* presumably because fibrinolysis is depressed. This may explain certain cases of bilateral cortical necrosis after septic abortions.

Another explanation (135): both local and general Shwartzman reactions are due to oversecretion of interferon gamma, and both are inhibited by antibody against interferon gamma. Once again, time will tell.

WHY TYPE I, II, III, OR IV?

In other words: given an antigenic challenge, why should the immune system choose to respond with hypersensitivity of one type rather than another?

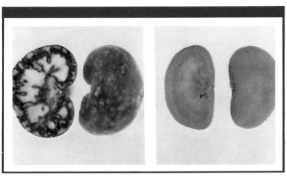

FIGURE 17.53
Generalized Shwartzman reaction. *Left:* Kidney of rabbit that received two intravenous injections of a meningococcal toxin 20 hours apart. Necrosis and hemorrhage involve large parts of the medulla and cortex. *Right:* Normal rabbit kidney. (Reproduced with permission from [178].)

There is no short answer to this important question. The first point is that one type does not exclude another. Rabbits that are sensitized intravenously to produce serum sickness (Type III, complex-mediated) when rechallenged may develop anaphylactic symptoms (Type I). In fact, you may recall that the arteritis of serum sickness is thought by some to require the cooperation of Types I and III (p. 536). Some degree of cell-mediated hypersensitivity may also develop at the same time. *Mycobacterium tuberculosis* induces delayed-type (cell-mediated) hypersensitivity but also plenty of antibodies (especially if injected with Freund's adjuvant) but, somehow, these antibodies seem to play no role in the pathogenesis of the disease.

This being said, it is true that a given type tends to prevail in a given setting. Several factors are involved: the nature of the antigen, the route and manner of administration, and the animal species. For example, rubbing an antigen into the skin (across the epidermis) favors the development of cell-mediated response, that is, delayed-type hypersensitivity. Giving an antigen intrave-nously (so that antigen and antibody mix in high concentrations) favors the formation of complexes; inhalation across the mucous membranes of the respiratory system, where IgE-forming plasma cells are lurking, favors an anaphylactic mechanism. Injecting an antigen mixed with Freund's adjuvant enhances the sensitization and includes a delayed response; and different adjuvants favor different pathways.

The Last Word to a Cobra

On 21 June, 1995, the Director of the Reptile World Serpentarium in St. Cloud, Florida, was bitten by a 12-foot king cobra (178a). That was not a new experience: he had been bitten by a king cobra once before, in 1987; antiserum had saved him. To any well-trained physician who might have been present at the scene of the accident it should have been obvious that there were *two* urgent problems: this latest bite was bad enough, but what about the effect of the earlier bite? Had it left the body protected, like a vaccination (by the IgG/IgM pathway), or hypersensitive and ready for anaphylaxis (by the IgE pathway)? Alas, theory could not help. As the serpentarium director was being rushed to the hospital, I doubt that even a seasoned immunologist could have advised him on the basis of theory alone. Luckily the patient knew what to do: herpetologists may not know about IgM and IgE, but they do know by experience that immunization against snake venom requires multiple injections of venom, and that a single cobra bite leaves the body hypersensitive (160a). So he gave himself two shots of epinephrine. Although this was not enough to avert anaphylactic shock, he survived to tell the story—which tells us that we still have a lot to learn about the relationship between immunity and hypersensitivity.

References

Hypersensitivity Type I

1. Abbas AK, Lichtman AH, Pober JS. Cellular and molecular immunology. Philadelphia: WB Saunders, 1994.
2. Anderson SD. Exercise-induced asthma. In: Middleton E Jr, Reed CE, Ellis EF, Adkinson NF Jr, Yunginger JW, eds. Allergy principles and practice. St. Louis: CV Mosby, 1988:1156–1175.
3. Atherton DJ. Skin disorders and food allergy. J R Soc Med 1985;78(suppl 5):7–10.
4. Austen KF. The heterogeneity of mast cell populations and products. Hosp Pract 1984;19:135–146.
5. Barnes PJ. (From the Department of Thoracic Medicine, National Heart and Lung Institute, London, UK). Frontiers in medicine: new aspects of asthma. J Intern Med 1992;231:453–461.
6. Berke G. Functions and mechanisms of lysis induced by cytotoxic T lymphocytes and natural killer cells. In: Paul WE, ed. Fundamental immunology, 2nd ed. New York: Raven Press, 1989:735–764.
7. Bowen ID, Bowen SM. Programmed cell death in

tumours and tissues. London: Chapman and Hall, 1990.

8. Bochner BS, Lichtenstein LM. Anaphylaxis. N Engl J Med 1991;324:1785–1790.

9. Braquet P, Touqui L, Shen TY, Vargaftig BB. Perspectives in platelet-activating factor research. Pharmacol Rev 1987;39:97–145.

9a. Brutkiewicz RR, Welsh RM. Major Histocompatibility Complex Class I Antigens and the Control of Viral Infections by Natural Killer Cells. J Virol 1995;69:3967–3971.

10. Charlesworth EN, Hood AF, Soter NA, Kagey-Sobotka A, Norman PS, Lichtenstein LM. Cutaneous late-phase response to allergen: mediator release and inflammatory cell infiltration. J Clin Invest 1989;83:1519–1526.

11. Cohen JJ. The immune system: an overview. In: Middleton E Jr, Reed CE, Ellis EF, Adkinson NF Jr, Yunginger JW, eds. Allergy principles and practice. St. Louis: CV Mosby, 1988:3–11.

12. Coombs RRA, Gell GH. Classification of allergic reactions responsible for clinical hypersensitivity and disease. In Gell PGH, Coombs RRA, Lachmann PJ, eds. Clinical aspects of immunology, 3rd ed. Oxford: Blackwell Scientific Publications, 1975:761–781.

13. Corren J, Schocket AL. Anaphylaxis. A preventable emergency. Postgrad Med 1990;87:167–178.

14. de Weck AL. In: Pearce FL. Non-IgE-Mediated Mast Cell Stimulation (discussion). In: IgE, Mast Cells and the Allergic Response. Ciba Foundation Symposium 1989; 147:74–92.

15. DeWeese DD, Saunders WH. Textbook of otolaryngology. St. Louis: CV Mosby, 1982.

16. DiNome MA, Young JD-E. How lymphocytes kill tumor and other cellular targets. Hosp Pract 1987;22:59–66.

17. Dvorak AM, Schleimer RP, Lichtenstein LM. Human mast cells synthesize new granules during recovery from degranulation. In vitro studies with mast cells purified from human lungs. Blood 1988;71:76–85.

18. Dvorak AM, Schuulman ES, Peters SP, et al. Immunoglobulin E-mediated degranulation of isolated human lung mast cells. Lab Invest 1985;53:45–56.

19. Duke RC, Chervenak R, Cohen JJ. Endogenous endonuclease-induced DNA fragmentation: an early event in cell-mediated cytolysis. Proc Natl Acad Sci USA 1983;80:6361–6365.

20. Espevik T, Kildahl-Andersen O, Nissen-Meyer J. The role of monocyte cytotoxic factor in monocyte-mediated lysis of tumour cells. Immunology 1986;57:255–259.

21. Foulds L. Neoplastic development, vol 1. London: Academic Press, 1969.

22. Fuller RW. Macrophages. Br Med J 1992;48:65–71.

23. Glauert AM, Butterworth AE. Morphological evidence for the ability of eosinophils to damage antibody-coated schistosomula. Trans R Soc Trop Med Hyg 1977;71:392–395.

24. Glauert AM, Butterworth AE, Sturrock RF, Houba V. The mechanism of antibody-dependent, eosinophil-mediated damage to schistosomula of Schistosoma mansoni in vitro: a study by phase-contrast and electron microscopy. J Cell Sci 1978;34:173–192.

25. Golstein P. Cytolytic T-cell melodrama. Nature 1987;327:12.

26. Ha T-Y, Reed ND. Systemic anaphylaxis in mast-cell-deficient mice of W/W^v and Sl/Sl^d genotypes. Exp Cell Biol 1987;55:63–68.

27. Hanifin JM. Atopic dermatitis. J Allergy Clin Immunol 1984;73:211–222.

28. Hildreth EA. Anaphylactoid reactions to iodinated contrast media. Hosp Pract 1987;22:77–95.

29. Holmes FL, Richet CR. In: Gillispie CC, ed. Dictionary

of scientific biography, vol XI. New York: Charles Scribner's Sons, 1975:425–432.

30. Jacoby W, Cammarata PV, Findlay S, Pincus SH. Anaphylaxis in mast cell-deficient mice. J Invest Dermatol 1984;83:302–304.

31. Kaliner MA. The late-phase reaction and its clinical implications. Hosp Pract 1987;22:73–83.

32. Kaplan AP. Urticaria and angioedema. In: Middleton E Jr, Reed CE, Ellis EF, Adkinson NF Jr, Yunginger JW, eds. Allergy. Principles and practice. St. Louis: CV Mosby, 1988:1377–1401.

33. Lachmann PJ. A common form of killing. Nature 1986;321:560.

34. Lagunoff D, Martin TW, Read G. Agents that release histamine from mast cells. Annu Rev Pharmacol Toxicol 1983;23:331–351.

35. Larsen GL. The pulmonary late-phase response. Hosp Pract 1987;22:155–169.

36. Leiferman KM, Fujisawa T, Gray BH, Gleich GJ. Extracellular deposition of eosinophil and neutrophil granule proteins in the IgE-mediated cutaneous late phase reaction. Lab Invest 1990;62:579–589.

37. Lichtenstein LM. The nasal late-phase response—an in vivo model. Hosp Pract 1988;23:105–128.

38. Lopez DM, Blomberg BB, Padmanabhan RR, Bourguignon LYW. Nuclear disintegration of target cells by killer B lymphocytes from tumor-bearing mice. FASEB J 1989;3:37–43.

39. MacQueen G, Marshcall J, Perdue M, Siegel S, Bienenstock J. Pavlovian conditioning of rat mucosal mast cells to secrete rat mast cell protease II. Science 1989;243:83–85.

40. Maitai CK, Talalaj S, Njoroge D, Wamugunda R. Effect of extract of hairs from the herb Urtica massaica, on smooth muscle. Toxicon 1980;18:225–229.

41. Maitai CK, Talalaj S, Talalaj D, Njoroge D. Smooth muscle stimulating substances in the stinging nettle tree Obetia pinnatifida. Toxicon 1981;19:186–188.

42. Majno G. The healing hand: man and wound in the Ancient World. Cambridge, MA: Harvard University Press, 1975.

43. Matsuda H, Watanabe N, Kiso Y, et al. Necessity of IgE antibodies and mast cells for manifestation of resistance against larval Haemaphysalis longicornis ticks in mice. J Immunol 1990;144:259–262.

44. Matthews N. Production of anti-tumour cytotoxin by human monocytes. Immunology 1981;44:135–142.

45. McFadden ER Jr. Pathogenesis of asthma. J Allergy Clin Immunol 1984;73:413–424.

46. McNeill WH. Plagues and peoples. Garden City, NY: Anchor Press/Doubleday, 1976.

47. Metcalfe DD, Samter M, Condemi JJ. Reactions to foods. In: Samter M, Talmage DW, Frank MM, Austen KF, Claman HN, eds. Immunological diseases, 4th ed. Boston: Little, Brown, 1988:1149–1171.

48. Middleton E Jr, Reed CE, Ellis EF, Adkinson NF Jr, Yunginger JW, eds. Allergy. Principles and practice. St. Louis: CV Mosby, 1988.

49. Morrow JD, Margolies GR, Rowland J, Roberts LJ II. Evidence that histamine is the causative toxin of scombroid-fish poisoning. N Engl J Med 1991;324:716–720.

50. Mrazek DA. Asthma: psychiatric considerations, evaluation, and management. In: Middleton E Jr, Reed CE, Ellis EF, Adkinson NF Jr, Yunginger JW, eds. Allergy. Principles and practice. St. Louis: CV Mosby, 1988: 1176–1196.

51. Nathan C, Cohn Z. Role of oxygen-dependent mechanisms in antibody-induced lysis of tumor cells by activated macrophages. J Exp Med 1980;152:198–208.

52. Norman PS. Immunotherapy of IgE-mediated disease. Hosp Pract 1990;25:81–92.

53. Owen RL. Macrophage function in Peyer's patch epithelium. Adv Exp Med Biol 1982;149:507–513.

54. Owen RL, Ermak TH. Structural specializations for antigen uptake and processing in the digestive tract. Springer Semin. Immunopathol 1990;12:139–152.

55. Patterson R, McKenna JM, Suszko IM, et al. Living histamine-containing cells from the bronchial lumens of humans. Description and comparison of histamine content with cells of rhesus monkeys. J Clin Invest 1977;59:217–225.

56. Patterson R, Pruzansky JJ, Dykewicz MS, Lawrence ID. Basophil-mast cell response syndromes: a unified clinical approach. Allergy Proc 1988;9:611–620.

57. Pearce FL. Non-IgE-mediated mast cell stimulation. Ciba Found Symp 1989;147:74–92.

58. Podack ER. Granule-mediated cytolysis of target cells. Curr Top Microbiol Immunol 1988;140:1–9.

59. Podack ER, Olsen KJ, Lowrey DM, Lichtenheld M. Structure and function of perforin. Curr Top Microbiol Immunol 1988;140:11–17.

60. Podack ER. Molecular assemblies in complement- and lymphocyte-mediated cytolysis. In: Steinman RM, North RJ, eds. Mechanisms of host resistance to infectious agents, tumors, and allografts. New York: Rockefeller University Press, 1986:217–230.

61. Portier P. Recherches sur les venins de coelentéréd. Découverte de l'anaphylaxie. In: Notice sur les titres et travaux scientifiques de P. Portier. Paris: A. Maretheux et L. Pactat, 1936.

62. Portier P, Richet C. De l'action anaphylactique de certains venins. C R Acad Sci [D] Paris 1902;54:170–172, 548–551, 837–838.

63. Prausnitz C, Küstner H. Studien über die Ueberempfindlichkeit. Zentralbl Bakteriol 1921;86:160–169.

64. Pretolani M, Ferrer-Lopez P, Vargaftig BB. From anti-asthma drugs to PAF-acether antagonism and back. Present status. Biochem Pharmacol 1989a;38:1373–1384.

65. Pretolani M, Lefort J, Dumarey C, Vargaftig BB. Role of lipoxygenase metabolites for the hyper-responsiveness to platelet-activating factor of lungs from actively sensitized guinea pigs. J Pharmacol Exp Ther 1989b;248:353–359.

66. Pretolani M, Lellouch-Tubiana A, Lefort J, Bachelet M, Vargaftig BB. PAF-acether and experimental anaphylaxis as a model for asthma. Int Arch Allergy Appl Immunol 1989c;88:149–153.

67. Reisman RE. Insect allergy. In: Middleton E Jr, Reed CE, Ellis EF, Adkinson NF Jr, Yunginger JW, eds. Allergy. Principles and practice, 3rd ed. St. Louis: CV Mosby, 1988:1345–1364.

68. Richet C, Portier P. Recherches sur la toxine des Coelentérés et les phénomènes d'anaphylaxie. Résultats des Campagnes Scientifiques Accomplies sur Son Yacht par Albert Ier Prince Souverain de Monaco. Monaco, 1936.

69. Rocklin RE, Rosen FS, David J, Fearon D, Piessens WF. Clinical immunology. In: Rubenstein E, Federman DD, eds. Scientific American Medicine. New York: Scientific American, 1991:1–35.

70. Roitt IM. Essential immunology, 6th ed. Oxford: Blackwell Scientific Publications, 1988.

71. Rosen FS, Steiner LA, Unanue ER. Dictionary of immunology. New York: Stockton Press, 1989.

72. Russell JH, Dobos CB. Mechanisms of immune lysis. II. CTL-induced nuclear disintegration of the target begins within minutes of cell contact. J Immunol 1980;125:1256–1261.

73. Russell JH, Masakowski V, Rucinsky T, Phillips G. Mechanisms of immune lysis. III. Characterization of the nature and kinetics of the cytotoxic T lymphocyte-induced nuclear lesion in the target. J Immunol 1982;128:2087–2094.

74. Russell M, Dark KA, Cummins RW, et al. Learned histamine release. Science 1984;225:733–734.

75. Sampson HA. Late-phase response to food in atopic dermatitis. Hosp Pract 1987;22:111–128.

76. Samter M, Talmage DW, Frank MM, Austen KF, Claman HN, eds. Immunological diseases, 4th ed. Boston: Little, Brown, 1988.

77. Sanderson CJ. The mechanism of T cell mediated cytotoxicity. II. Morphological studies of cell death by time-lapse microcinematography. Proc R Soc Lond B 1976;192:241–255.

78. Schadewaldt, H. La croisière du Prince Albert Ier de Monaco en 1901 et la découverte de l'anaphylaxie. In: Colloque International sur L'Histoire de la Biologie Marine. Paris: Masson & Cie, 1965:305–313.

79. Selye H. Anaphylactoid edema. St. Louis: Warren H. Green, 1968.

80. Serafin WE, Austen KF. Mediators of immediate hypersensitivity reactions. N Engl J Med 1987;317:30–34.

81. Smith PL, Kagey-Sobotka A, Bleecker ER, et al. Physiologic manifestations of human anaphylaxis. J Clin Invest 1980;66:1072–1080.

82. Steeves EBT, Allen JR. Basophils in skin reactions of mast cell-deficient mice infested with Dermacentor variabilis. Int J Parasitol 1990;20:655–667.

83. Takafuji S, Suzuki S, Muranaka M, Miyamoto T. Influence of environmental factors on IgE production. Ciba Found Symp 1989;147:188–204.

84. Tovey ER, Chapman MD, Platts-Mills TAE. Mite faeces are a major source of house dust allergens. Nature 1981;289:592–593.

85. Trenn G, Takayama H, Sitkovsky MV. Exocytosis of cytolytic granules may not be required for target cell lysis by cytotoxic T-lymphocytes. Nature 1987;330:72–74.

86. Turner KJ. Epidemiology of the allergic response. Ciba Found Symp 1989;147:205–209.

87. Ucker DS. Cytotoxic T lymphocytes and glucocorticoids activate an endogenous suicide process in target cells. Nature 1987;327:62–64.

88. Wasserman SI. Platelet-activating factor as a mediator of bronchial asthma. Hosp Pract 1988;23:49–58.

89. Wasserman SI, Marquardt DL. Anaphylaxis. In: Middleton E Jr, Reed CE, Ellis EF, Adkinson NF Jr, Yunginger JW, eds. Allergy. Principles and practice, 3rd ed. St. Louis: CV Mosby, 1988:1365–1376.

90. Wyllie AH, Morris RG, Smith AL, Dunlop D. Chromatin cleavage in apoptosis: association with condensed chromatin morphology and dependence on macromolecular synthesis. J Pathol 1984;142:67–77.

91. Young JD-E, Cohn ZA. How killer cells kill. Sci Am 1988;258:38–44.

92. Zachariae R, Bjerring P, Arendt-Nielsen L. Modulation of type I immediate and type IV delayed immunoreactivity using direct suggestion and guided imagery during hypnosis. Allergy 1989;44:537–542.

93. Ziegler-Heitbrock HWL, Möller A, Linke RP, Haas JG, Riebe EP, Riethmüller G. Tumor necrosis factor as effector molecule in monocyte mediated cytotoxicity. Cancer Res 1986;46:5947–5952.

Hypersensitivity Types II and III

94. Andres GA, Seegal BC, Hsu KC, Rothenberg MS, Chapeau ML. Electron microscopic studies of experimental nephritis with ferritin-conjugated antibody. J Exp Med 1963;117:691–704.

95. Arthus M. Injections répétées de sérum de cheval chez le lapin. C R Soc Biol (Paris) 1903;55:817–820.

96. Benveniste J, Henson PM, Cochrane CG. Leukocyte-dependent histamine release from rabbit platelets. The role of IgE, basophils, and a platelet-activating factor. J Exp Med 1972;136:1356–1377.

97. Cairns J. The history of mortality. In: Carroll KK, ed. Diet, nutrition, and health. Montreal: McGill-Queen's University Press, 1989:309–344.

98. Caulfield JP, Korman G, Butterworth AE, Hogan M, David JR. The adherence of human neutrophils and eosinophils to schistosomula: evidence for membrane fusion between cells and parasites. J Cell Biol 1980;86:46–63.

99. Caulfield JP, Lenzi HL, Elsas P, Dessein AJ. Ultrastructure of the attack of eosinophils stimulated by blood mononuclear cell products on schistosomula of Schistosoma mansoni. Am J Pathol 1985;120:380–390.

100. Cochrane CG. The Arthus reaction. In: Zweifach BW, Grant L, McCluskey RT, eds. The inflammatory process. New York: Academic Press, 1965:613–648.

101. Cochrane CG, Koffler D. Immune complex disease in experimental animals and man. Adv Immunol 1973;16:185–264.

102. Cochrane CG, Weigle WO, Dixon FJ. The role of polymorphonuclear leukocytes in the initiation and cessation of the Arthus vasculitis. J Exp Med 1959;110:481–494.

103. Cotran RS. Pathogenesis of vasculitis: an update. In: Fenoglio-Preiser C, ed. Advances in pathology, vol 3. St. Louis: Mosby-Year Book, 1990:301–310.

104. Cotran RS, Kumar V, Robbins SL. Robbins pathologic basis of disease, 4th ed. Philadelphia: WB Saunders, 1989:1025.

105. Crawford JP, Movat HZ, Ranadive NS, Hay JB. Pathways to inflammation induced by immune complexes: development of the Arthus reaction. Fed Proc 1982;41:2583–2587.

106. Dixon FJ. Mechanisms of immunologic injury. In: Good RA, Fisher DW, eds. Immunobiology. Stamford, CT: Sinauer Associates, 1971:161–173.

107. Dixon FJ, Cochrane CG, Theofilopoulos AN. Immune complex injury. In: Samter M, Talmage DW, Frank MM, Austen KF, Claman HN, eds. Immunological diseases, 4th ed. Boston: Little, Brown, 1988:233–259.

108. Dixon FJ, Feldman JD, Vazquez JJ. Experimental glomerulonephritis. The pathogenesis of a laboratory model resembling the spectrum of human glomerulonephritis. J Exp Med 1961;113:899–920.

109. Emancipator SN, Lamm ME. IgA nephropathy: pathogenesis of the most common form of glomerulonephritis. Lab Invest 1989;60:168–183.

110. Giglioli G. Malaria and renal disease, with special reference to British Guiana. II. The effect of malaria eradication on the incidence of renal disease in British Guiana. Ann Trop Med Parasitol 1962;56:225–241.

111. Hall CL, Colvin RB, McCluskey RT. Human immune complex diseases. In: Cohen S, Ward PA, McCluskey RT, eds. Mechanisms of immunopathology. New York: John Wiley & Sons, 1979:203–245.

112. Heckbert SR, Stryker WS, Coltin KL, Manson JE, Platt R. Serum sickness in children after antibiotic exposure: estimates of occurrence and morbidity in a Health Maintenance Organization population. Am J Epidemiol 1990;132:336–342.

113. Humphrey JH. The mechanism of Arthus reactions. II. The role of polymorphonuclear leucocytes and platelets in reversed passive reactions in the guinea-pig. Br J Exp Pathol 1955;36:283–289.

114. Kniker WT, Cochrane CG. Pathogenic factors in vascular lesions of experimental serum sickness. J Exp Med 1965;122:83–98.

115. Kusner DJ, Ellner JJ. Syphilis—a reversible cause of nephrotic syndrome in HIV infection. N Engl J Med 1991;324:341–342.

116. Lawley TJ, Bielory L, Gascon P, Yancey KB, Young NS, Frank MM. A prospective clinical and immunologic analysis of patients with serum sickness. N Engl J Med 1984;311:1407–1413.

117. LoBuglio AF, Cotran RS, Jandl JH. Red cells coated with immunoglobulin G: binding and sphering by mononuclear cells in man. Science 1967;158:1582-1585.

118. Metchnikoff E. Lectures on the comparative pathology of inflammation. (Translated from the French by Starling FA, Starling, EH, 1891.) New York: Dover Publications, 1968.

119. Moyer CF, Strandberg JD, Reinisch CL. Systemic mononuclear-cell vasculitis in MRL/Mp-lpr/lpr mice. A histologic and immunocytochemical analysis. Am J Pathol 1987;127:229–242.

120. Ranadive NS, Movat HZ. Tissue injury and inflammation induced by immune complexes. In: Movat HZ, ed. Inflammation, immunity and hypersensitivity, 2nd ed. Hagerstown: Harper & Row, 1979:409–443.

121. Rocklin RE, Rosen FS, David J, Fearon D, Piessens WF. Clinical immunology. In: Rubenstein E, Federman DD, eds. Scientific American Medicine. New York: Scientific American, 1991:1–35.

122. Samter M, Talmage DW, Frank MM, Austen KF, Claman HN, eds. Immunological diseases, 4th ed. Boston: Little, Brown, 1988.

123. Schmidt H. Grundlagen der spezifischen Therapie und Prophylaxe bakterieller Infektions-krankheiten. Berlin-Grünewald: Bruno Schultz, 1940:505–506.

124. Stankus RP, Salvaggio JE. Infiltrative lung disease: hypersensitivity pneumonitis, allergic bronchopulmonary aspergillosis, and the inorganic dust pneumoconioses. In: Samter M, Talmage DW, Frank MM, Austen KF, Claman NH, eds. Immunological diseases, 4th ed. Boston: Little, Brown, 1988:1561–1585.

125. von Pirquet C, Schick B. Die Serumkrankheit. Leipzig: Franz Deuticke, 1905.

126. von Pirquet C, Schick B. Serum Sickness. Baltimore: The Williams & Wilkins Company, 1951.

127. Ward PA, Cochrane CG. Bound complement and immunologic injury of blood vessels. J Exp Med 1965;121:215–234.

128. Zabriskie JB. New concepts in post-streptococcal glomerulonephritis. In: Neter E, Milgrom F, eds. The immune system and infectious diseases. Basel: S. Karger, 1975:282–293.

Hypersensitivity Type IV

129. Allison AC, Byars NE. An adjuvant formulation that selectively elicits the formation of antibodies of protective isotypes and of cell-mediated immunity. J Immunol Methods 1986;95:157–168.

130. Ando M, Dannenberg AM Jr, Sugimoto M, Tepper BS. Histochemical studies relating to activation of macrophages to the intracellular destruction of tubercle bacilli. Am J Pathol 1977;86:623–633.

131. Baumgarten A, Wilhelm DL. Vascular permeability responses in hypersensitivity. I. The tuberculin reaction. Pathology 1969;1:301–315.

132. Beck JS. Skin changes in the tuberculin test. Tubercle 1972;72:81–87.

133. Bendiner E. Albert Calmette: a vaccine and its vindication. Hosp Pract 1992;10:113–132.

134. Bendiner E. Baron von Pirquet: the aristocrat who discovered and defined allergy. Hosp Pract 1981;16:137–158.

135. Billiau A. Gamma-interferon: the match that lights the fire? Immunol Today 1988;9:37–40.

136. Bothamley GH, Granger JM. The Koch phenomenon and delayed hypersensitivity: 1891–1991. Tubercle 1991;72:7–11.

137. Chedid L. Muramyl peptides as possible endogenous immunopharmacological mediators. Microbiol Immunol 1983;27:723–732.

138. Colvin RB, Johnson RA, Mihm MC Jr, Dvorak HF. Role of the clotting system in cell-mediated hypersensitivity. I. Fibrin deposition in delayed skin reactions in man. J Exp Med 1973;138:686–698.

139. Cotran RS, Pober JS. Cytokine-endothelial interactions in inflammation, immunity, and vascular injury. J Am Soc Nephrol 1990;1:225–235.

140. Dannenberg AM Jr. Immune mechanisms in the pathogenesis of pulmonary tuberculosis. Rev Infect Dis 1989;11(suppl 2):S369–S378.

141. Dannenberg AM Jr. Immunopathogenesis of pulmonary tuberculosis. Hosp Pract 1993;1:51–58.

142. Dannenberg AM Jr. Delayed-type hypersensitivity and cell-mediated immunity in the pathogenesis of tuberculosis. Immunol Today 1991;12:228–233.

143. Dannenberg AM Jr, Meyer OT, Esterly JR, Kambara T. The local nature of immunity in tuberculosis, illustrated histochemically in dermal bcg lesions. J Immunol 1968;100:931–941.

144. Dannenberg AM Jr, Sugimoto M. Liquefaction of caseous foci in tuberculosis. Am Rev Respir Dis 1976;113:257–259.

145. Dannenberg AM Jr, Tomashefski JF Jr. Pathogenesis of pulmonary tuberculosis. In: Fishman AP, ed. Pulmonary diseases and disorders, 2nd ed. New York: McGraw-Hill, 1988:1821–1842.

146. Dienes L. Further observations concerning the sensitization of tuberculous guinea pigs. J Immunol 1928;15:153–174.

147. Dubos R, Dubos J. The white plague: tuberculosis, man, and society. New Brunswick, NJ: Rutgers University Press, 1952.

148. Dvorak HF. Cutaneous basophil hypersensitivity. J Allergy Clin Immunol 1976;58:229–240.

149. Dvorak AM, Mihm MC Jr, Dvorak HF. Morphology of delayed-type hypersensitivity reactions in man. II. Ultrastructural alterations affecting the microvasculature and the tissue mast cells. Lab Invest 1976;34:179–191.

150. Dvorak HF, Mihm MC Jr, Dvorak AN, et al. Morphology of delayed type hypersensitivity reactions in man. I. Quantitative description of the inflammatory response. Lab Invest 1974;31:111–130.

151. Freund J, McDermott K. Sensitization to horse serum by means of adjuvants. Proc Soc Exp Biol Med 1942;49:548–553.

152. Gheorghiu M. The present and future role of BCG vaccine in tuberculosis control. Biologicals 1990;18:135–141.

153. Good RA, Thomas L. Studies on the generalized Shwartzman reaction. II. The production of bilateral cortical necrosis of the kidneys by a single injection of bacterial toxin in rabbits previously treated with thorotrast or trypan blue. J Exp Med 1952;96:625–641.

154. Gregoriadis G. Immunological adjuvants: a role for liposomes. Immunol Today 1990;11:89–97.

154a. Hunter D. The Diseases of Occupations. London, The English Universities Press Ltd., 1969.

155. Kabat EQ, Mayer MM. Experimental immunochemistry, 2nd ed. Springfield, IL: Charles C. Thomas, 1964.

156. Kambara T, Yasaka T, Nakamura T. The role of polymorphonuclear leukocytes in delayed hypersensitivity skin reactions: suppressive effects of anti-polymorphonuclear leukocyte serum. Virchows Arch [B] 1981;37:191–198.

157. Koch R. Fortsetzung der Mittheilungen über ein Heilmittel genen Tuberculose. Dtsch Med Wochenschr 1891a;17:101–102.

158. Koch R.I. Weitere Mittheilung über das Tuberkulin. Dtsch Med Wochenschr 1891b;17:1189–1192.

159. Lagranderie M, Ravisse P, Marchal G, et al. BCG-induced protection in guinea pigs vaccinated and challenged via the respiratory route. Tubercle Lung Dis 1993;74:38–46.

160. May ME, Spagnuolo PJ. Evidence for activation of a respiratory burst in the interaction of human neutrophils with Mycobacterium tuberculosis. Am Soc Microbiol 1987;55:2304.

160a. Minton Jr., SA, Minton MR. Venomous Reptiles. New York: Charles Scribner's Sons, 1969.

161. Movat HZ, Fernando NVP. I. The earliest fine structural changes at the blood-tissue barrier during antigen-antibody interaction. Am J Pathol 1963;42:41–59.

162. Movat HZ, Jeynes BJ, Wasi S, Movat KW, Kopaniak MM. Quantitation of the development and progression of the local Shwartzman reaction. In: Agarwal MK, ed. Bacterial endotoxins and host response. Amsterdam: Elsevier-North Holland Biomedical Press, 1980:179–201.

163. Pober JS, Cotran RS. Cytokines and endothelial cell biology. Physiol Rev 1990;70:427–451.

164. Pober JS, Cotran RS. Immunologic interactions of T lymphocytes with vascular endothelium. Adv Immunol 1991;50:261–302.

165. Reichman LB. Tuberculin skin testing. The state of the art. Chest 1979;76(suppl):764S–770S.

166. Rich AR. The pathogenesis of tuberculosis, 2nd ed. Springfield, IL: Charles C. Thomas, 1951.

167. Rook GAW, Attiyah RA. Cytokines and the Koch phenomenon. Tubercle 1991;72:13–20.

168. Rosen FS, Steiner LA, Unanue ER. Dictionary of immunology. New York: Stockton Press, 1989.

169. Sakula A. BCG: who were Calmette and Guérin? Thorax 1983;38:806–812.

170. Sell S. Immunology immunopathology and immunity, 4th ed. New York: Elsevier, 1987.

171. Shapiro E. Robert Koch and his tuberculin fallacy. Pharos 1983;9:19–22.

172. Shima K, Dannenberg AM Jr, Ando M, Chandrasekhar S, Seluzicki JA, Fabrikant JI. Macrophage accumulation, division, maturation, and digestive and microbicidal capacities in tuberculous lesions. Am J Pathol 1972;67:159–180.

173. Shwartzman G. A new phenomenon of local skin reactivity to B. typhosus culture filtrate. Proc Soc Exp Biol Med 1928;25:560–561.

174. Shwartzman G. Phenomenon of local tissue reactivity and its immunological, pathological and clinical significance. New York: Paul B. Hoeber, Inc., 1937.

175. Simon HB. Infections due to mycobacteria. In: Rubenstein E, Federman DD, eds. Scientific American Medicine, 7, VIII. New York: Scientific American, 1989:1–18.

176. Stetson CA Jr. Similarities in the mechanisms determin-

ing the Arthus and Shwartzman phenomena. J Exp Med 1951;94:347–358.

177. Taft P, Edgar B. 1991, personal communication (Dr. Piri Taft is daughter of Dr. L. Dienes).

178. Thomas L, Good RA. Studies on the generalized Shwartzman reaction. I. General observations concerning the phenomenon. J Exp Med 1952;96:605–624.

178a. Thomas M. Cobra Atttack! In: Reader's Digest, December 1995, pp. 128–133.

179. Tidjani O, Amedome A, ten Dam HG. The protective effect of BCG vaccination of the newborn against childhood tuberculosis in an African community. Tubercle 1986;67:269–281.

180. Tripathy SP. The case for BCG. Ann Natl Med Sci (India) 1983;19:11–21.

181. von Pirquet C. Allergie. Münch Med Wochenschr 1906;30:1–4.

182. Willms-Kretschmer K, Flax MH, Cotran RS. The fine structure of the vascular response in hapten-specific delayed hypersensitivity and contact dermatitis. Lab Invest 1967;17:334–349.

183. Youmans GP. Tuberculosis. Philadelphia: WB Saunders, 1979.

Rejection of Grafts

CHAPTER 18

The Basic Dogma: Graft Rejection is an Immune Response

The Histocompatibility Antigens

Mechanisms of Graft Rejection

Graft-Versus-Host Reaction

Grafts and the Concept of Tolerance

I t is a fact of life that the body is generally unwilling to accept extraneous spare parts. We owe this discovery to the ever-daring surgeons (36), who have tried to overcome it for some 3000 years. The first on record are the *vaidya* of ancient India, who knew how to rebuild a lost nose with a graft of skin from the forehead of the same patient but not from another person (18). *From the same patient:* this was the key to successful grafts. In the late 1500s the Italian surgeon Gaspare Tagliacozzi was successfully rebuilding noses using a flap of skin from the arm (42), but he made the right choice (by taking the graft from the arm of the same patient) for the wrong reason: pure convenience. In fact he was quite sure that grafts from one person to another would take. After all, he argued, it is known since Roman times that grafts can be exchanged between fig trees and olive trees, and no two people are as different as such trees. And so the surgeons kept trying. John Hunter reported in the late 1700s that he had managed to graft the spur of one cock onto the comb of another cock (we shall return to this alarming report later). The year 1906 saw the first successful grafting of a cornea from one human to another (Figure 18.1) (47); thereafter this practice became standard, although a theoretical background was not available. In 1902 Alexis Carrel, surgeon and biologist, found a method for reconnecting severed blood vessels, and used the procedure to attempt experimental grafts of limbs, kidneys, and other organs. Grafts of one part to another part of the same individual succeeded, but all others failed (5). Carrel won the Nobel prize for his surgical procedure; but after him, by and large, organ transplantation was branded hopeless. Only a "liquid" graft, blood transfusion, took hold; the ABO system was worked out in 1910, and it was soon recognized as a key to success in transfusing blood.

Why did the organ grafts fail? As early as 1910 Da Fano puzzled over the fact that the inflammatory response under rejected skin grafts consisted mainly of lymphocytes, though dead tissue is usually surrounded by polymorphonuclear leukocytes (6). He could do little with his observation because the function of lymphocytes remained a mystery until the late 1940s. During World War II, a young British zoologist, Peter Medawar, began to work out the mechanisms of graft rejection. His work was prompted, once again, by a surgical need: a covering for extensive burn injuries. Skin grafts from uninjured donors would have been ideal in wartime, but they would not take. Medawar discovered that the mechanism was an immune response (21–24) and won the Nobel prize in 1960.

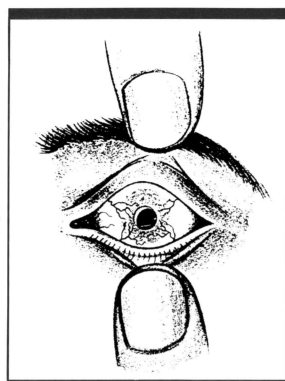

FIGURE 18.1
The first successful corneal graft, in 1906. The graft was provided by an 11-year-old boy whose eye had to be enucleated because of trauma; recipient was a 45-year-old man whose eyes had been burned by quicklime 16 months earlier. (Reproduced with permission from [48].)

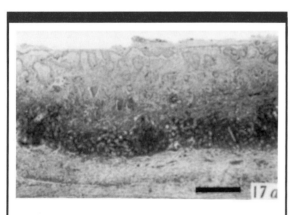

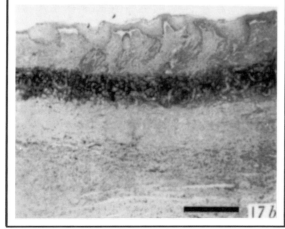

FIGURE 18.2
Allografts from the pioneer study by Peter B. Medawar in 1944. *Top:* Rabbit allograft at 8 days; the "black band" corresponds to lymphocytes. *Bottom:* Allograft at 16 days. **Bars =** 500 μm. (Reproduced with permission from [21].)

Now is the time for some vocabulary.

- **Autograft:** graft for which donor and recipient are the same individual.
- **Isograft:** graft between individuals of identical genetic makeup (**syngeneic**), such as identical twins or inbred animals.
- **Allograft:** graft between individuals of the same species but with different genetic makeup (**allogeneic**), such as grafts from one human being to another, or between different animals of noninbred strains. (The term *homograft* is obsolete.)
- **Xenograft:** graft between individuals of different species, such as human to mouse or baboon to human.

The Basic Dogma: Graft Rejection is an Immune Response

Just by observing the clinical course of graft rejection one should suspect that the underlying mechanism is an immune response; in fact this was suggested in the early 1900s by tumor researchers (36), but nobody drew the general conclusion until Peter Medawar. He and his research group, working mainly with mice bearing small patches of skin from other mice (Figure 18.2), formulated the following basic principles, which are valid for all grafts:

- Autografts and isografts are accepted; allografts and xenografts are rejected, xenografts sometimes in a matter of minutes (32).
- A first allograft begins by behaving properly: its vessels connect with those of the surrounding skin, and circulation is reestablished. However, starting from day one, lymphocytes and macrophages begin to appear and rapidly increase in numbers; soon the small vessels are thrombosed, necrosis sets in, and the dead graft is cast off. The initial "take" indicates that the host does not immediately recognize the graft as foreign; this requires a few days. Such is the so-called **first-set rejection,** which requires 7–10 days.
- A second allograft *from the same donor* is rejected much faster and with a livelier inflammation; the drama is over in 3–4 days. Some polymorphs and plasma cells are also involved. This is **second-set rejection.**
- A third allograft *taken from a different donor* produces a first-set rejection, providing evidence that the rejection response is specific

to the donor's tissue and therefore is consistent with an immune response.

T-lymphocytes are essential to rejection. Mice that have been deprived neonatally of their thymuses, and are therefore incapable of educating their T-cells, lose the capacity to reject grafts. Conversely, if lymphocytes of a mouse that has rejected a skin graft from donor X are injected intravenously into another mouse, that mouse becomes ready to develop a second-set rejection to a first graft from donor X.

All this tells us that the rejection is based on immunologic mechanisms. To understand what it is that the host recognizes as foreign, we will briefly explain the "identity cards" carried by all cells, namely the histocompatibility antigens.

The Histocompatibility Antigens

Because cells have no eyes and no ears, they must recognize each other by sniffing (i.e., by chemical messengers) and by feeling each other's surfaces. If cells were covered by a pure and simple phospholipid bilayer, life would be impossible; we would be just a pile of disoriented cells. Surface identity-markers are essential. Interestingly, *while cells are choosy with regard to their outer contacts, they are poorly equipped to recognize anything foreign that has managed to get inside them.* A human cell will accept the microsurgical intrusion of a tobacco plant nucleus without a blink. A number of intracellular parasites make their living from this biological loophole; viruses, for example, have discovered that the inside of any cell and even of a bacterium is a safe place. It has been hinted that some viruses have evolved the ability to cause cell fusion so that they can pass from one cell to another without being exposed to the dangers of the outer world, where antibodies may lurk. *There are no intracellular antibodies.* Lewis Thomas wrote one of his beautiful essays on this topic: "Symbiosis as an immunological problem" (44).

Back to the surface identity-markers: All cells have a choice of two sets of surface markers (Class I and Class II), both of which are glycoproteins (Figure 18.3). Because immunologists (like lymphocytes) understand proteins as antigens, these surface glycoproteins are called histocompatibility antigens. But do remember that these surface markers have important functions when they are

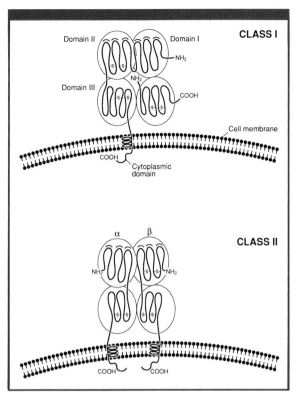

FIGURE 18.3 Two sets of surface markers for cells. *Top:* Class I MHC molecule; killer T-cells only attack cells marked by this molecule. *Bottom:* Class II MHC molecule displayed on the surface of antigen-presenting cells; it enables helper T-cells to recognize these cells. (Adapted from [20].)

"at home," besides waiting to be grafted onto someone else. Because geneticists (like DNA) understand proteins only as gene products, Class I and Class II histocompatibility antigens are usually explained in terms of the genes that code for them. We will follow these trends, but to remind the reader that "gene products" and "antigens" are just two other ways to say "proteins," we will temporarily confine "histocompatibility antigens" between quotation marks.

THE MAJOR HISTOCOMPATIBILITY COMPLEX

Now, it so happens that, in humans, the proteins that function as "histocompatibility antigens" are the products of a cluster of genes on a short segment of chromosome 6; this cluster is known as the Major Histocompatibility Complex (MHC), or as the HLA complex (Figure 18.4).

The term HLA is short for human leukocyte antigens, and dates from a time when it was believed that these "histocompatibility antigens" were present only on leukocytes. In mice the MHC is called H2 and it is on chromosome 17.

One factor that drastically complicates transplantation is that *the proteins coded by the HLA complex come in many variants;* in other words, for each gene in the complex there are a number of

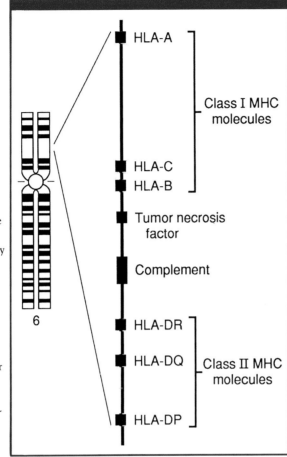

FIGURE 18.4
The best characterized loci of the human major histocompatibility complex (MHC) located in the HLA region of the short arm of chromosome 6. Inserted among the HLA genes are two genes for tumor necrosis factor and three genes for complement components. Adapted from (4)

possible alleles (**alleles** are variants of a gene at a particular genetic locus).

Class I "histocompatibility antigens" are present on the surfaces of virtually all cells, including platelets, a factor that must be considered in platelet transfusions. These antigens are coded in adjacent genetic loci labeled A, B, and C (HLA-A, HLA-B, HLA-C).

Class II "histocompatibility antigens" are normally limited to cells of the immunologic family: monocytes/macrophages, dendritic cells, Langerhans cells of the epidermis, B-cells and some activated T-cells (and, for unknown reasons, spermatozoa). However, gamma-interferon (secreted by activated T-cells) causes other cells to express Class II antigens, for instance, endothelial cells and fibroblasts. Class II antigens are coded in a region of the MHC complex known as HLA-D, which includes three clusters of genes called DR, DP, and DQ.

From what we have said, it follows that *all cells that carry Class II antigens also carry Class I antigens.* This fact has its consequences: in a graft, the most antigenic cells are likely to be those that carry

both classes of "histocompatibility antigens," such as macrophages.

Note: allografts can take even if HLA matching is not perfect. In a series of 20,000 transplants of cadaveric kidney, one-year survival was 83.3% for grafts with no HLA antigens mismatched, and 77.0 for kidneys with 4 mismatches (15a).

FUNCTIONS OF THE MAJOR HISTOCOMPATIBILITY COMPLEX

An elaborate system such as the HLA complex must have some profound reasons for its existence besides complicating the lives of students, teachers and surgeons. We might speculate, for example, that the tremendous variety fostered by the HLA system helps the survival of the species; if every human being carried the same HLA type, a cunning parasite able to exactly match that HLA type would escape detection and possibly wipe out the entire species. Another purpose might be to prevent mother and fetus from invading each other's tissues.

Much remains to be understood, but we can conclude that the HLA antigens are relevant (if not always useful) to three areas.

Regulation of the Immune Response In several interactions between effector cells of the immune response, Class I or Class II antigens are used as "passports" (i.e., recognition molecules).

- Cytotoxic (killer) T-cells that have been sensitized against a given virus are programmed to kill cells infected with that virus, but only if those cells carry the same Class I antigen as the killer cell.
- Helper T-cells recognize antigen presented to them only if the presenting cells carry Class II antigens (which tell them: "yes, I am an authorized antigen-presenting cell").

Association with Disease As soon as HLA typing became possible, it turned out that many of the Class I and Class II HLA antigens are statistically associated with specific diseases. For example, people who carry the HLA B27 antigen are 175 times more likely than normal to develop ankylosing spondylitis, a crippling disease of the spine. The known number of such associations continues to grow (9). There is even an association between the HLA antigen DR2 and narcolepsy, a disease consisting of an abnormal tendency to fall asleep (19). Most of the diseases related to HLA antigens are either inflammatory, autoimmune, or metabolic; how the correlation works is still not known, but one can speculate (46): (1) because up- or down-regulation of the immune response is a function of Class II antigens, malfunction of these antigens could lead to autoimmunity; (2) an HLA antigen might conceivably function as a receptor a virus and therefore favor infection by that virus.

You may now wonder whether you should run to the nearest hospital and obtain your HLA type as a more reliable, albeit more expensive, substitute for palm reading. But many correlations between HLA type and disease are rather weak, and we can only estimate the relative risks because not everybody who is DR2-positive tends to fall asleep and not all sleepy individuals are DR2-positive. And anyway, do we really want to know what *might* be in store for us?

Paternity Testing The HLA system was not created for this purpose, but in practice it has become an invaluable asset for paternity testing. The principle is to compare the peripheral blood lymphocytes of mother, putative father, and child with regard to surface (HLA) antigens. The same complexity of the HLA system that decreases the chance of success of a graft increases the chances of identifying the father. However, in legal matters, the HLA makeup is currently not acceptable as a sole source of evidence; it must be backed by other genetic markers such as red blood cell antigens and DNA.

HLA testing is a complex matter, but in essence human chromosome 6 carries, on each of its two strands, a string of seven HLA genes (called a haplo-type, from haploid genotype). Each of us therefore expresses two haplotypes. If we are heterozygous, we can express 14 possible HLA gene products, and the polymorphism of these genes means a great variety of product combinations (Figure 18.5). To identify the HLA makeup of a given individual, blood-derived lymphocytes of that individual are exposed to one of a series of specific anti-HLA antibodies (commercially available), and then complement is added. If the antigen is present, the lymphocytes are killed by complement; then the number of dead lymphocytes is counted by exposing the cell suspension to a dye (dye exclusion test, p. 190).

Transplantation The very notion of HLA antigens was worked out in relation to organ transplants, and these antigens remain a great difficulty facing the transplant team. The closer the HLA match between donor and recipient, the greater the chance of success; but unfortunately, in real life, it is very difficult to wait for a good match (41). In the context of a graft, the HLA recognition molecules truly function as antigens, resulting in antibody formation and cell-mediated hypersensitivity.

Mechanisms of Graft Rejection

Grafts are rejected by a combination of mechanisms that we discussed under hypersensitivity reactions, notably Types II, III, and IV. In other words, both

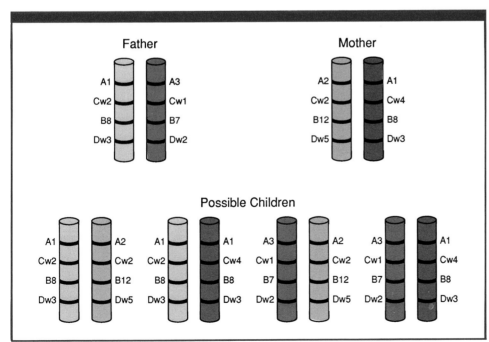

FIGURE 18.5
Haplotype combinations that may occur in the offspring of a mating. Note that the five alleles of a haplotype are always passed on together. Only five possible alleles are shown for each haplotype, but the total number recognized today is seven for any given haplotype. (Reproduced with permission from [26].)

cell-mediated and antibody-mediated mechanisms are at work; only the anaphylactic mechanism is left out. In addition, NK cells may participate in acute rejection, at least in mice (28).

The presence of an incompatible graft is perceived by two pathways: *peripherally,* that is, by cells of the host's immune system as they travel through the blood vessels of the graft; and *centrally,* that is, by host lymph nodes draining the territory of the graft. In mice, the local lymph nodes double or triple their size, and their blood flow increases fourfold (15); this helps to increase the outflow of sensitized lymphocytes.

The basic principles of rejection that have been worked out with grafts of skin are valid for grafts of other organs; details vary from organ to organ (15). However, it will probably come as a surprise to learn that the step-by-step sequence of graft rejection is still not fully understood.

CELL-MEDIATED MECHANISMS OF REJECTION.

Another surprise: the first killer cells to appear on the scene of the graft have been reported to be NK cells (38). Strictly speaking, NK cells do not belong to the immune system in the sense that they are nonspecific. They kill cells of the graft on first encounter, in the same way they kill virus-infected cells (p. 332); in renal allografts they reach a peak on day 5 and then decline (Figure 18.6).

Both T- and B-lymphocytes also appear on the scene, but the first step of an immune response must be the ritual of antigen presentation. It is not yet clear where the presenting cell comes from (15). One theory favors the dendritic cells of the donor, present in the graft as "passenger leukocytes," and strongly antigenic (7, 17). The endothelial cells of the graft may also be involved.

Of course, the cells to which antigen is being presented are the host's lymphocytes. Both T- and B-lymphocytes gather locally in varying proportions and then multiply, so that a large population of "immunoblasts" develops (the term includes any type of activated, replicating lymphocytes). Eventually the task of rejection is accomplished by various types of specialized cells; besides the NK cells there will be lymphocytes capable of killing by an antibody-dependent mechanism (ADCC, p. 527); most of the T-lymphocytes appear to be of the killer/suppressor phenotype, which can kill directly. Smaller numbers of macrophages also mix in the crowd; it is possible that they, too, take part in the killing, by means of cytokines or free radicals.

What cells are the targets and what type of killing can they expect? The strategies of this offensive are not fully understood, but the targets appear to depend on the antigenic anatomy (15) of the tissue, and especially on the distribution of MHC antigens. Strangely, *many parenchymal cells such as liver cells are safe from cytotoxic attack.* The endothelium, on the other hand, tends to be destroyed by one mechanism or another. There are organ as well as species differences.

ANTIBODY-MEDIATED MECHANISMS OF REJECTION

Antibody-mediated rejection is especially vicious against the endothelial lining of the vessels in the graft; it leads to thrombosis and therefore to accelerated graft failure. As soon as B-cell antibody production has reached high enough levels (5–7 days), the rejection is initiated: antibodies coating the endothelial surface activate complement (11, 12) and attract the wrath of cells bearing Fc receptors (the ADCC mechanism). Endothelial cells that survive the onslaught become activated, express adhesion molecules and trap more leukocytes (1).

The histopathology of rejection varies from one organ to another; rejection may occur within minutes, days, months, or years. The timing corresponds to various tissue events. Most is known about the kidney, as follows.

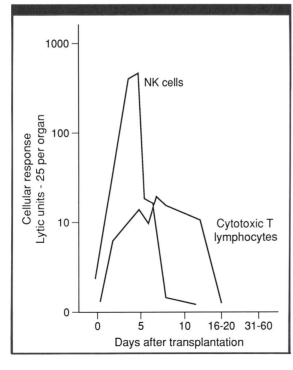

FIGURE 18.6 NK cells participate in graft rejection. In the study here shown, their numbers exceed those of cytotoxic lymphocytes. What attracts them to the allograft is not known. (Adapted from [15].)

Hyperacute Rejection Rejection of a kidney transplant may occur while the patient is still on the operating table. It is now known that some hosts have preformed antibodies against the graft endothelium. When this occurs, the kidney becomes swollen and purple as soon as the blood is allowed to flow into it, and must be removed immediately. One wonders how these individuals acquired their antiendothelial antibodies: possible mechanisms include previous infection with cross-reacting bacterial or viral agents, pregnancy, or transfusions. The latter concept is rather paradoxical because, on the whole, a history of previous blood transfusions seems to improve the survival of human grafts (45). Today, hyperacute rejection can be avoided by suitable preoperative tests.

Acute Rejection Rejection within weeks or months (Figure 18.7) is a combination of two unfortunate developments: (1) destruction of parenchyma by cytotoxic lymphocytes (Figure 18.8); in the kidney this is known as "tubulitis"; and (2) diffuse vascular changes, which presumably occur because the endothelium is being attacked by antibody as well as by cellular mechanisms. A strange thing happens in the small arteries; foam cells appear in the intima, quite similar to those seen in atherosclerosis, but the reason for the lipid storage remains a mystery (Figure 18.9) (33).

Chronic Rejection Chronic rejection is due to similar mechanisms, complicated by a progres-

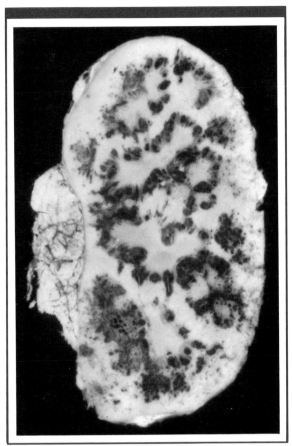

FIGURE 18.7
See color plate 17. Acutely rejected human kidney. The vessels are dilated and thrombosed; the parenchyma is white due to coagulation necrosis. Slightly reduced.

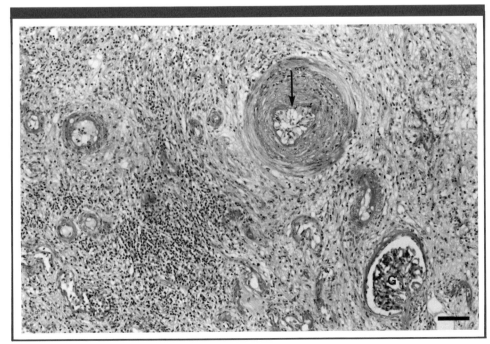

FIGURE 18.8
A kidney that suffered chronic rejection. Vascular changes: Arteriole with intimal hyperplasia, and subendothelial foam cells (**arrow**) with almost complete obliteration of the lumen. Parenchymal changes: Diffuse mononuclear cell infiltration and almost total disappearance of the renal parenchyma. A glomerulus (**G**) remains recognizable. **Bar** = 100 μm.

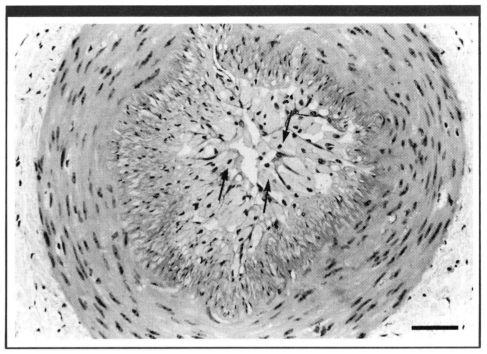

FIGURE 18.9
A typical but unexplained arterial change found in transplanted tissues: foam cells (**arrows**) in the intima. From a 90 day liver transplant. **Bar** = 250 μm. (Reproduced with permission from [33].)

sive, concentric narrowing of the arteries by intimal thickening with very few inflammatory cells, presumably the scarring stage of the earlier lesions. However, much remains unclear, especially about human grafts, which are complicated by immunosuppressive therapy, cytotoxic mechanisms (cyclosporine is nephrotoxic), and superimposed disease (Figure 18.10). It is fair to conclude that *the failure of a graft is ultimately due to a combination of at least two mechanisms: immune responses and vascular shutdown* (14).

Many tricks have been tried to reduce the immune attack against the graft. For small grafts such as those of endocrine tissues, it was found that organ culture for 2 weeks prior to transplantation in an

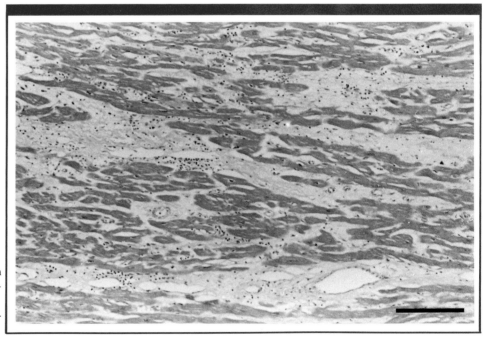

FIGURE 18.10
Rejection of a transplanted heart in a patient who chose to stop taking immunosuppressive medication. Note diffuse edema and inflammatory infiltrate. **Bar** = 200 μm.

atmosphere of 95 percent oxygen and 5 percent carbon dioxide greatly extends the survival (17). This fascinating phenomenon is not fully understood. It could be a matter of antigen modulation, or of loss of endothelium or possibly of "passenger leukocytes" and/or dendritic cells. Another imaginative trick that offers hope for treating diabetes: allografts of rat pancreatic islets survive if they are grafted in the thymus (31).

Graft-Versus-Host Reaction

By and large, the problems encountered in grafting organs are limited to the graft itself: vasculitis, inflammation, necrosis, and fibrosis. The host tends to reject the graft. The graft, however, has its own lymphoid cells; would they not fight the host? This does happen with *bone marrow grafts*, such as those for replenishing the hematopoietic system in a variety of conditions: aplastic anemia, leukemia, and immunodeficiency diseases. The result is a serious complication, a disease of the whole body called graft-versus-host disease (GVHD); it occurs in 40–45 percent of the patients (42). GVHD develops because a graft of bone marrow includes all the cell types of the immune system; injected into a new host these cells find themselves in a foreign environment and attempt to reject the host by cell-mediated mechanisms, especially if the host is immunosuppressed. A life-threatening rejection develops in one-fourth to one-third of the patients (16); it manifests itself by *selective epithelial damage of target organs* (10), especially in the epidermis as manifested by skin rashes (Figure 18.11) in the liver which becomes enlarged, and in the gut which develops ulcerations and diarrhea. In the meantime the ability to resist infection is depressed because the host bone marrow becomes aplastic. Treatment has somewhat improved the outlook of GVH disease; in some cases the two immune systems strike a balance and succeed in living side by side—the patient becomes a chimera—that is, an individual made up of cells of different genotype. Note, however, that *some degree of two-way chimerism occurs in successful organ grafts*: the graft adopts selected immune cells of the host, and vice versa. The antigen-presenting (dendritic) cells of the graft that migrate into the host appear to reprogram its immune system, acting as "veto cells" (39a). In essence, chimerism is part of the uneasy truce between graft and host.

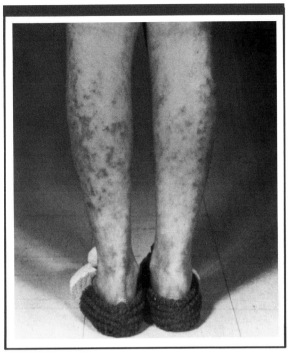

FIGURE 18.11 Graft-versus-host disease. Skin lesions in a patient who underwent a bone marrow transplant. (Courtesy of Dr. J.L. Sullivan, University of Massachusetts Medical Center, Worcester, MA.)

PATHOGENESIS

The pathogenesis of GVH disease is taking a surprising turn. It was once believed to be a typical cell-mediated effect, with cytotoxic T-cells destroying their various targets. It seemed so logical. However, a number of observations has cast doubts on this simple mechanism; most significantly, *many target cells seem to die in the absence of any significant T-cell infiltration* (Figure 18.12) (30, 37). Could cytokines be the culprits? Many lines of

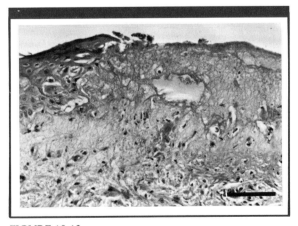

FIGURE 18.12
Biopsy of a skin lesion in graft-versus-host disease. Note the necrosis of the epidermis. The disproportion between this necrosis and the amount of inflammatory infiltrate fits the notion that such lesions are of "toxic" nature (an effect of TNF). **Bar** = 100 μm. (Reproduced with permission from [37].)

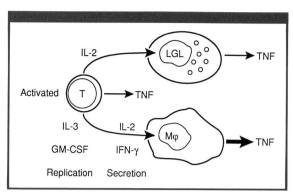

FIGURE 18.13

Three pathways to the secretion of tumor necrosis factor (TNF) as a consequence of T lymphocyte activation. **LGL:** Large granular lymphocyte (NK cell). Overproduction of TNF may lead to general and to local damage in a variety of situations, including graft-versus-host disease, malaria, tuberculosis, and toxic insults (e.g., lung fibrosis elicited by bleomycin). (Adapted from [31].)

evidence point to tumor necrosis factor alpha (TNF-α): for example, GVHD in humans is associated with elevated serum levels of TNF-α (16); and in mice, treatment with an antibody against TNF-α attenuates GVHD (30, 31). A likely sequence would therefore be that activated T-lymphocytes secrete interferon gamma, which induces macrophages and other leukocytes to secrete TNF-α (Figure 18.13).

Thus, GVHD turns out to be a disease of cytokine dysregulation (10) and comes to overlap with endotoxemia, because endotoxin produces many of its effects by inducing macrophages to secrete TNF-α (p. 701). So, GVHD is another classic case of basic research providing new insights to the clinician.

Grafts and the Concept of Tolerance

For the surgeons who transplant organs, and for their patients, the ideal solution to grafting would be some means to abolish rejection without immunosuppressing the individual altogether. Under certain conditions this ideal situation does exist; it is called tolerance.

Immunologically tolerant is an individual incapable of responding to a given antigen. Tolerance exists in nature, if you know where to look; in fact, this notion was born, as other concepts in immunology, of an observation in veterinary

medicine (12, 29). R.D. Owen reported in 1945 that the blood of nonidentical twin calves sometimes contained red blood cells of two blood groups, one from each twin, with no pathologic effect. A twin pregnancy in cows is unusual, but when it does occur the circulation of the two placentas is mixed, so that there is free exchange of blood cells. Shortly thereafter, Burnet and Fenner (3) used this observation in an attempt to explain why the body does not build antibodies against itself; they argued that during embryonic development the body learns to recognize its own constituents and also learns how to phagocytize and digest its obsolete components without making antibodies against them. They also predicted (one wonders why they did not try the critical experiment) that if an embryo were injected with an antigen, as an adult it would not respond to that antigen. Two years later Peter Medawar proved them right: twin calves (nonidentical) would accept grafts from each other's skin. Later work showed that mice would accept skin allografts if they had been injected with the allogeneic cells in fetal life (2). (Incidentally, red cells of two blood groups, A and O, have been found in human twins [8].)

Medawar argued that the biological significance of immune tolerance may be to prevent autoimmune reactions. This is probably true, but to explain how tolerance works at the level of cells, and how it can be broken, is a difficult matter; several theories have been proposed. We will explore some of these concepts in relation to autoimmune disease.

Xenografts—and an Afterthought on John Hunter's Experiment Xenografts are not supposed to take. However, the reader will be surprised to learn that *the immune response to xenografts is sometimes weaker than to allografts* (32, 35). True, some species combinations lead to hyperacute rejection—even within ten minutes—because the recipient carries "natural" antibodies against the red blood cells of the donor; these combinations are called *discordant*. The origin of the antibodies is not clear; we may be dealing with cross reaction by antibodies against intestinal bacteria or other environmental antigens. However, grafts between some closely related species (such as humans and chimpanzees) are tolerated for some time, because the antibodies are low or absent. These combinations are said to be *concordant*. In some xenografts, the T-lymphocyte reaction is weaker than against allografts; one of the reasons may be that different species do not respond to each other's cytokines (35). Xenografts are therefore coming under closer scrutiny for human use. Genetically engineered pigs may lead to a breakthrough (18a, 28a); a possible hazard of xenografts, however, could be the introduction of new pathogenic viruses.

In closing this section on supposedly "forbidden grafts," we should return to that historical allograft reported in the late 1700s by John Hunter: the cock's spur grafted in another cock's comb is still one of the prize exhibits of the Hunterian Museum in London. The implication of this exhibit is that we are witnessing a successful allograft. Experimental details are not available. Could this be an immunologic miracle? Or is this a 5-day result? Or maybe a horny spur is not very antigenic? In 1984 we consulted Sir Peter Medawar. His reply (25):

> I do not believe in the John Hunter story—and think it quite inconceivable that the two birds were so highly inbred as to make it possible for them to accept grafts from each other. I mean, I do not think that a natural law was suspended in Hunter's favour, though surgeons are normally quite ready to believe that such a thing can come to pass.
>
> I do think that you would be performing a public service if you persuaded a PhD student to go over the ground again.

We hope that someone will pick up that challenge. Until then, we will assume that the miraculous "graft" is just a dead spur stuck into a cock's comb, and tolerated as a thorn might be—for some time.

What Do Plants Tell Us About Grafts? In China the art of grafting plants was known around 1000 B.C., and also Aristotle (384–321 B.C.) knew a lot about it (13). The trees themselves, however, practiced grafting long before humans: in some species, branches pressed together tend to fuse; roots can establish grafts quite easily, sometimes even among different species. Stumps may be kept alive by this underground support, and some parasites—such as the fungus of Dutch elm disease—can spread by the same route (13). The relationship between host and graft (called *stock* and *scion*), is not the same in all cases, and anyway the rejection does not depend on phenomena that the "animal people" would call immunologic. A classic example: the quince rejects a graft of pear because the quince produces a glycoside that diffuses into the pear tissue, where it is broken down producing cyanide; so the pear cells die of cyanide poisoning (27).

Sometimes an impossible graft is made possible by an intermediate segment called *interstock*, which is compatible with both stock and scion (13); the comparison with the mammalian placenta is irresistible.

TO SUM UP: We still have a lot to learn about the mechanism of graft rejection. Perhaps one of the most surprising developments since Medawar's time has been the discovery that xenografts are not as hopeless as anticipated. However, in real life, the major obstacle to grafting is not biological but social: it is the shortage of organs. For the heart alone, the yearly shortage in the USA is on the order of 40,000 (28a).

References

1. Bacchi CE, Marsh CL, Perkins JD, et al. Expression of vascular cell adhesion molecule (VCAM-1) in liver and pancreas allograft rejection. Am J Pathol 1993;142:579–591.
2. Billingham RE, Brent L, Medawar PB. Quantitative studies on tissue transplantation immunity. III. Actively acquired tolerance. Philos Trans R Soc Lond (Biol) 1956;239:357–414.
3. Burnet FM, Fenner F. The production of antibodies, 2nd ed. Melbourne: MacMillan and Company Limited, 1949.
4. Carpenter CB, David J. Histocompatibility antigens and immune response genes. In: Rubenstein E, Federman DD, eds. Scientific American medicine, 6 immunology, V. Histocompatibility antigens. New York: Scientific American, 1991:1–10.
5. Carrel A. The transplantation of organs. NY Med J 1914;99:839–840.
6. Da Fano C. Zelluläre Analyse der Geschwulstimmunitätsreaktionen. Zeitschrift F. Immunitätsforsch 1910;5:1–74.
7. Demetris AJ, Qian S, Sun H, et al. Early events in liver allograft rejection. Delineation of sites of simultaneous intragraft and recipient lymphoid tissue sensitization. Am J Pathol 1991;138:609–618.
8. Dunsford I, Bowley CC, Hutchison AM, Thompson JS, Sanger R, Race RR. A human blood-group chimera. Br Med J 1953;2:81.
9. Dupont B. Immunobiology of HLA. New York: Springer-Verlag, 1989.
10. Ferrara JLM, Deeg HJ. Graft-versus-host disease. N Engl J Med 1991;324:667–674.
11. Forbes RDC, Guttmann RD. Evidence for complement-induced endothelial injury in vivo: a comparative ultrastructural tracer study in a controlled model of hyperacute rat cardiac allograft rejection. Am J Pathol 1982;106:378–387.
12. Gowans JL. The immunology of tissue transplantation. In: Florey HW, ed. General pathology, 4th ed. Philadelphia: WB Saunders, 1970:1160–1182.

13. Hartmann HT, Kester DE, Davis FT. Theoretical aspects of grafting and budding. In: Plant propagation: principles and practices, 5th ed. New Jersey: Prentice-Hall, 1990:305–332.

14. Häyry P. Intragraft events in allograft destruction. Transplantation 1984;38:1–6.

15. Häyry P, von Willebrand E, Parthenais E, et al. The inflammatory mechanisms of allograft rejection. Immunol Rev 1984;77:85–142.

15a. Held PJ, Kahan BD, Hunsicker LG, Liska D, Wolfe RA, Port FK, Gaylin DS, Garcia JR, Agodoa LYC, and Krakauer H. The impact of HLA mismatches on the survival of first cadaveric kidney transplants. N Engl J Med 1994;331:765–770.

16. Holler E, Kolb HJ, Möller A, et al. Increased serum levels of tumor necrosis factor α precede major complications of bone marrow transplantation. Blood 1990;75:1011–1016.

17. Lafferty KJ, Prowse SJ, Simeonovic CJ, Warren HS. Immunobiology of tissue transplantation: a return to the passenger leukocyte concept. Annu Rev Immunol 1983;1:143–173.

18. Majno G. The healing hand: man and wound in the ancient world. Cambridge, MA: Harvard University Press, 1975.

18a. Malouin R. Surgeons' quest for life: the history and the future of xenotransplantation. Perspect Biol Med 1994;37:416–428.

19. Matsuki K, Honda Y, Juji T. HLA antigens in 206 Japanese patients with narcolepsy and 46 patients with essential hypersomnia. In: Dupont B. Immunobiology of HLA. New York: Springer-Verlag, 1989:438–440.

20. McDevitt HO. Advances in genetic organization of the HLA transplantation system. In: Jamison RL, ed. Transplantation in the 1980s: recent advances. New York: Praeger, 1984:15–22.

21. Medawar PB. The behaviour and fate of skin autografts and skin homografts in rabbits. J Anat 1944;78:176–199.

22. Medawar PB. A second study of the behaviour and fate of skin homografts in rabbits. J Anat 1945;79:157–176.

23. Medawar PB. Immunity to homologous grafted skin. II. The relationship between the antigens of blood and skin. Br J Exp Pathol 1946;27:15–24.

24. Medawar PB. The homograft reaction. Proc R Soc London B 1958;149:145–166.

25. Medawar PB. Personal letter dated 7th September 1984.

26. Miller WV, Rodey G. HLA without tears. Chicago: American Society of Clinical Pathologists, Educational Products Division, 1981.

27. Moore R. Graft compatibility/incompatibility in higher plants. What's New in Plant Physiology 1981;12:13–16.

28. Murphy WJ, Kuman V, Bennett M. Acute rejection of murine bone marrow allografts by natural killer cells and T cells. Differences in kinetics and target antigens recognized. J Exp Med 1987;166:1499–1509.

28a. Nowak R. Xenotransplants set to resume. Science 1994;266:1148–1151.

29. Owen RD. Immunogenetic consequences of vascular anastomoses between bovine twins. Science 1945;102:400–401.

30. Piguet P-F. The graft-versus-host disease. A search of the pathogenesis of T lymphocyte induced tissue damage. Geneva, Switzerland: University of Geneva, 1990, Thesis.

31. Piguet P-F, Grau GE. Tumor necrosis factor (TNF) as an effector of immunopathological reactions elicited by T lymphocytes. In: Touraine JL, Traeger J, Bétuel H, Dubernard JM, Revillard JP, Daudon P, eds. Transplantation and clinical immunology, vol XXI. Amsterdam: Excerpta Medica, 1990:105–114.

32. Platt JL, Vercellotti GM, Dalmasso AP, et al. Transplantation of discordant xenografts: a review of progress. Immunol Today 1990;11:450–457.

33. Portmann BC. Histopathology of late liver graft failure: chronic rejection and other causes. In: Touraine JL, Traeger J, Bétuel H, Dubernard JM, Revillard JP, Daudon P, eds. Transplantation and clinical immunology, vol XXI. Amsterdam: Excerpta Medica, 1990:47–58.

34. Posselt AM, Barker CE, Tomaszewski JE, Markmann JF, Choti MA, Naji A. Induction of donor-specific unresponsiveness by intrathymic islet transplantation. Science 1990;249:1293–1295.

35. Sachs DH, Bach FH. Immunology of xenograft rejection. Hum Immunol 1990;28:245–251.

36. Silverstein AM. A history of immunology. San Diego: Academic Press, 1988.

37. Snover DC. The pathology of acute graft-vs.-host disease. In: Burakoff SJ, Deeg HJ, Ferrara J, Atkinson K, eds. Graft-vs.-host disease. New York: Marcel Dekker, 1990:337–353.

38. Soulillou JP. Functional characteristics of cells infiltrating rejected allografts. Immunol Today 1987;8:285–287.

39. Spital A. The shortage of organs for transplantation: where do we go from here? N Engl J Med 1991;325:1246.

39a. Starzl TE, Demetris AJ, Murase N, Trucco M, Thomson AW, Rao AS. The changing immunology of organ transplantation. Hospital Practice October 15, 1995;31–42.

40. Steinman RM, Inaba K. Stimulation of the primary mixed leukocyte reaction. CRC Crit Rev Immunol 1984–85;5:331–348.

41. Stevenson LW, Lake H, Terasaki PI, Kahan BD, Drinkwater DC. Cardiac transplantation—selection, immunosuppression, and survival [specialty conference]. West J Med 1988;149:572–582.

42. Storb R. Critical issues in bone marrow transplantation. Transplant Proc 1987;19:2774–2781.

43. Tagliacozzi G, 1597: Gasparis Taliacotii Bononiensis . . . De Curtorum Chirurgia per insitionem Libri Duo. Venetiis, MDXCVIII. Apud Gasparem Bindonum iuniorem. P. 59

44. Thomas L. Symbiosis as an immunologic problem. In: Neter E, Milgrom F, eds. The immune system and infectious diseases. Basel: S. Karger, 1975:2–11.

45. van Twuyver E, Mooijaart RJD, ten Berge IJM, et al. Pretransplantation blood transfusion revisited. N Engl J Med 1991;325:1210–1213.

46. Zabriskie JB, Gibofsky A. Genetic control of the susceptibility to infection with pathogenic bacteria. Curr Topics Microbiol Immunol 1986;124:1–20.

47. Zirm E. Eine erfolgreiche totale Keratoplastik. Albrecht von Graefes Arch Ophthalmol 1906;64:580–593.

Autoimmune Disease

CHAPTER 19

History and Nature of Autoimmune Disease

Pathogenesis of Autoimmune Disease

Some Lessons from Experimental Autoimmune Diseases

Over 40 human diseases are known or suspected to be **autoimmune:** that is, they seem to arise because the immune system turns against one or more bodily components, cellular or extracellular. Microscopically, their main feature is inflammation that has no apparent cause. The incidence of these diseases tends to increase with age, and females are much more susceptible than males by a factor of about six (30). However, this does not mean that females are less immunocompetent than males; the contrary is true. In fact, females are superior survivors immunologically and otherwise (43).

The Natural Superiority of Women is the title of a book published in 1954 by the eminent anthropologist Ashley Montagu (39). Current statistics and immunology wholly support Montagu. At birth there are about 5 percent more males than females, but females outlive males by an average of 8 years. Males are more susceptible to accidents, as well as to cancer and infectious diseases. Women have slightly higher IgG and 30 percent higher IgM serum antibody levels than men, and they respond more briskly to several antigens by antibody formation. They appear to enjoy the advantage of immunoregulatory genes located on the X chromosome, of which they have two copies. This may be an evolutionary adaptation that protects females from the immunosuppression associated with childbearing (immunosuppression occurs because a fetus is essentially an allograft that has to be kept alive "against the rules"). This adaptation may be a two-edged sword: though females are capable of a stronger immune response to infectious agents, they are also more prone to develop autoantibodies (43). However,

their tendency to develop autoimmune disorders is far outweighed by their "natural superiority." The updated 1992 edition of Montagu's book should be compulsory reading, for males anyway.

History and Nature of Autoimmune Disease

The concept of autoimmune disease gained respectability quite slowly. One reason was the fuzzy name—"collagen diseases"—that was applied to this group of diseases before the autoimmune mechanism was understood (see p. 256). This misnomer misled some very good scientists to search for—and to find—non-existing or irrelevant changes in the collagen fibers in hypersensitivity lesions (47). The alternative name "connective tissue diseases" is still used, although it is not much better. Another reason for skepticism toward the concept of the body turning against itself was that the mere presence of autoantibodies in the plasma is no proof of autoimmune disease. Autoantibodies are found in the plasma of people that are apparently normal, and they increase with age (53). Besides, autoantibodies could be a secondary phenomenon; the best-known case is the appearance of autoantibodies against myocardial tissue after an episode of myocardial infarction. It has been speculated that under such conditions autoantibodies might even perform a useful function (17, 21) by assisting in the normal scavenging process. For example, a coat of antibody on a bit of cell debris would make the debris stickier for macrophages and therefore easier to phagocytize. To certify an inflammation as autoimmune, it is necessary to prove that the autoantibodies are the primary mechanism of the disease and that no other cause is apparent.

The reader may be frustrated by the many uncertainties sprinkled over the following pages. Such is the state of the subject: autoimmune diseases are fascinating, and facts abound, but

mechanisms are hard to prove. We offer three generalizations:

- *The target organ is usually invaded by a chronic inflammatory infiltrate,* which can be very destructive.
- *Most autoimmune diseases are due to the antibody mechanism* rather than the cell-mediated mechanism. Indeed, the diagnosis is largely based on finding autoantibodies in the serum. This does not mean that cell-mediated

TABLE 19.1

Selected Autoimmune Diseases

Disease	Target of Autoantibody
Organ-specific diseases:	
Hashimoto's thyroiditis	Thyroglobulin and microsomal antigens
Myasthenia gravis	Antiacetylcholine receptor
Graves' disease (diffuse toxic goiter)	TSH receptor
Insulin-resistant diabetes, associated with acanthosis nigricans	Insulin receptor
Insulin-resistant diabetes associated with ataxia-telangiectasia	Insulin receptor
Juvenile insulin-dependent diabetes	Islet cells; insulin
Pernicious anemia	Gastric parietal cells; vitamin B_{12}-binding site of intrinsic factor
Allergic rhinitis, asthma, functional autonomic abnormalities	β_2-adrenergic receptors
Addison's disease	Adrenal cortical cells
Idiopathic hypoparathyroidism	Antigens of parathyroid cells
Spontaneous infertility	Sperm
Premature ovarian failure	Interstitial cells; corpus luteum cells
Pemphigus	Intercellular substance of skin and mucosae
Bullous pemphigoid	Basement membrane zone of skin and mucosae
Primary biliary cirrhosis	Mitochondrial antigens
Autoimmune hemolytic anemia	Red blood cells
Idiopathic thrombocytopenic purpura	Platelets
Idiopathic neutropenia	Neutrophils
Vitiligo	Melanocytes
Chronic active hepatitis	Nuclei; hepatocyte antigens
Ulcerative colitis	Colon mucosa
Systemic diseases (non–organ-specific)	
Goodpasture's syndrome	Basement membrane (lung, kidney)
Rheumatoid arthritis	γ-globulin; EBV-related antigens
Systemic lupus erythematosus (SLE)	DNA; nucleolus; histone; lymphocytes; red blood cells; platelets; neurons; other
Sjögren's syndrome	γ-globulin; other
Scleroderma	Topoisomerase; centromere; other
Polymyositis	Nuclei; histidyl-tRNA synthetase; other
Rheumatic fever	Myocardium; heart valves; choroid plexus; neurons

Adapted from (58)

mechanisms do not occur; we will point out some of these as we come across them.

Because the autoimmune mechanism is so often antibody-mediated, we conclude that the body can treat some of its own components as it would treat bacteria or other parasites. That is, if the target of the autoantibody is a structure, such as a cell, we can expect that target to be destroyed by complement or by leukocytes that have Fc receptors, as in Type II hypersensitivity. If, instead, autoantibody is formed against a soluble antigen, it will form complexes, and we can therefore expect the various types of complex-induced lesions described for Type III hypersensitivity.

- *Autoimmune diseases form a spectrum* from the single-organ type to the systemic and multiorgan type (Table 19.1). This is simply a fact of life. It has as yet no scientific explanation. It depends in part on the nature and specificity of the antibodies. Statistics show that *developing one autoimmune disease tends to increase the risk of developing another;* therefore, a single patient may "move" along this spectrum.

At one end of the range is *Hashimoto's thyroiditis,* in which antibodies are formed against thyroglobulin, and correspondingly this disease tends to remain limited to the thyroid. Also, *autoimmune infertility*—a fascinating topic—is due to antisperm antibodies in men or women (or antiovum antibodies in women) and is strictly limited to

reproduction (38, 55). At the other end of the spectrum is *systemic lupus erythematosus* (SLE), in which a variety of autoantibodies are formed and no organ is spared. *Rheumatoid arthritis* affects the joints primarily; however, because there are circulating antibodies against IgG, the disease has some features related to circulating complexes (as in serum sickness).

Here are sketches of a few typical autoimmune diseases in humans. Several have counterparts in other animals (6).

Hashimoto's Thyroiditis The mildest of all autoimmune diseases, Hashimoto's thyroiditis is usually recognized as a goitrous swelling accompanied by persistent fatigue (hypothyroidism), in middle-aged women; antithyroglobulin antibodies are present in the serum. Thyroid tissue is infiltrated and destroyed by a mononuclear infiltrate consisting mainly of lymphocytes and plasma cells (Figure 19.1). No other organ is affected. The plasma may also contain antibodies against gastric parietal cells in the absence of gastric disease; autoimmune gastritis may develop later, as well as pernicious anemia (because autoantibodies interfere with the absorption of vitamin B_{12}, and the lack of this vitamin leads to pernicious anemia). There is a slightly increased risk of developing lymphoma. Replacement hormone therapy enables these patients to lead normal lives.

Graves' Disease (Basedow's Disease in continental Europe), the most common form of hyperthy-

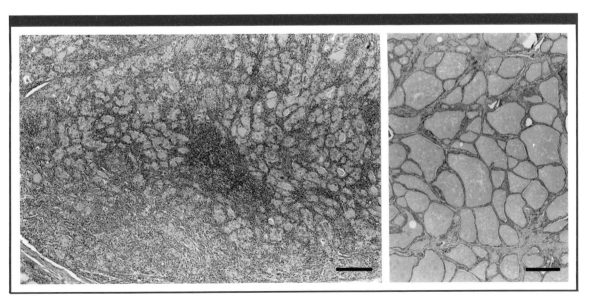

FIGURE 19.1 Comparison of diseased and normal thyroid. *Left:* Hashimoto's thyroiditis, an autoimmune disease; thyroid follicles, barely recognizable, have been destroyed by an intense mononuclear cell infiltrate consisting mainly of lymphocytes. *Right:* Normal thyroid. **Bars** = 250 μm.

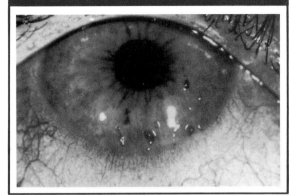

FIGURE 19.2 Cornea in severe Sjögren's syndrome has dried up and become vascularized (*keratitis filamentosa*). (Reproduced with permission from [26].)

roidism, is due to autoantibodies against the thyroid cell receptors for the thyroid-stimulating hormone (TSH) of the pituitary. Several types of autoantibodies have been described, but the prevailing result of antibody binding is that of stimulating the TSH receptor, resulting in oversecretion of thyroid hormone. Young women are more commonly affected; symptoms include sweating, palpitations, nervousness, diarrhea and loss of weight, and sometimes also connective tissue changes (especially periocular, retro-orbital and pretibial) which are not well understood (p. 266) (16a).

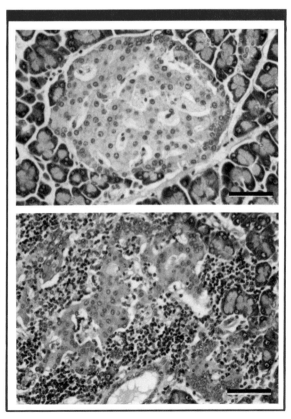

FIGURE 19.3 *Top:* Pancreatic islet of a nondiabetic, "normal" rat of the BB/W strain, which is prone to develop autoimmune diabetes. The islet is sharply defined; inflammatory cells are absent. *Bottom:* inflamed islet (insulitis) in an acutely diabetic BB/W rat. The cords of islet cells are separated and distorted by infiltrating lymphocytes. **Bars** = 50 μm. (Reproduced with permission from [37].)

Sjögren's Syndrome In this highly distressing disease, the eyes and mouth become extremely dry (*xerophthalmia, xerostomia*) because the lachrymal and salivary glands are destroyed by an infiltrate of lymphocytes, plasma cells, and fibrous tissue. Other mucosae may be involved (Figure 19.2), and other autoimmune diseases are often associated. Again, women are more often affected than men (9:1).

Diabetes Diabetes is not a single disease, but a group of disorders that have in common *hyperglycemia,* and affect about 5 percent of the population in Western societies (49). Over 90 percent of the patients suffer from one of two syndromes: insulin-dependent diabetes mellitus (IDDM) or diabetes Type I, and insulin-independent diabetes mellitus (NIDDM) or diabetes Type II. It is IDDM that concerns us here because a large body of evidence suggests that it is an autoimmune disease.

IDDM usually strikes before the age of 25; it is associated with abnormalities of peripheral lymphocytes and with inflammation of the pancreatic islets (*insulitis*). It is often familial and is associated with at least six HLA loci (42); insulin treatment is essential.

NIDDM also tends to be familial but is much more common and shows a preference for women; it usually appears after the age of 40. The pancreas shows no insulitis. Insulin treatment is not always required.

The insulitis of IDDM is histologically striking (Figure 19.3); it has been studied a great deal in an experimental model, the so-called BB rat. Because the insulin-secreting beta cells occupy the center of the rat islet (being surrounded by a rim of alpha and delta cells), autoimmune attack by T-lymphocytes appears to "hollow out" the islet (Figure 19.4) (37). The availability of various experimental models of IDDM is a major asset for the study of this disease (12, 14, 37, 42).

Systemic Lupus Erythematosus This disease (SLE) is usually diagnosed in a young woman who complains of fever, joint pains and skin rashes; typical is a "butterfly rash" over the nose and cheeks (Figure 19.5) (38a).

The name lupus *(wolf) is a leftover from the Middle Ages (56). Originally, it was applied to ulcers, especially of the face, that had the appearance of having been gnawed; the classic* lupus vulgaris *was tuberculosis of the face.*

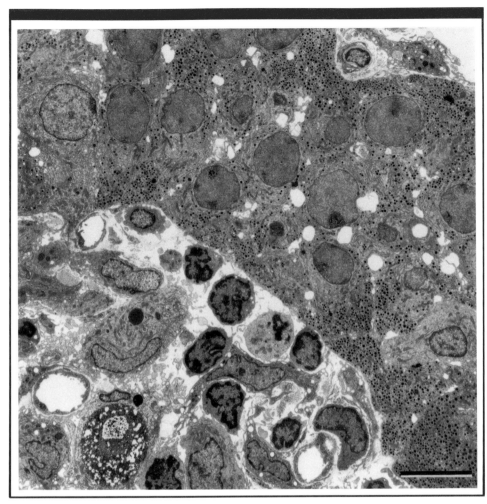

FIGURE 19.4
Low power electron micrograph of an inflamed islet from a diabetic BB/W rat. The B cells, usually set in the center of the islet, are absent. The core of the islet is "hollowed out" and filled with lymphocytes and macrophages. Some of the latter contain debris of phagocytized B cells. **Bar** = 10 μm. (Reproduced with permission from [37].)

The inflammatory lesions of SLE occur in the skin, kidneys, joints, serosal membranes, and practically any organ. Although the cause is not known, the amazing number and variety of autoantibodies suggest an underlying disorder in the mechanisms of self-tolerance. Circulating antinuclear antibodies are found in almost all patients. These antibodies cannot penetrate into normal cells, but they do react with exposed nuclei of damaged cells; complexes are found in the glomeruli and along the basal surface of the epidermis (Figure 19.6). In fact, much of the pathology is caused secondarily by vascular changes due to immune complexes ("immune complex disease", p. 529). There is no proof that the anti*nuclear* antibodies contribute as such to the pathogenesis of SLE. However, antiphospholipid antibodies have been implicated as a cause of thrombosis, lesions of heart valves, fetal loss, and thrombocytopenia; however, these antibodies are not specific to SLE (2, 3, 24).

Women are affected nine or ten times more often than men. A similar sex distribution is found in the New Zealand mice called NZB, a fine model for human SLE (30, 43).

Rheumatoid Arthritis About 1 percent of the population worldwide is affected by *rheumatoid arthritis* (23). This is a chronic inflammatory disease of the synovium that can also affect other tissues (skin, heart, eyes, lungs); knees and hands are most often affected. The inflamed synovium contains many plasma cells; it becomes tremendously hypertrophic, up to 100 times its original weight: a phenomenon that we have compared to the immunopathologic burgeoning of nasal polyps (p. 522). Eventually the articular cartilage is eroded and slowly replaced by a **pannus,** a sheet of connective tissue arising from the synovium. In 80 percent of these patients the blood contains an IgM autoantibody (called *rheumatoid factor*) against the patient's own IgG. The main portion

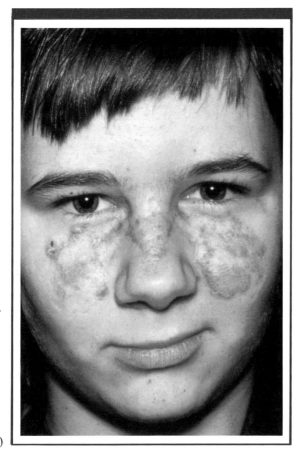

FIGURE 19.5
Typical butterfly-rash of systemic lupus in a young man aged 17. (Courtesy of Dr. J.L. Sullivan, University of Massachusetts Medical Center, Worcester, MA.)

IgG, and indeed it has been shown that the IgG immunoglobulins are abnormally glycosylated; however, this finding is not specific, as we will point out. Anticollagen (Type II) antibodies do develop, but they appear to be a secondary, "reinforcing" event that follows cartilage destruction. Infection with Epstein–Barr virus remains a possibility (23).

Goodpasture's Syndrome, most common in young *men* (quite unusual for an autoimmune disease), this syndrome is brought about by the sudden, unexplained appearance of autoantibodies against a collagen component of the glomerular basement membranes; the result is a necrotizing glomerulitis with spilling of blood into the urine. However, *lung* hemorrhage is often the first

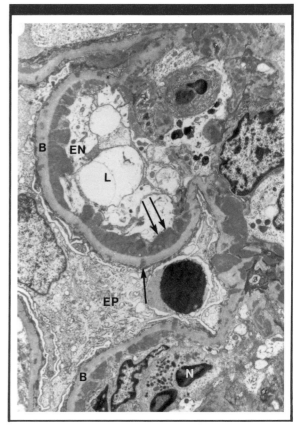

FIGURE 19.6
Deposits of antigen-antibody complexes in the capillary loops of a glomerulus, in a case of lupus nephritis (kidney biopsy). **B** = capillary basement membrane; **EN** = endothelial cell; **EP** = visceral epithelial cell; **L** = capillary lumen; **N** = nucleus of neutrophil; **double arrow:** subendothelial deposits of antigen-antibody complexes; **single arrow:** subendothelial deposits of antigen-antibody complexes. (Courtesy of Dr. H.G. Rennke, Brigham and Women's Hospital, Harvard Medical School, Boston, MA.)

of the IgG molecule that behaves as an antigen is the Fc segment (p. 272); large complexes form, consisting only of immunoglobulins that are "catching each other by the tail." The large circulating complexes are removed by the sinusoidal phagocytes and appear to be relatively harmless, but in the joints they activate complement and cause an influx of leukocytes, which destroy the articular cartilage. In 20–30 percent of seropositive patients *rheumatoid nodules* appear, usually in pressure areas of the skin (Figure 19.7). A nodule is essentially a huge granuloma with a necrotic center that is surrounded by palisading macrophages (Figure 19.8). It is difficult to relate all these events—especially considering the fact that rheumatoid factor, which is absent in some patients, is present in some normal individuals who never develop rheumatoid arthritis; it is also present in some unrelated diseases. The current opinion is that rheumatoid arthritis is an autoimmune disease with a genetic basis (it is associated with HLA-DR4 and HLA-DR1), but the peccant antigen remains unknown. The existence of rheumatoid factor suggests an abnormality of

clinical sign, presumably because the alveolar basement membranes contain the same antigen as the glomerular capillaries; some predisposing factor (such as influenza or heavy smoking) is required for the pulmonary hemorrhage to occur, suggesting that the pathogenic autoantibodies must be released from the pulmonary blood vessels in order to reach the alveolar membranes (in the kidney, circulating proteins normally have direct access to the capillary basement membrane through open endothelial fenestrae). Renal failure is frequent; with the help of immunosuppressive therapy and plasmapheresis to remove the autoantibodies, chances of survival are 50-50. Mysteriously, the autoantibodies tend to disappear after 6–12 months (11a).

Scleroderma The crippling disease *scleroderma* is unusual in that the basic lesion, seen especially in the skin, is a diffuse thickening by fibrosis; other organs may also be involved (e.g., the gastrointestinal tract and the muscles), thus justifying the name *systemic sclerosis*. Lymphocytes are present in the early stages, and the capillaries show a variety of abnormalities that are difficult to fit into a pathogenetic mechanism. Something appears to turn on the fibroblasts, but the mechanism is not understood; the collagen itself is normal, and the condition may represent hypersensitivity to collagen. A variety of antibodies against the cell nucleus, centromere, smooth muscle, and other targets are often present in the plasma, pointing to an autoimmune disorder. There is no comparable animal model, but the "tight skin mouse" comes close (40).

Myasthenia Gravis This disease manifests itself by profound weakness, often beginning with the muscles of the eye; histochemical studies have very precisely localized antibody attack against the acetylcholine receptors of the neuromuscular junction (Figure 19.9). Oddly enough, about 12 percent of these patients develop a tumor of the thymus (thymoma) containing cells that express an antigen similar to the acetylcholine receptor (32, 14a).

Vitiligo *Vitiligo* (a name of uncertain origin) is a condition in which patches of the skin lose their melanin (Figure 19.10); it can be psychologically very distressing. The mechanism is lymphocyte attack against melanocytes, although the keratinocytes can also be damaged (Figures 19.11 and 19.12) (4).

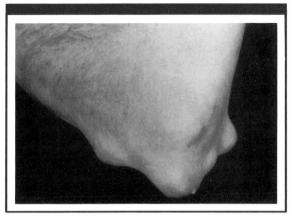

FIGURE 19.7
Elbow of a patient with rheumatoid arthritis, showing multiple subcutaneous nodules. (Reproduced with permission from [26].)

Pathogenesis of Autoimmune Disease

We now step into the realm of theory: no less than 14 mechanisms have been proposed to explain autoimmune diseases (Table 19.2). Some appear to the nonexpert as interesting intellectual exercises; others are based on more solid ground. The overall conclusion is that autoimmune diseases—like cancer—are multifactorial (58). Immunologic, genetic, viral, hormonal, environmental, and other mechanisms have been proposed.

Whatever mechanism may be involved in any particular disease, one fact must be kept in mind: *autoimmune mechanisms are not unnatural* and may even have a function (p. 569). Autoantibodies make up a substantial part of normal plasma immunoglobulins (13). There is ample evidence that autoreactive B-cells (B-cells programmed to make

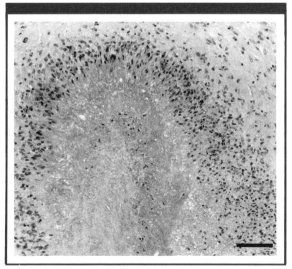

FIGURE 19.8
The mysterious rheumatoid nodule: a necrotic center surrounded by a crown of macrophages that tend to "palisade"—that is, to be radially oriented. The clinically visible nodules represent an aggregate of such structures, which tend to grow. **Bar** = 100 μm.

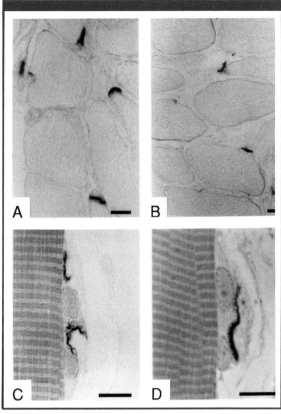

FIGURE 19.9

Evidence that myasthenia gravis is an autoimmune disease. Samples of striated muscle obtained from patients with myasthenia gravis. Light microscopic sections (**A & B**) were treated by an immunohistochemical method to demonstrate the presence of C3 (**A**) and C9 (**B**). In both cases the reaction product is sharply localized at the motor endplates. **C** and **D** are electron micrographs from tissues treated in a similar manner. Localization of complement components at the motor end-plate suggests that the latter are destroyed by an autoimmune mechanism, using the membrane attack complex (MAC) as an effector. **A & B bars** = 25 μm; **C & D bars** = 10 μm. (A & C reproduced with permission from [16] *and* B & D reproduced with permission from [50].)

autoantibody) are just sitting there waiting to be activated—but they are held in check (presumably) by suppressor mechanisms (19). Clones of autoreactive B-cells appear in mice injected with a polyclonal B-cell stimulant, such as endotoxin, PPD, some antibiotics (nystatin), some viruses, parasite components, and even some cytokines (20).

With this in mind, we now examine some of the best-known pathways to autoimmune disease.

RELEASE OF SEQUESTERED ANTIGENS

Because the immune system does not "see" antigens that are sequestered inside cells, it makes

sense that an immune response should develop if these antigens are suddenly released. This is the oldest theory of autoimmune disease, and it does fit a few facts (15, 53).

- *Sympathetic ophthalmia* is the best example, even though it is not fully understood. Weeks or months after injury to one uvea (the membrane that contains the iris), a granulomatous uveitis occasionally develops in the other eye (1, 11, 46). This is thought to be an immune response to uveal tissue or pigment, and it is prevented by enucleation of the useless injured eye within 2 weeks. Antibodies to uveal tissue are not found. The response seems to be the delayed hypersensitivity type, against a common antigen of various ocular tissues.
- *Injury of the crystalline lens* follows a similar pattern. If an eye is injured and lens protein is spilled, the resulting uveitis is thought to be partly autoimmune (*uveitis phacoanaphylactica*) and may flare up in the other eye (11). Here we run, once again, into the unsettling contradictions of autoimmune disease: over 50 percent of *normal* individuals have circulating antibodies against lens protein (27).
- *Vasectomized males* often develop antisperm antibodies, but autoimmune orchitis does not follow (38, 55). *Note:* The antigens of sperm are unusual in that they develop at puberty and therefore miss the chance of inducing tolerance during development *in utero* (38). This might help us understand the need for a blood–testis barrier.
- *Myocardial infarction* is often followed by the appearance of antimyocardial autoantibodies (35, 36), but they seem to do no harm. They do not correlate with the puzzling post–myocardial infarct syndrome that was once thought to be an autoimmune response occurring 1–5 weeks after an infarct in 1–4 percent of the patients. These patients experienced chest pain, fever, leukocytosis, and pericardial rub due to pericardial inflammation (36).

GENETIC FACTORS

That genes play a major role in autoimmune disease is obvious. You can actually buy mice guaranteed to develop autoimmune hemolytic anemia (called New Zealand Black) or chickens that develop autoimmune thyroiditis, to mention two examples. In humans there is a proven familial tendency to develop certain autoantibodies (48). If one identical twin develops systemic lupus, the other will be much more likely than normal to develop it (7).

For some autoimmune diseases, there is also an association with certain MHC haplotypes (54); this association has offered new hopes for therapy. If some autoimmune diseases, such as insulin-dependent diabetes, are associated with a certain Class II MHC molecule, would it be possible to devise a therapy based on antibodies against that molecule? Some positive experimental evidence is already available (59).

A pregnant woman affected by SLE can transfer some of her autoantibodies to her fetus: antibody attack against the heart may destroy the conduction system, resulting in fibrosis and congenital heart block. Other complications are possible, including placental damage (9).

A NONANTIGENIC BODY PROTEIN TURNS ANTIGENIC

Sometimes a nonantigenic body protein can become antigenic. A drug may be the culprit, and the list of possible drugs is long (5). Two examples: (a) prolonged treatment with *procainamide*, an antiarrhythmic agent, causes many patients to produce antinuclear antibodies, and even full-blown SLE; and (b) some mice develop autoimmune kidney disease if they are treated with a classic kidney poison, mercuric chloride.

The precise molecular change that makes the protein antigenic is known for rheumatoid arthritis: gamma globulins show an abnormal pattern of glycosylation, which causes them to be seen by the immune system as foreign (41). However, this finding comes with a bit of confusing news: the same protein abnormality has also been found in osteoarthritis ("degenerative" arthritis), which is not an autoimmune disease.

MOLECULAR MIMICRY

Imagine that a virus or a bacterium adopts—as a strategy for escaping host defenses—the device of mimicking a protein of the host. Two scenarios might follow:

- The worst case scenario leads to the demise of the host: the host's lymphocytes (T-helper cells), being tolerant toward the protein, fail to recognize the parasite, and the host is overwhelmed.
- A less disastrous outcome is autoimmunity.

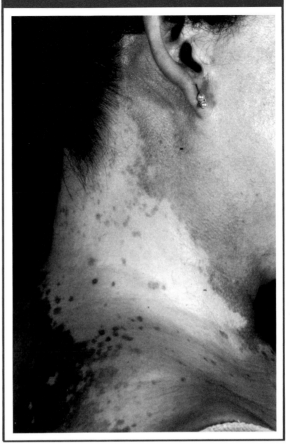

FIGURE 19.10 Vitiligo (loss of pigmentation) on the neck of a white woman. The dark dots within the area of vitiligo represent areas where repigmentation is beginning to develop; it arises from the hair follicles, under the effect of treatment (ultraviolet light plus psoralen [PUVA]). (Courtesy of Dr. J.D. Bernhard, University of Massachusetts Medical Center, Worcester, MA.)

Suppose that the parasite and the host share a hapten, for which host and parasite have different carriers (a hapten is a chemical substance that can induce an immune response only if it is bound to a carrier molecule; dinitrophenol is an example). Because the host lymphocytes are not tolerant toward the hapten-carrier complex, an immune response is initiated, and the resulting antibodies will react with parasite antigens as well as with host antigens. A similar result would occur if parasite and host carried similar, although not identical antigens.

The best-known human disease that is thought to arise by molecular mimicry is *acute rheumatic fever*, which is a heart disease that may follow a throat infection with group A streptococci. In this disease, several bacterial antigens cross-react with myocardial cells, with connective-tissue antigens of the heart valves (myocarditis and valvular damage do occur), and sometimes with antigens of the kidney and nervous tissues (Figure 19.13) (22, 63). The cross-reactions with nervous tissue are especially interesting. Symptoms of rheumatic

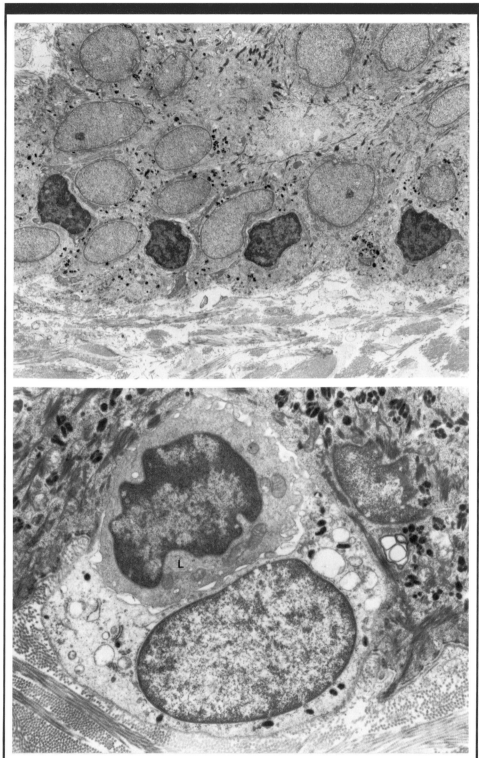

FIGURE 19.11
Skin biopsy of a dark-skinned patient affected by vitiligo. Biopsy was taken from the clinically normal skin next to the depigmented area. *Top:* Four lymphocytes invading the epidermis; they are in close contact with melanocytes. This may be interpreted as the first stage of immunologic attack. The melanocytes do not (yet) show signs of damage. *Bottom:* Lymphocyte (L) in close contact with a melanocyte, which shows signs of injury. (Courtesy of Dr. J. Bhawan, Boston University Medical Center, Boston, MA.)

fever include the uncontrolled movements of Sydenham's chorea, which originate from a disturbance in the subthalamic and caudate nuclei; antibodies in the serum of the patients react with the cytoplasm of neurons precisely in these nuclei.

In acute rheumatic fever the correlations between antibodies and anatomic lesions are quite obvious, but several puzzles remain: (a) To reach their targets, the antineuron antibodies have to cross the blood–brain barrier. How could they do it? (b) In an epidemic of

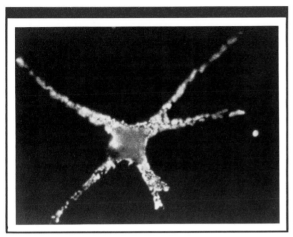

FIGURE 19.12

Human melanocyte in tissue culture, after exposure to serum from a patient with vitiligo. This immunofluorescence photomicrograph demonstrates that the melanocyte is covered with antibodies against a component of its surface. (Reproduced with permission from [10].)

Group A streptococcal throat infection, only 3 percent of the victims develop rheumatic fever. Why? (c) To produce acute rheumatic fever the streptococcal infection must be in the throat (skin infections may produce glomerulonephritis). Why? (63).

Although the best example of molecular mimicry between host and parasite is offered by Group A streptococci, a more general variant of this scenario is now under study; it involves stress proteins (heat-shock proteins, p. 175). Bacteria and host may be able to synthesize stress proteins of very similar structure. In the heat of an encounter, both host and parasite would express these proteins, and an immune attack directed against bacterial stress proteins may backfire and attack the host (31, 34, 57).

TABLE 19.2

Theories on the Origin of Autoimmunity

Release of sequestered antigens
Diminished suppressor T-cell function
Enhanced helper T-cell activity, T-cell bypass
Presence of abnormal clones, defects in tolerance induction
Polyclonal B-cell activation
Refractoriness of B-cells to suppressor messages
Defects on the thymus
Ectopic or altered expression of class II MHC molecules
Defects of macrophages
Defects of stem cells
Defects in the idiotype–anti-idiotype network
Genetic defects: abnormal immune response genes, immunoglobulin genes, T-cell receptor genes
Viral factors
Hormonal factors

Adapted from (58)

PERTURBATIONS OF THE IDIOTYPE–ANTI-IDIOTYPE NETWORK

The basic notion of idiotypes is that the variable segments of antibody molecules are themselves antigenic. In other words, the variable segments behave as epitopes, and as such they are called **idiotypes** (30). At first sight it seems absurd that an antibody should become antigenic, but remem-

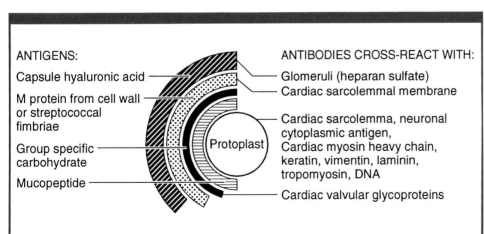

ANTIGENS:

Capsule hyaluronic acid
M protein from cell wall or streptococcal fimbriae
Group specific carbohydrate
Mucopeptide

Protoplast

ANTIBODIES CROSS-REACT WITH:

Glomeruli (heparan sulfate)
Cardiac sarcolemmal membrane

Cardiac sarcolemma, neuronal cytoplasmic antigen,
Cardiac myosin heavy chain, keratin, vimentin, laminin, tropomyosin, DNA

Cardiac valvular glycoproteins

FIGURE 19.13

Cross-reacting antigens of group A streptococci. These antigens cross-react with tissue antigens. Such reactions may explain damage to organs that are not infected. (Adapted from [63].)

ber that an antibody is after all a "unique" structure; so it stands to reason that it *could* behave like an antigen (54).

This topic is indeed as complicated as it sounds, but it was important enough to earn a Nobel prize (Niels K. Jerne, 1984), so the essentials should be understood (8, 28, 33).

The idiotype (i.e., variable segment) of an antibody molecule can be visualized as a sort of cast or negative image of the antigenic epitope. Therefore, an antibody against this idiotype (an anti-antibody) is a cast of a cast and thus should be similar to the original antigen; Jerne called it an internal image of the antigen. The series of idiotypes continues with anti-anti-antibodies, and so on. Each new antibody molecule becomes in turn an antigen; as such it combines with specific receptors on T- and B-cells, resulting in either stimulation or suppression. *In this way the entire immune system can be visualized as a network of interacting components.* The basic concept is illustrated in Figure 19.14.

Mind-boggling as it is, the anti-idiotype mechanism made it possible to devise an experimental model of myasthenia gravis. The principle was to inject rabbits with an acetylcholine analog, a large molecule that behaves as an antigen when injected with Freund's adjuvant into rabbits. Read slowly: because the analog (by definition) could react with the acetylcholine receptor, an antibody against the analog (being its negative image) should not fit into the receptor. However, myasthenia-like symptoms appeared in some rabbits (62). The explanation: the antibodies had given rise to anti-antibodies, which as negatives of negatives reproduced the "fitting shape."

Another intellectually satisfying product of the network concept: If anti-antibodies are made in the image of the original antigen, why not prepare vaccines consisting of anti-antibodies rather than of the original antigen? This would have several advantages, and experimentally the principle has been shown to work (8).

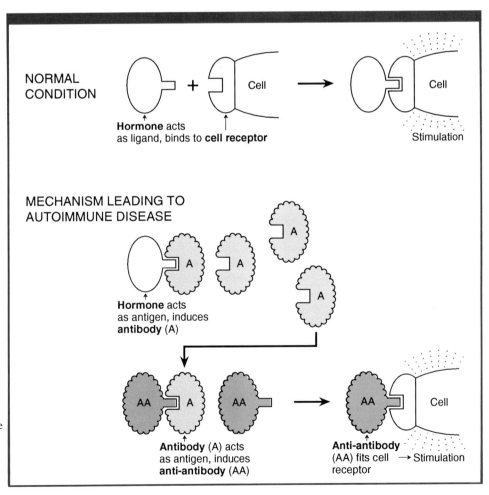

FIGURE 19.14
Idiotypes and anti-idiotypes. *Top:* Structural analogy between antigen and anti-antibody. *Bottom:* Because of the structural analogy, an anti-antibody can compete with a hormone for binding with its receptor. (Adapted from [8].)

NORMAL CONDITION

Hormone acts as ligand, binds to **cell receptor**

Cell

Cell

Stimulation

MECHANISM LEADING TO AUTOIMMUNE DISEASE

Hormone acts as antigen, induces **antibody** (A)

A

A

A

A

Antibody (A) acts as antigen, induces **anti-antibody** (AA)

AA   A

AA

Anti-antibody (AA) fits cell receptor

AA

Cell

→ Stimulation

Some Lessons from Experimental Autoimmune Diseases

Apart from the many natural examples of autoimmune diseases, it is a fairly simple matter to produce autoimmune diseases at will. The basic method is to inject homogenized tissue mixed with complete Freund adjuvant (p. 544) (tissue alone is much less effective). Most organs have been tested in this manner (29, 51) and have shown that within a week or two, almost miraculously, injected thyroid produces thyroiditis, uvea produces uveitis, adrenals produce adrenalitis, peripheral nerves produce peripheral neuritis (61), central nervous tissue produces encephalomyelitis (tantalizingly similar to multiple sclerosis) (Figure 19.15) (44), and so on. Sperm produces epididymitis, perhaps because the antibodies cannot violate the blood–testis barrier (60). Incidentally, Freund's adjuvant *alone*, in rats, produces an arthritic syndrome.

Such models have been useful for working out some basic mechanisms. For example:

- Experimental autoimmune thyroiditis can be transferred from one rabbit to another with either serum or white blood cells, proving that, in this model at least, antibody-mediated and cell-mediated mechanisms are involved.
- Experimental autoimmune encephalomyelitis (EAE) can be transferred only with cells (25).
- Rabbits can be given an autoimmune disease affecting their own central nervous system by injecting them with a single protein extracted from myelin, called myelin basic protein (MBP). MBP has been sequenced, and it turns out that it shares a sequence of six amino acids with a virus that produces encephalitis in rabbits. This suggests that a virus may initiate a brain lesion and then disappear; but nervous tissue has been damaged, and the lesion is perpetuated by endogenous MBP (18).

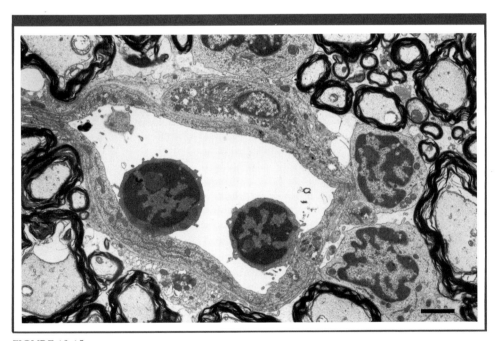

FIGURE 19.15
Early lesion of experimental allergic encephalomyelitis (EAE), the prime model for human multiple sclerosis. Two lymphocytes (probably T-cells) are attached to the endothelium of the blood vessel; three others (*top and right*) have traversed the wall of the vessel and lie among myelinated nerve fibers (black rings). Interpretation: the endothelial cells presented a brain-specific antigen or a lymphocyte recognition molecule on the luminal surface; T-cells with the appropriate receptors became attached, performed diapedesis, and secreted cytokines (gamma-interferon, interleukin-2) which recruited other lymphocytes. Recruited T-cells produced cytokines and antibodies against the nerve tissue. Monocytes will phagocytize the debris. Mouse EAE; 15 days after sensitization with myelin. **Bar** = 2 μm. (Reproduced with permission from [45].)

- Vaccination of humans against rabies is still performed in some countries with the older but cheaper method of injecting attenuated rabies virus that was grown in the brain or cords of adult animals (Semple vaccine). Roughly 1 in 400 patients develops neurologic complications, most likely due to cross-reaction between animal and human

MBP (25). In fact, this clinical complication was the stimulus for trying to produce experimental allergic encephalomyelitis with rabbit brain and Freund's adjuvant.

TO SUM UP: autoimmune disease is now an unquestionable reality, but its pathogenesis is still filled with enigmas.

References

1. Albert DM, Diaz-Rohena R. A historical review of sympathetic ophthalmia and its epidemiology. Surv Ophthalmol 1989;34:1–14.
2. Asherson RA. Antiphospholipid antibodies and "syndromes": many questions and few answers. Isr J Med Sci 1990;26:284–286.
3. Asherson RA, Lubbe WF. Cerebral and valve lesions in SLE: association with antiphospholipid antibodies. J Rheumatol 1988;15:539–543.
4. Bhawan J, Bhutani LK. Keratinocyte damage in vitiligo. J Cutan Pathol 1983;10:207–212.
5. Bigazzi PE. Mechanisms of chemical-induced autoimmunity. In: Dean JH, Luster MI, Munson AE, Amos H, eds. Immunotoxicology and immunopharmacology. New York: Raven Press, 1985:277–290.
6. Bigazzi PE. Anti-idiotypic immunity in autoimmunity. Ann NY Acad Sci 1986;475:66–80.
7. Block SR, Winfield JB, Lockshin MD, D'Angelo WA, Christian CL. Studies with twins with systemic lupus erythematosus. A review of the literature and presentation of 12 additional sets. Am J Med 1975;59:533–552.
8. Burdette S, Schwartz RS. Idiotypes and idiotypic networks. N Engl J Med 1987;317:219–224.
9. Buyon J, Szer I. Passively acquired autoimmunity and the maternal fetal dyad in systemic lupus erythematosus. Springer Semin Immunopathol 1986;9:283–304.
10. Bystryn J-C, Pfeffer S. Vitiligo and antibodies to melanocytes. Prog Clin Biol Res 1988;256:195–206.
11. Chan C-C. Relationship between sympathetic ophthalmia, phacoanaphylatic endophthalmitis, and Vogt-Koyanagi-Harada disease. Ophthalmology 1988;95:619–624.
11a. Cooggins CH, Rennke HG, Rose BD. Glomerulonephritis and the nephrotic syndrome. In: Dale DC, Gederman DD (eds) Scientific American Medicine. Chpt. 10 Nephrology 1995;1–18.
12. Crisá L, Mordes JP, Rossini AA. Autoimmune diabetes mellitus in the BB rat. Diabetes Metab Rev 1992;8:9–37.
13. Dighiero G, Lymberi P, Guilbert B, Ternynck T, Avrameas S. Natural autoantibodies constitute a substantial part of normal circulating immunoglobulins. Ann NY Acad Sci 1986;475:135–145.
14. Doukas J, Mordes JP. T lymphocytes capable of activating endothelial cells in vitro are present in rats with autoimmune diabetes¹. J Immunol 1993;150:1–11.
14a. Drachman DB. Myasthenia Gravis. N Engl J Med 1994;330–1797–1810.
15. Elkon KB. Autoantibodies: their nature and significance. In: Harris EN, Exner T, Hughes GRV, Asherson RA, eds. Phospholipid-binding antibodies. Boca Raton, FL: CRC Press, 1991:60–72.
16. Engle AG, Lambert EH, Howard FM Jr. Ultrastructural localization of the terminal and lytic ninth complement gravis. J Neuropathol Exp Neurol 1980;39:160–172.

16a. Federman DD. Thyroid. In: Dale DC, Federman DD (eds) Scientific American Medicine. Chpt. 3 Endocrinology 1994;2–27.
17. Finnegan A, Needleman BW, Hodes RJ. Function of autoreactive T cells in immune responses. Immunol Rev 1990;116:15–31.
18. Fujinami RS, Oldstone MBA. Amino acid homology between the encephalitogenic site of myelin basic protein and virus: mechanism for autoimmunity. Science 1985; 230:1043–1045.
19. Gibson J, Basten A, Walker KZ, Loblay RH. A role for suppressor T cells in induction of self-tolerance. Proc Natl Acad Sci USA 1985;82:5150–5154.
20. Goodman MG, Weigle WO. Role of polyclonal B-cell activation in self/non-self discrimination. Immunol Today 1981;2:54–57.
21. Grabar P. Autoantibodies and the physiological role of immunoglobulins. Immunol Today 1983;4:337–340.
22. Gulizia JM, Cunningham MW, McManus BM. Immunoreactivity of anti-streptococcal monoclonal antibodies to human heart valves. Am J Pathol 1991;138:285–301.
23. Harris ED Jr. Rheumatoid arthritis. Pathophysiology and implications for therapy. N Engl J Med 1990;322: 1277–1289.
24. Harris EN, Asherson RA, Hughes GRV. Antiphospholipid antibodies—autoantibodies with a difference. Annu Rev Med 1988;39:261–271.
25. Hemachudha T, Griffin DE, Giffels JJ, Johnson RT, Moser AB, Phanuphak P. Myelin basic protein as an encephalitogen in encephalomyelitis and polyneuritis following rabies vaccination. N Engl J Med 1987;316: 369–374.
26. Hughes GRV. Connective tissue diseases, 3rd ed. Oxford: Blackwell Scientific Publications, 1987.
27. Jaffe NS. Cataract surgery and its complications. St. Louis: CV Mosby, 1972.
28. Jerne NK. Towards a network theory of the immune system. Ann Inst Pasteur Immunol 1974;125C:373–389.
29. Kabat EA, Mayer MM. Experimental immunochemistry, 2nd ed. Springfield, IL: Charles C. Thomas, 1964.
30. Kantor FS. Autoimmunities: diseases of "dysregulation." Hosp Pract 1988;23:75–84.
31. Kaufmann SHE. Heat shock proteins and the immune response. Immunol Today 1990;11:129–136.
32. Kirchner T, Tzartos S, Hoppe F, et al. Pathogenesis of myasthenia gravis. Acetylcholine receptor-related antigenic determinants in tumor-free thymuses and thymic epithelial tumors. Am J Pathol 1988;130:268–280.
33. Klinman DM, Steinberg AD. Idiotypy and autoimmunity. Arthritis Rheum 1986;29:697–705.
34. Koga T, Wand-Württenberger A, DeBruyn J, et al. T cells against a bacterial heat shock protein recognize stressed macrophages. Science 1989;245:1112–1115.
35. Kuch J. Autoantibodies directed against heart antigens

and endocrine reactivity in patients with recent myocardial infarction. Cardiovasc Res 1973;7:649–654.

36. Liem KL, ten Veen JH, Lie KI, Feltkamp TEW, Durrer D. Incidence and significance of heart muscle antibodies in patients with acute myocardial infarction and unstable angina. Acta Med Scand 1979;206:473–475.

37. Like AA. Spontaneous diabetes in animals. In: Volk BW, Arquilla ER, eds. The diabetic pancreas. New York: Plenum Publishing, 1985:385–413.

38. Mandelbaum SL, Diamond MP, DeCherney AH. The impact of antisperm antibodies on human infertility. J Urol 1987;138:1–8.

38a. Mills JA. Systematic Lupus Erythematosus. N Engl J Med 1994;330:1871–1879.

39. Montagu A. The natural superiority of women. New York: Macmillan, 1954.

40. Muryoi T, Kasturi KN, Kafina MJ, et al. Antitopoisomerase I monoclonal autoantibodies from scleroderma patients and tight skin mouse interact with similar epitopes. J Exp Med 1992;175:1103–1109.

41. Parekh RB, Dwek RA, Sutton BJ, et al. Association of rheumatoid arthritis and primary osteoarthritis with changes in the glycosylation pattern of total serum IgG. Nature 1985;316:452–457.

42. Parham P. A diversity of diabetes. Nature 1990;345:662-664.

43. Purtilo DT, Sullivan JL. Immunological bases for superior survival of females. Am J Dis Child 1979;133:1251–1253.

44. Raine CS. Analysis of autoimmune demyelination: its impact upon multiple sclerosis. Lab Invest 1984;50:608–635.

45. Raine CS. In a biological cross-fire: neuroimmunology. Sci Focus 1987;2:3–5.

46. Reed CE, Friedlaender M. Immunologic aspects of diseases of the eye. JAMA 1982;248:2692–2695.

47. Rich AR, Voisin GA, Bang FB. Electron microscopic studies of the alteration of collagen fibrils in the Arthus phenomenon. Bull Johns Hopkins Hosp 1953;92:222–243.

48. Roitt IM. Essential immunology, 6th ed. Oxford: Blackwell Scientific Publications, 1988.

49. Rossini AA, Mordes JP, Like AA. Immunology of insulin-dependent diabetes mellitus. Annu Rev Immunol 1985;3:289–320.

50. Sahashi K, Engel AG, Lambert EH, Howard FM Jr. Immune complexes (IgG and C3) at the motor end-plate in myasthenia gravis. Mayo Clin Proc 1977;52:267–280.

51. Sell S. Immunology, immunopathology and immunity, 4th ed. New York: Elsevier, 1987.

52. Shoenfeld Y, Isenberg DA. Mycobacteria and auto-immunity. Immunol Today 1988;9:178–181.

53. Shoenfeld Y, Isenberg DA, eds. Natural autoantibodies. London: CRC Press, 1993.

54. Shoenfeld Y, Schwartz RS. Immunologic and genetic factors in autoimmune diseases. N Engl J Med 1984;311:1019–1029.

55. Shulman S. Autoimmune aspects of human reproduction. Concepts Immunopathol 1985;2:189–227.

56. Skinner HA. The origin of medical terms, 2nd ed. Baltimore: Williams & Wilkins, 1961.

57. Strober S, Holoshitz J. Mechanisms of immune injury in rheumatoid arthritis: evidence for the involvement of T cells and heat-shock protein. Immunol Rev 1990;118:233–255.

58. Theofilopoulos AN. Autoimmunity. In: Stites DP, Stobo JD, Wells JV, eds. Basic and clinical immunology, 6th ed. Norwalk, CT: Appleton & Lange, 1987:128–158.

59. Todd JA, Acha-Orbea H, Bell JI, et al. A molecular basis for MHC class II-associated autoimmunity. Science 1988;240:1003-1009

60. Tung KSK, Unanue ER, Dixon FJ. Pathogenesis of experimental allergic orchitis. II. The role of antibody. J Immunol 1971;106:1463–1472.

61. Waksman BH, Adams RD. A comparative study of experimental allergic neuritis in the rabbit, guinea pig, and mouse. J Neuropathol Exp Neurol 1956;25:293–333.

62. Wassermann NH, Penn AS, Freimuth PI, et al. Anti-idiotypic route to anti-acetylcholine receptor antibodies and experimental myasthenia gravis. Proc Natl Acad Sci USA 1982;79:4810–4814.

63. Williams RC Jr. Molecular mimicry and rheumatic fever. Clin Rheum Dis 1985;11:573–590.

64. Zabriskie JB, Gibofsky A. Genetic control of the susceptibility to infection with pathogenic bacteria. Curr Topics Microbiol Immunol 1986;124:1–20.

Immunosuppression

CHAPTER 20

Normal
Immunosuppression:
Pregnancy

Therapeutic
Immunosuppression

Congenital
Immunosuppression

Acquired
Immunosuppression

Coda: The Immune
Response at Its Best

The Pathogenesis of
Influenza

A state of immunosuppression can be a normal condition, a goal of therapy when the immune system overreacts, an unwanted side-effect of tumor therapy, a congenital disease, or an acquired disease.

Normal Immunosuppression: Pregnancy

Pregnant mammals have to break the rules: they must carry an allograft without rejecting it (although they do produce antifather antibodies, called paternal specific alloantibodies by purists). Exactly how mothers-to-be accomplish this feat is still puzzling (2, 14). It cannot be that the uterus is exempt from the rules of immunology because the uterine mucosa rejects experimental skin allografts (3). Establishing pregnancy is certainly not easy: in 60 percent of human pregnancies, the fetus aborts within 12 weeks. How many embryos (if any) are lost to immune attack is not known; however, it would be a gross oversimplification to equate natural birth with the rejection of a graft.

Overall, the baby-allograft (semi-allograft to be precise [6]) seems to be protected by barriers between itself and the mother, as well as by mechanisms that immunosuppress the mother (Table 20.1). The baby is so well protected that it can be carried for nine months even when it is a full allograft, obtained by fertilizing a human ovum *in vitro* and implanting it into a surrogate mother. In other species even xenogeneic pregnancies have been achieved: a mare can function as a surrogate mother to a zebra (6). The principal barrier between fetus and mother is the syncytiotrophoblast, a syncytial layer that derives from the ovum and forms a continuous sheet separating the mother's blood from the placental tissues. The syncytiotrophoblast expresses neither Class I nor Class II antigens of the MHC, which makes it an immunologic no-man's-land; this is not true, however, for the rest of the trophoblast (15).

Pregnant women are partly immunosuppressed. Their lymphocytes respond less vigorously to mitogens *in vitro* (25), and their cell-mediated immunity is reduced (precisely the type of immunity most involved in graft rejection). The total number of T-cells is reduced, and there is a relative loss of helper T-cells (T4+) (35), the same defect

TABLE 20.1

Why Is the Baby not Rejected? Some Proposed Mechanisms

Progesterone is immunosuppressive

Alpha-fetoprotein in amniotic fluid is immunosuppressive

Mother's plasma contains an immunosuppressive protein (PAPP-A, possibly produced by the endometrium)

Decidua and draining lymph nodes contain suppressor cells

Uterine macrophages are immunosuppressive

Endometrial epithelium loses Class I MHC antigens and replaces them with trophoblast antigens (called TLX)

Syncytiotrophoblast contains neither Class I nor Class II MHC antigens

Adapted from (2)

that occurs, much more severely, in AIDS. Certain cancers, and infections with intracellular parasites, carry a more severe prognosis if they occur in advanced pregnancy (25).

Therapeutic Immunosuppression

Immunosuppression as therapy is meant to protect allografts and to fight autoimmune diseases. The ideal procedure would be to render the patient tolerant to the antigen(s) of the graft or to the self-antigens in autoimmune disease, but that is still in the future.

The drugs used at present, such as corticoids, are nonspecific immunosuppressants; and some of these are antimitotics borrowed from cancer therapy. The rationale for antimitotics is that the immune response depends on a small number of cells that replicate to form large clones, and the antimitotics intervene at the early stage. Actually, the rationale was an afterthought; it followed the accidental observation that patients treated with antimitotics for cancer became immunosuppressed.

Cyclosporine, a fungal metabolite, is in a category of its own. One of its many effects is to prevent T-cells from secreting cytokines essential for the differentiation and proliferation of B-cells and cytotoxic T-cells (8, 16). This subtle mechanism has vastly improved the field of transplantation, even though the drug has its side effects, mainly nephrotoxicity.

Unfortunately, the long-term use of immunosuppressants increases the risk of developing cancer, mostly of the lymphoma type; why these particular tumors should be favored is not understood (17). Another risk, of course, is infection by one or more of the bacterial, viral, and fungal antigens in the environment. It is frightening to see, under the microscope, how fungi grow in the tissues of an immunosuppressed patient—as in a culture—without eliciting the slightest inflammatory response (Figure 20.1).

As mentioned earlier, blood transfusions produce immunosuppression and prolong the survival of allografts. Several explanations have been offered for this curious phenomenon, including the induction of suppressor cells, perhaps through a prostaglandin-dependent (PGE) pathway (30).

Congenital Immunosuppression

Congenital immunodeficiencies are uncommon but conceptually important. They are experiments of nature that confirmed, or led us to understand, basic mechanisms of the immune system—just as the lysosomal diseases helped us work out the functions of the lysosomes. Immunodeficiencies affect T-cell mechanisms, B-cell mechanisms, or both—in which case they are called severe

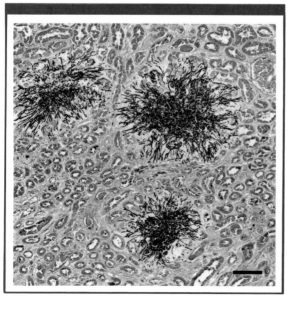

FIGURE 20.1 Three clusters of *Candida albicans*, a fungus, growing in the kidney of an immunosuppressed patient (after chemotherapy for a malignant tumor). Note the total lack of inflammatory response. (Grocott methenamine silver stain.) **Bar** = 100 μm.

combined immunodeficiency (SCID, pronounced skid) (11). They usually manifest themselves in infancy by an increased susceptibility to infections. The congenital lack of NK cells in humans leads to severe herpesvirus infections, as might be expected from the antiviral prowess of these cells (4). Descriptions of congenital immunodeficiencies can be found in specialized textbooks (28, Vol. I).

One of these congenital diseases was discovered in our department by the late Dr. David T. Purtilo and his collaborators. While on autopsy duty as a pathology resident, in 1969, Dr. Purtilo was called to examine a child who had died in the course of infectious mononucleosis, a viral infection not known to be lethal. No cause of death was apparent. Dr. Purtilo could have brushed off the case as a freak occurrence of death by mononucleosis, but he concluded that some important bit of information was missing and never forgot that child. Years later he autopsied another child with the same name (Duncan) who had died of lymphoma. This was the second clue on a trail that led to identifying the X-linked lymphoproliferative disease (XLP), also called Duncan's disease (12, 26). These children (all males) inherit a specific susceptibility to infection by the Epstein–Barr virus, the agent of infectious mononucleosis; when infected, they either succumb or develop a chronic infection (hypogamma-globulinemia) and in 25 percent of the cases a malignant lymphoma. The latter is probably a result of constant B-cell stimulation by the virus.

This episode was a sad development for the Duncan family, but it illustrates the importance of the autopsy even in our high-tech society.

Acquired Immunosuppression

Acquired immunodeficiency instantly evokes the image of AIDS, but there are other examples even closer to everyday life.

- *Aging* (which improves nothing, except perhaps wisdom in some cases) brings a decline also in the function of the immune system, especially of the T-cells (37).
- *Infant prematurity* tends to correlate with inadequate immune responses, especially if the infant's problems are compounded by malnutrition. Some immunodeficient infants have developed graft-versus-host disease after blood transfusions (5); in adults, the leukocytes in transfused blood can be neglected because they are almost always easily overcome by the host.
- *Severe malnutrition* is immunosuppressive,

but we must recall once again the extensive literature proving that mild undernutrition is the one and only sure way to prolong life (p. 51).

- *Cancer*, including its treatments, tends to suppress not only inflammation (p. 810) but also the immune response.
- *AIDS*, the prototype of immunosuppressive diseases, works in part by destroying helper T-cells. The mechanism is extraordinarily specific: to penetrate into the helper T-lymphocytes, the HIV virus uses the CD4 receptor typical of those cells (*in vitro*, monoclonal antibodies against the CD4 molecule block the infection of helper T-lymphocytes (13)). Normally, there are about two helper T-cells for each cytotoxic/suppressor T-cell; in AIDS this ratio can drop to less than one. The loss of CD4 cells seems to be enhanced by another complex mechanism, which can be simplified as "activation followed by apoptosis" (23). Due to the lack of helper T-lymphocytes, not enough cytotoxic T-lymphocytes can be produced to kill virus-infected cells. However, the immunosuppression of AIDS has more than one cause (31); the NK cells, although normal in number, do not function properly (31), and antigen-presenting cells may also be affected (19). On the other hand, we know that some antibody formation is maintained because it has been observed that some antigens are independent of T-cell help (T-independent antigens); in fact, AIDS patients may show *hyper*gammaglobulinemia.

AIDS victims seldom die of common bacterial infections. This can be explained as follows: T-independent antigens tend to be macromolecules with many copies of the same epitope. This feature is uncommon in proteins but common in carbohydrates, including those of bacterial capsules. Now, the resistance against encapsulated bacteria is highly dependent on antibodies; and because the B-cell mechanism of antibody formation is not destroyed by the AIDS virus, AIDS victims can defend themselves against those bacteria (9).

The last forms of acquired immunodeficiency that we will consider are stress and psychological stimuli.

Psychology and the Lymphocytes It is popular knowledge that labial herpes may remain dormant for years and then erupt under stress and that

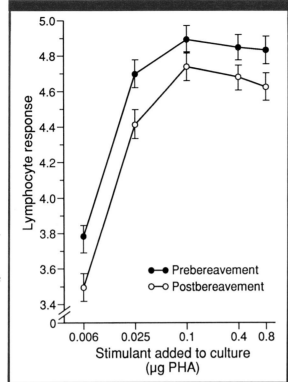

FIGURE 20.2 Depression of lymphocyte function during bereavement. The test measures the lymphocyte response after stimulation with phytohemagglutinin (PHA) Adapted from (29).

lupus and die within 8–14 months, unless treated with intraperitoneal injections of cyclophosphamide. If these are paired with a taste of saccharin in the drinking water, after some time just the drinks of saccharin—combined with an intraperitoneal injection of saline—prolong the life of the mice (7).

The mechanism of these conditioned responses is not well understood, but it does *not* depend on stress-induced steroids. Perhaps it is relevant that lymphatic organs receive sympathetic nerve fibers, and that neurons and leukocytes share neuroendocrine receptors (1).

What helps mice with lupus might, some day, help people with lupus.

Coda: The Immune Response at its Best

In the last four chapters we have portrayed the misdeeds of the immune response. To provide our readers with a more balanced view of this life-saving mechanism, we opted to close this section with a glimpse of the immune response at work in the course of an infectious disease. A fine example is influenza, because its pathogenesis involves an interplay of cell injury, inflammation, and regeneration, as well as T-cell and B-cell (antibody) responses. We will follow an excellent account recently published by P.A. Small, whose laboratory worked out many of the pertinent facts (33).

The Pathogenesis of Influenza

The name *influenza* is an echo of medieval Italy, when epidemics were attributed to the influence of stars and planets (32). On this planet it is indeed an uncontrolled killer; in the United States alone it claims 10–20 thousand victims a year (many more in years of pandemic) and the morbidity (ratio of number of people with the disease to the total population), as everyone knows, is far greater (33). Influenza includes the common cold, although most colds are caused by other viruses.

The first step of any infection is penetration into body. Experts on infectious disease tend to see the body as a container riddled with openings (Figure 20.3); each opening has its defenses and its habitual attackers. The influenza virus invariably chooses the respiratory pathway, and once it has

tuberculosis may flare up in depressed individuals. The mechanism is probably complicated, but it is proven that the immune system can be depressed by emotional factors. This is documented during bereavement. Mortality increases among widowers during the 10 years after the death of their spouses; their lymphocytes are significantly less responsive to mitogens for as long as 14 months (Figure 20.2) (29, 36). A similar depression of lymphocyte responsiveness was found in 16 psychiatry trainees taking final fellowship examinations (10). The link between stress and the immune system involves an endocrine–neuroendocrine network including ACTH, endorphins, and adrenal hormones (24).

Even more fascinating are studies showing that it is possible to "train" lymphocytes to respond to certain stimuli, recalling the pavlovian "mast cell conditioning" mentioned earlier (p. 519).

The key experiment: Cyclophosphamide, an immunosuppressant, injected intraperitoneally into rats, inhibits antibody formation and eventually kills the rats. If the rats are given saccharin-flavored water to drink in association with the injection of cyclophosphamide, after some time the saccharin drink alone—given once every three days—depresses antibody titers (7). This principle can be put to use for therapy: New Zealand mice develop systemic

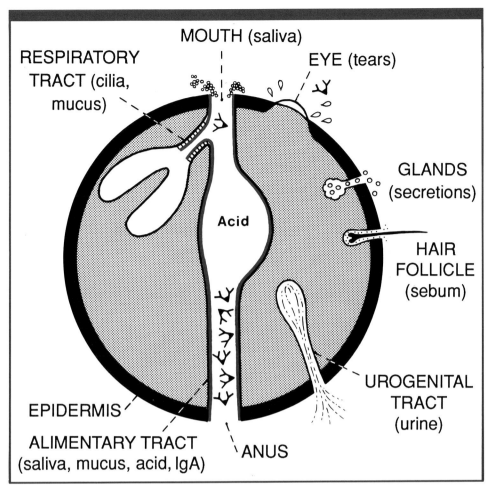

FIGURE 20.3
Schematic view of the body, indicating portals of entry for parasites, and key defenses displayed at body surfaces. (Adapted from [20].)

gained entrance it can cause three syndromes of increasing severity: (1) a simple, uncomplicated inflammation of the upper airways (*rhinotracheitis*); (2) a respiratory viral infection followed by a bacterial infection; and (3) a viral pneumonia.

1. *Rhinotracheitis.* Inflammation of the upper airways produces symptoms neatly explained by the pathologic events. Normally the epithelium of the upper respiratory tract contains mucus-secreting cells and ciliated cells (Figure 20.4); about one-third of the basement membrane is covered by basal cells, also known as *reserve cells.* Inhaled bacteria and viruses are trapped by the mucus, and the cilia sweep the whole mess, dead cells and mucus, up the trachea (we have referred to this as the "bronchial elevator") and eventually down the pharynx, unceremoniously called the tracheal toilet (33).

    Inhaled virus particles hit the mucosa, penetrate into the cells via special receptors, multiply inside them, and quickly

kill them. In three days the mucus-secreting cells and the ciliated cells are gone, and the basal cells spread over the basement membrane (Figure 20.4). In the meantime the underlying connective tissue (*lamina propria*) has become inflamed, and exudate oozes out through gaps between the basal cells. This explains the runny nose that is typical of this phase; the fluid is not mucus because the mucus-secreting cells are no longer there. Between 5 and 10 days after infection the basal cells differentiate into mature cells. The mucus-secreting cells reappear first; and without enough ciliated cells to move the mucus, it piles up. This explains the snorting, nose-blowing, and coughing of this stage. The repair is complete after 2 weeks, a little earlier if the patient (as is usually the case) has suffered a previous infection. Memory cells are doing their job (to be described shortly).

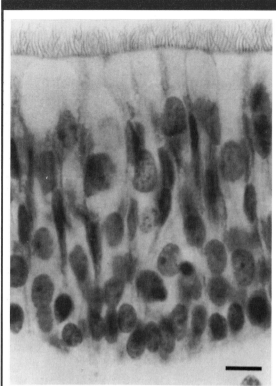

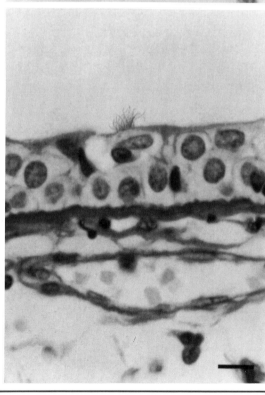

FIGURE 20.4 Effect of influenza on the epithelium of the human trachea. **Top:** Normal, mucus-producing ciliated epithelium. **Bottom:** After 2 days of influenza infection, most of the epithelium has sloughed off; it is replaced by cuboidal, less-differentiated cells with no mucous secretion and very few cilia. One advantage of the replacement: the regenerating epithelial cells have no receptors for the influenza virus. Cilia are enhanced. **Bar** = 10 μm. (Reproduced with permission from [22].)

Note that the regenerating basal cells seem to have escaped the lethal attack of the influenza virus. The reason seems to be that *they have no receptors for the virus* (33). This is what saves them,

and perhaps also the patient. You may recall that in discussing regeneration we mentioned that newly regenerated cells are not as "good" as mature cells (p. 29); but in the present case, immaturity is an advantage.

There is no specific cure for the rhinotracheitis of influenza, but timeless tradition prescribes rest, warmth, and lots of fluids. As it happens, this is very sensible advice: it fosters the therapeutic goal of preventing the virus from spreading beyond the upper respiratory tract. *Rest*, during which breathing is shallow, reduces the risk of inhaling the virus deeper into the lungs; *warmth* helps maintain the deeper respiratory epithelia at body temperature, which is not the optimal temperature (35°C) for influenza virus replication; and *fluid* helps mucous secretion and the elevator–toilet mechanism. Note that in this scenario fever should also help— and the traditional aspirin should not (p. 488).

2. *Viral infection is followed by bacterial pneumonia.* The usual sequence of events is that when the patient is beginning to recover, the malaise returns, the cough worsens, and the infection becomes purulent. Pus indicates the presence of leukocytes and, usually, bacterial infection. Indeed, the lack of a covering tracheo-bronchial epithelium causes bacteria to be retained (pneumococci, staphylococci, and *Haemophilus influenzae* are common offenders). Furthermore, the phagocytic function of alveolar macrophages is impaired after a bout of influenza (33).

3. *Viral pneumonia* occurs when the virus gains the upper hand and destroys the precious epithelial cells of the pulmonary alveoli, plasma leaks out of the capillaries, and pulmonary edema develops. Individuals with high capillary pressure are especially at risk—for example, in cases of mitral stenosis. A full-blown pneumonia develops.

Experiments on mice have revealed other interesting mechanisms. If the influenza virus is given as nose drops to mice anesthetized to abolish cough and gag reflexes, much of the fluid reaches the lungs directly; and the mice die in a week. If the nose drops are given to conscious mice, the virus reaches the trachea in 3 days and the lungs in 5; thus, the lethal dose (LD50) is 2000 times greater. This experiment suggests that the slow, downward progress of the virus gives the immune system time to respond.

Blood-borne antibodies appear in infected mice, and cell-mediated immunity also develops; but

TABLE 20.2

Components of the Immune Response Affecting Influenza

| | PREVENTION | | RECOVERY | |
COMPONENT	UPPER RESPIRATORY TRACT	LUNG	UPPER RESPIRATORY TRACT	LUNG
Secretory IgA	Essential	?	?	?
Systemic antibody	No role	Essential	Contributory	Contributory
Cell-mediated immunity	No role	No role	Essential	Essential

Adapted from (33)

neither can prevent the upper respiratory tract infection. This makes sense: the virus hides inside the epithelial cells where it is safe from antibodies. As to cell-mediated immunity, T cells would not be expected to migrate out of the vessels to kill free virus; their proper target is represented by virus-infected cells. On the other hand, blood-borne antibodies do prevent the viral pneumonia (27); the mechanism is probably serum IgG antibody in the alveolar fluid. This type of protection is the purpose of vaccination.

We have carefully used the expression *blood borne antibodies*. Although it is true that these antibodies do not prevent the infection of the upper respiratory tract, this does not mean that all those critical epithelia go through life unprotected. They secrete their own shield as a *secretory antibody*: that is, as IgA, a special form of immunoglobulin found in almost all secretions (including those of the intestine) and is highly resistant to proteolytic attack.

What is the role of cell-mediated immunity in influenza? A good way to find out is to infect nude mice, which lack cell-mediated immunity. The result is a prolonged state of infection. Treatment with serum antibodies offers temporary help but does not cure (33). The results from many laboratories showed that cell-mediated immunity is essential for recovery from influenza infection. This fact may help us understand the much greater mortality from influenza in persons of advanced age, whose cell-mediated immunity tends to be depressed. The higher mortality of infants is due to the lack of immunity from previous exposure.

The protective roles of the immune system in influenza are summarized in Table 20.2.

Such is, in capsule form, the pathophysiology of this viral disease. It tells us that the balance betweeen host and parasite can be tipped by a number of factors besides the immune response—even by regeneration.

References

1. Ader R, Cohen N. Conditioned immunopharmacologic effects on cell-mediated immunity. Int J Immunopharmac 1992;14:323–327.
2. Beer AE. Immunology of reproduction. In: Samter M, Talmage DW, Frank MM, Austen KF, Claman HN, eds. Immunological diseases, 4th ed. Boston: Little, Brown, 1988:329–360.
3. Beer AE, Billingham RE. Host responses to intra-uterine tissue, cellular and fetal allografts. J Reprod Fertil 1984;(suppl)21:59–88.
4. Biron CA, Byron KS, Sullivan JL. Severe herpesvirus infections in an adolescent without natural killer cells. N Engl J Med 1989;320:1731–1735.
5. Chandra RK. Influence of nutrition-immunity axis on perinatal infections. In: Ogra PL, ed. Neonatal infec-tions. Nutritional and immunologic interactions. Orlando, FL: Grune & Stratton, 1984:229–245.
6. Chaouat G. The roots of the problem; the fetal allograft. In: Immunology of pregnancy. New York: CRC Press, 1993:1–17.
7. Cohen DJ, Ader R. Immunomodulation by classical conditioning. Adv Biochem Psychopharmacol 1988;44:199–202.
8. Cohen DJ, Loertscher R, Rubin MF, et al. Cyclosporine: a new immunosuppressive agent for organ transplantation. Ann Intern Med 1984;101:667–682.
9. Cohen JJ. The immune system: an overview. In: Middleton E Jr, Reed CE, Ellis EF, Adkinson NF Jr, Yunginger JW, eds. Allergy principles and practice, 3rd ed. St. Louis: CV Mosby, 1988:3–11.

10. Dorian B, Garfinkel P, Brown G, et al. Aberrations in lymphocyte subpopulations and function during psychological stress. Clin Exp Immunol 1982;50:132–138.

11. Fulop GM, Phillips RA. The *scid* mutation in mice causes a general defect in DNA repair. Nature 1990;347:479–482.

12. Grierson H, Purtilo DT. Epstein-Barr virus infections in males with the X-linked lymphoproliferative syndrome. Ann Intern Med 1987;106:538–545.

13. Ho DD, Pomerantz RJ, Kaplan JC. Pathogenesis of infection with human immunodeficiency virus. N Engl J Med 1987;317:278–286.

14. Hunt JS, Orr HT. HLA and maternal-fetal recognition. FASEB J 1992;6:2344–2348.

15. Kabawat SE, Mostoufi-Zadeh M, Driscoll SG, Bhan AK. Implantation site in normal pregnancy. A study with monoclonal antibodies. Am J Pathol 1985;118:76–84.

16. Kahan BD. Cyclosporine. N Engl J Med 1989;321:1725–1738.

17. Locker J, Nalesnik M. Molecular genetic analysis of lymphoid tumors arising after organ transplantation. Am J Pathol 1989;135:977–987.

18. MacQueen G, Marshall J, Perdue M, Siegel S, Bienenstock J. Pavlovian conditioning of rat mucosal mast cells to secrete rat mast cell protease II. Science 1989;243:83–85.

19. Miedema F, Tersmette M, van Lier RAW. AIDS pathogenesis: a dynamic interaction between HIV and the immune system. Immunol Today 1990;11:293–297.

20. Mims CA. The pathogenesis of infectious disease. London: Academic Press, 1976.

21. Moynihan JA, Breer GJ, Ader R, Cohen N. The effects of handling adult mice on immunologically relevant processes[a]. Ann NY Acad Sci 1992;650:262–267.

22. Mulder J, Hers JFP. Influenza. Groningen, The Netherlands: Wolters-Noordhoff Publishing, 1972.

23. Pantaleo G, Graziosi C, Fauci AS. The immunopathogenesis of human immunodeficiency virus infection. N Engl J Med 1993;328:327–335.

24. Plotnikoff NP, Murgo AJ. Enkephalins-endorphins: stress and the immune system. Introduction. Fed Proc 1985;44:91.

25. Purtilo DT, Hallgren HM, Yunis EJ. Depressed maternal lymphocyte response to phytohaemagglutinin in human pregnancy. Lancet 1972;1:769–771.

26. Purtilo DT, Yang JPS, Cassel CK, et al. X-linked recessive progressive combined variable immunodeficiency (Duncan's disease). Lancet 1975;1:935–941.

27. Ramphal R, Cogliano RC, Shands JW Jr, Small PA Jr. Serum antibody prevents lethal murine influenza pneumonitis but not tracheitis. Infect Immun 1979;25:992–997.

28. Samter M, Talmage DW, Frank MM, Austen KF, Claman HN, eds. Immunological diseases, 4th ed. Boston: Little, Brown, 1988.

29. Schleifer SJ, Keller SE, Camerino M, Thornton JC, Stein M. Suppression of lymphocyte stimulation following bereavement. JAMA 1983;250:374–377.

30. Shelby J, Marushack MM, Nelson EW. Prostaglandin production and suppressor cell induction in transfusion-induced immune suppression. Transplantation 1987;43:113–116.

31. Sirianni MC, Tagliaferri F, Aiuti, F. Natural killer cell deficiency in AIDS. Immunol Today 1990;11:81–82.

32. Skinner HA. The origin of medical terms, 2nd ed. Baltimore: Williams & Wilkins, 1961.

33. Small PA Jr. Influenza: pathogenesis and host defense. Hosp Pract 1990;25:51–62.

34. Solomon GF. Emotions, immunity, and disease. In: Cooper EL. Stress, immunity, and aging. New York: Marcel Dekker, 1984.

35. Sridama V, Pacini F, Yang S-L, et al. Decreased levels of helper T cells. A possible cause of immunodeficiency in pregnancy. N Engl J Med 1982;307:352–356.

36. Stein M. Bereavement, depression, stress, and immunity. In: Guillemin R, Cohn M, Melnechuk T, eds. Neural modulation of immunity. New York: Raven Press, 1985:29–44.

37. Weigle WO. Effects of aging on the immune system. Hosp Pract 1989;24:112–119.

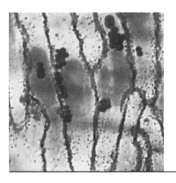

Disturbances of Fluid Exchange

CHAPTER 21

Endothelium: The
Primal Frontier

Normal Fluid
Exchanges Across
Capillary Endothelium

Hyperemia

Edema

Cells that lead solitary lives, such as amoebae in a swamp, must survive at the mercy of their environment. At the opposite extreme are the cells of vertebrates: they live enclosed in a fluid environment that they maintain and control. This implies that vertebrates have the ability to produce a liquid with very complex properties (namely blood) that is contained in a closed system of vessels equipped with a pump, and assisted by another complete system of vessels, the lymphatics. That this is not an easy task is proven by human mortality statistics. In industrialized countries most people die of failures of the system's tubing, such as atherosclerosis, or of the pump, such as myocardial infarcts (Figure 21.1). Furthermore, blood vessels are involved, directly or indirectly, in almost every disease: inflammation is largely a vascular phenomenon, and tumors survive on their blood supply. This is why vessels deserve a section of their own in General Pathology.

Seen from the perspective of function, the vascular system consists, broadly speaking, of two parts, both made essentially of tubing lined with endothelium. One part, visible to the naked eye, consists of large tubing (arteries and veins) and a pump. This part is a plumbing system for delivering blood to the other part, the microcirculation, where the exchanges between blood and tissues take place; this has been called the "business end" of the vascular system. Correspondingly, some types of malfunction—such as obstruction—can happen to either part of the vascular system, whereas other malfunctions are characteristic of one part or the other. For example: problems of wall maintenance (atherosclerosis) prevail in large arteries, which are unique in having thick walls that are devoid of "maintenance equipment" such as capillaries and macrophages; valvular failures are prominent in the heart, which is unique in being a pump with chambers separated by valves; and disorders of fluid exchange are a major feature of microcirculatory pathology.

Endothelium: The Primal Frontier

Before plunging into vascular pathology we should acknowledge the key function of the endothelium, which lines the entire container of the blood (Figure 21.2). It is so thin that its existence was denied up to 1865 (21), yet it has become one of the most studied cell types, and new books about it appear every year (31, 40, 41). It can secrete an amazing variety of products, and since its total weight has been estimated at one kilogram (37), it is by far the largest endocrine gland. The molecules it secretes (46) include collagen and elastin, factors opposing or favoring the clotting of blood,

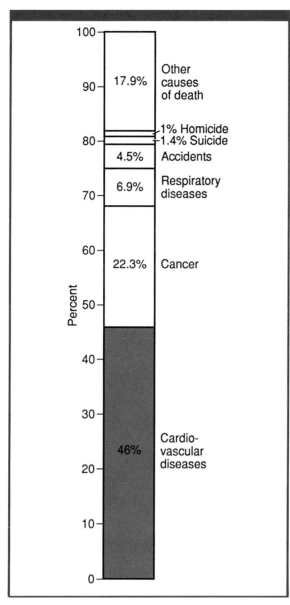

FIGURE 21.1 Cardiovascular disease is the single most important cause of death in the United States. (Adapted from [25].)

morphologic facts not fitting with neat mathematical calculations. It all began in 1953 when George Palade proposed that the vesicles seen by electron microscopy in endothelial cells are engaged in transport, picking up fluid from one side of the endothelium and releasing it on the other. This active process was thoroughly incompatible with the permeability mechanism that physiologists had just calculated, and based on purely physical exchanges across hypothetical "pores" (21).

The dust has not yet entirely settled (29), but those who believe in demonstrable facts agree that endothelial cells do perform active transport, or better, *transcytosis*, to use the term introduced in 1979 by Nicolae Simionescu (Figure 21.3) (39). This mechanism enables molecules as large as low-density lipoproteins to be ferried across the endothelial barrier, whereas fluid and molecules up to about 20 Å pass through the intercellular junctions (26). The intercellular junction is the main pathway involved in edema. To broach that topic we must quickly review some capillary physiology.

Normal Fluid Exchanges Across Capillary Endothelium

All extracellular fluids exist in a state of equilibrium with the plasma; exchanges between the two compartments occur across the "capillary" wall. (The quotation marks are there to remind us that in this particular instance the term *capillary* is meant to include the venules; although venules differ from capillaries with regard to pharmacologic responses, their walls are about as thin as those of capillaries and are in fact more permeable [42, 43].) The physiologic exchanges of fluid between blood and tissues are governed by Starling's law, now a century old. This law assumes that the capillary wall behaves essentially as a semipermeable membrane (i.e., it is capable of retaining proteins). We have illustrated this law on p. 415, and we urge the reader to review Table 12.1.

A capsule summary of Starling's law: The amount of fluid that filters out of the arterial end of a capillary is about equivalent to the amount of fluid reabsorbed at the venous end. *The forces involved are four:* the main force pushing fluid out is the hydrostatic pressure of the blood, which drops along the capillary from about 30 to 10 mm Hg; the

prostaglandins, cytokines, vasodilators and vasoconstrictors including the powerful endothelins (30), free radicals, and the adhesion molecules already discussed (p. 393). Much of this was learned from endothelial cells grown *in vitro.* One of the current endothelial dogmas, supported by overwhelming structural and functional evidence, is that *the endothelium in vivo differs from one organ to another, and even along the same vessel from arteriole to capillary to venule* (42, 43); but whether these differences are always maintained in tissue culture is not yet clear.

A controversy of nearly epic proportions raged for decades concerning the endothelium as a permeability barrier; it was a classic example of ugly

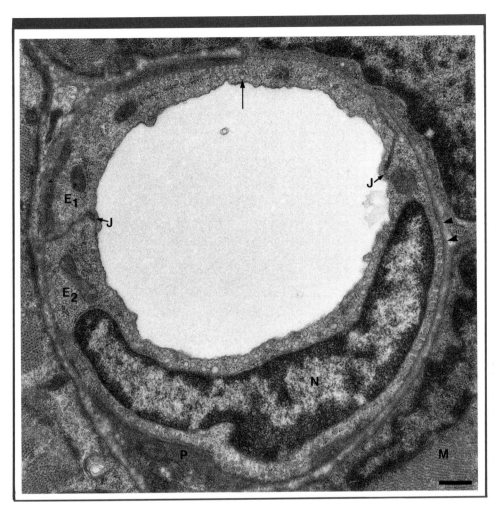

FIGURE 21.2
Capillary in rat striated muscle, fixed by perfusion under physiologic pressure. The capillary is lined by two endothelial cells (E_1, E_2); J = junctions between E_1 and E_2; N = nucleus of endothelial cell; P = part of a pericyte; M = striated muscle cell; **arrow** = micropinocytic vesicle; **arrowheads** = pericapillary basement membrane. **Bar** = 0.5 μm.

main force pulling fluid in is the osmotic pressure of the plasma proteins, which is constant at 28 mm Hg; a lesser force pulling fluid out is the osmotic pressure of extravascular proteins, about 6 mm Hg; the fourth and contentious item is the hydrostatic pressure of the interstitial fluid, which is usually given as low and negligible, but is actually negative, as we will explain next (12).

Our purpose now is to point out three lesser known facts about the Starling equilibrium.

The Phenomenon of Negative Tissue Pressure It is certainly not intuitive that there should be a vacuum in the tissues (i.e., a pressure lower than atmospheric pressure); in fact, practically all textbooks to this day define the tissue pressure as negligible or positive with a value of a few mm Hg. Yet the evidence for negative pressure is crystal clear. To prove the point, one has to find a suitable experimental model: namely, a tissue space large enough so that a fine needle connected to a

manometer can obtain a reliable measurement. A simple solution was found in 1960 by A.C. Guyton and his co-workers (Dr. Guyton is a surgeon turned physiologist) (11, 13, 14). They took standard ping-pong balls or other hollow plastic spheres, perforated them with some 200 holes (Figure 21.4), and implanted them aseptically into the subcutaneous tissue or other tissues of dogs. Several weeks' later, when inflammation had subsided, granulation tissue had developed around the spheres; it had also lined the inner surface of the spheres, leaving the central space permanently free and filled with fluid (Figure 21.5). At this point the central cavity could be considered as an expansion of the normal tissue spaces and in equilibrium with them. A *needle inserted into that cavity consistently found a negative pressure* with readings of −4 to −6 mm Hg. Strange as this may seem, this fits a number of other observations; for example, note the pressures measured in other expanded tissue spaces (12):

FIGURE 21.3
Endothelial transcytosis, demonstrated in pulmonary capillaries of a rat. The lungs were perfused with a solution of albumin molecules bound to particles of colloidal gold; the latter are visible here as black dots. *Top:* At 3 minutes, the albumin–gold particles are adsorbed to uncoated pits and to plasmalemmal vesicles open to the surface. *Center:* After 5 minutes, some particles are being ferried across by transcytosis, others are being unloaded toward the albuminal surface. *Bottom:* At 35 minutes, many gold particles have been discharged across the endothelium into the abluminal space. **Bars** = 0.1 μm. (Top reproduced with permission from [38]. Center and bottom reproduced with permission from [8].)

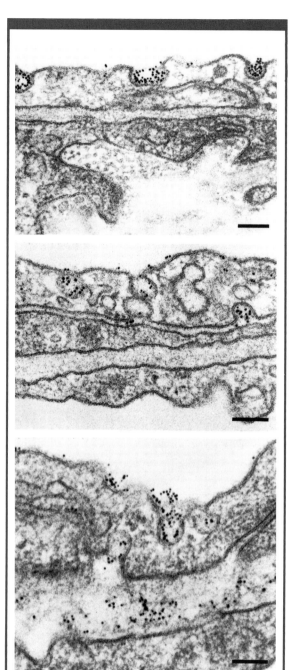

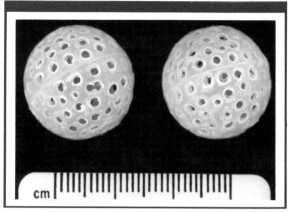

FIGURE 21.4
One of many types of perforated plastic spheres used by Guyton and collaborators for their measurements of hydrostatic pressure in the interstitial fluid. Scale in mm. (Courtesy of Dr. A.C. Guyton, University of Mississippi School of Medicine, Jackson, MS.)

pleural space	−8 mm Hg;
joints	−4 to −8 mm Hg;
epidural space	−4 to −7 mm Hg.

Exceptions to the rule of negative interstitial pressure include the very special environments of the eye and of the cerebrospinal fluid (14).

This partial vacuum is maintained by two forces: the osmotic suction of the plasma and the pumping action of the lymphatics, which remove fluid as well as osmotically active proteins. As we will see, the vacuum is an important safety factor against edema.

Guyton's concept is gaining acceptance only very slowly, even though it is nothing new in the big picture of biology. The negative pressures in animal tissues are minuscule compared with those in the sap of desert plants, which are of the order of −40 to −60 atmospheres (36). If a drop of liquid is placed on a cut in the xylem of a transpiring tree, the drop will be sucked in. The negative pressures recorded in the sap are 1000 times greater overall than those recorded in animal tissues (36).

Role of the Lymphatics Starling's law implies that the fluid escaping along the arterial end of the capillary is reabsorbed along the venous end. This is true for about 90 percent of the filtered fluid; the remaining 10 percent is drained away by the lymphatics. But how can the lymphatics act as a drain in an environment with a negative pressure?

In fact, the tissue spaces are under negative pressure *because* they are drained by the lymphatics. The lymphatic capillaries are equipped with valves. Every time the tissue is squeezed by body movement, a tiny amount of fluid is squirted downstream across the valves, which snap shut as soon as the pressure abates. Active contraction of the lymphatic itself is thought to be another pumping device (12).

The Concept of Edema Safety Factor Starling's law, narrowly interpreted, suggests that fluid

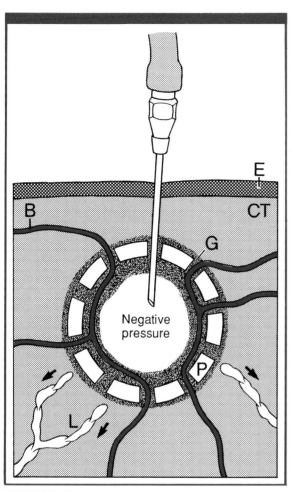

FIGURE 21.5
Demonstrating the negative interstitial pressure, using one of the perforated capsules (**P**) in the preceding figure. Over 3 weeks the capsule becomes covered and partly lined with granulation tissue (**G**), which includes a network of blood capillaries (**B**). Lymphatics have not been demonstrated in this granulation tissue, but of course they exist (**L**) in the surrounding tissues. The negative pressure is maintained by a combination of forces: removal of fluid and proteins by the lymphatics (**arrows**), and the suction provided by the oncotic pressure of the plasma proteins. (**T** = connective tissue, **E** = epidermis. (Adapted from [12].)

exchanges in the tissues are in precarious equilibrium. The capillaries ooze a little more fluid than they can reabsorb, but the providential lymphatics carry away the excess. This situation suggests that the slightest increase in venous pressure would upset the balance; more fluid would escape, less would be reabsorbed, and edema would develop. In reality, negative pressure comes to the rescue: no fluid can accumulate in the tissues as long as the interstitial pressure is negative. The excess fluid is sucked away by the lymphatics and by the oncotic pressure of the plasma proteins, and edema

cannot begin to develop until the interstitial pressure rises from −6 or −5 mm Hg to zero (12).

This is why the reader, who is presumably in a sitting position while perusing these lines, is not developing edema of the buttocks.

All these mechanisms will help understand the pathophysiology of hyperemia and edema.

Hyperemia

Although blood is life-giving, vessels overfilled with blood spell trouble. This fact was recognized, however dimly, by the Hippocratic physicians, who blamed "congestion" for many ills and bled their patients accordingly. **Hyperemia** is the term used to mean that *the vessels of the microcirculation contain more blood than normal.*

Hyperemia can be of two kinds. A red face is hyperemic and so are the dusky blue fingernails of a patient in congestive heart failure. In both cases the vessels are overfilled, but the redness and the blueness point to different situations: blood flow is either increased (active hyperemia) or decreased (passive hyperemia-congestion). Correspondingly, the temperature of hyperemic skin is abnormally warm or abnormally cool.

ACTIVE HYPEREMIA

Active hyperemia is often harmless or even beneficial. In fact, it is taught as a part of physiology that the arterioles dilate either because of a nervous impulse (as in blushing) or as a result of functional demand (as in exercising muscle). In both cases, the microcirculation is flushed with more blood under higher pressure; all the capillaries are perfused whereas normally they take turns. The raised pressure causes an increase in the amount of fluid filtering out of the capillaries (*transudation*), but without necessarily leading to edema because the situation is transient and the lymphatics can take care of it. We do not puff up every time we blush.

However, even hyperemia offers plenty of pathophysiology.

- Strenuous exercise, such as running a marathon, brings about an intense and prolonged muscular hyperemia. Transudation increases and may exceed the draining capacity of the lymphatics. Under these conditions, tissue pressure can rise enough to impair blood flow, with results that are sometimes irreversible. This scenario is called the *compartment syndrome* (p. 641).

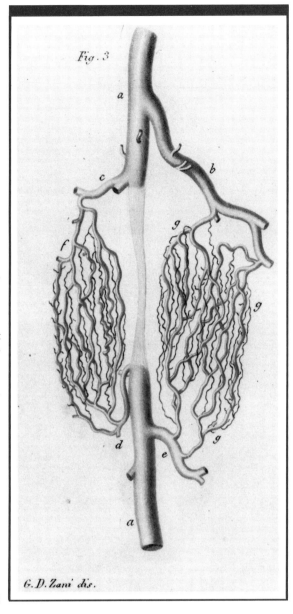

FIGURE 21.6 Development of collateral circulation, demonstrated by an 1845 experiment. A segment of the femoral artery (**a**) of a dog was tied off; 3 months later, dissection shows how the collateral circulation has developed. Branches (**b, c**) upstream from the tie have enlarged or acquired connections (**f, g**) with branches distal to the ligature (**d, e**). (Reproduced from [28].)

creased in the skin, retina and kidney, and capillary pressure is pathologically raised (45). This hyperemia is brought about by hyperglycemia, as can be proven experimentally by infusing glucose to normal humans or animals for 4–5 hours (48). The mechanism sounds paradoxical (48); tissues perceive hyperglycemia as hypoxia ("pseudohypoxia"), and react accordingly by vasodilatation and increased blood flow.

> *In hypoxic tissues the ratio NADH/NAD is increased: NADH increases because there is not enough oxygen to oxidize it to NAD. In diabetes the ratio of NADH/NAD is also increased, because more NADH is produced—due to the increased oxidation of sorbitol coupled to the reduction of NAD to NADH.*

This persistent vasodilatation in diabetics is important, because the microvascular pathology typical of diabetes, including a thickened capillary basement membrane, may be a consequence of this early malfunction (45).

- Bone fractures in children, especially those between the ages of 2 and 10, may cause an increase in the length of the fractured bone (22). This is attributed to increased blood flow to the fractured bone; indeed, a similar overgrowth can occur as a result of a congenital or accidental arteriovenous fistula (an abnormal communication between an artery and vein) or of large hemangiomas (tumors composed of blood vessels) (6).

PASSIVE HYPEREMIA (CONGESTION)

Passive hyperemia, also known as **congestion,** is much more damaging. Reduced blood flow means less oxygen, less substrates, and less removal of waste products. Congested tissues may develop edema (18). Causes can be local, such as an obstructed vein, or general, such as congestive heart failure.

Congested organs enlarge due to overfilling with blood. Eventually, over weeks and months, they become firmer because of diffuse fibrosis.

> *The fibrosis of chronic congestion is especially obvious in the liver and lung. Why it should develop is not clear, except that fibroblasts function optimally in a slightly anoxic environment (p. 457). It is also a fact that persistent edema of the skin leads to fibrosis.*

The color of congested organs is bluish or purple rather than red; *cyanotic* is the technical term (Greek *kyanós*, blue). The blueness is due in

- Persistent active hyperemia appears to be a stimulus for vascular growth. Increased flow places a mechanical stress on the microcirculation, and the small vessels respond by enlarging and adapting to the increased function (34,35). The arterioles become arteries, some capillaries become arterioles, and the venules become small veins. This may be one of the mechanisms whereby collateral circulation develops (Figure 21.6). We have seen this mechanism at work also in the active hyperemia of acute inflammation (p. 379).
- In poorly controlled diabetes, hyperemia is one of the earliest and possibly the earliest vascular change (48). Blood flow is in-

part to a change in the color of the blood; sluggish flow leads to greater oxygen extraction, and thus to a decrease in the ratio of bright red oxyhemoglobin to dusky red carboxyhemoglobin. Cyanosis of the skin, however, calls for a more complex physical explanation.

Congested white skin appears blue for the same basic reason that the sky is blue; so the experts tell us (2,7). The color of the skin normally depends on the light absorbed by various pigments (mainly melanins, plus oxidized and reduced hemoglobin) and on the light returned to the viewer by reflection and diffraction ("remittance"). A vein under the skin appears blue because most of the light is absorbed by the red blood cells, and the component that remains visible is mainly the blue light diffracted by the epidermis and dermis by a Tyndall effect. A similar phenomenon explains the blueness of deep-seated melanotic nevi ("blue nevi"). The normal color of the skin would actually be much redder were it not for the superimposed bluish diffraction just mentioned. Reduced hemoglobin has an absorption spectrum slightly displaced toward the red, which allows the remittance of more blue. It is the absolute concentration of reduced hemoglobin that appears as cyanosis; it must be at least 5 gm per 100 ml (normal total hemoglobin is 14 gm per 100 ml). This means that a severely anemic person will surely be pale but may never have enough reduced hemoglobin, in absolute amounts, to become cyanotic.

The effects of chronic congestion on the structure and function of organs depend on the tissues. To illustrate this, we will discuss conges-tion in three organs of very different structures: liver, lungs, and spleen.

Congested Liver Liver congestion is a classic result of heart failure (Figure 21.7). Normally, the liver lies against the diaphragm, just centimeters below the heart; if the right ventricle fails, blood is backed up in the liver, which can swell to 3000 g, double its weight. The pathologic effect on liver tissue is best understood by remembering that the liver lobule, in the traditional interpretation of liver structure, functions like a funnel in the sense that the blood flows toward the central vein. In this system, sluggish flow means that only the cells at the periphery of the lobule receive an adequate amount of oxygen and nutrients; these cells will show no change. The cells in the middle third of the lobule will be anoxic, and the reader will hopefully remember that the classic effect of anoxia on liver cells is steatosis (p. 81). The centrolobular cells become atrophic or just die, leaving space for a pool of blood under pressure.

In extreme cases only the cells surrounding the portal spaces survive, because life-supporting arterial blood comes from there; all the rest of the liver is necrotic. At this point the liver still appears as if it were made of discrete lobules, but these new lobules are actually centered around the portal spaces, not around the central veins. This pattern is called inverted liver.

To the naked eye, the cut surface of the congested liver shows a mottled pattern of red dots

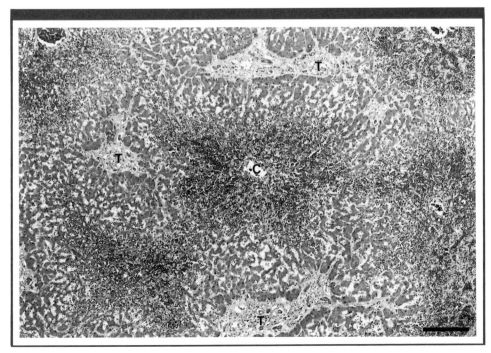

FIGURE 21.7
Severe congestion of the liver due to heart failure. **T**: Portal triad. **C**: Central vein of a liver lobule. Blood flows from **T** to **C**. Impaired outflow through the central vein caused stasis in the sinusoids feeding into it; hence the liver cords in the center of the lobule have disappeared. In contrast, the liver cords are well preserved around the portal triads, which have better access to nutrients and oxygen. **Bar** = 250 μm.

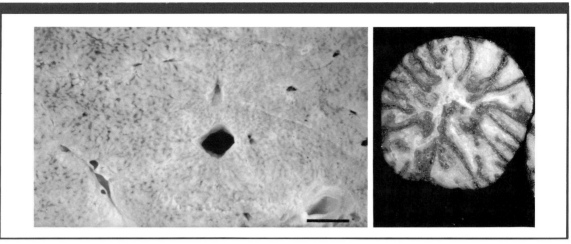

FIGURE 21.8
See color plate 18. The "nutmeg liver" typical of chronic congestion. The liver is filled with blood (hence the dark background) and studded with yellow dots and streaks corresponding to the centers of the lobules. The steatosis responsible for the yellow discoloration is caused by anoxia. Scale in mm. *Inset:* the polished surface of a nutmeg justifies the comparison.

on a yellowish background, hence the name *nutmeg liver*, a very appropriate term to anyone who has seen the cut surface of a nutmeg (Figure 21.8). In the long run, a mild degree of fibrosis creeps in (*cardiac cirrhosis*).

Overall, congestion in the liver causes mainly parenchymal changes, with a fairly minor connective tissue response.

Congested Lungs Lungs become congested when a malfunction of the left heart causes the blood to back up in the pulmonary circulation. A typical acute setting (hours) is the sudden failure of the left ventricle due to an extensive myocardial infarct.

As blood backs up in the pulmonary circulation, the congested capillaries bulge into the alveoli, allowing transudate to escape, at first into the connective tissue spaces. Luckily for the patient, the lymphatics of the lung are extremely efficient and can drain away a great deal of fluid, preventing further trouble. However, if congestion persists, the transudate eventually spills into the air spaces. The bulging alveolar capillaries can also burst, thereby mixing the transudate with plasma and red blood cells (Figure 21.9). The result is a frothy pink edema fluid that can suffocate the patient.

With these facts in mind, one can anticipate the effects of chronic congestion: a classic setting

FIGURE 21.9
Left: Normal lung (control). *Right:* Lung with severe acute congestion of the alveolar capillaries, with hemorrhage into the alveolar spaces. **Bars = 50 μm.**

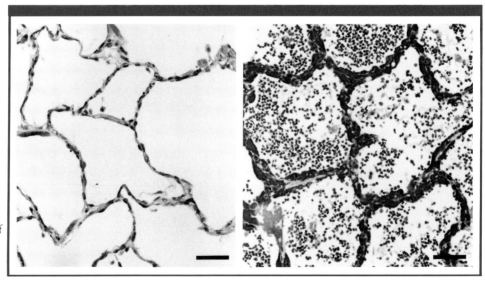

is stenosis (constriction) of the mitral valve, which causes a persistent backing up of blood in the lungs. The alveolar walls respond to chronic interstitial edema by developing a *diffuse fibrosis*. Spilled red blood cells are picked up by the resident alveolar macrophages, which become loaded with typical rusty-colored granules of hemosiderin (Figure 21.10). These helpful macrophages—there may be several in each alveolus—are known for obvious reasons as *heart failure cells*; eventually, they can be coughed out by the patient, who will notice a rusty-colored sputum.

Congested lungs become clinically less compliant (stiffer) and at autopsy appear firm and brown (brown induration).

Congested Spleen This is a wholly different matter, because—when it is chronic—congestion of the spleen leads to hypertrophy and thereby to *increased* function. Recall that the spleen vein empties into the portal vein; so whenever the portal flow through the liver is impaired (e.g., by cirrhosis), the increased venous pressure in the portal vein is transmitted to the splenic vein. Over months and years, the "overblown" spleen responds by increasing its mass: It undergoes true hypertrophy. This enlargement of the spleen leads to the syndrome called *hypersplenism*: reduced numbers of circulating red cells, white cells, and platelets. The precise mechanism is not clear, but it appears to involve an excessive trapping of circulating blood cells in the splenic sinusoids and an excessive number of splenic macrophages ready to devour these cells.

The main point here is the interesting paradox of congestion leading to increased function, to no advantage.

Lower Limbs Chronic congestion of the lower limbs due to heart failure causes a vicious circle: the large veins, submitted to increased hydrostatic pressure, dilate to such a point that their valves become incompetent, thus producing varicose veins and worsening the congestion. The chronically congested skin becomes edematous, ulcers develop about the ankles (and heal poorly), and the surrounding skin tends to become brownish from microscopic hemorrhages (19). Fibrin cuffs develop around some capillaries, presumably from chronic seepage of plasma (47); but overall, the pathogenesis of stasis ulcers is not yet well understood (27).

Migraine headaches may be somehow related to hyperemia, but the mechanism is still not clear (32).

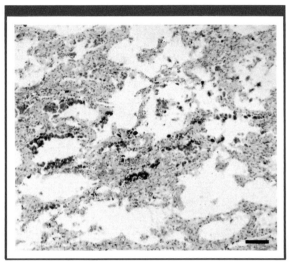

FIGURE 21.10
See color plate 19. Human lung with two typical changes of chronic passive congestion: (1) macrophages loaded with hemosiderin (the dark cells), (2) fibrosis of the alveolar walls, many of which are greatly thickened. **Bar** = 100 μm.

Edema

Edema is an excess of extracellular fluid—except in the brain, where the excess may be either intra- or extracellular.

For some reason, intracellular edema is not known in the "lower organs," as neuropathologists are apt to call anything below the brain. Intracellular edema of these organs may exist, but its consequences would not be as drastic as for the brain, which is locked in a box of bone and cannot afford to expand.

The body of a normal adult contains about 40 liters of water (12); most of it (25 liters) is sequestered in cells, including 2 liters in red blood cells; about 12 liters are in the extracellular spaces and 3 more in the plasma. The volume of water retained in each of these three spaces depends closely on a particular solute: *potassium* in the intracellular space, *sodium* in the extracellular space, and *proteins* (mainly albumin) in the plasma (Figure 21.11). Incidentally, the main electrolytes in plasma maintain roughly the same relative concentrations as in seawater, our ancestral plasma (Table 21.1).

Extracellular water is held in the tissue almost entirely as a gel by large, feathery, proteoglycan molecules (p. 265). As mentioned earlier, without these molecules all the extracellular fluid would run into the legs and feet in a matter of hours; in fact, when the amount of extracellular fluid exceeds the reserve capacity of the proteoglycans (they can imbibe an additional 30–50%

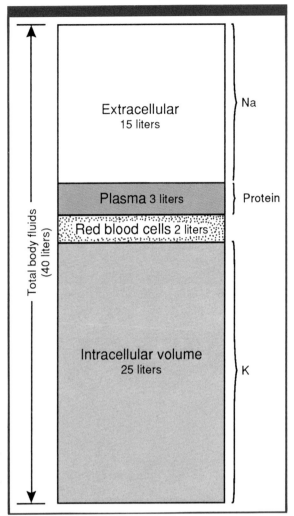

FIGURE 21.11 Body fluids. Diagram shows volumes of intracellular and extracellular fluid, blood, and total body fluids. (Adapted from [12].)

TABLE 21.2

Concentration and Osmotic Pressure of Plasma Proteins

PROTEIN	CONCENTRATION (G %)	OSMOTIC PRESSURE (MM HG)
Albumin	4.5	21.8
Globulins	2.5	6.0
Fibrinogen	0.3	0.2
Total	7.3	28.0

Adapted from (12).

above normal), it floods any available space. It can accumulate in the *loose connective tissue* and cause it to swell; in fact the ancient Greek *óidema* means swelling. It can also fill preformed spaces and create pockets of fluid called *effusions*; these pockets also have special names according to the organ in which they occur (effusions in the pleura, pericardium, or joints are called *hydrothorax, hydropericardium,* or *hydrarthrosis;* however, an effusion in the peritoneum is called *ascites*). A severe generalized edema is called *anasarca* or *dropsy,* the latter from the ancient Greek *hydrops.*

A protein-poor fluid resulting from ultrafiltration of plasma across the capillary wall is called a **transudate.** A protein-rich fluid due to increased endothelial permeability is called an **exudate** (Table 21.2) (p. 416). When the nature of a collection of fluid is not clear, clinicians use the convenient and noncommital term **effusion.**

LOCAL EDEMA

From the basic rules of capillary filtration and reabsorption and of endothelial permeability it is not difficult to understand the various clinical settings of edema. The mechanisms, however, are often multiple.

Local edema can be due to venous obstruction, lymphatic obstruction, or acute inflammation.

Local Venous Obstruction Venous obstruction can be produced, for example, by a tight cast or by a venous thrombus, particularly in the lower limbs. In terms of the Starling equilibrium, this type of edema is due to increased venous pressure leading to excessive filtration (*transudative edema*).

TABLE 21.1

Blood and Seawater: Salt Content

ELECTROLYTE	PERCENT OF TOTAL SALTS	
	IN SEAWATER	IN BLOOD SERUM
Na	30.59	39
Mg	3.79	0.4
Ca	1.20	1
K	1.11	2.7
Cl	55.27	45
SO_4	7.66	—
CO_3	0.21	12
Br	0.19	—
P_2O_5	—	0.4

Adapted from (15).

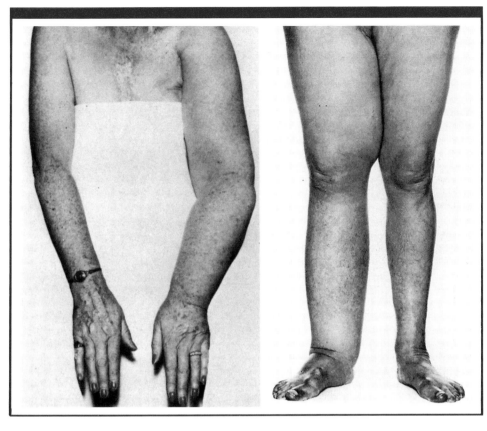

FIGURE 21.12
Two examples of iatrogenic lymphedema. *Left:* Lymphedema of the left arm after mastectomy; edema had been mild for 9 years, then increased suddenly. *Right:* Lymphedema after inguinal dissection and irradiation for a malignant melanoma that involved regional nodes; edema increased gradually over 30 years and was then treated surgically. (Reproduced with permission from [17].)

The edema is recognized clinically by pressing a finger firmly on the skin: a little depression or "pit" is produced (p. 608).

Lymphatic Obstruction *Lymphedema* is a reminder of the low-key but essential task of the lymphatic vessels. The obstruction can be purely functional: paraplegics sometimes suffer from edema of the paralyzed limbs, presumably because the lymphatics cannot perform their draining function without the pumping effect of muscular contraction. More commonly, the obstacle along the lymphatic pathways is iatrogenic. Treatment for breast tumor often includes removal or irradiation of the axillary lymph nodes; the lymphatic pathways are therefore interrupted (in the case of radiation therapy, by fibrosis) and lymphedema of the arm is a distressing consequence (Figure 21.12).

An extreme example of chronic lymphatic obstruction is the tropical disease filariasis, which is caused by the nematode *Wuchereria bancrofti* and presently affects over 250 million people. It is appropriately called *elephantiasis* (Figure 21.13) (5,23). The threadlike worms live coiled together in human lymphatics, where they somehow choose to dwell (Figure 21.14); there they cause a chronic

inflammatory reaction, especially when they die, leading to obstruction and lymphedema. The swollen tissues respond by permanent expansion, therefore this edema is nonpitting. In temperate climates a venereal disease, *lymphogranuloma venereum*, that destroys the local and regional lymph nodes can lead to genital elephantiasis in

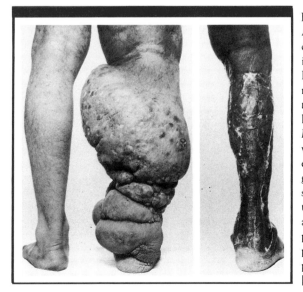

FIGURE 21.13
Advanced tropical elephantiasis in a native of Iraq. *Left:* Normal left leg. *Center:* Affected right leg before surgery. *Right:* Right leg 6 weeks after an operation using free grafts of healthy skin taken from the patient's back and from the opposite thigh. (Reproduced with permission from [17].)

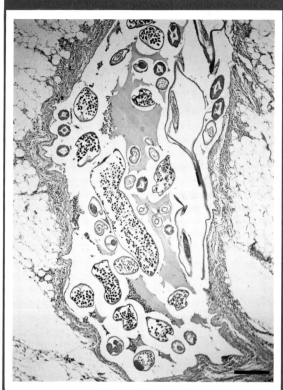

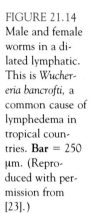

FIGURE 21.14 Male and female worms in a dilated lymphatic. This is *Wuchereria bancrofti*, a common cause of lymphedema in tropical countries. **Bar** = 250 µm. (Reproduced with permission from [23].)

both men and women. It is due to a chlamydia, an intracellular organism larger than a virus.

Congenital malformations of the lymphatics lead to lymphedema in rare conditions.

Acute Inflammatory Edema This edema can be recognized by the cardinal signs of acute inflammation: redness, heat, pain, and swelling. The pitting phenomenon is absent, presumably because the fibrin network of inflammation acts as a gel and traps the fluid. This type of local edema is caused, as we already know, by increased microvascular permeability (p. 374).

GENERAL EDEMA

Body-wide mechanisms of edema can operate in two principal ways: by raising the pressure in the entire venous tree, either pulmonary or systemic, which happens when the heart fails; or by decreasing the oncotic pressure of the plasma proteins.

Cardiogenic Edema This is by far the most common. The basic mechanics are easily grasped by considering a map of the circulatory system (Figure 21.15). Consider a failure of the left side

FIGURE 21.15
Map of the greater and lesser circulations. For clarity, the two sides of the heart are shown as separated. **LA:** Left atrium. **LV:** Left ventricle. **RA:** Right atrium. **RV:** Right ventricle. **M:** Mitral valve. **T:** Tricuspid valve. Dotted lines connecting the atria indicate that the wall between the atria in that area is a thin fibrous membrane, called the *foramen ovale*. In 6% of all individuals the fibrous membrane acts as a flap-valve. This is the route taken by paradoxical emboli. (Courtesy of Dr. H.F. Cuénoud, University of Massachusetts Medical Center, Worcester, MA.)

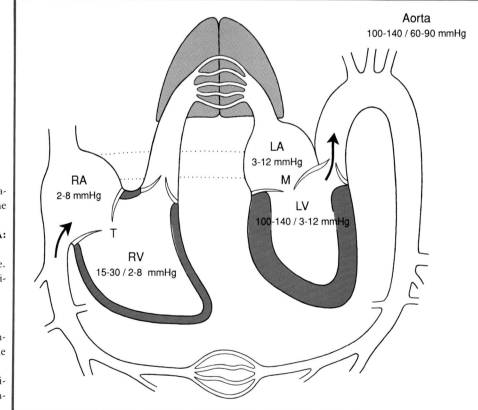

due to an infarct of the left ventricle; edema develops only in the lungs because the right heart pumps blood into the lungs but the left heart cannot forward it adequately. When the failure is bilateral, it leads to generalized congestion and edema. In this case the edema is related to overfilling the large veins; the pressure in the venules is highest where the column of blood is the tallest. Therefore, excess fluid begins to seep out into the lower or "dependent" parts of the body (*dependent edema*): the ankles in walking patients, the skin of the lower back in bedridden patients.

The pathogenesis of cardiogenic edema is complicated by many factors. First of all, remember (Figure 21.11) that the extracellular space is "sodium space," and it can remain expanded only if more sodium is provided. More sodium is indeed provided, and by several mechanisms. To begin, the kidney is involved. Reduced renal blood flow leads to more complete reabsorption of the glomerular filtrate by the proximal tubules; furthermore, being inadequately perfused, the kidney responds by secreting renin; the renin–angiotensin system in turn causes the adrenals to secrete more aldosterone, leading to further sodium retention and thus to expanded blood volume and more edema. Although not all the details are worked out, it should be clear that cardiogenic edema is more than a hydrostatic disturbance.

Nephrogenic Edema Edema can be induced by the kidney in several ways, depending on the underlying disease:

- *By a glomerular mechanism.* Protein (principally albumin) is lost through leaky capillary loops, thereby reducing the oncotic pressure of the plasma. Because albumin is the smallest of the plasma proteins, it contributes most to the oncotic pressure of the plasma (see Table 21.2). Leaky glomeruli occur in any inflammatory disease of the glomerulus (glomerulonephritis).
- *By constriction of the afferent arterioles.* Constriction reduces the glomerular filtrate and leads to greater reabsorption of sodium and water by the proximal convoluted tubules.
- *By secreting renin.* This causes the adrenals to secrete more aldosterone, which increases the reabsorption of sodium; the retained sodium produces edema by expanding the blood volume.

- *By failing to excrete salt and water.* As fluid intake continues, the blood volume expands. This occurs in acute renal failure, which has a variety of causes including ischemia, massive infection, and obstruction of the urinary pathways.

Nephrogenic edema is rarely severe; it tends to affect the eyelids first and then the genitalia and ankles. This is usually explained by the fact that the subcutaneous tissue in these sites is loose.

Edema Associated with Liver Cirrhosis This edema is a combination of local and general causes (3). The cirrhotic liver is criss-crossed by a meshwork of fibrous strands that slowly contract and strangle the parenchyma; the result is that fluid weeps from the liver surface and accumulates in the peritoneal cavity, producing the condition called **ascites.** The belly can protrude to grotesque proportions.

> Interestingly, the name ascites comes from askós for "wine bag." The Greeks carried wine and water in pouches made of animal skins; the method is still used in Africa, and we are told that it works very well. The protruding belly of cirrhotic (and perhaps alcoholic) patients reminded the Greeks of their wine-bags. They also knew that the belly was full of fluid; in fact, a Hippocratic book explains how to drain it.

Here are some of the mechanisms proposed to explain the ascites of liver cirrhosis:

- The lymphatics of the liver are strangled.
- The roots of the portal veins are also strangled, which increases portal pressure.
- Portal pressure is further increased by arteriovenous anastomoses; nodules of regenerating liver do develop, but they do not have the proper vascular architecture, with the result that arterial blood feeds directly into the roots of the portal vein.
- Insufficient albumin is synthesized by the liver.
- Aldosterone is inadequately inactivated by the malfunctioning liver cells, which normally conjugate it; this results in salt and water retention.
- The kidney responds by activating the renin–angiotensin system, as if blood volume were reduced (the mechanism is still debated).

As if all this were not enough, high abdominal pressure from the ascitic fluid can create an obstacle to venous return from the lower limbs, where edema may also develop.

Note: Ascites can also develop without liver cirrhosis if the peritoneal cavity is seeded with tumors (carcinomatosis of the peritoneum). This type of ascites is best explained by the fact that tumors produce permeability-increasing factors (p. 745), which presumably affect the entire peritoneal surface. Some experimental tumors are maintained by transplantation in the peritoneum, precisely because they have a special tendency to produce ascites, in which they grow (p. 743); their capacity to increase vascular permeability in the peritoneum can be comparable to an intraperitoneal injection of a potent inflammatory mediator, serotonin (24).

Hypoalbuminemia Insufficient albumin can lead to edema if the concentration of albumin drops to 2.5 percent or less from the normal 4.5 percent. There is a normal loss of albumin to the gastrointestinal tract, and this fraction can be increased in many diseases. These protein-losing enteropathies can be inflammatory, neoplastic, infectious, or of cardiac origin. The edema of malnutrition was originally thought to reflect hypoalbuminemia, but the mechanism is probably more complex (9).

Edema from Sundry Causes Edema due to *glucocorticoid treatment* has several causes, including salt retention and possibly a change in the connective tissue ground substance; the typical localization to the face ("moon face") is not explained. *High altitude* causes cerebral as well as pulmonary edema (mountain sickness); the pathogenesis is still debated (4,16). An even greater mystery is *idiopathic cyclic edema* whereby a patient suffers from periodic episodes of local or generalized edema that can be severe enough to cause shock if untreated.

EFFECTS OF EDEMA ON TISSUES

Skin Edema of the skin can cause a great deal of discomfort, but it is painless unless it is caused by inflammation. In subcutaneous tissue, the excess fluid is initially free to move about, hence the clinical phenomenon of pitting; a finger pressed firmly on edematous skin for a few seconds leaves a depression that disappears in less than a minute (Figure 21.16). This free-moving fluid facilitates infection. Bacteria, even if suspended in fluid, can easily perform their aggressive functions such as multiplying and producing toxins, whereas leukocytes are helpless because they crawl but do not swim. For these reasons, injuries of edematous skin, even minor ones, can lead to severe and rapidly spreading infections. If edema persists for weeks or longer, connective tissue produces new cells and new fibers to fill the extra spaces, and the swelling becomes permanent.

Edema is critically dangerous in two organs: the lung and the brain.

Lung Edema of the lung has a pathophysiology of its own. It can be transudative as well as exudative; its causes, besides heart failure, include infection, toxic agents, pure oxygen, and paradoxically, anoxia, as in high-altitude disease. Most of these agents damage the alveolar capillary, which becomes leaky and produces a protein-rich edema.

Physiologists have calculated that the edema safety factor in the lung is higher than in other tissues: 21 mm Hg, a reassuring fact, considering that pulmonary edema, unlike edema in most other organs, can be quickly fatal (12). Due to the large capacity of the lung's lymphatics and to the pumping action of respiratory movements, the efficiency of lymphatic drainage is very high and can increase tenfold in chronic edema. At first the edema fluid accumulates in the narrow space between the capillary and the alveolar

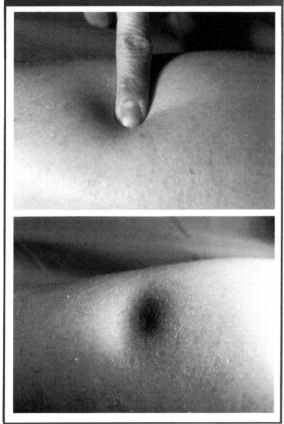

FIGURE 21.16 Pitting edema in the leg of a patient suffering from right ventricular heart failure. Firm pressure with a finger, sustained for a few seconds, leaves a depression that disappears within a few minutes. If the edema is the result of chronic lymphatic obstruction (lymphedema), the pitting phenomenon cannot be elicited. (Courtesy of Dr. H.F. Cuénoud, University of Massachusetts Medical Center, Worcester, MA.)

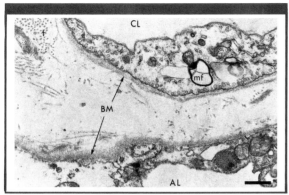

FIGURE 21.17
Edema of the alveolar wall, in the lung of a patient who had breathed oxygen at high concentration for 3 days (oxygen pneumonitis or respirator-lung syndrome). The basement membranes (**BM**), which are normally very close or in direct contact, are separated by edema. Note damage in the endothelium and epithelium. **CL:** Capillary lumen, **AL:** Alveolar lumen, **mf:** myelin figure. **Bar** = 1 μm. (Reproduced with permission from [10].)

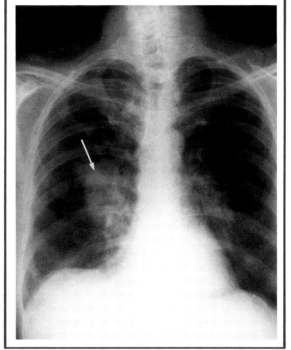

FIGURE 21.18
The only type of edema that can be seen by X-rays is pulmonary edema. **Arrow:** a patch of pulmonary edema caused by high altitude, in the typical pattern of a "cotton ball." A side effect of a lecture delivered at 14,000 feet in Cuzco, Peru.

epithelium (interstitial edema) (Figure 21.17) (10); then it pours out into the alveolar space (alveolar edema). If the patient survives, the alveolar fluid may become secondarily infected from inhaled bacteria.

Incidentally, pulmonary edema is the only form of edema directly visible by X-rays, because it replaces air with water, which is much more radio-opaque (Figure 21.18).

Cerebral Edema The brain has no lymphatic drainage and little room to expand within the skull. Thus, if it does swell, the increased volume of the brain produces dramatic shifts of tissue, with compression of blood vessels and distortion of vital centers. Parts of the brain may protrude (herniate) through several anatomical openings, such as the foramen magnum leading to the spinal cord. After head injury, acute cerebral edema develops almost immediately and can be lethal. Early symptoms include headache, nausea, and vomiting. Neuropathologists recognize many forms of cerebral edema (1), but for our purposes it suffices to mention two major mechanisms:

- *Intracellular edema* (also called cytotoxic edema), which is typically seen as a result of ischemia; this corresponds to the hypoxic cellular swelling already discussed (p. 191).
- *Vasogenic edema*, which is due to diffuse damage to the blood–brain barrier (e.g., after trauma or around focal lesions such as tumors or abscesses).

The fluid accumulates mainly in the extracellular spaces of the white matter and can sometimes lead to myelin breakdown. Cerebral edema can be recognized by computerized tomography and by magnetic resonance imaging (MRI) even when mild, such as in early mountain sickness (20).

References

1. Adams JH, Corsellis JAN, Duchen LW, eds. Greenfield's neuropathology, 4th ed. New York: John Wiley & Sons, 1984.
2. Anderson RR, Parrish JA. The optics of human skin. J Invest Dermatol 1981;77:13–19.
3. Arroyo V, Bernardi M, Epstein M, Henriksen JH, Schrier RW, Rodés J. Pathophysiology of ascites and functional renal failure in cirrhosis. J Hepatol 1988;6:239–257.
4. Bäertsch P, Maggiorini M, Ritter M, Noti C, Vock P, Oelz W. Prevention of high-altitude pulmonary edema by nifedipine. N Engl J Med 1991;325:1284–1289.
5. Binford CH, Connor DH, eds. Pathology of tropical and extraordinary diseases, vol 2. Washington, DC: Armed Forces Institute of Pathology, 1976.
6. Coleman SS. Lower limb length discrepancy. In: Lovell

WW, Winter RB, eds. Pediatric orthopaedics, vol 2, 2nd ed. Philadelphia: JB Lippincott, 1986:781–863.

7. Edwards EA, Duntley SQ. The pigments and color of living human skin. Am J Anat 1939;65:1–33.

8. Ghitescu L, Fixman A, Simionescu M, Simionescu N. Specific binding sites for albumin restricted to plasma-lemmal vesicles of continuous capillary endothelium: receptor-mediated transcytosis. J Cell Biol 1986;102:1304–1311.

9. Golden MHN, Golden BE, Jackson AA. Albumin and nutritional oedema. Lancet 1980;1:114–116.

10. Gould VE, Tosco R, Wheelis RF, Gould NS, Kapanci Y. Oxygen pneumonitis in man. Ultrastructural observations on the development of alveolar lesions. Lab Invest 1972;26:499–508.

11. Guyton AC. A concept of negative interstitial pressure based on pressures in implanted perforated capsules. Circ Res 1963;12:399–414.

12. Guyton AC. Textbook of medical physiology, 7th ed. Philadelphia: WB Saunders, 1986.

13. Guyton AC, Armstrong GG, Crowell JW. Negative pressure in the interstitial spaces. Physiologist 1960;3:70.

14. Guyton AC, Granger HJ, Taylor AE. Interstitial fluid pressure. Physiol Rev 1971;51:527–563.

15. Henderson LJ. The fitness of the environment; an inquiry into the biological significance of the properties of matter. Boston: Beacon Press, 1958.

16. Johnson TS, Rock PB. Acute mountain sickness. N Engl J Med 1988;319:841–845.

17. Kinmonth JB. The lymphatics. London: Edward Arnold, 1982.

18. Landis EM, Jonas L, Angevine M, Erb W. The passage of fluid and protein through the human capillary wall during venous congestion. J Clin Invest 1932;11:717–734.

19. Leu HJ. Morphology of chronic venous insufficiency—light and electron microscopic examinations. VASA Band 1991;20:330–342.

20. Levine BD, Yoshimura K, Kobayashi T, Fukushima M, Shibamoto T, Ueda G. Dexamethasone in the treatment of acute mountain sickness. N Engl J Med 1989;321:1707–1713.

21. Majno G. The capillary then and now: an overview of capillary pathology. Mod Pathol 1992;5:9–22.

22. McCullough FL. Skeletal trauma in children. Orthop Nurs 1989;8:41–46.

23. Meyers WM, Neafie RC, Connor DH. Bancroftian and Malayan filariasis. In: Binford CH, Connor DH, eds. Pathology of tropical and extraordinary diseases, vol 2. Washington, DC: Armed Forces Institute of Pathology, 1976:340–355.

24. Nagy JA, Herzberg KT, Masse EM, Zientara GP, Dvorak HF. Exchange of macromolecules between plasma and peritoneal cavity in ascites tumor-bearing, normal, and serotonin-injected mice. Cancer Res 1989;49:5448–5458.

25. National Cancer Institute. Cancer statistics review 1973-1986. Washington, DC: US Department of Health and Human Services, National Institutes of Health, 1989.

26. Palade GE The microvascular endothelium revisited. In: Simionescu N, Simionescu M, eds. Endothelial cell biology in health and disease. New York: Plenum Press, 1988:3–22.

27. Partsch H. Investigations on the pathogenesis of venous leg ulcers. Acta Chir Scand Suppl 1988;544:25–29.

28. Porta L. Delle Alterazioni Patologiche delle Arterie per la Legatura e la Torsione. Esperienze ed Osservazioni. Milano: Tipografia di Giuseppe Bernardoni di Gio, 1845.

29. Renkin EM. Transport pathways and processes. In: Simionescu N, Simionescu M, eds. Endothelial cell biology in health and disease. New York: Plenum Press, 1988:51–68.

30. Rubanyi GM, Botelho LHP. Endothelins. FASEB J 1991;5:2713-2720.

31. Ryan US. Endothelial cells, vol 1. Boca Raton, FL: CRC Press, 1988.

32. Sacks O. Migraine. Understanding a common disorder. Berkeley, CA: University of California Press, 1985.

33. Schaper W. Tangential wall stress as a molding force in the development of collateral vessels in the canine heart. Experientia 1967;23:595–596.

34. Schaper W, Sharma HS, Quinkler W, Markert T, Wünsch M, Schaper J. Molecular biologic concepts of coronary anastomoses. J Am Coll Cardiol 1990;15:513–518.

35. Scheel KW, Fitzgerald EM, Martin RO, Larsen RA. The possible role of mechanical stresses on coronary collateral development during gradual coronary occlusion. A simulation study. In: Schaper W, ed. The pathophysiology of myocardial perfusion. Amsterdam: Elsevier/North-Holland Biomedical Press, 1979:489–518.

36. Scholander PF, Hargens AR, Miller SL. Negative pressure in the interstitial fluid of animals. Science 1968;161:321–328.

37. Simionescu M. Receptor-mediated transcytosis of plasma molecules by vascular endothelium. In: Simionescu N, Simionescu M, eds. Endothelial cell biology in health and disease. New York: Plenum Press, 1988:69–104.

38. Simionescu M, Ghitescu L, Fixman A, Simionescu N. How plasma macromolecules cross the endothelium. News Physiol Sci 1987;2:97–100.

39. Simionescu N. The microvascular endothelium: segmental differentiations, transcytosis, selective distribution of anionic sites. In: Weissmann S, Samuelson B, Paoletti R, eds. Advances in inflammation research, vol 1. New York: Raven Press, 1979:61–70.

40. Simionescu N, Simionescu M, eds. Endothelial cell biology in health and disease. New York: Plenum Press, 1988.

41. Simionescu N, Simionescu M, eds. Endothelial cell dysfunctions. New York: Plenum Press, 1992.

42. Simionescu N, Simionescu M, Palade GE. Structural basis of permeability in sequential segments of the microvasculature of the diaphragm. I. Bipolar microvascular fields. Microvasc Res 1978a;15:1–16.

43. Simionescu N, Simionescu M, Palade GE. Structural basis of permeability in sequential segments of the microvasculature of the diaphragm. II. Pathways followed by microperoxidase across the endothelium. Microvasc Res 1978b;15:17–36.

44. Tooke JE, Östergren J, Adamson U, Fagrell B. The effects of intravenous insulin infusion on skin microcirculatory flow in type 1 diabetes. Int J Microcirc Clin Exp 1985;4:69–83.

45. Tooke JE, Shore AC. The regulation of microvascular function in diabetes mellitus. In: Pickup JC, Williams G, eds. Textbook of diabetes, vol 2. Oxford: Blackwell Scientific Publications, 1991:546–553.

46. Vane JR, Änggård EE, Botting RM. Regulatory functions of the vascular endothelium. N Engl J Med 1990;323:27–36.

47. Vanscheidt W, Laaff H, Wokalek H, Niedner R, Schöpf E. Pericapillary fibrin cuff: a histological sign of venous leg ulceration. J Cutan Pathol 1990;17:226–268.

48. Williamson JR, Chang K, Frangos M, et al. Hyperglycemic pseudohypoxia and diabetic complications. Diabetes 1993;42:801-813.

Hemostasis and Thrombosis

I njury, as we mentioned earlier, creates three kinds of problems: destruction of tissues, infection, and bleeding. Nature counters with three processes: regeneration, inflammation, and hemostasis (Figure 8.1). *Hemostasis ("stopping of hemorrhage") is the fastest:* it has to act within seconds because blood is the essence of life. One of the hemostatic devices provided by evolution is clotting, a process by which blood becomes a solid mass as soon as it makes contact with connective tissue, *while remaining fluid in the container itself.* Now imagine the engineering problem of creating a fluid with these properties. To be effective, the clotting mechanism must be hair-triggered; but at the same time it must be kept from firing inappropriately because then the whole mass of circulating blood might clot. This feat is achieved by means of an intricate system of checks and balances in which clotting agents are controlled by inhibitors that are controlled by inhibitors of inhibitors—while a parallel system (fibrinolysis) destroys the clots as fast as they are forming. The intricacy of this system for Nature, and for those who attempt to understand it, is measured by the fact that the plasma concentration of control molecules, both anticlotting and antifibrinolysis, is much greater than that of the clotting factors (103). Again, because the system is so complicated it can misfire and create unwanted and dangerous intravascular clots, called *red thrombi*. Before we proceed any further, it is essential to learn the basic terminology of this field:

- **A clot** is the end-product of the activated clotting mechanism, which can operate *in vitro* as well as *in vivo*.

> *Blood clotting is based upon the generation of fibrin filaments, which imprison the red blood cells. For blood to coagulate the clotting system must be activated to produce the enzyme thrombin, which acts on fibrinogen, a plasma protein, thereby generating fibrin.*

- **A thrombus** *is any solid object developing from the blood in vivo and within the vascular system.* This includes the same type of red clot that can be obtained *in vitro*; we will call such masses *red thrombi*, to emphasize that they were formed *in vivo* (p. 633).
- **Thrombosis** *includes more than clotting:* the "solid objects derived from the blood *in vivo*" include clumps of pure platelets, masses of fibrin, or mixtures of platelets and

fibrin, which develop during hemostasis but not when whole blood coagulates in a test tube. It may be helpful to remember that thrombosis has been defined as "*hemostasis in the wrong place*" (71).

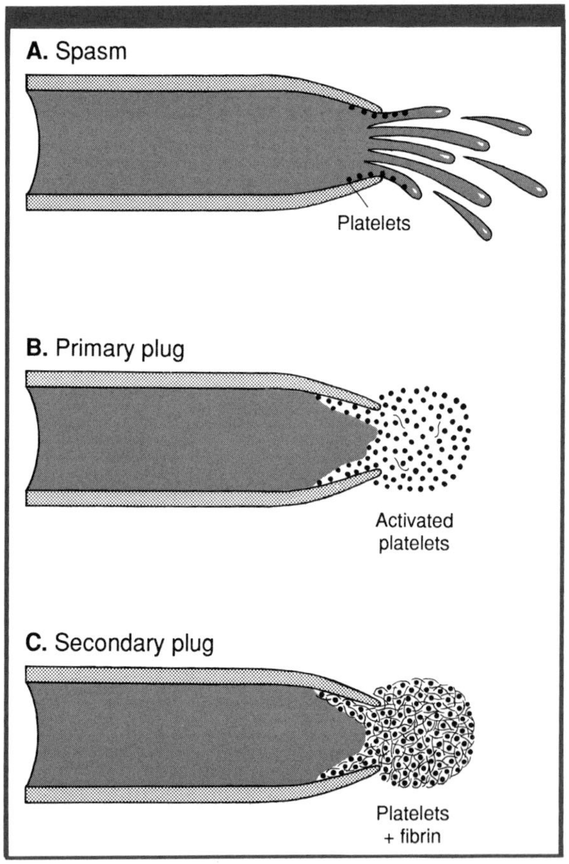

Hemostasis: The Control of Bleeding

Let us perform a simple experiment. We will sever a small artery (50–500 μm in diameter) in the omentum of a rat and follow what happens by light and electron microscopy. The reason for choosing an artery is that high-pressure vessels are the most critical for the process of hemostasis. What we will see requires lengthy explanations, but let us begin with the facts (25, 46, 47, 61, 87). We will witness a three-step process (Figure 22.1):

1. *The severed artery contracts immediately*— not enough to stop the bleeding, but enough to lower the pressure downstream. (In severed veins this contraction is virtually absent, but it is also unnecessary, because venous blood pressure is much lower.) This response is important: in rabbits treated with an anticoagulant, hemostasis in a wound depends solely on vasoconstriction; bleeding abates but then resumes as soon as the vasoconstriction has worn off (25).

Arterial constriction is probably due at first to trauma. Later it is reinforced or maintained by products of the platelets deposited on the mouth of the severed vessel, especially serotonin and thromboxane A_2.

2. *A plug of platelets develops at the mouth of the vessel and beyond* (47). As the hemorrhage continues, red blood cells stream by, but platelets stick to the traumatized part of the artery and to the connective tissue outside it. This creates a fragile but quickly growing *platelet plug*, which may become thick enough to occlude the vessel and contain the bleeding (Figure 22.2). At this stage the plug consists almost entirely of platelets. Although a few fibrin filaments begin to develop on the surface of the platelet plug, they are still too thin to stabilize the mass (110). This is the *pri-*

A. Spasm

Platelets

B. Primary plug

Activated platelets

C. Secondary plug

Platelets + fibrin

FIGURE 22.1
The three steps of hemostasis in a small artery that has just been severed. The entire sequence occurs in a few minutes.

mary hemostatic plug; it forms within seconds and minutes after the trauma (15, 56, 99).

3. *Fibrin filaments stabilize the platelet plug and the mass of red blood cells in the tissues beyond it.* The crumbly platelet plug is now reinforced by a network of fibrin and becomes a *secondary hemostatic plug.* In human volunteers this stage was reached at 30 minutes (110). The emergency is over.

From this point on the stage is set for a process similar to wound healing: this secondary hemostatic plug is destined to be organized, that is, destroyed and replaced by granulation tissue, and eventually by a tiny scar. The fibrin and debris are cleared away by macrophages.

All three steps of hemostasis are essential (103), especially steps 2 and 3. Patients with platelet counts below 10,000 or with nonfunctional platelets lack step 2, the pure platelet plug. Hemophiliacs lack step 3; they have normal platelets but impaired blood clotting and therefore cannot produce fibrin.

This overview of hemostasis taught us that three actors are involved in hemostasis: the platelet, the process of blood clotting, and the vascular wall. We will now consider each in some detail.

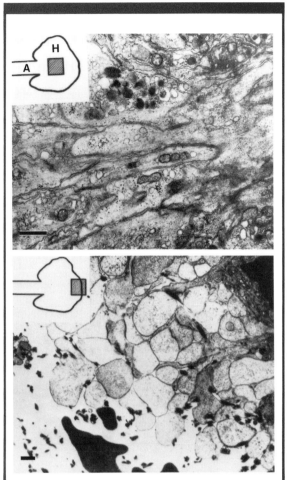

FIGURE 22.2
Hemostatic plug from a severed enteric artery of a dog; electron micrographs. The sites from which the sections were taken are shown in the diagrams of the plug in the upper left-hand corners. **A:** Severed artery. **H:** Hemostatic plug. *Top:* This part of the plug consists of packed platelets. *Bottom:* At the periphery of the plug the platelets in contact with collagen are swollen and degranulated. The small dark patches represent fibrin. **Bars** = 0.5 μm. (Reproduced with permission from [87].)

The Platelet in Hemostasis

Considering that platelets are just flat little discs a micron or two in diameter and without a nucleus, they are extraordinarily complex (Figure 22.3). Normal platelets are stiff and do not stick, but their secret is that they can be activated within seconds to an almost explosive performance, which includes becoming sticky and helping the blood to clot (Figure 22.4). Platelet activators include, first of all, collagen surfaces—which makes sense because injury brings platelets in contact with the extravascular world where collagen abounds. There are also soluble activators: thrombin, which signals to the platelets that the clotting sequence is activated; adenosine diphosphate (ADP), which is released by activated platelets and injured red cells and helps amplify the platelet response; epinephrine; and some prostaglandins.

Fully activated platelets swell into sticky, branching spheres and die (61). This process depends on the coordinated action of membrane, granules, and cytoskeleton; it can be subdivided somewhat artificially into four phases, which tend to overlap:

1. adhesion (to other surfaces)
2. aggregation (with other platelets)
3. swelling
4. secretion

The first part of the activation program, adhesion and early aggregation, is reversible; the subsequent steps are not. Platelet response varies somewhat depending on the stimulus, but ADP causes platelets to swell maximally in 5–10 seconds (61).

ADHESION

Adhesion refers to the sticking of platelets to certain tissue surfaces, not to each other (91). Platelets do not stick except fleetingly to normal endothelium, and it is uncertain whether they will stick to it if it is injured. However, they are

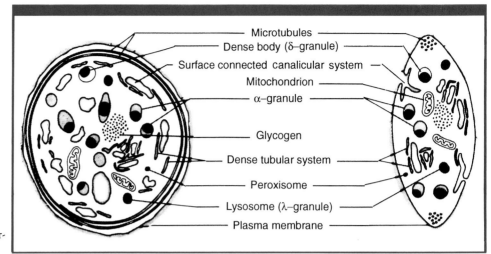

FIGURE 22.3
Diagram of a human platelet (face and profile) showing components visible by electron microscopy and cytochemistry. (Reproduced with permission from [13].)

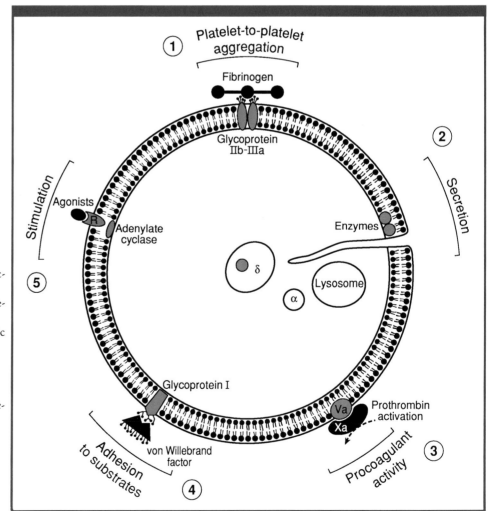

FIGURE 22.4
Platelets, small as they are, are equipped to perform at least five functions: (1) Binding to fibrinogen, which acts as a glue with other platelets (*aggregation*). (2) *Secretion* originates from the membrane (enzymatic production of thromboxane) as well as by extrusion of granule contents through the canalicular system. (3) *Prothrombin activation,* a key step in the clotting mechanism. (4) *Adhesion to nonplatelet surfaces,* by means of specific receptors for von Willebrand factor. (5) *Stimulation by agonists,* such as thrombin, epinephrine, or ADP which lead to aggregation and secretion. (Adapted from [104].)

equipped with ligands that make them stick instantly to subendothelium: that is, to the basement membrane or the collagenous tissue that is exposed if the endothelium is removed. The ligands are also receptors for molecules of von Willebrand factor (vWF) adsorbed to the subendothelial structures (Figure 22.5). Recall that von Willebrand factor is concentrated in the Weibel–Palade bodies of the endothelium; endothelial cells secrete some of it toward their basement membrane (94), where it becomes bound to collagen, ready to attract a layer of platelets in case of endothelial damage. Almost instantly after adhesion the platelets spread and begin to degranulate.

AGGREGATION

Aggregation is the sticking of platelets to each other, which is how a hemostatic plug grows.

It has been very instructive to study aggregation with the aggregometer, proposed by the British pharmacologist G.V.R. Born (17). This is actually a turbidometer. A ray of light is passed through a suspension of platelets, and an aggregating agent such as ADP is added to the suspension. The intensity of the light transmitted by the suspension increases as platelets aggregate. On the same principle, fog seen out of a window is opaque, rain is not (61). With a low dose of ADP the aggregation is reversible, and with a higher dose the aggregation curve is biphasic. That is, the first wave of aggregation is caused by the added ADP, the second by the ADP released by the aggregating platelets themselves (Figure 22.6).

Depending on the activator, platelet aggregation can be accompanied by a change in the shape of platelets: without increasing its volume a platelet turns into a spiny or hairy little sphere. Adhesion molecules are exposed on its threadlike extensions. How the platelets sometimes aggregate without changing shape is not well understood.

SWELLING

Seen by electron microscopy the swelling of platelets is obvious (Figure 22.2). As the membrane is stretched, its charges spread out, decreasing the repulsion between platelets, and *fibrinogen* adhesion receptors are exposed. These receptors consist of a pair of glycoproteins and are known by the inconvenient name of GP-IIb-IIIa complex (Figure 22.4) (93). This complex (on one platelet) seizes a fibrinogen molecule while another part of the same fibrinogen molecule is seized by a GP-IIb-IIIa complex of another platelet. Each platelet has about 50,000 of these sites, possibly a record concentration of adhesion receptors (29). In essence, *the main glue among platelets is fibrinogen between platelets and endothelium it is von Willebrand factor* (Figure 22.5).

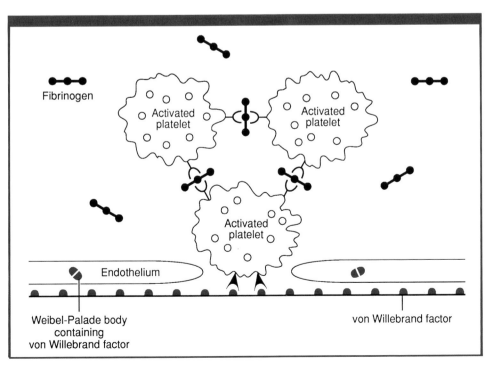

FIGURE 22.5
Mechanisms of platelet adhesion and aggregation are mediated by different receptors. Adhesion to the subendothelium by receptors for von Willebrand factor, which is produced by the endothelium, stored in the Weibel–Palade bodies, and captured in part by the basement membrane. Aggregation among platelets is mediated by receptors for fibrinogen, which acts as a glue. (Adapted from [33].)

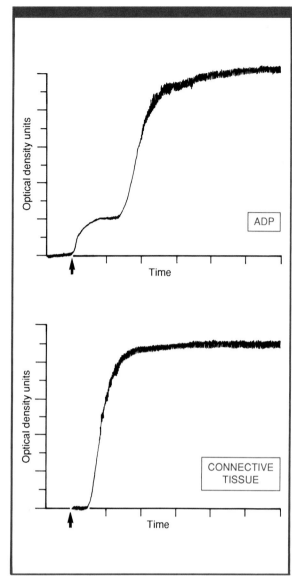

FIGURE 22.6
Two typical
curves obtained
with a platelet
aggregometer.
Top: Biphasic
aggregation
induced with a
high dose ADP.
Bottom: Mono-
phasic aggre-
gation caused
by collagen.
(Adapted from
[92].)

some ready-made fibrinogen (which will add to the fibrin ultimately produced by the clotting cascade) and an anti-anticoagulant, namely platelet factor 4. *Delta granules* (delta for *dense* see Figure 22.3) release ADP, which activates more platelets.

In addition, the dying platelet manages, in its last gasp, to actively synthesize and secrete an arachidonic acid metabolite: *thromboxane* A_2, a powerful aggregator of platelets.

In the context of a hemostatic plug, these latest events help the plug to grow. Both ADP and thromboxane A_2 induce aggregation and thereby recruit more platelets; the secretion of fibrinogen and the assistance given to clotting by platelet factor 3 make sure that fibrin filaments appear right inside the plug, where they are needed for mechanical strengthening, rather than in the extracellular spaces at random.

Such is the story of the platelet plug in the hemostatic process. Now we can examine the other major contributor to the hemostatic process: the blood clotting mechanism.

The Clotting Mechanism

Like the complement system, clotting is a system of fine-tuned checks and balances. We will sketch the essentials; specialized textbooks (30, 61) will satisfy any further appetite.

In clotting, the blood is stiffened into a solid mass by a three-dimensional network of fibrin (Figure 9.32), which derives from a circulating precursor, fibrinogen. The basic purpose of the clotting cascade is to produce fibrin. Each unit of the fibrin polymer is a fibrinogen molecule from which four short peptides have been cleaved (Figure 9.33) (p. 344); the enzyme responsible for the cleaving is thrombin. Therefore, the basic reaction of the clotting system is

$$\text{fibrinogen} \xrightarrow{\text{thrombin}} \text{fibrin}$$

Obviously, thrombin cannot circulate in its active state or blood would be a solid. The critical point, then, is how to activate thrombin. This is achieved by an array of circulating molecules that are numbered from I to XIII in the order of discovery, not in the order of function: experts have no pity for the outsiders. Most of these molecules, incidentally, were identified in

Another component becomes exposed on the platelet membrane as the platelet swells: platelet factor 3 (PF3), which is a phospholipid that takes part in the clotting mechanism. Now the activated platelet is helping the clotting sequence, which produces thrombin, which in turn activates more platelets.

SECRETION

Finally, the cytoskeleton of the platelet gathers itself into a "noose"—or rather, a basket that tightens around a cluster of granules in the center of the platelet. As a result, the content of the granules is squeezed out through the tubular system. The alpha granules contribute, among much else, two factors that help clotting:

patients who congenitally lacked one or another. Most but not all are proenzymes, which must be activated; each proenzyme activates the next in line and amplifies the effect, much as happens with the complement system. This is why the coagulation mechanism is also referred to as a cascade. (We will just comment that the term *cascade,* "waterfall," is not very proper; no waterfall becomes thousands of times larger as it plunges.)

A simplified version of the clotting cascade, Figure 22.7, shows the following characteristics:

- *Clotting occurs by either of two converging pathways;* note the analogy with activation of the complement system.
- *Besides the clotting factors there are some cofactors, notably phospholipids and calcium.* The phospholipids act as surfaces. The advantage of assembling the reagents on a surface, as usual, is to favor the reaction by concentrating and positioning the reagents. An example: to produce thrombin (factor IIa) factors Va and Xa attach to a special domain on the surface of an activated platelet (Figure 22.8). In this favorable position and with the help of calcium, factor X can activate in 2 minutes the amount of prothrombin that it could activate in 1 year if it were floating free (61).

The complement cascade has no lipid factors, but it uses the "surface trick" from the very start: C1 becomes attached to the surface of the cell destined to be perforated (p. 339).

At several steps there are feedback loops that either inhibit or accelerate the reaction. This maddening complication is part of the essential fine tuning of the clotting/anticlotting balance.

Blood can clot also in the absence of platelets, but not as well. The surface of activated platelets exposes a lipid domain, platelet factor 3, that greatly accelerates the clotting process (it intervenes at two steps of the cascade). If platelet-rich plasma is watched as it clots under the microscope, filaments of fibrin seem to emerge from platelet clumps (Figures 22.9, 22.10, 22.11).

Modern photographs of this event are virtually identical to the drawing published in 1882 by Bizzozero, in the paper that first proposed the name platelet. *Macrophages can also act as centers of fibrin formation, by means of fibrin receptors on their plasma membrane (Figure 22.11).*

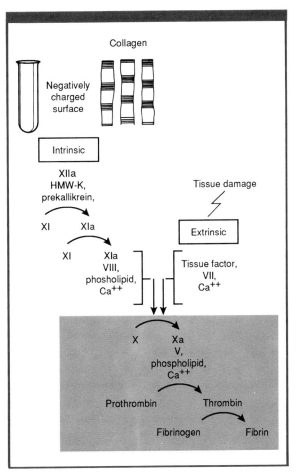

FIGURE 22.7 The coagulation cascade. The intrinsic and extrinsic pathways meet at the level of factor X.

Why Are There Two Pathways for Clotting? It is important to realize that the two pathways were discovered and defined *in vitro.* Early studies showed that blood clotting could be triggered experimentally in two ways: (a) By pouring the blood into a glass container. It turned out that the property of the glass responsible for this effect was its negative surface charge; other surfaces with that property would have the same effect, including collagen. (b) By mixing blood with tissue extracts. These extracts contained a clotting "tissue factor," later identified as thromboplastin. When the entire clotting sequence was worked out, it became apparent that the two clotting mechanisms set in motion different clotting factors, leading to chain reactions that converge at the level of factor X (Figure 22.7).

It is traditional to point out that the longer pathway, activated by negative surfaces, functions with factors that are contained in the blood: hence its name, *intrinsic pathway.* The shorter pathway needs an extra "tissue factor" supplied from outside; hence it is called the *extrinsic pathway.* But

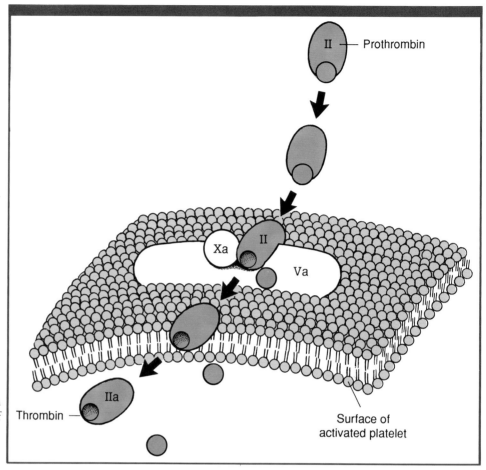

FIGURE 22.8
A critical step near the end of the clotting cascade: activation of prothrombin to thrombin. This reaction is greatly accelerated by the surface of activated platelets, which holds in place the activating complex formed by Xa and Va. (Adapted from [89].)

this distinction is not sharp at all. For instance, the typical activator of the extrinsic mechanism—the complex [thromboplastin + factor VII]—also activates factor IX of the intrinsic pathway.

How Are the Two Pathways Triggered *In Vivo?*
The intrinsic pathway requires a negatively charged surface, a condition that can be fulfilled without breaking open any vessel if the endothelium is lost by trauma or some other mechanism. The subendothelium is strongly thrombogenic, thanks especially to its collagen fibers and basement membrane, although not everybody agrees about the latter (65). It follows that the Hageman factor (factor XII, p. 338) becomes fixed and activated on de-endothelialized surfaces.

If blood is spilled out of the vessels, which is by far the most common situation, the extrinsic pathway is triggered by injured cells, which release thromboplastin; while the Hageman factor operates alongside, being activated by collagen.

Thromboplastin (tissue factor) is a membrane-spanning protein; some tissues produce it constitutively (fibroblasts, smooth muscle cells, cardiac valve stromal cells, placental trophoblast, probably brain), some produce it if properly stimulated (endothelium, monocytes, and macrophages, stimulated for example by endotoxin), and some produce little or none (lymphocytes, neutrophils) (6, 38, 88). Thromboplastin is present in high concentra-

FIGURE 22.9
Clot developing *in vitro* from platelet-rich plasma (scanning electron micrograph). A cluster of platelets appears to be tugging at the surrounding network of fibrin. **Bar** = 5 μm. (Reproduced with permission from [12].)

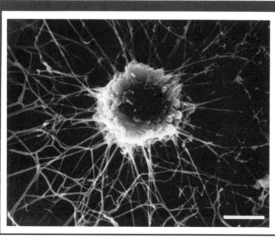

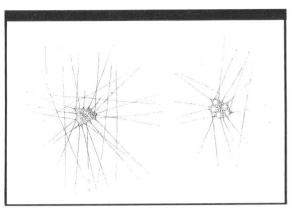

FIGURE 22.10
Role of platelets in coagulation as illustrated by G. Bizzozero in 1882. Dog blood examined for 2–3 minutes: platelets have aggregated into clumps from which radiate fine filaments of fibrin. This was the paper in which platelets were first called by that name. (Reproduced from [15].)

tion in the brain, perhaps because in this organ even the slightest hemorrhage can be hazardous (37). Histochemistry shows thromboplastin in many extravascular cells, especially in the outer vascular coat (adventitia)—as if constituting a hemostatic envelope ready to activate clotting (37).

How Do the Two Pathways Share the Job In Vivo? There is much evidence that they always operate together. Indeed, bleeding disorders develop in patients deficient with regard to one or the other pathway (61).

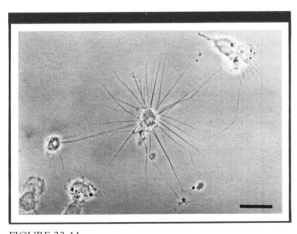

FIGURE 22.11
Needles of fibrin arising from the surface of cultured human monocytes after 10 minutes of incubation with plasma. Receptors for fibrin and fibrinogen are present on the surface of monocytes. Phase microscopy. **Bar** = 10 μm. (Reproduced with permission from [58].)

Given that the two pathwyas, in vivo, work in unison, we do not know if either one contributes differently from the other in any particular situation. The extrinsic pathway is shorter and may be slightly faster; perhaps it is called upon when the blood mixes with a great deal of crushed tissue that supplies tissue factor. Note the difference between the two pathways of clotting and the two pathways of complement; those of complement really have two separate functions. The alternative pathway offers the advantage of killing bacteria in the absence of antibody (p. 342).

RETRACTION OF THE CLOT

After a clot forms, it contracts (contraction and retraction in this context mean the same thing). This amazing phenomenon, also called **syneresis,** is easily observed *in vitro*. If you pour fresh blood into a test tube, it will clot; and within about 2 hours the red mass will shrink while oozing out a yellowish fluid called serum (not plasma!). We illustrated this event while discussing erythrocyte sedimentation rate (Figure 15.6). The clotted red mass shrinks to about half its original volume; it cannot shrink further because red blood cells take up almost half of the total blood volume. In contrast, if plasma that contains platelets is poured into a test tube, it will form a diffuse whitish clot, which will shrink to about one-tenth of the fluid volume. *In the absence of platelets, the plasma will clot but not contract.*

These experiments tell us that retraction must have something to do with platelets. Indeed, electron microscopy has shown that while platelets are dying they cling to the filaments of fibrin by their membrane receptors, and their inner actin–myosin system keeps pulling (Figure 22.12) (28).

HOW CLOTS CONTRACT

The mechanism of clot contraction is basically the same as in muscle contraction; in fact, a blood clot shaped like a strip can be made to respond *in vitro* very much like smooth muscle (72). There is a puzzle, however. Although the contractile mechanism is based on actin–myosin as in muscle, no known muscle can contract to one-tenth of its original length. Perhaps the platelets twist the filaments around themselves (Figure 22.13) (85), but we are more inclined to believe in a hand-over-hand type of pull such as we have described for fibroblasts (p. 474) (12). As a matter of fact, platelets can be replaced by

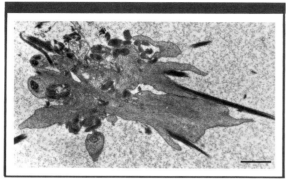

FIGURE 22.12

Platelet during clot formation (electron micrograph). The dark filaments of fibrin appear to be firmly attached to the platelet. **Bar** = 1 µm. (Reproduced with permission from [12].)

fibroblasts for inducing the retraction of the fibrin clot (90).

What Is the Purpose of Clot Retraction? Common sense suggests that retraction may toughen the hemostatic plug by squeezing out fluid; it might conceivably help in pulling together the sides of small wounds, but firm evidence is lacking (96).

> *There is an experiment of Nature in this regard: rare individuals are born with platelets that lack receptors for fibrinogen (Glanzmann's thrombasthenia, which means "platelet weakness"). Clot retraction is*

impaired, and the patients do suffer from bleeding disorders and prolonged bleeding after surgery (61).

An Odd Alliance: The Clotting–Kinin Connection

In describing the mediators of inflammation, we mentioned a blood-borne kinin precursor that binds to negative surfaces just like the Hageman factor does: high molecular weight kininogen (HMWK) (p. 337). Therefore, when a negatively charged surface is exposed to plasma, two types of molecules will attach to it: Hageman factor and HMWK (Figure 9.24). The point of this peculiar association becomes obvious when we learn that HMWK floats around in plasma loosely bound to two other molecules. One type is factor XI of the clotting system, precisely the molecule that the Hageman factor is supposed to activate: so HMWK very helpfully delivers substrate to the Hageman factor. The other molecule that is bound to HMWK is prekallikrein; this is the precursor of kallikrein, the enzyme that HMWK needs for cleaving kinins. The result is that we have Hageman factor and prekallikrein side by side, and they are programmed to activate each other with a double effect: the clotting cascade is activated and kinins are released.

We still need to explain why Nature has chosen to combine these two functions, clotting and kinin generation. Kinins do not clot blood; they are inflammatory mediators (p. 337). As such they are

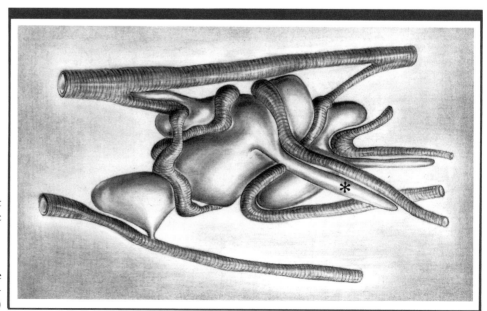

FIGURE 22.13

Reconstruction, from serial sections, of platelet–fibrin contacts during clot retraction. This electron microscopic image suggests that clot retraction may occur by shortening platelet pseudopodia (**asterisk**) and by adhesion of twisted fibrin filaments to the body of the contracting platelet. (Reproduced with permission from [85].)

also potent stimulators of smooth muscle, including the medial smooth muscle of severed arteries. We therefore venture to guess that the two molecules delivered by HMWK carry a double message to the Hageman factor: "clot the blood, but also turn off the spouts."

A Hageman puzzle. For readers with strong nerves, here is a maddening but interesting fact. It is dogma that the Hageman factor (factor XII) triggers the intrinsic pathway, together with the kinin and fibrinolytic cascades. This factor was named after a gentleman who lacked it: Mr. John Hageman, a railroad brakeman whose bleeding time was unusually long but who was otherwise asymptomatic (96). Besides the puzzling fact that he did not suffer from spontaneous bleeding problems, Mr. Hageman confused posterity by dying of thromboemboli (97), thereby proving that his intrinsic clotting cascade was functional. Clearly, besides the Hageman factor, there must be some other way to trigger the intrinsic mechanism in vivo. One possibility: the surfaces of activated platelets activate factor XI independently of the Hageman factor (61).

FACTORS THAT OPPOSE CLOTTING

Clotting is potentially dangerous. Here are some of the mechanisms that tend to limit it (Table 22.1).

- *Dilution of clotting factors by blood flow* is the most important. Consider a successful hemostatic plug; the clotting mechanism has

worked, but some mechanism must stop the plug from working its way back to fill the entire vascular system. Local blood flow does this by washing away and diluting the clotting factors, which are eventually removed by the liver and other provinces of the RES/MPS (p. 297).

- *Natural anticoagulants,* namely factors that oppose the formation of fibrin, in contrast with others that destroy it after it has formed (fibrinolysis; see later). Understandably, these anticlotting agents are designed to be especially effective on the surface of the endothelium, which must be protected from being embroiled in clotting. The major anticoagulants are antithrombin III and proteins C and S. Their story is complex but important: individuals who lack one or the other suffer from episodes of thrombosis. We will briefly describe these two anticoagulants as an example of Nature's complex ways.

Antithrombin III *(AT III), also called heparin cofactor, is made by the endothelium, the liver, and megakaryocytes. In contact with heparin, or with heparinlike molecules such as those that coat the endothelium, AT III becomes 1000 times more effective, blocking thrombin as well as four other activated clotting factors (Figure 22.14). Anti-*

TABLE 22-1

Natural Plasma Inhibitors of Coagulation (*) and Fibrinolysis

INHIBITORS	NORMAL PLASMA CONCENTRATION (MG/DL)	MAJOR ENZYMES INHIBITED	HEREDITARY DEFICIENCY STATES
*Antithrombin III (heparin cofactor)	18–30	Factor IX_a, Factor X_a, thrombin	Thrombosis
*Protein C	0.4	Factor Va_1, VIII_a	Thrombosis
α-macroglobulin	150–350	Kallikrein, thrombin, plasmin	?
$α_1$-antitrypsin	200–400	Factor X, elastase	Pulmonary emphysema
$α_2$-plasmin inhibitor ($α_2$-antiplasmin)	5–7	Plasmin	Bleeding tendency
C1 inactivator (C1 esterase inhibitor)	15–35	Factor XII_a, Factor XII kallikrein	Hereditary angioneurotic edema

Adapted from (31) and (103).

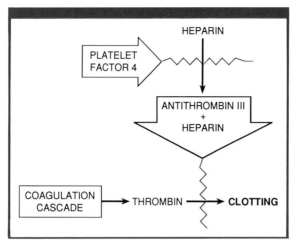

FIGURE 22.14

Inhibition of thrombin generated by the coagulation cascade. "Heparin" combines with antithrombin III to oppose the clotting effect of thrombin ("heparin" includes heparin-like molecules bound to the surface of the endothelium). Note that thrombin has an ally in platelet factor 4 (released by stimulated platelets), which prevents heparin from combining with antithrombin III. (Adapted from [74].)

thrombin III has its own opponents: platelet factor 4 (not surprising because platelets on the whole favor coagulation) and three adhesive proteins that bind heparin (von Willebrand factor, thrombospondin, and laminin).

Note: **heparin,** *a proteoglycan, is extensively used for therapeutic purposes; but whether it is present in normal plasma is not certain (19). It is the major constituent of mast cell granules, and it is released during degranulation (p. 516). Its molecular size and properties vary a great deal in different preparations. For our purposes it is important to remember that, in the clotting process, the "heparinlike" molecules on the surface of the endothelium (heparan sulfate) behave in the same manner as heparin.*

Protein C *is a proenzyme that circulates, waiting for its chance; this comes when thrombin hits the endothelial surface and is bound by thrombomodulin. The complex (thrombomodulin + thrombin) activates protein C, which selectively inactivates factors V and VIII (Figure 22.15) (6a, 27, 43) whereby the generation of thrombin is reduced.* **Protein S** *(for Seattle) is made by the endothelium and modulates the process.*

FIBRINOLYSIS

Fibrin is a precious stop-gap material, but it is never there to stay. It has a built-in, short-term obsolescence. Macrophages recognize it as something to eliminate and break it down. It is also destroyed by free-floating enzymes: this is fibrinolysis. Interestingly, the split products of fibrin inhibit blood clotting.

The simplest way to demonstrate fibrinolysis is to let some blood stand in a test tube at room temperature: within minutes it clots; within hours the clot retracts, and by the end of the day it dissolves and becomes unclottable. The same sequence occurs in the blood vessels after death.

"Animals who are run very hard, and killed in such a state, have not . . . their blood coagulated; and the effect . . . is in proportion to the cause" (66). So wrote John Hunter in 1794, in his famous treatise *On the Blood, Inflammation, and Gun-shot Wounds.* It is now well-established that the fibrinolytic activity of plasma is increased by exercise (115); perhaps this is related to the beneficial effect of exercise in decreasing the risk of coronary thrombosis. Fibrinolysis is also increased in venous blood when flow is sluggish (stasis), another logical arrangement. For these effects we must be grateful, as we will see, to the endothelium.

Note: The stress of surgery also increases fibrinolysis, but after surgery fibrinolytic activity drops and remains low for 7–10 days (fibrinolytic shutdown [61]); this coincides with the increased postoperative risk of thrombosis.

The enzyme responsible for fibrinolysis is **plasmin,** a very active serine protease that is also capable of hydrolyzing many other substrates. Plasmin circulates as an inactive precursor, plasminogen (a liver product), together with its activator (tissue plasminogen activator, tPA), which is also inactive. tPA is synthesized by a number of cells, including the endothelium.

Plasminogen must be activated. In the blood-

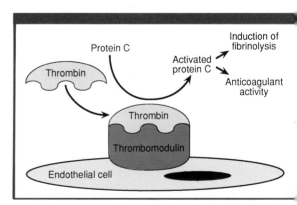

FIGURE 22.15

Contributions of the endothelium to anticlotting mechanisms. Thrombin is inactivated by binding to thrombomodulin; the complex then activates protein C, which initiates both anticoagulation and fibrinolysis. (Adapted from [32].)

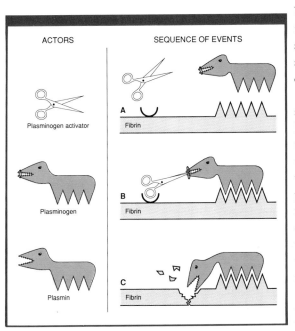

ACTORS

Plasminogen activator

Plasminogen

Plasmin

SEQUENCE OF EVENTS

A Fibrin

B Fibrin

C Fibrin

FIGURE 22.16
A cartoon version of some molecular interactions in fibrinolysis. **A:** Both plasminogen and its activator settle on a filament of fibrin. The animal-like features of plasminogen are fanciful, but the "paws" symbolize the lysin-binding sites critical in binding to fibrin. **B:** Plasminogen activator transforms plasminogen into an active enzyme, plasmin. **C:** Plasmin breaks down the fibrin. (Simplified from [69].)

stream this happens automatically, and most conveniently, when tPA attaches to fibrin filaments, where it also finds its substrate: both plasminogen and its activator have a high affinity for fibrin (Figure 22.16). Another mechanism for activating plasminogen is the Hageman factor, which switches on the two opposing processes: clotting and fibrinolysis.

Plasminogen activator (tPA) is secreted by the endothelium, especially and very appropriately under conditions of stasis; it is released from a complex with tPA-inhibitor (61). Other cell types also produce tPA:

- *Mesothelial cells and activated macrophages* (24, 69); this may be important in the dissolution of fibrinous adhesions in the inflamed peritoneum and pleura (102).
- *The lining of the uterus.*
- *Many malignant tumors*, which may also do the opposite, that is, secrete thromboplastic factors.

A different protein is urokinase, a plasminogen activator found in urine, where it may have the function of keeping the renal tubules open (63).

Urokinase is synthesized by a variety of cells including cultured endothelium (16). Both tPA and urokinase are also different from streptokinase, another plasminogen activator (but not an enzyme) obtained from streptococci.

The current great interest in plasminogen activators is due to their therapeutic use: they all lead to the dissolution of fibrin and therefore of thrombi and thromboemboli. The first activators to be tried were streptokinase and urokinase; both work, but they also attack fibrinogen in its fluid phase and therefore cause a general depletion of fibrinogen, which is a hazard. Another drawback of streptokinase is that it is antigenic. In contrast, tPA has a much higher affinity for fibrin and therefore acts much more specifically where it is needed (14); it can be given intravenously, and it is not antigenic. This is why the production of recombinant tPA for antithrombotic therapy was hailed as a major step forward. It was obtained from a human melanoma, a rare therapeutic use of a malignant tumor (106).

Nothing is perfect, however; tPA cannot distinguish between fibrin in a thrombus and fibrin in a purposeful hemostatic clot. Therefore, a major complication is hemorrhage (70, 79).

To demonstrate fibrinolysis microscopically, a simple method is to cut a section of fresh tissue, overlay it with a thin layer of fibrin (which always has plasminogen adsorbed to it), and incubate it at 37°C. Wherever tPA is present, a hole is digested in the fibrin overlay, which is easily shown by staining (Figure 22.17). According to this test the endothelium induces fibrinolysis—but strangely, not everywhere. Even in the cross section of a single vessel, one side may produce fibrinolysis, the other not. The reason is not known (57).

Inhibitors of fibrinolysis are mainly alpha-2-antiplasmin, alpha-1-antitrypsin, alpha-2-macroglobulin, and plasminogen activator inhibitor (PAi). The endothelium, which secretes tPA, also secretes a tPA inhibitor.

Role of the Vascular Wall in Hemostasis

If we think of the vascular system in terms of container and content, the content performs the main tasks in hemostasis: platelets form a plug, the

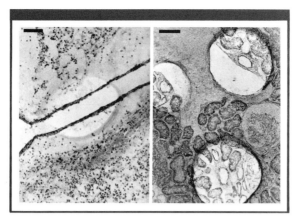

FIGURE 22.17

Demonstration of fibrinolysis by the endothelium in frozen sections of unfixed rat tissues. Each section is overlaid with a thin layer of fibrin, incubated at 37°C for 20 minutes, and stained with hematoxylin and eosin. Clear circular zone indicates fibrinolysis. *Left:* Longitudinal section of a small vein. Why the fibrinolysis is limited to one segment of the vein (a common finding) is not known. **Bar** = 100 μm. *Right:* Renal cortex. The three circles of fibrinolysis are centered on veins. **Bar** = 100 μm. (Reproduced with permission from [48].)

blood clots. However, the vascular wall is not passive. As we have seen, the arterial media contracts (little is known about contraction of veins and capillaries), and the subendothelium acts as a trap for platelets. We still need to discuss the key role of the endothelium in clotting (49, 50).

Normally, of course, the endothelium does not favor clotting. Indeed, it is one of the very few cell types that can live with the blood without clotting it; only the leukocytes, platelets, and red blood cells can do the same. This property frustrates the makers of artificial blood vessels, who have found it very difficult to copy.

The endothelial surface is extremely complex. It turns out that the endothelium performs a *balancing act* between opposing and favoring the clotting mechanism. At first sight it seems mind-boggling that the endothelium should ever be programmed to favor clotting and thrombosis (Figure 22.18); this conflicting behavior has even been labeled schizophrenic (33). However, such are the facts, and there are times when intravascular clotting might be life-saving—for example, to limit the spread of infection.

In adopting M. Gimbrone's diagram of the endothelial balancing act concept (Figure 22.18) (50), we have taken the liberty of tilting the balance toward the anticlotting action because we

find it difficult to accept that the endothelium is always on the verge of betrayal. We will now briefly comment on these opposing endothelial tendencies, using Figure 22.18 as a guideline.

ENDOTHELIAL MECHANISMS THAT INHIBIT INTRAVASCULAR CLOTTING AND THROMBOSIS

At least six protective mechanisms are known (see Figure 22.18). They inhibit key steps of the thrombotic process, beginning with platelet aggregation.

The Endothelium Opposes Platelet Aggregation

- Secretion of prostacyclin (PGI$_2$) begins as soon as the endothelial cell is exposed to thrombin, a platelet aggregator. Prostacyclin is a powerful inhibitor of platelet aggregation and the most powerful vasodilator known. Vasodilatation increases blood flow, which tends to wipe away the platelets. PGI$_2$ is secreted by the endothelium when it is injured or stimulated by a number of agents (p. 359).
- Adenosine diphosphate (ADP), a strong aggregator secreted by platelets, is converted by the endothelium to adenine nucleotides, which inhibit platelet aggregation (18).
- Secretion of endothelium-derived relaxing factor (EDRF), which is thought to be NO (nitric oxide) (76).

The Endothelium Opposes Thrombin

- Thrombin is captured by thrombomodulin, a protein on the endothelium, and the resulting complex activates plasma protein C, a powerful anticoagulant.
- Thrombin generation is reduced: heparin-like molecules on the endothelial surface conspire with plasma antithrombin II to inactivate all clotting factors from IXa to IIa.

The Endothelium Favors Fibrinolysis It secretes two plasminogen activators, tPA and urokinase.

ENDOTHELIAL MECHANISMS THAT FAVOR INTRAVASCULAR CLOTTING

The *clotting activities* of the endothelium are aimed at the same targets as above, but with opposite intent.

The Endothelium Favors Platelet Aggregation

- von Willebrand factor (vWF), stored in the Weibel–Palade bodies, is the "glue" that enables platelets to stick to the subendothelium.

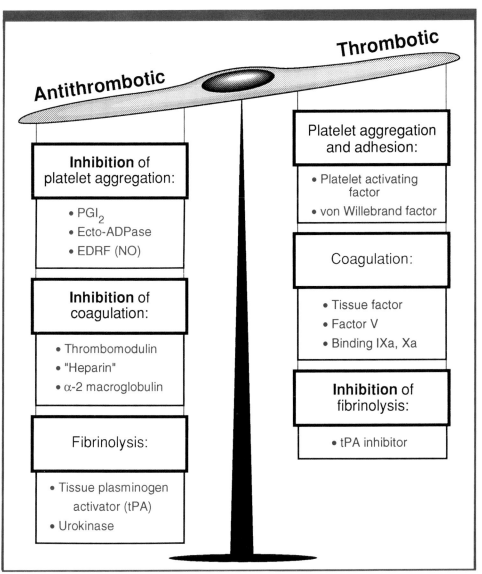

FIGURE 22.18
The endothelial balance. The surface of the endothelial cells can either favor or inhibit thrombosis, depending on its functional condition. (Modified from [50].)

- The endothelium can be induced to secrete that omnipotent inflammatory mediator platelet activating factor (PAF), at least *in vitro*.

The Endothelium Favors the Coagulation Cascade

- Factors V, IX, and X bind to the endothelial surface.
- Tissue factor (thromboplastin), the very source of the extrinsic coagulation mechanism, is expressed by endothelial surfaces. This response is induced by agents such as interleukin-1 and tumor necrosis factor; it requires some time (hours) to take effect because it requires protein synthesis.

The Endothelium Opposes Fibrinolysis

- The accumulation of fibrin is encouraged by an endothelium-derived inhibitor of tPA, called plasminogen activator inhibitor (PAi).

THE HEMOSTATIC MECHANISM: A CAPSULE OVERVIEW

In summary, here is the sequence of events that stop bleeding:

- Blood comes in contact with connective tissue.
- Hageman factor is activated by collagen.
- Hageman factor activates the clotting, fibrinolytic and kinin cascades.
- Fibrin is formed.

- Platelets adhere to collagen and become activated.
- Activated platelets help the clotting process.
- Platelets pile up to form a mechanical plug.
- Severed arteries contract (due to platelet products, probably also kinins).
- Fibrin binds plasminogen and plasminogen activator (tPA).
- tPA is activated by binding and digests fibrin.
- Fibrin may or may not continue to form, depending on the relative rates of clotting and fibrinolysis.

Such is, greatly simplified, the intricate story of hemostasis. There are still many holes to fill. For example, anyone who sees—for the first time—a surgical scalpel parting human skin is impressed by the scanty hemorrhage, other than a couple of "bleeders" that may require a hemostat. Millions of capillaries are severed; yet after the cut has been dabbed with a swab or two, it remains dry. Exactly how the capillaries are plugged is not clear; an old light-microscopic study suggests that many are sealed much as a plastic tube is sealed by heat (62).

We will close with a clotting episode that we find especially interesting, also because it links the beach and the laboratory, in the tradition of Metchnikoff.

The horseshoe crab (*Limulus polyphemus*) lives on the eastern seaboard of North America (Figure

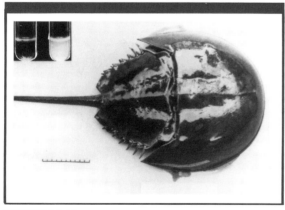

FIGURE 22.19
A dorsal view of *Limulus polyphemus*, the horseshoe crab, much reduced (scale in cm.). The inset illustrates the Limulus test: the test tube at left contains a lysate of Limulus amebocytes; it does not clot. The test tube at right shows clotting after the addition of endotoxin. (Adapted from [67].)

22.19). Its blood contains only one type of cell, called amebocyte. Amebocytes congregate at a site of injury and degranulate, recalling the behavior of platelets; they release a protein that (by itself) does not cause limulus blood to coagulate (Figure 11.11) (68). One day, about 1956, the biologist F.B. Bang had the opportunity to autopsy some horseshoe crabs that had died of an unknown cause. He noticed that the blood had massively coagulated; the crabs were also infected by an endotoxin-producing vibrio. Pursuing the matter, Levin and Bang showed that the protein secreted by the amebocytes had been clotted by endotoxin. The current practice of testing plasma and cerebrospinal fluid for endotoxin by assaying them with limulus blood (the limulus test) was born in this manner.

Thrombosis

Sometimes the normal hemostatic mechanisms are turned on inappropriately, and solid clumps (**thrombi**) develop in the blood vessels or in the heart. The basic components of thrombi and those of hemostatic plugs are the same—platelets, fibrin, and red and white blood cells—but they are put together differently because they form under different conditions.

Today this interpretation of a thrombus seems self-explanatory, but in Virchow's time it seemed logical that a thrombus was an inflammatory secretion of the vascular wall. The first illustration showing that thrombi and emboli could be formed by platelets came from the hand of Bizzozero in 1882 in the paper in which he proposed the term *platelet* (Figure 22.20) (15). Shortly thereafter, elegant experiments in Germany showed that a puncture in a vein is sealed by a small clot that is prolonged toward the lumen by a small thrombus (Figure 22.21) (41): an excellent illustration of the concept that thrombosis is hemostasis in the wrong place. Many of these experiments were done on living transparent membranes, and improved optics showed that the phenomenon of margination, known for leukocytes, also occurs with platelets (Figure 22.22).

To qualify as a thrombus, a solid intravascular clump must fulfill three conditions: it must be formed (a) within the heart or vessels, (b) from constituents of the blood, and (c) during life.

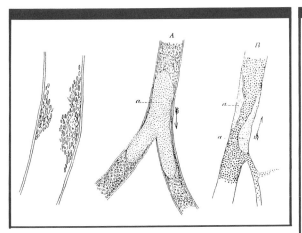

FIGURE 22.20
First illustration of thrombosis as observed in living guinea pig mesentery by Bizzozero (1882). *Left:* Parietal thrombus consisting of platelets and occasional leukocytes, in an arteriole after it was gently pressed with a needle. *Center:* Arteriole embolized at the level of a bifurcation; this embolus (**a**) later disintegrated and vanished (compare with the retinal embolus shown in Figure 23.12). *Right:* Two parietal thrombi consisting of platelets, in a small vein. (Reproduced with permission from [15].)

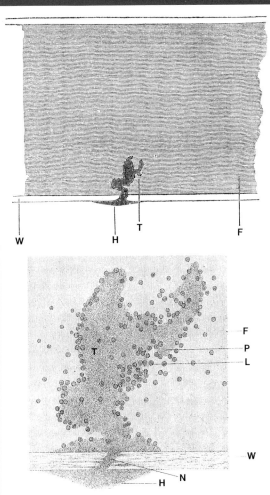

FIGURE 22.21
This early study of thrombosis (1886–1888) contributed to prove the role of platelets. *Top:* Enlarged sketch of a jugular vein of a dog, punctured with a needle, excised and fixed 25 minutes later. A small thrombus (**T**) has formed over the puncture site. **W** = wall of vein; **H** = hemorrhage; **F** = flowing blood. *Bottom:* Microscopic preparation of the thrombus. Its surface is covered with leukocytes (**L**). **P** = granular mass of platelets (individual platelets are not visible at this power); **N** = needle track. (Adapted from [40]. Lettering modified.)

The purpose of these qualifications is to exclude extravascular clots that develop from spilled blood and the clots that form in many vessels after death.

What kinds of solid masses could arise from the blood? Because a thrombus represents a malfunction of the clotting mechanism, we can expect—alone or in combination—(a) platelet aggregates, (b) clotted blood, and (c) fibrin. They will be called, respectively, platelet thrombi, red thrombi, and fibrin thrombi.

> *A perennial source of confusion to students is that an honest red clot, formed in the living vascular system by the regular clotting mechanism, is not called a clot; it is a red thrombus. This terminology was introduced by pathologists working in autopsy rooms, where it is essential to find out whether "clots" happened before or after death. The word thrombus is meant to convey instantly the notion "formed in vivo." An acceptable alternative to red thrombus might be a red clot formed while the patient was still alive, but red thrombus is shorter.*
>
> *Many physicians who need to explain an occluded coronary artery in lay terms, will tell their patients "you had a clot." This is acceptable for purposes of communication.*

Pathogenesis of Thrombosis: Virchow's Triad

It was Virchow, once again, who adopted the ancient term *thrómbos* ("lump" or "clot") to represent a modern concept. Tradition also credits Virchow with pronouncing, in 1845, the law that thrombosis depends on three kinds of changes:

- changes in the vascular wall (endothelial damage)
- changes in flow (slow or turbulent flow)
- changes in the blood (hypercoagulability)

This is the famous **triad of Virchow**, still perfectly valid, and now firmly rooted in National Board multiple choice exams.

> *For the record, there is no mention of a "triad" as such in any of Virchow's papers. This arcane term seems to have been an improvement by posterity.*

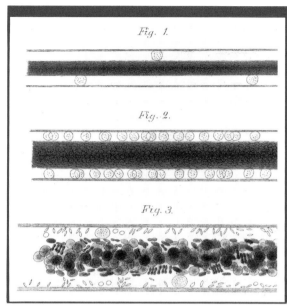

FIGURE 22.22
Early vascular changes in inflammation observed in the omentum of a living dog "about one foot high," as studied in 1886. *Top:* "A vessel" (probably a venule) with accelerated blood flow. The axial stream is obvious; it flows so fast that the individual red blood cells cannot be identified. In the clear plasma zone, occasional leukocytes can be seen rolling along. *Center:* Small vein in which flow is beginning to slow; the red blood cells are now identifiable. Many white blood cells adhere to the wall. *Bottom:* More advanced stasis in another venule. Not only leukocytes but also platelets adhere to the wall (early thrombosis). These observations were made 21 years after Cohnheim and just after the discovery of platelets. Cohnheim (1867) had missed the platelets; perhaps his microscope was not as powerful. (Reproduced with permission from [40].)

FIGURE 22.23
Extraction of an arterial embolus with the Fogarty catheter. **A:** Catheter is pushed through the embolus. **B:** Balloon is inflated. **C:** Catheter is retrieved, pulling the embolus with it. (Adapted from [45].)

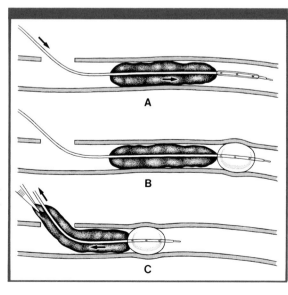

However, Virchow did discuss each of the three elements in various writings, beginning with the second lecture he ever gave, at age 23. The manuscript of this 1845 lecture, which was perceived as revolutionary, was rediscovered in Germany in 1966 by two American scholars, Kenneth Brinkhous and Elizabeth Sommer. As far as we know, it has not been translated (21, 22). Anyway, this episode confirms that whatever Virchow said tended to become a law.

What is still not so clear is how the triad theory should be interpreted. Does it mean that all three elements are necessary? Endothelial damage alone, for example, starts a platelet "carpet"; this thin coating of platelets does not continue to grow into a substantial thrombus, but it will do so if endothelial damage is followed by stasis (82). Stasis alone does not work either; however, stasis combined with hypercoagulability can create a thrombus even without apparent endothelial damage. It seems fair to conclude that thrombosis may occur even if the triad is not complete; just two of the conditions suffice.

The best proof is the strange story of the "ball thrombus." If the mitral valve becomes stenotic, blood is retained in the left atrium, where it forms an eddy. In the long run a free, spherical thrombus can form in this eddy: under these conditions a change in the endothelial surface is probably not involved (the ball thrombus, incidentally, can become a source of emboli or lead to sudden death by plugging the mitral valve, but it can also be removed by surgery).

Endothelial Damage That endothelial damage has a role is easily proven by studying what happens when the endothelium is mechanically removed. A favorite method is to slip a Fogarty catheter into the chosen vessel (Figure 22.23) and inflating the tiny balloon in its tip. As the catheter is pulled back, the balloon wipes away the endothelium (since 1966 this experimental procedure has been called "ballooning") (8). Within minutes the denuded intima is carpeted with platelets (Figure 22.24), which promptly swell and degranulate (Figure 22.25).

The reader may wonder how a tool chosen by experimenters to produce vascular damage can also be used on humans for a therapeutic purpose. It is a fact that an embolectomized artery is also necessarily ballooned. However, in practice this does not seem to matter too much because the coating of platelets does not grow; anticoagulants are given, and eventually the endothelium regenerates. New endothelial cells grow out of the mouths (ostia) of arterial branches, as well as from the intima upstream and downstream.

Platelets adhere to the arterial subendothelium for the same reason they form hemostatic plugs: their surface receptors interlock with factor VIII (vWF) bound to the matrix. In arteries these carpetlike platelet thrombi do not grow because the swift current washes away the platelets and the chemical mediators that activate them; small clusters of platelets that are torn off become emboli downstream. Thrombi can be obtained *in vitro* by perfusing a ballooned artery at a low rate of flow (Figure 22.26).

In real life, endothelial damage occurs in many settings: after trauma or surgery, in inflamed tissues, in immune responses (such as in grafts), and on the surfaces of atherosclerotic plaques when they break open.

> *In the heart, when a myocardial infarct reaches close to the endocardium (the thin layer that lines the heart cavities), endocardial thrombosis is the rule. But in this case the mechanism is complex: the myocardial tissue that dies beneath the endocardium releases inflammatory mediators as well as thromboplastin (tissue factor), whereby the clotting mechanism is triggered on the endothelial surface.*

Sluggish Flow The effect of sluggish flow is self-evident: it gives platelets a better chance to stick and clotting factors a better chance to accumulate. Low flow helps us understand why thrombosis is much more frequent in veins than in arteries (there is even a special word for venous thrombosis, *phlebothrombosis*); furthermore, the valves in the veins favor thrombosis because they produce eddies and pockets of stagnant blood (Figure 22.27).

Serum-induced thrombosis. We can demonstrate the importance of flow in relation to thrombosis by a classic experiment on rabbit veins (34,111, 114). The first step is to find out what happens when blood in the vein does not flow at all. Anesthetize a rabbit, and carefully expose about 5 cm of a jugular vein. Gently apply two clamps on the vein about 4 cm apart. An hour or so later, slit the vein between the clamps: surprise! The blood in the isolated segment is still fluid. This shows that stasis alone cannot initiate the clotting process. Any clotting factors that were released into the vein by the surgical procedure have been successfully opposed by the anticlotting mechanisms of the vein's endothelium. Remember that stasis induces the endothelium to

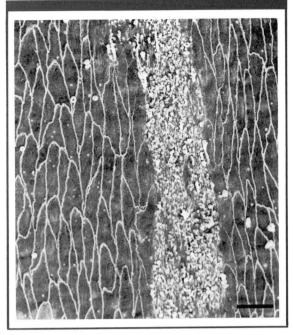

FIGURE 22.24 Changes in the surface of a rat aorta after ballooning. *Left:* Carpet of platelets has been deposited on the denuded surface 15 minutes after it was scratched with a nylon filament. Scanning electron microscopy after staining with silver. **Bars** = 25 μm. (Reproduced with permission from [98].)

favor fibrinolysis by secreting more plasminogen activator, tPA.

> *It may have been a surprise for the newcomer to learn that the blood between two ligatures is still fluid after 1 hour, but F. Zahn knew in 1875 that it is still fluid after 5 days (116).*

Now let us create a combination of two of Virchow's three elements: stasis plus hypercoagulable blood. In another rabbit, expose the jugular

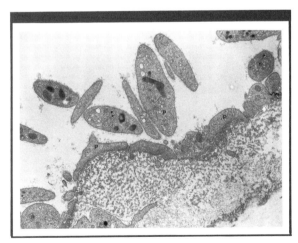

FIGURE 22.25
Electron microscopy of a rat aorta, 15 minutes after it was gently scratched with a nylon thread, removing the endothelium. A carpet of platelets (**P**) has covered the denuded intima; a second, incomplete layer of platelets has formed just above the first. **Bar** = ~1 μm. (Courtesy of Dr. Michael A. Reidy, University of Washington, Seattle, WA.)

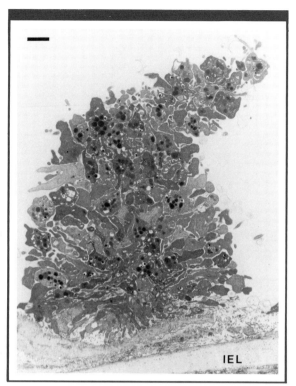

FIGURE 22.26
Typical platelet thrombus, produced *in vitro* by circulating blood for 10 minutes over a rabbit aorta deprived of its endothelium. Note that the platelets at the surface of the thrombus still contain some granules, whereas the platelets that were first in contact with the internal elastic lamina (**IEL**) have degranulated. **Bar** = 1 μm. (Reproduced with permission from [7].)

injected serum have no effect where the blood is circulating; but where the blood is held in complete stasis, they make it clot. This method can be used also for producing experimental pulmonary emboli, using two clamps on a peripheral vein (113). It is conceivable that this serum-induced thrombosis might operate also in clinical conditions, for example after an accident, when the blood is temporarily hypercoagulable (112).

An interesting addendum: if fresh serum is injected intravenously in a rabbit with the portal vein tied off, venous thrombosis will occur throughout the body. This proves that the liver is very active in removing clotting factors from the blood (34, 64).

Clinically, the combination of stasis plus another element of Virchow's triad occurs classically in pregnancy. Pressure on the large veins of the pelvis creates stasis, and the blood is hypercoagulable, conditions that favor thrombosis in the lower limbs (64). The same is true for bedridden patients, especially after surgery; their leg veins suffer from stasis and their blood is notoriously hypercoagulable.

Concerning the dangers of immobilization, it has been suggested that even sitting on chairs can be hazardous; chairless cultures are said to enjoy a very low incidence of thromboembolism (1). However, there are many other differences between sitting and squatting cultures, including the amount of dietary fiber eaten and the way toilets are constructed. According to the theory of Dr. Burkitt, a low-fiber diet requires more effort for defecating; this results in increased pressure on the veins of the lower limbs,

vein without clamping it, and inject into the bloodstream (using a different vein) 1.3 ml of fresh serum per kg of body weight (human serum will do). This serum is loaded with activated clotting factors. However, no adverse reaction occurs in the rabbit even though the rabbit's blood, if tested, is more prone than normal to clot (34). Then, within 1 minute, apply the two clamps to the jugular vein; 10 minutes later the blood in the vein is clotted. Why? Because the clotting factors contained in the

FIGURE 22.27
Stages in the progression of a venous thrombus. **A:** Typically, the thrombus begins in the recess behind a valve. **B,C:** the thrombus grows downstream by a succession of white layers (platelets) and red layers (fibrin with entrapped red blood cells). If the lumen is occluded (**D**) the blood clots proximally and/or distally to the obstruction. At this point the thrombus consists of a mixed white and red "head" attached to the wall and one or two red "tails" loose in the lumen. The formation of tails depends on the local conditions of flow as determined by the vein's branching pattern. (Adapted from [11].)

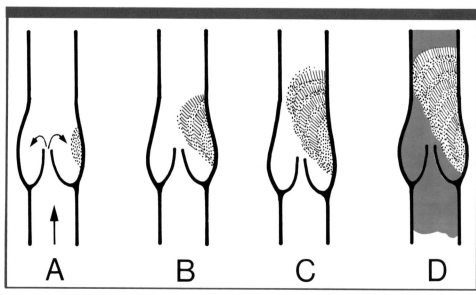

especially when sitting on toilets. These circumstances favor the extreme degree of venous dilatation called varicose veins. Primal cultures do not suffer from this condition (p. 823).

Hypercoagulability

The third item of Virchow's triad is obvious but hard to define. There is no doubt that hypercoagulability exists. Indeed, there are at least 48 conditions—ranging in seriousness from cancer through pregnancy to prolonged air travel—known to be associated with an increased risk of thrombosis (6a, 64). Considering the large number of clotting and anticlotting agents that could malfunction, this list of risky situations should not come as a surprise. However, no single blood change can account for all the hypercoagulable states; there is no single laboratory test for hypercoagulability.

A few mechanisms are clear, especially among the inherited disorders, such as lack of antithrombin III (84) or proteins C or S (27). Among the acquired disorders, increased platelet stickiness or platelet hyperreactivity is best known. Increased aggregability of platelets in the morning is associated with an increased frequency of myocardial infarction in the morning (107). Smoking activates the Hageman factor (factor XII) (9); pregnancy and recent surgery are accompanied by increased levels of fibrinogen and factor VIII (both are acute-phase reactants, p. 491). The pathogenesis of atherosclerosis appears to include a unique pathway to thrombosis: a high level of the plasma protein lipoprotein(a), which interferes with fibrinolysis (54, 81).

Birth and Growth of a Thrombus

Knowing the three basic conditions that favor thrombosis, we will now follow, step by step, the development of an actual thrombus, as well as we understand it, in a deep vein in the calf of a bedridden, postsurgical patient.

PLATELET AGGREGATION

As platelets flow along the vein, they are (as usual) more concentrated along the endothelium, because they are the smallest formed elements in the blood. Recall the river analogy: rocks flow in the center of the stream, sand is deposited along the banks (see Figure 22.22). Because we are dealing with a postoperative patient, the platelets are not normal; *in vitro* tests show that platelets of such patients aggregate more easily than normal. As they flow past a valve in a vein, they are caught in the eddy behind it, form an aggregate, and settle on the wall. This step is not well understood.

Here we pause for an admission of ignorance. Nobody has ever proven that the endothelium is really damaged in the veins of the calf in a bedridden patient. To the contrary, histology and even electron microscopy (5) of early venous thrombi show that the endothelium is structurally intact (59). This finding is rather disturbing because platelets are not supposed to adhere to normal endothelium; perhaps in a bedridden patient the endothelium of some large veins is functionally abnormal or somehow activated by the mild trauma of continued pressure (activated endothelium expresses tissue factor and starts the clotting cascade, p. 625).

Once attached to the wall, the platelets are activated, swell, spread out, and become sticky; more platelets pile over them, favored by the eddy. A few leukocytes also adhere, trapped by chemotactic factors released by the platelets.

FIBRIN FORMATION

Then comes an odd event: threads of fibrin grow out of the platelet layer just as in a hemostatic plug; visualize them swaying in the lazy current, trapping red blood cells (Figure 22.28). In this way a fluffy, red carpet is laid over the platelets (red because of the entrapped red blood cells). The surface of this fibrin layer is thrombogenic because platelets stick to nascent fibrin, so the fibrin layer

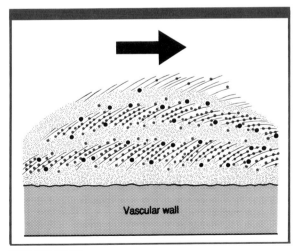

Vascular wall

FIGURE 22.28
Layered growth of a mixed thrombus. The first layer, whitish to the naked eye, consists of platelets (**P**); its surface favors coagulation and gives rise to filaments of fibrin that entrap red blood cells and a few white blood cells. This new (red) layer is thrombogenic and causes the deposition of a new layer of platelets; and so the cycle repeats.

FIGURE 22.29 **See color plate 20.** Occluding thrombi in the popliteal and femoral veins. The thrombi are mixed (red and white). Note that the artery (**arrow**) is spared. From a patient who died of adenocarcinoma of the stomach. Scale in mm.

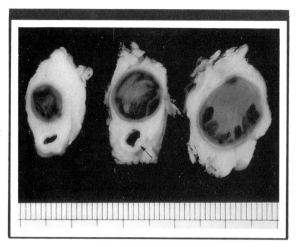

is soon buried under another layer of platelets; then these platelets generate their own carpet of fibrin filaments and red cells; and so the process continues. Note the behavior of the leukocytes, which tend to stick to the surfaces of the platelet layers, perhaps in response to chemotactic factors released by the platelets (20).

> *Platelets stick to fibrin while it is being generated, but not when it is fully cross-linked. Neutrophils inhibit platelet activation, while red blood cells enhance it— mechanisms unclear (76).*

LINES OF ZAHN

In the way just described, *the thrombus develops as a laminated structure*, which makes it very different from clots after death or *in vitro*. The layering is rarely as perfect as shown in our diagram because flow conditions are irregular, but red and white parts are always recognizable, hence the old name *mixed thrombus* (Figure 22.29). The two components are visible to the naked eye on a cut surface of a thrombus; the layers of platelets are whitish, and sandwiched between them are red layers of fibrin and entrapped red blood cells. These layers are now known worldwide as the **lines of Zahn** (Figure 22.30). Sometimes the lines run perpendicular to the surface; in this case the white layers of platelets stand out as white ripples alternating with sunken red lines (the latter have undergone clot retraction or syneresis, p. 619). It has been aptly said that the white ripples of compacted platelets on the surface of a thrombus are "not unlike geological strata which reach the surface of a thrombus as an outcrop" (59). This gross aspect has earned the name of coralline thrombus in the British literature (53) (Figure 22.31). Some thrombi have few if any orderly lines, but it is still clear that they are composed of white and red parts.

> *Friedrich Zahn described his ripples, if not his lines, over a century ago at the Institute of Pathology in Geneva, Switzerland. Zahn was probably the first to define thrombi as red, white, or mixed (116). On cross sections of mixed thrombi he noticed that white and red material formed irregular layers rather than a neat onion-skin pattern, "perhaps due to disturbed*

FIGURE 22.30 Lines of Zahn (**Z**) in a parietal venous thrombus. The lines of Zahn consist of aggregated platelets; they are connected by festoons of fibrin filaments with entrapped red blood cells. **L:** Lumen. **G:** Granulation tissue. **W:** Wall of the vein. **Bar** = 500 μm.

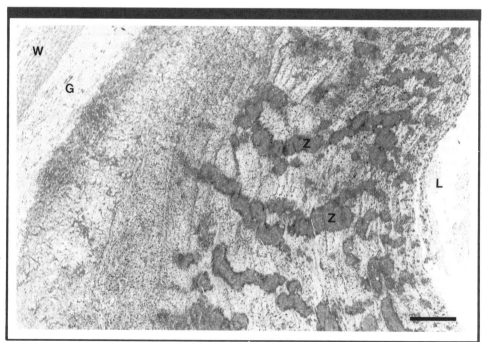

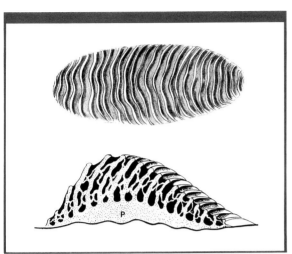

FIGURE 22.31
Layered thrombus. *Top:* Surface of a thrombus as it appears through a magnifying glass. The ridges, perpendicular to the direction of flow, are the original "ripple lines" of Zahn and consist of aggregated platelets. *Bottom:* Cross section shows that the layers of platelets (**P**) are interconnected; between them are strands of fibrin containing red blood cells (**black areas**). Thrombi of this appearance are called coralline. (Reproduced with permission from [53].)

axial direction of blood flow" (Figure 22.32). Later he observed that the surfaces of some mixed thrombi were rippled. He compared these ripples with the ripples in the mud on the bank of the river Arve, along which he walked on the way to work. He actually suggested that the ripples on the thrombi and on the river bank might develop by the same hydrodynamic mechanism. The great German pathologist Ludwig Aschoff tried to prove the hydrodynamic explanation, but his experiments were inconclusive (4). The mechanism of layering, as we now see it, is a result of platelet physiology interacting with blood flow. From what we have said, it should be clear that the surface rippling is a continuation of the layering of the thrombotic mass.

THE MANY FATES OF A THROMBUS

The thrombus continues to grow until the vessel is occluded or until antithrombus forces gain the upper hand. If the thrombus merely restricts the lumen, the thrombus is called **parietal** (Figure 22.33); if it fills the lumen completely it is called **occlusive** (Figure 22.29). The heartening feature of thrombosis, however, is that it is self-limiting. It is fortunately rare for a thrombus to spread into several communicating veins; such *propagating thrombi* represent failure of the control systems.

The most important mechanism for limiting the spread of thrombosis is blood flow, as illustrated by the serum-induced thrombosis mentioned earlier.

Another example: if a thrombus becomes occlusive, flow stops; the clotting factors oozing from the mass, if they are not washed away, will cause the static blood to clot. Therefore, the laminated head of the thrombus is prolonged by a tail of red **thrombus** (53). The clotting stops at the level of the nearest branch, where flow dilutes the clotting factors. The red tail points downstream, upstream, or both ways, depending on the location of the branches and the course of blood flow. Note: The head of a thrombus is the only part that is attached to the wall, often to a valve; the tail is free, especially after contraction has occurred (*syneresis,* p. 619), which makes it especially prone to break loose. A thrombus filling a superficial vein, especially in a leg, can sometimes be palpated through the skin.

The possible fates of a thrombus are many (Figure 22.34). The following description applies to both venous and arterial thrombi.

- *A thrombus may be dissolved* in a matter of hours, probably with the help of enzymes from trapped leukocytes; fibrinolysis is accomplished by plasmin adsorbed to the fibrin filaments. The mass breaks up into microscopic lumps that cause no significant damage as they embolize the lungs.

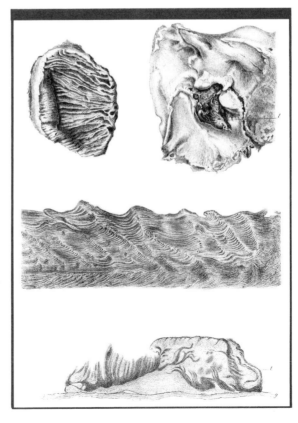

FIGURE 22.32
Structure of a thrombus as illustrated by Zahn in 1891. *Top and center:* Thrombi with a typical rippled surface. *Bottom:* Cross section shows banded structures (lines of Zahn). (Reproduced from [117].)

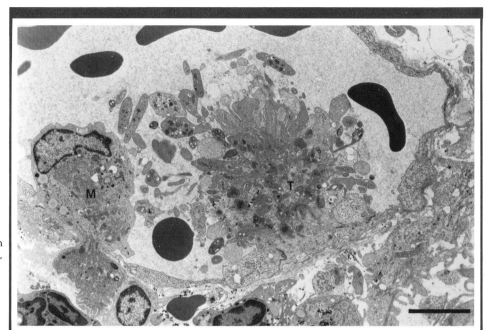

FIGURE 22.33
Microscopic parietal thrombus (**T**) in a rat venule, in a focus of aseptic inflammation 48 hours old. Thrombi are common in inflamed tissues; the mechanism is not clear. Note the macrophage (**M**) performing diapedesis. **Bar** = 5 μm.

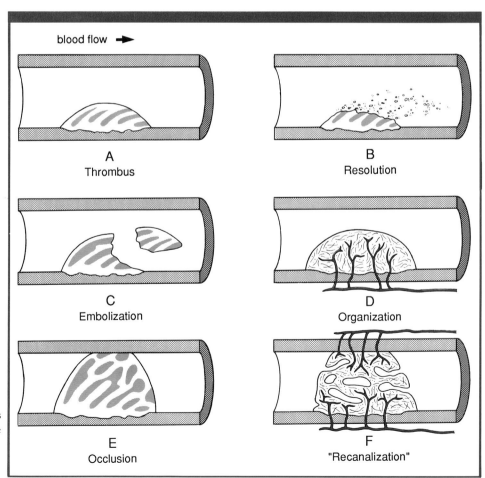

FIGURE 22.34
Fates of a thrombus. In **F,** no vessel is shown running all the way across the thrombus ("recanalizing" the occlusion) because this event is not proven.

- *A thrombus may break off* and become an embolus (see Chapter 23).
- *A thrombus may become covered by cells and be organized.* This process has not been adequately studied. It seems that the surface of the thrombus can be prevented from growing any further by the endothelial cells and monocytes that spread over it in a matter of hours (62a); monocytes too have an antithrombotic surface, as we can surmise from the fact that they circulate in the bloodstream without inducing clots. In the meantime, the thrombus is also attacked at its base: cells and vessels penetrate from the adventitia and reabsorb it, a process (*organization*) that requires several days at least. This means that some chemical message from the thrombus has diffused across the wall of the vein and alerted the surrounding tissues (it has been suggested that a thrombus can be entirely organized by mononuclear cells circulating in the blood, that is, monocytes and possibly stem cells capable of giving rise to connective tissue [43a, 66]. This heretical but fascinating mechanism needs to be confirmed). Once organized, a parietal thrombus leaves on the wall of the vessel a fibrous scar, pigmented for some time with hemosiderin. An organized occluding thrombus appears in cross section like a fibrous mass perforated by vessels (see Figure 22.34) (35, 59).

From the few studies available, the cells that organize thrombi seem to be a mixture of blood-derived monocytes/macrophages (66), endothelial cells, medial and adventitial cells, and ingrowing adventitial vessels. The covering of the thrombus surface by cells is slow (weeks) (105). How the medial smooth muscle cells participate is not known. *Amyloid* is sometimes found in old thrombi, perhaps because plasma precursors of amyloid are deposited in the thrombus and macrophages turn them into amyloid (p. 270) (51, 52).

It is said that an occluding thrombus may be organized and "recanalized." Experimentally, venous thrombi are said to recanalize much more extensively than arterial thrombi (44). **Recanalization** is supposed to mean that new channels, lined with endothelium, are running across the occlusion and restoring blood flow. This fa-

vorable outcome may well occur, but it could be demonstrated only by studying serial sections of a thrombus; as far as we know, this has not been done. The presence of many small vessels in a thrombus suggests that we are looking at adventitial vessels that have simply organized the thrombus. It is unlikely that adventitial vessels would communicate with the lumen of the occluded vessel (35), especially if it is an artery: the ingrowing adventitial capillaries would have a pressure of roughly 20 mm Hg against a pressure about four times greater in the artery.

- *A thrombus may partially calcify* like any mass of necrotic material.

For obscure reasons, little white beads of calcium salts 3 or 4 mm in diameter are commonly found in the small veins of the pelvis. They are called phleboliths and are presumed to be calcified thrombi. How they become spherical and lie loose, yet trapped, in the veins nobody knows. Pathologists and radiologists have learned to discount them as insignificant oddities.

DIFFERENCES BETWEEN ARTERIAL AND VENOUS THROMBI

Arterial thrombi develop under conditions of high shear; they are smaller, more compact, white, and tend to remain parietal. Lamination may therefore be missing. Thrombi in small arteries are more dangerous than venous thrombi because arteries are much less anastomosed than veins. In arteries, occlusive thrombi usually form over an atherosclerotic plaque that has cracked open; they are not much larger than the head of a match, but in a coronary artery they can kill (Figure 22.35).

Arterial thrombi lead us to a brief discussion on aneurysms. An **aneurysm** is a local dilatation of an artery due to a weakening of the arterial wall. The weakening mechanism in large arteries is almost always atherosclerosis. Similar local dilatations occur in veins, but they are known as **varices.** Aneurysms can be shaped like a sac (*saccular*) or like a spindle (*fusiform*). Saccular aneurysms of the aorta may appear as huge, bulging, hemispherical pockets 10–15 cm in diameter; they are usually lined, and sometimes filled, with thrombus.

Dissecting aneurysms are mentioned here for completeness but they are of special nature. They

FIGURE 22.35
Cross section of
a human coro-
nary artery se-
verely affected by
atherosclerosis;
the lumen (**L**) is
reduced to about
⅓ of the original
diameter. **C** =
calcifications;
I = thickened
intima; **asterisk**
= a thrombus
which was the
cause of death;
two dark areas =
hemorrhage. **Bar**
= 500 μm.

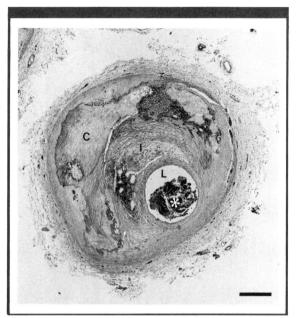

occur virtually only in the aorta and its major branches. The inner layer of the arterial wall suddenly tears open; blood rushes into the tear and proceeds to dissect (separate) the media into two layers, sometimes along the entire length of the aorta. The blood may then find its way back into the lumen through a second tear. All this may take place in a matter of minutes. Survival is rare but possible.

The thrombus in a saccular aneurysm is a compact, firm, rubbery mass that has patently been there for months or years. Bits of it can be carried off as emboli, but the mass itself may help survival because it prevents the thin aneurysmal pocket from bursting under the aortic pressure. These massive thrombi have one unusual charac-teristic: they never become organized, they simply "sit" on the thinned arterial wall, which tolerates them with the utmost indifference. Why? Platelets are loaded with inflammatory mediators, and organization could be helpful by reinforcing the paper-thin wall and anchoring the thrombus. The answer, we believe, is that no chemical message ever reaches the adventitia in concentrations large enough to be perceived. As the aneurysm begins to form, over months if not years, all mediators arising in the thrombus are washed away by the torrential arterial flow; furthermore, the muscular media of large arteries is a major obstacle to outward diffusion. Later the wall thins, but by then the thrombus has grown so thick (up to several centimeters) that outward diffusion from freshly deposited platelets becomes negligible.

GROSS ASPECTS OF THROMBI

A thrombus can cause death; a clot formed postmortem obviously cannot. It can be critical to distinguish the two, especially in the setting of a medicolegal autopsy.

Differences Between Thrombi and Postmortem Clots Typical thrombi are laminated with lines of Zahn and are apposed to the intimal surface; even if the lamination is not present, a mixture of red and white parts is the signature of a mixed thrombus. Pure platelet thrombi are whitish and tend to crumble. Red thrombi are the real challenge to pathologists, but usually they are attached at some point to a mixed thrombus. Postmortem clots are rubbery, shiny, and usually red. They are never laminated because lamination requires blood flow, and nowhere are they at-tached to the intima.

A peculiar feature of postmortem clots is that they can be made of two superimposed layers, one red and one white. This is a result of erythrocyte sedimenta-tion after death. When the heart stops, the blood within it clots very slowly, and the red blood cells have the time to settle, perhaps more so if the patient's sedimentation rate was high. When clotting finally occurs, the upper part of the blood mass, which is free of red blood cells, clots into a yellowish, gelatinous mass that has the time-honored but somewhat repulsive name of **chicken fat clot.** *The point of this distinction is to prevent confusion of this peculiar postmortem artifact with a white thrombus.*

Vegetations Traditionally, a thrombus on a cardiac valve is called a vegetation. The name is appropri-ate because large vegetations are attached to the valve by a base from which they expand, rather like a bush (Figure 22.36). A vegetation may grow to a length of 2–3 cm, with branches that easily break off and embolize. Vegetations develop most fre-quently on the valves of the left heart; the reason is that the mitral and aortic valves slam shut under pressures that are at least four times greater than those of the corresponding valves on the right side. This makes them liable to suffer microtrauma and loss of endothelium, especially if they are mis-shapen due to congenital or acquired disease. The exposed subendothelial tissue is thrombogenic and becomes covered with platelets.

Infected Thrombi Infected thrombi can occur anywhere, but the prototypes are infected vegeta-tions, especially on the mitral valve. The bacteria grow in the thrombus as in a culture medium

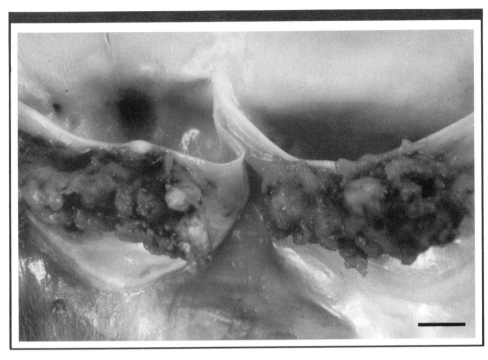

FIGURE 22.36
"Vegetations": Thrombi on the aortic valves in a debilitated leukemic patient who had undergone a bone marrow transplant. This is noninfectious endocarditis. **Bar** = 5 mm. (Courtesy of Dr. W.D. Edwards, Department of Laboratory Medicine and Pathology, The Mayo Clinic, Rochester, MN.)

(Figure 22.37); tucked away between the platelets, and perhaps also under a cap of fibrin (3, 39), they are fairly well shielded from leukocytes (Figure 22.38). It has also been suggested that platelets may stick to certain bacteria and help disseminate them (55). *Bland thrombus*, incidentally, is the term used for a noninfected thrombus.

Clinical Aspects of Thrombosis

The yearly incidence of thrombosis in the United States, including symptomless cases, could be of the order of half a million to a million, possibly more (86); firm figures are not available. One way to reach an estimate is to start with pulmonary thromboembolism, which is a reflection of thrombosis. The number of new cases of pulmonary thromboembolism per year in the United States is estimated at 170,000, plus 99,000 cases of recurrent disease (2). Yearly deaths from pulmonary emboli are estimated at 50,000 to 200,000 (10). Considering that there are many times more pulmonary emboli than fatal ones and that some thrombi never embolize, the high estimate seems reasonable.

Most dangerous as sources of emboli are the thrombi in the *large veins of the lower limbs: femoral, iliac, and popliteal*. The deep veins of the calf thrombose easily but seem to pose less threat; the superficial veins, including the large saphenous vein, can thrombose but rarely produce emboli. Many thrombi are symptomless.

A study of symptomless thrombosis was carried out, using radioactive fibrinogen, on patients who had had two common, low-risk operations: hernia and prostatectomy. In the legs of patients over 50, thrombi developed in 25 and 50 percent, respectively (101).

Pain Pain could be a useful warning sign of thrombosis, but it is not always present. Occasionally, thrombosis of a superficial vein is accompanied by dramatic symptoms: edema, sometimes redness, pain, and fever. This is thrombophlebitis, an enigmatic condition described by Trousseau in Paris as *phlegmasia alba dolens* (white painful inflammation) (108). There are in fact two enigmas: why does thrombosis occur in the first place? and why does the vein become inflamed?

There is usually a predisposing factor such as lying in bed after surgery, a malignant tumor, or pregnancy. As to the inflammation, bacteria are rarely involved. We will propose an explanation: platelets are loaded with inflammatory mediators (20). If the thrombus becomes occlusive and the platelets continue to degranulate, their mediators would no longer be washed away but should be able to diffuse through the thin venous wall and cause inflammation, including pain. This would account for the aseptic nature of the process. This hypothesis should not be too difficult to test.

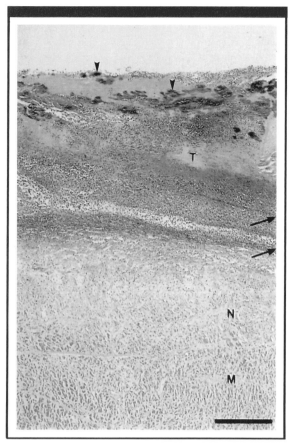

FIGURE 22.37

See color plate 21. An infected thrombus on the inner surface of the heart (left ventricle). Such thrombi may give rise to septic emboli. **T** = thrombus, almost free of red blood cells, and consisting mainly of platelets and fibrin; **arrowheads** point to colonies of bacteria, appearing as granular clouds. **M** = myocardium, **N** = necrotic myocardium; this layer may have been killed by bacterial toxins and/or by deprivation of oxygen and nutrients by the overlying thrombus. The layer between arrows corresponds to the endocardium (former inner lining of the heart). **Bar** = 500 μm.

Aspirin and Thrombi Among the many virtues of aspirin is that of being antithrombogenic. It irreversibly acetylates in platelets an enzyme of prostaglandin metabolism (prostaglandin G/H synthase), with the result that platelets can no longer produce thromboxane A_2, a platelet activator. Inevitably, the same enzyme is inhibited also in the endothelium, which uses it to produce prostacycline, an *inhibitor* of platelet aggregation. However, platelets cannot synthesize new enzyme for as long as they live (8–10 days), so the inhibition is permanent, whereas the endothelium can quickly recover (91a). As a result, the anti-platelet effect of aspirin prevails, the formation of the hemostatic plug is inhibited, and bleeding time is prolonged.

Still, much effort is concentrated on finding drugs that inhibit thromboxane synthesis without affecting the helpful endothelial production of prostacyclin (26, 83).

Anticoagulants, which block the clotting cascade, are the most effective antithrombotic agents, especially for venous thrombi, because fibrin is the glue that stabilizes thrombi. There is, of course, a trade-off between the dangers of hemorrhage and those of thrombosis and its complications. The anticoagulants most used are heparin (109) and warfarin (which has no connection with warfare; it stands for Wisconsin Alumni Research Foundation, Inc.).

Disseminated Intravascular Coagulation

Imagine the blood clotting throughout the circulatory system. This catastrophe occurs almost daily in hospitals, as a life-threatening event known as disseminated intravascular coagulation (DIC). It never occurs as a disease in itself but as a complication to some primary event that triggers generalized blood clotting. This primary event can be sepsis, especially gram-negative sepsis (Gram-negative bacteria produce endotoxin, which activates the intrinsic clotting cascade); severe trauma (especially to the brain, which is especially rich in thromboplastin); a complication of childbirth (amniotic fluid embolism, a retained dead fetus); shock; a tumor; the bite of a rattlesnake; and much else. The mechanism leading to generalized coagulation is not always the same and not always clear.

Of course, if a large amount of thromboplastin is introduced into the circulation, the blood clots everywhere and death is almost immediate. This is what a Frenchman reported to the Paris Academy of Medicine in 1834 (96). He had injected a generous amount of mashed brain intravenously into experimental animals, thereby triggering the extrinsic pathway of coagulation. Later, with smaller doses of intravenous tissue, it was found that the animal could survive; but then the blood was incoagulable. It had been, as we now say, defibrinated. This is a key feature of DIC: a combination of clotting and nonclotting, leading to thromboembolic problems as well as to hemorrhage. Hence DIC is also known by the oxymoronic name (as Jandl puts it) of *hemorrhagic microthrombosis* (61). Bleeding is inevitable because the clotting factors are being used up, which accounts for another name, **consumption coagulopathy** (Figure 22.39) (77).

DIC is a complicated and varied syndrome, but in the acute form *the cascade of events is initiated when an activator of the clotting system finds its way into the blood*. It may be an endogenous factor, such as thromboplastin, or an exogenous factor, such as endotoxin. In either case, thrombin is produced on a large scale, with three main effects:

1. Loose aggregates of fibrin develop in the bloodstream and embolize the arterioles and capillaries throughout the body (large thrombi do not form [96]). Some microthrombi may originate in the capillaries, but this is not clear.

2. Platelets are activated and form aggregates that become microemboli. Some of these are removed by the littoral phagocytes of the liver, but others occlude arterioles and capillaries throughout the body. In parallel, *thrombocytopenia* develops.

3. Endothelial cells exposed to thrombin and to fibrin filaments respond by secreting a plasminogen activator. So the plasmin (fibrinolytic) system is also activated, and fibrin/fibrinogen degradation products (FDP) are released; in fact they are the

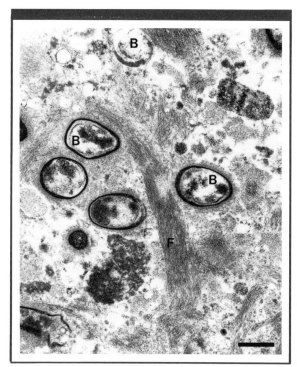

FIGURE 22.38 Electron micrograph of an infected thrombus on a mitral valve, from a case of bacterial endocarditis. **F** = fibrin strands; **B** = bacteria. The platelets that originally constituted this thrombus have long since broken up. **Bar** = 0.5 μm.

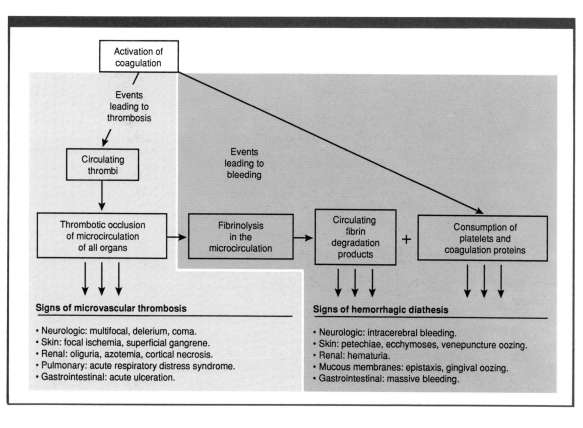

FIGURE 22.39 During disseminated intravascular coagulation (DIC), two conflicting sets of events develop: one set leads to coagulation and thrombosis (*left*); the other to fibrinolysis and bleeding (*right*). (Adapted from [77].)

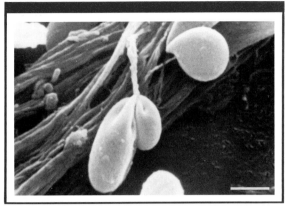

FIGURE 22.40
Fibrin threads in capillaries can slice red blood cells. This scanning electron micrograph shows a red blood cell being "hanged" across a fibrin strand. From a clot prepared *in vitro*. **Bar** = 2 μm. (Reproduced with permission from [23].)

classic markers of DIC. FDP have further pernicious effects: some act as anticoagulants or damage the endothelium and increase vascular permeability.

The red cells are not spared. Imagine them ramming at high speed into capillaries partially clogged by meshes of fibrin filaments. Some red cells may break up, and others are sliced into smaller pieces, which continue to circulate as "schistocytes," "helmet cells," or the like (Figure 22.40).

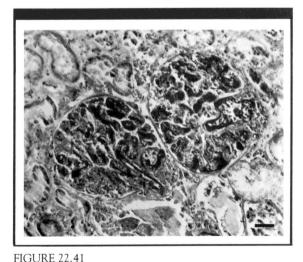

FIGURE 22.41
A result of disseminated intravascular coagulation: fibrin deposits in the glomerular capillaries, in the kidney of a 55-year-old woman who died in 3½ days of fulminant meningococcemia. (Phosphotungstic acid-hematoxylin fibrin stain. **Bar** = 25 μm.) (Reproduced with permission from [80].)

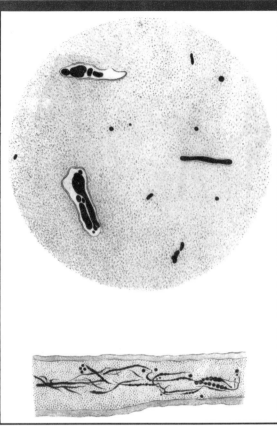

FIGURE 22.42
Fibrin thrombi in brain capillaries of a patient who died of meningitis and bronchopneumonia, presumably accompanied by terminal sepsis and disseminated intravascular coagulation. This illustration appeared in Virchows Archiv in 1892. *Top:* Brain tissue with vessels occluded by fibrin thrombi (either formed locally or embolized). *Bottom:* Detail showing vessel containing filaments of fibrin. (Reproduced from [73].)

This complication is known as microangiopathic hemolytic anemia. *The same predicament can befall red blood cells in other situations, such as when they are forced through an angioma or a malignant tumor.*

A great deal of damage is caused by microthrombi and microemboli. Most affected is the kidney because of its function as a filter (Figure 22.41). In the brain, microthrombi or emboli of fibrin (which were seen as early as 1892) often cause death (Figure 22.42). In the skin, large patches of hemorrhagic infarction may turn to gangrene. In the gastrointestinal tract, ulceration and hemorrhage are common (78). The infarcted tissues release thromboplastin and thereby create a vicious circle. The platelets, which might check the bleeding, are severely depleted by aggregation and by adhesion to the fibrin thrombi. Other clotting factors are also depleted. This anomalous mixture of clotting and hemorrhage is a therapeutic nightmare. Indeed, trying to think up a way to stop the vicious circle is an interesting intellectual challenge.

The solution is another paradox. To stop the bleeding, the best weapon is an anticoagulant; a controlled infusion of heparin, together with other measures such as the replenishment of exhausted clotting factors, may sometimes be effective. We will return to DIC in relation to shock.

In this section we have learned that thrombi are dangerous as obstacles to flow: they tend to occlude the vessels in which they develop; they can also break off and occlude arteries downstream. Before we go on to study the effects of vascular occlusion, namely ischemia and infarction, we will review some other causes of obstructed blood flow.

References

1. Alexander, C.J. Chair-sitting and varicose veins. *Lancet, 1*:822–824, 1972.
2. Anderson, F.A., Jr., Wheeler, H.B., Goldberg, R.J., Hosmer, D.W., Patwardhan, N.A., Jovanovic, B., Forcier, A., and Dalen, J.E. A population-based perspective of the hospital incidence and case-fatality rates of deep vein thrombosis and pulmonary embolism. The Worcester DVT Study. *Arch. Intern. Med., 151*:933–938, 1991.
3. Archer, G.L. Experimental endocarditis. In Duma, R.J. (ed.), *Infections of Prosthetic Heart Valves and Vascular Grafts*. Baltimore, University Park Press, 1977, pp. 43–59.
4. Aschoff, L. *Lectures on Pathology*. New York, Paul B. Hoeber, Inc., 1924.
5. Ashford, T.P., and Freiman, D.G. The role of the endothelium in the initial phases of thrombosis. *Am. J. Pathol., 50*:257–273, 1967.
6. Bach, R.R. Initiation of coagulation by tissue factor. *CRC Crit. Rev. Biochem, 23*:339–368, 1988.
6a. Bauer, K.A. Hypercoagulability - A New Cofactor in the Protein C Anticoagulant Pathway. *N. Engl. J. Med., 330*:566–567, 1994.
7. Baumgartner, H.R. The role of blood flow in platelet adhesion, fibrin deposition, and formation of mural thrombi. *Microvasc. Res., 5*:167–179, 1973.
8. Baumgartner, H.R., and Muggli, R. Adhesion and aggregation: morphological demonstration and quantitation in vivo and in vitro. In Gordon, J.L. (ed.), *Platelets in Biology and Pathology*. Amsterdam, North-Holland Publishing Company, 1976, pp. 23–60.
9. Becker, C.G., and Dubin, T. Activation of factor XII by tobacco glycoprotein. *J. Exp. Med., 146*:457–467, 1977.
10. Becker, D.M. Venous thromboembolism: epidemiology, diagnosis, prevention. *J. Gen. Intern. Med., 1*:402–411, 1986.
11. Beckering, R.E., Jr., and Titus, J.L. Femoral-popliteal venous thrombosis and pulmonary embolism. *Am. J. Clin. Pathol., 52*:530–537, 1969.
12. Behnke, O. The blood platelet. A potential smooth muscle cell. In Perry, S.V., Margreth, A., and Adelstein, R.S. (eds.), *Contractile Systems in Non-Muscle Tissues*. Amsterdam, North-Holland Publishing Company, 1976, pp. 105–115.
13. Bentfeld-Barker, M.E., and Bainton, D.F. Identification of primary lysosomes in human megakaryocytes and platelets. *Blood, 59*:472–481, 1982.
14. Bergmann, S.R., Fox, K.A.A., Ter-Pogossian, M.M., Sobel, B.E., and Collen, D. Clot-selective coronary thrombolysis with tissue-type plasminogen activator. *Science, 220*:1181–1183, 1983.
15. Bizzozero, J. Ueber einen neuen Formbestandtheil des Blutes und dessen Rolle bei der Thrombose und der Blutgerinnung. *Virchows Arch. Pathol. Anat., 90*:261–332, 1882.
16. Booyse, F.M., Osikowicz, G., Feder, S., and Scheinbuks, J. Isolation and characterization of a urokinase-type plasminogen activator (M_r = 54,000) from cultured human endothelial cells indistinguishable from urinary urokinase. *J. Biol. Chem., 259*:7198–7205, 1984.
17. Born, G.V.R., and Cross, M.J. The aggregation of blood platelets. *J. Physiol., 168*:178–195, 1963.
18. Born, G.V.R., Honour, A.J., and Mitchell, J.R.A. Inhibition by adenosine and by 2-chloroadenosine of the formation and embolization of platelet thrombi. *Nature, 202*:761–765, 1964.
19. Brandt, K.D. Glycosaminoglycans. In Kelley, W.N., Harris, E.D., Ruddy, S., and Sledge, C.B. (eds.), *Textbook of Rheumatology*, vol. 1, 2nd ed. Philadelphia, W.B. Saunders Company, 1985.
20. Braunstein, P.W., Cuénoud, H.F., Joris, I., and Majno, G. Platelets, fibroblasts and inflammation. Tissue reactions to platelets injected subcutaneously. *Am. J. Pathol., 99*:53–62, 1980.
21. Brinkhous, K.M. The problem in perspective. In Sherry, S., Brinkhous, K.M., Genton, E., and Stengle, J.M. (eds.), *Thrombosis*. Washington, DC, National Academy of Sciences, 1969, pp. 335–338.
22. Brinkhous, K.M., and Sommer, E. Why Virchow became a physician. *Arch. Pathol., 85*:331–334, 1968.
23. Bull, B.S., and Kuhn, I.N. The production of schistocytes by fibrin strands (a scanning electron microscope study). *Blood, 35*:104–111, 1970.
24. Chapman, H.A., Jr., Vavrin, Z., and Hibbs, J.B., Jr. Macrophage fibrinolytic activity: identification of two pathways of plasmin formation by intact cells and of a plasminogen activator inhibitor. *Cell, 28*:653–662, 1982.
25. Chen, T.I., and Tsai, C. The mechanism of haemostasis in peripheral vessels. *J. Physiol., 107*:208–288, 1948.
26. Clarke, R.J., Mayo, G., Price, P., and FitzGerald, G.A. Suppression of thromboxane A_2 but not of systemic prostacyclin by controlled-release aspirin. *N. Engl. J. Med., 325*:1137–1141, 1991.
27. Clouse, L.H., and Comp, P.C. The regulation of hemostasis: the protein C system. *N. Engl. J. Med., 314*:1298–1304, 1986.
28. Cohen, I., Gerrard, J.M., and White, J.G. Ultrastructure of clots during isometric contraction. *J. Cell Biol., 93*:775–787, 1982.
29. Coller, B.S. Platelets and thrombolytic therapy. *N. Engl. J. Med., 322*:33–42, 1990.

30. Colman, R.W., Hirsh, J., Marder, V.J., and Salzman, E.W. (eds.). *Hemostasis and Thrombosis: Basic Principles and Clinical Practice*, 2nd ed. Philadelphia, J.B. Lippincott Company, 1987.

31. Colman, R.W., Marder, V.J., Slazman, E.W., Hirsh, J. Overview of hemostasis. In Colman, R.W., Hirsh, J., Marder, V.J., Salzman, E.W. (eds.), *Hemostasis and Thrombosis: Basic Principles and Clinical Practice*, 2nd ed., Philadelphia, J.B. Lippincott Company, 1987, pp. 3–17.

32. Comp, P.C., Jacocks, R.M., Ferrell, G.L., and Esmon, C.T. Activation of protein C in vivo. *J. Clin. Invest.*, 70:127–134, 1982.

33. Cotran, R.S., Kumar, V., and Robbins, S.L. *Robbins Pathologic Basis of Disease*, 5th ed. Philadelphia, W.B. Saunders Company, 1994.

34. Deykin, D. The role of the liver in serum-induced hypercoagulability. *J. Clin. Invest.*, 45:256–263, 1966.

35. Dible, J.H. *The Pathology of Limb Ischaemia*. St. Louis, Warren H. Green, Inc., 1966.

36. Donati, M.B., Curatolo, L., Borgia, R., Balconi, G., and Morasca, L. Fibrin clot retraction by cultured human fibroblasts. In de Gaetano, G., and Garattini, S. (eds.), *Platelets: A Multidisciplinary Approach*. New York, Raven Press, 1978, pp. 149–158.

37. Drake, T.A., Morrissey, J.H., and Edgington, T.S. Selective cellular expression of tissue factor in human tissues. Implications for disorders of hemostasis and thrombosis. *Am. J. Pathol.*, 134:1087–1097, 1989.

38. Drake, T.A., and Pang, M. Effects of interleukin-1, lipopolysaccharide, and streptococci on procoagulant activity of cultured human cardiac valve endothelial and stromal cells. *Infect. Immun.*, 57:507–512, 1989.

39. Durack, D.T., and Beeson, P.B. Experimental bacterial endocarditis. I. Colonization of a sterile vegetation. *Br. J. Exp. Pathol.*, 53:44–49, 1972.

40. Eberth, C.J., and Schimmelbusch, C. Experimentelle Untersuchungen über Thrombose. *Virchows Arch. Pathol. Anat. Physiol. Klin. Med.*, 103:39–87 and 105:331–350, 1886.

41. Eberth, C.J., and Schimmelbusch, C. *Die Thrombose nach Versuchen und Leichenbefunden*. Stuttgart, Ferdinand Enke, 1888.

42. Esmon, C.T. Regulation of protein C activation by components of the endothelial cell surface. In Gimbrone, M.A., Jr. (ed.), *Vascular Endothelium in Hemostasis and Thrombosis*. Edinburgh, Churchill Livingstone, 1986, pp. 99–119.

43. Esmon, C.T. The regulation of natural anticoagulant pathways. *Science*, 235:1348–1352, 1987.

43a. Feigl, W. Susani, M., Ulrich, W., Matejka, M. Losert, U., and Sinzinger, H. Organisation of experimental thrombosis by blood cells: Evidence of the transformation of mononuclear cells into myofibroblast and endothelial cell. *Virchow Arch (Pathol Anat) 406:133–148*, 1985.

44. Flanc, C. An experimental study of the recanalization of arterial and venous thrombi. *Br. J. Surg.*, 55:519–524, 1968.

45. Fogarty, T.J., Cranley, J.J., Krause, R.J., Strasser, E.S. and Hafner, C.D. A method for extraction of arterial emboli and thrombi. *Surg. Gynecol. Obstet.*, 116:241–244, 1963.

46. French, J.E. The structure of natural and experimental thrombi. *Ann. R. Coll. Surg. Engl.*, 36:191–200, 1965.

47. French, J.E., MacFarlane, R.G., and Sanders, A.G. The structure of haemostatic plugs and experimental thrombi in small arteries. *Br. J. Exp. Pathol.*, 45:467–474, 1964.

48. Fuchs, U., and Graff, J. Gefässwand und Fibrinolyse— Pathologische Aspekte. *Folia Haematol.*, 113:176–183, 1986.

49. Gimbrone, M.A., Jr. (ed.), *Vascular Endothelium in Hemostasis and Thrombosis. Contemporary Issues in Haemostasis and Thrombosis*, vol. 2. Edinburgh, Churchill Livingstone, 1986a.

50. Gimbrone, M.A., Jr. Vascular endothelium: nature's blood container. In Gimbrone, M.A., Jr. (ed.), *Vascular Endothelium in Hemostasis and Thrombosis. Contemporary Issues in Haemostasis and Thrombosis*, vol. 2. Edinburgh, Churchill Livingstone, 1986b, pp. 1–13.

51. Glenner, G.G., Osserman, E.F., Benditt, E.P., Calkins, E., Cohen, A.S., and Zucker-Franklin, D. (eds.), *Amyloidosis*. New York, Plenum Press, 1986.

52. Goffin, Y.A., Gruys, E., Sorenson, G.D., and Wellens, F. Amyloid deposits in bioprosthetic cardiac valves after long-term implantation in man. A new localization of amyloidosis. *Am. J. Pathol.*, 114:431–442, 1984.

53. Hadfield, G. Thrombosis. *Ann. R. Coll. Surg. Engl.*, 6:219–234, 1950.

54. Hajjar, K.A., Gavish, D., Breslow, J.L., and Nachman, R.L. Lipoprotein a modulation of endothelial cell surface fibrinolysis and its potential role in atherosclerosis. *Nature*, 339:303–305, 1989.

55. Hawiger, J. Adhesive interactions of blood cells and the vessel wall. In Colman, R.W., Hirsh, J., Marder, V.J., and Salzman, E.W. (eds.), *Hemostasis and Thrombosis*, 2nd ed. Philadelphia, J.B. Lippincott Company, 1987, pp. 182–209.

56. Hayem, G. Sur le mécanisme de l'arrêt des hémorrhagies. *C. R. Acad. Sci. (Paris)*, 95:18–21, 1882.

57. Hedner, U., and Nilsson, I.M. The role of fibrinolysis. *Clin. Haematol.*, 10:327–342, 1981.

58. Hogg, N. Human monocytes are associated with the formation of fibrin. *J. Exp. Med.*, 157:473–485, 1983.

59. Hume, M., Sevitt, S., and Thomas, D.P. *Venous Thrombosis and Pulmonary Embolism*. Cambridge, Harvard University Press, 1970.

60. Hunter, J. *A Treatise on the Blood, Inflammation, and Gun-Shot Wounds*. London, John Richardson, 1794.

61. Jandl, J.H. *Blood: Textbook of Hematology*. Boston, Little, Brown and Company, 1987.

62. Jorgensen, L., and Borchgrevink, C.F. The platelet plug in normal persons. 1. The histological appearance of the plug 15 to 20 minutes and 24 hours after the bleeding and its rôle in the capillary haemostasis. *Acta Pathol. Microbiol. Scand.*, 57:40–56, 1963.

62a. Joris, I., and Braunstein Jr., P.W. Platelets and endothelium: Effect of collagen-induced platelet aggregates on pulmonary vessels. *Exp. & Molec. Pathol.*, 37:393–405, 1982.

63. Kane, K.K. Fibrinolysis—a review. *Ann. Clin. Lab. Sci.*, 14:443–449, 1984.

64. Kitchens, C.S. Concept of hypercoagulability: a review of its development, clinical application, and recent progress. *Semin. Thromb. Hemost.*, 11:293–315, 1985.

65. Kozin, F., and Cochrane, C.G. The contact activation system of plasma: biochemistry and pathophysiology. In Gallin, J.I., Goldstein, I.M., and Snyderman, R. (eds.), *Inflammation: Basic Principles and Clinical Correlates*. New York, Raven Press, 1988, pp. 101–120.

66. Leu, H.J., Feigl, W., and Susani, M. Angiogenesis from mononuclear cells in thrombi. *Virchows Arch. A*, 411:5–14, 1987.

67. Levin, J. The history of the development of the limulus amebocyte lysate test. *Prog. Clin. Biol. Res.*, 189:3–28, 1985.

68. Levin, J., and Bang, F.B. Clottable protein in limulus: its localization and kinetics of its coagulation by endotoxin. *Thromb. Diath. Haemorrh.*, 19:186–197, 1968.

69. Lijnen, H.R., and Collen, D. Interaction of plasminogen

activators and inhibitors with plasminogen and fibrin. *Semin. Thromb. Hemost., 8:*2–10, 1982.

70. Loscalzo, J., and Braunwald, E. Tissue plasminogen activator. *N. Engl. J. Med., 319:*925–931, 1988.

71. Macfarlane, R.G. Haemostasis: introduction. *Br. Med. Bull., 33:*183–185, 1977.

72. Majno, G., Bouvier, C.A., Gabbiani, G., Ryan, G.B., and Statkov, P. Kymographic recording of clot retraction: effects of papaverine, theophylline and cytochalasin B. *Thromb. Diath. Haemor., 28:*49–53, 1972.

73. Manasse, P. Ueber hyaline Ballen und Thromben in den Gehirnegefässen bei acuten Infectionskrankheiten. *Virchows Arch. Pathol. Anat. Physiol. Klin. Med., 130:*217–233, 1892.

74. Mann, K.G., and Fass, D.N. The molecular biology of blood coagulation. In Fairbanks, V.F. (ed.), *Current Hematology,* vol. 2. New York, John Wiley & Sons, Inc., 1983.

75. Marcus, A.J. Platelets and their disorders. In Ratnoff, O.D., and Forbes, C.D. (eds.), *Disorders of Hemostasis.* Philadelphia, W.B. Saunders Company, 1991.

76. Marcus, A.J., and Safier, L.B. Thromboregulation: multicellular modulation of platelet reactivity in hemostasis and thrombosis. *FASEB J., 7:*516–522, 1993.

77. Marder, V.J. Microvascular thrombosis. In Lichtman, M.A. (ed.), *Hematology and Oncology.* New York, Grune & Stratton, 1980, pp. 230–234.

78. Marder, V.J., Martin, S.E., and Colman, R.W. Clinical aspects of consumptive thrombohemorrhagic disorders. In Colman, R.W., Hirsh, J., Marder, V.J., and Salzman, E.W. (eds.), *Hemostasis and Thrombosis: Basic Principles and Clinical Practice.* Philadelphia, J.B. Lippincott Company, 1982, pp. 664–693.

79. Marder, V.J., and Sherry, S. Thrombolytic therapy: current status. (Second of two parts). *N. Engl. J. Med., 318:*1585–1595, 1988.

80. McGehee, W.G., Rapaport, S.I., and Hjort, P.F. Intravascular coagulation in fulminant meingococcemia. *Ann. Intern. Med., 67:*250–260, 1967.

81. Miles, L.A., Fless, G.M., Levin, E.G., Scanu, A.M., and Plow, E.F. A potential basis for the thrombotic risks associated with lipoprotein(a). *Nature, 339:*301–303, 1989.

82. Millet, J., Theveniaux, J., and Pascal, M. A new experimental model of venous thrombosis in rats involving partial stasis and slight endothelium alterations. *Thromb. Res., 45:*123–133, 1987.

83. Mills, J.A. Aspirin, the ageless remedy? *N. Engl. J. Med., 325:*1303–1304, 1991.

84. Moake, J.L. Hypercoagulable states: new knowledge about old problems. *Hosp. Pract., 26:*31–42, 1991.

85. Morgenstern, E., Korell, U., and Richter, J. Platelets and fibrin strands during clot retraction. *Thromb. Res., 33:*617–623, 1984.

86. Moser, K.M. Pulmonary embolism: where the problem is not. *JAMA, 236:*1500, 1976.

87. Mustard, J.F., and Packham, M.A. Normal and abnormal haemostasis. *Br. Med. Bull., 33:*187–192, 1977.

88. Nemerson, Y., and Bach, R. Tissue factor revisited. *Prog. Hemost. Thromb., 6:*237–261, 1982.

89. Nesheim, M.E., Hibbard, L.S., Tracy, P.B., et al. Participation of factor Va in prothrombinase. In Mann, K.G., and Taylor, F.B., Jr. (eds.), *The Regulation of Coagulation.* New York, Elsevier North-Holland, 1980.

90. Niewiarowski, S., Regoeczi, E., and Mustard, J.F. Adhesion of fibroblasts to polymerizing fibrin and retraction of fibrin induced by fibroblasts. *Proc. Soc. Exp. Biol. Med., 140:*199–204, 1972.

91. Packham, M.A., and Mustard, J.F. Platelet adhesion. *Prog. Hemost. Thromb., 7:*211–288, 1984.

91a. Patrono, C. Aspirin as an antiplatelet drug. *N. Engl. J. Med., 330:*1287–1294, 1994.

92. Puszkin, E.G., and Aledort, L.M. Platelets: biochemistry and physiology. In Root, W.S., and Berlin, N.I. (eds.), *Physiological Pharmacology,* vol. 5. New York, Academic Press, 1974, pp. 177–198.

93. Pytela, R., Pierschbacher, M.D., Ginsberg, M.H., Plow, E.F., and Ruoslahti, E. Platelet membrane glycoprotein IIb/IIIa: member of a family of Arg-Gly-Asp-specific adhesion receptors. *Science, 231:*1559–1562, 1986.

94. Rand, J.H., Gordon, R.E., Sussman, I.I., Chu, S.V., and Solomon, V. Electron microscopic localization of factor-VIII-related antigen in adult human blood vessels. *Blood, 60:*627–634, 1982.

95. Ratnoff, O.D. The evolution of knowledge about hemostasis. In Ratnoff, O.D., and Forbes, C.D. (eds.), *Disorders of Hemostasis.* Orlando, Grune & Stratton, Inc., 1984, pp. 1–21.

96. Ratnoff, O.D. Disseminated intravascular coagulation. In Ratnoff, O.D., and Forbes, C.D. (eds.), *Disorders of Hemostasis.* Orlando, Grune & Stratton, Inc., 1984, pp. 289–319.

97. Ratnoff, O.D., Busse, R.J., Jr., and Sheon, R.P. The demise of John Hageman. *N. Engl. J. Med., 279:*760–761, 1968.

98. Reidy, M.A., and Schwartz, S.M. Endothelial regeneration. III. Time course of intimal changes after small defined injury to rat aortic endothelium. *Lab. Invest., 44:*301–308, 1981.

99. Robb-Smith, A.H.T. Why the platelets were discovered. *Br. J. Haematol., 13:*618–637, 1967.

100. Roberts, H.R., and Lozier, J.N. New perspectives on the coagulation cascade. *Hosp. Pract., 1:*97–112, 1992.

101. Rubenstein, E. Thromboembolism. In Rubenstein, E., and Federman, D.D. (eds.), *Scientific American Medicine,* pt. 1 Cardiovascular Medicine, Sect. XVIII. New York, Scientific American, Inc., 1991, pp. 1–10.

102. Ryan, G.B., Grobéty, J., and Majno, G. Mesothelial injury and recovery. *Am. J. Pathol., 71:*93–112, 1973.

103. Saito, H. Normal hemostatic mechanisms. In Ratnoff, O.D., and Forbes, C.D. (eds.), *Disorders of Hemostasis.* Orlando, Grune & Stratton, Inc., 1984, pp. 23–42.

104. Shattil, S.J., and Bennett, J.S. Platelets and their membranes in hemostasis: physiology and pathophysiology. *Ann. Intern. Med., 94:*108–118, 1980.

105. Tanaka, K., Hirst, A.E., and Smith, L.L. Rate of endothelialization in venous thrombi. *Arch. Surg., 117:*1045–1048, 1982.

106. The TIMI Study Group. Comparison of invasive and conservative strategies after treatment with intravenous tissue plasminogen activator in acute myocardial infarction. Results of the thrombolysis in myocardial infarction (TIMI) phase II trial. *N. Engl. J. Med., 320:*618–627, 1989.

107. Trip, M.D., Cats, V.M., van Capelle, F.J.L., and Vreeken, J. Platelet hyperreactivity and prognosis in survivors of myocardial infarction. *N. Engl. J. Med., 322:*1549–1554, 1990.

108. Trousseau, A. Phlegmatia alba dolens. In *Clinique Médicale de Hôtel-Dieu de Paris,* vol. 3, 2nd ed. Paris, Balliere, 1865, pp. 654–712.

109. Turpie, A.G.G., Robinson, J.G., Doyle, D.J., Mulji, A.S., Mishkel, G.J., Sealey, B.J., Cairns, J.A., Skingley, L., Hirsh, J., and Gent, M. Comparison of high-dose with low-dose subcutaneous heparin to prevent left ventricular mural thrombosis in patients with acute transmural anterior myocardial infarction. *N. Engl. J. Med., 320:*352–357, 1989.

110. Wester, J., Sixma, J.J., Geuze, J.J., and Heijnen,

H.F.G. Morphology of the hemostatic plug in human skin wounds. Transformation of the plug. *Lab. Invest.*, 41:182–192, 1979.

111. Wessler, S. Studies in intravascular coagulation. III. The pathogenesis of serum-induced venous thrombosis. *J. Clin. Invest.*, 34:647–651, 1955.

112. Wessler, S., Cohen, S., Fleischner, F.G.: The temporary thrombotic state. *N. Engl. J. Med.*, 254:413–419, 1956.

113. Wessler, S., Freiman, D.G., Ballon, J.D., Katz, J.H., Wolff, R., Wolf, E.: Experimental pulmonary embolism with serum-induced thrombi. *Am. J. Pathol.*, 38:89–101, 1961.

114. Wessler, S., Reiner, L., Freiman, D.G., Reimer, S.M., and Lertzman, M. Serum-induced thrombosis. Studies of its induction and evolution under controlled conditions in vivo. *Circulation*, 20:864–874, 1959.

115. Williams, R.S., Logue, E.E., Lewis, J.L., Barton, T., Stead, N.W., Wallace, A.G., and Pizzo, S.V. Physical conditioning augments the fibrinolytic response to venous occlusion in healthy adults. *N. Engl. J. Med.*, 302:987–991, 1980.

116. Zahn, F.W. Untersuchungen über Thrombose. Bildung der Thromben. *Virchows Arch. Pathol. Anat. Physiol. Klin. Med.*, 62:81–124, 1875.

117. Zahn, F.W. Ueber die Rippenbildung an der freien Oberfläche der Thromben. *Int. Beitr. Wissenschaftlichen Med.*, 2:201–215, 1891. Festschrift Rudolf Virchow, Berlin, 1891.

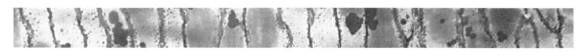

Obstacles to Blood Flow

CHAPTER 23

Obstacles Arising in the Lumen: Emboli

Obstruction by Changes in the Vascular Wall

Obstruction by Compression

Obstructions at the Capillary Level

Inadequate blood flow—**ischemia**—is one of the major threats to life; ischemic tissues become atrophic or die (infarction). It is therefore important to understand the many causes of impaired flow. No other topic, incidentally, illustrates better Virchow's definition of pathology as "physiology with obstacles" (p. 14).

Blood flow through a vessel can be impaired by three local mechanisms (Figure 23.1): an obstacle arising in the lumen; a thickening of the vessel's wall; and compression of the vessel from outside. A fourth, body-wide calamity—failure of the pump, leading to circulatory shock—will be discussed later. We will now review the three local mechanisms (Table 23.1).

Obstacles Arising in the Lumen: Emboli

Obstacles to flow that arise in the lumen can be thrombi (already discussed) or emboli. **Emboli** are solid, liquid, or gaseous objects carried by the blood that cannot mix with the blood and that are large enough to become impacted in the arterial or capillary lumen. It follows that an embolus can exist as such only for five or six seconds: the time it takes to develop and to become impacted.

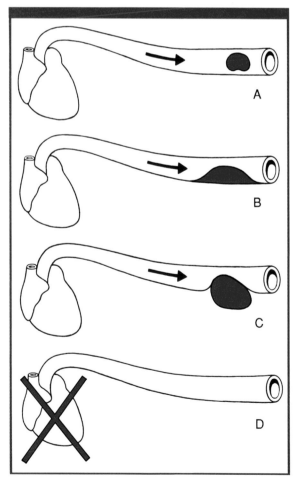

FIGURE 23.1 Four mechanisms that impair blood flow. **A:** Obstruction carried by the bloodstream (embolus). **B:** Obstacle due to a change in the vascular wall. **C:** Extrinsic obstacle compressing the vessel. **D:** Malfunction of the cardiac pump.

TABLE 23.1

Obstacles to Blood Flow

OBSTRUCTIONS ARISING IN THE
LUMEN
Thrombi
—arterial thrombi
—venous thrombi
Emboli
—thromboemboli
—paradoxical emboli
—emboli of atheroma
—emboli of fat or bone marrow
—gas emboli
—amniotic fluid emboli
—therapeutic emboli
—sundry emboli
OBSTRUCTIONS BY CHANGES IN
THE VASCULAR WALL
—Arteriosclerosis
—atherosclerosis
—arteriolosclerosis
—Mönckeberg's disease
—Arterial spasm
OBSTRUCTIONS BY EXTERNAL
COMPRESSION
—Increased tissue pressure
—compartment syndrome
—Torsion
—Increased pressure on body parts
—pressure sores

Embolism is the impaction of an embolus. Needless to say, embolism cannot occur in veins because venous blood flows from small to ever larger vessels.

The concept of embolism is attributed to Virchow, but it actually surfaced soon after Harvey published his discovery of the circulation in 1628 (15). Observations made at autopsies led the Swiss physician Jakob Wepfer (1620–1695) to conclude that solid bodies formed in the blood could break loose and obstruct arteries; and the Florentine physician–scientist Francesco Redi (1626–1698) showed experimentally that animals can be killed by introducing air into their circulation, thereby "interrupting the pulse." There were many other pioneers. However, it was certainly Virchow who codified the notion that thrombi can become emboli. (A **thrombus**—recall—is any solid mass that arises in the bloodstream *in vivo* from components of the blood.) Virchow also chose the ancient word *embolus* (from the Greek *en-bállein*, in-throw).

Virchow did not know about the observations of his ancient predecessors, but he certainly became the champion of embolism, as we are about to prove. The fateful year 1848 saw him as a young revolutionary in Berlin (he was 26), siding with those who were fighting on the barricades in the name of democracy. One day of that same year, working as a prosector, he happened to meet Schoenlein, court physician and a political adversary, to discuss an autopsy. The cause of death was supposed to have been cerebral hemorrhage, but Virchow pointed out an embolus that had obstructed a cerebral artery. Whereupon Schoenlein, only half in jest, retorted: "Really, you see barricades everywhere!" (104).

Most emboli arise from thrombi (hence the term **thromboembolism**); however, a single red or white blood cell can also embolize a capillary under some circumstances (p. 667). Emboli can also be droplets of body fat, fragments of bone marrow (usually moblized by trauma), the content of atheromatous plaques, fragments of tumors, parasites, bubbles of air or other gases, debris injected intravenously, trophoblast cells, bits of brain or liver after accidents, runaway cardiac catheters (137), and even bullets.

Where is an embolus likely to become impacted? The rules are simple. Remember that there are two circulations, the systemic and the pulmonary, arranged in series (Figure 21.15); emboli can arise and become impacted in either circuit, depending where they originate:

- *Emboli coming from the peripheral veins or from the right heart end up in the lungs*, the rare exception being paradoxical emboli (to be discussed later). Drug addicts, who inject their veins with all manner of unclean suspensions, fill their lungs with microscopic granulomas.
- *Emboli arising in the left heart or in the aorta can end up anywhere in the body* (this includes the lungs, because theoretically at least they could be embolized also through the bronchial arteries—although we have never heard of such an event).

THROMBOEMBOLI IN PULMONARY ARTERIES

Pulmonary thromboemboli in human pathology are common. Clinically, the yearly incidence in the United States is of the order of 650,000 cases (4a); about 10 percent of these patients die within 1 hour (117). Pulmonary emboli are commonly found postmortem (Figure 23.2): in our experience, about once every 8–10 autopsies. Large emboli that become lodged astride the bifurcation

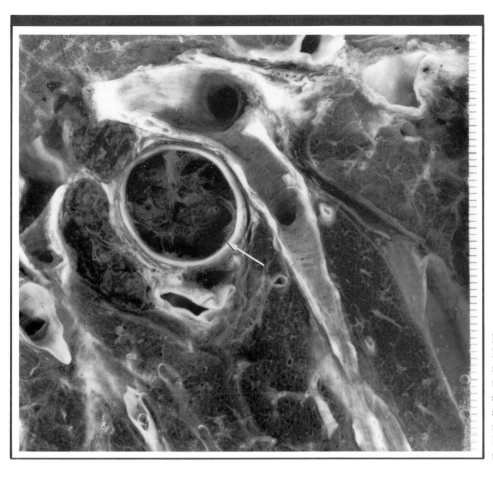

FIGURE 23.2
Embolic occlusion of the right pulmonary artery (**arrow**) in an 86-year-old man. The gray, branching, laminated structures within the embolus represent layers of platelets, typical of mixed thrombi. The embolism was bilateral and instantly lethal. Scale in mm.

of the pulmonary artery (**saddle emboli**) are usually lethal (Figure 23.3).

About 80 percent of all thromboemboli arise from thrombi in the deep veins of the thigh and from the popliteal vein (9, 55); the main risk factors for developing the initial thrombosis include a history of (previous) pulmonary embolism, cancer, congestive heart failure, surgery, obesity and old age (4a). Visualize these thrombi as soft, oblong masses of clotted blood mixed with irregular whitish layers of platelets; such thrombi often fill a vein and form a cast of its lumen, even extending into its branches. Pieces of such thrombi can become detached; these emboli can be longer and thicker than pencils. Because of their size, it is possible to stop them in their tracks by placing an umbrella-shaped metal filter in the inferior vena cava (Figure 23.4). When emboli become impacted in the pulmonary arteries, they are often doubled up or coiled. After the impact, some blood flow can usually trickle past (90); in so doing it may deposit fresh platelets on the embolus, until it becomes fully occlusive.

The various fates of an embolus are indicated in Figure 23.5. As has been proven with serial

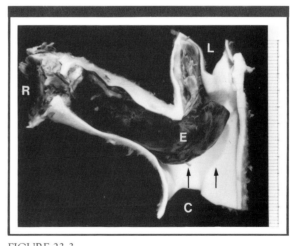

FIGURE 23.3
Saddle embolus occluding both branches of the pulmonary artery. The size and shape of this large embolus indicate that it came from a large vein of the lower limb. **Arrows:** Direction of flow. **E:** Embolus. **C:** Common pulmonary artery. **R:** Right pulmonary artery. **L:** Left pulmonary artery. Scale in mm.

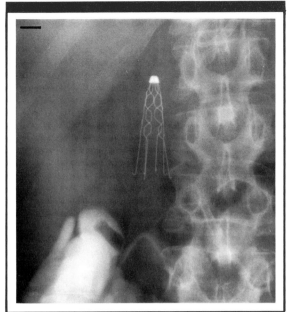

FIGURE 23.4 X-ray of the abdomen in a patient who had been implanted with a metallic "umbrella" (Greenfield filter) in the vena cava as a protection against thromboemboli. **Bar** = 1 cm.

arteriograms, *most pulmonary emboli undergo complete lysis and disappear* within 2–3 weeks (38, 137). The next most common fate is organization. An embolus is organized very much like a thrombus: the embolus is covered first by a carpet of flattened monocytes and later by endothelium (63); the underlying mass is then slowly reabsorbed, probably with the assistance of monocytes turned into macrophages. Smooth muscle cells are thought to creep out of the arterial media, colonize

the embolus, and secrete collagen, elastin, and ground substance; the final result is a special kind of scar that is probably without fibroblasts because there are none in the arterial intima and media. The overall shape of the scar may be that of a patch flattened against the arterial wall, a solid plug perforated by canals, or a free strand (called a **web**) crossing the lumen (Figure 23.6). Webs are often found at autopsy in the larger branches of the pulmonary arteries (72); they are harmless but interesting as evidence of previous emboli.

THROMBOEMBOLI IN SYSTEMIC ARTERIES

To become impacted in the systemic circulation, an embolus must arise from the left heart or from lesions of the aorta (e.g., thrombi in aneurysms). The left heart is a rich source of thromboemboli for four reasons:

- Infarcts affect especially the left ventricle, and a common complication of these infarcts is thrombosis in the ventricular cavity (p. 689). Thrombi inside a beating heart are of course easily turned into emboli.
- Thrombosis affects the mitral valve much more frequently than the tricuspid; these thrombi, called vegetations, are extremely prone to break off and embolize.
- Atrial fibrillation leads to decreased atrial contraction, dilatation of the left atrium, and stagnation of the blood with formation of thrombi. Fibrillation is a condition of disorderly contraction of the myocardial fibers, leading to ineffective pulsation.
- Loose thrombi can develop in a dilated left atrium. The classic example is the so-called **ball thrombus.** Imagine a stenotic, stiffened mitral valve that can neither open nor close properly (Figure 23.7); under these conditions, at each systole of the left ventricle blood is pumped back into the left atrium through the insufficient mitral valve. The left atrium expands, and the systolic reflux creates a permanent eddy in which a free-standing thrombus can develop and grow to a diameter of several centimeters. As mentioned earlier, this is the best proof that thrombosis can occur in the absence of endothelial injury because the ball thrombus is loose in the lumen.

All these sources of thrombi can produce emboli that are pumped into the aorta; their journey can end anywhere, but especially in the lower limbs (32).

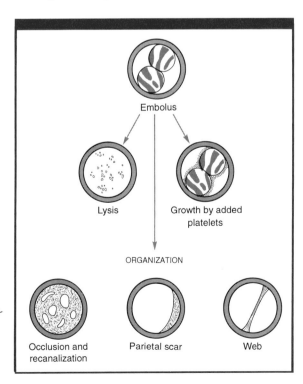

FIGURE 23.5 Fates of an embolus consisting of thrombotic material (thromboembolus).

Embolus

Lysis

Growth by added platelets

ORGANIZATION

Occlusion and recanalization

Parietal scar

Web

It is sometimes feasible to remove an embolus impacted in an artery, using the Fogarty catheter (Figure 22.23) (36). Note the paradox: the Fogarty catheter is also used experimentally to produce endothelial damage (denudation). The medical rationale is that the embolus is much more dangerous than endothelial denudation by the catheter.

PARADOXICAL EMBOLI

These rule-breaking emboli arise in the systemic veins; but instead of ending in the lungs, they embolize the systemic arteries. They bypass the lung in one of two ways:

- Small emboli pass through the arteriovenous anastomoses in the pulmonary circulation. Experiments using intravenous injections of microspheres have shown that normal lungs contain arteriovenous shunts that are 20–40 times the diameter of a capillary (49). This pathway is certainly used by embolic fat droplets and probably also by small air bubbles (68).

- Larger emboli must find a right-to-left passage in the heart (62, 77). A congenital defect (a gap) in the interventricular septum can provide such a pathway; this is rare, but about 6 percent of all normal hearts have a *foramen ovale* patent enough to allow the passage of a probe (77).

> The *foramen ovale is a leftover from the intricacies of cardiac embryology. Imagine an oval gap between the atria about the size of a small coin. Now close that gap with a fibrous membrane a little wider than the gap, applied in the left atrium and soldered all around. The membrane remains pressed against the rim of the gap by the slightly higher pressure in the left atrium. However, in about 6 percent of humans, the rim and the membrane are not wholly soldered; thus, at autopsy, a probe can be slipped across the gap; this is called a* **patent foramen ovale.**

If the pressure in the right heart is momentarily raised, such as by coughing or straining, some blood can be ejected across a patent *foramen ovale*, together with any embolus that may be floating by. Some emboli trapped in the passage have actually been caught in the act, either at autopsy or *in vivo* by echocardiography (148) (Figure 23.8). This calamity is rare, but its incidence is probably underestimated because *patients with stroke are four times more likely to have a patent foramen ovale*, compared with the general population (76).

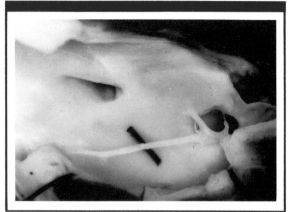

FIGURE 23.6
Webs in a pulmonary artery. These stringlike structures represent the end-stage of organized, healed emboli. A metal rod (black) was slipped beneath the longest web. Slightly enlarged.

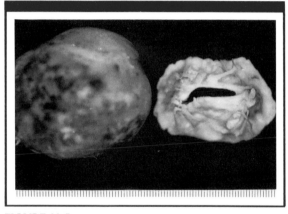

FIGURE 23.7
Left: Ball thrombus about the size of a plum. This free thrombus was removed surgically from the left atrium of a patient who suffered from stenosis and insufficiency of the mitral valve, which was also excised (*right*). Scale in mm. (Courtesy of Dr. H.F. Cuénoud, University of Massachusetts Medical Center, Worcester, MA.)

Astute clinicians have made the diagnosis during life (100); a suspicious setting is an ischemic stroke in a young adult (62, 76).

Paradoxical emboli are rare, but they do occur; it is well to remember that even a small bubble of air injected intravenously has a chance of ending in the brain or in a coronary.

EMBOLI OF ATHEROMA

Atheroma is the gruel-like necrotic material contained in atherosclerotic plaques; it is released into the blood when a plaque breaks open. This accident happens spontaneously and during catheterization or surgery on atherosclerotic arteries, whereby plaques are inevitably traumatized (Figure 23.9). Cholesterol crystals and necrotic debris usually embolize small arteries of the order of 1–2 mm or less (157); an infarct may follow (Figure

FIGURE 23.8
The mechanism of paradoxical embolism. *Left:* the four chambers of a normal heart. **RA** and **LA** = right and left atrium; **VC** = inferior vena cava. The atria are separated in part by a thin fibrous membrane called *foramen ovale;* in 6% of the population this membrane behaves as a flap valve. Normally the pressure in the two atria is within the same range, as indicated. *Right:* a pencil-shaped embolus is caught in the act of crossing the patent foramen ovale. For the flap valve to open, the pressure in the right side of the heart must be momentarily raised (**large arrow**), as might occur during the physical effort of lifting. (Adapted from [6].)

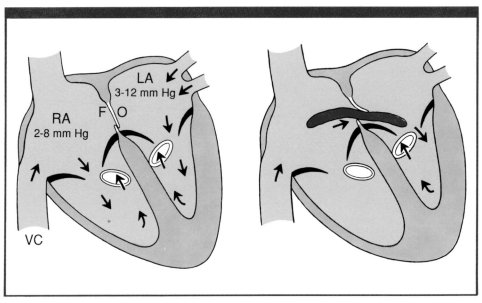

FIGURE 23.9
Emboli from atheroma. *Top:* Mesenteric arterioles embolized by crystals of cholesterol (**arrows**) after surgery on the aorta. In three dimensions these crystals are actually thin rhomboidal plates. **Bar** = 200 μm. *Bottom:* Branch of a mesenteric artery occluded by an embolus of atheroma 4 days after an arteriogram of the aorta. The occlusion has caused an inflammatory response in the adventitia (**A**). **Arrow:** Crystal of cholesterol. **Bar** = 500 μm.

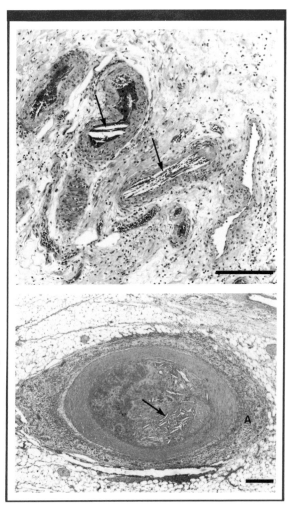

23.10). Favorite target organs are the kidney, spleen, brain, intestine (Figure 23.11), and skin. Many cholesterol emboli are symptomless; but when symptoms do arise, they are often misinterpreted because they can mimic a number of unrelated conditions (27) from belly pain to a skin disease.

Note: Ulcerated plaques can also thrombose and shed microemboli consisting mainly of platelets (73, 159).

Transient Ischemic Attacks It was the notion of microscopic atheroembolism to the brain that led to the concept of the transient ischemic attack (TIA). TIAs are episodes of neurologic dysfunction that appear suddenly, last minutes or hours, and disappear. Originally they were attributed to transient spasm of cerebral arteries, until an ophthalmologist in the early 1960s happened to examine the retina of a patient during an episode of transient monocular blindness (**amaurosis fugax**). He saw a whitish material plugging a retinal arteriole; as it was cleared away, the blackout also disappeared (Figure 23.12) (164). This observation suggested that TIAs are also due to microscopic atheromatous emboli or platelet emboli arising from thrombi in the carotid arteries or the left heart. Apparently, these emboli are small enough to break up before any lasting harm is done.

EMBOLI OF FAT AND BONE MARROW

Fat embolism is common, being largely a complication of bone fractures: that is, fat cells in the bone marrow break up; oily droplets float around and coalesce; and some droplets are sucked into gaping venules torn by the fracture, from which they begin a complicated journey—with a first stop in the lung. All this happens within the time of a few heartbeats, as was documented in victims of a helicopter crash (107).

> *Fat embolism has also occurred after bone surgery, after trauma or surgery involving adipose tissue including liposuction, in fat necrosis from acute pancreatitis (107, 119), and even from fatty livers of chronic alcoholics (Figure 23.13) (31, 83). The development of microemboli from intravenous fat emulsions used for parenteral nutrition has been contested (122).*

Almost every fracture is accompanied by some degree of fat embolism; but clinically, only about 1 percent of patients with a single fracture develop pulmonary and systemic symptoms (the proportion rises to 5–10 percent of patients with pelvic or multiple long-bone fractures) (129). The symptoms—typically delayed by 1–3 days—are mainly respiratory distress and lethargy or other signs pointing to brain damage. The mortality from systemic fat embolism is of the order of 10–15 percent. It is clearly important to work out the pathogenesis in order to plan a rational therapy.

One part of the story of fat embolism is simple: namely, the mechanical part. The oily droplets

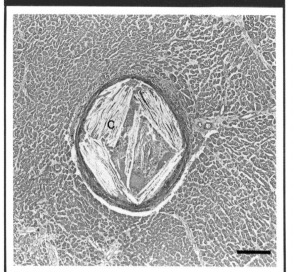

FIGURE 23.10 Branch of a coronary artery within the myocardium obstructed by an embolus of atheromatous material. **C:** Crystals of cholesterol. The patient died of a myocardial infarct 2 days after coronary bypass surgery. **Bar** = 200 μm.

embolize the lung, where they cause subclinical hypoxemia (109, 115) and sometimes overt respiratory distress; then some droplets emerge from the lung and embolize the systemic circulation. Some of these systemic droplets may have squeezed through the alveolar capillaries, but the larger ones surely have passed through the arteriovenous anastomoses mentioned earlier. Thanks to this second pathway, it is quite possible that many droplets repeat their circular journey over and over until they are broken up (127). In the meantime,

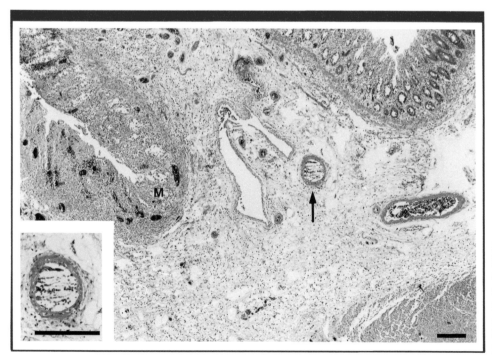

FIGURE 23.11 Embolus of atheroma in one of the arterioles (**arrow**) supplying the cecum. Widespread embolism caused the mucosa of this cecum (**M**) to become necrotic, and the cecum had to be resected. **Bars** = 200 μm. *Inset:* Detail of embolized arteriole.

FIGURE 23.12
Left: Small thromboembolus photographed as it slowly passed through the retinal circulation (**arrow**). The patient was having an attack of *amaurosis fugax* (transient blindness). The embolus moved along for a few minutes, paused at a bifurcation, and became smaller as it reached the retinal periphery. Such emboli usually arise from thrombi in the carotid artery or from a thrombosed mitral valve. *Right:* Similar embolus pausing at a bifurcation. (Reproduced with permission from [120].)

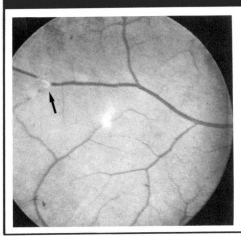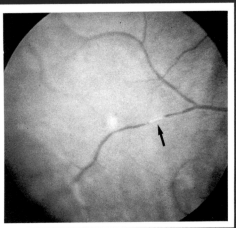

the lung, showered with microemboli, can develop a capillary leak syndrome—or *adult respiratory distress syndrome* (ARDS) (p. 703)—which explains the clinical respiratory failure and hypoxemia (115).

In the systemic circulation, the main target organs of emboli are: the *brain*, where each embolus can produce a tiny infarct surrounded by a "ring hemorrhage" (127), enough to prove that fat embolism can produce serious damage; the *kidney* (droplets of fat are commonly found in the urine, showing that some glomeruli have been damaged by the emboli); and the *skin*, where the presence of

emboli may be betrayed by small petechiae (minute round spots of hemorrhage) recalling those of the brain: the conjunctiva is a good place to look for them. Droplets of fat can also be found in the sputum.

Purely mechanical explanations in biology are often too simple to be true; so this simple theory of fat embolism has been complicated by a few ugly facts (48, 59). (a) Fatty acids have been drawn into the picture. In the lung, digestion of the fat emboli by macrophages could release fatty acids, which are toxic and could contribute to the local damage (108). Normally the plasma fatty acids are carried by albumin, but after trauma the load of free fatty acids could exceed the carrying capacity of circulating albumin (96). (b) It has been suggested that fatty acids could arise systemically (even in the absence of trauma) because stress releases adrenaline, which increases lipolysis and thereby the amount of circulating free fatty acids. All this is possible but unproven. (c) Occasional fat emboli have been reported in nontraumatic settings such as diabetes and inhalation anesthesia (129). It seems that lipoproteins can become unstable and aggregate. Rabbits treated with cortisone develop fat emboli (84). Perhaps occasional fat emboli arise by this physico-chemical mechanism.

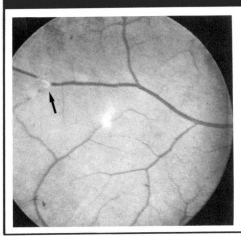

FIGURE 23.13
Multiple fat emboli (black masses) in a small pulmonary artery (section of lung stained with osmium tetroxide). This patient, an alcoholic, had a 2600-g fatty liver and died from a superimposed carbon tetrachloride intoxication. The fat globules were presumably released by necrotic liver cells. (Drawing reproduced with permission from [83].)

Bone marrow emboli arise like fat emboli: whole chunks of hemopoietic bone marrow are mobilized from the site of a fracture, sometimes with spicules of bone. Today, marrow emboli are a routine histologic finding in the small pulmonary arteries of patients who died after vigorous efforts at cardiopulmonary resuscitation (CPR) (Figure 23.14). These emboli are clinically insignificant. However, we saw one case in which an unrecognized hepatoma (liver tumor) had showered the lungs with microscopic metastases, apparently as a result of CPR (Figure 23.15).

GAS EMBOLI

Air and other gases introduced into the bloodstream are dangerous because gas bubbles have enough surface tension to behave like solid beads.

Air Embolism There are hints in Morgagni's work that in past centuries air was blown into the jugular veins to dispatch large animals (137).

A number of medical maneuvers can lead to accidental air embolism. Medical students should keep in mind at least two critical settings:
- *There is negative pressure in the veins of the chest and head during inspiration in the upright position;* therefore, these veins can draw in air. Trauma of the neck and chest can be fatal for this reason. It is believed that the fatal amount of air is about 100 ml; the bubbles gather in the right heart as a frothy mass that stops the circulation.
- During labor, air can find its way into the uterus; then it can be forced into open veins by uterine contractions.

The Caisson Syndrome This is a special type of gas embolism better known as *the bends* (51). It is a serious problem for professional divers as well as those amateur scuba divers who flout prescribed times for underwater decompression at the end of a dive. The french word *caisson* refers to a boxlike chamber large enough to hold one or more workers; it is lowered into the water open side down, so that it remains filled with compressed air. Whoever is inside it can walk, for example, on the bottom of the sea while most of the body is in air (Figure 23.16). The physiologic principle exploited by the caisson is sound and is now applied to scuba diving: *in order to breathe under water, air must be delivered to the lungs at the same pressure as that of the surrounding water.* Thus, all body tissues and blood become saturated with gas at high pressure (about one additional atmosphere for every ten meters of depth). If a diver resurfaces too quickly, the dissolved gases come out of solution and are released massively within the body as bubbles (much the same happens when you open a bottle of champagne). The bubbles distort the tissues and act as emboli in the blood, causing endothelial damage and platelet aggregation (158), as happens with fat emboli. Nitrogen is the main culprit because it is fat-soluble but poorly

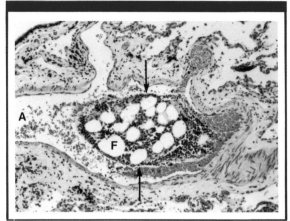

FIGURE 23.14 Embolus of bone marrow (between **arrows**) in the lumen of an artery (**A**) as a result of cardiopulmonary resuscitation (CPR). **F:** Fat cells.

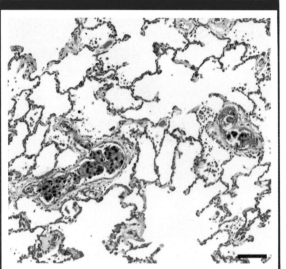

FIGURE 23.15 Emboli of a hepatoma in two pulmonary arterioles. These emboli were pumped into the lung by vigorous efforts at cardiopulmonary resuscitation (CPR) in a patient whose liver was found later to contain a large hepatoma. **Bar** = 100 μm.

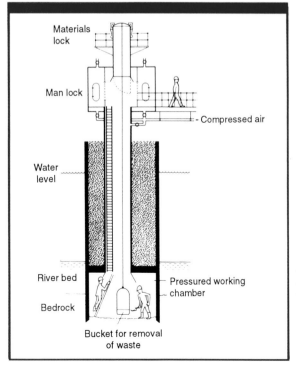

FIGURE 23.16 Modern version of the caisson, a pressurized chamber for working under water. (Reproduced with permission from [146].)

soluble in tissue fluids; thus, it creates persistent bubbles in lipid-rich tissues, most importantly the central nervous system. Treatment is prompt recompression in a special chamber, but without rushing the diver to a hospital by helicopter, which would make the bubbles grow larger. Chronic effects are mainly epiphyseal necrosis in some long bones, resulting in secondary osteoarthrosis. The pathogenesis is still not completely understood, and the disease is still with us, since modern versions of the ancient caissons are used for deep-sea drilling (51, 147).

AMNIOTIC FLUID EMBOLISM

Amniotic fluid embolism is a rare but catastrophic event that occurs as a complication of labor and cesarean section. Its clinical presentation is the mother's sudden respiratory distress, cyanosis, and collapse (94, 111). The syndrome is unleashed by penetration of amniotic fluid into the circulation, presumably through a tear in the amniotic membranes. Microscopic emboli of fetal origin are found in the lung (epithelial squames, lanugo hair, fat and mucus droplets, meconium) but not in quantities to cause cardiorespiratory failure. It is more likely that the syndrome depends on other mechanisms such as disseminated intravascular coagulation and/or pulmonary arterial spasm due to a prostaglandin of the spasmogenic F series (PGF$_2$ alpha), which is found in the amniotic fluid (94).

SUNDRY AND THERAPEUTIC EMBOLI

Embolism by microscopic foreign bodies in the lung is a common complication of drug addiction.

Drugs on the illicit market are diluted with inert fillers such as talcum, which is innocuous if taken by mouth but becomes a foreign body when injected intravenously. Less dangerous are microscopic fragments of filters and other materials related to cardiopulmonary bypass surgery, hemodialysis, and other interventions (102, 137, 154). Pulmonary emboli of placental cells are a normal and harmless occurrence (Figure 23.17).

The ultimate fate of these small foreign objects has a peculiar twist. They become covered by monocytes and eventually create a granuloma, and the arterial elastica interna beneath the granuloma breaks up. Then, it is thought, the granuloma is slowly extruded into the lung tissue, perhaps aided by arterial pressure, while the arterial wall rebuilds itself behind it (137).

Therapeutic emboli have been attempted for a variety of conditions. Favorite targets have been carcinomas of the kidney. Emboli introduced by catheter into the renal artery have varied from minced autologous muscle to plastic microspheres, and even lead shot. Pain is a major problem, and the complications are many (91). However, there is one hopeful lead: it seems that embolization of a renal carcinoma may favor the regression of metastases (141). We are drawn to speculate that the necrosis of a tumor within the body is a very different biological process from the sudden disappearance of a tumor by surgical removal.

Another therapeutic use of emboli, still at the experimental stage, has been conceived for diabetes: normal pancreatic islets (embolized into the liver of a diabetic rat via the portal vein), survived for some time and secreted insulin (Figure 23.18) (160).

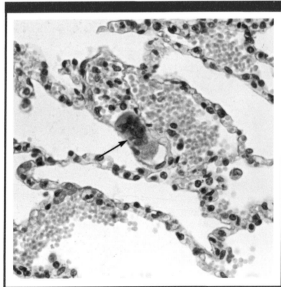

FIGURE 23.17
A normal event: placental giant cell (syncytiotrophoblast) (**arrow**) that embolized to the lung. Autopsy finding in a young woman who died of infected abortion at 16 weeks. (Courtesy of Dr. K. Benirschke, University of California, San Diego, CA.)

Obstruction by Changes in the Vascular Wall

Impaired blood flow can result from changes in the vascular wall. The two main culprits are atherosclerosis and arterial spasm. Both lead to stenosis of the arterial lumen.

Biophysicists have given us a general and somewhat reassuring law about stenosis: *flow through a stenosed tube or artery is not significantly affected until the lumen is reduced by 70–80 percent* (Figure 23.19) (81, 92). This does not mean that a 65 percent stenosis of a coronary artery has no

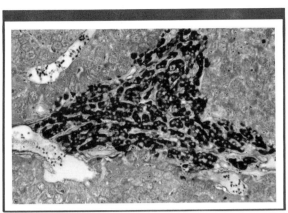

FIGURE 23.18

Embolism applied to a therapeutic purpose: a rat pancreatic islet embolized into the liver. Rat islets, cultured for 7 days at 24°C to destroy antigen-presenting cells, were injected into the portal vein of a rat from another strain. The recipient rat, made diabetic by an injection of streptozotocin, was immunosuppressed with cyclosporin A for 3 days prior to the islet injection. After this transplantation the blood glucose became normal, and remained so until the animal was killed at 62 days. In untreated control rats injected with untreated islets, the islets were rejected in 15–20 days. Aldehyde fuchsin stain to demonstrate the granules of the beta cells. (Courtesy of Dr. P.E. Lacy, Washington University School of Medicine, St. Louis, MO.)

effect; the functional reserve is decreased. Should the heart require more blood as a result of exercise, that extra demand may not be met—also because at higher flow rates a stenosis produces a relatively greater flow reduction (81).

ATHEROSCLEROSIS

Although special diseases are not considered in this book, we will touch briefly on two forms of arteriosclerosis, because—as a cause of ischemia—they are common enough to represent a basic problem.

Arteriosclerosis is a broad term that means "hardening of the arteries." It includes three diseases that decrease arterial elasticity in different ways (Table 23.1):

- *atherosclerosis*, a disease of the large and medium-sized arteries; it begins in the intima, where it produces "plaques" filled with a necrotic, gruel-like material (*athére* is Greek for gruel or porridge); *this is the disease that laymen mean when they say "arteriosclerosis"*;
- *arteriolosclerosis*, affecting the small arteries, to be discussed later; and
- *Mönckeberg's disease*, rather uncommon, a calcification of the media of large arteries.

The following discussion refers to atherosclerosis. In the Western world, no disease kills more people; its impact on the adult population in terms of myocardial infarcts and stroke has no match. Among the risk factors that predispose to atherosclerosis, nutrition and high blood cholesterol rank highest; in fact, almost all experimental models of atherosclerosis are animals (even birds) maintained on a high cholesterol diet. Although a high level of blood cholesterol should affect all blood vessels, pathologic changes develop only in large and medium-sized arteries, and then only parts of those arteries: the basic lesion is a *plaque*, typically a centimeter or so in diameter. Therefore, to understand atherosclerosis, we must understand the genesis of a plaque.

Pathogenesis of Atherosclerosis The natural history of atherosclerosis is summarized in Figure 23.20. The disease develops in patches of the intima, often where flow is disturbed, such as around the opening of a branch. The key event is a focal accumulation of lipid and cells beneath the endothelium; ultimately this creates a raised, flat plaque 1–2 mm thick that can be a major obstacle to flow in arteries with a lumen of about 3 mm, such as the coronaries. In cross section (Figure 23.21), the plaque shows a necrotic core called *atheroma*, which consists of dead cells, debris, and cholesterol crystals.

Experimental Models and Mechanisms To explain atherosclerosis we must explain which lipid and which cells accumulate, why they do so, and why they are found in a particular patch of

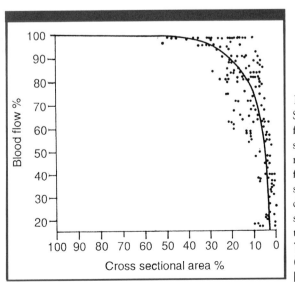

FIGURE 23.19 Surprisingly, the flow through a stenotic artery is not seriously affected until the stenosis has reduced the cross-sectional area of the lumen by 70–80 percent. (Adapted from [92].)

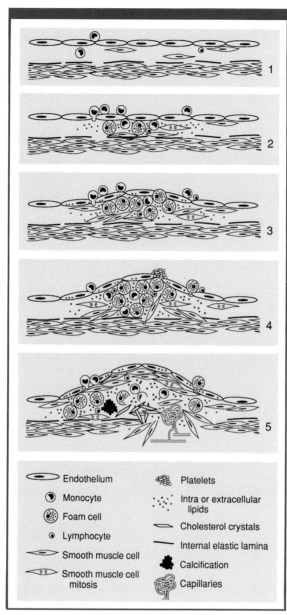

FIGURE 23.20

Birth, growth, and development of an atherosclerotic plaque as seen in experimental hypercholesterolemic animals. *1:* Normal arterial wall with endothelial cells, subendothelial space, interrupted elastic lamina, and smooth muscle cells of the media. Occasional macrophages and lymphocytes migrate into the subendothelial space. *2:* The two earliest events detectable: the transendothelial passage of lipid droplets (which accumulate as liposomes) and the transendothelial migration of monocytes (which turn into foam cells). *3:* Crowded foam cells cause the endothelium to bulge. Some foam cells may return to the bloodstream. Smooth muscle cells arise from the media. *4:* Growth of the plaque by increase in the number of foam cells and smooth muscle cells. Platelets adhere where endothelial cells allow gaps to develop. *5:* Necrosis occurs in the plaque, followed by development of cholesterol crystals, calcification, and vascularization from the adventitia. (Adapted from [86].)

intima. Much was learned in the 1980s, and now it is generally agreed that the lipid comes from plasma lipoproteins, mainly low-density lipoproteins (LDL, which carry cholesterol) and that high plasma cholesterol is a major factor. Experimental models of atherosclerosis are based largely on feeding animals a high cholesterol diet.

The very first event in the birth of a plaque seems to be the appearance of submicroscopic lipid droplets (liposomes) and LDL particles beneath the endothelium (Figure 23.22). This can be seen in rabbits and hamsters after only 1–2 weeks on a high-cholesterol diet (93, 132, 133). Because the endothelium is intact, the likeliest interpretation is that LDL particles are being transcytosed into the subendothelial space, where they come to lie, either intact or degraded to liposomes.

Promptly thereafter, monocytes and a few lymphocytes become attached to the endothelial surface (Figure 23.23); then they migrate into the intima (Figure 23.24), where the monocytes become macrophages, pick up much of the lipid, and turn into foam cells (p. 87) (Figure 23.25) (66, 118). The cellular population of the plaque is further increased by smooth muscle cells that migrate from the media into the intima.

At this point, seen by scanning electron microscopy, the intimal lesion appears as a hill stretched in the direction of flow; it is covered with endothelium and may have a few mononuclear cells sticking to it (Figure 23.26). This is called a **fatty streak.**

The fatty streak continues to grow, by continued immigration of monocytes and lymphocytes and by proliferation of intimal and medial smooth muscle cells. Some of these join the foam cells and even phagocytize lipid (Figure 23.27). Others grow as a layer beneath the endothelium, constituting a sort of roof, reinforced by collagen, elastin, and other matrix proteins; this becomes the so-called fibrous cap. At this stage the lesion is called a **fibrofatty plaque.** Eventually, the core of the plaque, filled with foam cells and smooth muscle cells, becomes necrotic and turns into atheroma.

As to the time frame: with the extremely high levels of hypercholesterolemia that can be reached in experimental animals, the process just described can occur over several months. In humans it takes years, probably many years.

This long sequence of events raises some basic questions, and some answers are now available. First of all: *why do the monocytes stick to the arterial endothelium?* The sticking followed by diapedesis is

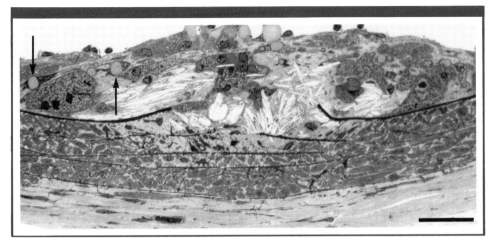

FIGURE 23.21
Miniature atherosclerotic plaque in the aorta of a rat maintained for 11 months on a high-cholesterol diet. In the center, the intima has become thicker than the media; mononuclear cells are attached to the surface. Among the subendothelial foam cells, those with few large lipid droplets (**arrows**) are derived from smooth muscle cells. Note crystals of cholesterol in the core of the plaque. **Bar** = 25 μm.

reminiscent of inflammation, and the similarity extends to the mechanism: in rabbits on a high-cholesterol diet, the endothelial cells covering early fatty streaks express a vascular endothelium adhesion molecule, VCAM-1, that is selective for monocytes and appears also in inflammation (25, 35, 80). The expression of this molecule is focal, which brings us to the next question: *why are the sticking, and the accumulation of lipid, selective for certain places?* It is long known that areas of disturbed flow and especially of *low* shear stress (166) favor lipid deposition and plaque formation; recent findings show that the endothelial cells are able to transduce shear stress into messages that

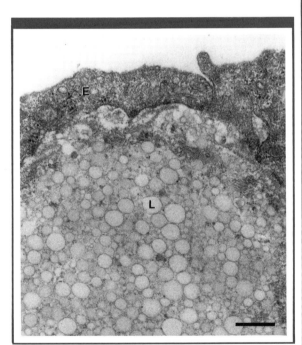

FIGURE 23.22
Evidence of transendothelial transport in early atherosclerosis. Electron micrograph of a guinea pig aortic valve after 1 week on a hypercholesterolemic diet. **L:** Mass of rounded bodies called liposomes composed of lipid that must have crossed the intact epithelium. **E:** Endothelium. **Bar** = 0.5 μm. (Courtesy of Drs. M. and N. Simionescu, Institute of Cellular Biology and Pathology, Bucharest, Romania.)

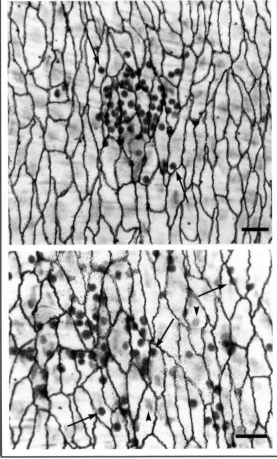

FIGURE 23.23
Inner surface of the aorta of a rat after 8 weeks on a hypercholesterolemic diet. The network of black lines represents junctions between endothelial cells. Many mononuclear cells (**arrows**) are sticking to the endothelial surface; those that are faintly stained (**arrowheads**) have migrated beneath the endothelium. Silver nitrate and hematoxylin. **Bars** = 25 μm.

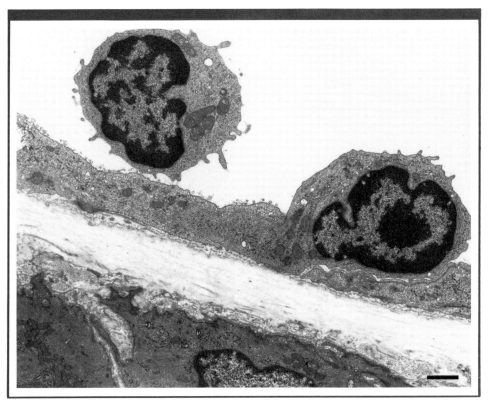

FIGURE 23.24
Margination and diapedesis of monocytes along the aortic intima of a rat after 11 weeks on a high-cholesterol diet. **Bar** = 1 μm. (Reproduced with permission from [66].)

turn on certain genes (28, 29, 113). We expect important developments along these lines. Besides adhesion molecules, cytokines and growth factors abound in fatty streaks and plaques, as would be expected for lesions filled with activated cells, especially monocytes (23).

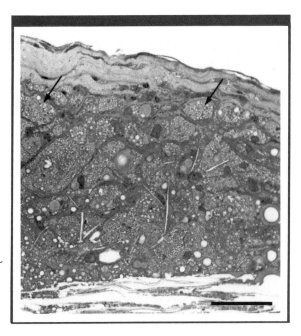

FIGURE 23.25
Typical macrophage-derived foam cells (**arrows**) packed in the intima of a human atherosclerotic artery. The fine slits correspond to crystals of cholesterol. **Bar** = 50 μm.

Foam Cell Puzzles Foam cells are at center stage in atherosclerosis, but their role is not entirely clear. Are they part of the problem or part of the solution? Electron microscopy has suggested that some of them migrate back into the bloodstream (44), in which case they would be performing a laudable function. But what would they do in the bloodstream? Their size is such that they would become microemboli and break up. Nor is it clear why foam cells die in the plaque. Perhaps the core of the plaque suffers from anoxia, or perhaps some lipid has a toxic effect. Another puzzle is that monocytes incubated with particles of native LDL do not phagocytize them. They do so only if the particles are oxidized or otherwise modified (p. 88)—hence the theory that the endothelium modifies (oxidizes) the LDL particles as it transmits them to the subendothelium (107a). This oxidation mechanism is important scientifically (oxidized lipoproteins are related to monocyte sticking [20]) and practically, as a possible target for therapy of atherosclerosis by means of antioxidants (11).

Complications Plaques can develop complications, a series of accidents that mar the clinical course (34a). The following list does not imply a necessary sequence. (1) *Ulceration;* the fibrous cap is eroded from underneath, the core is exposed, and (2) *thrombosis* (Figure 23.28) may develop on the ulcerated plaque. (3) *Thrombosis may develop even on structurally intact endothelium.* This possibility was long debated, but it now seems well supported: abnormally high levels of a lipoprotein called LP(*a*) can lead to thrombosis by the mechanism shown in Figure 23.28 (57). (4) Thrombi may release vasoconstrictors that induce *spasm* at the site of the plaque. (5) The exposed atheroma may break up and shed *atheromatous emboli.* (6) *Calcification* may develop in and around the plaque, making the artery even stiffer. (7) *Vascularization* occurs; the plaque may be invaded by vessels from the adventitia. This in itself is not particularly bad, but one of those vessels may break and cause (8) *hemorrhage in the plaque;* the pressure of the hemorrhage may break the plaque open (Figure 22.35). (9) *Local dilatation (aneurysm)* may also be caused by a local weakening of the wall. (10) *Rupture of the atherosclerotic artery and bleeding* may be caused by a weakening of the medial layer; this is a common event in cerebral arteries especially with associated hypertension.

Reversibility Up to a point the process of atherosclerosis as described is reversible: fatty streaks can disappear and plaques can shrink (49a). The mechanisms of reversal are still uncertain, but there is hope for those who abandon a high-cholesterol diet. This hope is tempered by another set of facts: what dieting may want to do, genes may undo. Genetically induced high cholesterol is difficult to deal with. Conversely, "good genes" protect some lucky individuals against a high-cholesterol diet.

In closing, we should point out a distressing characteristic of atherosclerosis. For most of its course it is a totally silent disease; when symptoms appear as a result of plaque complications—a myocardial infarct, a cerebral hemorrhage—it is often too late to do much about it. Prevention is the answer.

ARTERIOLOSCLEROSIS

This "hardening of the arterioles" is common but poorly understood. It has little or no connection with atherosclerosis. Two varieties are known.

Hyaline arteriolosclerosis means that the arteriolar wall is stuffed with extracellular material, such as blood-borne macromolecules (Figure 7.1); this condition is common in the kidney, spleen, and other organs, it increases with age, and it is

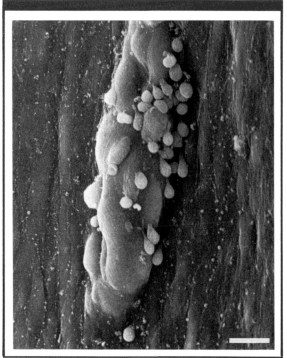

FIGURE 23.26 Early fatty streak in the aorta of a rat after 8 weeks on a hypercholesterolemic diet (scanning electron micrograph). The elongated bulge is due to foam cells packed beneath the endothelium. Its surface appears to be selectively sticky for other leukocytes, which are mostly monocytes. **Bar** = 25 μm. (Reproduced with permission from [87].)

aggravated by hypertension; it has little clinical significance, although it can produce small foci of atrophy in the kidney. Why the arteriolar endothelium becomes leaky is not known.

Hyperplastic arteriolosclerosis means that the

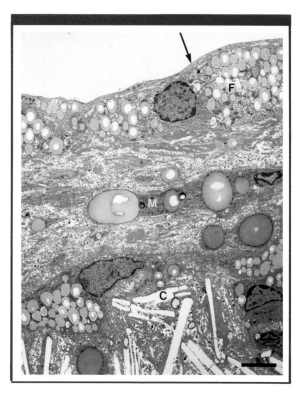

FIGURE 23.27 Various aspects of lipid deposition in the aortic intima of a rat after 1 year of hypercholesterolemia. **Arrow:** Very thin endothelial layer. **F:** Macrophage-derived foam cell. **M:** Smooth muscle cell, containing fewer and larger droplets. **C:** Crystals of cholesterol among necrotic debris. **Bar** = 5 μm. (Reproduced with permission from [66].)

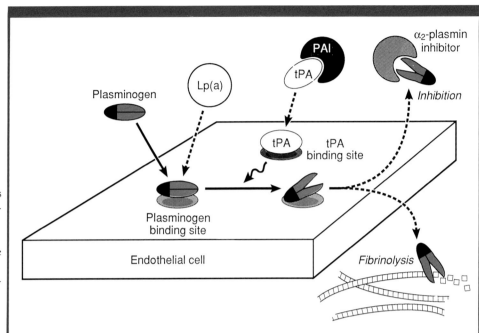

FIGURE 23.28

A proposed mechanism of thrombosis in atherosclerosis. The initiating factor is an excess of the lipoprotein called Lp(a). Lp(a) competes with plasminogen for a shared binding site on the surface of endothelial cells; this interferes with the normal activation of the fibrinolytic pathway. Impaired fibrinolysis leads to fibrin formation and thrombosis. (Adapted from [124].)

arteriolar muscular cells have undergone hyperplasia at the expense of the lumen and stiffening the wall (Figure 23.29). This condition is usually the result of severe hypertension; it affects arterioles throughout the body but especially those of the kidney.

Arterioles are the principal resistance vessels, hence diffuse arteriolosclerosis can cause hypertension; conversely, hypertension is known to cause or aggravate arteriolosclerosis. Despite these important connections, this aspect of vascular pathology has received little attention.

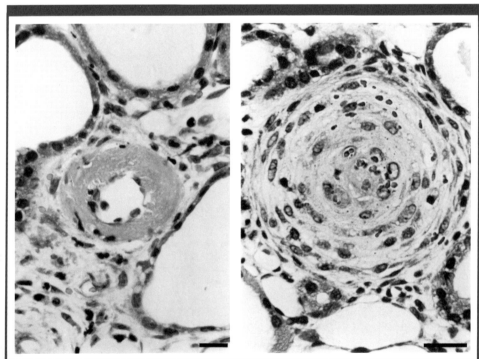

FIGURE 23.29

Two types of arteriolar changes in rat "remnant kidneys" (after removal of one kidney and ⅚ of the other). *Left:* Necrosis of the wall. *Right:* Hyperplastic thickening of the vascular wall with great reduction of the lumen. **Bars** = 25 μm. (Reproduced with permission from [123].)

ARTERIAL SPASM

There is no standard definition of spasm, but we may consider it as "persistent vasoconstriction." The time frame may be hours or days. Arterial spasm can be useful as a first line of defense against hemorrhage, but then, why should an artery become spastic to the point of creating an infarct?

> *This aberrant behavior of arteries occurred in epidemic proportions during the Middle Ages. After rye bread came into the general diet, tens of thousands of people saw their nose, hands, and feet shrivel up and blacken with dry gangrene and burning pain, "as if charred by St. Anthony's fire." The reason was that the rye was contaminated with the fungus ergot (Claviceps purpurea), and it so happens that ergot alkaloids are potent vasoconstrictors (14). The modern equivalent of St. Anthony's fire may be cocaine abuse; it also can induce (among other damage) necrosis of the skin, presumably by vasospasm (Figure 23.30) (165).*
>
> *We should mention that arteriolar spasm is at the root of at least one physiologic infarct: the monthly shedding of the endometrium (21, 128).*

Pathophysiology of Spasm Arterial lumen is easily restricted. Because the volume of the arterial media remains constant, the media becomes thicker as it contracts; therefore a mild reduction of the outer diameter of the artery corresponds to a proportionately greater reduction of the lumen (Figure 23.31) (131).

> *An intriguing possible cause of spasm was suggested by a single autopsy: a patient known to suffer from coronary spasm had 5–6 times more mast cells in the adventitia of the spastic artery, compared with controls (37). Mast cells produce at least three kinds of coronary constrictors: histamine, prostaglandin D$_2$, and leukotrienes.*

A major link in the pathogenesis of spasm was discovered in 1980 and is known as the **Furchgott phenomenon:** the media cannot relax in the absence of endothelium. The first inkling came from experiments *in vitro*. Acetylcholine, a powerful vasodilator, could not relax the media if the endothelium was absent. Then the mechanism was found. When the endothelium is stimulated by acetylcholine (or by many other agents), it produces a relaxing factor, nitric oxide (NO) (Figure 23.32). Now it is possible to understand the spasm of an artery denuded of its endothelium and lined with platelets (151).

Other surprising facts turned up later. In experimental hypercholesterolemia and in athero-

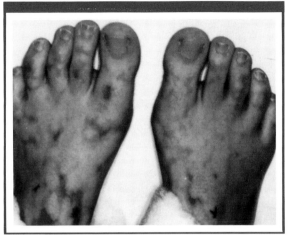

FIGURE 23.30
Effect of spasm in the small arteries: necrotizing lesions in the skin of a patient after inhalation of cocaine (crack). (Reproduced with permission from [165].)

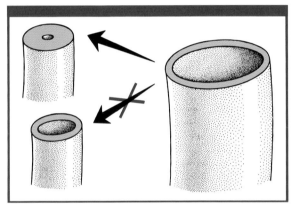

FIGURE 23.31
When an artery contracts the lumen shrinks proportionately more than the outer diameter. The reason: as the media contracts, it also becomes thicker. (Adapted from [131].)

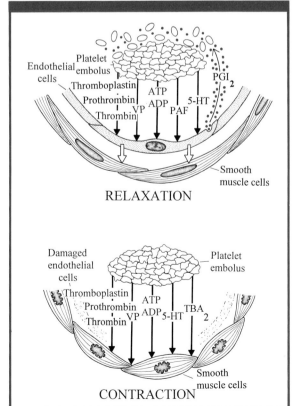

FIGURE 23.32
The Furchgott phenomenon: *Top:* Factors released by platelet thrombi cause a normal artery to relax; the endothelium also responds by secreting PGI$_2$, which opposes thrombus formation. *Bottom:* If the same factors are released in an artery lacking endothelium, contraction results. (Adapted from [151].)

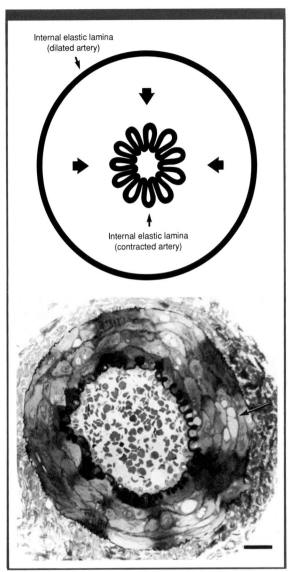

FIGURE 23.33

Top: Diagram of the internal elastic lamina of a small artery, and its change after full contraction. Because the elastic membrane cannot shorten, it is thrown into tight longitudinal folds. *Bottom:* Arterial spasm, shown in cross section of a spermatic artery of a rat, contracted by a local application of norepinephrine. The wavy black line along the inner surface is the internal elastic lamina, thrown into folds by the medial contraction. The cartwheel pattern of the media is due to zones of hypercontraction alternating with noncontracted vacuolated zones. The vacuoles (**arrow**) represent herniations of one cell into another. **Bar** = 25 μm.

sclerosis, the endothelial response is perverted. That is, *when the media is stimulated with vasodilators, it contracts instead of relaxing* (151), in pigs as well as in humans (82). This may explain why coronary spasm tends to occur in segments already stenosed by atherosclerotic plaques (41, 130).

Electron microscopy has shown that spasm has a built-in potential for a vicious circle. We have found experimentally that a tightly contracted artery traumatizes its own endothelium (64). Indeed, there seems to be a flaw in the design of the arterial wall. When the media contracts concentrically, the intima cannot reduce its caliber except by forming many longitudinal folds, rather like an accordion (Figure 23.33). As a result, the endothelium inside the folds is unavoidably squeezed (Figure 23.34), and some endothelial damage occurs (10, 64).

Another self-inflicted injury develops in the spastic media: smooth muscle cells develop cell-to-cell herniae that appear as vacuoles (65) (p. 73). This is not a serious injury but it is certainly a marker of spasm, at least in rat arteries.

Spasm in Human Disease Spasm is a known cause of disease, especially in the heart and brain.

- *Coronary spasm.* Some individuals suffer from severe chest pain (angina pectoris) even at rest without any stress. This so-called variant angina or Prinzmetal angina has been convincingly shown to be the result of coronary spasm (13) (Figure 23.35). Myocardial infarcts due to spasm are rare but well documented (10, 13, 22, 153). Interestingly, the vasoconstrictor ergonovine, currently used by cardiologists for coronary testing, is a direct descendant of ergot, the cause of St. Anthony's fire.
- *Cerebral arterial spasm.* This is a feared complication of subarachnoid hemorrhage; it occurs with a delay of 4–14 days and can cause severe neurologic deficits (3). One of its peculiar features is its long duration, which is probably due to the fact that free hemoglobin, released at the site of hemorrhage, inhibits the endothelium-dependent relaxation of the arteries. In addition, hemoglobin itself is a vasoconstrictor (69).
- *Raynaud's phenomenon* is a three-stage event seen most often in young women (50). First, a feeling of cold or an emotional upset triggers a bilateral spasm in the fingers, which become white; then the fingers become cyanotic; finally, the event comes to an end with a phase of reactive hyperemia (redness) (Figure 23.36). This may be the only trouble, but occasionally there is an underlying disease, such as rheumatoid arthritis or a hematologic abnormality (2, 17).

- Transient blindness of one eye can be due to arterial spasm (16).
- Sudden death by cocaine abuse may be related to coronary spasm (70, 95).
- A genetically induced cardiomyopathy of the hamster produces scattered foci of necrosis, attributed to spasm in small arteries (33).
- The pathogenesis of acute stress ulcers of the stomach probably includes a component of vasoconstriction, but the mechanism is more complex (78).
- Venous spasm may occur (75), but it is not a known cause of disease.

Obstruction by Compression

Obstacles to flow due to compression affect primarily the veins because they have the lowest pressure and the thinnest walls. This means that the pathogenesis of pressure damage begins in the veins. Veins may be squeezed either when edema increases the interstitial tissue pressure or when physical pressure is exerted on a part of the body.

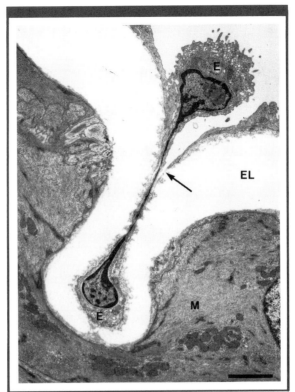

FIGURE 23.34 Intima of a spastic artery; electron microscopic detail. Endothelial cell (**E**) squeezed almost to vanishing thinness in a tight fold of the internal elastic lamina (**EL**). Endothelial breaks can develop under such conditions; a small break is shown by the **arrow. M:** Part of a smooth muscle cell. **Bar** = 2 μm. (Reproduced with permission from [64].)

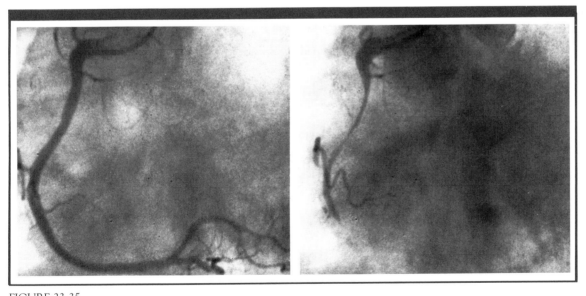

FIGURE 23.35
Arterial spasm can be intense enough to stop the flow of blood. *Left:* Arteriogram of the right coronary artery in a patient who suffered from episodes of chest pain due to coronary spasm (the so-called Prinzmetal angina). The image shows only mild narrowings, insufficient to cause ischemia. *Right:* Four minutes after an intravenous injection of a vasoconstrictor (ergonovine), the same artery shows a long segment of severe narrowing followed by total obstruction. At this point the patient experienced chest pain; after administration of a vasodilator (nitroglycerine) the artery dilated and the pain disappeared. (Courtesy of Dr. F.A. Heupler, Director, Cardiac Catheterization Laboratory, The Cleveland Clinic Foundation.)

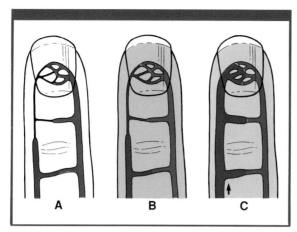

FIGURE 23.36
Three phases of Raynaud's phenomenon: **A:** White phase, due to spasm of the small arteries. **B:** Blue phase, when limited arterial flow permits pooling of poorly oxygenated blood. **C:** Red phase, when the spasm ends and oxygenated blood flows back into the finger (arrow). (Adapted from [138].)

COMPRESSION BY INCREASED TISSUE PRESSURE: THE COMPARTMENT SYNDROME

The compartment syndrome is a painful ischemic accident that happens, as the name implies, to organs contained within a tight "container" with little leeway for expansion—typically the muscles of the limbs, which are snugly packed in fibrotendinous wrappings (fasciae) (Figure 23.37) (88,

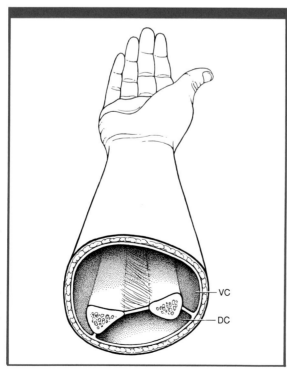

FIGURE 23.37
The two compartments of the forearm, which explain the development of compartment syndromes in this area. **DC:** Dorsal compartment. **VC:** Volar (anterior) compartment. (Adapted from [88].)

98, 110). The fasciae create anatomic and functional compartments. Whenever the content of a compartment swells rapidly because of edema, inflammation, or hemorrhage, tissue pressure can rise above venous pressure, and a vicious circle is set in motion.

The Case of the Marathon Runner The nature of the compression problem is best illustrated by the case of an inexperienced runner determined to win a marathon. Right from the start the muscles of the calf call for more blood. This is perfectly normal; the arterioles dilate, and the microcirculation is perfused more fully and under higher pressure (hyperemia). Now the volume of the muscle has increased a little, but there is still room for it in the distended fascia. Because capillary pressure has increased, more transudate is formed; for a time the lymphatics are able to drain it. The runner presses on. The hyperemia increases, the transudate increases. Tissue pressure begins to rise, but the fascia surrounding the muscle cannot be distended any further. The small veins and the lymphatics begin to be squeezed. The muscle begins to ache. Now a vicious circle sets in:

increased tissue pressure → compression of the veins and lymphatics (while high-pressure arterial inflow continues) → congestion of the tissues → increased transudation from the capillaries → anoxic swelling of the muscle fibers → increased tissue pressure → more compression of the veins → . . .

Pain is the warning. If the runner takes heed, the situation is reversible; if not, the vicious circle can be interrupted only by releasing the tissue pressure. This means surgery: the fascia has to be slit open (fasciotomy) (97).

> We have heard about a well-known athlete whose performance was greatly improved after bilateral fasciotomy of the calf. Apparently, the operation created more space also for muscle hypertrophy.

> The term shin splints, *incidentally, covers a number of injuries, including compartment syndromes (7, 61).*

Clinical signs are a throbbing, unrelenting pain, out of proportion with the clinical setting; weakness of the muscles affected, and, eventually, numbness of the part due to compression of the nerves. The muscles feel tense and swollen; in some orthopedic services the degree of tissue pressure is evaluated with manometric devices; criteria vary, but a value above 35–45 mm Hg usually calls for decompression.

The Case of the Tight Cast Another classic setting for the compartment syndrome is a tight cast on a fractured limb. *Severe pain should sound the alert.* If the pressure is not released, the muscle is infarcted and replaced by a slowly contracting fibrous mass. The notorious deformation of the forearm called Volkmann's contracture, with a forced flexure of the wrist, is shown in Figure 23.38 (45, 74). Needless to say, such deformation should never happen after any fracture; the case here illustrated was due to a bleeding disorder, and the increased tissue pressure was due to deep hemorrhage (there was no fracture). It is of some interest to notice that many of the published illustrations of Volkmann's contracture after a fracture of the forearm represent children; it is well established that children complaining about pain tend to receive less attention than adults (116, 155a).

Other Settings of the Compartment Syndrome When Richard von Volkmann described his contracture in 1881, he meant to draw attention to the danger of excessively tight bandages (42). He would have been surprised to learn about the compartment syndrome and its settings in the late twentieth century:

- Drug addicts who lie asleep or in coma for many hours without moving can develop a compartment syndrome. The constant weight of the body on a limb or of one leg over another is enough to set off the vicious circle (Figure 23.39) (105, 106). Blood trickles into the muscles through arteries while venous outflow is blocked; so the tissue pressure rises. At some point, tissue pressure is high enough to impair venous flow even if the weight on the muscle is relieved.
- Patients in shock are now clad in tight-fitting pneumatic garments to squeeze more blood into the general pool. The venous blood is certainly squeezed out, but some arterial flow persists. Thus, the tissue pressure rises. When the garment is removed hours later, the price may be a bilateral, overwhelming compartment syndrome (143, 144).

In both these settings the triggering mechanism is not active hyperemia as it is for runners, but passive hyperemia caused by pressure on the veins.

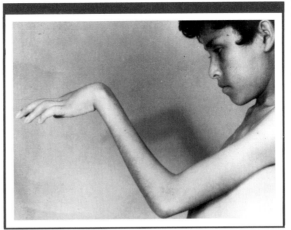

FIGURE 23.38 Volkmann's ischemic contracture of the forearm of an 8-year-old boy. Note the typical posture. The child is a hemophiliac; the ischemia resulted from an untreated hemorrhage in the forearm. (Reproduced with permission from [43].)

The pathogenesis is probably complicated by the damage that occurs when reflow is established in ischemic tissues (p. 684).

Capture myopathy *is a wildlife equivalent of the marathon syndrome. It is usually seen in animals running for their lives, even from fear of a well-meaning ranger. A running deer, a moose, a bighorn sheep may suddenly keel over, and its limbs will become stiff (8, 53, 79, 89). The same type of accident can happen to a dolphin struggling to escape a net (Figure 23.40).*

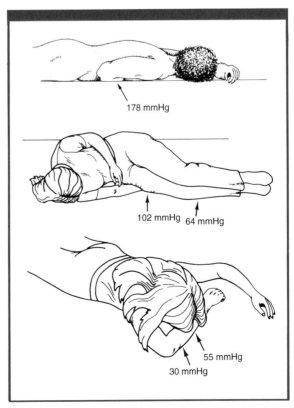

FIGURE 23.39 Tissue pressures that can be generated by the weight of the body in various positions. Drug addicts who lie for many hours in one position may develop a compartment syndrome upon reperfusion of the ischemic muscles. (Reproduced with permission from [105].)

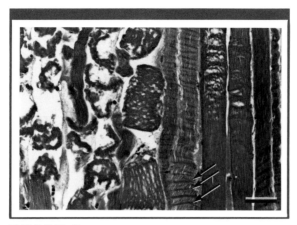

FIGURE 23.40

"Capture myopathy" in a bottlenose dolphin: an example of the compartment syndrome. This unfortunate dolphin was caught in a net, and struggled to free itself; within 2 days it became stiff and unable to swim; after 2 weeks it died. Histology of the muscle shows fibers that are beginning to break up into a series of contraction bands (**arrows**) and fibers that are completely broken up (*left*). **Bar** = 50 μm. (Preparation kindly provided by Dr. L. Johnson, Armed Forces Institute of Pathology, Washington, DC.)

VENOUS COMPRESSION BY TORSION

In organs that have a stalk, ischemia can develop if the stalk is twisted. The technical name for a stalk is *peduncle*; the twisting itself is *volvulus*. The mechanism: when twisting begins, the vein in the stalk is first occluded because its internal pressure is low, but the artery continues to function. As a result, the tissue downstream becomes congested with noncirculating blood and becomes a hemorrhagic infarct.

One of the oddities of medicine is that the testicle can twist itself around its vascular stalk and become infarcted; this very painful accident can occur at birth, at puberty, and in young men (135). Both cold weather and a hot climate have been implicated (6, 103). More rarely, ovaries suffer the same fate (155). And in volvulus of the intestine, which is also rare, the entire intestinal mass can be infarcted by twisting of the mesentery around its root.

A similar but more cheerful event is a tumor that twists itself out of existence: a benign tumor of smooth muscle (myoma) can grow out of the intestinal wall like a pedunculated appendage and never give any inkling of its existence until it accidentally twists on its stalk and becomes infarcted (see Figure 26.44).

PRESSURE SORES

Tissue pressure high enough to stop blood flow occurs in the buttocks every time we sit. We do not develop infarcts because we tend to squirm. Necrosis and pressure ulcers (*pressure sores*) do develop in patients who lie in the same position for many hours; sitting has the same effect in chair-bound patients. These ulcers are associated with a fourfold increase in the risk of death (4, 67).

Microscopic studies have shown that the damage occurs first in dermal and subdermal structures (fat and muscle) even though the epidermis remains intact (26, 163). Damage is greater over bony prominences. Remember that capillary pressure averages 20 mm Hg; in patients lying on a mattress, the pressure over the sacrum or the greater trochanter can reach 100–150 mm Hg (4).

> In the rat and rabbit, the skin is resistant to ischemia; it does not break down before 8–9 hours (162). In healthy pigs, a pressure of 200 mm Hg takes 16 hours to produce full-thickness necrosis. In debilitated patients the critical time is much shorter.

The critical period for producing a decubitus ulcer in bedridden patients is about a couple of hours (114). Nurses are advised to turn patients at risk at least every 1–2 hours (142), but this interval is often stretched because of other priorities. The principal danger of pressure sores is infection, which can lead to bacteremia and sepsis (40), with the compounded hazard that circulating bacteria tend to localize in the ulcer (26). Modern alternating-air mattresses or water beds are a partial answer to this distressing problem.

Obstructions at the Capillary Level

Obstacles to flow can develop, obviously, also in the capillaries; however, little is known about capillary pathology altogether (85). Here are some highlights.

THE HYPERVISCOSITY SYNDROMES

Flow in the microcirculation, and especially in the capillaries, can be hampered by increased viscosity of the blood, a problem that does not affect larger vessels. Hyperviscous blood interferes with the function of virtually every organ. The symptoms are therefore quite varied: fatigue, blurred vision, headache, dizziness, and bleeding from the gums and nose. The ophthalmoscope can show quite strikingly the congested microcirculation (Figure 23.41) (121).

How does the blood become too viscous? It may contain too many red blood cells (polycythemia), too many white blood cells (leukemia), or high concentrations of proteins that tend to aggregate (60):

- *Polycythemia* can be secondary (to anoxia, as in chronic mountain sickness, or in cases of renal carcinomas secreting an excess of erythropoietin); or it can be primary, a red-cell equivalent of leukemia, although it is not as malignant.
- The role of *leukemia* as a cause of hyperviscosity will be discussed below.
- *Plasma proteins that increase viscosity* are found in multiple myeloma, especially when the product of the monoclonal neoplastic plasma cells is IgG3, which tends to form complexes (especially at cool temperatures), or IgA, which tends to form elongated polymers. Waldenström's macroglobulinemia is another B-cell malignancy in which the hypersecreted protein is IgM; in many cases the IgM precipitates develop in the cold, which explains the clinical appearance of Raynaud's phenomenon in cold weather (p. 662).

CAPILLARY PATHOLOGY

Complete obstruction can occur in capillaries as in any other vessel, but little is known about it. In fact, little is known about capillary pathology altogether (85). The capillaries have long been considered to be privileged vessels, spared by most diseases except diabetes. It used to be said that "blood never clots in capillaries," which is surely wrong; but it is a fact that clots in capillaries are rarely found *postmortem*, probably because the fibrinolytic activity of the endothelium destroys them. It is also true that no known vasoactive agent affects capillary function, be it contractility, caliber, or permeability. Perhaps evolution has deprived them of the necessary receptors because they should remain aloof: their unimpeded function is critical.

We have summarized in Figure 23.42, and in the following list, the principal mishaps known to occur in capillaries; most of them are obstacles to flow (85):

1. *Impaction of leukocytes*. It seems strange that nature should have made leukocytes larger than most capillaries; this can be of help in inflammation (p. 397), but it can

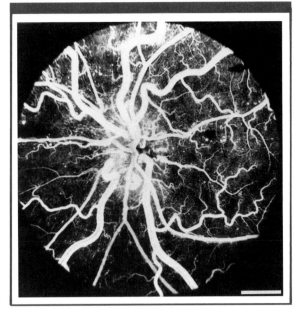

FIGURE 23.41 Dilated retinal arteries and veins in a case of hyperviscosity syndrome. **Bar** = 1 mm (Reproduced with permission from [121].)

also lead to capillary plugging and cause leukostasis. This is common in leukemia, especially myelocytic leukemia; in such cases it may cause complications in the brain and lungs, and even death from microcirculatory failure (99, 121). *Leukostasis* is now receiving much attention because it is implicated in the pathogenesis of reflow after ischemia (p. 686), shock (p. 689) (19), and other conditions (46, 58, 112). The normal tendency of leukocytes to become temporarily impacted in the capillaries can be exaggerated by several mechanisms: trapping by adhesion proteins, increased stiffness due to activation (164a), and increased size (in leukemia).

2. *Impaction of red blood cells*. Red blood cells can become impacted when their rigidity and volume are increased by acidosis (24, 30, 126). Ischemic tissues are acid. The red blood cells of diabetics are stiffer than normal and may cause flow disturbances (134).

3. *Impacted sickle cells*. These are involved in the pathogenesis of sickle cell anemia (140). Sickled red blood cells are deformed by the internal crystallization of the abnormal hemoglobin S. Under normal circumstances, red blood cells flowing through the microcirculation of the spleen have to squeeze through very tight passages; sickled cells are held up and can impede flow to the point of causing complete infarction of the spleen (*autosplenectomy*) (Figure

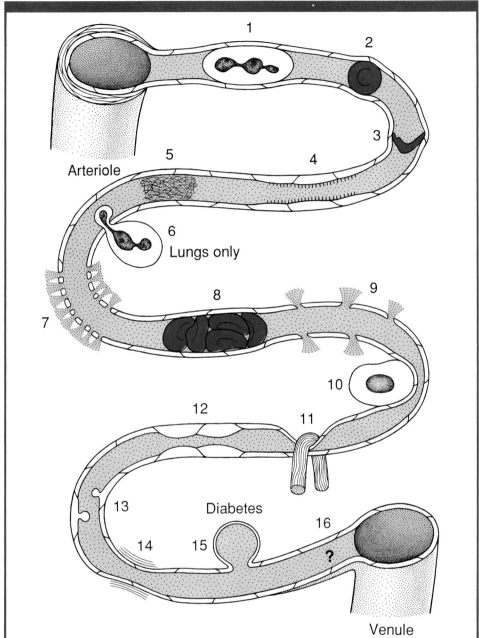

FIGURE 23.42
Pathologic mechanisms that may affect capillary structure and function. *1:* Plugging by leukocytes. *2:* Plugging by stiffened erythrocytes, as in acidosis. *3:* Plugging by abnormally shaped erythrocytes, such as in sickle cell disease. *4:* Activation of the endothelium, with expression of adhesion molecules. *5:* Obstruction by fibrin, either embolized or locally generated. *6:* Sticking of leukocytes followed by diapedesis, in lung capillaries only. *7:* Direct injury of the capillary wall. *8:* Stasis by red blood cells, such as occurs when fluid is lost. *9:* Late capillary leakage as it occurs in inflammation. *10:* Compression by swelling extravascular cells, such as astrocytes. *11:* Kinking over a collagen fiber. *12:* Swelling of endothelial cells, as occurs in eclampsia. *13:* Blebbing of endothelial cells. *14:* Stenosis by a multilayered, thickened basement membrane. *15:* Microaneurysms, as found in diabetes. *16:* For future discoveries.

23.43). A similar sequence can lead to multiple organ failure (101).

4. *Activation of the endothelium.* In venules and capillaries, this may lead to leukocyte sticking, clotting, and other changes (p. 397).

5. *Intracapillary clotting or embolization by fibrin clots,* as in disseminated intravascular coagulation (DIC, p. 683).

6. *Diapedesis* may occur in the capillaries of the lung (elsewhere it occurs in the venules). Activated leukocytes may cause capillary damage.

7. *Direct injury to the capillary* (as produced by oxygen overdose in the lungs) leads to diffuse, prolonged capillary leakage.

8. *Stasis of red blood cells (massive impaction)* due to fluid loss.

9. *Capillary leakage of the delayed type,* as seen after 24–48 hours of inflammation (p. 381).

10. *Extrinsic compression by swollen cells,* such as in ischemic brain (p. 686).

11. *Kinking over a collagen fiber,* in tissues swollen by edema.

12. *Endothelial swelling,* as in the renal glomeruli in eclampsia (56).

13. *Endothelial blebbing* (p. 125), as seen in ischemia.

14. *Repeated duplication of basement membranes,* which may lead to capillary stenosis in diabetes and other conditions (p. 264).

15. *Microaneurysms,* as occur in diabetes; it seems that the endothelial wall is "blown out" because the pericytes have died (Figure 23.44) (39, 149, 161).

16. Open for new discoveries.

Let it be clear that flow through a single capillary may be impaired by several defects of structure and function. The microcirculation in diabetes offers a sorry example: its causes of malfunction include changes in the endothelium (increased permeability, increased production of von Willebrand factor, decreased production of plasminogen activator), a thickened and biochemically abnormal basement membrane, microaneurysms due to pericyte loss, increased stickiness of the platelets, stiffening of the red blood cells, and the list is not complete (72a, 155b).

VASCULAR PLUGGING IN PLANTS

Obstacles can develop also in the vessels of apple trees and tomato plants (47, 156), and infarcts develop, although plant pathologists do not call them by that name ("wilting" is one of the alternatives). Infection and other types of injury cause vessels to become occluded by a mechanism that seems to be purposeful, like thrombosis in animals; this type of vascular occlusion is achieved by large cellular protrusions called tyloses (from the Greek *tylos,* lump or knob) (Figure 23.45). These **tyloses** resemble what animal pathologists call blebbing: the capillary-occluding mechanism listed as #13 in the figure just described. Nature plays themes and variations.

TO SUM UP: The variety of obstacles that may develop in the circulatory system reflects the problems that may develop in any plumbing system, but there are some oddities due to the subdivision of the vascular system into three sections—arteries, veins, and capillaries. In arteries, flow runs from large to smaller vessels, so that a variety of objects carried by the blood in large arteries will become impacted into smaller arteries. In veins, the blood runs from smaller to larger vessels, hence embolization cannot occur; objects carried by the blood will go through the heart and

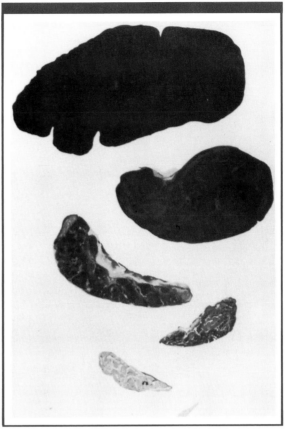

FIGURE 23.43 Human spleens illustrating the progressive atrophy that occurs in sickle cell anemia. The sickle cells become jammed in the microcirculation and impair blood flow; this may lead to autosplenectomy. Slightly enlarged. (Reproduced with permission from [125].)

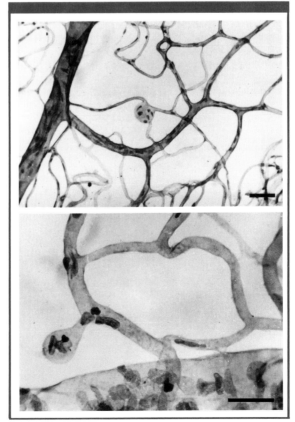

FIGURE 23.44 Microaneurysms in the retina of a diabetic patient. The entire vascular network of the retina was freed from other tissues by trypsinization, then laid out flat and photographed. *Top:* **Bar** = 500 µm. *Bottom:* **Bar** = 50 µm. The aneurysmal dilatations are thought to represent areas of weakness due to loss of pericytes. (Reproduced with permission from [39].)

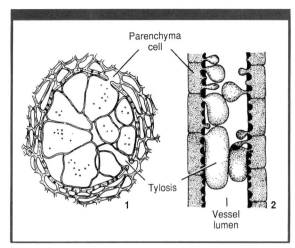

FIGURE 23.45

Example of plant pathology reminiscent of human pathology: namely, the blebbing and herniation of perivascular cells into the lumen, resulting in vascular occlusion. These plant protrusions are called tyloses. *Left:* Cross section of a vessel of *Robinia pseudacacia*. *Right:* Longitudinal section of a vessel of the vine tree *Vitis vinifera*. (Reproduced with permission from [34].)

embolize the pulmonary arteries. Venous flow is slow, which favors thrombosis. Capillary circulation is threatened by many types of malfunction, including obstruction by white or red blood cells, all of which are normally larger than the capillary lumen. In the microcirculation, several obstructive mechanisms can be at work at the same time, notably in diabetes.

Arteries suffer from a major disease related to age and to plasma cholesterol: atherosclerosis. We cannot explain why it has no counterpart in veins, but we can speculate. The arterial wall (notably the media) is designed for maximal toughness; the main components of the media are elastin and collagen, plus smooth muscle cells to synthesize both. When the media is infiltrated by plasma cholesterol it has no means to get rid of it: the media contains no macrophages and no capillaries to carry it away. Cholesterol cannot be broken down. The result is atherosclerosis.

It seems that the arterial wall was not designed for our current diet.

References

1. Agrios GN. Plant pathology, 3rd ed. New York: Academic Press, 1988.
2. Allen EV, Barker NW, Hines EA Jr. Peripheral vascular diseases, 3rd ed. Philadelphia: WB Saunders, 1962.
3. Allen GS, Ahn HS, Preziosi TJ, et al. Cerebral arterial spasm—a controlled trial of nimodipine in patients with subarachnoid hemorrhage. N Engl J Med 1983; 308:619–624.
4. Allman RM. Pressure ulcers among the elderly. N Engl J Med 1989;320:850–853.
4a. Anderson FA, Wheeler HB, Goldberg RJ, Hosmer DW, Patwardham NA, Jovanovic B, Forcier A, and Dalen JE. A population-based perspective of the hospital incidence and case-fatality rates of deep vein thrombosis and pulmonary embolism: the Worcester DVT study. Arch. Intern. Med. 1991;151:933–938.
5. Anderson JB, Williamson RCN. Testicular torsion in Bristol: a 25-year review. Br J Surg 1988;75:988–992.
6. Anderson RH, Wilcox BR, Becker AE. Anatomy of the normal heart. In: Hurst JW, Anderson RH, Becker AE, Wilcox BR. Atlas of the heart. New York: Gower Medical Publishing, 1988:1.1–1.20.
7. Armstrong RB. Muscle damage and endurance events. Sports Med 1986;3:370–381.
8. Bartsch RC, McConnell EE, Imes GD, Schmidt JM. A review of exertional rhabdomyolysis in wild and domestic animals and man. Vet Pathol 1977;14:314–324.
9. Beckering RE Jr, Titus JL. Femoral-popliteal venous thrombosis and pulmonary embolism. Am J Clin Pathol 1969;52:530–537.
10. Benacerraf A, Scholl JM, Achard F, Tonnelier M, Lavergne G. Coronary spasm and thrombosis associated with myocardial infarction in a patient with nearly normal coronary arteries. Circulation 1983;67:1147–1150.
11. Bocan TMA, Mueller SB, Brown EQ, Uhlendorf PD, Mazur MJ, Newton RS. Antiatherosclerotic effects of antioxidants are lesion-specific when evaluated in hypercholesterolemic New Zealand white rabbits. Exp Mol Pathol 1992;57:70–83.
12. Bove FJ. The story of ergot. Basel: S. Karger, 1970.
13. Braunwald E, ed. Heart disease. A textbook of cardiovascular medicine, 3rd ed. Philadelphia: WB Saunders, 1988.
14. Brazeau P. Oxytocins. Oxytocin and ergot alkaloids. In: Goodman LS, Gilman A, eds. The pharmacological basis of therapeutics, 4th ed. New York: Macmillan, 1970:893–907.
15. Buess H. Zur Geschichte des Embolie-Begriffs bis auf Virchow. In: Leuch O, Merkelbach O, eds. Schweizerisches Medizinisches Jahrbuch 1946. Basel: Benno Schwabe & Co., 1946:57–69.
16. Burger SK, Saul RF, Selhorst JB, Thurston SE. Transient monocular blindness caused by vasospasm. N Engl J Med 1991;325:870–873.
17. Cardelli MB, Kleinsmith DM. Raynaud's phenomenon and disease. Med Clin North Am 1989;73:1127–1141.
18. Cheitlin MD, McAllister HA, de Castro CM. Myocardial infarction without atherosclerosis. JAMA 1975;231:951–959.
19. Chien S, Sung K-LP, Schmid-Schönbein GW, Skalak R, Schmalzer EA, Usami S. Rheology of leukocytes. Ann NY Acad Sci 1987;516:333–347.
20. Chisolm GM. Oxidized lipoproteins and leukocyte-endothelial interactions: growing evidence for multiple mechanisms. Lab Invest 1993;68:369–371.
21. Christiaens GCML, Sixma JJ, Haspels AA. Hemostasis in menstrual endometrium: a review. Obstet Gynecol Surv 1982;37:281–303.
22. Cipriano PR, Koch FH, Rosenthal SJ, Baim DS,

Ginsburg R, Schroeder JS. Myocardial infarction in patients with coronary artery spasm demonstrated by angiography. Am Heart J 1983;105:542–547.

23. Clinton SK, Libby P. Cytokines and growth factors in atherogenesis. Arch Pathol Lab Med 1992;116:1292–1300.

24. Crandall ED, Critz AM, Osher AS, Keljo DJ, Forster RE. Influence of pH on elastic deformability of the human erythrocyte membrane. Am J Physiol 1978;235:C269–C278.

25. Cybulsky MI, Gimbrone MA Jr. Endothelial expression of a mononuclear leukocyte adhesion molecule during atherogenesis. Science 1991;251:788–791.

26. Daniel RK, Priest DL, Wheatley DC. Etiologic factors in pressure sores: an experimental model. Arch Phys Med Rehabil 1981;62:492–498.

27. Darsee JR. Cholesterol embolism: the great masquerader. South Med J 1979;72:174–180.

28. Davies PF, Robotewskyj A, Griem ML, Dull RO, Polacek DC. Hemodynamic forces and vascular cell communication in arteries. Arch Pathol Lab Med 1992;116:1301–1306.

29. DePaola N, Gimbrone MA Jr, Davies PF, Dewey CF Jr. Vascular endothelium responses to fluid shear stress gradients. Arterioscler Thromb 1992;12:1254–1257.

30. Dintenfass L. Microrheology of blood in health and disease. In: Onogi S, ed. Proceedings of the Fifth International Congress on Rheology, vol 2. Tokyo: University of Tokyo Press, 1970:27–59.

31. Durlacher SH, Meier JR, Fisher RS, Lovitt WV Jr. Sudden death due to pulmonary fat embolism in chronic alcoholics with fatty livers. J Forensic Sci 1959;4:215–228.

32. Elliott JP Jr, Hageman JH, Szilagyi DE, Ramakrishnan V, Bravo JJ, Smith RF. Arterial embolization: problems of source, multiplicity, recurrence, and delayed treatment. Surgery 1980;88:833–845.

33. Factor SM, Minase T, Cho S, Dominitz R, Sonnenblick EH. Microvascular spasm in the cardiomyopathic Syrian hamster: a preventable cause of focal myocardial necrosis. Circulation 1982;66:342–354.

34. Fahn A. Plant anatomy. Oxford: Pergamon Press, 1967.

34a. Falk E, Shah PK, Fuster V. Coronary plaque disruption. Circulation 1995;92:657–671.

35. Faruqi RM, DiCorleto PE. Mechanisms of monocyte recruitment and accumulation. Br Heart J 1993:S19–S29.

36. Fogarty TJ, Cranley JJ, Krause RJ, Strasser ES, Hafner CD. A method for extraction of arterial emboli and thrombi. Surg Gynecol Obstet 1963;116:241–244.

37. Forman MB, Oates JA, Robertson D, Robertson RM, Roberts LJ II, Virmani R. Increased adventitial mast cells in a patient with coronary spasm. N Engl J Med 1985;313:1138–1141.

38. Fred HL, Axelrad MA, Lewis JM, Alexander JK. Rapid resolution of pulmonary thromboemboli in man. JAMA 1966;196:121–123.

39. Fuchs U, Tinius W, vom Scheidt J, Reichenbach A. Morphometric analysis of retinal blood vessels in retinopathia diabetica. Graefe's Arch Clin Exp Ophthalmol 1985;223:83–87.

40. Galpin JE, Chow AW, Bayer AS, Guze LB. Sepsis associated with decubitus ulcers. Am J Med 1976;61:346–350.

41. Ganz P, Alexander RW. New insights into the cellular mechanisms of vasospasm. Am J Cardiol 1985;56:11E–15E.

42. Garfin SR. Historical review. In: Mubarak SJ, Hargens AR, eds. Compartment syndromes and Volkmann's contracture. (Saunders monographs in clinical orthopaedics, vol III). Philadelphia: WB Saunders, 1981:6–16.

43. Gelberman R. Volkmann's contracture of the upper extremity: pathology and reconstruction. In: Mubarak SJ, Hargens AR, eds. Compartment syndromes and Volkmann's contracture. (Saunders monographs in clinical orthopaedics, vol III). Philadelphia: WB Saunders, 1981:183–193.

44. Gerrity RG, Naito HK. Lipid clearance from fatty streak lesions by foam cell migration. Artery 1980;8:215–219.

45. Gershuni DH. Volkmann's contracture of the lower extremity: pathology and reconstruction. In: Mubarak SJ, Hargens AR, eds. Compartment syndromes and Volkmann's contracture. (Saunders monographs in clinical orthopaedics, vol III). Philadelphia: WB Saunders, 1981:194–208.

46. Goldblum SE, Cohen DA, Gillespie MN, McClain CJ. Interleukin-1-induced granulocytopenia and pulmonary leukostasis in rabbits. J Appl Physiol 1987;62:122–128.

47. Goodman RN, Király Z, Wood KR. The biochemistry and physiology of plant disease. Columbia, MO: University of Missouri Press, 1986.

48. Gossling HR, Donohue TA. The fat embolism syndrome. JAMA 1979;241:2740–2742.

49. Gossling HR, Pellegrini VD Jr. Fat embolism syndrome. A review of the pathophysiology and physiological basis of treatment. Clin Orthop 1982;165:68–82.

49a. Gott AM. Lipid lowering, regression, and coronary events. Circulation 1995;92:646–656.

50. Greenfield H. Raynaud's phenomenon: the cold facts. Harvard Health Letter 1992;17(3):1–2.

51. Gregg PJ, Walder DN. Caisson disease of bone. Clin Orthop 1986;210:43–54.

52. Gutstein WH, Anversa P, Guideri G. Spasm of small coronary arteries and ischemic myocardial injury induced by hypothalamic stimulation in the rat. Am J Pathol 1987;129:287–294.

53. Haigh JC, Stewart RR, Wobeser G, MacWilliams PS. Capture myopathy in a moose. J Am Vet Med Assoc 1977;171:924–926.

54. Hajjar KA, Gavish D, Breslow JL, Nachman RL. Lipoprotein(a) modulation of endothelial cell surface fibrinolysis and its potential role in atherosclerosis. Nature 1989;309:303–305.

55. Havig O. Deep vein thrombosis and pulmonary embolism. An autopsy study with multiple regression analysis of possible risk factors. Acta Chir Scand Suppl 1977;477:1–120.

56. Heaton JM, Turner DR. Persistent renal damage following pre-eclampsia: a renal biopsy study of 13 patients. J Pathol 1985;147:121–126.

57. Howard GC, Pizzo SV. Biology of disease: lipoprotein (a) and its role in atherothrombotic disease. Lab Invest 1993;69:373–386.

58. Howard RJ, Crain C, Franzini DA, Hood I, Hugli TE. Effects of cardiopulmonary bypass on pulmonary leukostasis and complement activation. Arch Surg 1988;123:1496–1501.

59. Hulman G. Pathogenesis of non-traumatic fat embolism. Lancet 1988;1:1366–1367.

60. Jandl JH. Blood. Boston: Little, Brown, 1987.

61. Jones DC, James SL. Overuse injuries of the lower extremity: shin splints, iliotibial band friction syndrome, and exertional compartment syndromes. Clin Sports Med 1987;6:273–290.

62. Jones HR Jr, Caplan LR, Come PC, Swinton NW Jr, Breslin DJ. Cerebral emboli of paradoxical origin. Ann Neurol 1983;13:314–319.

63. Joris I, Braunstein PW Jr. Platelets and endothelium: effect of collagen-induced platelet aggregates on pulmonary vessels. Exp Mol Pathol 1982;37:393–405.

64. Joris I, Majno G. Endothelial changes induced by arterial spasm. Am J Pathol 1981a;102:346–358.

65. Joris I, Majno G. Medial changes in arterial spasm induced by L-norepinephrine. Am J Pathol 1981b;105:212–222.

66. Joris I, Zand T, Nunnari JJ, Krolikowski FJ, Majno G. Studies on the pathogenesis of atherosclerosis. I. Adhesion and emigration of mononuclear cells in the aorta of hypercholesterolemic rats. Am J Pathol 1983;113:341–358.

67. Judson R. Pressure sores. Med J Aust 1983;1:417–422.

68. Jungbluth A, Erbel R, Darius H, Rumpelt H-J, Meyer J. Paradoxical coronary embolism: case report and review of the literature. Am Heart J 1988;116:879–885.

69. Kanamaru K, Waga S, Kojima T, Fujimoto K, Niwa S. Endothelium-dependent relaxation of canine basilar arteries. Part 2: inhibition by hemoglobin and cerebrospinal fluid from patients with aneurysmal subarachnoid hemorrhage. Stroke 1987;18:938–943.

70. Karch SB, Billingham ME. The pathology and etiology of cocaine-induced heart disease. Arch Pathol Lab Med 1988;112:225–230.

71. Kerstell J, Hallgren B, Rudenstam C-M, Svanborg A. I. The chemical composition of the fat emboli in the postabsorptive dog. Acta Med Scand Suppl 1969;499:3–18.

72. Korn D, Gore I, Blenke A, Collins DP. Pulmonary arterial bands and webs: an unrecognized manifestation of organized pulmonary emboli. Am J Pathol 1962;40:129–151.

72a. Korthius RJ, Fuselier SP, Jerome SN. Diabetic microangiopathy. In: Mortillaro NA, and Taylor AE. The pathophysiology of the microcirculation. Boca Raton: CRC Press, Inc., 1994:141–160.

73. Lam JYT, Chesebro JH, Steele PM, Badimon L, Fuster V. Is vasospasm related to platelet deposition? Relationship in a porcine preparation of arterial injury in vivo. Circulation 1987;75:243–248.

74. Lapuk S, Woodbury DF. Volkmann's ischemic contracture. A case report. Orthop Rev 1988;17:618–624.

75. Lawrie GM. Spasm of saphenous veins used as conduits for aortocoronary bypass grafting. Am J Cardiol 1988;61:675.

76. Lechat P, Mas JL, Lascault G, et al. Prevalence of patent foramen ovale in patients with stroke. N Engl J Med 1988;318:1148–1152.

77. Leonard RCF, Neville E, Hall RJC. Paradoxical embolism. A review of cases diagnosed during life. Eur Heart J 1982;3:362–370.

78. Levinson MJ. Gastric stress ulcers. Hosp Pract 1989;24:59–68.

79. Lewis RJ, Chalmers GA, Barrett MW, Bhatnagar R. Capture myopathy in elk in Alberta, Canada: a report of three cases. J Am Vet Med Assoc 1977;171:927–932.

80. Li H, Cybulsky MI, Gimbrone MA Jr, Libby P. An atherogenic diet rapidly induces VCAM-1, a cytokine-regulatable mononuclear leukocyte adhesion molecule, in rabbit aortic endothelium. Arterioscler Thromb 1993;13:197–204.

81. Logan SE. On the fluid mechanics of human coronary artery stenosis. IEEE Trans Biomed Eng BME 1975;22:327–334.

82. Ludmer PL, Selwyn AP, Shook TL, et al. Paradoxical vasoconstriction induced by acetylcholine in atherosclerotic coronary arteries. N Engl J Med 1986;315:1046–1051.

83. MacMahon HE, Weiss S. Carbon tetrachloride poisoning with macroscopic fat in the pulmonary artery. Am J Pathol 1929;5:623–630.

84. Mahley RW, Gray ME, LeQuire VS. Role of plasma lipoproteins in cortisone-induced fat embolism. Am J Pathol 1972;66:43–64.

85. Majno G. The capillary then and now: an overview of capillary pathology. Mod Pathol 1992;5:9–22.

86. Majno G, Cuénoud HF, Joris I. Arteriosclerosis 1988: the cellular events. New Trends in Arrhythmias 1989;5:33–40.

87. Majno G, Zand T, Nunnari JJ, Kowala MC, Joris, I. Intimal responses to shear stress, hypercholesterolemia, and hypertension. Studies in the rat aorta. In: Simionescu N, Simionescu M, eds. Endothelial cell biology in health and disease. New York: Plenum Press, 1988:349–367.

88. Matsen FA III, Winquist RA, Krugmire RB Jr. Diagnosis and management of compartmental syndromes. J Bone Joint Surg 1980;62A:286–291.

89. McEwen SA, Hulland TJ. Histochemical and morphometric evaluation of skeletal muscle from horses with exertional rhabdomyolysis (typing-up). Vet Pathol 1986;23:400–410.

90. McIntyre KM, Sasahara AA. The hemodynamic response to pulmonary embolism in patients without prior cardiopulmonary disease. Am J Cardiol 1971;28:288–294.

91. Miller FJ, Mineau DE. Transcatheter arterial embolization—major complications and their prevention. Cardiovasc Intervent Radiol 1983;6:141–149.

92. Moore WS, Malone JM. Effect of flow rate and vessel calibre on critical arterial stenosis. J Surg Res 1979;26:1–9.

93. Mora R, Lupu F, Simionescu N. Prelesional events in atherogenesis: colocalization of apolipoprotein B, unesterified cholesterol and extracellular phospholipid liposomes in the aorta of hyperlipidemic rabbit. Atherosclerosis 1987;67:143–154.

94. Morgan M. Amniotic fluid embolism. Anaesthesia 1979;34:20–32.

95. Morris DC. Cocaine heart disease. Hosp Pract 1991;26:83–92.

96. Moylan JA, Birnbaum M, Katz A, Everson MA. Fat emboli syndrome. J Trauma 1976;16:341–347.

97. Mubarak SJ. Etiologies of compartment syndromes. In: Mubarak SJ, Hargens AR, eds. Compartment syndromes and Volkmann's contracture. (Saunders monographs in clinical orthopaedics, vol III). Philadelphia: WB Saunders, 1981:71–97.

98. Mubarak SJ, Hargens AR, eds. Compartment syndromes and Volkmann's contracture. (Saunders monographs in clinical orthopaedics, vol III). Philadelphia: WB Saunders, 1981.

99. Myers TJ, Cole SR, Klatsky AU, Hild DH. Respiratory failure due to pulmonary leukostasis following chemotherapy of acute nonlymphocytic leukemia. Cancer 1983;51:1808–1813.

100. Nellessen U, Daniel WG, Matheis G, Oelert H, Depping K, Lichtlen PR. Impending paradoxical embolism from atrial thrombus: correct diagnosis by transesophageal echocardiography and prevention by surgery. J Am Coll Cardiol 1985;5:1002–1004.

101. Noguchi CT, Schechter AN. The intracellular polymerization of sickle hemoglobin and its relevance to sickle cell disease. Blood 1981;58:1057–1068.

102. Orenstein JM, Sato N, Aaron B, Buchholz B, Bloom S. Microemboli observed in deaths following cardiopulmonary bypass surgery: silicone antifoam agents and polyvinyl chloride tubing as sources of emboli. Hum Pathol 1982;13:1082–1090.

103. Osegbe DN. Testicular torsion in a hot country. N Engl J Med 1988;318:1129–1130.

104. Osler W. Rudolf Virchow, the man and the student. Boston Med Surg J 1891;125:425–427.

105. Owen CA. Clinical diagnosis of acute compartment syndromes. In: Mubarak SJ, Hargens AR, eds. Compartment syndromes and Volkmann's contracture. (Saunders monographs in clinical orthopaedics, vol III). Philadelphia: WB Saunders, 1981a:98–105.

106. Owen CA. The crush syndrome. In: Mubarak SJ, Hargens AR, eds. Compartment syndromes and Volkmann's contracture. (Saunders monographs in clinical orthopaedics, vol III). Philadelphia: WB Saunders, 1981b:166–182.

107. Palmovic V, McCarroll JR. Fat embolism in trauma. Arch Pathol 1965;80:630–635.

107a. Parthasarathy S. Modified lipoproteins in the pathogenesis of atherosclerosis. Austin, RG In Landis Company, 1994.

108. Peltier LF. Fat embolism. III. The toxic properties of neutral fat and free fatty acids. Surgery 1956;40:665–670.

109. Peltier LF. Fat embolism. A perspective. Clin Orthop 1988;232:263–270.

110. Perry MO. Compartment syndromes and reperfusion injury. Surg Clin North Am 1988;68:853–864.

111. Price TM, Baker VV, Cefalo RC. Amniotic fluid embolism. Three case reports with a review of the literature. Obstet Gynecol Surv 1985;40:462–475.

112. Redl H, Dinges HP, Schlag G. Quantitative estimation of leukostasis in the posttraumatic lung—canine and human autopsy data. Prog Clin Biol Res 1987;236A:43–53.

113. Resnick N, Collins T, Atkinson W, Bonthron DT, Dewey CF Jr. Platelet-derived growth factor B chain promoter contains a cis-acting fluid shear-stress-responsive element. Proc Natl Acad Sci 1993;90:4591–4595.

114. Reuler JB, Cooney TG. The pressure sore: pathophysiology and principles of management. Ann Intern Med 1981;94:661–666.

115. Riseborough EJ, Herndon JH. Alterations in pulmonary function, coagulation and fat metabolism in patients with fractures of the lower limbs. Clin Orthop 1976;115:248–267.

116. Rogers MC. Do the right thing. Pain relief in infants and children. N Engl J Med 1992;326:55–56.

117. Rosenow EC III, Osmundson PJ, Brown ML. Pulmonary embolism. Mayo Clin Proc 1981;56:161–178.

118. Ross R. Atherosclerosis: a problem of the biology of arterial wall cells and their interactions with blood components. Arteriosclerosis 1981;1:293–311.

119. Ross RM, Johnson GW. Fat embolism after liposuction. Chest 1988;93:1294–1295.

120. Russell RWR. Carotid artery disease and *Amarousis Fugax*. In: Miller S, ed. Clinical ophthalmology. Bristol: Wright, 1987:524–532.

121. Sanders MD, Graham EM. Ocular disorders associated with systemic diseases. In: Vaughan D, Asbury T, Tabbara KF, eds. 1989 General ophthalmology, 12th ed. Norwalk, CT: Appleton & Lange, 1989:279–319.

122. Schröder H, Paust H, Schmidt R. Pulmonary fat embolism after intralipid therapy—a post-mortem artifact? Light and electron microscopic investigations in low-birth-weight infants. Acta Paediatr Scand 1984;73:461–464.

123. Schwartz MM, Bidani AK, Lewis EJ. Glomerular epithelial cell function and pathology following extreme ablation of renal mass. Am J Pathol 1987;126:315–324.

124. Scott J. Thrombogenesis linked to atherogenesis at last? Nature 1989;341:22–23.

125. Serjeant GR. Sickle cell disease. Oxford: Oxford University Press, 1985.

126. Sevick EM, Jain RK. Effect of red blood cell rigidity on tumor blood flow: increase in viscous resistance during hyperglycemia. Cancer Res 1991;51:2727–2730.

127. Sevitt S. The significance and pathology of fat embolism. Ann Clin Res 1977;9:173–180.

128. Shaw ST Jr, Roche PC. Menstruation. In: Finn CA, ed. Oxford reviews of reproductive biology. Oxford: Clarendon Press, 1980:41–96.

129. Shier MR, Wilson RF. Fat embolism syndrome: traumatic coagulopathy with respiratory distress. Surg Annu 1980;12:139–168.

130. Shimokawa H, Tomoike H, Nabeyama S, et al. Coronary artery spasm induced in atherosclerotic miniature swine. Science 1983;221:560–562.

131. Shipley RE, Gregg DE. The effect of external constriction of a blood vessel on blood flow. Am J Physiol 1944;141:289–296.

132. Simionescu N. Prelesional changes of arterial endothelium in hyperlipoproteinemic atherogenesis. In: Simionescu N, Simionescu M, eds. Endothelial cell biology in health and disease. New York: Plenum Press, 1988:385–429.

133. Simionescu N, Mora R, Vasile E, Lupu F, Filip DA, Simionescu M. Prelesional modifications of the vessel wall in hyperlipidemic atherogenesis. Extracellular accumulation of modified and reassembled lipoproteins. Ann NY Acad Sci 1990;598:1–16.

134. Simpson LO. Intrinsic stiffening of red blood cells as the fundamental cause of diabetic nephropathy and microangiopathy: a new hypothesis. Nephron 1985;39:344–351.

135. Skoglund RW, McRoberts JW, Ragde H. Torsion of the spermatic cord: a review of the literature and an analysis of 70 new cases. J Urol 1970;104:604–607.

136. Snyder AB, Barone JG, DiGiacomo JC, Barone JE. Postoperative pulmonary leukostasis. Crit Care Med 1990;18:116–117.

137. Spencer H. Pathology of the lung, 4th ed. Oxford: Pergamon Press, 1985.

138. Stephenson J. Raynaud's phenomenon: the cold facts. Harvard Health Letter 1992;17(3):1–4.

139. Strock PE, Majno G. Vascular responses to experimental tourniquet ischemia. Surg Gynecol Obstet 1969;129:309–318.

140. Stuart J, Johnson CS. Rheology of the sickle cell disorders. Baillieres Clin Haematol 1987;1:747–775.

141. Swanson DA, Wallace S. Surgery of metastatic renal cell carcinoma and use of renal infarction. Semin Surg Oncol 1988;4:124–128.

142. Taylor C, Lillis C, LeMone P. Fundamentals of nursing: the art and science of nursing care. Philadelphia: JB Lippincott, 1989.

143. Taylor DC, Salvian AJ, Shackleton CR. Crush syndrome complicating pneumatic antishock garment (PASG) use. Injury 1988;19:43–44.

144. Templeman D, Lange R, Harms B. Lower-extremity compartment syndromes associated with use of pneumatic antishock garments. J Trauma 1987;27:79–81.

145. Thomas DP, Gurewich V, Ashford TP. Platelet adherence to thromboemboli in relation to the pathogenesis and treatment of pulmonary embolism. N Engl J Med 1966;274:953–956.

146. Thomas IH. Studies relating to the aetiology of caisson disease of bone. Newcastle-upon-Tyne, UK: University of Newcastle-upon-Tyne, 1983a, thesis.

147. Thomas IH. Caisson disease of bone. The seed and the soil. J R Coll Surg Edinb 1983b;28:347–360.

148. Thompson T, Evans W. Paradoxical embolism. Q J Med 1930;23:134–150.

149. Tilton RG, Faller AM, Hoffmann PL, Kilo C, Williamson JR. Acellular capillaries and increased pericyte degeneration in the diabetic extremity. Front Diabetes 1987;8:186–189.

150. van Buchem MA, te Velde J, Willemze R, Spaander PJ. Leucostasis, an underestimated cause of death in leukaemia. Blut 1988;56:39–44.

151. Vanhoutte PM. The endothelium and control of coronary arterial tone. Hosp Pract 1988;23:67–84.

152. Vanhoutte PM, Shimokawa H. Endothelium-derived relaxing factor and coronary vasospasm. Circulation 1989;80:1–9.

153. Vincent GM, Anderson JL, Marshall HW. Coronary spasm producing coronary thrombosis and myocardial infarction. N Engl J Med 1983;309:220–223.

154. Vogler C, Sotelo-Avila C, Lagunoff D, Braun P, Schreifels JA, Weber T. Aluminum-containing emboli in infants treated with extracorporeal membrane oxygenation. N Engl J Med 1988;319:75–79.

155. Wakamatsu M, Wolf P, Benirschke K. Bilateral torsion of the normal ovary and oviduct in a young girl. J Fam Pract 1989;28:101–102.

155a. Walco GA, Cassidy RC, Schechter NL. Pain, hurt, and harm: the ethics of pain control in infants and children. New Engl J Med 1994;331:541–544.

155b. Walker JD, Viberti GC. Pathophysiology of microvascular disease: an overview. In: Pickup JC, Williams G, (eds) Textbook of diabetes. Oxford: Blackwell Scientific Publications 1992;2:526–533.

156. Wallis FM, Truter SJ. Histopathology of tomato plants infected with *Pseudomonas solanacearum*, with emphasis on ultrastructure. Physiol Plant Pathol 1978;13:307–317.

157. Warren BA. Atheroembolism. Boca Raton, FL: CRC Press, 1986.

158. Warren BA, Philp RB, Inwood MJ. The ultrastructural morphology of air embolism: platelet adhesion to the interface and endothelial damage. Br J Exp Pathol 1973;54:163–172.

159. Willerson JT. Clinical diagnosis of acute myocardial infarction. Hosp Pract 1989;24:65–77.

160. Williamson JR, Chang K, Rowold E, Kilo C, Lacy PE. Islet transplants in diabetic Lewis rats prevent and reverse diabetes-induced increases in vascular permeability and prevent but do not reverse collagen solubility changes. Diabetologia 1986;29:392–396.

161. Williamson JR, Chang K, Tilton R, Kilo C. Etiopathogenesis of diabetic microangiopathy. An integrated view. Front Diabetes 1987;8:58–66.

162. Willms-Kretschmer K, Majno G. Ischemia of the skin. Electron microscopic study of vascular injury. Am J Pathol 1969;54:327–353.

163. Witkowski JA, Parish LC. Histopathology of the decubitus ulcer. J Am Acad Dermatol 1982;6:1014–1021.

164. Wolf PA. Transient ischemic attacks locating the source. Hosp Pract 1985;20:35–43.

164a. Worthen GS, Schwab III B, Elson EE, and Downey GP. Mechanics of simulated neutrophils: cell stiffening induces retention in capillaries. Science 1989;245:183–186.

165. Zamora-Quezada JC, Dinerman H, Stakecker MJ, Kelly JJ. Muscle and skin infarction after free-basing cocaine (crack). Ann Intern Med 1988;108:564–566.

166. Zand T, Majno G, Nunnari JJ, et al. Lipid deposition and intimal stress and strain: a study in rats with aortic stenosis. Am J Pathol 1991;139:101–113.

Ischemia and Shock

Having run through a long list of obstacles to blood flow, we are ready to examine the effect of those obstacles, namely inadequate blood flow or *ischemia*. Inadequate flow may be limited to a small part of an organ; it may also affect the body as a whole, in which case the result is called *shock*. We will begin with local ischemia.

Local Ischemia

Not surprisingly, it was Virchow—the barricade expert—who coined the word *ischemia* by combining the Greek *iskho*, I hold back, with *háima*, blood. He wisely chose the verb "to hold back" rather than "to stop" because the concept of ischemia includes inadequate blood flow as well as lack of blood flow.

Ischemia Versus Anoxia. Our first concern is to distinguish ischemia and anoxia. The latter is often used loosely to mean *hypoxia*. Anoxia and hypoxia refer only to lack of oxygen. Ischemia does have a component of anoxia, but ischemia and anoxia can be entirely separate. Villagers who live high in the Andes are chronically hypoxic and develop hypertrophic hearts, but they are not ischemic (103). In victims of drowning, as long as the heart beats, the brain and all other organs are hypoxic, not ischemic. Similarly, pearl and sponge divers, who hold their breath for prolonged periods, may suffer anoxic (but not ischemic) brain damage.

In the Polynesian islands the pearl divers' disease has many names including Nou-nou parau *(pearl shell insanity); it ranges from transient functional impairments to permanent paralysis and dementia (25).*

Anoxia plays an important role in brain pathology because neurons are especially sensitive to oxygen deprivation (1).

A tissue deprived of oxygen suffers *one* loss; a tissue deprived of its blood supply suffers *three*:

- *The supply of oxygen*, which is not stored in significant amounts.

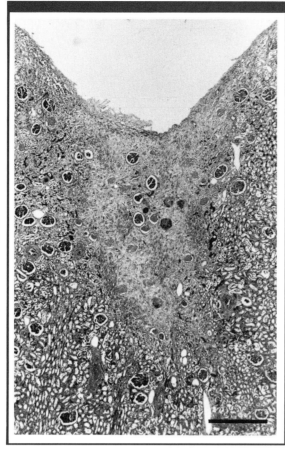

FIGURE 24.1 Small scar in the renal cortex from chronic ischemia due to arteriolosclerosis. *Top:* The surface of the kidney is depressed because renal parenchyma has disappeared and was replaced by connective tissue; some glomeruli have survived. **Bar** = 500 μm.

- *The supply of substrates* for metabolic and synthetic processes.
- *Means of removing waste products,* including acid metabolic products.

It follows that the effects of ischemia are much worse than those of anoxia alone. The difference is dramatized in tissue cultures. We have grown bovine endothelial cells *in vitro* under conditions of complete anoxia for as long as 4 days with no visible adverse effects; the tissues were presumably surviving on anaerobic glycolysis. But if we also removed glucose to obtain a kind of "ischemia *in vitro,*" cells began to die within an hour (29a).

Ischemia continues to attract an enormous amount of research, not only because it often paves the way to death by strokes or myocardial infarcts, but also because cardiac surgery and organ transplantation hinge on keeping organs alive for several hours in the absence of blood flow. Also, in newborns, asphyxia suffered in the uterus or during birth causes many forms of hypoxic-ischemic brain damage, including motor deficits (cerebral palsy), seizures, and mental retardation (61).

Tissue Changes Caused by Local Ischemia

Local ischemia causes damage, but it also triggers corrective responses. We shall begin with the latter.

Development of collateral circulation The basic fact was clear already in 1845 (Figure 21.6): when flow through a given artery is stopped, alternative channels develop in and around the ischemic tissue (110a). Some of these channels arise by enlargement and remodeling of previously existing vessels, while others are entirely new, and therefore represent *angiogenesis.* Just how all this growth is brought about is not so clear. Increased blood pressure and flow are probably involved; furthermore, it has been shown that, *under conditions of ischemia, angiogenic factors are produced by several cell types*—macrophages, retinal cells (99a), myocardial cells, and several tumors (30a). This feedback (ischemia ⟶ angiogenesis) makes good sense; perhaps it will turn out to be true for all or most cell types. There is a model for such a feedback: the secretion of erythropoietin depends on an oxygen-sensitive gene (30a).

Damage caused by local ischemia Mild, chronic local ischemia induces atrophy (Figure 24.1); but

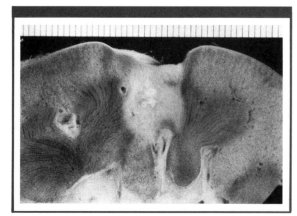

FIGURE 24.2
Cut surface of a kidney; the white area indicates infarction. The depressed surface indicates that removal of necrotic tissue has been taking place for several weeks. Some necrotic tissue is still present. From a patient with a defective prosthetic aortic valve that had been shedding thromboemboli. Scale in mm.

acute ischemia may lead to ischemic necrosis, that is, **infarction** (Figure 24.2). Within an infarct, *the most specialized cells are the first to die.* It would be intellectually satisfying if the service structures (microcirculatory vessels) were the most resistant; and indeed, for the ischemic heart there is some evidence that vessels survive longer than myocardial cells (73).

Because infarcts are basically dead tissue, we would expect them to be white, firm masses (p. 192), roughly shaped like wedges, corresponding to the treelike vascular territory. In reality, some infarcts are white, and some are red because the dead tissue is soaked with blood; hence the old terms *white infarct* and *red infarct.* As for the shape of a wedge, it is best seen with the help of a little wishful thinking.

At the start, to the naked eye, all infarcts are red (or at least reddish) (Figure 24.3). *Later—within days—they turn white,* because the red blood cells hemolyze, and the hemoglobin diffuses away (Figure 5.16).

The apparent paradox of ischemic tissue being filled with blood is easily explained. The blood pools, at first, in dilated, "paralyzed" capillaries (48); later it spills into the tissue spaces. The redness means that some blood is trickling into the ischemic tissue—not enough to keep it alive but enough to stuff it with red blood cells. In fact, the word *infarct* comes from the Latin *infarcire,* to stuff in.

How does blood trickle into the vessels of a recent infarct? There are at least five mechanisms.

- *In an infarct due to venous obstruction,* the redness is self-explanatory: the veins and capillaries are distended with blood that has no way out.
- *In an infarct due to an embolized artery,* the embolus may not be completely occlusive; or it may be a thromboembolus that shrank secondarily by clot retraction. In either case some blood may trickle past the obstacle.
- *In a recent infarct the pressure in the vessels drops to zero,* and blood therefore tends to seep in through capillaries from the surrounding tissues. Eventually these capillaries, at the point where they enter the infarct, become plugged by thrombi and seal off.
- *In infarcts of the lung, which has double circulation,* the influx of blood into the dead tissue comes from the bronchial circulation (p. 682).
- *Infarcts in tissues with a collateral circulation*

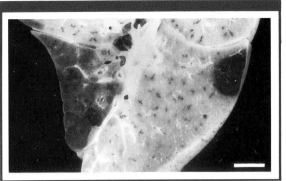

may fill with blood, but not enough to rescue the infarcted tissue.

The reddest of red infarcts are found in the lung, presumably because of the double source of blood (see Figure 24.3). Later these infarcts become white, like any other; as followed by X-rays, signs of shrinkage begin to appear in 2–4 weeks. Fifty percent of such infarcts disappear without trace within 3 months, although some leave a fine scar, an adhesion, or a pleural thickening (58, 88).

In the heart, the red stage of infarction is barely recognizable as congested, vaguely purplish tissue, so infarcts appear pale almost from the start. Older

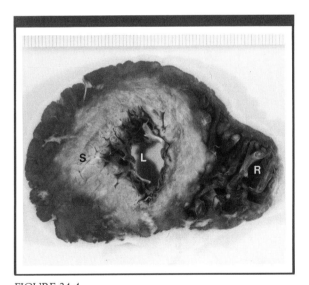

FIGURE 24.4
Cross section of a human heart with an extensive subendocardial infarct (**S**) of the left ventricle, demonstrated by the TTC stain; the pale (unstained) area corresponds to the infarct. This type of infarct (without coronary occlusion) develops when the heart suffers from coronary hypoperfusion, a situation that can occur in shock. **L:** Left ventricle. **R:** Tip of the right ventricle. Scale in mm. (Courtesy of Dr. H.F. Cuénoud, University of Massachusetts Medical Center, Worcester, MA.)

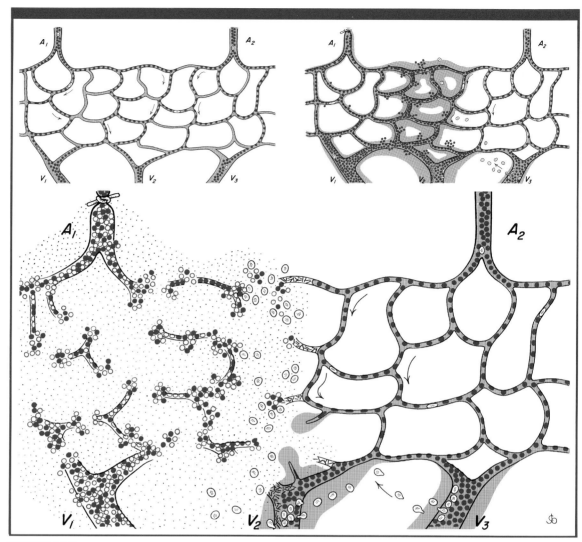

FIGURE 24.5

Microcirculatory events during infarction. *Top left:* A normal microcirculatory network fed by two arterioles, **A1, A2.** *Top right:* Arteriole **A1** has been obstructed, and blood pressure downstream falls to zero. Through connections with the network of **A2,** some blood drifts into the ischemic area, which therefore becomes purplish to the naked eye. The ischemic capillaries lose their tone, dilate, and allow some red blood cells to escape into the tissues. *Bottom:* The capillaries that connected **A1** to **A2** are occluded by platelet thrombi; the dying tissue attracts leukocytes which break down the connections between the two networks. In the infarct, red blood cells hemolyze. Eventually all the dead tissue will be reabsorbed.

myocardial infarcts are white with a greenish tinge due to the breakdown of hemoglobin. In the brain, the red phase may be missing for reasons that are unclear.

> At autopsy, the gross diagnosis of a recent infarct is a recurrent problem because visible changes do not appear until many hours or even a day after infarction. In the heart, the diagnosis can be helped by dipping slices of tissue in triphenyltetrazolium chloride, a dye that stains normal myocardium brick red (TTC test). Infarcts older than 3 hours remain unstained, and so do 50 percent of 30-minute

infarcts (130). The principle is that a myocardial dehydrogenase becomes nonfunctional in the infarcted area (Figure 24.4). The TTC test is a gift from botany: it was devised in 1942 to distinguish live and dead parts of seeds (56, 77).

The microscopic events that follow infarction are largely predictable. As the tissue dies, its capillaries and other vessels appear "paralyzed," overdilated, and filled with compacted red blood cells (Figure 24.5). Within hours the infarct evokes an acute inflammatory response, spearheaded by a

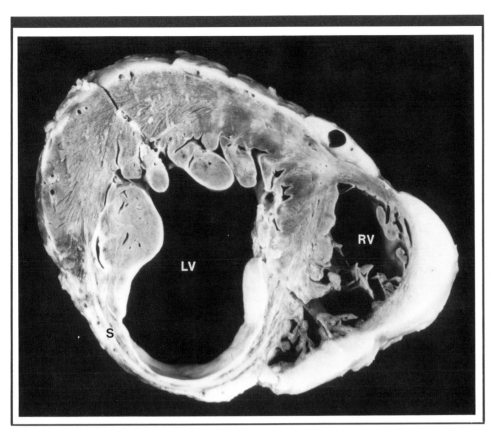

FIGURE 24.6
Cross section of a heart showing the scar (**S**) of a myocardial infarct in the wall of the left ventricle (**LV**). Normally the thickness of the ventricular wall should be the same all around. The scar consists of fibrous tissue that tends to give way over the years and may bulge like an aneurysm. **RV:** right ventricle. (Courtesy of Dr. W.D. Edwards, Mayo Clinic, Rochester, MN.)

wave of polymorphs (p. 440). Capillaries connected with the infarcted tissue seal off by thrombosis, while the ischemic tissue releases factors that stimulate endothelial growth (44). Within a few days, a layer of granulation tissue surrounds the necrotic mass, which is slowly reabsorbed. The ultimate result is a fibrous scar (Figure 24.6).

In the brain, the sequence is somewhat different. The debris of liquefying tissue are picked up by microglial cells, the local representatives of the macrophage family, which become stuffed with lipid droplets and come to resemble foam cells (Figure 5.53). The result is a cavity filled with fluid or a scar consisting of astrocytes.

The Pathogenesis of Ischemic Damage

Ischemic damage can occur also in the presence of blood flow if the flow is inadequate. In general, whether damage develops or not depends on several factors: type of vessel occluded (artery, vein), local vascular pattern, intensity and duration of ischemia, nature of the tissue involved, temperature of the tissue, viscosity and glucose content of the blood, and whether there is a double source of blood. Electron microscopy shows that early changes of cell membranes and mitochondria are reversible (Figures 24.7, 24.8).

Oddly enough, some of the molecular damage can be traced to oxygen-derived free radicals that develop despite the hypoxic conditions (102a).

ISCHEMIA WITHOUT OBSTACLES TO FLOW

Some examples:

- A *myocardial infarct* can occur with patent coronaries. If the aortic valve is constricted (aortic stenosis), the left ventricle pumps against increased resistance and becomes hypertrophic. Meanwhile, the coronary arteries that arise from the aorta just beyond the stenosis receive less blood. Now, if the left ventricle is placed under a strain and needs more blood than it can receive, it may develop an infarct (20).
- *Shock,* as we will see, is a condition of *generalized inadequate perfusion.* Blood flows in all tissues, but not enough. This condition may lead to brain damage and coma; the

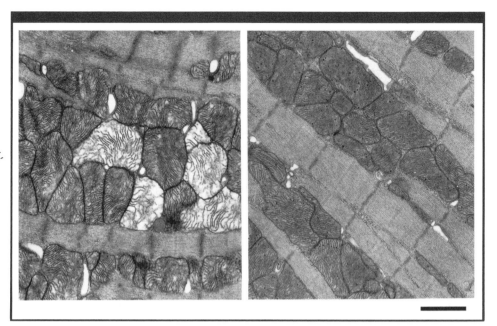

FIGURE 24.7
Left: Anoxic rat heart cell 1 hour after incubation in culture medium. Note some mitochondrial swelling, loss of matrix granules, and shortening of the sarcomeres. *Right:* Recovery from 60 minutes of anoxia after 30 minutes of reoxygenation. The mitochondria appear normal and have reacquired their matrix granules. The sarcomeres are more relaxed. **Bar** = 1 μm. (Reproduced with permission from [114].)

Purkinje cells of the cerebellum are especially sensitive. The renal cortex can develop massive tubular necrosis; the liver may also develop large patches of ischemic necrosis.

• *Watershed lesions* are fairly common in the brain and the colon; as the name suggests,

they are areas of ischemia at the junction of territories supplied by two arteries (125a). In the brain, watershed lesions are seen in survivors of cardiac arrest (Figure 24.9). The mechanism of this infarction is unclear; perhaps, when the heart resumes pumping, two adjacent cerebral arteries do

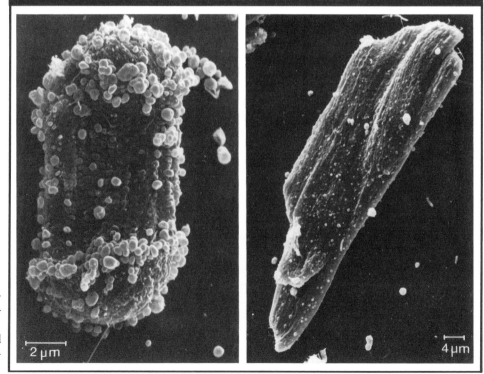

FIGURE 24.8
Left: Anoxic rat heart cell after 2 hours of incubation with nitrogen. Note many microscopic blebs and contraction of the cell. *Right:* Recovery from 2 hours of anoxia by 30 minutes of reoxygenation. The blebs have almost disappeared, and the cell has become more elongated. (Reproduced with permission from [114].)

not immediately supply the periphery of their territories. In the colon ischemic damage tends to develop at the junction of the transverse and the descending colon, the watershed between the territories of the superior and inferior mesenteric arteries (108).

ROLE OF VASCULAR PATTERNS

Occlusion of an Artery Given an obstacle to flow in an artery, say an embolus, the first question that arises is whether ischemia will or will not occur downstream of that obstacle. This depends on the pattern of blood distribution. *Occlusion of a nonterminal artery causes no damage, but occlusion of a terminal artery causes ischemia and infarction.* This is what happens in the retina (Figure 24.10), the kidney (see Figure 24.2), the heart, and the brain.

The heart has its own way of escaping damage from occlusion of a terminal artery. Imagine that a myocardial territory suffers a period of chronic ischemia due to stenosis in an artery that we will call X. Being a branch of a coronary artery, X is a terminal vessel. Now, chronic ischemia in the territory that X supplies may have the effect of attracting blood flow from the nearby myocardium; over months, collateral vessels develop, including bridges from neighboring arteries. A sudden obstruction of X now will find the myocardium equipped with an emergency blood supply.

Occlusion of Veins The effect of venous occlusion follows similar rules, except that the damage is upstream rather than downstream. However, veins are much more numerous and interconnected than arteries, so infarction by venous occlusion is not as common. It occurs, for example, after occlusion of the renal vein.

FACTORS THAT MODULATE ISCHEMIC DAMAGE

Degree and Duration of Ischemia If a tissue is *chronically* blood-starved, it does not die outright but atrophies; its cells shrink a little and then succumb discretely in a hierarchical order. Parenchymal cells, which have the more complex and demanding functions, are the first to shrivel and disappear (p. 42); they die by apoptosis (p. 200). The final result of chronic ischemia is a tissue with few or no parenchymal cells and more connective tissue. A classic example is the renal cortex that is made chronically ischemic by stenosis of its small arteries (see Figure 24.1).

At the other extreme, *acute* total ischemia

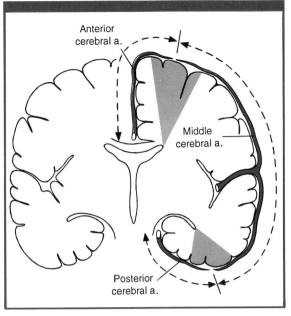

FIGURE 24.9 Parts of the brain most susceptible to ischemia and infarction: the so-called watershed zones (pink) between the territories supplied by the anterior, middle, and posterior cerebral arteries. (Adapted from [2].)

causes cells to swell and die by the process that we called *oncosis* (p. 191) followed by massive necrosis. The corresponding sequence of cellular events was described earlier (p. 191).

Nature of the Tissue The outcome of ischemia depends on the type of tissue involved, for obvious reasons. Some cell types are sturdier than others, the toughest of all being the fibroblasts and the most sensitive the neurons (p. 693).

Temperature of the Tissue Higher temperature increases tissue damage. This is why many sur-

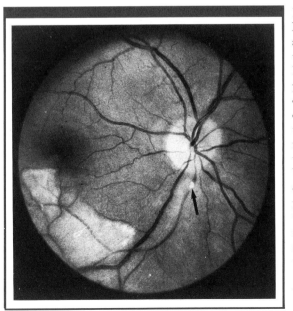

FIGURE 24.10 Retinal vessels are a natural window to the microcirculation. The **arrow** points to a small calcified embolus, originating from a thrombus on the mitral or aortic valve (subacute bacterial endocarditis). The white patch at the bottom left represents the corresponding zone of retinal infarction. (Reproduced with permission from [109].)

geons choose to cool the heart during surgery for bypass (87) and why drowning in cold water can be followed by recovery if the submersion lasted 40 minutes, or even longer (28, 40). Children are the best survivors of drowning, probably because they cool faster; but it is a fact that immature brains are more resistant to anoxia (128).

Abnormally Viscous Blood Whatever the cause, blood that is too thick can lead to brain damage; a hematocrit above 46 percent increases the risk (14). Conversely, a low leukocyte count (in dogs) reduces the size of myocardial infarcts (105).

Blood Glucose Hypoglycemia causes brain lesions similar to those of anoxia. The effects of hyperglycemia are somewhat controversial. Intuitively, one might think that—for ischemic cells—glycolysis, although inefficient, would be better than nothing in terms of energy production. On the other hand, glycolysis produces lactic acid, and local acidosis is said to be detrimental (66, 96, 120). The damage may be self-limiting because acidosis poisons the glycolytic mechanism (74, 101). Local acidosis also increases the rigidity of red blood cells, making the blood more viscous (99). There are occasional dissenting voices: under certain conditions, acidosis is said to protect against ischemic damage (79, 116).

Myocardium that is depleted of glycogen before ischemia makes a better recovery (96). Clinical studies concluded that the outcome of cerebrovascular accidents was worse in hyperglycemic patients, but experimental results have been contradictory (30).

> The hour of the day *bears some relationship to myocardial infarction, which is much more frequent at 8–9 AM than at 5 PM. It seems that the blood level of catecholamines is higher and that the platelets are stickier in the early morning (94). Insomniacs may want to read an article on the dangers of going to bed (7).*

Induction of Angiogenesis There is growing evidence that tissues respond to hypoxia by producing angiogenic factors, thereby tending to correct the hypoxia. Hypoxic macrophages certainly behave in this fashion, as we mentioned in relation to wound healing (p. 469). Hypoxia causes the retina to secrete the potent angiogenesis factor VEGF (vascular endothelial growth factor), thereby inducing inappropriate and damaging vascularization (99a), and tumor cells may also respond to hypoxia by secreting VEGF (99a).

Obviously this angiogenic response to hypoxia can be harmful (as in diabetic retinopathy), but its primary role must be to assist the process of cellular adaptation to ischemia.

ISCHEMIA IN ORGANS WITH DOUBLE BLOOD SUPPLY

The two main examples are the lungs and liver. The lungs receive most of their blood under low pressure from the pulmonary arteries and some blood under high pressure from the bronchial arteries. The two networks are connected at their distal ends. For this reason, occlusions in the bronchial arteries do not produce ischemia (the bronchial arteries are not reconnected in the course of lung transplants). Occlusions of the pulmonary arteries by emboli are commonplace. Depending on the size of the occluded artery and on the function of the heart, *occlusion may produce a transient hemorrhage, an infarct, or no effect at all.* Here are the somewhat bewildering facts:

- *Massive bilateral embolism.* If 60 percent or more of the pulmonary flow is cut off, the result is instant death. Many clinicians have experienced the shock of seeing a patient rise from bed only to keel over without uttering a sound. The cause is usually a single massive embolus astride the pulmonary artery bifurcation (*saddle embolus*) (Figure 23.3). Death being so sudden, there is of course no infarction. (The mechanism of death: occlusion of the pulmonary arteries interrupts the circulation, whereby the heart stops beating.)
- *Sudden obstruction of a single, main pulmonary artery.* The sudden and total occlusion or constriction of the right or left pulmonary artery produces only minimal cardiocirculatory effects (107). There is no infarction. Virchow was the first to face this rather surprising effect (29), and he correctly argued that the lung has two circulations: when the pulmonary flow is cut off, the bronchial arteries take over. This has been abundantly confirmed.
- *Emboli in peripheral branches of the pulmonary arteries.* Emboli in arteries that are less than 3 mm in diameter (126) can produce two kinds of lesions: intraalveolar hemorrhage without necrosis (Figure 24.11) or hemorrhagic infarct.

So we are faced with a paradox: emboli in the smaller pulmonary arteries are more dangerous to lung tissue than occlusion of the large arteries. We

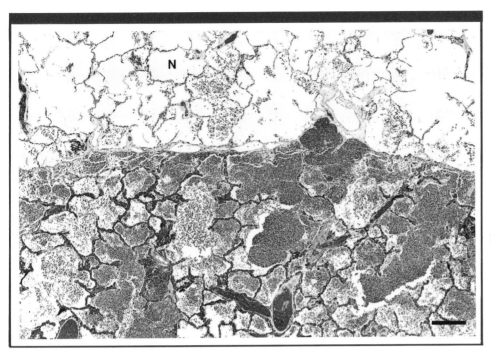

FIGURE 24.11
Lung tissue just after embolism. Diffuse congestion and hemorrhage into the alveolar spaces may or may not proceed to necrosis. The sharp edge between hemorrhagic and normal (**N**) lung tissue corresponds to an interlobular septum. **Bar** = 250 μm.

are embarrassed to say that, despite much thinking by the experts (27), there is no proven explanation.

We need to understand the nature of the pulmonary hemorrhage and how it relates to a hemorrhagic infarct. Schematically, we see the problem as follows (55):

- *Pathogenesis of the hemorrhage.* A branch of the pulmonary artery is occluded; the tissue downstream begins to suffer, but the bronchial circulation succeeds, just barely, in keeping it alive. Some ischemic capillaries break down, hence the hemorrhage, but eventually the bronchial circulation improves (arterial dilatation?) and the tissue survives. Macrophages clean up the spilled blood.

- *Pathogenesis of a hemorrhagic infarct.* A branch of the pulmonary artery is occluded, and the tissue downstream dies because the bronchial circulation is unable to rescue it; bronchial artery blood just trickles into the dead tissue, so the infarct is hemorrhagic.

In other words, the hemorrhage represents an early and reversible stage of infarction; it is an *incomplete infarct* (55). These purely hemorrhagic and reversible lesions really exist (see Figure 24.11); the best proof is supplied by serial chest X-rays after a pulmonary embolism, which show an infiltrate in the lung that fades away within a week or less. This cannot represent an infarct (27) because only 50 percent of infarcts clear within 3 months (88).

A pulmonary infarct and a hemorrhage are clinically indistinguishable except by following their progression on chest films: a shadow that disappears in 2–4 days must be a hemorrhage (55). Many lung infarcts are silent; the classic symptoms are chest pain, dyspnea, hemoptysis, and systemic hypotension (106). The pain is probably due to an acute inflammatory response in the parietal pleura. Remember that deep lesions (within the lung itself) are painless: people walk around without feeling their pneumonia.

Why do some emboli in normal lungs produce hemorrhage and others an infarct, even though they lodge in arteries of similar caliber? Nobody knows. We can only suggest that the difference may depend on the completeness of occlusion. In an angiographic study, the degree of occlusion varied between 13 and 68 percent (mean 37%) (89). Infarcts are reportedly more common than hemorrhage in cases of shock, pulmonary edema, pneumonia, and malignancy (126).

- *In the lungs of patients with heart disease, infarcts are much more frequent than hemorrhages.* This can be explained. In a patient with left ventricular failure, an embolus in a branch of a pulmonary artery creates downstream a territory of congested vessels, perhaps even some hemorrhage; if the heart were functioning normally, the bronchial circulation would intervene to relieve this congestion, but since the left heart is failing, the bronchial circulation is also failing and cannot rescue the embolized territory, which becomes an infarct (27).

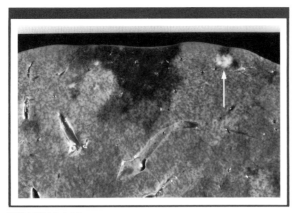

FIGURE 24.12
Typical Zahn infarct of the liver in a patient with generalized carcinoma. Such infarcts are caused by thrombosis in a branch of the portal vein; in this case thrombosis was probably related to the carcinoma. **Arrow:** Small metastasis. Scale in mm.

A teaser: what happens when an embolus lands in a grafted lung? In lung transplants, the bronchial circulation is not reconnected; therefore all emboli should produce infarcts. So far nobody has reported a higher incidence of infarcts in grafted lungs, and there may be a good reason: in dogs with grafted lungs, the neglected bronchial artery seems to reconnect itself on its own (90).

The liver receives arterial blood from the hepatic artery and venous blood from the portal vein; blood from the two sources is mixed at the microcirculatory level. Because some oxygen and all necessary nutrients can be supplied by the portal vein, infarcts by arterial occlusion are rare; but they do occur. If a small branch of the portal vein is occluded, necrosis does not develop; liver tissue simply becomes atrophic. Smaller cells and wider sinusoids produce a red, depressed area called a *Zahn infarct* (10, 135). The venous obstruction is usually a thrombus of the kind that may develop in the presence of generalized cancer or other debilitating condition (Figure 24.12). Clinically it is not significant.

The Pathophysiology of Reperfusion

To anyone interested in healing, the local catastrophe called infarct poses a challenge: how to rescue the tissue before it dies, by reperfusing the vessels. This means, first of all, removing the obstacle: an embolus can be surgically extracted (embolectomy); a coronary thrombus can be dissolved by enzymes (thrombolysis). After the obstacle is removed, however, functional problems arise. Reperfusion of an ischemic territory turns out to be a complex subject.

Experimentally, the study of reperfusion (reflow) is straightforward. You choose a part of the body (a limb, a kidney, a part of the liver), clamp off its blood supply, and then restore it at various times to see what happens. This approach has led to two rather startling discoveries:

- Reflow may be incomplete (no-reflow phenomenon).
- Reflow triggers a wave of damage to ischemic tissue.

THE NO-REFLOW PHENOMENON

Reflow after a short period of ischemia (seconds or minutes, depending on the organ) is a simple matter: nothing bad happens beyond functional changes, and accordingly the topic is taught by physiologists. Consider a tourniquet: if the circulation is cut off for a few minutes and then released, there is a phase of active hyperemia, which is attributed to metabolic products acting on the arterioles, especially adenosine (67). This is a fine arrangement: the ATP of ischemic tissues cannot be regenerated; instead, it is degraded to adenosine diphosphate, then to monophosphate, and finally to simple adenosine, which is a vasodilator that tends to correct the ischemia. Note that *prolonged* ischemia, to the contrary, leads to the formation of *vasoconstrictor* eicosanoids (93).

Reflow after prolonged ischemia involves a great deal of pathophysiology. The first rule is that reflow through *dead* tissue is not possible.

The pioneer experiments on reflow were done by Cohnheim in 1872 (22, 23). His procedure was to tie off the tongue of a frog; if the ligature is released after more than 3 days—he writes—"the blood . . . barely forces its way into the commencement of the arteries and a little distance in advance of the point of ligature, and . . . no more blood reaches the small arteries to say nothing of the capillaries and veins" (23). After shorter periods of ischemia (12–60 hours) reflow did occur; but the tongue became swollen, congested, and inflamed. With ischemic rabbit ears the results were the same, but the sequence was much faster.

To demonstrate the lack of reflow through dead tissue, let us repeat the experiments of Sheehan and Davis of Liverpool, performed almost a century after Cohnheim (119). First, clamp the artery and vein of a rabbit kidney for 3 hours; at this point the kidney is dead (the limit for irreversible renal ischemia in the rat is 1 hour for two-thirds of the animals [84]). Now release the clamp; the kidney quickly becomes congested and stuffed with blood. There is a trickle of blood out of the renal vein, but after half an hour or so it stops, and the kidney looks like a typical red infarct. What stops the flow of blood? Sheehan and Davis listed seven possibilities and were pleased with none. In retrospect, the basic mechanisms may be fairly straightforward. We would expect our readers to work it out before reading the answer.

The answer: the ischemic endothelium breaks down; when blood flow returns, plasma escapes from the vessels, which remain filled with a sludge of red blood cells that cannot be pushed along. Tissue pressure rises (the kidney is wrapped in a tight capsule); the veins are thereby compressed, while the overfilled capillaries expand and even bleed. In the meantime, thromboplastin is released by all the dead cells, and whatever plasma is left in the vessels clots, permanently blocking the path to reflow.

So much for the reperfusion of a *dead* tissue.

Reperfusion of ischemic tissue that is still alive can be tested with the same experimental models. We explored this topic in the 1960s by testing reflow in the globally ischemic rabbit brain. To visualize reflow we infused a suspension of carbon black. We could see with our naked eyes that reperfusion was not complete even after a period of ischemia as short as 5 minutes (Figure 24.13). The hind limb of the rat, made ischemic by a tourniquet, showed patchy reflow after 30 minutes. We called this incomplete reperfusion *the no-reflow phenomenon* (4, 75, 83, 122, 123, 132). Similar results were obtained by others with the kidney (124), the heart (50, 51, 72), the skin (85), and other organs. We conclude that *some obstacle or obstacles develop in the vessels of ischemic tissues.*

It is now clear that the obstacles can be many and that they vary from tissue to tissue. The topic is of great practical interest because therapeutic measures against the no-reflow phenomenon would have to be aimed at the specific mechanisms. It is likely, though not proven, that the obstacles lie at the capillary level. In the list shown in Figure 23.42 three items stand out as most relevant: compression by cellular swelling, plugging by granulocytes, and endothelial damage.

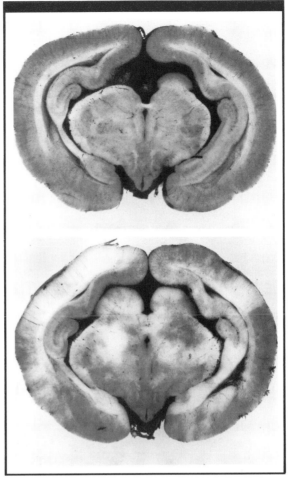

FIGURE 24.13
The no-reflow phenomenon illustrated in the rabbit brain. *Top:* Section through a normal rabbit brain after perfusion with carbon black. The white matter stands out clearly because it contains fewer capillaries. *Bottom:* Rabbit brain submitted to 7.5 minutes of ischemia followed by carbon perfusion 30 minutes later. Notice the spotty distribution of non-perfused white areas representing the no-reflow phenomenon. Scale in mm. (Reproduced with permission from [4].)

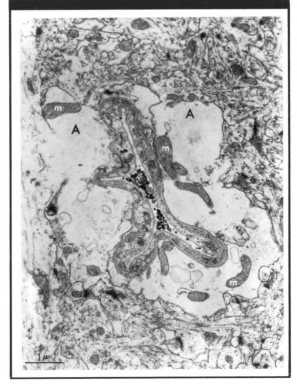

FIGURE 24.14
A mechanism of no-reflow in the brain of a rabbit infused with carbon and killed after 15 minutes of ischemia. The "feet" of astrocytes (**A**) surrounding a capillary are greatly swollen; the lumen, which contains some carbon black particles, is reduced to a slit. **m:** Astrocytic mitochondria. **Bar** = 1 μm. (Reproduced with permission from [21].)

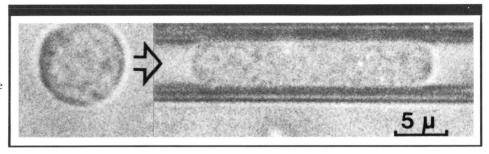

Compression by Cellular Swelling This reflects a typical cellular effect of anoxia (p. 74). In the brain, the perivascular glia and the endothelium seem to be exquisitely sensitive to anoxia or ischemia (21, 47a); they swell selectively and thereby compress capillaries (Figure 24.14). Evidence for capillary compression by cellular swelling was also found in the heart (51); in the kidney the swelling involved all cell types, including the endothelium (41). An increase in volume should be especially dangerous for the kidney, which is enclosed in a tight fibrous capsule. Therapeutically, cellular swelling can be opposed by infusing hypertonic solutions into the vascular system (134).

Plugging of Capillaries by Granulocytes The trapping of granulocytes during reflow has been demonstrated in the myocardium (33–36, 64, 70, 102, 111–113). Passing through a capillary is a tight squeeze even for a normal granulocyte (141) (Figure 24.15); this was elegantly shown also *in vivo* (Figure 24.16) (152), and we have already discussed the possible role of this phenomenon in inflammation (p. 397). Why are the leukocytes trapped in the capillaries during reflow? It seems that ischemia can cause both the endothelium (42a) and the leukocytes to become more sticky. A fascinating new development: in cats, it has been possible to inhibit the damage of reflow after ischemia by pretreating the cat *with an antibody* against the leukocyte adhesion complex CD18, the same complex that we encountered in discussing margination and diapedesis (p. 393) (59). Now it is understandable why myocardial infarcts in dogs depleted of neutrophils are 43 percent smaller than those in controls (105).

> *Incidentally, if leukocytes that stick in capillaries interfere with blood flow, we can understand why diapedesis in inflammation is programmed to occur in the venules. Because venules are wider than capillaries, blood flow can be maintained while the leukocytes remain attached to the walls.*

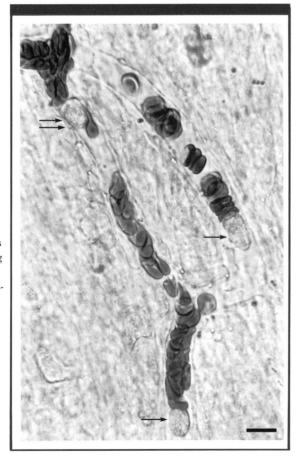

FIGURE 24.16
Three leukocytes (**arrows**) holding up the red cell traffic in skin capillaries of a human volunteer. **Double arrows:** Red cell squeezing past the impacted leukocyte. **Bar** = 10 μm. (Reproduced with permission from [152].)

Endothelial Damage Damage to the ischemic endothelium can certainly occur at a functional level (78), but by electron microscopy we found it unimpressive in rat muscles, even after 2.5 hours of ischemia (123). Perhaps the endothelium is more resistant to ischemia than parenchymal cells, which would show good engineering because the plumbing should be the last mechanism to fail. Changes observed in endothelial cells include blebbing, swelling or thinning (123) and the formation of gaps.

Therapeutic intervention against the no-reflow phenomenon is by definition a thorny problem because it calls for the delivery of drugs to a tissue that has little or no blood flow. However, on the assumption that cellular swelling is an especially important aspect of no-reflow, hypertonic mannitol was tried in several systems; and it worked (19, 41, 134). Ironically, it may have worked for the wrong reasons: mannitol is also a free-radical scavenger, and we now know that the damage of reflow is due primarily to free radicals. This discovery opened new possibilities for therapy, as we will explain later.

THE DAMAGE CAUSED BY REFLOW

It may be conceptually repulsive that reflow should cause damage, but the facts speak for themselves. For example, a rabbit ear detached from the body and therefore ischemic for 3 hours would appear histologically almost normal; but if it were reattached and reperfused, it would become congested, edematous, and inflamed.

We therefore conclude that the damage to a reperfused organ has two components: damage by ischemia and damage by reperfusion.

Damage due to ischemia was described in the chapter on cell death. In essence (101), the cells of ischemic tissue, or most of them, swell, lose potassium, acquire sodium, sustain injury to their membranes, and their cytoplasm is flooded by an excess of calcium. Mitochondria and other organelles swell, and protein denaturation sets in.

The damage due to reflow is probably triggered by several mechanisms. Metabolites accumulated in the cells during ischemia are ready to cause a further burst of osmotic swelling as soon as reflow provides fluid. Much of the reflow damage is due to "unnecessary" inflammation (37, 93): ischemic tissue releases platelet activating factor (91), and platelets are loaded with inflammatory mediators (p. 328). The endothelium becomes leaky; the plasma that seeps out coagulates and the clotting mechanism releases more inflammatory mediators. Many capillaries are plugged by leukocytes, and activated leukocytes may cause more damage; however, a major source of reflow-damage is attributed to free radicals. Reflow brings oxygen, the cornerstone of free-radical genesis. This topic deserves a closer look.

Free Radicals and Reperfusion Damage The breakthrough paper came from Alabama in 1981 (52). D.N. Granger and co-workers were studying ischemic damage to the intestine of the cat, using a model of low-flow (i.e., local reduction

of blood pressure to 30–40 mm Hg). After 1 hour of low-flow, the vessels became leaky. The experimenters tried to protect them by *pretreatment* with antihistamines: no effect. They tried an inhibitor of prostaglandin synthesis: no effect. They tried a free-radical scavenger, superoxide dismutase (SOD): it worked.

The Alabama group then proposed an hypothesis to explain the generation of free radicals in their system; this mechanism is now widely accepted as the principal key to reperfusion damage (Figure 24.17) (15, 39, 86).

The theory is fairly simple. Ischemic cells accumulate an excess of a substrate and of an enzyme, which—if they reacted together—would destroy the cells. However, the reaction cannot take place because it requires oxygen which, by definition, is absent in ischemic tissue. When oxygen is supplied by reflow, the time bomb goes off.

The substrate accumulated by ischemic cells is hypoxanthine. During ischemia, ATP breaks down to ADP, then to AMP, then to adenosine, to inosine, and finally to hypoxanthine (67). The enzyme is xanthine oxidase, generated as follows: the ischemic cell imbibes an excess of calcium, which activates proteolytic enzymes set free by ischemia. These proteases act on the innocuous enzyme xanthine dehydrogenase and convert it to xanthine oxidase.

When reflow comes, molecular oxygen comes with it. The xanthine oxidase then acts on hypoxanthine and produces uric acid, with superoxide (O_2-) as a by-product. Superoxide is not very dangerous, but as we learned earlier, superoxide dismutase acts on superoxide to produce H_2O_2, whereupon superoxide and H_2O_2 react to produce the highly toxic hydroxyl radical (p. 184).

A vast number of facts fit this theory (3a, 9). In experimental models, it has been found during the past few years that free-radical scavengers prevent or reduce all manner of ischemic injuries such as myocardial infarcts (16), ischemic necrosis of the kidney, hemorrhagic shock ("global ischemia"), and necrosis of skin flaps (a method of plastic surgery); they also help maintain cadaver organs taken for transplantation (39, 121). Another compelling bit of evidence is that xanthine oxidase appears in the blood reflowing from human limbs after surgery under tourniquet for 1–2 hours (43).

Many questions remain. You will have noticed that, experimentally, free-radical scavengers do

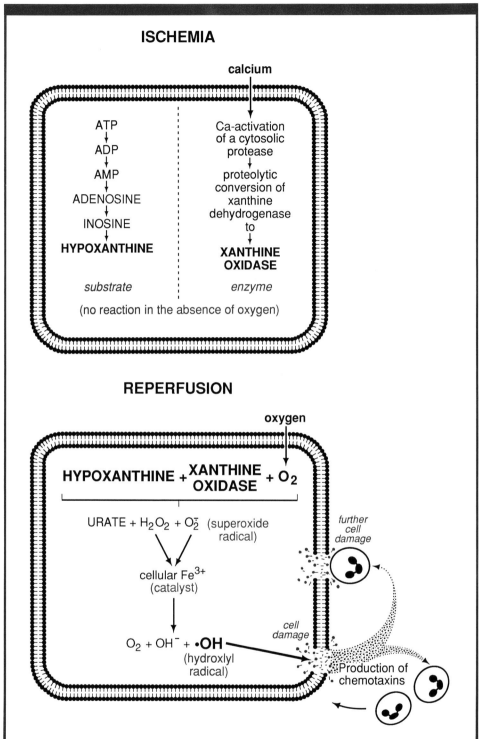

FIGURE 24.17
A mechanism to explain the tissue damage produced by reperfusion after ischemia. *Top:* Ischemia. During the ischemic interval the cells (endothelial and other cells) produce an enzyme and a substrate that cannot react with each other in the absence of oxygen. *Bottom:* Reperfusion. When flow returns, and oxygen is supplied, the enzyme (an oxidase) attacks the substrate and produces injurious free radicals.

protect against the damage of reflow if they are present in the vessels before ischemia starts. In the setting of human disease this is obviously not feasible. However, understanding the mechanism of damage is an important step. Ischemic injury is not as irreversible as it once seemed.

By now the reader may be ready to accept the notion that a little blood flow may be worse than no flow at all (65, 104), something that pathologists long suspected. If blood flow is reduced to a trickle (low flow), ischemic damage and reflow damage take place at the same time.

Some Examples of Infarction

The natural history of an infarct varies depending on the organ involved. It makes a great difference whether the organ beats, thinks, or conveys feces.

MYOCARDIAL INFARCTS

Myocardial infarcts are special for many reasons, besides the fact that they kill many humans, and correspondingly more is known about them. Here is a partial list.

(1) *Infarction occurs in a contractile tissue.* Therefore, one of the earliest effects of acute myocardial ischemia is local paralysis. This phenomenon can be witnessed as it occurs in the exposed heart of a dog or pig: the ischemic area becomes purplish within 5–15 seconds, then ceases to beat and bulges passively at every systole (101). Within 40 minutes most of the myocardial cells are irreversibly injured (101). (Release of enzymes by myocardial infarcts was discussed on p. 219.)

Because the heart beats, the paralyzed myocardial fibers become stretched and wavy. Wavy fibers therefore become a sign of infarction before necrosis sets in. The traditional way to diagnose a myocardial infarct histologically was to look for signs of necrosis, which means that the infarct could not be detected before it was at least 8 hours old. The wavy fibers develop much earlier, possibly within 30 minutes of the onset of ischemia (Figure 24.18) (12).

We observed the wavy fibers in Geneva as a result of a challenge by the World Health Organization, which needed a histological marker more sensitive than outright necrosis to establish worldwide statistics of death by myocardial infarction. We simply looked at many sections of clinically recent myocardial infarcts and noticed that many of these hearts contained foci of thin and wavy fibers. The mechanism: as ischemia sets in, the ischemic fibers stop contracting; but they are connected to the living fibers outside of the infarct, which continue to beat. Therefore, the paralyzed fibers are rhythmically tugged; in the process they become long, thin, and wavy, while still retaining their nuclei. Preliminary work on dogs showed that wavy fibers are present at 3 hours (26). The wavy fibers seem to have escaped recognition because they look "more beautiful" than normal straight ones. Yet a moment's reflection is enough to realize that a wavy fiber could not possibly beat to produce contraction. By shortening, it would just straighten.

Contraction bands are another hallmark of ischemic damage in contractile cells; they are

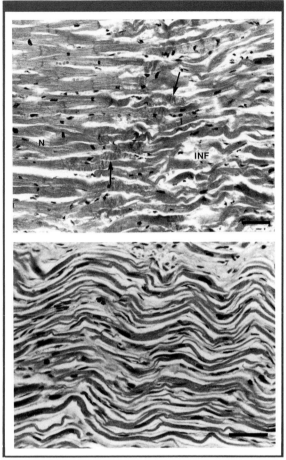

FIGURE 24.18
Myocardial wavy fibers and their pathogenesis. *Top:* Development of wavy fibers at the edge of a myocardial infarct. Imagine the tissue on the left as pulsating and tugging at the paralyzed fibers on the right-hand side, which become thin and wavy. Contraction bands have developed (**arrows**), a hallmark of ischemia, between the normal and the infarcted myocardium. Clinical symptoms suggested a 12-hour infarct, but this area probably represents a more recent extension. Very few neutrophils are present; the nuclei are still well-defined. **N:** Normal myocardium. **INF:** Infarcted area. *Bottom:* Typical wavy fibers from a recent myocardial infarct. The fibers are not only wavy but are stretched very thin. Nuclei are still present. **Bars** = 50 μm. (Reproduced with permission from [11].)

transverse bands of hypercontracted sarcomeres (Figure 24.19). By electron microscopy, groups of sarcomeres appear to be packed together almost as if telescoped (Figure 24.20). The pathogenesis is not clear (3, 45), but it requires ATP (127) and it is related to calcium overload. A similar change occurs in ischemic striated muscle.

(2) *Infarcted myocardium may come in contact with flowing blood.* This usually happens when infarction affects the whole thickness of the left

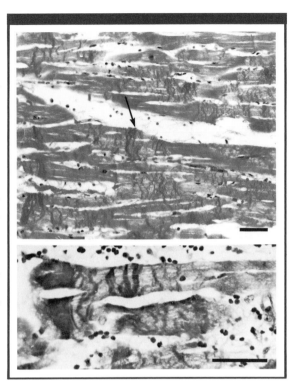

FIGURE 24.19 Contraction bands (**arrow**) in the myocardium at the periphery of an infarct. Contraction bands are a hallmark of ischemia; they can develop only in living tissue as in this case. *Top:* The edema and the inflammatory cells between the myocardial fibers are related to the nearby infarct. *Bottom:* Closer view of contraction bands. **Bars** = 50 μm.

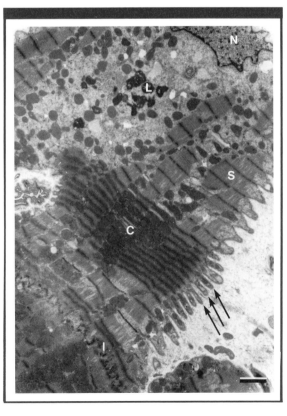

FIGURE 24.20 Contraction bands are typical of ischemia; this one (**C**) was found in a biopsy of human heart (electron micrograph). The sarcomeres (**S**) on either side are relatively normal; in the contraction band they appear to be telescoped. Note the corresponding tight folds in the sarcolemma (**arrows**). **L**: lipofuscin, **I**: intercalated disk, **N**: nucleus. **Bar** = 2 μm.

detached and produce emboli in the systemic arteries.

(3) *An infarct in the wall of a ventricle is under pressure and may burst,* leading to **cardiac tamponade** (French term meaning that blood spilling into the pericardium acts as a "tampon" or "stopper" on the heart). This happens because the infarcted tissue becomes soft; in fact an old name for a myocardial infarct was *myomalacia,* muscle softening (136). This tenderizing of dead myocardial cells is helped by the enzymes of leukocytes, which rush to the scene. There is no apparent usefulness to the acute phase of this inflammatory response (p. 420); it finds no bacteria to destroy. One could argue that it does more harm than good.

In dogs, some antiinflammatory agents (inhibitors of prostaglandin metabolism) do reduce the size of myocardial infarcts; they also inhibit the local release of the leukotriene LTB$_4$, a powerful leukotactic agent (110).

(4) *Myocardial infarcts become hemorrhagic if reperfused.* Usually the red phase of a myocardial infarct is mild and brief; but if the infarct is reperfused 45 minutes or more after coronary occlusion, the infarct becomes hemorrhagic (47). The mechanism: reperfusion came too late, and the reflow of blood simply spills into dead tissue (Figure 24.21). Whether this makes things worse—as regards local healing—is not certain (81).

Reperfusion of a recent myocardial infarct can be attempted by two means: coronary bypass surgery and thrombolysis (60, 129). Thrombolysis is achieved by injecting tissue plasminogen activator (tPA) or streptokinase intravenously within 3–6 hours (62, 131). To the nonexpert it may seem futile to attempt reperfusion after several hours when it is known that myocardial cells are dead after 40 minutes. The experts have two answers: there may be a salvageable border zone around the infarct (this is controversial) (8); and experiments on dogs show that infarction starts beneath the endocardium and proceeds like a wavefront toward the endocardium (64), a process that takes 3–6 hours (Figure 24.22). Therefore, the window of opportunity for thrombolysis lasts much longer than 40 minutes. Ultimately, the rationale for thrombolysis stands on the bare fact that—statistically—it helps (53, 68).

Normally, capillary perfusion is most difficult beneath the endocardium. In the left ventricle of the dog

ventricle. Dying cells release thromboplastin, with the result that a thrombus may cover the infarcted area. Imagine the fate of a thrombus on the wall of a beating left ventricle: fragments may become

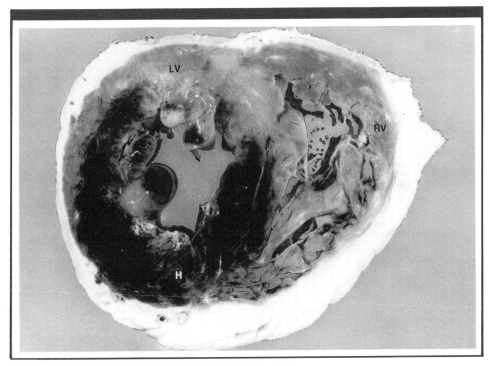

FIGURE 24.21
Cross section of a heart, showing an unusual and extensive hemorrhagic infarction (**H**) of the left ventricular wall (**LV**). The hemorrhagic filling of the necrotic tissue is due to the special circumstances of this infarction, as explained by the clinical history. Ten hours after surgery for triple bypass, the blood pressure of the patient dropped. When resuscitation efforts failed, the chest was reopened. One of the grafts was found to be occluded, and a new anastomosis was performed. The patient died 20 hours after the second operation. The hemorrhagic aspect of the infarct is clearly due to reperfusion of nonviable myocardium. **RV**: right ventricle.

during systole, the interstitial pressure averages 121 ± 10 mm Hg compared with 93 ± 7 beneath the epicardium (6). It follows that an acute reduction in coronary flow will affect first the subendocardial capillaries. This explains why the subendocardial zone in humans is so susceptible to infarction (see Figure 24.4).

(5) *Myocytolysis:* This is one more twist to myocardial ischemia (Figure 24.23). Patches of myocardial fibers that are *chronically* ischemic become greatly swollen (perhaps over weeks and months); gradually they appear to lose their content of fibrils and other organelles, become empty-looking, and eventually disappear, leaving their basement membrane as a ghost of what was once a myocyte. There is no inflammatory response. Contrast this slow process (accompanied by swelling and lysis) with the shrinking and coagulation typical of myocardial cells in sudden infarcts (Figure 24.24).

The calcium paradox and the "stone heart."
Experimentally, if a heart is first perfused with a calcium-free medium and then reperfused with calcium, the return of the calcium initiates massive, explosive tissue disruption, enzyme release, and a firm contracture of the whole heart (72, 100, 137). The mechanism is uncertain, but it seems likely that the first perfusion with calcium-free medium causes mild membrane damage; then when calcium returns, it penetrates the fibers and sets off the response:

contraction bands develop (127). This calcium paradox recalls the oxygen paradox set off by returning oxygen to ischemic tissue (57). There is, alas, a clinical equivalent to the calcium paradox: sometimes a patient undergoing a cardiopulmonary bypass dies on the operating table with the heart irreversibly contracted in systole. This has been called the "stone heart" (24).

The stunned myocardium *is a related phenomenon. If a coronary artery in a dog is occluded for less than 20 minutes, no necrosis develops; but after reperfusion the myocardium remains depressed or "stunned" for hours or days. The mechanism is unclear (100). The same disturbance can occur in humans after thrombolytic therapy (70).*

Therapy for myocardial infarction has taxed the imagination of many researchers (18). Attempts to counteract different steps in the pathogenesis have included antiinflammatory drugs (42), calcium channel blockers (not useful), aspirin and anticoagulants (useful) (5), hyaluronidase (rationale unclear), and even retrograde perfusion through the veins (54). Other remedies for ischemic cell death have been discussed earlier (p. 208).

INFARCTION OF OTHER TISSUES

Infarcts can occur in any organ, including the very small hypophysis. The following selection

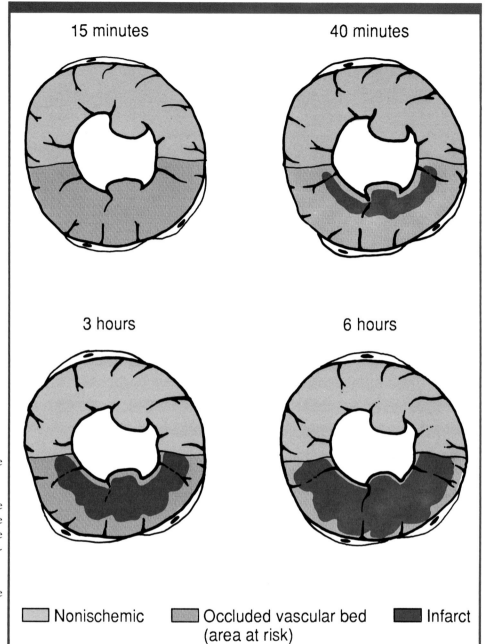

FIGURE 24.22
Wave-front phenomenon in myocardial infarction. After occlusion of the left circumflex coronary artery, cell death always occurs first in the subendocardial myocardium; later the zone of infarction extends to involve the middle and outer portions of the myocardium. The full extent of myocardial infarction is achieved by 6 hours. Because of this phenomenon, it makes sense to attempt to reperfuse a myocardial infarct even after 40 minutes, the time it takes for a myocardial cell to die of ischemia. (Adapted from [64].)

illustrates the many possible consequences of infarction.

Nervous Tissue Infarcts of the brain differ from infarcts of other tissues in their tendency to liquefy (p. 214). They can be seen by nuclear magnetic resonance imaging even before that stage (Figure 24.25). The extent of brain destruction can be impressive (Figure 24.26), yet brain infarcts, dreadful as they may be, are painless.

Some cerebral infarcts are hemorrhagic (Figure 24.27). Experimental work suggests that this happens when a phase of ischemia (~6 hr) is followed by reperfusion (115). In human infarcts reperfusion could be due to a sudden rise of blood pressure or to lysis or contraction of a thromboembolus. In other words, the mechanism of damage in hemorrhagic infarction in the brain is the same as in myocardial red infarcts after iatrogenic reperfusion.

Ischemia of the nervous tissue is special for two reasons: (a) *ischemia is currently recognized as an important complication of trauma, especially to the spinal cord,* a tissue that is very sensitive to ischemia. This means that the treatment of such injuries must also address an ischemic component. (b) *The pathogenesis of ischemic damage to nervous tissue involves biochemical agents called excitotoxins, which are neurotransmitters with excitatory properties (95) (p. 214).*

For brain cells the order of decreasing vulnerability to ischemia is as follows (76):

1. neurons (with local variations)
2. oligodendroglia
3. astroglia
4. microglia (i.e., macrophages)
5. connective tissue structures

> We mentioned earlier that the influence of cerebral infarction was reported to be greater if the hematocrit is higher than 46 percent (normal values are 45–52 percent in males, 37–48 percent in females) (125). Of the 500,000 strokes per year in the United States, 75 percent are infarcts; the others are due to hemorrhage, that is, rupture of atherosclerotic arteries (1).

Nerve ischemia is thought to be the mechanism of diabetic neuropathy, a result of microcirculatory derangements including increased blood viscosity (Figure 24.28) (17, 31).

Intestine Infarcts of the intestine can be the result of arterial occlusion (emboli, atherosclerosis) or venous thrombosis. They are especially dangerous because the whole thickness of the wall is affected: peristalsis stops; bacterial growth in the lumen goes unchecked, producing gas, which dilates the intestine and dangerously stretches its inert wall; eventually bacteria cross the wall, even before it breaks down, causing peritonitis.

Kidneys and Spleen Embolization of these organs causes red infarcts that soon become white (see Figures 5.16 and 24.2). These infarcts may cause pain, but many are clinically silent and have little significance. Computed tomography can visualize 75 percent of splenic infarcts (38, 63).

Lung The lung is a special case because it has double circulation. We have already discussed the topic and its mysteries (p. 682).

Bones Bones suffer infarcts in caisson disease (p. 653). In sickle cell anemia one of the many targets of infarction, by impacted red blood cells, are the vertebrae and the head of the femur, which may slowly cave in under pressure and become deformed.

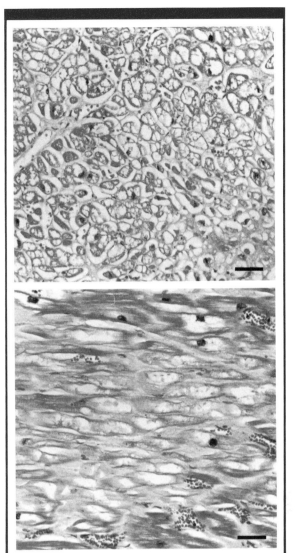

FIGURE 24.23
Myocytolysis, the effect of chronic ischemia on myocardial cells. The cells swell, their organelles are dissolved; eventually only an empty basement membrane remains. *Top:* Cross section. *Bottom:* Longitudinal section. **Bars** = 50 μm. Compare with Figure 24.22.

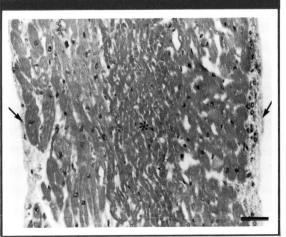

FIGURE 24.24
Coagulation necrosis (**asterisk**), typical of sudden ischemic death of myocardial cells. Longitudinal section of a human infarcted papillary muscle. The cells near the surface (**arrows**) are kept alive by blood flowing in the ventricle. **Bar** = 50 μm.

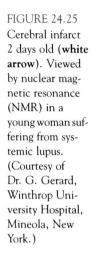

FIGURE 24.25 Cerebral infarct 2 days old (**white arrow**). Viewed by nuclear magnetic resonance (NMR) in a young woman suffering from systemic lupus. (Courtesy of Dr. G. Gerard, Winthrop University Hospital, Mineola, New York.)

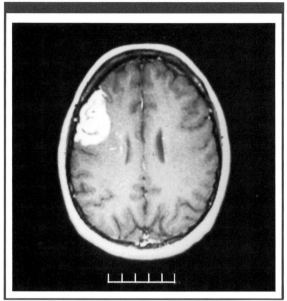

Whole Limbs Almost invariably, lower limbs are affected. The most common cause is atherosclerosis (often complicated by diabetes), and the precipitating factor is a thrombus over an atherosclerotic plaque. When a limb is affected in this manner, the dead tissue is exposed to the outer world; the possible consequences, you may recall (p. 209) are two. (a) The tissue may dry out and turn into *dry gangrene*, a relatively benign development because bacteria do not grow in dried tissue; this allowed the Hippocratic physicians—who did

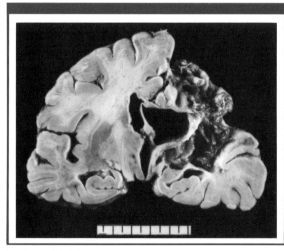

FIGURE 24.26
Extensive infarction of the right hemisphere due to occlusion of the middle cerebral artery. The destruction and reabsorption of cerebral tissue occurred over months and years. Scale in cm. (Courtesy of Dr. T.W. Smith, University of Massachusetts Medical Center, Worcester, MA.)

not amputate—to watch a blackened limb fall off bit by bit over 2–3 months (82). (b) If the limb becomes infected, it turns greenish and foul-smelling; this is the sinister *wet gangrene*.

To close: Overall, ischemia is bad news, but there are a couple of exceptions. Anecdotally, we might mention that retinal tumors have been destroyed by infarction: the retinal artery is terminal. More significantly, although most cells suffer when their blood supply is diminished, some anoxic cells secrete helpful angiogenic factors, and anoxic fibroblasts are stimulated to produce more collagen: mechanisms that contribute to wound healing. There is also a vitally important physiologic infarct: the monthly shedding of the uterine lining, which is due to a spasm of the so-called spiral arterioles of the mucosa.

General Ischemia: Shock

Shock is a whole-body event resulting from the general failure of the circulatory system. In the preceding section we studied ischemia at the local level; here we will examine its effects on a larger scale (178). In shock, *all organs are perfused inadequately*; as a result, all tissues suffer—some more, some less—from a massive attack by four and often five agents:

- lack of oxygen
- lack of substrates
- lack of waste removal
- damage from low flow
- bacteria (in septic shock)

The first three items are also involved in the damage caused by local ischemia; damage from low flow requires some explanation. Low flow is the main characteristic of shock. As mentioned earlier, low flow can be more damaging than no flow at all because it has two components: because the flow is *inadequate,* there is ischemic damage (items 1, 2, 3 in the list above); and because *some flow persists,* the perfused ischemic tissue also develops reperfusion damage (e.g., leukocyte plugging and free-radical damage).

Shock is therefore a cardiovascular problem, at least initially; it is not to be confused with coma, which concerns the nervous system. *Coma is a sleeplike condition with unresponsiveness to stimuli, however intense.* No patient could ever say "I am in coma," whereas many patients in shock are alert.

It is true, however, that prolonged shock can lead to coma.

> The concept of shock as inadequate perfusion was slow in developing. As first used, the word shock was the translation of the French secousse, used in 1731 to describe the impact of a bullet as a "jarring of the nervous system." As late as World War I, wound-related shock was attributed to a toxin. Finally, in 1940, Minot and Blalock opened the era of shock as "a peripheral circulatory failure resulting from a discrepancy in the size of the vascular bed and the volume of intravascular fluid" (178).

To understand the concept of *inadequate generalized perfusion*, consider the cardiovascular system as consisting of a pump, a fluid, and two tubes connected to a microvascular network (Figure 24.29): insufficient flow through this system can result from one of three principal mechanisms.

- THE FLUID LEVEL IS LOW due to loss of blood volume.
- THE PUMP IS WEAK due to heart malfunction.
- THE CONTAINER IS TOO LARGE by vasodilatation.

These three basic factors are purely mechanical. However, they perform in a biological system, and their ultimate biological effect is *microvascular failure*. In shock, the microcirculation fails by three mechanisms of its own: plugging by leukocytes, plugging by disseminated intravascular coagulation (DIC), and endothelial injury. This microvascular catastrophe is the final *common pathway: it may occur in any form of shock.*

This broad picture (represented in Figure 24.29) allows us to understand the three major clinical settings of shock (the term "clinical" has human connotations, but experimental animals can also lapse into any one of the three following predicaments):

- *Hypovolemic shock* is due to low blood volume in the system; the underfilling may be the effect of losing whole blood (hemorrhagic shock), plasma alone (e.g., by severe burns), or fluid alone by persistent vomiting or diarrhea.
- *Cardiogenic shock* (pump failure) occurs when the function of the heart is impaired. The heart itself may have suffered an infarct, or the pulmonary circulation may be severely impaired by an embolus in the pulmonary artery, which acts like a clamp on the entire circulatory system.

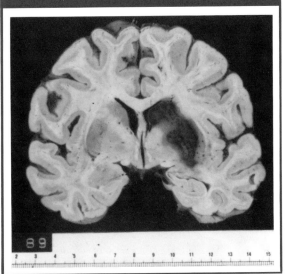

FIGURE 24.27
Hemorrhagic infarct of the right hemisphere, due to obstruction of small branches arising from the middle cerebral artery. Scale in cm. (Courtesy of Dr. T.W. Smith, University of Massachusetts Medical Center, Worcester, MA.)

- *Shock by generalized vasodilatation*, also called "distributive shock" (201), effectively makes the "container" too large. It occurs in three settings: as **septic shock,** the most common, a result of sepsis by gram-negative bacteria and sometimes other organisms; as **anaphylactic shock;** and as **neurogenic shock,** which can develop, for instance, as a complication of general anesthesia or of spinal cord injury.

From what we have said it should be clear that *shock is not a disease of its own but a complication of some other disease.* **Anyone suffering from shock is also suffering from some other major problem.** This makes shock difficult to diagnose and to

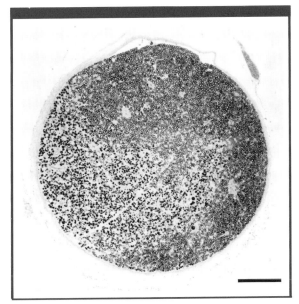

FIGURE 24.28
Cross section of a rat sciatic nerve, showing the effect of infarction 7 days after experimental embolization. Microspheres were injected into the arteries supplying the nerve. Note loss of myelinated fibers. Stain was phenylenediamine. **Bar** = 200 μm. (Reproduced with permission from [97].)

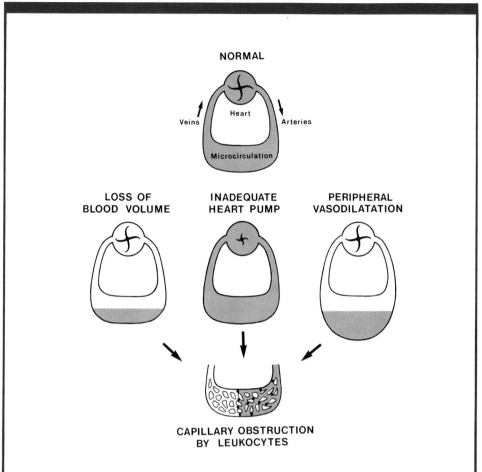

FIGURE 24.29
Explaining the decreased perfusion in shock. *Top:* Normal circulatory system, represented as a pump connected to two channels (arteries and veins) leading to a container (the peripheral circulation). *Center:* Three mechanisms that cause low blood flow. *Left to right:* (1) The blood volume is too small (hemorrhage), (2) the pump is inadequate (typically due to myocardial infarct), (3) the container has become too large (peripheral vasodilatation, typical of sepsis or neurogenic shock). *Bottom:* In all three situations, decreased perfusion leads to capillary obstruction by leukocytes, which further aggravates the low blood flow condition—one of the many vicious circles that occur in shock.

treat; its clinical picture must be seen through the signs and symptoms of the precipitating disease, be it myocardial infarct, trauma, surgery, sepsis, or other. The typical clinical picture of shock includes rapid, shallow breathing; cold, clammy, and cyanotic skin; constricted veins; fast, shallow pulse; low blood pressure; and low or nil urine output; the patient may be fully conscious (226). This is the stage of compensated hypotension (163).

> Reversible versus irreversible shock. *Some years ago it was fashionable to attempt to define the "point of no return" of shock; the favorite experimental model was hemorrhagic shock in the dog, followed by reinfusion of the blood (164). Under these experimental conditions it was easy to establish whether a dog could survive after a given amount of blood loss. In clinical practice, however, there is no way to decide whether a given situation is irretrievable, and the concept of irreversible shock has lost much of its relevance. Until recently there was no blood "marker" for the severity of shock. Now one has been proposed:* the platelet-derived *plasminogen-activator inhibitor-1. High levels of this factor correlate with hypercoagulability and poor prognosis (202).*

Pathophysiology of Hemorrhagic Shock

This is the best understood variety of shock; it also helps understand the other forms. Much of what follows in this section applies to all forms of shock because we are dealing essentially with the pathophysiology of hypoperfusion.

About 10 percent of the blood volume can be lost without a decrease in blood pressure or cardiac output, but with greater losses both functions drop; they reach zero with a blood loss of 35–45 percent. As hypotension develops, correcting reflexes intervene immediately (Figure 24.30). A sympathetic response is initiated by the baroreceptors (pressure sensors): (a) the arterioles constrict (hence the cold skin), thereby increasing the peripheral resistance; (b) the veins constrict helping to restore blood volume; and (c) the heart rate increases. The vasomotor reflexes do not affect the heart and the brain, which are therefore the main beneficiaries of the protective reflexes (175).

These immediate reflexes are followed, in a matter of hours, by slower corrective responses. The kidney, for example, responds to anoxia by activating the renin–angiotensin–aldosterone system, leading to salt and water conservation; the secretion of vasopressin, a vasoconstrictor, helps correct the hypotension.

At this point it is still possible to reverse the process by restoring the blood volume, even with a plasma substitute. If this is not done, and if the compensatory mechanisms fail to stop the process, the circulatory functions begin to deterio-rate: the vasomotor center is depressed, the peripheral vessels dilate, and blood pressure drops. All tissues suffer. Now a number of vicious circles are set in motion, so that shock breeds more shock (176).

VICIOUS CIRCLES IN SHOCK

Vicious circles are typical of shock of all kinds (Figure 24.31). Here are some examples:

- *Poor perfusion of the heart* impairs myocardial function, with further impairment of cardiac output, and therefore reduced perfusion of all organs including the heart itself.
- *Poor perfusion of the pancreas* induces the pancreas to produce peptides that further depress cardiac function (186); a circulating myocardial depressant factor (MDF) has actually been demonstrated in shock patients (Figure 24.32) (199).

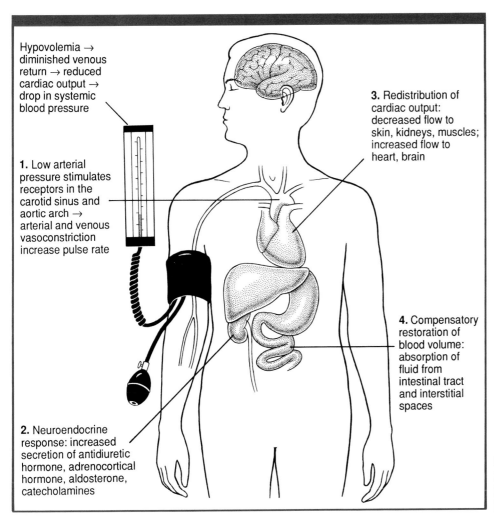

Hypovolemia → diminished venous return → reduced cardiac output → drop in systemic blood pressure

1. Low arterial pressure stimulates receptors in the carotid sinus and aortic arch → arterial and venous vasoconstriction increase pulse rate

2. Neuroendocrine response: increased secretion of antidiuretic hormone, adrenocortical hormone, aldosterone, catecholamines

3. Redistribution of cardiac output: decreased flow to skin, kidneys, muscles; increased flow to heart, brain

4. Compensatory restoration of blood volume: absorption of fluid from intestinal tract and interstitial spaces

FIGURE 24.30
Major compensating mechanisms in hypovolemic shock. (Adapted from [154].)

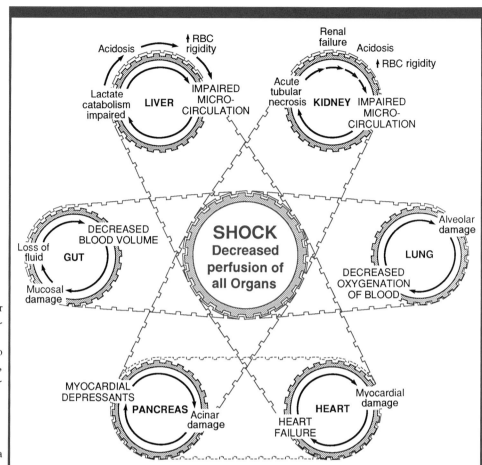

FIGURE 24.31

Some of the vicious circles that occur in shock. The condition of shock (decreased perfusion) is represented in the center; when this wheel begins to turn, it activates many other wheels, creating conditions that in turn aggravate shock. Some of the secondary wheels activate each other (*bottom*). Other vicious circles can be proposed, such as microvascular occlusion by leukocytes as a result and as a cause of decreased perfusion.

• *Poor perfusion of the liver* places it in double jeopardy because the liver receives its blood from two sources: 40 percent from the hepatic artery and 60 percent from the portal vein (210). The liver is the site where most

of the lactic acid is broken down; now it is presented with an excess of it, but being anoxic it cannot handle it, so the liver becomes a producer of lactate (187); this worsens the acidosis, which impairs cardio-

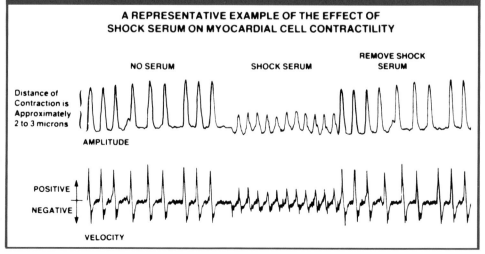

FIGURE 24.32

Demonstrating a myocardial depressant substance in serum from a patient during the acute phase of septic shock. The serum was applied to a culture of rat myocardial cells contracting spontaneously in a petri dish: it depressed both the extent (*top*) and the velocity (*bottom*) of cell shortening. (Adapted from [200].)

vascular function (178, 210a). Under these conditions the liver becomes unable to inactivate all the chemical mediators that flood the circulation, thus creating another vicious circle.

- *Poor perfusion of the gut* causes a breakdown of the mucosal barrier (the gut is very sensitive to ischemia); bacteria reach the blood (164, 209), setting the stage for septic shock; sloughing of the mucosa causes bleeding and further fluid loss, aggravating the poor perfusion throughout the body.
- *Poor perfusion of the kidneys* impairs renal function and thereby the excretion of acid metabolites, which worsens the acidosis; reduced blood perfusion may lead to tubular necrosis, with further retention of toxic metabolites.
- *Poor perfusion of the lungs* contributes to the genesis of the "shock lung" (see later), which further impairs the oxygenation of the blood.

THE CHEMICAL MEDIATORS OF SHOCK

Practically all the chemical mediators of inflammation have been found in the blood of shock patients, including histamine, serotonin, kinins and nitric oxide (NO) (149, 150, 151, 158, 161). According to current thinking, the key is injured tissue—be it tissue injured by poor perfusion or by the condition that caused the shock (such as trauma). Injured cells respond by secreting prostaglandins and leukotrienes. Dying and dead cells can activate complement (p. 437) and also release lysosomal proteolytic enzymes as well as thromboplastin; these in turn can activate the kinin, complement (196), clotting, and fibrinolytic cascades. The activation of the complement cascade is critical (177). The complement-derived anaphylatoxins (C3a, C4a, C5a) activate the leukocytes, which respond by aggregating and producing microemboli, as well as by sticking to the endothelium and causing damage; correspondingly, the number of circulating leukocytes drops. Other chemotaxins (platelet activating factor, leukotriene B$_4$) contribute to these leukocyte responses. The microvascular endothelium is made leaky by permeability-increasing mediators as well as by injury due to activated leukocytes.

Philosophically, it is rather puzzling to find that all these mediators, so helpful in a local response, inflammation, are conspiring to induce a potentially lethal general condition. It is difficult to know precisely what roles each mediator plays in shock. The list includes even endorphins (vasodilators) (146), the presence of which has caused opiate antagonists to be added to the list of drugs tried against shock. In addition, at least nine myocardial depressant factors (MDFs) have been described, some of them originating in the pancreas (185); circulating proteases such as lysosomal cathepsins may be involved in their release (180). Tumor necrosis factor and interleukin-1 are primarily involved in septic shock (see below).

> *That lysosomal enzymes have a role in shock is taken for granted (138, 178), but the idea is based on work by only a few (174, 180, 184, 185). The level of lysosomal enzymes in the blood is not used as a measure of shock. However, the therapy of shock should include (according to some) the use of corticosteroids for "stabilizing cell membranes and lysosomes" (227).*

A FINAL COMMON PATHWAY: PLUGGING OF CAPILLARIES BY LEUKOCYTES

This phenomenon is simply an extension of the leukocyte plugging that develops in ischemic tissues (p. 686). Because shock implies generalized ischemia, it is not too surprising that it should also entail generalized plugging by leukocytes. It was long known that leukocytes become sticky in hemorrhagic shock and are trapped, especially in the lung (205, 225). Recent studies showed that this phenomenon is a major step in the pathogenesis of hemorrhagic shock (140, 142, 144, 218, 220) (Figure 24.33). The most convincing experimental proof is that animals submitted to hemorrhagic shock could be saved by treatment with an antibody against a leukocyte adhesion protein, CD18 (192, 219). Capillary plugging by leukocytes creates another vicious circle by aggravating the ischemia.

THE ULTIMATE COMPLICATIONS OF SHOCK

As shock progresses, more complications are in store. Extensive cell death may activate the clotting system to the point of triggering disseminated intravascular coagulation (DIC) which can be the fatal blow (p. 638). Septicemia is another grim possibility: the ischemic mucosa of the gut begins to slough off and becomes an open highway for bacteria to travel from the lumen of the gut into the tissue spaces; there they find little opposition because inflammation depends on the blood supply, which is of course inadequate. In shock, the inflammatory response is depressed

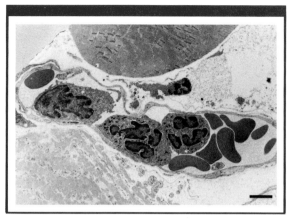

FIGURE 24.33
Three leukocytes plugging a small postcapillary venule after 3 hours of hemorrhagic shock (rat maintained at a mean arterial pressure of 40 mm Hg). **Bar** = 2 μm. (Courtesy of Drs. J. Barroso-Aranda and G.W. Schmid-Schönbein, University of California, San Diego, La Jolla, CA.)

throughout the body, presumably because the delivery of leukocytes is drastically reduced (191). The way is therefore open for the bacteria to pass into the blood, and there too the usual defenses are inefficient, the RES/MPS (p. 297) being depressed (139). Now hemorrhagic shock may lapse into septic shock.

Pathophysiology of Septic Shock

Septic shock has been defined as the ultimate disease of medical progress (227). It now kills about 100,000 patients per year in the United States, and the rate is increasing; it rose about 15-fold between 1977 and 1987 (160). The reason: patients can be rescued from conditions that used to be rapidly fatal (e.g., tumors, multiple trauma, extensive burns, and respiratory failure); but those who survive, often immunosuppressed or debilitated, can now become prey to bacteria. The most common victims are elderly patients with genitourinary, abdominal, or pulmonary infections. The mortality by septic shock is about 50 percent (160).

The microorganisms involved are gram-negative aerobes in 60 percent of the cases, gram-positive bacteria in 20–40 percent, and anaerobes and fungi in the remaining cases. We will describe the sequence of events in gram-negative sepsis, the most common and best understood.

Endotoxin, that amazing molecule, is the critical bacterial agent (Figure 24.34) (207a). Experimentally injected intravenously, it reproduces the main features of septic shock. In patients at risk, the advent of septic shock can be suspected if pulse and respiration accelerate and are accompanied by fever, warm skin, and a flush; hence the name *warm shock* at this stage. The change may occur from one day to the next. Diastolic pressure drops as the peripheral vessels dilate; cardiac output is increased, although not enough to compensate for the vasodilatation.

At the same time a number of metabolic disturbances occur, amounting to impaired utilization of substrates, first of glucose, then of fat and protein (227). Because oxygen is lacking, mitochondrial respiration is down, and correspond-

FIGURE 24.34
Endotoxin (lipopolysaccharide, LPS). Inset: a molecule of LPS, consisting of a polysaccharide moiety of variable length (**P**), two disaccharide units (**D**) and a lipid moiety (**L**: four fatty acids). The main figure shows the position of LPS in the wall of gram-negative bacteria; the wall of gram-positive bacteria is shown for comparison. (Adapted from [215a])

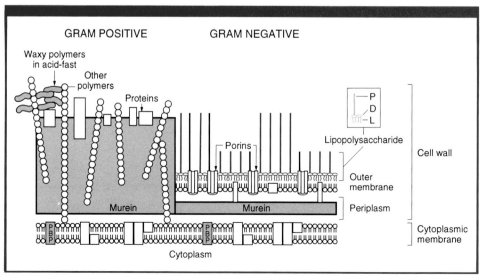

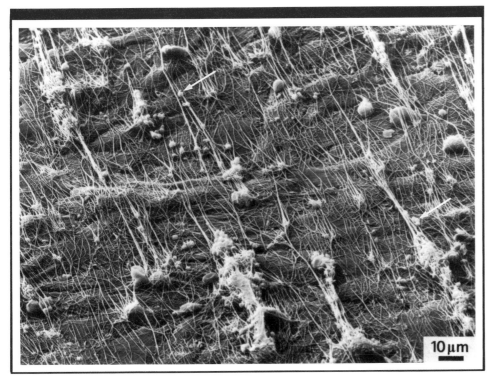

FIGURE 24.35
Cultured human endothelium perverted by endotoxin into producing clots. Scanning electron micograph. The filaments are fibrin. Endothelial cultures were incubated 4–18 hours with endotoxin and then superfused with freshly drawn human blood for 5 minutes. Fibrin strands are deposited only at low shear rates, such as could occur in veins. Platelets (**arrows**) adhere to the fibrin. (Reproduced with permission from [157].)

ingly, anaerobic glycolysis is up, leading to acidosis. Muscle proteolysis is greatly increased. Drastic events occur in the blood: endotoxin activates platelets, which clump and embolize the lung capillaries, where they release their arsenal of inflammatory mediators; granulocytes follow a similar path, contributing to lung damage and edema. Liver damage by endotoxin is reduced in rats depleted of leukocytes (181). A series of mishaps occur in the microcirculation, largely as a result of circulating endotoxin (see below); most importantly, the fine blood vessels (capillaries?) become leaky everywhere; the permeability to albumin is increased (Figure 24.36) (216); the corresponding loss of blood volume can only aggravate the shock. This phase may be sustained for a week or longer; patients who survive may be severely emaciated.

A *paradoxical aspect of this catastrophe is that it is largely self-inflicted: it is due not to endotoxin itself but to cellular or molecular responses triggered by endotoxin.* Indeed "the most unique feature of endotoxin . . . is its almost ubiquitous capacity to elicit the entire spectrum of host effector molecules" (193). The most powerful effector molecules are probably tumor necrosis factor (TNF) and interleukin-1 (IL-1). This fact pins most of the blame on the macrophages, which respond to endotoxin by producing TNF, IL-1, and tissue

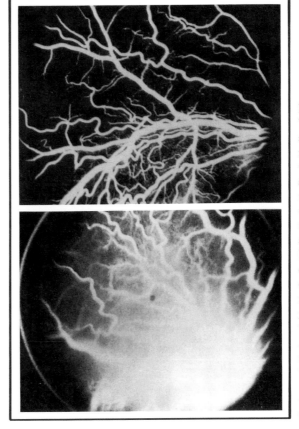

FIGURE 24.36
Top: Retinal angiogram of a normal dog. The vessels, demonstrated by an intravenous injection of fluorescein, are sharply outlined because the dye does not leak out. *Bottom:* Fluorescein was injected 6 hours after infusion of *Escherichia coli:* note extensive vascular leakage. (Reproduced with permission from [216].)

factor, which is the trigger of the extrinsic clotting cascade. However, endotoxin induces so many factors that attempting to counteract any single one would not be sufficient.

The evidence incriminating a variety of endogenous mediators is powerful (160, 192a): an infusion of TNF reproduces the syndrome of shock (217) (Figure 24.37); a strain of mice that is resistant to endotoxin shock (208) is congenitally unable to produce TNF (147); mice given antibodies against TNF are partially protected against endotoxin (148); rabbits given a specific antagonist to the IL-1 receptor are protected against shock by E. coli infused intravenously (222); in dogs with E. coli peritonitis, two inhibitors of prostaglandin synthesis restored normal hemodynamics (166); depletion of complement is also advantageous (165, 167); the severity of meningococcemia in children correlates with the blood levels of TNF and IL-1 (172); endotoxin activates the kinin system (183).

Why should endotoxin elicit such a disastrous series of events? Endotoxin means the archenemy: gram-negative bacteria; and millions of years have taught vertebrates to fight it off in the tissues with a potent inflammatory response (195). But here is the hitch. If endotoxin is released by bacteria *within the tissues*, it triggers inflammation, which serves a useful purpose in fighting the infection; but if endotoxin is released *in the blood*, the programmed response becomes inappropriate; think of histamine liberation in local inflammation versus massive release in anaphylaxis. Indeed the properties of endotoxin are disastrous when applied to circulating blood. Although the molecule itself has little or no toxicity for most cells, except for the endothelium in relatively high doses (179, 207), it binds to endotoxin receptors of monocytes/macrophages and many other cells (203) and stimulates them to produce cytokines on a large scale. It activates the endothelium throughout the body, inducing it to become leaky (perhaps some of the leakiness reflects outright damage), and to express various adhesion molecules (162, 169, 206, 224); as a result, monocytes and other leukocytes become inappropriately stuck in the microcirculation, hampering blood flow. The endothelium is also induced to express tissue factor, whereby circulating fibrinogen is polymerized into purposeless and troublesome filaments of fibrin (Figure 24.35). Another effect of endotoxin is almost diabolical: low density lipoprotein (LDL) tends to protect the endothelium against endotoxin, which is fat-soluble and dissolves into the LDL particles; but then, endothelial cells transport the endotoxin-loaded LDL particles to the tissue spaces, where they can trigger an inflammatory response (197). Yet this is not all. *Endotoxin activates the complement cascade (221), the coagulation cascade, the kinin cascade, the fibrinolytic cascade, and the platelets.* A molecule that can do all this does not "need" to be directly toxic to kill (173).

Note: The same cascades are activated in the non-septic forms of shock, but as a result of secondary cell injury; in septic shock the cascades are activated first by endotoxin and then again by injured tissues.

Nobody has explained endotoxin better than Lewis Thomas, who was known for his work on this subject even before he achieved literary fame. Concerning the local effect of endotoxin, he wrote:

Lipopolysaccharide is read by our tissues as the very worst of bad news. When we sense lipopolysaccharide, we are likely to turn on every defense at our disposal; we will bomb, defoliate, blockade, seal off, and destroy all the tissues in the area. Leukocytes become more actively phago-

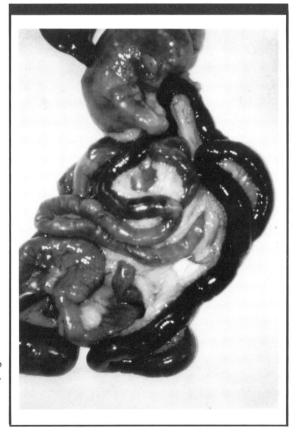

FIGURE 24.37 Effect of tumor necrosis factor (TNF) on the gastrointestinal tract of a rat. These hemorrhagic changes, typical of shock, were present 4 hours after infusion of TNF into the tail vein. (Reproduced with permission from [217].)

cytic, release lysosomal enzymes, turn sticky, and aggregate together in dense masses, occluding capillaries and shutting off the blood supply. Complement is switched on . . . to release chemotactic signals, calling in leukocytes from everywhere. Vessels become hyperreactive to epinephrine so that physiologic concentrations suddenly possess necrotizing properties. Pyrogen is released from leukocytes, adding fever to hemorrhage, necrosis and shock. It is a shambles. All this seems unnecessary, panic-driven. There is nothing intrinsically poisonous about endotoxin, but it must look awful, or feel awful, when sensed by cells. Cells believe that it signifies the presence of gram-negative bacteria, and they will stop at nothing to avoid this threat (212).

Concerning endotoxin in the blood:

The center of the puzzle is that endotoxin is really not much of a toxin, at least in the ordinary sense of being a direct poisoner of cells. Instead, it seems to be a sort of signal, a piece of misleading news. When injected into the bloodstream, it conveys propaganda, announcing that typhoid bacilli in great numbers (or other related bacteria) are on the scene, and a number of defense mechanisms are switched on, all at once. When the dose of endotoxin is sufficiently high, these defense mechanisms, acting in concert or in sequence, launch a stereotyped set of physiological responses, including fever, malaise, hemorrhage, collapse, shock, coma and death. It is something like an explosion in a munitions factory (213).

Multiple Organ Failure

The full-blown picture of advanced shock has earned the name of **multiple organ failure** (MOF), also known as multiple systems organ failure (MSOF) (150). The gut, always loaded with gram-negative bacteria, can be seen as the "motor of multiple organ failure" (165, 167); but any organ or function can be hit: the heart, the kidneys, the lungs, the liver, the system of mononuclear phagocytes (139), inflammation, the immune system. Eventually, the brain also can fail and lead to coma (145). Few patients survive the failure of three organs. Each failing system calls for support, leading to a therapeutic nightmare. In fact, there is no definitive treatment (155).

The cost of multiple organ failure (MOF) to society is enormous. It is worth mentioning, even in a textbook of basic science, that MOF is the most common cause of death in intensive care units; a recent study found that the average stay of a patient with MOF is 21 days, at a cost of about $85,000 for those who do not survive, compared with $300,000 for those who do. The latter expense relates to months of rehabilitation (155).

Toxic shock syndrome in women, *prominent in the press in recent years due to an outbreak related to the use of certain brands of vaginal tampons, is not due to endotoxin but to toxin 1 of* Staphylococcus aureus. *This toxin is not produced in the presence of magnesium. Because magnesium was efficiently absorbed by the fibers of the tampons, the bacteria were free to produce large amounts of toxin (182).*

ORGAN CHANGES IN SHOCK

All organ changes in shock are potentially reversible, except those of the brain (178).

- *In the kidney, the structures most sensitive to anoxia are the convoluted tubules, and* **acute tubular necrosis** (ATN) is the result. If not extensive, ATN can heal within several weeks; but polyuria develops during that time because the regenerating cells are incapable of adequate reabsorption.
- *The lungs develop diffuse alveolar damage (DAD) and becomes a "shock lung," the anatomic substrate for a clinical condition known as the* **adult respiratory distress syndrome** (ARDS). This is a major complication that encompasses more than shock and deserves special attention. ARDS is anatomically a situation in which gas exchanges in the lung are severely curtailed because the alveoli (including their capillary network) are diffusely damaged. Clinically, the patient develops an acute respiratory insufficiency, the heart rate accelerates, and cyanosis appears. Oxygen therapy is of little help. X-rays show a diffuse infiltration, and at autopsy the lung appears heavy and congested.

Microscopically, part of the alveolar lining is replaced by hyaline membranes (Figure 24.38), which consist of fibrin and debris of dead alveolar epithelium. The capillaries in the alveolar wall are damaged and leaky, hence the fibrin in the membranes.

The mechanism of alveolar damage

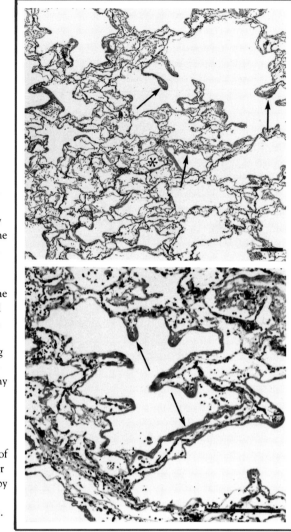

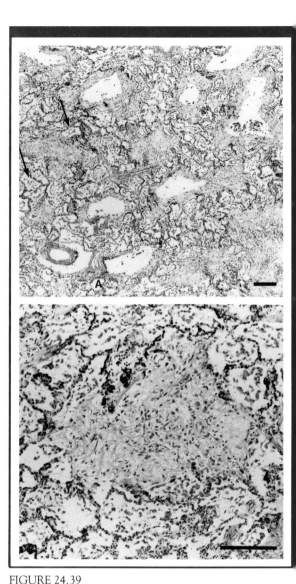

FIGURE 24.38 *Top:* Lung in an early stage of adult respiratory distress syndrome (ARDS) caused in this case by oxygen therapy for 4 days. Some alveoli are lined by thick, hyalin membranes (**arrows**) consisting of necrotic cells and fibrin. Many alveoli contain inflammatory cells (**asterisk**). **Bar** = 200 μm. *Bottom:* Detail of alveoli wholly or partially lined by hyalin membranes (**arrows**). **Bar** = 200 μm.

FIGURE 24.39
Advanced ARDS. *Top:* Few alveoli contain air (**A**); most are filled with cells (**arrows**), not identifiable at this enlargement. *Bottom:* Detail showing that the alveoli contain fibroblasts (elongated cells) as well as macrophages. The exudate has been organized, resulting in obliteration of the air space. **Bars** = 200 μm.

(both epithelial and capillary) is probably multiple (198). When ARDS develops in the course of oxygen therapy ("*respirator*" *lung*), the mechanism is thought to be toxic: oxygen-derived free radicals are generated by the high concentration of O_2. In septic shock the injury appears to originate within the alveolar capillaries: activated neutrophils are trapped and release free radicals and enzymes, and the endothelial and epithelial cells are damaged or killed. Neutrophils are activated by endotoxin itself, as well as by activated complement and other chemotaxins (leukotriene B_4, platelet activating factor). Remember that activated leukocytes tend to aggregate, and therefore to

become microemboli; the tendency of leukocytes to stick is also increased (214, 215, 223).

What happens next? The alveoli become filled with semifluid exudate; fibroblasts migrate into it and organize it (Figure 24.39). Surprisingly, some patients recover even from this stage: the alveolar filling is reabsorbed and air flows back into the alveoli.

• *The gut* becomes congested, edematous, and hemorrhagic (see Figure 24.37); the mucosa tends to slough off and bleed. As mentioned, the breakdown of the mucosal barrier can initiate sepsis and septic shock.

- *The liver* shows necrosis, which is centrolobular at first but can also be massive; more than one-fourth of the liver may die (160). Jaundice may develop (211) and liver enzymes seep into the blood.

- *The heart* shows subendocardial hemorrhages (mechanism unclear); in addition, pathologists at Duke University have described a myocardial change in hemorrhagic shock that is almost specific: the "zonal lesion" (Figure 24.40) (188–190, 204). The change affects a small "zone" of the myocardial cell; the fibrils normally attached to the intercalated disc seem to have torn away from it, and the adjacent sarcomeres are supercontracted. In dogs this occurred within 15–45 minutes of hemorrhagic shock. In humans it has been seen only "in situations where the heart is beating strongly and rapidly" (156). It may be related to high levels of circulating catecholamines, a typical event of early shock.

- *The pancreas* can develop small patches of self-digestion with the typical fat necrosis (p. 213). Occasionally the full-blown picture of acute pancreatic necrosis is a surprise finding at autopsy: this is usually an extremely dramatic and painful episode, but it can escape notice if the patient is terminally ill.

- Damage to the *brain* can be generalized and result in coma, but localized lesions can develop in the watershed areas mentioned earlier (170). The main problem is that hypoxia and ischemia of the brain lead to cellular swelling (i.e., to intracellular

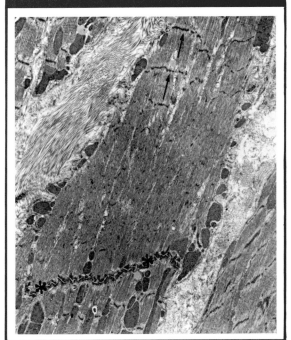

FIGURE 24.40 Myocardial zonal lesion, typical of shock. **Arrows:** Z bands. The sarcomeres above the intercalated disk (**asterisks**) are no longer distinguishable because the Z bands have been pulled out of shape. From a papillary muscle of a cat in hemorrhagic shock. (Courtesy of Dr. N.B. Ratliff Jr., The Cleveland Clinic Foundation, Cleveland, OH.)

edema). This raises the intracranial pressure, which creates a further obstacle to blood flow, which causes more ischemic swelling, and so on: another vicious circle. The ultimate anatomic catastrophe is the "respirator brain," a swollen, semiliquid mass that represents essentially autolysis of the brain *in vivo*; fragments of cerebellum float away in the cerebrospinal fluid and can be found attached to the spinal cord.

TO SUM UP: With the syndrome of shock we have reached a level of disease that encompasses virtually all organs and tissues. And yet, in each facet of its pathogenesis, shock teaches us that the underlying problem is always a problem of the cell, the elementary patient.

References

Ischemia

1. Adams JH, Corsellis JAN, Duchen LW, eds. Greenfield's neuropathology, 4th ed. New York: John Wiley & Sons, 1984.

2. Adams JH, Graham DI. An introduction to neuropathology. Edinburgh: Churchill Livingstone, 1988:72.

3. Adomian GE, Laks MM, Billingham ME. The incidence and significance of contraction bands in endomyocardial biopsies from normal human heart. Am Heart J 1978;95: 348–351.

3a. Al-Mehdi A, Shuman H, Fisher AB. Fluorescence microtopography of oxidative stress in lung ischemia-reperfusion. Lab Invest 1994;70:579–587.

4. Ames A III, Wright RL, Kowada M, Thurston JM, Majno G. Cerebral ischemia. II. The no-reflow phenomenon. Am J Pathol 1968;52:437–453.

5. Antman EM, Braunwald E. Acute MI management in the 1990s. Hosp Pract 1990;25:65–82.

6. Armour JA, Randall WC. Canine left ventricular intramyocardial pressures. Am J Physiol 1971;220:1833–1839.

7. Asher RAJ. The dangers of going to bed. Br Med J 1947;2:967–968.

8. Axford-Gately RA, Wilson GJ. The "border zone" in myocardial infarction. An ultrastructural study in the dog using an electron-dense blood flow marker. Am J Pathol 1988;131:452–464.

9. Babbs CF, Cregor MD, Turek JJ, Badylak SF. Endothelial

superoxide production in the isolated rat heart during early reperfusion after ischemia. A histochemical study. Am J Pathol 1991;139:1069–1080.

10. Bellesi G, Santini F. Sull'atrofia congestizia circoscritta del fegato (cosidetto infarto di Rattone-Zahn). Profilo anatomo-patologico e problematica della patogenesi. Arch De Vecchi Anat Patol 1966;47:913–930.

11. Bouchardy B, Majno G. Histopathology of early myocardial infarcts. Am J Pathol 1974;74:301–318.

12. Bouchardy B, Majno G. A new approach to the histologic diagnosis of early myocardial infarcts. Cardiology 1971/72;56:327–332.

13. Braunwald E. Mechanism of action of calcium-channel-blocking agents. N Engl J Med 1982;307:1618–1627.

14. Brierley JB, Graham DI. Hypoxia and vascular disorders of the central nervous system. In: Adams JH, Corsellis JAN, Duchen LW, eds. Greenfield's neuropathology, 4th ed. New York: John Wiley & Sons, 1984:125–207.

15. Bulkley GB. Free radical-mediated reperfusion injury: a selective review. Br J Cancer 1987;55(suppl VIII):66–73.

16. Burton KP. Evidence of direct toxic effects of free radicals on the myocardium. Free Radic Biol Med 1988;4:15–24.

17. Cahill BE, Kerstein MD. Ischemic neuropathy. Surg Gynecol Obstet 1987;165:469–474.

18. Campbell CA, Przyklenk K, Kloner RA. Infarct size reduction: a review of the clinical trials. J Clin Pharmacol 1986;26:317–329.

19. Cantu RC, Ames A III. Experimental prevention of cerebral vasculature obstruction produced by ischemia. J Neurosurg 1969;30:50–54.

20. Cheitlin MD, McAllister HA, de Castro CM. Myocardial infarction without atherosclerosis. JAMA 1975;231:951–959.

21. Chiang J, Kowada M, Ames A III, Wright RL, Majno G. Cerebral ischemia. Am J Pathol 1968;52:455–465.

22. Cohnheim J. Untersuchungen üeber die Embolischen Processe. Berlin: Verlag von August Hirschwald, 1872.

23. Cohnheim J. Lectures on general pathology, sect I. The pathology of the circulation. London: The New Sydenham Society, 1889.

24. Cooley DA, Reul GJ, Wukasch DC. Ischemic contracture of the heart: "stone heart." Am J Cardiol 1972;29:575–577.

25. Cross ER. Taravana. Diving syndrome in the Tuamotu diver. In: Rahn H, ed. Physiology of breath-hold diving and the AMA of Japan. Washington, DC: National Academy of Sciences, 1965:207–219.

26. Cuénoud HF. Unpublished data.

27. Dalen JE, Haffajee CI, Alpert JS, Howe JP III, Ockene IS, Paraskos JA. Pulmonary embolism, pulmonary hemorrhage and pulmonary infarction. N Engl J Med 1977;296:1431–1435.

28. Daviss B. Cold water to the rescue. Science 1985;85(June):72.

29. Dexter L. A brief history of venous thrombosis and pulmonary embolism. In Dalen JE, ed. Pulmonary embolism. New York: Medcom Press, 1972:1–5.

29a. Doukas J, Cutler AH, Boswell CA, Joris I, Majno G. Reversible endothelial cell relaxation induced by oxygen and glucose deprivation. Am J Pathol 1994;145:211–219.

30. Duverger D, MacKenzie ET. The quantification of cerebral infarction following focal ischemia in the rat: influence of strain, arterial pressure, blood glucose concentration, and age. J Cereb Blood Flow Metab 1988;8:449–461.

30a. Dvorak HF, Brown LF, Detmar M, Dvorak AM. Vascular permeability factor/vascular endothelial growth factor, microvascular hyperpermeability, and angiogenesis. Am J Pathol 1995;146:1029–1039.

31. Dyck PJ. Hypoxic neuropathy: does hypoxia play a role in diabetic neuropathy? The 1988 Robert Wartenberg Lecture. Neurology 1989;39:111–118.

32. Editorial. Haemorrhagic myocardial infarction. Lancet 1983;1:802–803.

32a. Edwalds GM, Said JW, Block MI, Herscher LL, Siegel RJ, Fishbein MC. Myocytolysis (vacuolar degeneration) of myocardium: immunohistochemical evidence of viability. Hum Pathol 1984;15:753–756.

33. Engler R. Granulocytes and oxidative injury in myocardial ischemia and reperfusion. Introduction. Fed Proc 1987a;46:2395–2396.

34. Engler R. Consequences of activation and adenosine-mediated inhibition of granulocytes during myocardial ischemia. Fed Proc 1987b;46:2407–2412.

35. Engler RL, Dahlgren MD, Morris DD, Peterson MA, Schmid-Schönbein GW. Role of leukocytes in response to acute myocardial ischemia and reflow in dogs. Am J Physiol 1986;251:H314–H322.

36. Engler RL, Schmid-Schönbein GW, Pavelec RS. Leukocyte capillary plugging in myocardial ischemia and reperfusion in the dog. Am J Pathol 1983;111:98–111.

37. Entman ML, Michael L, Rossen RD, et al. Inflammation in the course of early myocardial ischemia. FASEB J 1991;5:2529–2537.

38. Federle M, Moss AA. Computed tomography of the spleen. CRC Crit Rev Diagn Imaging 1983;19:1–16.

39. Fehér J, Csomós G, Vereckei A. Free radical reactions in medicine. Berlin: Springer-Verlag, 1987.

40. Felix WR, MacDonnell KF, Jacobs L. Resuscitation from drowning in cold water. N Engl J Med 1981;304:843–844.

41. Flores J, DiBona DR, Beck CH, Leaf A. The role of cell swelling in ischemic renal damage and the protective effect of hypertonic solute. J Clin Invest 1972;51:118–126.

42. Flynn PJ, Becker WK, Vercellotti GM, et al. Ibuprofen inhibits granulocyte responses to inflammatory mediators. A proposed mechanism for reduction of experimental myocardial infarct size. Inflammation 1984;8:33–44.

42a. Formigli L, Manneschi LI, Adembri C, Orlandini SZ, Pratesi C, Novelli GP. Expression of E-selectin in ischemic and reperfused human skeletal muscle. Ultrastruct Pathol 1995:19:193–200.

43. Friedl HP, Smith DJ, Till GO, Thomson PD, Louis DS, Ward PA. Ischemia-reperfusion in humans. Appearance of xanthine oxidase activity. Am J Pathol 1990;136:491–495.

44. Galloway AC, Pelletier R, D'Amore PA. Do ischemic hearts stimulate endothelial cell growth? Surgery 1984;96:435–439.

45. Ganote CE. Contraction band necrosis and irreversible myocardial injury. J Mol Cell Cardiol 1983;15:67–73.

46. Ganote CE, Worstell J, Iannotti JP, Kaltenbach JP. Cellular swelling and irreversible myocardial injury. Effects of polyethylene glycol and mannitol in perfused rat hearts. Am J Pathol 1977;88:95–118.

47. Garcia-Dorado D, Théroux P, Solares J, et al. Determinants of hemorrhagic infarcts. Histologic observations from experiments involving coronary occlusion, coronary reperfusion, and reocclusion. Am J Pathol 1990;137:301–311.

47a. Garcia JH, Liu K-F, Yoshida Y, Chen S, Lian J. Brain microvessels: factors altering their patency after the occlusion of a middle cerebral artery (Wistar rat). Am J Pathol 1994;145:728–740.

48. Garcia JH, Lowry SL, Briggs L, et al. Brain capillaries expand and rupture in areas of ischemia and reperfusion. In: Reivich M, Hurtig HI. Cerebrovascular diseases. New York: Raven Press, 1983:169–179.

49. Garfin SR. Historical review. In: Mubarak SJ, Hargens

AR, eds. Compartment syndromes and Volkmann's contracture. (Saunders monographs in clinical orthopaedics, vol III). Philadelphia: WB Saunders, 1981:6–16.

50. Gavin JB, Humphrey SM, Herdson PB. The no-reflow phenomenon in ischemic myocardium. Int Rev Exp Pathol 1983a;25:361–383.

51. Gavin JB, Thomson RW, Humphrey SM, Herdson PB. Changes in vascular morphology associated with the no-reflow phenomenon in ischaemic myocardium. Virchows Arch (Pathol Anat) 1983b;399:325–332.

52. Granger DN, Rutili G, McCord JM. Superoxide radicals in feline intestinal ischemia. Gastroenterology 1981;81:22–29.

53. Gusto Angiographic Investigators. The effects of tissue plasminogen activator, streptokinase, or both on coronary-artery patency, ventricular function, and survival after acute myocardial infarction. N Engl J Med 1993;329:1615–1622.

54. Haendchen RV, Corday E, Meerbaum S. Hypothermic synchronized retroperfusion of the coronary veins for the treatment of acutely ischemic myocardium. Compr Ther 1982;8:7–15.

55. Hampton AO, Castleman B. Correlation of postmortem chest teleoroentgenograms with autopsy findings with special reference to pulmonary embolism and infarction. Am J Roentgenol Rad Ther 1940;43:305–326.

56. Hartmann HT, Kester DE, Davies FT Jr. Plant propagation: principles and practices, 5th ed. Englewood Cliffs, NJ: Prentice Hall, 1990.

57. Hearse DJ, Humphrey SM, Bullock GR. The oxygen paradox and the calcium paradox: two facets of the same problem? J Mol Cell Cardiol 1978;10:641–668.

58. Heitzman ER. The lung. Radiologic-pathologic correlations, 2nd ed. St. Louis: C.V. Mosby, 1984.

59. Hernandez LA, Grisham MB, Twohig B, Arfors KE, Harlan JM, Granger DN. Role of neutrophils in ischemia-reperfusion-induced microvascular injury. Am J Physiol 1987;253:H699–H703.

60. Higginson LAJ, White F, Heggtveit HA, Sanders TM, Bloor CM, Covell JW. Determinants of myocardial hemorrhage after coronary reperfusion in the anesthetized dog. Circulation 1982;65:62–69.

61. Hill A, Volpe JJ. Pathogenesis and management of hypoxic-ischemic encephalopathy in the term newborn. Neurol Clin 1985;3:31–46.

62. ISAM Study Group. A prospective trial of intravenous streptokinase in acute myocardial infarction (ISAM). Mortality, morbidity, and infarct size at 21 days. N Engl J Med 1986;314:1465–1471.

63. Jaroch MT, Broughan TA, Hermann RE. The natural history of splenic infarction. Surgery 1986;100:743–749.

64. Jennings RB, Reimer KA. Pathobiology of acute myocardial ischemia. Hosp Pract 1989;24:89–107.

65. Kalimo H, Garcia JH, Kamijyo Y, Tanaka J, Trump BF. The ultrastructure of "brain death." II. Electron microscopy of feline cortex after complete ischemia. Virchows Arch B Cell Pathol 1977;25:207–220.

66. Kalimo H, Rehncrona S, Söderfeldt B, Olsson Y, Siesjö BK. Brain lactic acidosis and ischemic cell damage: 2. Histopathology. J Cereb Blood Flow Metab 1981;1:313–327.

67. Katori M, Berne RM. Release of adenosine from anoxic hearts. Relationship to coronary flow. Circ Res 1966;19:420–425.

68. Kennedy JW. Streptokinase for the treatment of acute myocardial infarction: a brief review of randomized trials. J Am Coll Cardiol 1987;5:28B–32B.

69. Klein HH, Puschmann S, Schaper J, Schaper W. The mechanism of the tetrazolium reaction in identifying

experimental myocardial infarction. Virchows Arch A Pathol Anat 1981;393:287–297.

70. Kloner RA. Do neutrophils mediate the phenomenon of stunned myocardium? J Am Coll Cardiol 1989;13:1164–1166.

71. Kloner RA, Przylklenk K. Recent advances in stunned myocardium. Cardiovasc Rev Reports 1987;8:25–29.

72. Kloner RA, Przylkenk K, Campbell CA. Coronary reperfusion following experimental myocardial infarction. J Cardiol Surg 1987;2:291–297.

73. Kloner RA, Rude RE, Carlson N, Maroko PR, DeBoer LWV, Braunwald E. Ultrastructural evidence of microvascular damage and myocardial cell injury after coronary artery occlusion: which comes first? Circulation 1980;62:945–952.

74. Kost GJ. Surface pH of the medial gastrocnemius and soleus muscles during hemorrhagic shock and ischemia. Surgery 1984;95:183–190.

75. Kowada M, Ames A III, Majno G, Wright RL. Cerebral ischemia. An improved experimental method for study; cardiovascular effects and demonstration of an early vascular lesion in the rabbit. J Neurosurg 1968;28:150–157.

76. Krainer L. Pathological effects of cerebral anoxia. Am J Med 1958;25:258–266.

77. Lakon G. The topographical tetrazolium method for determining the germinating capacity of seeds. Plant Phys 1949;24:389–394.

78. Lefer AM, Tsao PS, Lefer DJ, Ma X-L. Role of endothelial dysfunction in the pathogenesis of reperfusion injury after myocardial ischemia. FASEB J 1991;5:2029–2034.

79. Levene CI, Kapoor R, Heale G. The effect of hypoxia on the synthesis of collagen and glycosaminoglycans by cultured pig aortic endothelium. Atherosclerosis 1982;44:327–337.

80. Levine RL. Ischemia: from acidosis to oxidation. FASEB J 1993;7:1242–1246.

81. Little WC, Rogers EW. Angiographic evidence of hemorrhagic myocardial infarction after intracoronary thrombolysis with streptokinase. Am J Cardiol 1983;51:906–908.

82. Majno G. The healing hand: man and wound in the ancient world. Cambridge, MA: Harvard University Press, 1975.

83. Majno G, Ames A III, Chiang J, Wright RL. No reflow after cerebral ischaemia. Lancet 1967;2:569–570.

84. Marshall V, Jablonski P, Howden B, Leslie E, Rae D, Tange J. Recovery of renal function in the rat after warm ischaemia: functional and morphological changes. In: Pegg DE, Jacobsen IA, Halasz NA, eds. Organ preservation: basic and applied aspects. Lancaster: MTP Press Limited, 1982:69–76.

85. May JW Jr, Chait LA, O'Brien BM, Hurley JV. The no-reflow phenomenon in experimental free flaps. Plast Reconst Surg 1978;61:256–267.

86. McCord JM. Oxygen-derived free radicals in post-ischemic tissue injury. N Engl J Med 1985;312:159–163.

87. McDonagh PF, Laks H. Use of cold blood cardioplegia to protect against coronary microcirculatory injury due to ischemia and reperfusion. J Thorac Cardiovasc Surg 1982;84:609–618.

88. McGoldrick PJ, Rudd TG, Figley MM, Wilhelm JP. What becomes of pulmonary infarcts? Am J Roentgenol 1979;133:1039–1045.

89. McIntyre DM, Sasahara AA. The hemodynamic response to pulmonary embolism in patients without prior cardiopulmonary disease. Am J Cardiol 1971;28:288–294.

90. Mégevand R, Cruchaud A, Kapanci Y. Etude de l'action

de différents médicaments immuno-suppresseurs appliqués aux allogreffes pulmonaires chez le chien. Helv Chir Acta 1968;35:327–330.

91. Montrucchio G, Alloatti G, Mariano F, et al. Role of platelet-activating factor in the reperfusion injury of rabbit ischemic heart. Am J Pathol 1990;137:71–83.

92. Mubarak SJ. Exertional compartment syndromes. In: Mubarak SJ, Hargens AR, eds. Compartment syndromes and Volkmann's contracture. (Saunders monographs in clinical orthopaedics, vol III). Philadelphia: WB Saunders, 1981:209–226.

93. Mullane KM. Eicosanoids in myocardial ischemia/reperfusion injury. Adv Inflam Res 1988;12:191–214.

94. Muller JE, Tofler GH. Circadian variation and cardiovascular disease. N Engl J Med 1991;325:1038–1039.

95. Nedergaard M. Mechanisms of brain damage in focal cerebral ischemia. Acta Neurol Scand 1988;77:81–101.

96. Neely JR. Metabolic disturbances after coronary occlusion. Hosp Pract 1989;24:81–96.

97. Nukada H, Dyck PJ. Microsphere embolization of nerve capillaries and fiber degeneration. Am J Pathol 1984; 115:275–287.

98. Owen CA. The crush syndrome. In: Mubarak SJ, Hargens AR, eds. Compartment syndromes and Volkmann's contracture. (Saunders monographs in clinical orthopaedics, vol III). Philadelphia: WB Saunders, 1981:166–182.

99. Paljärvi L, Rehncrona S, Söderfeldt B, Olsson Y, Kalimo H. Brain lactic acidosis and ischemic cell damage: quantitative ultrastructural changes in capillaries of rat cerebral cortex. Acta Neuropathol 1983;60:232–240.

99a. Pe'er J, Shweiki D, Itin A, Hemo I, Gnessin H, Keshet E. Hypoxia-induced expression of vascular endothelial growth factor by retinal cells is a common factor in neovascularizing ocular diseases. Lab Invest 1995;72: 638–645.

100. Przyklenk K, Kloner RA. Superoxide dismutase plus catalase improve contractile function in the canine model of the "stunned myocardium." Circ Res 1986;58: 148–156.

101. Reimer KA, Jennings RB. Myocardial ischemia, hypoxia, and infarction. In: Fozzard HA, Jennings RB, Haber E, Katz AM, Morgan HE, eds. The heart and cardiovascular system, vol 2. New York: Raven Press, 1986:1133–1201.

102. Reynolds JM, McDonagh PF. Early in reperfusion, leukocytes alter perfused coronary capillarity and vascular resistance. Am J Physiol 1989;256:H1–H8.

102a. Rifind JM, Abugo O, Levy A, Monticone R, Heim J. Formation of free radicals under hypoxia. In: Hochachka PW, Lutz PL, Sick T, Rosenthal M, van den Thillart G. (eds). Surviving hypoxia: mechanisms of control and adaptation. Boca Raton: CRC Press Inc., 1993, pp. 509–525.

103. Riley RL. Historical review of hypoxia. Bull Eur Physiopathol Respir 1982;18(suppl 4):13–19.

104. Roberts JP, Perry MO, Hariri RJ, Shires GT. Incomplete recovery of muscle cell function following partial but not complete ischemia. Circ Shock 1985;17:253–258.

105. Romson JL, Hook BG, Kunkel SL, Abrams GD, Schork MA, Lucchesi BR. Reduction of the extent of ischemic myocardial injury by neutrophil depletion in the dog. Circulation 1983;67:1016–1023.

106. Rosenow EC III, Osmundson PJ, Brown ML. Pulmonary embolism. Mayo Clin Proc 1981;56:161–178.

107. Sabiston DC Jr. Pathophysiology, diagnosis, and management of pulmonary embolism. Am J Surg 1979;138: 384–391.

108. Saegesser F, Roenspies U, Robinson JWL. Ischemic diseases of the large intestine. Pathobiol Annu 1979;9: 303–337.

109. Sanders MD, Graham EM. Ocular disorders associated with systemic diseases. In: Vaughan D, Asbury T, Tabbara KF, eds. General ophthalmology, 12th ed. Norwalk, CT: Appleton & Lange, 1989:279–319.

110. Sasaki K, Ueno A, Katori M, Kikawada R. Detection of leukotriene B_4 in cardiac tissue and its role in infarct extension through leucocyte migration. Cardiovasc Res 1988;22:142–148.

110a. Schaper W, Schaper J. (eds). Collateral circulation. Boston: Kluwer Academic Publishers, 1993.

111. Schmid-Schönbein GW. Capillary plugging by granulocytes and the no-reflow phenomenon in the microcirculation. Fed Proc 1987;46:2397–2401.

112. Schmid-Schönbein GW. Granulocyte: friend and foe. NIPS 1988;3:144–147.

113. Schmid-Schönbein GW, Engler RL. No-reflow in the microcirculation. The granulocyte tragedy. In: Hartmann A, Kuschinsky W, eds. Cerebral ischemia and hemorheology. Berlin: Springer-Verlag, 1987:464–471.

114. Schwartz P, Piper HM, Spahr R, Spieckermann PG. Ultrastructure of cultured adult myocardial cells during anoxia and reoxygenation. Am J Pathol 1984;115: 349–361.

115. Seki H, Yoshimoto T, Ogawa A, Suzuki J. Hemodynamics in hemorrhagic infarction—an experimental study. Stroke 1985;16:647–651.

116. Shanley PF, Johnson GC. Calcium and acidosis in renal hypoxia. Lab Invest 1991;65:298–305.

117. Sheehan HL, Davis JC. Complete permanent renal ischaemia. J Pathol Bacteriol 1958;76:569–587.

118. Sheehan HL, Davis JC. Patchy permanent renal ischaemia. J Pathol Bacteriol 1959a;77:33–48.

119. Sheehan HL, Davis JC. Renal ischaemia with failed reflow. J Pathol Bacteriol 1959b;78:105–120.

120. Siesjö BK. Acidosis and ischemic brain damage. Neurochem Pathol 1988;9:31–88.

121. Simpson PJ, Mickelson JK, Lucchesi BR. Free radical scavengers in myocardial ischemia. Fed Proc 1987;46: 2413–2421.

122. Strock PE, Majno G. Vascular responses to experimental tourniquet ischemia. Surg Gynecol Obstet 1969a; 129:309–318.

123. Strock PE, Majno G. Microvascular changes in acutely ischemic rat muscle. Surg Gynecol Obstet 1969b;129: 1213–1224.

124. Summers WK, Jamison RL. The no reflow phenomenon in renal ischemia. Lab Invest 1971;25:635–643.

125. Tohgi H, Yamanouchi H, Murakami M, Kameyama M. Importance of the hematocrit as a risk factor in cerebral infarction. Stroke 1978;9:369–374.

125a. Torvik A. The pathogenesis of watershed infarcts in the brain. Stroke 1984;15:221–223.

126. Tsao M-S, Schraufnagel D, Wang N-S. Pathogenesis of pulmonary infarction. Am J Med 1982;72:599–606.

127. Vander Heide RS, Angelo JP, Altschuld RA, Ganote CE. Energy dependence of contraction band formation in perfused hearts and isolated adult myocytes. Am J Pathol 1986;125:55–68.

128. van Hof MW, Wildervanck de Blécourt EMW. Early brain damage due to hypoxia. In: Almli CR, Finger S, eds. Early brain damage, vol 1. Research orientations and clinical observations. New York: Academic Press, 1984:81–91.

129. Vander Salm TJ, Pape LA, Price J, Burke M. Hemorrhage from myocardial revascularization. J Thorac Cardiovasc Surg 1981;82:768–772.

130. Vivaldi MT, Kloner RA, Schoen FJ. Triphenyltetra-

zolium staining of irreversible ischemic injury following coronary artery occlusion in rats. Am J Pathol 1985;121:522–530.

131. White HD, Norris RM, Brown MA, et al. Effect of intravenous streptokinase on left ventricular function and early survival after acute myocardial infarction. N Engl J Med 1987;317:850–855.

132. Willms-Kretschmer K, Majno G. Ischemia of the skin. Electron microscopic study of vascular injury. Am J Pathol 1969;54:327–353.

133. Wise BL, Cockayne S. Enzymes. In: Bishop ML, Duben-Von Laufen JL, Fody EP, eds. Clinical chemistry. Philadelphia: JB Lippincott, 1985:205–239.

134. Zager RA, Mahan J, Merola AJ. Effects of mannitol on the postischemic kidney. Biochemical, functional, and morphologic assessments. Lab Invest 1985;53:433–442.

135. Zahn FW. Ueber die Folgen des Verschlusses der Lungenarterien und Pfortaderäste durch Embolie. Verh Ges Dtsch Naturforsch Ärzte 1898;69:9–11.

136. Ziegler E. Ueber Myomalacia cordis. Virchows Arch Pathol Anat Physiol Klin Med 1882;90:211–212.

137. Zimmerman ANE, Daems W, Hülsmann WC, Snijder J, Wisse E, Durrer D. Morphological changes of heart muscle caused by successive perfusion with calcium-free and calcium-containing solutions (calcium paradox). Cardiovasc Res 1967;1:201–209.

Shock

138. Abboud FM. Pathophysiology of hypotension and shock. In: Hurst JW, ed. The heart, 6th ed. New York: McGraw-Hill, 1986:370–382.

139. Altura BM, Hershey SG. RES phagocytic function in trauma and adaptation to experimental shock. Am J Physiol 1968;215:1414–1419.

140. Bagge U, Amundson B, Lauritzen C. White blood cell deformability and plugging of skeletal muscle capillaries in hemorrhagic shock. Acta Physiol Scand 1980;180:159–163.

141. Bagge U, Skalak R, Attefors R. Granulocyte rheology. Experimental studies in an in vitro micro-flow system. Adv Microcirc 1977;7:29–48.

142. Barroso-Aranda J, Schmid-Schönbein GW. Transformation of neutrophils as indicator of irreversibility in hemorrhagic shock. Am J Physiol 1989;257:H846–H852.

143. Barroso-Aranda J, Schmid-Schönbein GW. Pentoxifylline pretreatment decreases the pool of circulating activated neutrophils, in-vivo adhesion to endothelium, and improves survival from hemorrhagic shock. Biorheology 1990;27:401–418.

144. Barroso-Aranda J, Schmid-Schönbein GW, Zqeifach BW, Engler RL. Granulocytes and no-reflow phenomenon in irreversible hemorrhagic shock. Circ Res 1988;63:437–447.

145. Baue AE, Chaudry IH. Prevention of multiple systems failure. Surg Clin North Am 1980;60:1167–1178.

146. Bernton EW, Long JB, Holaday JW. Opioids and neuropeptides: mechanisms in circulatory shock. Fed Proc 1985;44:290–299.

147. Beutler B, Krochin N, Milsark IW, Luedke C, Cerami A. Control of cachectin (tumor necrosis factor) synthesis: mechanisms of endotoxin resistance. Science 1986;232:977–980.

148. Beutler B, Milsark IW, Cerami AC. Passive immunization against cachectin/tumor necrosis factor protects mice from lethal effect of endotoxin. Science 1985;229:869–871.

149. Bond RF. Mediator mechanisms in shock. Fed Proc 1985;44:273–274.

150. Bone RC. Multiple system organ failure and the sepsis syndrome. Hosp Pract 1991a;26:101–126.

151. Bone RC. The pathogenesis of sepsis. Ann Intern Med 1991b;115:457–469.

152. Brånemark PI. Intravascular anatomy of blood cells in man. Basel: S. Karger, 1971.

153. Bull BS, Kuhn IN. The production of schistocytes by fibrin strands (a scanning electron microscope study). Blood 1970;35:104–111.

154. Carey LC. Shock: differential diagnosis and immediate treatment. Hosp Med 1975;11:68–93.

155. Cerra FB. The multiple organ failure syndrome. Hosp Pract 1990;25:169–176.

156. Chang J, Hackel DB. Comparative study of myocardial lesions in hemorrhagic shock. Lab Invest 1973;28:641–647.

157. Clozel M, Kuhn H, Baumgartner HR. Procoagulant activity of endotoxin-treated human endothelial cells exposed to native human flowing blood. Blood 1989;73:729–733.

158. Colman RW. The role of plasma proteases in septic shock. N Engl J Med 1989;320:1207–1209.

159. Cybulsky MI, Chan MKW, Movat HZ. Acute inflammation and microthrombosis induced by endotoxin, interleukin-1, and tumor necrosis factor and their implication in gram-negative infection. Lab Invest 1988;58:365–378.

160. Dal Nogare AR. Southwestern Internal Medicine Conference: septic shock. Am J Med Sci 1991;302:50–65.

161. Dinarello CA. The proinflammatory cytokines interleukin-1 and tumor necrosis factor and treatment of the septic shock syndrome. J Infect Dis 1991;163:1177–1184.

162. Doherty DE, Zagarella L, Henson PM, Worthen GS. Lipopolysaccharide stimulates monocyte adherence by effects on both the monocyte and the endothelial cell. J Immunol 1989;143:3673–3679.

163. Ferguson DW, Abboud FM. The pathophysiology, recognition, and management of shock. In: Hurst JW, ed. The heart, 7th ed. New York: McGraw-Hill Information Services Company, 1990:442–461.

164. Fine J. The bacterial factor in traumatic shock. Springfield, IL: Charles C. Thomas, 1954.

165. Fink MP, Cohn SM, Lee PC, et al. Effect of lipopolysaccharide on intestinal intramucosal hydrogen ion concentration in pigs: evidence of gut ischemia in a normodynamic model of septic shock. Crit Care Med 1989a;17:641–646.

166. Fink MP, MacVittie TJ, Casey LC. Inhibition of prostaglandin synthesis restores normal hemodynamics in canine hyperdynamic sepsis. Ann Surg 1984;200:619–626.

167. Fink MP, Rothschild HR, Deniz YF, Cohn SM. Complement depletion with Naje haje cobra venom factor limits prostaglandin release and improves visceral perfusion in porcine endotoxic shock. J Trauma 1989b;29:1076–1085.

168. Frank HA, Jacob S, Friedman EW, et al. Traumatic shock XXII. Irreversibility of hemorrhagic shock and VDM hypothesis. Failure of Ferritin to affect arterial pressure and survival period of hepatectomized-nephrectomized dogs. Am J Physiol 1952;168:150–155.

169. Fries JWU, Williams AmJ, Atkins RC, Newman W, Lipscomb MF, Collins T. Expression of VCAM-1 and E-selectin in an in vivo model of endothelial activation. Am J Pathol 1993;143:725–737.

170. Garcia JH. Morphology of global cerebral ischemia. Crit Care Med 1988;16:979–987.

171. Gimbrone MA, Aster RH, Cotran RS, Corkery J, Jandl

JH, Folkman J. Preservation of vascular integrity in organs perfused in vitro with a platelet-rich medium. Nature 1969;222:33–36.

172. Girardin E, Grau GE, Dayer J-M, Roux-Lombard P, The J5 Study Group, Lambert P-H. Tumor necrosis factor and interleukin-1 in the serum of children with severe infectious purpura. N Engl J Med 1988;319:397–400.

173. Ghosh S, Latimer RD, Gray BM, Harwood RJ, Oduro A. Endotoxin-induced organ injury. Crit Care Med 1993;21:S19–S24.

174. Goldstein IM. Lysosomes and their relation to the cell in shock. In: The proceedings of a symposium on recent research developments and current clinical practice in shock: the cell in shock. Kalamazoo, MI: The Upjohn Company, 1975:30–34.

175. Guyton AC. Textbook of medical physiology, 7th ed. Philadelphia: WB Saunders, 1986.

176. Hackel DB, Ratliff NB, Mikat E. The heart in shock. Circ Res 1974;35:805–811.

177. Hammerschmidt DE. Activation of the complement system and of granulocytes in lung injury: the adult respiratory distress syndrome. Adv Inflam Res 1983;5:147–172.

178. Hardaway RM. Shock: the reversible stage of dying. Littleton, MA: PSG Publishing Commpany, 1988.

179. Harlan JM, Harker LA, Reidy MA, Gajdusek CM, Schwartz SM, Striker GE. Lipopolysaccharide-mediated bovine endothelial cell injury in vitro. Lab Invest 1983;48:269–274.

180. Herlihy BL, Lefer AM. Selective inhibition of pancreatic proteases and prevention of toxic factors in shock. Circ Shock 1974;1:51–60.

181. Hewett JA, Schultze AE, VanCise S, Roth RA. Neutrophil depletion protects against liver injury from bacterial endotoxin. Lab Invest 1992;66:347–361.

182. Kass EH. Magnesium and the pathogenesis of toxic shock syndrome. Rev Infect Dis 1989;11(suppl 1):S167–S175.

183. Katori M, Majima M, Odoi-Adome R, Sunahara N, Uchida Y. Evidence for the involvement of a plasma kallikrein-kinin system in the immediate hypotension produced by endotoxin in anaesthetized rats. Br J Pharmacol 1989;98:1383–1391.

184. Lefer AM. The role of lysosomes in circulatory shock. Life Sci 1976;19:1803–1810.

185. Lefer AM. Properties of cardioinhibitory factors produced in shock. Fed Proc 1978;37:2734–2740.

186. Lefer AM. Interaction between myocardial depressant factor and vasoactive mediators with ischemia and shock. Am J Physiol 1987;252:R193–R205.

187. Lindberg B. Liver circulation and metabolism in haemorrhagic shock. Acta Chir Scand Suppl 1977;476:1–18.

188. Martin AM Jr, Green WB, Simmons RL, Soloway HB. Human myocardial zonal lesions. Arch Pathol 1969;87:339–342.

189. Martin AM Jr, Hackel DB. The myocardium of the dog in hemorrhagic shock. A histochemical study. Lab Invest 1963;12:77–91.

190. Martin AM Jr, Hackel DB, Kurtz SM. The ultrastructure of zonal lesions of the myocardium in hemorrhagic shock. Am J Pathol 1964;44:127–140.

191. Miles AA, Niven JSF. The enhancement of infection during shock produced by bacterial toxins and other agents. Br J Exp Pathol 1949;31:73–95.

192. Mileski WJ, Winn RK, Vedder NB, Pohlman TH, Harlan JM, Rice CL. Inhibition of CD18-dependent neutrophil adherence reduces organ injury after hemorrhagic shock in primates. Surgery 1990;108:206–212.

192a. Mohler KM, Sleath PR, Fitzner JN, Cerretti DP, Alderson M, Serwar SS, Torrance, DS, Otten-Evans C, Greenstreet T, Weerawarna K, Kronhelm SR, Petersen M, Gerhart M, Kozlosky CJ, March CJ, Black RA. Protection against a lethal dose of endotoxin by an inhibitor of tumour necrosis factor processing. Nature 1994;370:218–220.

193. Morrison DC, Ryan JL. Endotoxins and disease mechanisms. Annu Rev Med 1987;38:417–432.

194. Moss GS. Pulmonary involvement in hypovolemic shock. Annu Rev Med 1972;23:201–228.

195. Movat HZ. Microcirculation in disseminated intravascular coagulation induced by endotoxins. In: Renkin EM, Michel CC, eds. Handbook of physiology, sect 2: The cardiovascular system. Bethesda, MD: American Physiological Society, 1984:1047–1076.

196. Müller-Eberhard HJ. The significance of complement activity in shock. In: Proceedings of a symposium on recent research developments and current clinical practice in shock: the cell in shock. Kalamazoo, MI: The Upjohn Company, 1975:35–38.

197. Navab M, Hough GP, Van Lenten BJ, Berliner JA, Fogelman AM. Low density lipoproteins transfer bacterial lipopolysaccharides across endothelial monolayers in a biologically active form. J Clin Invest 1988;81:601–605.

198. Ognibene FP, Martin SE, Parker MM, et al. Adult respiratory distress syndrome in patients with severe neutropenia. N Engl J Med 1986;315:547–551.

199. Parrillo JE. The cardiovascular pathophysiology of sepsis. Annu Rev Med 1989;40:469–485.

200. Parrillo JE, Burch C, Shelhamer JH, Parker MM, Natanson C, Schuette W. A circulating myocardial depressant substance in humans with septic shock. J Clin Invest 1985;76:1539–1553.

201. Parrillo JE, Parker MM, Natanson C, et al. Septic shock in humans: advances in the understanding of pathogenesis, cardiovascular dysfunction, and therapy. Ann Intern Med 1990;113:227–242.

202. Pralong G, Calandra T, Glauser M-P, et al. Plasminogen activator inhibitor 1: a new prognostic marker in septic shock. Thromb Haemost 1989;61:459–462.

203. Raetz CRH, Ulevitch RJ, Wright SD, Sibley CH, Ding A, Nathan CF. Gram-negative endotoxin: an extraordinary lipid with profound effects on eukaryotic signal transduction. FASEB J 1991;5:2652–2660.

204. Ratliff NB, Kopelman RI, Goldner RD, Cruz PT, Hackel DB. Formation of myocardial zonal lesions. Am J Pathol 1975;79:321–334.

205. Ratliff NB, Wilson JW, Mikat E, Hackel DB, Graham TC. The lung in hemorrhagic shock. IV. The role of neutrophilic polymorphonuclear leukocytes. Am J Pathol 1971;65:325–334.

206. Redl H, Dinges HP, Buurman WA, et al. Expression of endothelial leukocyte adhesion molecule-1 in septic but not traumatic/hypovolemic shock in the baboon. Am J Pathol 1991;139:461–466.

207. Reidy MA, Bowyer DE. Scanning electron microscopy: morphology of aortic endothelium following injury by endotoxin and during subsequent repair. Atherosclerosis 1977;26:319–328.

207a. Rietschel ET, Kirikae T, Schade FU, Mamat U, Schmidt G, Loppnow H, Ulmer AJ, Zähringer U, Seydel U, Di Padova F, Schreier M, Brade H. Bacterial endotoxin: molecular relationships of structure to activity and function. FASEB J 1994;8:217–225.

208. Rosenstreich DL, Glode LM, Wahl LM, Sandberg AL, Mergenhagen SE. Analysis of the cellular defects of endotoxin-unresponsive C3H/HeJ mice. In: Schlessinger

D, ed. Microbiology—1977. Washington, DC: American Society for Microbiology, 1977:314–320.

209. Schweinburg FB, Frank HA, Fine J. Bacterial factor in experimental hemorrhagic shock. Evidence for development of a bacterial factor which accounts for irreversibility to transfusion and for the loss of the normal capacity to destroy bacteria. Am J Physiol 1954;179:532–540.

210. Seeley HF. Pathophysiology of haemorrhagic shock. Br J Hosp Med 1987;37:14–20.

210a. Shapiro JI. Functional and metabolic responses of isolated hearts to acidosis: effects of sodium bicarbonate and carbicarb. Am J Physiol 1990;258:H1835–H1839.

211. Sherlock S. Diseases of the liver and biliary system, 8th ed. Oxford: Blackwell Scientific Publications, 1989.

212. Thomas L. The lives of a cell. New York: The Viking Press, 1974.

213. Thomas L. The youngest science. New York: The Viking Press, 1983.

214. Till GO, Hatherill JR, Tourtellotte WW, Lutz MJ, Ward PA. Lipid peroxidation and acute lung injury after thermal trauma to skin. Evidence of a role for hydroxyl radical. Am J Pathol 1985;119:376–384.

215. Till GO, Morganroth ML, Kunkel R, Ward PA. Activation of C5 by cobra venom factor is required in neutrophil-mediated lung injury in the rat. Am J Pathol 1987;129:44–53.

215a. Tipper DJ. Antibiotic inhibitors of bacterial cell wall biosynthesis. In: Encyclopedia of Human Biology, Volume 1. New York: Academic Press Inc. 1991;271–285.

216. Tom WW, Villalba M, Szlabick RE, Walsh M, Margherio R, Lucas RJ. Fluorophotometric evaluation of capillary permeability in gram-negative shock. Arch Surg 1983;118:636–641.

217. Tracey KJ, Beutler B, Lowry SF, et al. Shock and tissue injury induced by recombinant human cachectin. Science 1986;234:470–474.

218. Vedder NB, Fouty BW, Winn RK, Harlan JM, Rice CL. Role of neutrophils in generalized reperfusion injury associated with resuscitation from shock. Surgery 1989a;106:509–516.

219. Vedder NB, Winn RK, Rice CL, Chi EY, Arfors K-E, Harlan JM. A monoclonal antibody to the adherence-promoting leukocyte glycoprotein, CD18, reduces organ injury and improves survival from hemorrhagic shock and resuscitation in rabbits. J Clin Invest 1988;81:939–944.

220. Vedder NB, Winn RK, Rice CL, Harlan JM. Neutrophil-mediated vascular injury in shock and multiple organ failure. Prog Clin Biol Res 1989b;299:181–191.

221. Vukajlovich SW, Hoffman J, Morrison DC. Activation of human serum complement by bacterial lipopolysaccharides: structural requirements for antibody independing activation of the classical and alternative pathways. Mol Immunol 1987;24:319–331.

222. Wakabayashi G, Gelfand JA, Burke JF, Thompson RC, Dinarello CA. A specific receptor antagonist for interleukin 1 prevents Escherichia coli–induced shock in rabbits. FASEB J 1991;5:338–343.

223. Ward PA, Till GO, Hatherill JR, Annesley TM, Kunkel RG. Systemic complement activation, lung injury, and products of lipid peroxidation. J Clin Invest 1985;76:517–527.

224. Whisler RL, Cornwell DG, Proctor KVW, Downs E. Bacterial lipopolysaccharide acts on human endothelial cells to enhance the adherence of peripheral blood monocytes. J Lab Clin Med 1989;114:708–716.

225. Wilson JW. Leukocyte sequestration and morphologic augmentation in the pulmonary network following hemorrhagic shock and related forms of stress. Adv Microcirc 1972;4:197–232.

226. Wyngaarden JB, Smith LH, eds. Cecil textbook of medicine, vol 1, 16th ed. Philadelphia: WB Saunders, 1982.

227. Zimmerman JJ, Dietrich KA. Current perspectives on septic shock. Pediatr Clin North Am 1987;34:131–163.

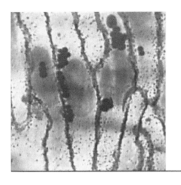

TUMORS

Introduction

CHAPTER 25

Tumors: A Working
Definition

Benign and Malignant:
Points of View

Names and
Classification of
Tumors

Tumors Have
Personalities

In multicellular animals and plants, all organs live and function thanks to the planned, harmonious, highly disciplined cooperation of different types of cells. One of the accidents that can disrupt this harmony is the focal, purposeless overgrowth of one of the cellular components: this is, in essence, a **tumor.**

It is fortunate that we are writing this chapter well after 1976. Before that year, the world of tumors—as seen by the nonexpert—was quite depressing. Tumor cells were outlaws, cells gone mad. They seemed to follow no rules. The subject of tumors contrasted sharply with other topics of general pathology, which have a neat internal logic of their own: vascular disturbances are almost as logical as plumbing problems, inflammation reads like an epic of self-defense, diapedesis is beautiful and we know what it means. Nothing was intellectually beautiful about tumors, and little was predictable; in fact, the eminent Mexican pathologist Ruy Pérez Tamayo once said very aptly that no generalization can be made about tumors, except this one—namely, that no generalization can be made.

Then it was realized, almost overnight, that many tumors are driven by normal genes that are expressed inappropriately (**oncogenes**); and other tumors are triggered by the loss of normal genes (**suppressor genes**). So, tumor cells are neither outlaws nor mad; they are ordinary cells that are simply obeying the wrong orders. In some cases they are even ready to mend their ways if the internal driving message can be corrected. Because there are so many types of cells—about 200 in humans—and so many genes as sources of orders, the variety of tumors is so great that the underlying unity is hard to discern; but now we know where to look for it, and molecular biologists are hard at work.

The novice will probably continue to be struck more by the variety than by the unity. Pérez Tamayo's quip is still largely true. In humans, the number of tumors that the microscope can distinguish is of the order of 600 (Table 1.1), and each has its own natural history. Other animals are afflicted by tumors that are homologous, but not identical, to those of humans. This means that there is no "universal tumor" to serve as a model, and correspondingly, there can be no universal rules about tumors. Therefore, our text will be replete with dissatisfying restrictions such as "often," "usually," "in one strain of mice," and the irritating "tends to be" in place of "is."

Nonetheless, the story of tumors has developed into a fascinating saga, overlapping all other chapters of general pathology and reaching, more than any other type of disease, into all facets of human life, from the embryo and genetics to worldly professions, nutrition, toxicology, and the environment of our planet.

Tumors: A Working Definition

As a start, we must be content with a working definition of tumor because a flawless one does not exist. We will be better prepared to answer the question "What is a tumor?" at the end of this section (p. 921).

Henry Pitot, author of an excellent book on tumors (17), proposed this sober statement: *A tumor is a heritably altered, relatively autonomous growth of tissue.* Everyone would accept that tumors represent a *growth*, as long as we add that some tumors stop growing for years. *Heritable* means passed on from cell to daughter cell, not from parents to children, although that happens too. The reference to *tissue* is meant to imply that tumors are a curse of multicellular creatures, be they animals or plants (19). Nature imposes a "tumor burden" (a standard expression of oncologists) even on corals (2), oysters, fruit flies (Figure 25.1) (10, 11), and salmon (Figure 25.2).

Is it really true that unicellular organisms are spared? Paramecia exposed to carcinogens develop peculiar shapes (7, 15). Also, we could visualize a science-fiction horror story of amoebae in a pond proliferating out of control like a monstrous leukemia and perhaps metastasizing to other ponds. Somehow this does not happen, but we consulted some yeast experts, and learned the following. Normal yeast cells are very sensitive to food deprivation; when food supplies become scarce, they withdraw from the cell cycle and

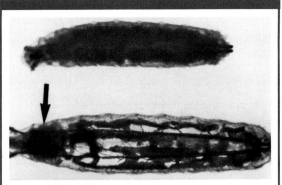
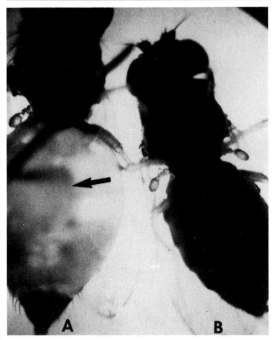

FIGURE 25.1 Tumor in the fruit fly, *Drosophila melanogaster.* Top: Normal larva and a larger mutant larva containing a tumorous mass in the frontal part (neuroblastoma, **arrow**). *Bottom* **A:** Bloated adult, which has been injected with tumorous brain tissue (*Drosophila* neuroblastoma) that is now growing in the abdomen (**arrow**), as was confirmed by histology. **B:** Control. (Reproduced with permission from [10].)

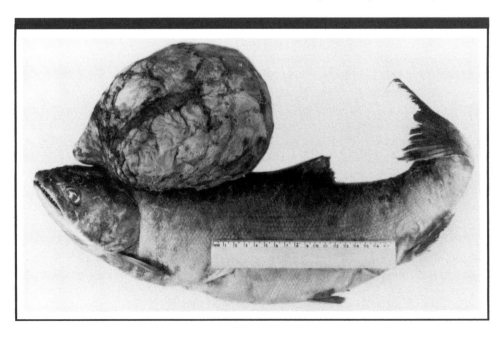

FIGURE 25.2
Coho salmon with a fibrolipoma. (Courtesy of Dr. J.C. Harshbarger, Smithsonian Institute, Washington, DC.)

dramatically reduce their metabolic activity. If they are transfected with the ras2 oncogene (homologous to the various human ras oncogenes) they proliferate out of control, and when nutrients run out they just die. It seems to us that this condition is not far removed from a yeast leukemia. Paramecia exposed to carcinogens develop peculiar shapes (7, 15).

Tumors in general, including benign and malignant varieties, differ from other types of growth in at least four ways:

- *They are purposeless,* meaning that, in the human perspective, they are of no conceivable use to the host. In the perspective of certain viruses, of course, a tumor serves a vital purpose.
- *They tend to be atypical,* which means that their microscopic patterns and their individual cells are structurally and functionally abnormal in varying degrees.
- *They tend to be autonomous;* that is, they escape the controls that regulate growth (they only *tend* to escape; fortunately for many patients, some tumors do respond to controlling hormones).
- *They tend to be aggressive;* that is, they invade the host.

In summary,

TUMORS ARE PURPOSELESS GROWTHS OF TISSUE THAT TEND TO BE ATYPICAL, AUTONOMOUS, AND AGGRESSIVE.

Benign and Malignant: Points of View

The reader should be ready for a surprise. Whereas "everybody knows" that some tumors are benign and others are malignant, experts in tumor biology do not. They mostly ignore benign tumors and almost never talk about them. The experimental production of a tumor is called **carcinogenesis,** which means production of **cancer,** a malignant tumor. To our knowledge, there is not even a book about benign tumors. We consulted some experts, and the upshot was that when they speak of tumors in general they are referring to malignant tumors. So-called benign tumors do not have a clear-cut place in the current theory of carcinogenesis. They are not well explained (p. 927).

However, we must advise worried readers that benign tumors are a clinical if not a biological reality. From the clinical point of view, there is no question that some tumors behave predictably as benign; fibroadenomas of the breast and most lipomas fall into this category. After they have been removed, the patients can forget about them (exceptions are extremely rare).

Regarding the text that follows, we want our position to be clear. *When discussing human tumors,* we will use the traditional distinction between benign tumors (slowly growing, noninfiltrating, not fatal) and malignant tumors (more rapidly growing, infiltrating, metastasizing, and—if untreated—fatal). When discussing experimental carcinogenesis, we will follow the party line of the experts: tumors are malignant or on the way to malignancy. In the end, we will attempt to reconcile these views.

Names and Classification of Tumors

The science of tumors is **oncology** (from the Greek *ónkos,* a mass). As oncologists know well, talking about tumor causes great anxiety because the world at large still believes that tumors are mysterious and incurable killers. Therefore, the technical terms *neoplasm* or *neoplasia* (new growth) are sometimes used professionally in the hope that bystanders will not understand. In antiquity, of course, the term *tumor* was much less frightening because it meant a swelling of any kind, including the pregnant abdomen; remember that *tumor* is one of the four cardinal signs of inflammation. Indeed, this is the time to point out that a *swelling or lump may correspond to a variety of disturbances other than a tumor,* such as:

- a bacterial infection (e.g., abscess, tuberculosis)
- an inflammatory response to other pathogens (e.g., parasites, fungi, viruses)
- a rheumatic nodule
- an enlarged lymph node
- a hematoma
- an aneurysm
- a hernia
- a bone callus
- a malformation

Cancer is synonymous with malignant tumor; the Latin *cancer* is actually a literal translation of the Greek *karkínos* for crab, a common creature on Mediterranean shores. In the Hippocratic books, *karkínos* and *karkínoma* are used for conditions that

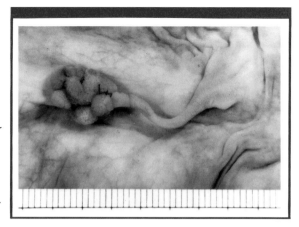

FIGURE 25.3 Typical polyp of the colon found incidentally at autopsy. Note the long peduncle, which favors twisting and thereby bleeding. Scale in mm.

In the second century A.D., Galen explained that "cancer of the breast is so called because of the fancied resemblance to a crab given by the lateral prolongations of the tumor and the adjacent distended veins" (18). Radiating dilated veins often do appear over and around a bulging tumor. In the sixteenth century, Gabriele Falloppio (of Fallopian tube fame) reviewed the ancient origins of the name, gave all the explanations that we have listed, and added one more: cancers are "extremely hard, rough tumors, resembling a crab in this respect as well" (18). Today the claws of the Greek crab describe just as effectively what we see of breast cancer through the microscope or on mammograms: ominous offshoots with which a cancerous mass seems to "grab" the surrounding tissues.

we would almost certainly call *carcinoma* (epithelial cancer) or, more generally, *cancer.* There seem to have been many reasons for borrowing the image of the crab, and the choice was extraordinarily successful: the name of the innocent crustacean became a sinister metaphor, even for the destructive ills ("cancers") of society (22).

The nomenclature of tumors is as untidy as might be expected of a collection of names that began 2500 years ago. After it was accepted— around 1885 (18)—that each type of tumor represents one type of cell, an effort was made to name all tumors accordingly; but tradition could not be wholly displaced. What follows is the ABC of tumors; we cannot discuss them without calling them by their names.

Note first that the ending *-oma* usually denotes a tumor, just as *-itis* denotes inflammation. The inevitable exceptions include granuloma, atheroma, glaucoma, and neuroma (p. 26). Then consider that each of the four basic types of tissue— epithelial, connective, muscular, and nervous— has its own benign and malignant tumors.

TUMORS OF EPITHELIA

Tumors of epithelial origin represent about 80 percent of all tumors.

Benign Benign tumors of epithelium can arise from glands or surface linings. Those that arise *from glands*, whether exocrine or endocrine, are called **adenomas** (from *adén*, gland). Examples are pancreatic adenoma, salivary gland adenoma, and sweat gland adenoma (the last two also have more fanciful, Greek names: *sialoadenoma* and *hydroadenoma*). Adenomas riddled with cavities (cysts) are called *cystadenomas.*

Benign epithelial tumors arising *from surfaces* are more readily seen and have earned colorful descriptive names referring to their shapes. A club-shaped tumor arising (or dangling) from a surface by means of a stalk is called a **polyp** (Figures 25.3, 25.4); if the polyp lacks a stalk it is called a *sessile polyp,* which means "sitting" (as in the word *session*). In either case the neoplastic part is only the covering epithelium; the core is just connective tissue stroma. If a polyp also

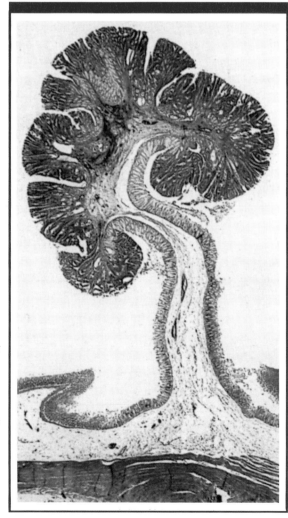

FIGURE 25.4 Cross section of a typical colorectal polyp (pedunculated adenoma). The polyp is normally lying on the mucosa; its head tends to be dragged along by the stools, hence it is stretched and may easily bleed. (Reproduced with permission from [8].)

contains some glandular growth, we speak of an *adenomatous polyp*.

Polyps appear as soft, fleshy masses growing out of the skin or a mucosa. Their appearance explains the name, which takes us back to the sunny shores of Greece: it means octopus (*poly*-pus, many feet, is an imprecise version of *octo*-pus, eight feet). Figure 25.5 shows an ancient Greek representation of an octopus; its body even recalls the peduncle of a typical polyp.

A **papilloma** is also an outgrowth from an epithelial surface, but it has long, thin branches (papillae) (Figures 25.6, 25.7, 25.8). There is a good reason for distinguishing polyps from papillomas. Simple geometry tells us that a papilloma has more epithelial surface and therefore more tumor mass than a polyp of comparable size. This means that papillomas tend to grow more actively than polyps; indeed, malignant tumors arise from papillomas more often than from polyps.

Note: If the papillae are packed tightly together, a papilloma may look like a polyp (Figure 25.9). A fitting comparison is that of a cauliflower; only a lengthwise cut reveals its branching structure.

You may wonder why the epithelium of a papilloma should grow outward and create branches, rather than grow downward and create blind canals. The latter does happen, and the result is called an *inverted papilloma*, a rare occurrence. Such papillomas can be found in the nose and in the bladder.

Malignant Malignant epithelial tumors are called **carcinomas;** those that arise from glands are **adenocarcinomas.** The basic names carcinoma and adenocarcinoma are often qualified by descriptive terms that indicate the cell of origin (basal cell carcinoma, squamous cell carcinoma), the structure (papillary carcinoma, cystadenocarcinoma, cystic papillary adenocarcinoma), or the function (mucus-secreting adenocarcinoma).

TUMORS OF CONNECTIVE TISSUES

Tumors of connective tissues have acquired a more orderly set of names. For benign tumors, the basic rule is to add *-oma* to the proliferating cell type:

fibroblasts	fibroma
fat cells	lipoma
blood vessels	hemangioma
lymphatic vessels	lymphangioma
bone	osteoma
cartilage	chondroma
embryonal fibroblasts	myxoma
bone marrow	myeloma

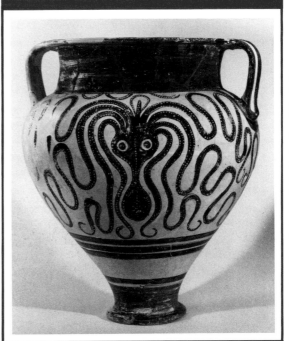

FIGURE 25.5
Polyp comes from the Greek word for octopus. This is how the Greeks saw an octopus; the oblong, pear-shaped body is actually very similar to what we now call a pedunculated polyp. From a Mycaenean vase, about 1350 BC. (Courtesy of the Trustees, British Museum, London, England.)

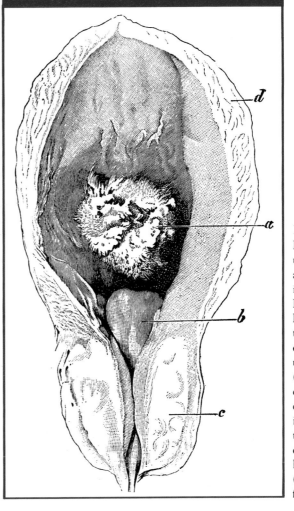

FIGURE 25.6
Papilloma of the urinary bladder as illustrated in 1908. **a:** Papilloma. **b, c:** Enlarged prostate. **d:** Thickened wall of the urinary bladder (the smooth muscle layer develops hypertrophy in response to the resistance caused by the enlarged prostate). (Reproduced from [23].)

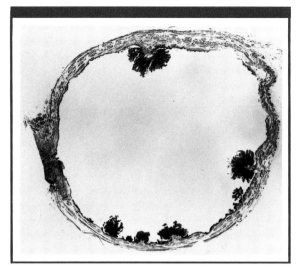

FIGURE 25.7
Section through an entire human bladder showing multiple papillary carcinomas of the "recurrent" type (recurrence does not necessarily occur at the same site as the primary tumor). (Courtesy of Dr. R.O.K. Schade, Dr. L.G. Koss and of the Armed Forces Institute of Pathology. (Reproduced with permission from [14].)

Myelomas are malignant; this is the inevitable exception to the rule. In Figure 25.10, a myeloma of the tibia appears on cross section as a soft lump—soft but capable of eroding its bony casing.

A *hemangioma* of the liver (Figure 25.11) appears as a dark-red mass embedded in the liver; the single thin-walled vessels are obvious on the cut surface. *Myxomas* are so called because they produce a "myxoid," i.e., "mucuslike" ground substance.

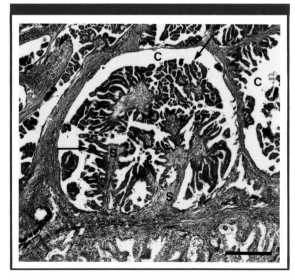

FIGURE 25.8
Papillary cyst-adenocarcinoma of the ovary.
C: Cystic space.
S: Vascular stalk from which many papillae arise (**arrows**).
Bar = 250 μm.

Malignant tumors of connective tissues are called **sarcomas**: hence fibrosarcoma, liposarcoma, chondrosarcoma, and so on. The tumors of lymphoid organs have special names such as *leukemias* (which deserve a special name as the only "liquid" tumors); *lymphomas*, so named even though they are malignant (they used to be called lymphosarcomas); *Hodgkin's disease*; and so on (see Table 25.1).

TUMORS OF MUSCLE TISSUES

Muscle tumors are camouflaged by Greek names. A *leiomyoma* is a benign tumor of smooth muscle (*léios*, smooth; *mys*, muscle); the very common *leiomyomas* of the uterus appear in cross section as pale, firm, spherical masses embedded in the uterine wall (Figure 25.12). A benign tumor of striated muscle is called a *Rhabdomyoma* on the grounds that the striations are equated microscopically to little bars or rods; *rhàbdos* means rod or wand (as in rhabdomancy). The malignant counterparts are *leiomyosarcoma* and *rhabdomyosarcoma*.

TUMORS OF NERVOUS TISSUES

Tumors of nervous tissue are easily understood from Table 25.1. You will be shocked to discover that there exists a *ganglioneuroma*, a tumor of neurons (which are supposed to be nondividing cells). Actually, this tumor occurs mainly in children or young adults; we will return to it later because it has a fascinating natural history (p. 898). Note that a malignant glial tumor is not called a gliosarcoma but a *glioblastoma*; the ending *-blastoma* usually refers to a poorly differentiated cell of embryonic type (which is correspondingly more malignant).

TUMORS OF MIXED CELL TYPES

Tumors of more than one cell type (mixed tumors) are not uncommon; we must assume that they derive from immature cells that can still differentiate in several directions. Some classic examples:

- The benign, mosaic-like tumors of connective tissue, which can appear as fibrolipomas, angiofibrolipomas, and so on.
- The puzzling mixed tumors or *pleomorphic adenomas* of the salivary glands, which contain mixtures of epithelium, connective tissue, and cartilage (pleomorphic is just another way of saying polymorphic).
- The common *fibroadenoma of the breast;* here the proliferating glands are surrounded

TABLE 25.1.

Nomenclature of Tumors

CELL/TISSUE OF ORIGIN	BENIGN TUMOR	MALIGNANT TUMOR
Tumors of Epithelia		
Covering epithelia	**Polyp, papilloma**	**Carcinoma, papillary carcinoma**
Squamous stratified	Squamous cell papilloma	Squamous cell carcinoma
Basal cells	Seborrheic keratosis(*)	Basal cell carcinoma
Mesothelial cells	Fibrous mesothelioma (*rare*)	Mesothelioma
Urinary (transitional epithelium)	Transitional cell papilloma	Transitional cell carcinoma
Glandular epithelia	**Adenoma**	**Adenocarcinoma**
	Cystadenoma	**Cystadenocarcinoma**
	Papillary adenoma	**Papillary adenocarcinoma**
Liver cells	Liver cell adenoma	Hepatoma
Renal tubules	Renal cell adenoma	Renal cell carcinoma (formerly hypernephroma)
Testicular tubules	■■■■■	Seminoma
		Embryonal carcinoma
Placental epithelium	Hydatidiform mole	Choriocarcinoma
Tumors of Connective Tissues		
Fibroblasts	Fibroma	Fibrosarcoma
Immature (fetal) fibroblasts	Myxoma	Myxosarcoma
Fat cells (lipoblasts)	Lipoma	Liposarcoma
Chondrocytes	Chondroma	Chondrosarcoma
Osteoblasts	Osteoma	Osteosarcoma
Meningeal cells	Meningioma	Malignant meningioma
Synovial cells	■■■■■	Synoviosarcoma
Endothelium: blood vessels	Hemangioma	Hemangiosarcoma
Endothelium: lymphatics	Lymphangioma	Lymphangiosarcoma
Erythroblasts	■■■■■	Erythroleukemia
Myeloblasts		Myeloblastic leukemia
Monoblasts		Monocytic leukemia
Lymphocytes		Lymphomas, myeloma, lymphocytic leukemia
Tumors of Muscular Tissues		
Striated muscle	Rhabdomyoma (*rare*)	Rhabdomyosarcoma
Smooth muscle	Leiomyoma	Leiomyosarcoma
Tumors of Neural Origin		
Astrocytes	Astrocytoma	Glioblastoma
Oligodendrocytes	Oligodendroglioma	Malignant oligodendroglioma
Ependymal cells	Ependymoma	Malignant ependymoma
Schwann cells	Schwannoma	Malignant schwannoma
Neuroblasts	Ganglioneuroma (**)	Neuroblastoma
Melanocytes	Nevus	Melanoma
Mixed Tumors (2 or more cell types but from one germ layer)		
Salivary glands	Pleomorphic adenoma ■■	Malignant mixed tumor of salivary gland
Renal blastema		Wilms' tumor (nephroblastoma)
Teratomas (several cell types representing all 3 embryonal germ layers)		
Totipotential cells	Mature teratoma, dermoid cyst	Teratocarcinoma

A display of the somewhat erratic tumor terminology. The red blocks emphasize the peculiar fact that some malignant tumors have no benign counterpart; other benign counterparts are indicated as rare.

(*) Strange names are common in dermatology. This one applies to a very common warty growth that has actually nothing to do with seborrhea.

(**) Ganglioneuroma as a benign tumor is unusual: instead of being a precursor of the corresponding malignant tumor (as many benign tumors are), it arises by differentiation of the malignant form.

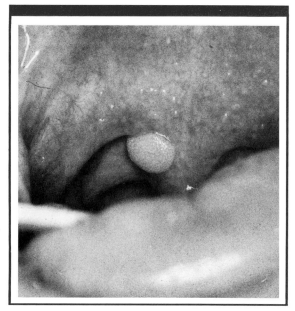

FIGURE 25.9
Papilloma of the soft palate in a 59-year-old man. The papillae appear as tiny white dots; they are too tightly packed to be seen as separate branches. (Courtesy of Dr. G. Fiore-Donno, School of Dentistry, Geneva, Switzerland.)

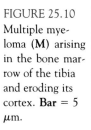

FIGURE 25.10
Multiple myeloma (**M**) arising in the bone marrow of the tibia and eroding its cortex. **Bar** = 5 μm.

by a mantle of special connective tissue that many believe to be a layer of benign mesenchymal tumor surrounding the sheets of benign epithelial tumor (Figure 25.13). There is no doubt that something similar occurs in another and more worrisome breast tumor called *cystosarcoma phyllodes*, which means leaflike; sheets of neoplastic (benign) epithelium intersect a sarcomatous mass, so that the tumor (when cut open) displays a leaflike structure, as if it were made of compressed papillae. This is but one of the infinite and bizarre patterns that tumors create.

Teratomas are the most startling of all the mixed tumors. It was Virchow who coined this name, which means "monster-oma." Imagine cutting through a mass in the ovary of a young woman and finding a mass of hair and sebum, a couple of teeth, some bone, bits of brain, or even a fully functional thyroid (Figure 25.14). This amazing assortment is explained by assuming that teratomas derive from a cell type so primitive that it produces daughter cells representing all three of the embryonal leaflets (ectoderm, mesoderm, endoderm). Such tumors may be benign or malignant; the malignant growth arises from a single cell type. These tumors are probably related to developmental errors. Consider, for instance, the peculiar fact that they tend to arise along the midline: at the base of the skull, in the anterior mediastinum (space in the middle of the chest), along the aorta, and in the gonads.

FIGURE 25.11
Hemangioma of the liver, discovered accidentally at autopsy. This is a typically benign tumor, despite the obvious lack of encapsulation. The original color was of course bright red. Scale in mm.

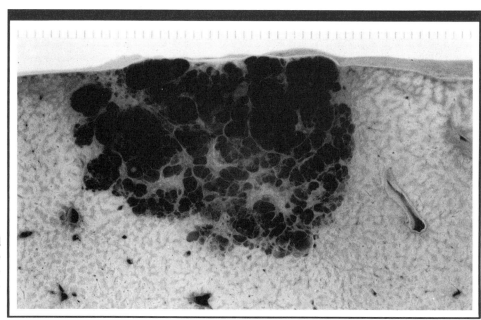

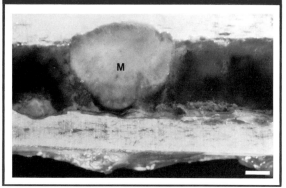

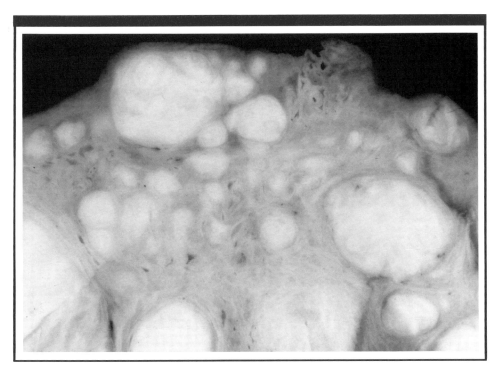

FIGURE 25.12
Cross section of the muscular wall of a uterus containing multiple leiomyomas (this condition is known as *leiomyomatosis* of the uterus). Magnification approximately 2×.

TUMOR-LIKE LUMPS

A **hamartoma** is not really a tumor, although it may appear so to the naked eye; it is a lump of tissues that belong to the organ in which the lump is found but have been "wrongly assembled" in the course of development. We still recall the sudden anxiety of a 22-year-old student, a heavy smoker, when a routine chest X-ray showed a round 3-cm mass in the left lung. Surgery produced a firm, sharply limited mass, of cartilage, smooth muscle, and epithelium, which you will recognize as typical components of bronchi (Figure 25.15). Hamartomas are present at birth and grow with the individual. Their name derives from *hamartia*,

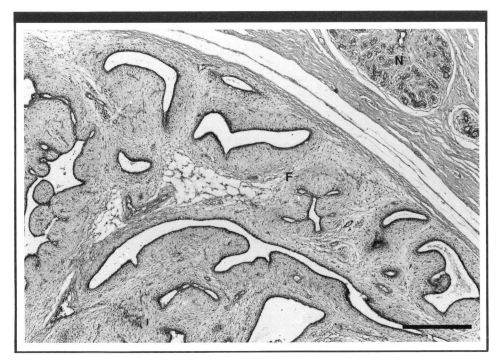

FIGURE 25.13
Fibroadenoma of the breast (**F**). Its pattern bears only a vague resemblance to the glandular pattern of the normal breast (**N**). An extremely thin fibrous layer is present between the tumor and the normal tissue. **Bar** = 500 μm.

FIGURE 25.14
Typical thyroid
follicles in a
teratoma of the
ovary (*struma
ovarii*). Such in-
clusions of thy-
roid tissue can be
functional and
can even pro-
duce hyperthy-
roidism. **Bar** =
100 μm.

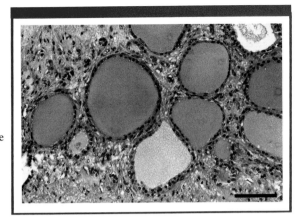

is being replaced by the more understandable
expression *ectopic tissue*.

At this point it will help to review Table 25.1
and related comments. Note two oddities: there is
a *nearly total lack of benign tumors of lymphoid tissue.*
As to *fibromas*, they are listed, but these cells,
which are so ready to multiply in healing tissues,
rarely produce benign tumors.

scribal error or mistake, as if the body, while
assembling the lung, ended up with a lump of
leftovers and buried them. Another type of
hamartoma worries surgeons who, while operating
on the abdomen, discover a sprinkling of small,
round, whitish, slightly raised spots on the liver,
which suggest metastases from an unknown cancer. A biopsy will show the reassuring image of
hamartoma made of peaceful-looking bile ducts.

Choristomas are little lumps of normal tissue
that do not belong in the organ where the lump is
found. For example, a small mass of pancreatic
tissue may be found in the duodenal mucosa (often
called a pancreatic inclusion); or tiny accessory
spleens may be found in the abdominal cavity. The
term *choristoma* seems to be going out of fashion; it

Tumors Have Personalities

Being able to name a tumor is important, but it is
not enough for predicting the tumor's biology and
behavior (in other words, "adenoma" or "carcinoma" are not as fully descriptive as "daisy" or
"sparrow"). Tumors of one morphologic type—
such as papillomas or adenocarcinomas—behave
differently in different organs, which surely reflects
differences in the tissue of origin. For example:

- An angioma of the liver is a quiet neoplasm
  that almost never disturbs its bearer. It is
  usually discovered at autopsy. By contrast, an
  angioma of the skin in the newborn may
  develop into an awful-looking mass (p. 898)
  and then regress and disappear. Other angiomas persist and are very difficult to treat.
- A papilloma should be benign (indeed, a
  papilloma of the skin is utterly benign). But
  a papilloma of the larynx is a worrisome tu-

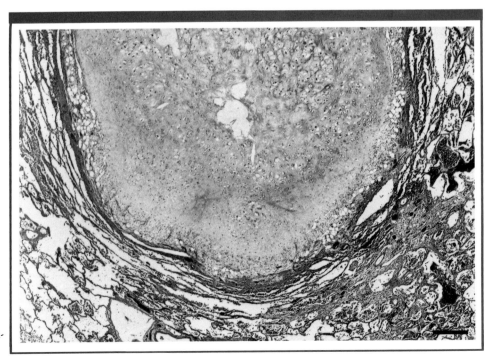

FIGURE 25.15
Typical hamartoma of the lung: a
sharply defined mass of hyalin cartilage. The surrounding lung is somewhat compressed, but there is no invasion. **Bar** = 500 μm.

mor that tends to recur; it may kill by suffocation even if benign, but it may also heal by itself. A papillomatous tumor of the urinary bladder is often malignant.

- An adenocarcinoma is a malignant tumor of a gland. However, if it arises from the prostate, the patient may live for years; if it concerns the pancreas, most patients die within 3 months of the diagnosis.

Even the part of the organ in which a tumor arises can make a difference in a tumor's behavior, especially for tumors of the skin. A pigmented mole almost anywhere on the body is of no concern, except perhaps cosmetic reasons, whereas a pigmented mole on the palms of the hands or on the soles of the feet is prone to undergo malignant transformation and must be removed, preferably in childhood if it is observed.

Why the part of an organ should make a difference is probably explained by the fact that normal cells of the same type can differ according to their location. This is well proven for endothelial cells, mast cells (p. 329), fibroblasts (6, 9, 16), adipocytes (3, 5, 12, 21), and liver cells in the lobule.

To the medical student, this means that it will be necessary to learn the personality of the most common human tumors, as determined statistically, while keeping in mind that the aggressiveness of a tumor in any particular case may vary unpredictably. A mesothelioma of the pleura may kill one patient within a year and allow another patient to survive 5 years. These differences are not yet explainable, but they are compatible with current knowledge of tumors: *the original molecular defect need not be identical,* and the body's responses are also variable. Even the attitude of the patient is a factor (20). All of this amounts to saying that at the molecular as well as the clinical level, *each tumor must be thought of as a potentially different disease.*

For this reason, predicting the life span of a patient is unwise to say the least, and robbing a patient of hope is inexcusable.

References

1. Angel A, Hollenberg CH, and Roncari DAK eds. The adipocyte and obesity: cellular and molecular mechanisms. New York: Raven Press, 1983.
2. Bigger CH, Hildemann WH. Cellular defense systems of the coelenterata. In Cohen N, and Sigel MM eds. The Reticuloendothelial System. A Comprehensive Treatise, vol. 3, Phylogeny and Ontogeny. New York: Plenum Press, 1982; 59–87.
3. Björntorp P. Development of adipose tissue *in vivo* and *in vitro*. In Angel A, Hollenberg CH, and Roncari DAK eds. The Adipocyte and Obesity: Cellular and Molecular Mechanisms. New York: Raven Press, 1983; 33–39.
4. Burck KB, Liu ET, Larrick JW. Oncogenes. An Introduction to the Concept of Cancer Genes. New York: Springer-Verlag, 1988.
5. Cahill GF Jr, Renold AE. Adipose tissue: a brief history. In Angel A, Hollenberg CH, Roncari DAK eds., The adipocyte and obesity: cellular and molecular mechanisms. New York: Raven Press, 1983; 1–7.
6. Conrad GW, Hart GW, Chen Y. Differences *in vitro* between fibroblast-like cells from cornea, heart, and skin of embryonic chicks. J Cell Sci 26:119–137, 1977.
7. El-Mofty MM, Abdelmeguid N, Michael AE, El-Marhouni KM. A quick test for screening the carcinogenity of certain chemicals, using various protozoan parasites. Folia Morphol 36:350–356, 1988.
8. Fenoglio-Preiser CM, Hutter RVP. Colorectal polyps: pathologic diagnosis and clinical significance. CA 35:322–344, 1985.
9. Gabbiani G, Hirschel BJ, Ryan GB, Statkov PR, Majno G. Granulation tissue as a contractile organ. A study of structure and function. J Exp Med 135:719–734, 1972.
10. Gateff E. Malignant neoplasms of genetic origin in *Drosophila melanogaster*. Science 200:1448–1459, 1978a.
11. Gateff E. The genetics and epigenetics of neoplasms in *Drosophila*. Biol Rev 58:123–168, 1978b.
12. Hollenberg CH, Roncari DAK, Djian P. Obesity and the fat cell: future prospects. In Angel A, Hollenberg CH, and Roncari DAK eds. The adipocyte and obesity: cellular and molecular mechanisms. New York: Raven Press, 1983; 291–300.
13. Kaiser HE. Animal neoplasms—a systematic review. In Kaiser HE ed. Neoplasms—comparative pathology of growth in animals, plants, and man. Baltimore: Williams & Wilkins, 1981; 747–812.
14. Koss LG. Atlas of tumor pathology, 2nd ser, fasc 11. Tumors of the urinary bladder. Washington, DC: Armed Forces Institute of Pathology, 1975.
15. Mottram JC. The problem of tumours. London: HK Lewis & Co Ltd, 1942.
16. Phipps RP. Pulmonary fibroblast heterogeneity. Boca Raton: CRC Press Inc, 1992.
17. Pitot HC. Fundamentals of oncology, 3rd ed. New York: Marcel Dekker Inc, 1986.
18. Rather LJ. The genesis of cancer. Baltimore: The Johns Hopkins University Press, 1978.
19. Scharrer B, Lockhead MS. Tumors in the invertebrates: a review. Cancer Res 10:403–419, 1950.
20. Siegel BS. Love, medicine and miracles. New York: Harper & Row, 1986.
21. Smith U. Regional differences and effect of cell size on lipolysis in human adipocytes. In Angel A, Hollenberg CH, Roncari DAK eds. The adipocyte and obesity: cellular and molecular mechanisms. New York: Raven Press, 1983; 245–250.
22. Sontag S. Illness as metaphor and AIDS and its metaphors. New York: Doubleday, 1990.
23. Ziegler E. General pathology. New York: William Wood and Company, 1908.

Anatomy and Biology of Tumors

CHAPTER 26

> The Tumor Cell
>
> The Structure of Tumors
>
> Birth and Growth of a Tumor
>
> Life Inside a Tumor

The Tumor Cell

Tumors were once thought to consist of nondescript "deposits." The news that they were made of cells was rushed into print by Johannes Müller (Virchow's teacher) in 1838, the very same year that saw the birth of cell theory (Figure 26.1). That was no coincidence: Theodor Schwann, father of cell theory, was working in Müller's laboratory (170,171). The next most urgent question, then, became: What is the difference between a normal cell and a tumor cell? The better part of two centuries has gone by, but nobody has rushed into print with an answer valid for all tumors; the few who have tried were proven wrong. We know that tumor cells suffer from trouble in their DNA—and we will discuss this later (p. 921)—but beyond this fact we cannot mention a single structural, functional, or biochemical characteristic that is common to all tumor cells. There may be none.

We do have a long catalog of differences between normal and neoplastic cells, each difference being applicable to a certain number of malignant tumors. Notice that we said *malignant* tumors. Very little is known about the cells of benign tumors; one reason is that carcinogenesis *in vitro* appears to occur without a recognizable intermediate benign stage. The leap from normal to malignant as observed in cultured cells is often called **transformation.** We must briefly discuss this useful but fuzzy expression.

THE MEANING OF "TRANSFORMATION"

To the average person, *transformation* is a very vague term, hence it is rather exasperating to see it used in tumor language to mean a concept as definitive as *switch to malignancy of cultured cells.* However, a vague term is appropriate because the change itself—in a population of growing cells— is difficult to pinpoint (66,87).

It was a long step forward to discover that transformed cells (malignant cells) can be produced *in vitro*. In the 1940s, W.R. Earle and collaborators treated fibroblast cultures with methylcholanthrene and found that some cells took on a malignant phenotype; when implanted into mice these cells formed sarcomas that killed the host (61,62). This pioneer work was forgotten for 20 years (175), partly because it seemed to have a flaw: fibroblasts from untreated cultures also produced sarcomas in 8 percent of the animals. Today this would not surprise anybody: it is a mysterious but accepted fact that a malignant phenotype may occasionally spring up spontaneously in cultures of cell lines. Experimental transformation *in vitro* by X-rays has become commonplace (p. 826); human cells, however, are very reluctant to transform. This is good news for all of us, but the reason is unknown.

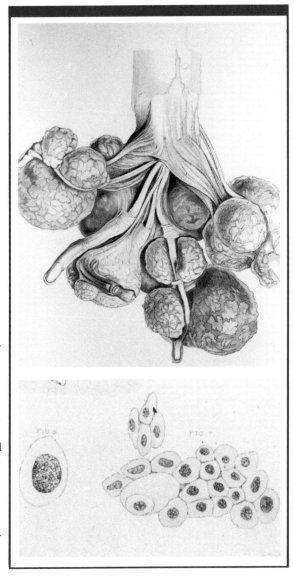

FIGURE 26.1
The first illustration of tumor cells. In 1840, Johannes Müller took samples from a museum specimen (*top*) showing multiple cartilaginous tumors of the hand (enchondromas). *Bottom:* The microscope showed that the tumors consisted of cells with irregular nuclei. (Adapted from [154].)

their normal counterparts" (66). So much for theory. However, in practice, there is a classic study on recognizing transformed cells by Barbara Barker and Katherine Sanford (10), who watched a variety of cell lines as they grew in culture and identified a sequence of five cytologic features that announce transformation: when injected *in vivo*, the cultures that had tested positive under the microscope (on the scale from 1 to 5) gave rise to sarcomas, in increasing numbers. The progressive changes were:

1. increased cytoplasmic basophilia
2. increased number and size of nucleoli
3. increased nuclear-cytoplasmic ratio
4. retraction of the cytoplasm
5. formation of clusters and cords of cells.

The concept of transformation is imprecise enough, but beware of another source of confusion: *the so-called transforming growth factors (TGFs) do not transform*, at least not in the sense of causing malignancy. These polypeptides, originally discovered as products of tumors, are able to induce some types of normal cells to grow dispersed in agar, as anchorage-independent cells (most normal cells prefer to grow safely anchored to a surface) (Figure 26.2) (133). We now know that TGFs are produced also by normal tissues, that other growth factors such as PDGF can induce anchorage-independent growth, and that the change is always reversible. Thus platelets, for example, contain large amounts

When cultured fibroblasts are irradiated, transformation is announced here and there by foci of cells that overgrow and pile up, as normal cells never do (p. 834). This is most interesting, but it does not tell us what has happened to the transformed cells. Should we decide that the turning point is immortalization? Not really: it is now clear that immortal cell lines sometimes appear in cell cultures, and they are not malignant. They may even revert to being mortal. On the other hand, it is generally agreed that immortalization is a step toward malignancy.

Hear the words of an expert, M.R. Escobar: "In theory, transformation is defined as a stable, heritable alteration in the growth control of cells in culture. In practice . . . no set of characteristics invariably distinguishes transformed cells from

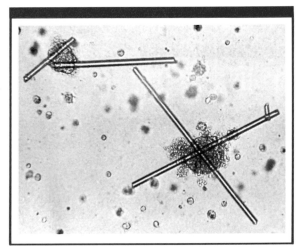

FIGURE 26.2
The phenomenon of anchorage-dependent growth of normal cells. Cells of a hamster cell line, freely suspended in agar, fail to grow (note lack of free clusters); but those cells that take a foothold on microscopic glass fibrils succeed in forming colonies. (Reproduced with permission from [194].)

of TGF-beta—which does not mean, of course, that platelets are carcinogenic; TGF-beta induces fibrogenesis, and this may play a role in wound healing (122).

In practice, when cells have to be tested experimentally for malignancy, many criteria have to be met (165), but two are essential: immortality, which is an absolute requirement (although not all immortal cell lines are transformed) and the ability to form tumors when the cells are transplanted into a suitable host.

THE MALIGNANT PHENOTYPE

The following is a composite portrait of the malignant cell. The details vary from one cancer to another and in the same cancer they may change with time: as a pessimist might guess, the change is usually from bad to worse, although a rare malignant tumor, as we will see, may turn benign. Malignant features can be found in all aspects of cell biology: structure, behavior, function, and biochemistry.

STRUCTURAL DIFFERENCES

To visualize a cancer cell, begin with the corresponding normal cell and make it
- less differentiated,
- with some features of a rapidly growing cell, and
- with some additional bizarre features (*atypia*)

Lack of Differentiation Lack of differentiation means that the special features of the normal cell are imperfectly expressed: a ciliated cell will have fewer cilia, a secretory cell less secretion, and so on. This fact has given rise to the common and synonymous terms *anaplasia* and *dedifferentiation*, both implying that the cancer cell has somehow regressed to a lesser state of differentiation. However, it seems very unlikely that tumors consist of mature cells that regress. The current concept of carcinogenesis is that tumors contain undifferentiated stem cells whose progeny fail to mature. In other words, the tumor cell is born in a state of low differentiation and does not become immature by dedifferentiating itself.

This concept needs to be qualified. (a) Some kind of "backward differentiation" does indeed occur in many malignant tumors as they change from bad to worse, a phenomenon known (backwardly) as tumor progression (p. 762). (b) In some malignant tumors, such as squamous cell carcinoma of the epidermis, full differentiation does occur here and there; in fact, this observation gave rise to the theory that cancer may be a disease of differentiation (p. 924).

Fast Growth Features of fast-growing cells are easy to grasp:
- *Cytoplasmic basophilia is increased*, which means more RNA and thus more active protein synthesis (Figure 26.3). Needless to say, slow-growing malignant tumors do not follow this rule. The electron microscope shows many free ribosomes, which correspond to the fact that the cell is busy making "more of itself" rather than producing proteins for export.
- *Nucleoli increase in size and number* (remember that RNA is synthesized within them).

A recent nucleolar development: the interphase nucleolus contains Ag-NOR proteins (stainable with silver), which correspond to ribosomal genes (NOR stands for nucleolar organizer proteins). They appear as black granules, and their quantity parallels the cell duplication rate; they can be quantitated to estimate the tumor proliferation rate (51,52) (Figure 26.4).

- *Mitoses are increased, and the mitotic figures may be normal*. Tri- and tetrapolar mitoses are not uncommon (Figure 26.5). Because the number of mitoses is roughly parallel to the rate of growth, and therefore to aggressiveness, pathologists' reports sometimes refer to the number of mitoses per high-power field as a measure of malignancy.
- *Glycogen content is high*, as it is in embryonic cells. This abundance of glycogen correlates with the anaerobic glycolysis typical of embryonic as well as of tumor cells (see later).

Bizarre Features The features of atypia are especially important because *atypia tends to parallel the degree of aggressiveness*. It can hit virtually every aspect of cellular structure. For example:
- *Size and shape of the cell are abnormal*. Typically, a malignant cell is more rounded and tends to be irregular. Today these changes begin to make sense: malignancy is linked to cytoskeletal disturbances, which lead to internal disarray as well as to mechanical effects on cell shape (p. 845). The same

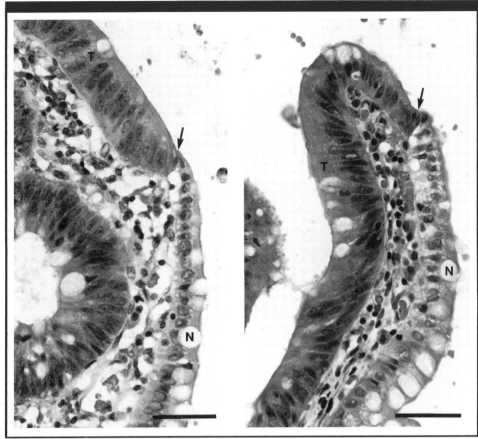

FIGURE 26.3
Two details of a benign polyp in a case of polyposis coli. **Arrows:** Junction between the tumor tissue (**T**) and normal epithelium (**N**). Note the differences between normal and neoplastic tissue, regarding size, shape, and basophilia of the cells, size and shape of the nuclei and function as shown by the secretion of mucus. **Bar** = 50 μm.

FIGURE 26.4
Histologic section of an adenocarcinoma of the colon (**AC**), stained with silver to demonstrate the nucleolar organizer region (NOR). **N:** Normal gland. Neoplastic cells contain more NORs than normal epithelial cells or cells within the stroma (**S**). The quantitative difference between normal and cancerous cells, however, is not always as clear-cut as in this example. **Bar** = 25 μm. (Courtesy of Dr. M. Derenzini, Department of Experimental Pathology, University of Bologna, Italy.)

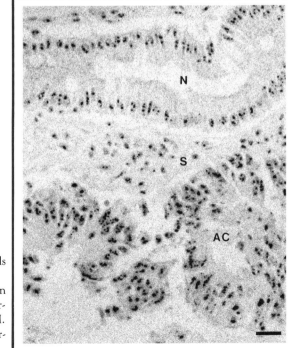

mechanism accounts for disturbed cell-to-stroma attachments (16).

- *The nucleus is too large for the cell.* In other words, there is an increase in the nuclear-cytoplasmic ratio. This too can be explained: many tumor nuclei are polyploid and therefore enlarged. They look even larger in cells that are more rounded and therefore smaller.

- *The cell surface often bristles with a large number of microvilli* (Figure 26.6) (54), perhaps another manifestation of cytoskeletal disturbances.

- *Cell-specific organelles are distorted or lost,* as best seen by electron microscopy. A good example are the sarcomeres of striated muscle: in rhabdomyosarcomas they are rudimentary (Figure 26.7) or disappear altogether.

> The case for "mitochondriomas." *We refer the reader to p. 132, where we discussed the bizarre intracellular tumors consisting of mitochondria that proliferate until they fill the cell. No other organelle shows this behavior, presumably because no other organelle shares the parasitic bacterial ancestry of mitochondria. And correspondingly, no other organelle besides the nucleus contains DNA.*

- *Secretion becomes irregular,* as best seen in mucus-secreting cells. Mucus may not be produced at all, or it may be retained as a large droplet that distends the cell (Figure 26.8); it may also be secreted indiscriminately into the tissue spaces, so the cells find themselves floating in their own product (Figure 26.9).

- *Sundry abnormalities may appear,* too many to list. For example, epithelial cells that normally surround a glandular lumen can develop an internal lumen (Figure 26.10) (185). Occasionally, a new type of organelle appears, which is unexplained but may be useful as a marker for a particular type of tumor; such is the *ribosome–lamella complex* of the so-called hairy-cell leukemia (Figure 26.11) (121). Another classic example is the Auer rod of acute myelogenous leukemia; it represents an abnormal neutrophil granule (Figure 26.12).

BEHAVIOR IN CULTURE

A number of behavioral changes characterize transformed cells.

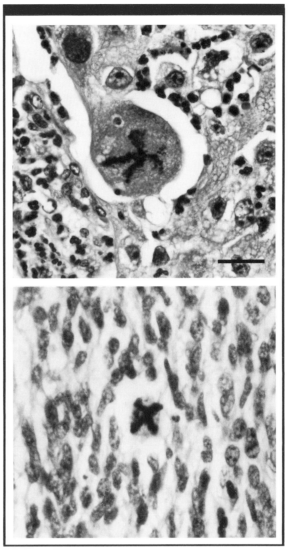

FIGURE 26.5
Tetrapolar mitoses. *Top:* In a squamous cell carcinoma of the cervix. **Bar** = 25 μm. *Bottom:* In a very malignant brain tumor (glioblastoma).

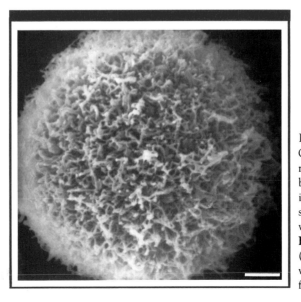

FIGURE 26.6
Cell from a carcinoma of the breast, suspended in a pleural effusion, covered with microvilli. **Bar** = 500 μm. (Reproduced with permission from [54].)

FIGURE 26.7
Bundles of fibrils representing sketchy sarcomeres in a cell from a rhabdomyosarcoma (in the nasal cavity of a 26-year-old woman). The family history of this patient was intriguing: a sister had died of an osteosarcoma at age 12; both parents had worked in a uranium reprocessing plant for 9 years. **Bar** = 0.2 μm. (Reproduced with permission from [107].)

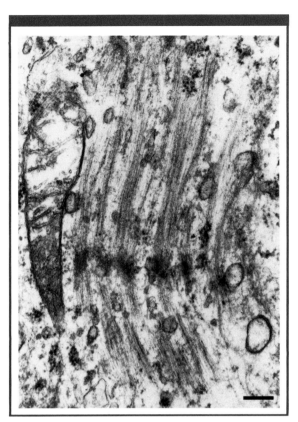

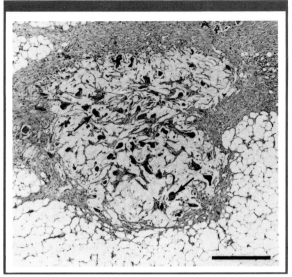

FIGURE 26.9
Mucus-secreting carcinoma of the breast: Clumps of deeply basophilic carcinomatous cells (**arrows**) are surrounded by pools of mucus that they have secreted. In other parts of this tumor mucus secretion was absent. **Bar** = 500 μm.

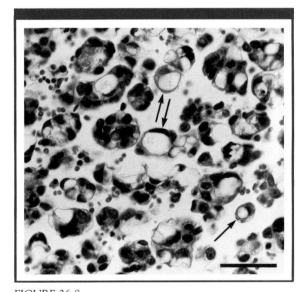
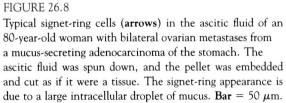

FIGURE 26.8
Typical signet-ring cells (**arrows**) in the ascitic fluid of an 80-year-old woman with bilateral ovarian metastases from a mucus-secreting adenocarcinoma of the stomach. The ascitic fluid was spun down, and the pellet was embedded and cut as if it were a tissue. The signet-ring appearance is due to a large intracellular droplet of mucus. **Bar** = 50 μm.

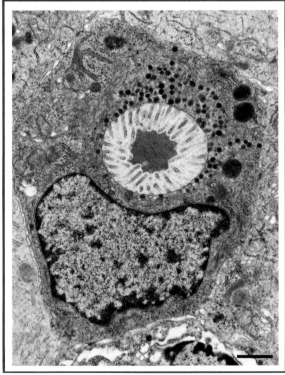

FIGURE 26.10
A bizarre form of cellular atypia: An intracellular lumen, complete with microvilli, in an epithelial cell of an invasive lobular carcinoma of the breast. **Bar** = 1 μm. (Reproduced with permission from [185].)

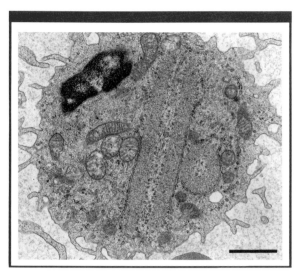

FIGURE 26.11

The "ribosome–lamella complex," one of the peculiar inclusions found in some malignant cells. This rod-shaped structure (shown in longitudinal and in transverse section) is typical, although not entirely characteristic, of hairy-cell leukemia. It can be seen also by light microscopy. **Bar** = 1 μm. (Reproduced with permission from [121].)

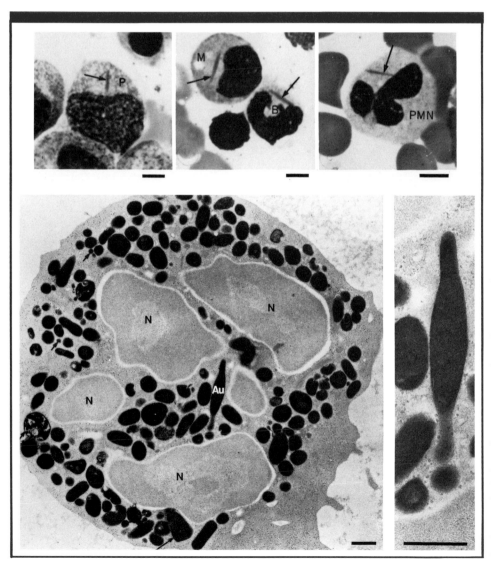

FIGURE 26.12

Abnormalities in the granules of neutrophils in acute myelogenous leukemia. *Top:* **Arrows** point to elongated azurophilic granules (Auer rods) in a promyelocyte (**P**), a myelocyte (**B**), a metamyelocyte (**M**), and a mature polymorphonuclear neutrophil (**PMN**). Wright stain; **bars** = 5 μm. *Bottom left:* Mature neutrophil reacted for peroxidase. The nucleus (**N**) is subdivided into five lobes. All granules are peroxidase-positive and thus azurophilic; some are abnormally small or defective (**arrows**); one is elongated (**Au:** Auer rod). Peroxidase-negative specific granules are missing. **Bar** = 0.5 μm. *Bottom right:* Detail of the Auer rod shown at left. **Bar** = 0.5 μm. (Reproduced with permission from [8].)

Immortality Transformed cells can grow forever, in stark contrast with normal animal cells, which can replicate only within the limit of their particular Hayflick number (p. 30). A sadly famous lady named Henrietta Lacks died in 1951 of a cervical carcinoma; cells from her tumor, the ubiquitous HeLa cells (p. 805), are still growing relentlessly in laboratories throughout the world. We will discuss how transformed cells escape from growth control in relation to oncogenes (p. 843). Note that this immortality does not compare with the immortality of bacteria: in real life, every strain of "immortal" malignant cells dies when it kills its host unless it is cultured like the HeLa cells. *Every case of cancer is therefore a "new" disease.*

Loss of Anchorage Dependence As mentioned earlier, normal cells prefer to grow on a surface; they become attached to it, spread out, and begin to replicate (see Figure 26.2) (194). In contrast, transformed cells can also do well in a fluid medium such as soft agar, in which they maintain a more rounded shape. Cytoskeletal changes are probably involved (175).

Loss of Contact Inhibition Transformed cells grow to cover all available space, then continue to grow and pile up over each other haphazardly (p. 834). Normal cells usually stop when they contact each other, at which point they constitute a confluent sheet with little or no cell overlap.

> *The term* contact inhibition *has been used in various ways; for some it has meant inhibition of movement and for others inhibition of growth, hence the current tendency to replace the phrase* loss of contact inhibition *with the cumbersome* decreased density-dependent inhibition of growth *(175).*

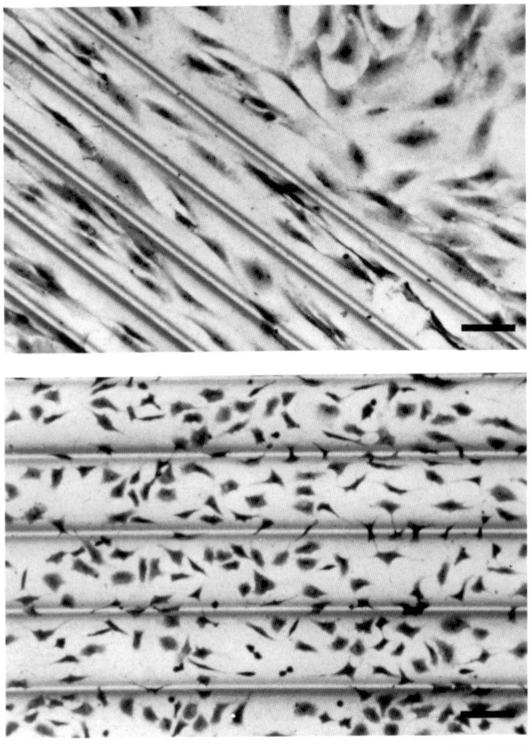

Loss of Orientation on an Oriented Substrate This lesser known feature is illustrated in Figure 26.13. In essence, malignant cells growing on a surface with a distinctive pattern have partially lost the ability to align themselves accordingly. This is, we presume, another consequence of a faulty cytoskeleton.

Decreased Requirement for Growth Factors Normal cells tend to be fussy about the medium in which they are nurtured; special mixtures of growth factors must be worked out for each type. Transformed cells are much easier to grow and require less serum (i.e., fewer growth factors). The reason is now apparent: malignant cells supply their own growth factors by a curious property known as autocrine secretion (p. 32).

BEHAVIOR UPON TRANSPLANTATION

For transplants to succeed they must be performed on animals that do not reject them. The choice lies between syngeneic, immunosuppressed, or congenitally immunodeficient animals. The latter include the SCID mice (p. 586) and the sorry-looking nude mice, which (besides having no hair) have no thymus and therefore lack the ability to reject a graft. The basic procedure is to inject a suspension of the tumor cells subcutaneously; one million is usually enough. If the cells are malignant, they form a palpable nodule usually within weeks. *Normal* adult cells injected in this manner either die or survive without significant growth; this is the general rule for all grafts of normal tissues, with one startling exception: one way to produce a very malignant teratoma in the mouse is to graft normal but embryonic tissue into the testis (p. 903).

FUNCTIONAL AND BIOCHEMICAL CHANGES

Motility and Chemotaxis Many types of cancer cells can move around rather like amoebae, although their normal counterparts may be station-

FIGURE 26.13
Top: Normal mouse fibroblasts that had been seeded 24 hours earlier on a surface, partly flat (*top right*) and partly etched (*lower left*). Where grooves were present, the fibroblasts oriented themselves accordingly. *Bottom:* Transformed fibroblasts show very little tendency to become oriented along the grooves. **Bars** = 50 μm. (Reproduced with permission from [210].)

ary. This characteristic helps us understand the mechanism of invasiveness; it was actually shown *in vitro* that the fastest moving cells are the most invasive (98). Moreover, some cancer cells secrete a factor that accelerates their motion and even directs it by chemotaxis (p. 797) (which sounds like a cellular version of "pulling oneself up by one's bootstraps").

Surface-Related Changes Such changes are many; they are summarized in Figure 26.14 and the following list. Of course, they vary from tumor to tumor.

- *Decreased adhesion between cells.* In a classic experiment, D.R. Coman of Philadelphia showed in 1944 that cells of a carcinoma are more easily pulled apart than their normal counterparts (Figure 26.15). The experiment was criticized as too simple, but since then it has been abundantly proven that malignant cells in general have fewer intercellular contacts and fewer attachments to the stroma (144,219) because actin-to-membrane attachments are one of the prime targets of transformation-related dis-

turbances (151). This reduced cohesion helps to understand the invasiveness of malignant cells (p. 795).

- *Altered intercellular communication.* No broad generalizations can be made, but some isolated facts are intriguing. For example, some carcinogens inhibit intercellular communication across gap junctions (129a), and there seems to be an inverse relationship between cell replication and cell-to-cell communication, in tumors as well as in regenerating liver (123). Accordingly, some transformed cells stop growing when they establish contact with normal cells (145); needless to say, if all tumor cells did this, there would be no tumors. Junctions between normal and neoplastic cells have long been observed by electron microscopy (208).

Of course, gap junctions (communicating junctions) also exist between the neoplastic cells of a given tumor. These channels allow the passage of molecules as large as 2 kilodaltons; growth-controlling signals might follow this route (145). This story is becoming more interesting since it turned out that the famed src oncogene regulates

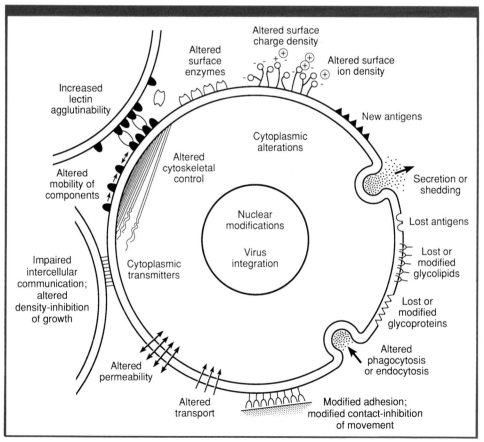

FIGURE 26.14
Some of the cell surface alterations found in tumor cells. (Adapted from [156].)

FIGURE 26.15
Coman's classic experiment demonstrating the loose connection between cancerous epithelial cells. *Left:* A pair of normal, living squamous epithelial cells from the lip; as they are drawn apart by microneedles they stretch because they cling to each other tenaciously. *Right:* A pair of living squamous epithelial cells from a carcinoma of the lip. As the needles just begin to move apart, the cells detach with little deformation. This experiment focused attention on the decreased adhesion between malignant cells. (Reproduced with permission from [43].)

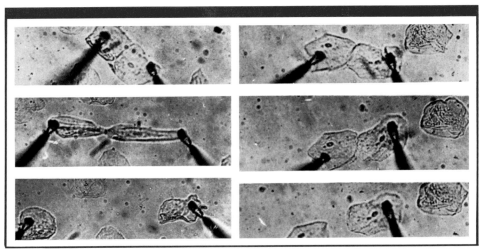

intercellular communication and growth (136). It has also been postulated that teratogens (chemicals producing malformations) disrupt intercellular communication (221). All in all, however, this field has not led to tumor-related breakthroughs (160).

- *Increased susceptibility to agglutination by lectins* (carbohydrate-binding proteins, p. 129) such as concanavalin A. In other words, lectins that recognize and agglutinate normal cells only after mild proteolytic digestion, agglutinate untreated malignant cells (15). This is merely a laboratory tool for detecting an abnormality of cancer cells; it tells us that specific carbohydrate sites on transformed cells are somehow more "exposed" than normal on the cell surface (15). Because surface carbohydrates are key factors in cell recognition, we can assume that a change in their arrangement affects the "social relations" of malignant cells.
- *Tendency to shed surface molecules,* including proteins, glycoproteins, and enzymes. This has many implications (25). Shedding enzymes such as collagenase can help the malignant cell work its way through the extracellular matrix (p. 797). Shedding tissue factor, fibronectin, or other macromolecules may lead to exaggerated clotting (57). Conversely, shedding plasminogen activator activates plasmin, a trypsin-like enzyme that digests fibrin and may perhaps extricate cells from fibrin clots; it is an old observation that malignant cells *in vitro* dissolve plasma clots whereas normal cells do not (Figure 26.16) (198). Plasminogen, incidentally, circulates with the blood and is always available in low concentration in the extracellular fluid.

Some of the shed molecules can be found in the blood and are therefore available as tumor markers, a useful device for diagnosing the presence of a particular type of tumor or for monitoring its response to therapy (p. 931). The shedding of tumor antigens may help the cell escape immune attack: the immune system is kept busy destroying these loose molecules while the tumor cells are left intact.

This type of shedding is a military strategy. During World War II, Allied airplanes shed clouds of metal leaflets, which looked like targets on radar and kept the flak busy, while the planes went on with their mission.

Biochemical Changes Such changes follow the general rule that there are no general rules—but a limited number of tumors show biochemical differences than can be exploited as a target for therapy. The classic example: some tumor cells require more exogenous asparagine than normal cells do. Treatment with L-asparaginase (obtained from bacteria) depletes the asparagine supply and starves the tumor cells. This works best for acute lymphocytic and myelocytic leukemias, but anaphylactic reaction to the enzyme limits its usefulness.

Another biochemical change that we find potentially important, and which seems to apply to many tumors, is that rhodamine 123, a fluorescent dye, localizes in the mitochondria of living cells; normal cells release it within a few hours whereas epithelial tumors retain it for 2–5

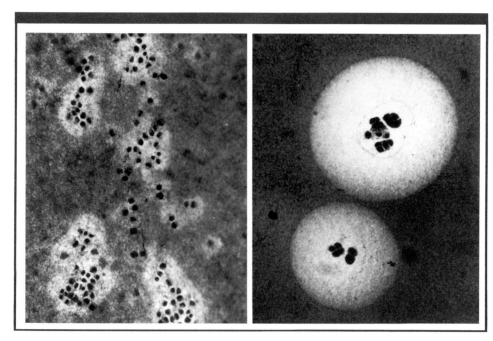

FIGURE 26.16
Demonstrating the secretion of tissue plasminogen activator (TPA) by tumor cells. Low and high power. The dark dots are rat ascites tumor cells seeded onto a fibrin film that contains plasminogen naturally adsorbed to the fibrin. The clear areas represent digested fibrin; they would not develop in the absence of plasminogen. (Courtesy of Dr. K. Tanaka, Kyushu University, Fukuoka, Japan.)

days (Figure 26.17) (21). Efforts are under way to exploit this phenomenon (38).

Other differences will be discussed in relation to oncogenes; a longer list can be found in specialized textbooks. Currently the bottom line is that *many of the biochemical and physiological differences described for malignant cells reflect accelerated growth or immaturity, not the neoplastic condition.* Tumor cells grow fast and tend to be immature: two properties that they share with embryonic, fetal, or fast-growing cells.

> *The classic proof of this point is the theory of Otto Warburg (215), a pioneer in the study of respiratory enzymes, which led him to the Nobel prize in 1931. In a monograph published in 1930 (214), Warburg pointed out that slices of* normal tissues *incubated in the presence of glucose produced lactic acid only if they were deprived of oxygen (anaerobic glycolysis), whereas slices of tumors produced lactic acid also if they were supplied with oxygen (aerobic glycolysis). He concluded that tumors suffered from an irreversible disturbance of their respiratory metabolism. The observations were perfectly correct, but the theory did not stand the test of time (110). It remains true that aerobic glycolysis is common in tumors, but it is merely one of many features that tumor cells share with immature cells (161,218). An extensive review of tumor mitochondria produced a long list of biochemical anomalies, but none was specific to tumors (161).*

TO SUM UP: the malignant phenotype of a cell is that of a different, but not radically different

or aberrant cell; electron microscopy in particular has failed to show any sensational differences apart from the occasional presence of viruses. Several structural and biochemical features of tumors are

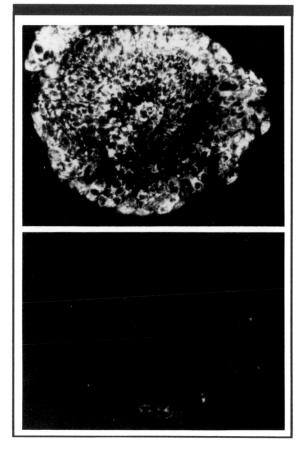

FIGURE 26.17
An abnormality of mitochondria in some tumors. *Top:* Fluorescence photomicrograph; culture of a human colon carcinoma stained with the fluorescent dye rhodamine 123 for 10 minutes and left in dye-free medium for 24 hours. Much dye is retained. *Bottom:* Lack of rhodamine 123 retention by a culture of normal human colonic epithelium, treated as above. (Reproduced with permission from [38].)

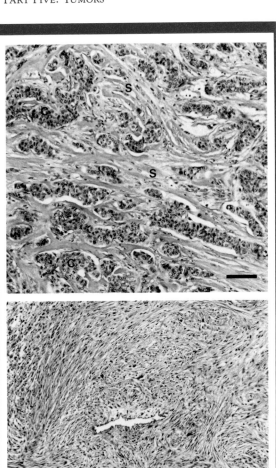

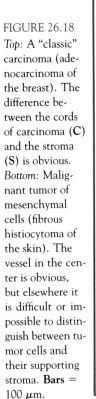

FIGURE 26.18
Top: A "classic" carcinoma (adenocarcinoma of the breast). The difference between the cords of carcinoma (**C**) and the stroma (**S**) is obvious. *Bottom:* Malignant tumor of mesenchymal cells (fibrous histiocytoma of the skin). The vessel in the center is obvious, but elsewhere it is difficult or impossible to distinguish between tumor cells and their supporting stroma. **Bars =** 100 μm.

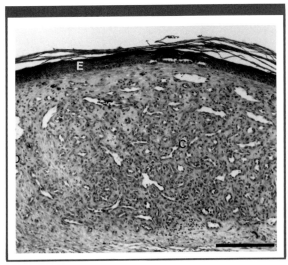

FIGURE 26.19
Capillary hemangioma of the skin, a benign tumor excised for cosmetic reasons. Essentially a tangle of capillaries (**C**) without a capsule. **E:** epidermis; **D:** dermis. **Bar =** 200 μm. (Slide courtesy of Dr. R. Malhotra, University of Massachusetts Medical School, Worcester, MA.)

those of immature embryonic-type cells. All this fits with the present notion that malignant cells, in some cases, can be artificially reprogrammed to resemble normal cells (p. 900).

The Structure of Tumors

To understand the gross and microscopic aspect of tumors, it is essential to realize that all tumors consist of two components: (a) a population of neoplastic cells that is supported and nourished by (b) connective tissue and vessels supplied by the host. In other words, every solid tumor contains a neoplastic **parenchyma** (the distinctive tissue of an organ) lying in a non-neoplastic **stroma** (the supporting framework of an organ). *Stroma* is a Greek word well suited to this use; it is related to *straw* and means *bed*: a bed for the parenchymal cells. This dual composition is best appreciated in microscopic sections; in epithelial tumors (such as adenomas and carcinomas) the parenchymal epithelial structures stand out quite clearly against the connective tissue stroma. It is not as easy to recognize the two components in sections of connective tissue tumors such as sarcomas; the contrast between tumor and stroma is minimal because both are mesenchymal (Figure 26.18).

> *With the naked eye the diagnosis of sarcoma versus carcinoma is not easy. Because sarcomas lack the contrast between epithelium and stroma, they appear smoother on cross sections; hence the traditional comparison of sarcomas with fish flesh (sarx is Greek for flesh).*

The concept that all tumors have a vascularized stroma that is supplied by the host means that, to a large extent, the body cooperates with the aggressor. Indeed, tumors have sophisticated means of enticing vessels to join the growth.

GROSS FEATURES OF TUMORS
Most tumors look like lumps, but there are some major exceptions. Some appear as hollow craters (ulcers); there are even some liquid tumors.

THE TUMOR–HOST INTERFACE
Regarding those tumors that do appear as lumps, it is a general rule that benign tumors tend to have sharply defined edges whereas malignant tumors tend to have branches reaching into their surround-

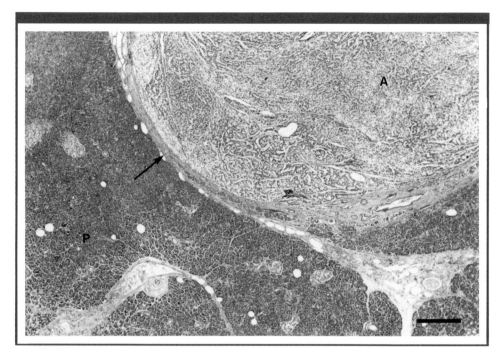

FIGURE 26.20
A benign tumor of the endocrine pancreas (adenoma, **A**). **P:** Pancreatic tissue. Note the thin fibrous capsule (**arrow**) surrounding the adenoma. **Bar** = 500 μm.

ings. However, there are many exceptions. Above all, beware of the legend that "benign tumors are encapsulated, malignant ones not." This is a gross oversimplication. Many benign tumors have no capsule at all, such as leiomyomas of the uterus, hemangiomas of the skin (Figure 26.19) or liver, and fibrohistiocytomas of the skin (which actually look infiltrating). It is also true that benign tumors are sometimes surrounded by a thin fibrous capsule, perhaps laid down by the surrounding tissues as a response to pressure (Figure 26.20). On the other hand, some very malignant tumors may have a capsule; it is usually incomplete and the tumor breaks through it (Figure 26.21). Fast-growing malignant tumors have a special way of surrounding themselves with a fibrous coat: as they rapidly expand within parenchymal organs such as the kidney or liver,

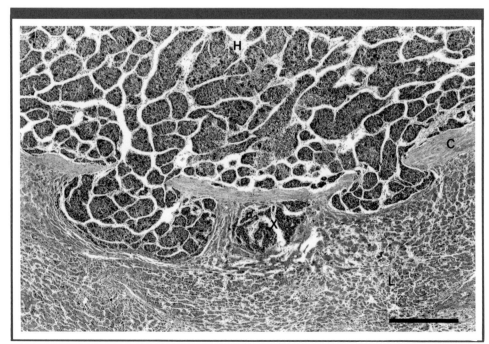

FIGURE 26.21
A primary carcinoma of the liver (hepatoma, **H**) expanding into liver tissue (**L**). The hepatoma is surrounded by a thin fibrous capsule (**C**); at two points this capsule is perforated by a mushroom-shaped mass of hepatoma. **X:** Mass of hepatoma tissue that has escaped through a gap in the capsule not visible in this section. Note atrophy of the liver tissue, probably due to compression. **Bar** = 500 μm.

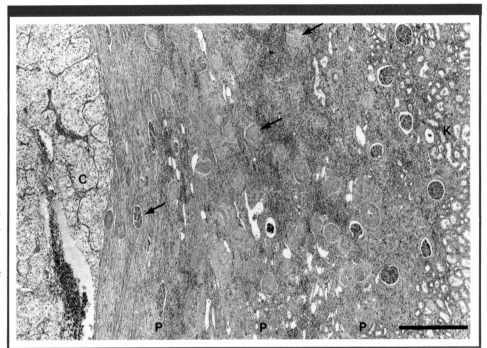

FIGURE 26.22
Pseudocapsule (**PPP**) separating a renal cell carcinoma (**C**) and kidney tissue (**K**). The pseudocapsule represents what is left of kidney tissue, squeezed out of existence by pressure from the advancing tumor. This is proven by the many atrophic or hyalinized glomeruli (**arrows**) contained in the pseudocapsule. **Bar** = 500 μm.

the parenchymal cells are squeezed out of existence, and their stroma alone remains to surround the tumor. This has been called a *pseudocapsule* (141). Its genesis is obvious in renal cell carcinomas because atrophic glomeruli remain to tell the story (Figure 26.22).

The capsule issue has practical relevance for surgery. Certain benign tumors such as the fibroadenoma of the breast can be removed with little or no surrounding tissue because they are surrounded by a capsule or by a clear-cut cleavage plane; occasionally they can even be "shelled out." In contrast, infiltrating malignant tumors must be removed along with a generous layer of the surrounding tissue.

Regarding the pseudocapsules of renal cell carcinomas and other large malignant tumors, their outer surface often carries large tortuous veins. Why these superficial veins grow so large is not clear. Perhaps they expand under the stimulus of growth factors in the blood that they drain out of the tumor. Needless to say, they do not even remotely recall a crab sitting on the tumor with claws extended, as someone fancied long ago (p. 718).

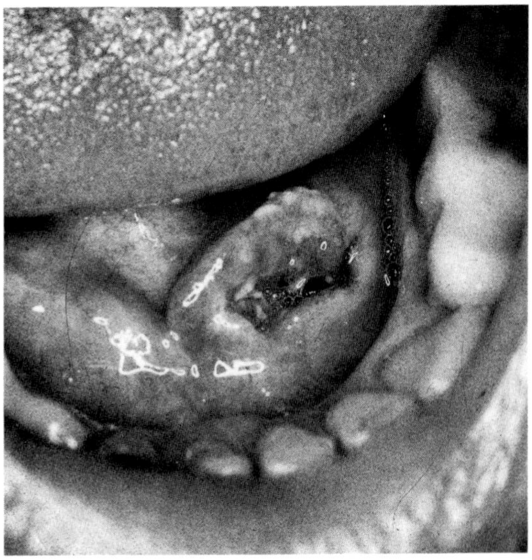

ULCERATED TUMORS

Tumors that arise from a bacterially contaminated surface (such as the skin or gut) tend to become ulcerated (Figure 26.23). In the gut this is due to bacterial infection, with some help from digestive enzymes. At first the surface of the tumor is eroded by mechanical friction; then bacteria colonize it, and persist (tumors have a poor blood supply and, thus, a poor inflammatory response). The result is an ulcer that does not heal. Malignant tumors are especially prone to ulcerate, and when they do, they can be difficult to recognize. Are we dealing with an ulcer or with an ulcerated tumor? A raised edge (also called a rolled edge), as shown in Figure 26.24, strongly suggests an ulcerated tumor. When radiologists examine X-rays of questionable gastric

FIGURE 26.23
Craterlike ulcerated carcinoma from the floor of the mouth in a 40-year-old-woman. The raised edges are characteristic of an ulcerated tumor as opposed to a simple ulcer. (Courtesy of Dr. G. Fiore-Donno, School of Dentistry, Geneva, Switzerland.)

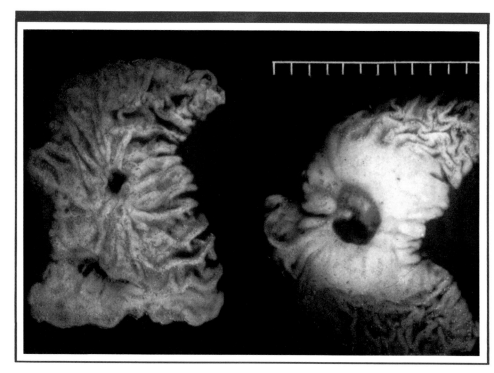

FIGURE 26.24
The nature of a gastric ulcer can be established only with the microscope. *Left:* Ulcer of the left curvature without "rolled edges" and with radiating gastric folds, suggestive of a chronic process. *Right:* Ulcer with greatly swollen margins. Microscopic examination of both specimens showed an ulcerated carcinoma (*left*) and a gastric ulcer (*right*). Scale in cm. (Courtesy of Dr. R. Lattes, Columbia University, New York, NY.)

ulcers, taken after a barium swallow, they can actually see the raised edge as a negative image. However, the diagnosis of tumor versus ulcer can be made only by the microscope. Witness Figure 26.24, which defies all classic teaching about raised edges.

Another site where tumors may typically be present as ulcers is the face, or any part of the skin exposed to the sun (Figure 26.25). Any skin ulcer that persists for longer than 3–4 weeks is suspect. An everyday example is the basal cell carcinoma of the face, a malignancy with a very distinctive personality: it grows slowly but tends to ulcerate so relentlessly that its ancient Latin name was *ulcus rodens*, the gnawing ulcer (Figure 26.26). Such persistent "ulcers" are best removed as a whole rather than biopsied; they almost invariably turn out to be basal cell carcinomas; and once removed, they pose no further threat.

THE CONSISTENCY OF TUMORS

Most tumors feel firm, even hard, especially those with a large amount of connective tissue stroma. The latter are called scirrhous carcinomas (from the Greek *skirrhòs*, hard). Epithelial tumors with little stroma are soft or medullary (which means marrowlike). Carcinomas of both kinds occur, for example, in the breast.

THE CUT SURFACE OF A TUMOR

A cut surface provides a lot of information:

- *Tumor tissue tends to be white* (Figure 26.27), whether benign or malignant, and even in areas that are clearly not necrotic. This is bizarre because no normal parenchyma is truly white, except for the brain on account of its high lipid content. As far as we know, the whiteness of tumors has not been explained.

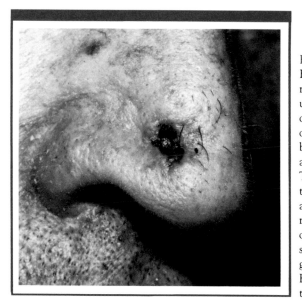

FIGURE 26.25
Basal cell carcinoma. The small ulcer on the nose of this 76-year-old man has been present for about 3 months. This presentation is typical of a basal cell carcinoma. (Courtesy of Dr. R.A. Johnson, New England Deaconess Hospital, Boston, MA.)

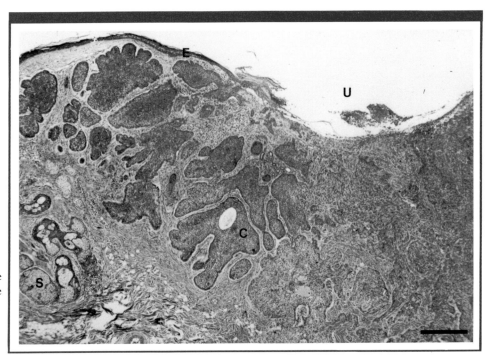

FIGURE 26.26
Ulcerated basal cell carcinoma of the face, similar to that shown in Figure 26.25. **E:** epidermis; **U:** ulcer; **C:** cords of the carcinoma invading the dermis; S = sebaceous gland near a hair follicle. **Bar** = 500 μm.

We have submitted this problem to several experts, who offered three excellent solutions. (a) The late biochemist Albert Szent-Györgyi, twice Nobel laureate, suggested that oxidative processes in tumors are low, and on the whole "oxidation tends to entail colored products." Indeed, anaerobic glycolysis, as we will see, is typical of tumors. (b) Quite independently, a similar suggestion was made by Dr. H. Pitot. In tumors, he wrote, there is a "relative lack of cytochromes which are tan, orange, beige or even brown and a dramatic increase in nucleic acids . . . which are white or very light yellow in visible light." (c) Dr. P. Gullino (who made important contributions to studies of the vascularization of tumors) noted that tumors are less vascularized than the normal corresponding tissue; this may be the principal mechanism (the interstitial pressure in tumors is high (p. 770); this would tend to compress the blood vessels). Note: The whiteness of tumor tissue is unrelated to the whiteness of necrosis. A liver adenoma, white to the naked eye, can be histologically very similar to normal liver tissue.

Of course, some tumors contain pigments. Melanomas can be extraordinarily black, even in fish (Figure 3.51); angiomas are red with blood; and hepatomas can be green with bile.

- *The margin of the tumor* may blend with the normal tissue around it; this suggests infiltration, an aggressive feature typical of malignancy. A sharp margin is compatible with benign behavior, albeit with the reservations mentioned earlier.

- *Foci of necrosis* usually mean bad news because *necrosis is much more common in malignant tumors and correlates statistically with poor prognosis* (Figure 26.28) (149). Necrosis is usually of the coagulative type and may be accompanied by hemorrhage. The mechanisms of necrosis in tumors will be discussed later (p. 749).

- *Large spaces filled with fluid (cysts) suggest that the tumor is epithelial (benign or malignant).* The mechanism: if the tumor contains secreting glands, the secretion has no

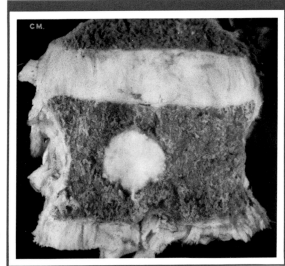

FIGURE 26.27
Metastasis of a carcinoma of the breast in a human vertebra.

way out and therefore expands the lumen of the glands (Figure 26.29).

THE SPECIAL CASE OF LIQUID TUMORS

It is sometimes said that leukemias are liquid tumors; this is not completely accurate because the circulating leukemic cells come from the bone marrow, which is very soft but not truly fluid, even though it can be aspirated with a needle. The term is quite appropriate, however, for the experimental tumors called **ascites tumors,** extensively studied by George and Eva Klein at the Karolinska Institute (124). Many transplantable tumors of rats and mice can be induced (some more easily than others) to grow freely in the peritoneal cavity where they induce an exudate (ascites) and thrive within it like bacteria in a broth, without invading the peritoneal surfaces, at least initially. The ascitic fluid is presumably caused by factors increasing vascular permeability that are secreted by the tumor cells (p. 769). The biological change of cells to ascites tumor behavior is irreversible; it may be a manifestation of tumor progression. Ascites tumors are an artefact, but they do have a major experimental advantage in that the malignant cells are easily harvested.

THE MICROSCOPIC STRUCTURE OF TUMORS

The basic principle of tumor structure, which is sufficiently established to resemble dogma, is that *tumors tend to reproduce the cellular type and the*

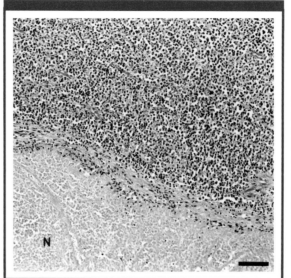

FIGURE 26.28 Coagulation necrosis (**N**) in a lymphoma. A thin fibrous layer has developed along the demarcation line. The lymphoma appears typically as a "sea of lymphocytes." **Bar** = 100 μm.

architectural pattern of the parent tissue. There is a corollary: Benign tumors are relatively faithful imitations of the original tissue, malignant tumors are rather caricatures.

Considering that the human body contains roughly 200 types of cells and that tumors tend to create fanciful variants, it is easy to grasp that the microscopic patterns of tumors number in the hundreds. Because pathologists must memorize them, they are sometimes teased as "stamp collectors." We will offer two examples, comparing a normal tissue with its benign and malignant counterpart (Figures 26.30, 26.31).

The first step in working out the structure of

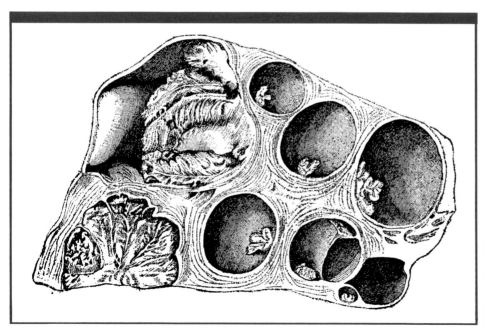

FIGURE 26.29
A papillary cystadenocarcinoma of the ovary seen in cross section. Drawn from a specimen ca. 1900. (Reproduced with permission from [227].)

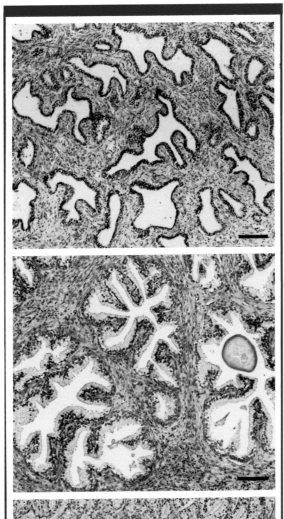

FIGURE 26.30 Comparing normal prostatic glands (*top*) with glands of prostatic hypertrophy (*center*) and with an adenocarcinoma of the prostate (*bottom*). In the latter, the glandular structure is preserved but barely apparent. **Bars** = 100 μm.

amount of each component varies greatly; the scirrhous tumors just mentioned are packed with collagen fibers but, oddly enough, also with elastic fibers (207).

> *Even more odd is the fact that some of the elastin in human breast cancers is produced by the neoplastic epithelial cells as well as by fibroblasts and microvascular endothelium. This was found by means of* in situ *hybridization of mRNA for human elastin (129).*

The intimate contact between tumor and stroma exposes the stromal cells to a variety of enzymes, growth factors, and other secretions of the tumor cells. The overproduction of collagen by the fibroblasts of scirrhous tumors is probably a response to tumor cell products (120). The stroma can also affect the tumor, for example by sequestering positive or negative growth factors (112a).

> *In colorectal carcinomas the c-myc gene is expressed by the tumor cells as well as by the stromal cells; the latter are probably responding in this manner to epidermal growth factor (EGF) produced by the tumor cells (142).*

Not only stromal cells but any tissue near a tumor is exposed to an overdose of growth factors; for example, the thickening of the gastric mucosa surrounding a gastric carcinoma is attributed to EGF secreted by the tumor (132).

The blood vessels of the stroma include vessels that have been incorporated by the growing tumor, and others have been newly developed by angiogenesis (163). As expected, the number of vessels varies greatly from tumor to tumor and within different areas of the same tumor. Values published for various rat and mouse tumors, concerning the relative volume occupied by vessels, range from 1 to 50 percent (4,73,103,223).

Because the vessels in tumors are provided by the normal host in response to chemically normal factors, we might expect them to be normal; in fact, they are a mixed bag of normal and abnormal vessels (60). The following are a few basic points:

- *Tumor vessels have a high mitotic rate*, as expressed by a labeling index (p. 766) that is 20–2000 times higher than normal (49,50) (Figure 26.32). This is good news for chemotherapy, which should be able to hit these "cycling" vessels as well as the "cycling" tumor cells (49).
- Electron microscopy has shown, in general,

tumors is to distinguish the non-neoplastic stroma from the tumor cells.

THE STROMA OF TUMORS

All tumors have a stroma consisting of connective tissue, vessels, a moderate inflammatory infiltrate (58), and sometimes, myofibroblasts (183). The

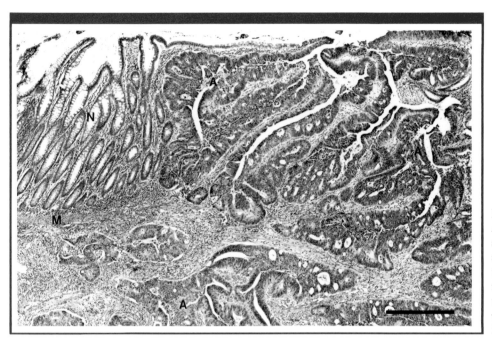

FIGURE 26.31
Adenocarcinoma (**A**) of the colon
arising from the normal (**N**) mucosa
at left. Note the difference between
the normal glands and the carcinomatous glands. There is tumor invasion beneath the *muscularis
mucosae* (**M**). **Bar** =
500 µm.

rather immature vessels, with few pericytes
and few smooth muscle cells; according to
one report, some of the newly developed
vessels are poorly formed, and their
endothelial lining is incomplete (216).

• Functionally, the vessels of tumors are not
normal; they react poorly to vasoactive
agents (162), and many are leaky (60). If
dyes are injected intravenously into tumor-
bearing mice, parts of the tumors can be

stained, especially the rims (97). The vessels leak, not only because their lining is
incomplete but also because tumor cells secrete factors that increase vascular permeability (33, 55a, 60). The leaky vessels are
mainly venules, but the mechanism of
leakage—as seen by electron microscopy—
does not resemble any type of leakage that
we described in inflamed tissues (p. 369)
(126a). It is noteworthy that the vascular

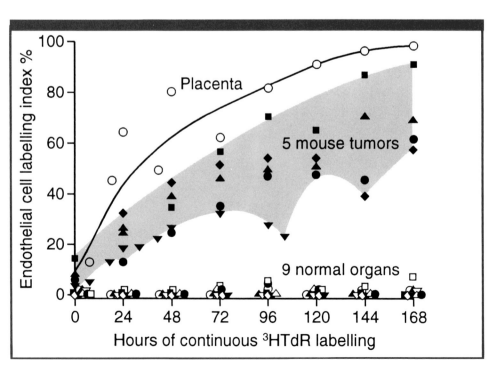

FIGURE 26.32
Comparing the turnover of endothelial cells in various mouse tissues
by injecting tritiated thymidine every
8 hours for 7 days. The rate is highest
for the placenta, high for five types of
mouse tumor, very low for nine normal adult tissues. (Adapted from
[49].)

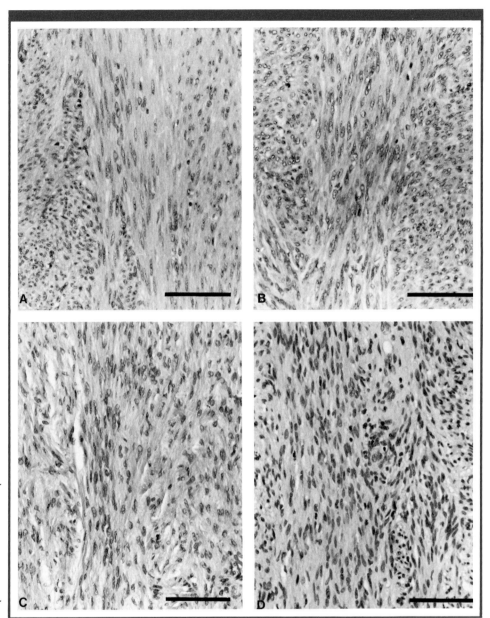

FIGURE 26.33
A panel of photographs illustrating the limits of normal histology in diagnosing tumors. **A:** Normal smooth muscle of the uterus (myometrium). **B:** Leiomyoma of the uterus. **C:** Fibroma of the ovary. **D:** Tumor of Schwann cells (schwannoma). The clinical and topographic context of each tumor assists in the diagnosis, but special stains provide a further degree of certainty. **Bars** = 100 μm.

permeability factor (VPF) described by Dvorak and collaborators in experimental tumors was later found to be also a potent *angiogenic* factor produced by many fetal and adult tissues, including human tissues, especially under anoxia: hence its double name VPF/VEGF (for vascular endothelial growth factor) (55a). We shall return to this topic in dealing with inflammation in tumors (58). Vascular leakage in tumors has its good side: it can help chemotherapy by allowing drugs to seep out (59).

- The vessels of brain tumors tend to maintain a partial blood–brain barrier, which means that they retain a significant level of normality. It also means that they complicate therapy because to reach brain tumors with chemotherapeutic agents it is necessary to break down the blood–brain barrier temporarily; this can be done, for example, by injecting hypertonic mannitol into the carotid artery.

- Whatever the number of vessels in a tumor, the key point to remember is that—in general—the blood supply of tumor tissue is less than normal (162, 163).

The process whereby tumor vessels are generated—tumor angiogenesis—is a story in itself; we will tell it in relation to tumor growth. Inflammation in tumors will be discussed on p. 768.

THE NEOPLASTIC COMPONENT OF TUMORS

After tumor cells are identified, two questions must be answered: where do they come from? and how aggressive are they?

The ancestry of tumor cells is often quite clear because tumors tend to reproduce the original cell and tissue. See, for example, an adenoma of the endocrine pancreas (Figure 26.20) or a leiomyoma of the uterus (Figure 25.12). Even if the tumor is so undifferentiated that it has lost all identifiable structural features, it usually retains some cell-specific antigen that can be recognized by a specific antibody. Antibodies can also be helpful for distinguishing look-alikes (Figure 26.33).

The question of aggressiveness can be answered by studying abnormalities of the cells and abnormalities of tissue architecture. These are the cornerstones of tumor diagnosis.

Cellular Abnormalities The malignant phenotype has already been portrayed; in summary, when diagnosing a tumor, the following criteria must be kept in mind.

- *Lack of differentiation.* Whereas normal cells have set characteristics that define their state of maturity (differentiation), tumor cells tend to be, and to look, less differentiated. For example, a mucus-secreting cell in a tumor may contain minimal amounts of mucus and a fat cell may contain many small droplets of fat (like embryonic fat) rather than a single larger drop (Figure 26.34). *Highly undifferentiated cells suggest a very aggressive tumor.* As a matter of fact, we will learn later that one way to treat malignant tumors is to encourage them to differentiate.
- *Cytologic atypia*, that is, abnormal size, shape, or content.
- *Pleomorphism (polymorphism).* Cellular atypia goes hand in hand with cellular pleomorphism because the degree of atypia tends to vary from one cell to another and from one microscopic field to another. The sight of a tissue with nuclei of different sizes and shapes is immediately worrisome (Figure 26.35). Assessing pleomorphism is often a subjective, almost artistic judgment. It can be made quantitative by deferring the

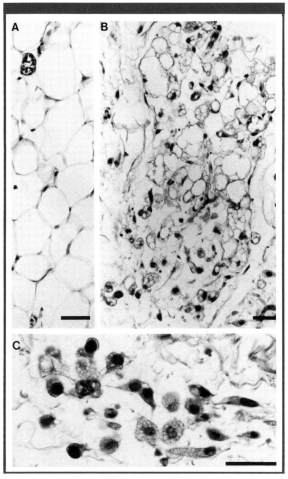

FIGURE 26.34
A: Normal adipose tissue. **B:** Malignant tumor of adipose tissue (liposarcoma). The cells are irregular; many contain small, multiple pockets of fat, as better shown at higher power in **C. Bars** = 50 μm.

judgment, for example, to the fluorescence-activated cell sorter (FACS) (p. 15); however, the verdicts of the FACS are time-consuming and expensive.

Abnormalities of Architecture *Architectural atypia.* By this we mean abnormal cellular pattern. This feature is best seen in glandular tumors, in which beautiful normal patterns give way to disorderly structures of varying degrees of ugliness and, correspondingly, of threat (Figure 26.36).

Infiltration (local invasion) means that tumor tissue invades its neighboring tissues. *Infiltration is a nearly absolute sign of malignancy* (Figures 26.37, 26.38).

SECONDARY CHANGES IN TUMORS

Because tumors are poorly planned structures, they tend to develop mishaps. One of these is ulceration (p. 740); others are listed below.

FIGURE 26.35 Malignant tumor of liver tissue (hepatoma). This tumor can be interpreted as a caricature of normal liver tissue: it consists of cords of epithelial cells separated by vascular spaces. **Bar** = 200 μm. *Left:* Note the variations in nuclear size and shape, better seen (*right*) at a higher power (**arrows**). **Bar** = 100 μm.

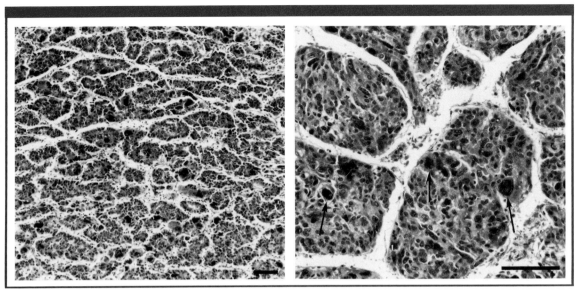

FIGURE 26.36 A simplified drawing of the so-called Gleason grading system for prostatic adenocarcinoma. As the glandular structure departs more and more from the original pattern (**1**) and as glandular atypia increases, the prognosis becomes worse. (Reproduced with permission from [96].)

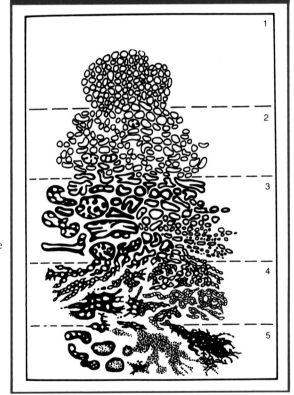

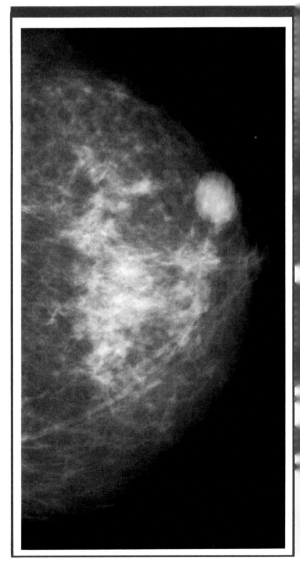

FIGURE 26.37   (*Right*)
Mammogram showing a benign tumor with sharp outlines (fibroadenoma). The diffuse mass at the left is normal glandular tissue. (Courtesy of Dr. C. D'Orsi, University of Massachusetts Medical Center, Worcester, MA.)

NECROSIS

Necrotic masses, so common in malignant tumors, develop in two ways (31):

- Ischemia is the reason for the massive central necrosis almost invariably seen in large malignant tumors, and sometimes in large benign tumors. It is best explained by the impairment of blood flow caused by high tissue pressure (p. 770).

- *Programmed cell death* may occur in tumors developing from cells with a built-in "death program" (30,149). Consider a stratified epithelium such as the skin; in normal life the basal cells proliferate, giving rise to cells that move upward and eventually die and slough off. The same basic program functions in tumors of this epithelium, except that the cells, once sloughed off, are trapped inside the tumor and pile up as a necrotic mass (Figure 26.39). When this occurs, the morphology of cell death is apoptosis (p. 200). The best example are the "epithelial pearls" of squamous cell carcinoma (Figure 26.40).

When tumor cells are killed by anticancer agents they often die by apoptosis.

CALCIFICATION

Calcification usually develops in dead cells or necrotic masses. For reasons unknown, the cells of some carcinomas have a special propensity to calcify (especially in the breast and ovary); the resulting tiny, gritty calcifications have suggested a comparison with sand, hence the name *psammomas* for these tumors (Greek *psámmos*, sand) (Figures 26.41, 26.42). In the breast, tiny calcifications are so common that mammography exploits them as an early warning of possible malignancy. Unfortunately, benign lesions also calcify, and there is no way yet to distinguish them.

The genesis of microscopic psammoma bodies needs more study; it may differ from tumor to tumor (23). A strange mechanism has been observed in carcinomas of the breast: the calcification of secretions within an intracellular lumen (Figure 26.43) (2).

Leiomyomas sometimes calcify, and this seems to have been true also 5000 years ago: a rounded calcified mass about 5 cm in diameter, found in a neolithic burial site in Switzerland, was diagnosed as "presumed calcified leiomyoma of the uterus" (128).

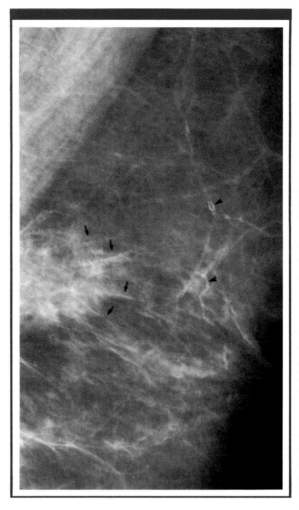

FIGURE 26.38 Mammogram showing a typical malignant tumor (carcinoma) in a 66-year-old woman. **Arrows:** Streaks suggestive of infiltration. *Top left:* Pectoral muscle to which the mass was clinically adherent. Note the calcified arteries (**arrowheads**). (Courtesy of Dr. C. D'Orsi, University of Massachusetts Medical Center, Worcester, MA.)

TORSION

Torsion is an accident that besets pedunculated tumors, be they benign or malignant. Ovarian tumors are especially susceptible. As might be expected, the veins in the twisted stalk are compressed first, while the arteries still manage to pump blood beyond the stricture. The result is a red infarct: the tumor has killed itself (Figure 26.44).

DIFFERENCES BETWEEN BENIGN AND MALIGNANT TUMORS: A SUMMARY

We have mentioned the key principles of distinguishing a malignant tumor: the degree of malignancy tends to correlate with atypia, local invasiveness suggests malignancy, metastasis *proves* malignancy. In addition to these guidelines, there are many finer criteria, which are summarized in Table 26.1. All are helpful, but they are simply suggestive and therefore must be interpreted with a grain of salt. Mitoses, for example, are plentiful

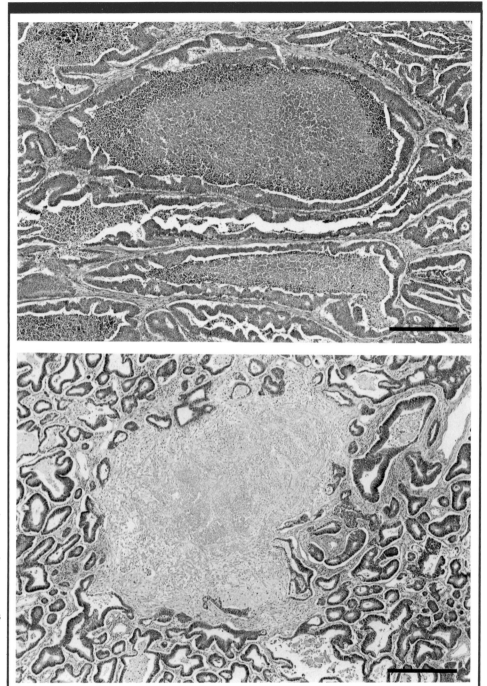

FIGURE 26.39

Two types of cell death in carcinomas. *Top:* Programmed cell death. The dead cells are contained in atypical glands lined by epithelium. As the epithelial cells lining the glands go through their cycle of constant renewal and replacement, those that slough off accumulate in the lumen. (Adenocarcinoma of the colon.) **Bar** = 500 μm. *Bottom:* Ischemic necrosis due to inadequate blood supply. A whole mass of tumor dies, including epithelium and stroma. (Adenocarcinoma of the lung.) **Bar** = 500 μm.

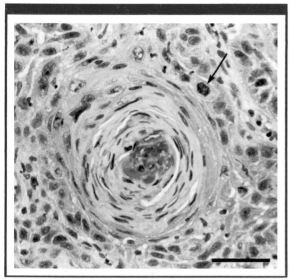

FIGURE 26.40
Typical epidermal "pearl" characteristic of squamous cell carcinoma of the skin. Pearls consist of squamous cells that have reached maturation (keratinization) but cannot slough off because they lie deep in the tumor. **Arrow:** A mitosis. **Bar** = 50 μm.

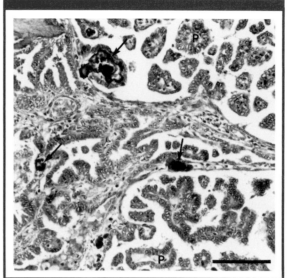

FIGURE 26.42
Focal calcifications (psammoma bodies, **arrows**) in a papillary cystadenocarcinoma of the ovary. The isolated structures (**P**) are actually cross sections of papillae. **Bar** = 100 μm.

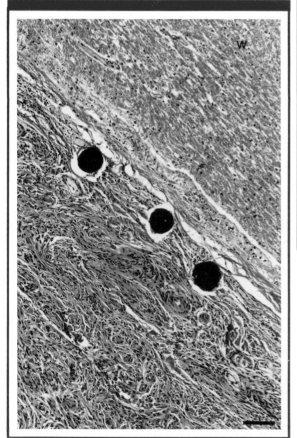

FIGURE 26.41
Microscopic calcifications in a tumor: Three psammoma bodies at the periphery of a meningioma (*lower left*). **W:** White matter. **Bar** = 100 μm. (Specimen courtesy of Dr. T.W. Smith, University of Massachusetts Medical Center, Worcester, MA.)

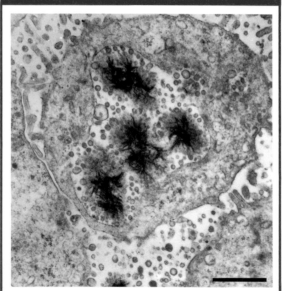

FIGURE 26.43
Example of calcification in carcinoma of the breast. Four clusters of apatite needles have formed in what appears to be an intracellular lumen. **Bar** = 1 μm. (Reproduced with permission from [2].)

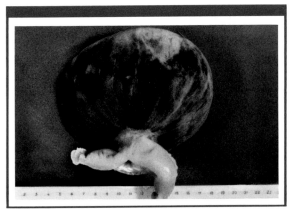

FIGURE 26.44

Infarction of a benign tumor by torsion. This leiomyoma, bulging from the outer wall of the small intestine, twisted itself around its peduncle; as it became necrotic it caused enough inflammation and pain to mimic appendicitis. (The original color was deep purple from venous congestion.) (Courtesy of the Department of Pathology, Geneva, Switzerland.)

not only in malignant tumors but in regenerating tissues.

Afterthoughts on Tumor Diagnosis *Identifying tumors under the microscope is more complex than matching a pattern with a name.* Earlier we resorted to the term *ugliness* in relation to malignant cells. We did so because the concepts of atypia and pleomorphism require a certain degree of aes-

thetic judgment, and to this degree the diagnosis is tinged by the personality of the observer. This is why pathology, like all of medicine, is science as well as art. Medical students traditionally anguish over tumor diagnosis: how much atypia is required for the verdict of malignancy? Only experience can tell. Pathologists anguish too over certain tumors. There are some known traps, such as leiomyomas that look perfectly benign and yet metastasize, thus earning the paradoxical name of metastasizing leiomyomas (45). There are bland-looking thyroid "adenomas" that have already metastasized to the bone when they are first seen. And then there are tumors that could be labeled either benign or malignant for equally valid reasons. The worried pathologist who studies such slides feels as if contemplating the intertwined angels and devils of Escher (Figure 26.45).

To maximize the reliability of microscopic diagnosis there are specific guidelines for each type of tumor, based on statistics and experience. The internationally recognized authority is represented by the fascicles published by the U.S. Armed Forces Institute of Pathology (A.F.I.P.) which also functions as a diagnostic consulting service worldwide. The A.F.I.P. has long been one of the most important, effective, peaceful, and welcome ambassadors of the United States.

TABLE 26.1

Comparison of Various Features in Benign and Malignant Tumors

FEATURE	IN BENIGN TUMORS	IN MALIGNANT TUMORS
Rate of growth	Slow	Fast
Mode of growth	Expansile	Infiltrative
General effects	Uncommon (except endocrine)	Common
Metastases (**)	—	Common
Recurrence after removal	Rare	Common
Gross:		
Capsule	Common	Pseudocapsule
Necrosis	Rare	Common
Ulceration	Rare	Common
Microscopic:		
Atypia	Mild	Severe
Pleomorphism	Mild	Severe
Mitoses	Few	Many
Nuclear/Cytoplasmic ratio	Normal	Increased
Nucleolus	Normal	Prominent
Ploidy	Often normal	Usually abnormal

**Most reliable criterion.

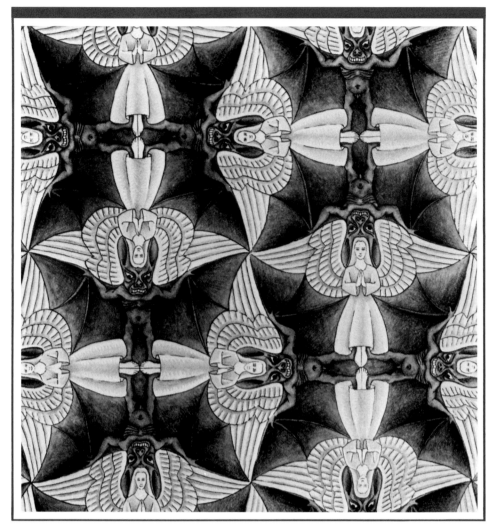

FIGURE 26.45
Interwoven angels and devils, the nightmare of the pathologist examining a tumor that appears neither benign nor malignant. The composition is by Dutch artist M.C. Escher (1941). (Reproduced with permission from [65].)

Birth and Growth of a Tumor

The key ingredient, in order to produce a tumor, is a cell type capable of dividing. Most cells fit this category, a few do not. Until recently, the cell types considered incapable of dividing (permanent cells) were those of the crystalline lens, the neurons, and possibly also the cells of the myocardium and striated muscle. The cells of the lens have finally yielded to the oncogene wizards, who have produced true carcinomas of the lens in transgenic mice, using the gene for the lens protein alpha-A-crystallin combined with a coding sequence from the oncogenic virus SV40 (Figures 26.46, 26.47) (138,155). Tumors containing mature neurons may sound like heresy, but they exist: *gangliogliomas*, for example, are mixed tumors of neurons and glia. Tumors of striated muscle and of the myocardium are rare, but they

also exist. The notion of permanent cells is not as strict as was once thought (p. 17); however, permanent status is not the main issue. Tumors containing mature cells such as neurons or myocardial cells probably do *not* arise from the multiplication of adult cells.

WHICH CELLS GENERATE TUMORS?
It is now thought that tumors, generally speaking arise from immature precursors, called stem cells,

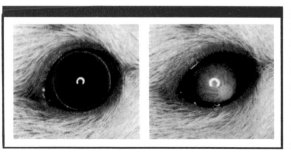

FIGURE 26.46
Left: Eye of a normal mouse. *Right:* Eye of a transgenic mouse developing a tumor of the lens. (Reproduced with permission from [138].)

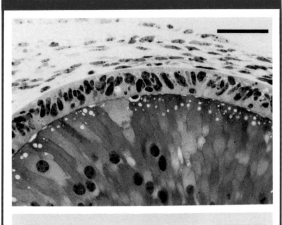

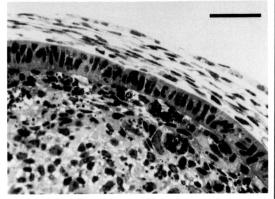

FIGURE 26.47
Top: Section through the normal crystalline lens of a mouse. *Bottom:* Lens of a transgenic mouse developing a malignant tumor. The overall structure is preserved, but there is extensive cellular atypia. **Bars** = 50 μm. (Reproduced with permission from [155].)

which then differentiate into mature forms. An obvious example is brain tissue contained in teratomas of the ovary (together with mature tissues of many other types). This aberrant brain tissue is not the product of neuronal mitoses; it develops by the differentiation of pluripotent cells of embryonic type. Significantly, tumors with permanent cells tend to appear in children and young adults. It is wiser to speak of tumors *with* permanent cells rather than tumors *of* permanent cells.

The concept of stem cells was applied to tumors almost a century ago; it was suggested by the study of teratomas, which contain a great variety of tissues, all of which can be proven to derive from a single cell (126,127). The basic idea is that tissues contain specialized cells dedicated to cell replacement by the mechanism of asymmetric division: that is, at each mitosis, one of the two daughter cells is exported for cell replacement and differentiation, while the other remains in place and persists in its role of immortal stem cell (127). The existence of stem cells is not difficult to prove in epithelia, where they can actually be seen as reserve cells squatting on the basement membrane. Besides teratomas, the concept fits with the pathogenesis of certain leukemias (71,175); but for most tissues the concept remains hypothetical. The main reason is

that it is extremely difficult to identify a cell that qualifies as a stem cell in connective tissues (some have been found in bone marrow and blood [133a]).

HOW MANY CELLS ARE NEEDED TO START A TUMOR?

Most tumors are born, like people, from one cell, which means that a 75-kg human being, made of somewhere near 75,000,000,000,000 cells, can be felled by the misbehavior of one single cell.

Note: the following discussion concerns only the monoclonal versus polyclonal birth of tumors. It has nothing to do with the fact that all malignant tumors tend to become polyclonal in their advanced stages, by the phenomenon of progression (p. 762).

The evidence for tumor monoclonality comes from several sources. In mice, leukemia can be transmitted by injecting one leukemic cell (188). Furthermore, if all the cells in a tumor (human or other) carry a specific, recognizable chromosomal defect that is not present in the normal cells of the same individual, they must have inherited it from a single ancestor. This is the case of the historic Philadelphia chromosome present in chronic myelogenous leukemia (p. 872).

Another approach to studying the clonality of tumors is offered by individuals who are chimeras; if their tumors are not chimeric, this suggests that the tumors derived from a single cell. Accordingly, there has been much interest in tumors of women who are heterozygous for glucose-6-phosphate dehydrogenase (G6PD), an experiment of nature that has been much used for studies of monoclonality. Simply stated, G6PD comes in many variants (isoenzymes) and is encoded by a gene on the X chromosome. Women have two X chromosomes, one of maternal and the other of paternal origin. Now it so happens that in all female embryos, at the blastocyst stage, all cells are submitted to a random inactivation of one X chromosome; in some cells the maternal chromosome is inactivated, in others the paternal. This means that all the adult woman's organs will be a mosaic of cells bearing either the maternal or the paternal X chromosome; and if, by chance, the isoenzymes encoded by the two chromosomes are different, as happens most often in women of African origin, all organs contain both enzymes. What about tumors? Most tumors, benign or malignant, produce only one enzyme, suggesting a monoclonal origin (71,222). However, this type of evidence is not flawless. It could also indicate that the tumor began as a polyclonal growth, but later a more successful clone crowded out the others.

A rather spectacular example of chimeras are the so-called allophenic mice, obtained by combining two blastocysts. If the embryos are selected from a white and a black mouse, the striped adults are chimeras even to the naked eye (Figure 26.48) (148). Most but not all tumors in these chimeric mice are monoclonal (44,112).

If methylcholanthrene is used to produce fibrosarcomas in mice, low and high doses tend to produce monoclonal and polyclonal tumors, respectively (222).

There is nothing intrinsically bizarre about tumors being polyclonal. Multiple tumors do exist side by side; one uterus may contain dozens of myomas. Therefore, a polyclonal tumor can be considered, conceptually, as the fusion of two adjacent tumors (106). A good example is the common basal-cell carcinoma of the skin, which when studied histologically is often multicentric; that is, it appears to start at several points along the epidermis (Figure 26.49). One venereal wart (*condyloma acuminatum*) was found to arise from 4000–5000 cells (71).

The best evidence for tumor monoclonality comes from hematologic or mesenchymal tumors; the best examples of polyclonality come from epithelia. This makes sense. Epithelia are located in the body as shields against chemical and physical carcinogens, which offers greater opportunities for clusters of mutagenic events (106). Remember that 80 percent of tumors are epithelial.

TUMOR GROWTH AND ANGIOGENESIS

Once a tumor cell is born, the path to developing an actual tumor is not yet open. Tumors cannot grow much beyond the size of a pinhead unless they become vascularized. The host must supply blood vessels. This "law" was first expressed in Cohnheim's lectures in 1889 (39). It has practical implications because if the formation of new vessels (**angiogenesis**) can be inhibited, then tumor growth should also be inhibited. However, the concept that vessels are essential for tumor growth was forgotten, and the vascularization of tumors came to be considered a secondary phenomenon, perhaps a reaction to necrosis.

THE REDISCOVERY OF ANGIOGENESIS

Tumor angiogenesis was rediscovered in the 1940s (217) and then became a science on its own,

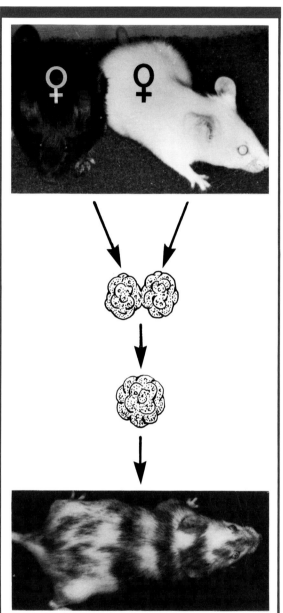

FIGURE 26.48
Bottom: Allophenic mouse derived from the fusion of two embryos, one from a black mouse, another from a white one. (Adapted from [147].)

thanks to the systematic studies of Dr. Judah Folkman, an extremely imaginative surgeon–biologist. This tale is worth recounting.

Dr. Folkman's first encounter with experimental tumors was not planned as such. His purpose at the time was to find some effective blood substitutes. To test the effectiveness of some candidates, he perfused isolated dog thyroids to find out how long they could be kept alive. Under the best conditions the thyroids seemed to survive longer than 1 week; but would the same blood substitutes also support growth? To check this point Dr. Folkman mixed some mouse melanoma cells into the perfusing fluid, thinking that the black melanoma cells would be good indicators of new

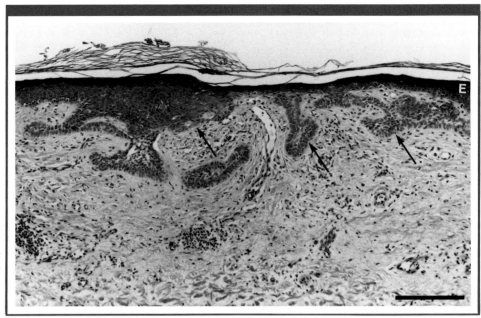

FIGURE 26.49
Multicentric origin of a basal cell carcinoma. **E:** epidermis; the **arrows**
point to separate outgrowths of tumor
cells. **Bar:** = 200 μm. (Slide courtesy
of Dr. R. Malhotra, University of
Massachusetts Medical Center,
Worcester, MA.)

*growth. Indeed, tiny black melanomas did appear on
the perfused thyroids. At first they grew very fast, but
then—surprisingly—they all stopped growing at the
same stage, when they reached a diameter of 1–2
mm (Figure 26.50) (76,77).*

*A fascinating by-product of this study was the
discovery that the endothelium of perfused capillaries
breaks down unless platelets are added to the medium
(91). How the platelets preserve the endothelial cells
is still not clear, but this is the best available proof of
their mysterious endothelium-supporting function.
Recall that, clinically, tiny hemorrhages (petechiae)
appear when the number of platelets per cubic
millimeter drops below 10,000.*

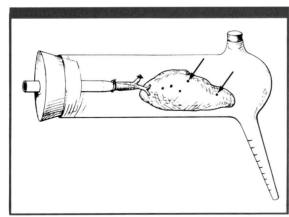

FIGURE 26.50
A thyroid gland maintained by perfusion *in vitro*, and metastasized with a suspension of melanoma cells. The metastases
(arrows) do not grow beyond 1–2 mm in diameter, because
under the conditions of this experiment new vessels cannot
develop. (Reproduced with permission from [76].)

Dr. Folkman then tested the following hypothesis: perhaps *tumors cannot grow beyond 1–2 mm
unless they are supported by ingrowth of new
capillaries*, which could not occur in the perfusion
system. To test this idea he had to find a living
system in which tumor cells could be made to grow
with or without blood vessels; his choice was the
anterior chamber of the rabbit eye. Rabbit tumor
cells injected into that space grew, within 2 weeks,
into free-floating spheroids with a volume of about
0.5 mm³; thereafter, the spheroids persisted without further growth. However, if they were manu-
ally seated against the iris, which is highly
vascularized, they grew in 3 days to 16,000 times
the original volume; their growth curve shot up
almost at a right angle (95) (Figure 26.51). The
behavior of the floating spheroids may be a clue to
the phenomenon of tumor dormancy observed
clinically (77,95); for example, a mastectomy scar,
may remain normal for years until suddenly a
cancerous nodule grows in it, presumably from
cells that had remained quiescent since surgery.

*Spheroids are an established tool for tumor research
(Figure 26.52) (1,55,81,196). Tumor cells maintained in stirred culture media tend to grow as
rounded aggregates. Under ideal conditions with
continuously renewed medium, these spheroids grow
to a maximal diameter of 3–4 mm, at which point
they contain a necrotic center surrounded by about 1
million cells. In contrast, the two-dimensional growth
of a standard tumor culture in vitro is limitless;
diffusion is not restricted. The spheroids serve as*

models of nodular tumors, minus the influence of the host; they can also be used to test the effects of chemotherapy.

Another model used by the Folkman group was the rabbit cornea (92), which has no blood vessels. Tiny bits of rabbit tumor inserted into a flat pocket created in the thickness of the cornea could not grow as spheres (due to the tight quarters) but formed a sheet; as the sheet advanced toward the edge of the cornea, capillaries began to grow toward it, advancing as much as 1 mm per day. When they reached the tumor, it began to grow so fast that in 4 weeks it was as large as the eye (80). This type of experiment suggested that the capillaries might be growing in response to a powerful call, perhaps a diffusible factor. Indeed, a tumor angiogenesis factor was soon obtained from a variety of tumors; it was tested by "loading" it into plastic pellets implanted into the cornea (Figure 26.53).

The modern industry of plastic pellets for slow delivery of drugs was greatly boosted as a by-product of this work (83). The idea to use pellets of plastic as slow-release devices came through a chance observation. As a resident, Dr. Folkman had noticed that the silicone rubber tubing of a laboratory pump became stained with a dye added to the fluid. Almost anyone else would have considered this a nuisance; to Dr. Folkman it meant that if the silicone rubber picked up the dye it might also pick up a drug, and also release it. It did both.

Now admire the latest, much simpler, and cheaper model for studies of angiogenesis on a large scale: fertilized eggs are incubated for 3–4 days and then poured out on a Petri dish, where the embryo continues to grow (admittedly rather flat) for up to 3 weeks (Figure 26.54). Small objects laid on the vascular chorioallantoic membrane can be tested for angiogenic and anti-angiogenic substances. In this way it was confirmed that cartilage produces an inhibitory factor to angiogenesis (Figure 26.55) (32,63,64,80). Cartilage was tested because it is usually spared by advancing tumors. Tradition held that the obstacle was mechanical, but the mechanism turned out to be more subtle: cartilage contains a protein that inhibits angiogenesis *in vivo* and *in vitro*; it also inhibits collagenases (152).

The natural history of tumor angiogenesis *in vivo* is much the same as that of wound healing (p. 469). Sprouts come from capillaries and venules whose

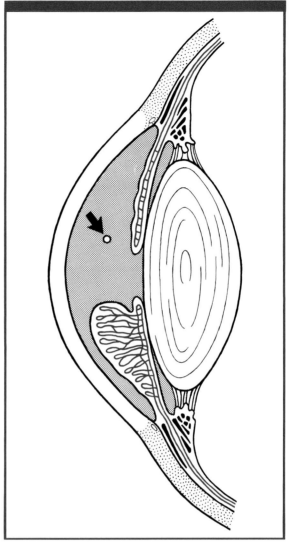

FIGURE 26.51 Malignant tumor cells, introduced into the anterior chamber of the rabbit's eye and left floating there, survive but stop growing before they reach the diameter of 1 mm (**arrow**). If this avascular "spheroid" is placed in contact with the iris (bottom), it is invaded by new vessels and grows. Diagram of an experiment by J. Folkman (1974). (Reproduced with permission from [73].)

endothelial cells secrete proteolytic enzymes, which help the sprouts escape their cage of basement membrane. Thus, the cells sprout, emigrate, and eventually multiply and form tubes (Figure 26.56). If the stimulus ceases, the vessels break up and disappear (7,75). *In vitro*, endothelial cells respond to angiogenic stimuli, in most cases, by moving around more actively (Figure 11.31) (224) and by dividing.

Different tumors produce different combinations of factors. For example, induction of angiogenesis may precede neoplastic transformation, so the appearance of blood vessels may be the first sign of malignancy; this fact was first established by implanting fragments of normal hyperplastic, preneoplastic, and malignant mouse mammary tissue in the rabbit eye, (77,84,85,93,195). Oddly enough, the stimulus to tumor angiogenesis may not come only from the tumor cells; anoxic

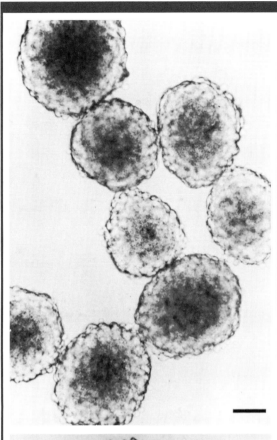

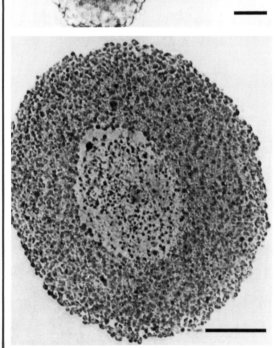

FIGURE 26.52
Spheroids that developed *in vitro* in a spinning suspension of hamster lung carcinoma cells. These spheroids can be used as models for the study of tumor growth. *Top:* Whole mount showing a "squash preparation" of spheroids. *Bottom:* Histological cross section through the center of the spheroid. The thickness of the viable rim is about 120 micrometers. **Bars** = 100 μm. (Reproduced with permission from [196].)

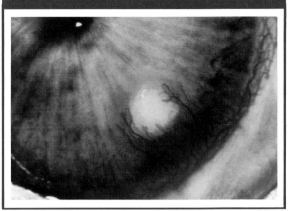

FIGURE 26.53
Tumor angiogenesis factor was impregnated into a 1 mm^3 slow-release plastic pellet. Implanted in the cornea, the pellet, 11 days later, has induced vascular growth. (Courtesy of Dr. J. Folkman, Harvard Medical School, Boston, MA.)

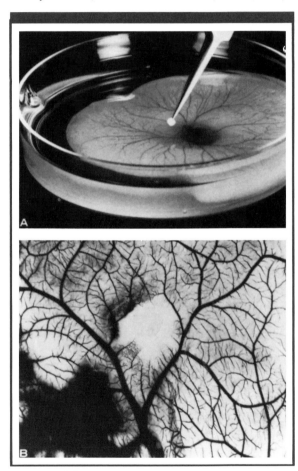

FIGURE 26.54
Chorioallantoic membrane method for studying the microcirculation. A yolk bearing a chick embryo is poured into a petri dish, where it becomes flat and convenient for microscopic study between days 6 and 10. The chick does not hatch. *Top:* Disc of methylcellulose loaded with an antiangiogenic substance is about to be implanted on the membrane. *Bottom:* Avascular zone that has developed 48 hours later. The vessels have been injected with India ink. The disc contained heparin and 11 α-epicortisol. (Reproduced with permission from [77].)

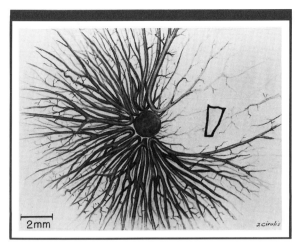

FIGURE 26.55
Inhibition of angiogenesis by cartilage: Diagram of an experiment in which a dose of tumor angiogenesis factor (**disk in center**) and a fragment of cartilage (*right*) were implanted on a chorioallantoic membrane. Growth of new vessels induced by TAF was inhibited around the cartilage. (Reproduced with permission from [32].)

macrophages, as we now know (p. 469), can also contribute. Hence the paradox that *the inflammatory response inside a tumor may help it grow.*

ANGIOGENESIS FACTORS AND INHIBITORS

When Folkman's studies began, polypeptide growth factors were almost unknown except for their forerunner, nerve growth factor. Today so many angiogenesis factors have been purified or otherwise described in so many laboratories that we are puzzled by their abundance (82,225). They have been obtained from tumors, activated macrophages, some classes of lymphocytes (77), platelets, endothelium, from ischemic tissues (89) and from many normal tissues (46)—but not from neutrophils (150). As a result, the original question—what makes angiogenesis start—is now reversed: why is it that blood vessels do *not* grow incessantly? Perhaps the endothelial cells of the capillaries and venules are kept in check by their wrapping of pericytes (p. 369); in mixed cell cultures, the pericytes do inhibit the growth of endothelium (159).

> *In the absence of tissue injury and repair, angiogenesis in the normal adult is minimal. It is part of normal function only in the female; menstruation, ovulation, and placentation are akin to physiologic wounds, which require new capillaries (72). We should add, however, that new capillaries are made whenever we build more tissue, such as adipose tissue by overeating or striated muscle by exercise.*

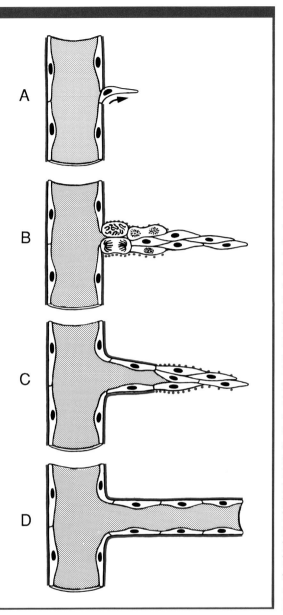

FIGURE 26.56
The basic steps of angiogenesis, originating from venules or capillaries. **A:** Pseudopod from an endothelial cell perforates the basement membrane (red line) and becomes the bridgehead for further growth. **B:** Endothelial cells multiply and a capillary sprout begins to form, surrounded by incomplete basement membrane. **C:** Lumen begins to appear in the sprout. **D:** Mature new blood vessel is formed. (Adapted from [11].)

Several angiogenesis factors are chemically bound by heparin, a property that is exploited for isolating them. There is much heparin in the extracellular matrix, notably in the basement membranes; perhaps angiogenesis factors are stored there, ready for release.

> *Angiogenic molecules include proteins that were already known for other properties: such are the acidic and basic fibroblast growth factors, and VEGF (vascular endothelial growth factor) which was originally described as a tumor-produced vascular permeability-increasing factor (VPF). Others induce "transformation" (p. 727), suggesting that they play a dual role in oncogenesis; such are the transforming growth factors alpha and beta, and the*

fibroblast growth factors, acidic and basic. Tumor necrosis factor alpha (TNFα) has a paradoxical behavior; injected intravenously it causes necrosis of tumors (as the name implies), but injected locally into normal tissues, it helps angiogenesis. Angiogenin, the first angiogenic factor to be sequenced, presents another paradox: it has no effect on endothelial cells growing in vitro; presumably it acts through an intermediary cell. Some prostaglandins are angiogenic, especially E_1 and E_2 (47,119,225).

The angiogenesis story moved a long step forward when it was found that the growth of new vessels depends on a *balance between stimulating and inhibiting factors.* Among the latter the prototype is now *angiostatin,* a small protein that appears in the circulation in the presence of a primary tumor and disappears within 5 days after the tumor is removed (79a,79b). Now we can begin to understand the occasional clinical observations of metastases that regress—or burst into growth—when a primary tumor is removed: the metastases may have been maintained by angiogenin, or held in check by angiostatin, secreted by the primary tumor. Other angiostatic molecules were discovered among proteins that were already well known for other reasons, such as Platelet Factor 4 (PF4) and thrombospondin (79b). All this opens new therapeutic possibilities, and indeed clinical trials are underway to test the anticancer potential of antiangiogenic therapy (79b). Hopes are high, not only from tests on animals, but also because this therapy is not significantly toxic and does not generate drug resistance.

Because many diseases besides tumors involve angiogenesis—such as arthritis, diabetic retinopathy, and psoriasis—work on angiogenesis continues to grow (78). And some day, artificial angiogenesis may help by bringing blood to blood-starved tissues (206).

THE THEORY OF TUMOR INITIATION, PROMOTION, AND PROGRESSION

As soon as it became possible to produce tumors experimentally by means of chemical carcinogens, in particular by painting tar on the back of mice, two facts became apparent: first, carcinogenesis in these models is an extremely slow process; in fact it is one of the slowest biological processes known. The reason is still unclear. Second, carcinogenesis occurs in these models by separate, sudden steps, from a reversible hyperplasia to a benign tumor to a malignant tumor of increasing aggressiveness.

The concept that tumors develop by steps was born in the 1930s, in the laboratory of Peyton Rous at the Rockefeller Institute. Working on rabbit tumors produced by a virus (173) or tar (174), Rous and his co-workers noticed that the path to malignancy was not a continuous slope. At first they obtained hyperplastic lesions that behaved as benign warts or papillomas; but then these papillomas did not become globally more and more atypical until they could be called cancers. Instead, most cancers arose quite suddenly and *only in a part of a papilloma, as a wholly new and different event.*

Intensive work on the multistep theory later produced a dogma: tumor production occurs in two main phases, *initiation* and *promotion,* followed by a relentless, stepwise increase in malignancy called *progression.* (The British oncologist Leslie Foulds who coined the term *progression* in the 1940s meant it to include the whole life history of the tumor; today it is restricted to the terminal phase.)

We will now analyze the multistep dogma. In so doing we will not forget that all biological dogmas must be interpreted with an open mind; in fact, we will have to revise this one before the chapter is closed.

INITIATION AND PROMOTION

A surprising fact had been reported off and on since the 1920s: if the skin of an experimental animal is painted with tar and then biopsied for microscopic study, tumors often arise at the site of the biopsy (137). This phenomenon was studied extensively in the 1940s, again in the laboratory of Peyton Rous. The basic plan was to tar rabbit ears "throughout a period somewhat less than is ordinarily required to elicit growths," and then to wound the ear. The results were clear; wounding was enough to encourage latent neoplastic cells. "The medicolegal bearing of these facts," wrote the authors, "is obvious." The tar had somehow initiated the neoplastic process, and the wound promoted it.

We must note in passing that the medicolegal implications (tumors elicited by trauma on a prepared tissue) did not really materialize. Human tumors following trauma are rare (p. 833).

Then came variations on the theme (20,27,29). The principle of initiation by a subcarcinogenic dose was retained, but wounding as a promoter was replaced with a local irritant; the choice was croton oil (17,153), a dreadfully irritating drug from India that had been used medically for centuries, if not millennia (p. 60). This technique of promotion became more "scientific" when two laboratories, one in Germany, the other in New York, independently isolated the irritating principle of croton oil and named it, respectively, *phorbol myristate acetate* (PMA) and *tetradecanoyl phorbol acetate* (TPA)—the latter name seems to have won over. Many other initiators and promoters were proposed, but the most popular of the promoters remains TPA (Figure 26.57).

Eventually the basic rules of the initiation–promotion routine were worked out; for example, promotion before initiation produces no tumors. The permutations are best explained graphically (Figure 26.58) (27).

What are the cellular and subcellular equivalents of initiation and promotion? This is not clear. The current interpretation is that the birth of a tumor cell requires at least two successive events. First, an initiator strikes the DNA of a cell and introduces a "suitable" defect. (At this point the cell is potentially a cancer cell but is somehow held in check.) Second, a promoter causes the cell to multiply and to generate a tumor, thus revealing the latent curse of the initiated cell. Note, however, the possible hitch: why didn't the DNA-repair enzymes correct the defect? The answer is that they will correct the defect—unless mitosis occurs promptly to make the defect "permanent" (42,68).

It is obvious that initiation and promotion are seen as very different processes:

• *Initiation* is conceived as a quick, almost instantaneous process; if it is repeated, the effect on the tissue is additive. It may take place even in minutes (18), and once it has happened the effect is nearly permanent. In the mouse the effect of initiation may last as long as a year (86). In the long run, however, the effect does wane (182). This should be good news for smokers, who continually initiate their bronchial mucosa. Those who quit can look forward to recovering a safe bronchial mucosa within a few years. Overall, these findings about initiation fit with the notion of an agent that damages DNA. Initiators can be chemical, physical, or biological. They do not cause cell proliferation; in fact, carcinogens in general are (somewhat paradoxically) inhibitors of cell proliferation (68). Initiated cells

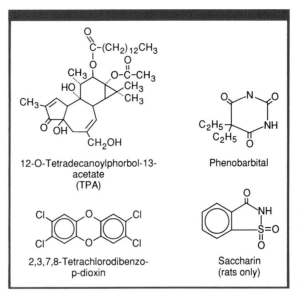

12-O-Tetradecanoylphorbol-13-acetate (TPA)

Phenobarbital

2,3,7,8-Tetrachlorodibenzo-p-dioxin

Saccharin (rats only)

FIGURE 26.57
Chemical structure of some typical tumor promoters. (Adapted from [5].)

are morphologically indistinguishable from normal cells, at least to the present.

• *Promotion* is viewed as a slow process; its effect is reversible and nonadditive. Many promoters cause cells to multiply; in fact, there is some consensus that hyperplasia is a typical effect of promoters (Figure 26.59) (125). However, it is not the only effect; it has been claimed that "most all" promoters (29) eliminate metabolic cooperation be-

■			Tumors
■	PPPPPPP		Tumors
▪	PPPPPPP		Tumors
▪		PPPPPPP	Tumors
▪			No tumors
None	PPPPPPPPPPPPPPPPPPPPPP		No tumors
PPPPPPP ▪			No tumors

■ Initiator, single large dose
▪ Initiator, subcarcinogenic dose
P = Promoter

FIGURE 26.58
Distinction between initiation and promotion. The effect of initiation depends in part on the dose of the initiator. **Large square:** Full carcinogenic dose. **Small square:** Subcarcinogenic dose, e.g. of methylcholanthrene. Each **P** represents one dose of promoter (such as phorbol ester, 2–5 applications per week). The scheme is largely derived from painting carcinogens on the skin of mice; the time is in the range of 1–2 years. (Adapted from [177].)

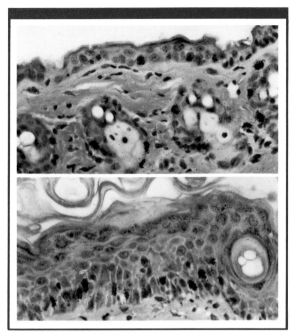

FIGURE 26.59
Demonstrating the hyperplastic effect of a classic tumor promoter, TPA. Histologic sections and autoradiographs of mouse skin. *Top:* Control; mitoses are indicated by clusters of black (silver) grains. *Below:* 48 hours after a local application of 2 micrograms of TPA. Note hyperplasia, increased cornification, and increased number of mitoses. (Courtesy of Dr. A.J.P. Klein-Szanto, Fox Chase Cancer Center, Philadelphia, PA.)

tween adjacent cells by destroying the gap junctions (209). Phorbol esters (the classic tumor promoters) have a vast array of effects. Quite a stir greeted the discovery that TPA activates protein kinase C; this gives TPA the key to a number of intracellular processes (p. 61). Some promoters have a certain degree of organ specificity: for example, saccharin (*in rats*) for the bladder (165,189). For saccharin, the carcinogenic mechanism in rat bladder is now understood (p. 927).

As regards our daily lives, the initiation–promotion theory means that we may be surrounded by "innocent" promoters that can play a nasty role if we have been unknowingly prepared by some toxin, radiation, or other initiating agent. Experimentally, promoters include mitogens as physiologic as hormones (134) and as innocuous as physiologic saline instilled into initiated bronchi (3,135).

All this being said, this neat scheme of initiation–promotion has a major flaw: *most carcinogens are initiators as well as promoters*, and are

therefore known as "complete carcinogens" (29, 165). Another hitch is that promoters alone can also produce a few tumors. These facts did cause some consternation, but many experts today believe that such flaws do not destroy the central dogma (29). However, the time may have come for some rethinking, as we will explain in due course (p. 926).

The original scheme of initiation–promotion was derived largely from experiments using mouse skin as a model. Later, the scheme was used to explain carcinogenesis in rat liver and other organs (164,168,169,182) as well as some human tumors, such as hepatomas (14,167).

> *Refinements on the mechanism of initiation and promotion continue to appear. Although inflammation is a major effect of TPA, inflammation itself does not seem to be a promoting agent (182). Another point of view holds that promoters induce cells to generate free radicals, which damage the DNA molecule (37,140). It has also been suggested that promotion includes two steps (19,28,29,88): (a) derepression, which would act at the level of a regulator gene and thus enable the cell to multiply, and (b) progression toward malignancy, involving membrane and cytoplasmic phenomena (19). This model would explain some benign tumors; they would be the result of derepression without progression.*

TUMOR PROGRESSION

Once malignant tumors have started to grow, they tend to "go from bad to worse": this is how Rous and Kidd described in 1941 what is now called *tumor progression* (174).

The likeliest mechanism of progression is what P.C. Nowell called the "genetic instability" of the neoplastic cell (157,158). This defect favors such accidents as chromosomal breaks and translocations that result in the appearance of new clones; and the selective survival of the most aggressive clones depends in part on evolutionary pressures due to the host's immune response and to chemotherapy. The overall result is clinically apparent as a trend toward an increased rate of growth, increased invasiveness and metastatization, reduce sensitivity to drugs and hormones, decreased antigenicity, decreased radiosensitivity, and so on.

It follows that malignant tumors and their metastases must be conceived as progressing toward an ever-increasing polyclonality. On rare occasions this evolution can be appreciated with the naked eye; a heavily pigmented melanoma may produce nonpigmented metastases, or a hepatoma may produce metastases that are greenish because they can still produce bile, as well as pale ones that have lost that ability.

The mechanisms of progression are beginning to be understood (pp. 885–886).

An interesting theory is that stability genes are involved; this would fit with the fact that chromosome instability syndromes exist (213). Another mechanism: Some tumor cells amplify the genes that relate to drug resistance; in fact they may amplify them so much that the pertinent chromosome may be visibly elongated (p. 873) (179). The secretion of growth factors can be switched from inducible to constitutive (178). The ability to induce angiogenesis seems to parallel neoplastic progression (226). Microscopically, with immunohistochemical methods, the overexpression of certain genes can be recognized: for example, Type IV collagenase and laminin, which are involved in metastatization (p. 799) (53).

Could cell fusion be involved in progression? The proponent of this somewhat heretical concept argues that the fusion of tumor cells with normal host cells appears to occur in vivo (p. 450). In vitro this fusion usually leads to loss of malignant properties, but under certain circumstances it may also produce increased malignancy (48).

After having read, a few pages back, that most tumors are born monoclonal, the notion that established malignant tumors are found to be typically polyclonal may seem to be something of a paradox. As a matter of fact, this concept was not easily accepted; in 1977 it was considered so outlandish that a manuscript proposing it was refused by a journal. The authors eventually won the battle; one of their arguments was that, after all, they themselves (just as the referees) were polyclonal creatures that had progressed from monoclonal beginnings (108).

The heterogeneity of tumor cell populations has major clinical implications. It means, for example, that tumors should be treated as early as possible, when their population is most homogeneous; drugs should be varied to discourage the development of specific drug resistance; and drugs given jointly should be chosen among those that induce different mechanisms of drug resistance—such as enhanced repair of DNA damage versus decreased transport across the cell membrane (181).

AFTERTHOUGHTS ON TUMOR INITIATION, PROMOTION, AND PROGRESSION

The view that carcinogenesis is a multistep process is not disputed; there is only one known exception: some retroviruses, such as the Rous sarcoma virus, can transform cells within one cell cycle (69). Multistep carcinogenesis fits well, for example, with liver tumors (69,70), melanomas (109), and carcinomas of the colon and rectum (118). Tumor progression is unfortunately an everyday reality in tumor wards. We must remember, however, that manmade schemes rarely explain all the facts of any biological event. The initiation-promotion scheme is no exception; it has flaws, which we will examine later (p. 926).

One unsolved problem is the role of the benign-tumor stage before the appearance of a malignancy. In most experimental tumors (especially skin tumors) a benign stage is evident; however, in some cases a carcinoma seems to appear directly from "normal" epidermis without an intermediate stage of papilloma (86); is this simply an accelerated variant of the usual scheme? In humans, a stepwise evolution of melanomas is sometimes seen (109); in other species the malignancy seems to strike out of the blue, without benign precursors (172). Indeed, many researchers still believe that most human cancers develop without a benign precursor. However, this may be due to our own inadequate observation; by the time an inner cancer is recognized, it may have erased its benign precursor, as happens with colonic polyps. When more facts are available, it may turn out that most human malignant tumors do indeed have benign precursors. We will return to this theme in relation to precancerous lesions (p. 879).

HOW FAST DO TUMORS GROW?

The rate of tumor growth is a question of great practical importance because most anticancer treatments now available suppress cell proliferation. Therefore, while we wait for more specific and really *anticancer* drugs (as opposed to antiproliferative drugs), therapy remains centered around the kinetics of tumor cell division. This is, incidentally, an area in which mathematics has contributed to biological understanding.

VOLUME DOUBLING TIME

The volume doubling time of a whole tumor is easily measured in mice; for transplanted tumors it is of the order of 1–5 days (204). For human tumors, it is convenient to remember a number that is 30 times greater: 1–5 months (Table 26.2). The record for short doubling time probably belongs to a mouse carcinoma called Ehrlich ascites tumor; when this tumor is seeded into the

TABLE 26.2

Doubling Times of Human Tumors (reported from six sources)

SITE	NUMBER OF MEASUREMENTS	MEDIAN VOLUME-DOUBLING TIME (DAYS)	RANGE (DAYS)
Lung metastases	86	40	4–745
Lung metastases	24	40	11–164
Lung metastases from colon or rectum	25	96	34–210
Primary bronchial carcinomas	22	105	27–480
Primary bronchial carcinomas	12	62	17–200
Primary skeletal sarcomas	6	75	21–366

Adapted from (191).

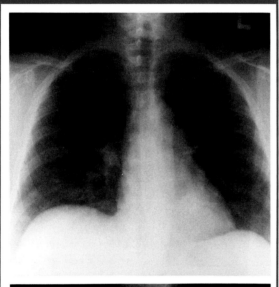
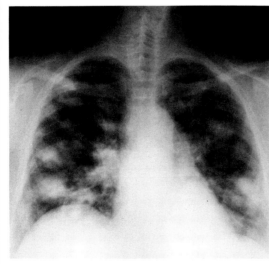

FIGURE 26.60 The growth of metastases in the lung can be exceedingly rapid: These two X-rays were taken only 43 days apart. Undifferentiated carcinoma of the ovary. (Courtesy of Dr. A. Davidoff, University of Massachusetts Medical Center, Worcester, MA.)

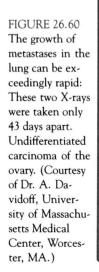

peritoneum, its cell population doubles in 21 hours (22). Nobody knows why tumors grow so fast in mice (p. 928).

The actual doubling times reported for humans are of the order of 50–100 days, with extremes of 1 week and 1 year (113,191). Note that we are referring to volumes, not diameters. Tumors that are highly sensitive to chemo- or radiotherapy are also those that grow fastest—which makes sense because both properties depend on a high mitotic rate. Data for human tumors have been difficult to obtain because the results can be affected by treatment. Most of the figures available were obtained by studying serial X-rays of primary and metastatic tumors of the lung, but keep in mind that metastases tend to grow faster than the primary tumor (Figure 26.60).

THE GOMPERTZIAN CURVE

The doubling times reported are in a sense misleading because the rate of growth of a tumor changes throughout its life. Until 1964, tumor growth rates offered a confusing picture. It was found that some tumors seemed to grow exponentially, like young bacterial cultures; but applying this exponential curve to certain slowly growing tumors led to the absurd conclusion that the tumors had started before conception (143). Clearly something was wrong with the measurements, or with the assumptions. A breakthrough came when Anna Laird of the Argonne National Laboratory found that *tumor growth is an exponential process that is limited by an exponential retardation*; this function was defined by the mathematician Benjamin Gompertz (1779–1865) (90) and is now widely known as the Gompertzian curve (130,131). Interestingly, this curve also describes the rate of growth of the human fetus (143,187) (Figure 26.61). In simple terms: tumor growth is fast at the outset, then it declines.

Why so?

In the fetus, the retarding force is probably differentiation (187). In tumors, it must be the decrease in blood supply relative to size; the tumor grows faster than the vessels. The respective growth rates of capillary endothelium and tumor cells have actually been compared in a mouse tumor. They show that as capillary growth falls behind, the mean intercapillary distance increases, whereby many tumor cells should become anoxic as well as starved and should die (201).

Now see the tangible implications of the Gompertzian curve. It has long been known that a tumor, starting from a cell about 10 μm in diameter, takes 30 doublings to reach a mass of roughly 1 g and another 10 doublings to reach 1 kg (40), a figure often quoted as the upper limit of the "tumor burden" that is compatible with life. This means that when we discover a tumor about 1 cm in diameter—an early tumor by clinical standards—it is indeed a small tumor; but *most of its growth in terms of cell doublings has already occurred.* It is high on the Gompertzian curve, and its cells are no longer multiplying very fast; for this reason the most propitious time for anticancer therapy has already gone by (Figure 26.62). Interestingly, if a few cells are taken from a tumor at an advanced stage of growth and implanted elsewhere, they start a new tumor that resumes growth according to a new Gompertzian curve (193).

The Gompertzian curve has also blown apart a dangerous myth: an overoptimistic idea (which we used to teach) that tumors, when discovered clinically, had been there for 10–20 years and that therefore there was no great urgency to remove them. Now it seems likely that most tumors detected clinically have developed in 2 years or less (193).

NUMBER OF REPLICATING CELLS

The study of tumor growth at the cellular level (as opposed to the tissue level) probes deeper into the biology of the tumor. The key is to measure the number of replicating cells, which can be done in several ways. The basic result is that *tumor cells grow—in general—more slowly than their normal counterparts* (12).

There are four standard methods for measuring cell growth in tumors.

- *Counting mitoses in histologic sections.* This procedure, when applied to experimental

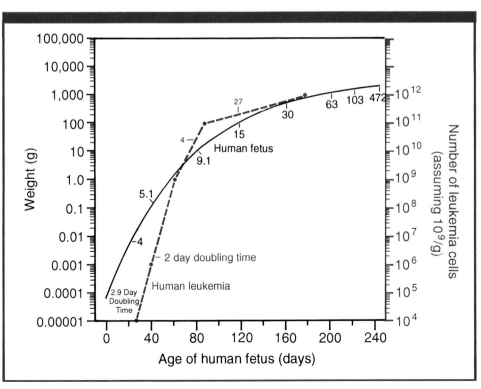

FIGURE 26.61
Demonstrating that the growth curve of tumor tissue (in this study, human leukemia) approaches the growth curve of the human fetus. In either case, the curve fits the so-called Gompertzian equation. (Adapted from [187].)

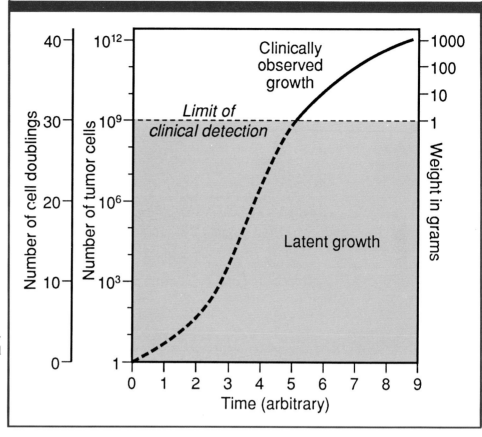

FIGURE 26.62
A depressing curve. To reach a palpable size (1 g), a tumor requires 30 cell doublings; only 10 more doublings are needed to reach one kilogram. Skin tumors are an exception: They can be detected well before they weigh 1 g. (Adapted from [204].)

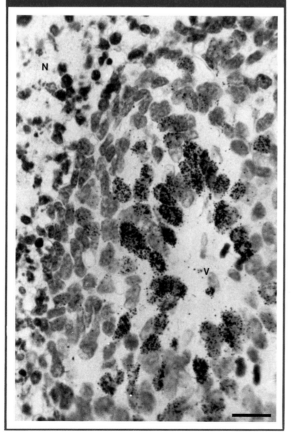

FIGURE 26.63
Autoradiograph from a malignant tumor labeled with thymidine; note the intense labeling adjacent to a blood vessel (**V**). This particular tumor, a mouse adenocarcinoma, contained regions of necrosis (**N**) through which ran cords of viable tissue such as the one shown here in cross section. **Bar** = 25 μm. (Reproduced with permission from [199].)

tumors, is easier if the animal is injected with a microtubular poison such as colchicine, which stops all mitoses in metaphase (p. 155). The percentage of cells in mitosis then provides the *mitotic index*.

- *Histochemical demonstration of dividing cells*, using antibodies against cell-cycle related proteins, such as cyclin (104).
- *Radioactive labeling of dividing cells* in vivo. A tumor-bearing animal is injected with tritiated thymidine, which is incorporated into the DNA of cells preparing to divide. Microscopic sections of the tumor are then overlaid with an X-ray emulsion, whereby autoradiographs are produced: silver grains develop over each dividing cell (Figure 26.63). The percentage of labeled cells found in this manner is the *labeling index*.
- *By the cell-sorter* (p. 15), which can be loaded with a suspension of tumor cells treated with a DNA stain and then instructed to count those that are in the S-phase of the cell cycle.

On histologic sections, the labeling method is more sensitive and more accurate than the mitotic

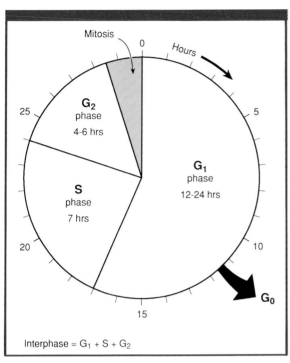

FIGURE 26.64

The cell cycle, shown here as requiring about 30 hours. This duration applies to most normal human cells but may not be applicable to abnormal cells. The G_1-phase corresponds to synthesis of enzymes and of "luxury proteins," the S-phase to replication of chromosomes (DNA and associated proteins), and the G_2-phase to synthesis of proteins for the spindle and mitotic apparatus. Cells may also escape into G_0 and become quiescent or "out of cycle." (Adapted from [180].)

count because labeled cells are easier to identify than mitoses. Labeled cells are also more numerous because the DNA synthesis (S-phase) of the cell cycle lasts much longer than mitosis. Furthermore, counting mitoses can be misleading. Suppose that the mitoses in a given tumor were normal in number but lasted twice as long as in the control tissue; the net result would be a doubling of the visible mitoses, which could falsely suggest an increased mitotic rate (12).

For tumors in rodents the percentage of replicating cells, as shown by the labeling index, is in the range of 2–8 percent. In human tumors the same index is generally lower than 10 percent, and lower than in normal epithelia such as the lining of the intestinal mucosa (index about 16 percent) (204). As to the cell cycle (Figure 26.64), studies available on human tumors also show times longer than normal: 20 hours for leukemias, 60 hours for superficial solid tumors (Table 26.3) (204). All this goes to say that cell replication inside a tumor (with a few exceptions) is far from a frenzy. It is

actually depressed but, unfortunately, not depressed enough.

CELL LOSS

Despite what we just said, the apparent slow growth of most tumors has little to do with the duration of the cell cycle: cell loss is a major factor. Plain histology shows that some areas of tumors are necrotic due to poor blood supply, and dead cells are scattered through the tumor. *A tumor grows because there is an excess of cell production over cell loss* (Figure 26.65). A small fraction of the cell loss is due to cells leaving the tumor via the blood vessels. The overall cell loss varies greatly but can be estimated: knowing (by experiment) the cycling time of the cells in a given tumor and the labeling index, it is possible to calculate the *theoretical* doubling time of the tumor. The *actual* doubling time is shorter. From the difference one can estimate the amount of cell loss, which can be of the order of 50 percent or more (191).

Whereas some cells are physically lost to tumor growth (by death or by metastatization), other cells are lost functionally, either because they have differentiated to a nonreplicating stage or because they are somehow mitotically impaired. It follows that, in terms of cell replication, tumors contain four populations of neoplastic cells (Figure 26.66) (187): population A, cycling cells; population B, cells that can be recruited into cycling but are

TABLE 26.3

Cell-Cycle Times of Various Normal Tissues and Tumors in Humans

Tissue	Cell-Cycle Time (hour)
Bone-marrow precursor cells	18
Colon, epithelium of crypt cells	39
Rectum, epithelium of crypt cells	48
Bronchus, epithelial cells	220
Carcinoma of stomach	72
Acute myeloblastic leukemia	80–84
Chronic myeloid leukemia	120
Carcinoma of bronchus	196–260

Adapted from (12).

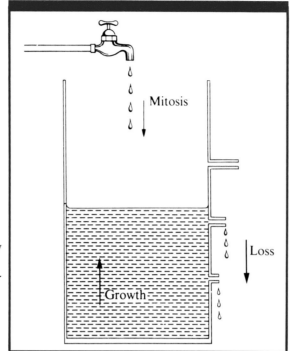

FIGURE 26.65
Simplified diagram showing that tumors grow by an imbalance between cell production and cell loss. (Reproduced with permission from [192].)

kill off the cells in population A and then move as many cells as possible from B to A. An empirical but effective way to do this is to reduce the mass of the tumor, a procedure known in surgery as "debulking." Somehow debulking prods the noncycling cells into a spurt of growth, and while they are cycling, they become targets for another therapeutic attack (193).

Growth of tumor cells can be inhibited by contact with normal cells, at least *in vitro* (24,145). We have already mentioned this curious phenomenon in relation to cell-to-cell communications (p. 735); for the time being it is an intriguing curiosity worthy of more study.

TO SUM UP: the popular image of a tumor tends to be that of a monstrous creature that grows unrestrained. This is a myth. Tumors grow fast enough to kill, but their growth is fraught with obstacles.

temporarily quiescent (at the G_o stage); population C, cells that are permanently unable to divide (e.g., because they have differentiated); and population D, dead and dying cells.

The existence of differing cell populations in a tumor is a key for planning therapeutic strategies. Population A is the main target of anticancer agents because they are most effective against cycling cells; therefore, the ideal procedure is to

Life Inside a Tumor

Tumor cells have to live and grow in their own self-made environment: an untidy assembly of connective tissue and vessels that they have extorted from the host but not properly planned. It turns out to be a hostile environment: like that of some fast-growing cities, it is haphazard, polluted, and lacking in services. Oncologists, whose aim is to wipe out its inhabitants, exploit these environmental faults as best they can.

What life must be like for the cells of a malignant tumor we can but dimly perceive. Most of their neighbors are other malignant cells; this means competition for scarce nutrients, but also a free supply of paracrine growth factors. Because a tumor's vessels are leaky, the surrounding milieu is rather similar to an inflammatory exudate, and some of the surrounding cells are in fact inflammatory cells.

INFLAMMATION IN TUMORS

Summoned by chemotactic messages, a variety of host cells migrate into the tumor. They include natural killer cells as well as T- and B-lymphocytes, all of which are potential enemies to the tumor cells. Many of the blood-derived cells, however, are macrophages, which are drawn into the tumor by specific mononuclear chemotactic proteins (MCP) of the chemokine family, secreted by the tumor

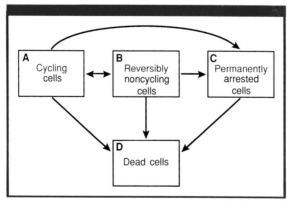

FIGURE 26.66
The neoplastic cells of a tumor belong to four growth populations (**A, B, C, D**). The purpose of current cancer therapy is to move the tumor cells from **B** to **A**, because chemotherapeutic agents are most effective against cycling cells. (Adapted from [193].)

itself (139a). How many macrophages? Counts in rodent tumors yielded numbers averaging 10–30 percent of the cell population within the tumor (67,197). What the macrophages contribute probably varies from one tumor to another. On the one hand, they are equipped to initiate an immune response against the tumor, and if activated they may even kill tumor cells; on the other hand, they may attract blood vessels and thereby do the tumor a favor (remember that anoxic macrophages stimulate angiogenesis). In essence, the macrophages establish with the tumor an ambivalent symbiotic relationship, a "macrophage balance" which may tip either way (139a). We should not forget that macrophages can also scavenge necrotic tumor cells, although this task is overwhelming when massive necrosis occurs. Indeed, the inflammatory response within the tumor is usually poor; true granulation tissue rarely if ever develops around a necrotic mass. Experiments on tumors of rats and mice have shown that a cotton thread placed in tumor tissue elicits a minimal response compared with that of normal tissues (139). True, some types of human tumors do elicit a hefty inflammatory (immune) response, but they are the exception; some tumors actually depress the inflammatory response (p. 810).

Tumor cells produce a variety of molecules that cause vascular leakage without necessarily inducing an inflammatory response (Figure 26.67) (33,56). For example, if a suspension of tumor cells is injected subcutaneously into an experimental animal, within hours the cells become embedded in a gel of fibrin. This means that fibrinogen leaked out of the vessels and then clotted, presumably as a result of a tumor procoagulant activity. What this fibrin "cocoon" may mean to the tumor cell, however, is not certain because tumor cells can also induce fibrinolysis.

THE INTERNAL MILIEU OF TUMORS

The basic data on the aqueous internal environment of tumors, their **internal milieu,** were obtained by P.M. Gullino and co-workers by means of a small plastic chamber permanently implanted into an experimental tumor (Figure 26.68); interestingly, no granulation tissue developed around the sampling device (99), confirming the inadequate inflammatory response within tumor tissue. These and later studies showed that the medium in which the tumor cells live is quite pathologic (99). Although derived basically from

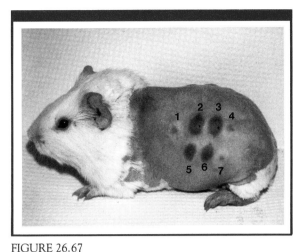

FIGURE 26.67
Evans blue test demonstrating vascular permeability factors (VPF) produced by an ascites tumor. The seven skin sites of this otherwise normal guinea pig were injected with 1: Antibody against VPF (control, negative); 2: VPF from Line 10 ascites tumor (strongly positive); 3: VPF plus an unrelated antibody (strongly positive); 4: VPF plus specific neutralizing antibody (negative, neutralized); 5: VPF from a different ascites tumor (Line 1) (strongly positive); 6: VPF plus unrelated antibody (strongly positive); 7: VPF plus specific antibody, again showing neutralization of the VPF factor. (Courtesy of Drs. D.R. Sanger and H.F. Dvorak, Department of Pathology, Beth Israel Hospital, Boston, MA.)

plasma, the medium is almost free of glucose (100) and is polluted with enzymes released from dead cells; it may therefore act as a tenderizer, dissociating the live tumor cells and thereby perhaps helping invasion (p. 796). It is also acid, in the

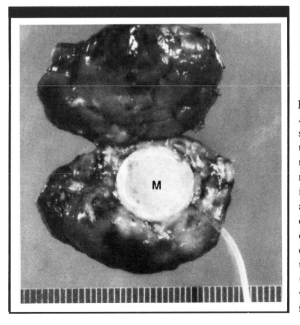

FIGURE 26.68
A method for studying the internal milieu of a tumor: A carcinoma of the rat is grown around a micropore chamber (**M**) equipped with a draining catheter. Scale in mm. (Reproduced with permission from [101].)

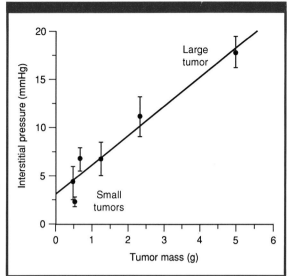

FIGURE 26.69
Values of tissue pressure measured in the center of mouse transplantable tumors (Walker 256 carcinoma). (Adapted from [26].)

range of pH 6.7–7.0 (99,212), and in many parts hypoxic due to the poor distribution of blood vessels (116).

Another peculiarity of this acid fluid is that it flows as a slow current toward the tumor's surface. The genesis of this current is twofold: lack of lymphatics, and leaky blood vessels.

LYMPHATICS ARE MISSING

Absence of lymphatic drainage is a basic problem of tumor tissue. Tumors can induce hemangiogenesis, but, somehow, lymphangiogenesis does not occur; so we can look at tumors as an experiment of nature to show what happens when lymphatics are missing. What does happen, as might be guessed, is that the fluid seeping out of the capillaries and venules into a confined environment distends the tissue spaces and raises the tissue pressure. In most normal tissues, the pressure is negative (p. 597). In tumors, especially the larger ones, tissue pressure is positive (36,99,111,114,117); the highest pressure is in the center (13,116b,117), where it can be as much as 30 mm Hg (Figure 26.69), even 45 mm in human melanomas (116). Due to the high tissue pressure, blood flow in the centers of the tumor is impaired (116a). This phenomenon is surely related to the typical central necrosis of malignant tumors, which is usually and rather glibly explained by stating that "tumors outgrow their vessels." Perhaps they do, but this is not the only mechanism of necrosis. The poor blood flow also helps explain the whiteness of most tumors when they are cut open (p. 741) (102).

BLOOD VESSELS ARE LEAKY

The source of the fluid that oozes from the tumor is, of course, the microcirculation: many vessels—as we have seen—are leaky. The amount of this fluid is considerable. A porous chamber inserted into an experimental tumor drains 4–5 times as much fluid as one inserted into normal skin (36). Obviously, this fluid has to go somewhere. In fact, the interstitial fluid inside a tumor continues to move toward the surface at a velocity calculated at 6–12 μm per minute, and it then drains out into the surroundings at the respectable rate of about 0.2 ml per hour per gram of tissue, as measured in a rat carcinoma (36,115).

These simple facts of hydraulics mean a lot to the oncologist (116a,116b). Because flow in the center of the tumor is poor (as well as uneven), chemotherapeutic agents have to diffuse into that zone from the well-perfused outer shell; but this diffusion is opposed by the outward convection (Figure 26.70) (13,116). This convection also flushes out any autocrine chemoattractants that the tumor may secrete (p. 797), with the result

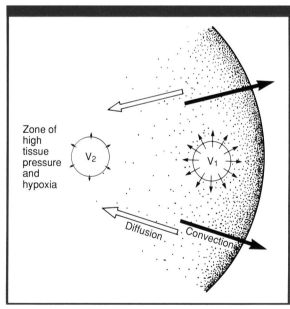

FIGURE 26.70
Schematic cross section of a tumor illustrating some aspects of tumor fluid dynamics. Interstitial pressure is assumed to decrease from the center to the periphery. The two circles (V_1 and V_2) represent microscopic vessels; **arrows** emerging from the vessels indicate filtration pressure. The pressure gradient leads to a radial, outward convection (**black arrows**), which opposes the radial, inward diffusion (**open arrows**). In the center of the tumor, the interstitial pressure being higher, the microvascular transudation of fluid and of macromolecules (**small dots**) is lower. (Adapted from [117].)

that mobile or mobilized tumor cells are attracted outward (this, however, is pure speculation).

> Brain tumors *should offer a special opportunity to study the oozing phenomenon because the lack of lymphatics in the brain itself should trap the edema fluid around the tumor. The topic is complicated by the blood–brain barrier, which is usually (but capriciously) incomplete in primary brain tumors. Edema of the white matter around a glioma is common; around meningiomas it is "classic" (176). This topic needs further study.*

The loss of plasma from the vessels into the tumor raises the intravascular hematocrit, which impairs flow by raising the viscosity of the blood (184). Other factors also conspire to increase the viscosity: sluggish flow favors the aggregation of red blood cells into rouleaux (p. 493), and the acidic tumor environment increases the rigidity of red blood cells (p. 667) (114).

HYPOXIA

Hypoxia threatens any tumor cell that moves too far away from the blood vessel(s). We will call this "hypoxia" to go along with current terminology, but actually cells that are too far from the blood supply suffer from lack of oxygen, lack of substrates, and loss of waste removal—that is, from ischemia. The critical distance is of the order of 100 μm; in one pioneer study no tumor cell was found alive at 180 μm distance from a vessel (205).

Tumor Cords The effects of ischemia are best studied, quantitatively, in some fast-growing tumors (mostly epithelial) that develop in the shape of cords. Each cord is made of a capillary surrounded by a sleeve of tumor cells. The reverse pattern is also possible: a cord of tumor cells surrounded by capillaries. In either case, mitoses occur close to the blood vessel(s) and decrease centrifugally, which means that there is a constant displacement of cells from the vascular core toward the necrotic never-never land (Figure 26.71) (192,199).

> *The radius of the cord depends on the partial pressure of oxygen, the diameter of the vessel, the coefficient*

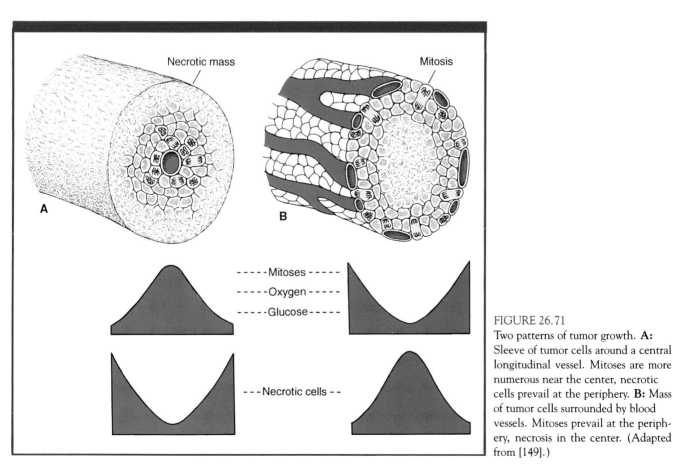

FIGURE 26.71
Two patterns of tumor growth. **A:** Sleeve of tumor cells around a central longitudinal vessel. Mitoses are more numerous near the center, necrotic cells prevail at the periphery. **B:** Mass of tumor cells surrounded by blood vessels. Mitoses prevail at the periphery, necrosis in the center. (Adapted from [149].)

of diffusion of oxygen, and the rate of oxygen consumption by the tumor cells. It was found to be 98.7 ± 11.9 μm in retinoblastomas and 104 μm in squamous cell carcinomas. The cord pattern, prevalent in retinoblastomas, occurs also in other tumors, such as squamous cell carcinomas of the lung (34 percent) and of the cervix (14 percent) (34).

This pathophysiology of tumor cords has practical consequences because most tumor therapies are cell-cycle dependent; therefore, they hit the cycling perivascular cells but tend to spare those beyond, which are alive but anoxic and not cycling. As the perivascular cells are killed by the treatment and disappear, their places in the cord are taken by the noncycling cells that have survived the "cure." Now these newcomers, having moved closer to the capillary, have a second chance to grow—and therefore to be hit by the next dose of therapy (202).

How do the necrotic tumor cells disappear? Do they all disappear? Do they completely disappear? This is not clear. All malignant tumors contain macrophages (220), but it is obvious that there are not enough macrophages around to phagocytize the whole necrotic mass. Our impression is that dead tumor cells undergo a combination of autolysis and denaturation, whereby a part of the mass shrivels away. This would explain the depressed surface of subcapsular tumor metastases in the liver (p. 000).

The growth of tumors has a lot to do with hypoxia. Because hypoxia is a typical "accident" in the life of a cell, we would expect hypoxic tumor cells to die by the mechanism typical of accidental cell death as seen in infarcts, namely with swelling (oncosis). Oddly enough, many hypoxic tumor cells die by suicide (apoptosis); as a result, hypoxia selects for survival those tumor cells that are *less* apt to commit suicide—thereby favoring the progression of the tumor toward ever greater malignancy. We shall return to this topic in discussing oncogenes.

Hypoxia poses another challenge for the oncologists: it makes the cells more resistant to radiation. It takes 2–3 times the normal dose of radiation to kill them compared with well-oxygenated cells (41); remember that the mechanism of cell killing by X-rays depends in part on the formation of *oxygen-derived* free radicals. Solving such problems requires a close collaboration between cell biologist, pathologist, and oncologist.

In summary, to understand a tumor one has to understand not only the tumor cells themselves but also the peculiar milieu in which they live. It is regrettable that this "hostile" microenvironment (211) is not sufficiently hostile to kill the tumor altogether.

References

1. Acker H, Carlsson J, Durand R, Sutherland RM, eds. Spheroids in cancer research. Recent results in cancer research, vol 95. Berlin: Springer-Verlag, 1984.
2. Ahmed A. Calcification in human breast carcinomas: ultrastructural observations. J Pathol 1975;117:247–251.
3. Akaza H, Murphy WM, Soloway MS. Bladder cancer induced by noncarcinogenic substances. J Urol 1984; 131:152–155.
4. Algire GH, Chalkley HW. Vascular reactions of normal and malignant tissues in vivo. I. Vascular reactions of mice to wounds and to normal and neoplastic transplants. J Natl Cancer Inst 1945;6:73–85.
5. Archer MC. Chemical carcinogenesis. In: Tannock IF, Hill RP, eds. The basic science of oncology. New York: Pergamon Press, 1987:89–105.
6. Armed Forces Institute of Pathology. Atlas of tumor pathology, 2nd series, fasc 1. Washington, DC: Universities Associated for Research and Education in Pathology, Inc, 1967.
7. Ausprunk DH, Falterman K, Foldman J. The sequence of events in the regression of corneal capillaries. Lab Invest 1978;38:284–294.
8. Bainton DF, Friedlander LM, Shohet SB. Abnormalities in granule formation in acute myelogenous leukemia. Blood 1977;49:693–704.
9. Baird A, Mormède P, Böhlen P. Immunoreactive fibro-

blast growth factor (FGF) in a transplantable chondrosarcoma: inhibition of tumor growth by antibodies to FGF. J Cell Biochem 1986;30:79–85.
10. Barker BE, Sanford KK. Cytologic manifestations of neoplastic transformation *in vitro*. J Natl Cancer Inst 1970;44:39–63.
11. Barnhill RL, Wolf JE Jr. Angiogenesis and the skin. J Am Acad Dermatol 1987;16:1226–1242.
12. Baserga R. The cell cycle. N Engl J Med 1981;304:453–459.
13. Baxter LT, Jain RK. Transport of fluid and macromolecules in tumors. I. Role of interstitial pressure and convection. Microvasc Res 1989;37:77–104.
14. Becker FF. Hepatoma—nature's model tumor. A review. Am J Pathol 1974;74:179–200.
15. Ben-Bassat H, Inbar M, Sachs L. Changes in the structural organization of the surface membrane in malignant cell transformation. J Membrane Biol 1971;6:183–194.
16. Ben-Ze'ev A. The cytoskeleton in cancer cells. Biochim Biophys Acta 1985;780:197–212.
17. Berenblum I. The cocarcinogenic action of croton resin. Cancer Res 1941;1:44–48.
18. Berenblum I. Sequential aspects of chemical carcinogenesis: skin. In: Becker FF, ed. Cancer. A comprehensive treatise, vol 1. New York: Plenum Press, 1975: 323–344.

19. Berenblum I, Armuth V. Two independent aspects of tumor promotion. Biochim Biophys Acta 1981;651: 51–63.
20. Berenblum I, Shubik P. A new, quantitative approach to the study of the stages of chemical carcinogenesis in the mouse's skin. Br J Cancer 1947;1:383–391.
21. Bernal SD, Lampidis TJ, McIsaac RM, Chen LB. Anticarcinoma activity in vivo of rhodamine 123, a mitochondrial-specific dye. Science 1983;222:169–172.
22. Bertalanffy FD, Schachter R, Ali J, Ingimundson JC. Mitotic rate and doubling time of intraperitoneal and subcutaneous Ehrlich ascites tumor. Cancer Res 1965; 25:685–691.
23. Berthezene F, Greer MA. Studies on the composition of the thyroid psammoma bodies of chronically iodine-deficient rats. Endocrinology 1974;95:651–659.
24. Bertram JS, Faletto MB. Requirements for and kinetics of growth arrest of neoplastic cells by confluent 10T½ fibroblasts induced by a specific inhibitor of cyclic adenosine 3':5'-phosphodiesterase. Cancer Res 1985;45: 1946–1952.
25. Black PH. Shedding from the cell surface of normal and cancer cells. Adv Cancer Res 1980;32:75–199.
26. Boucher Y, Baxter LT, Jain RK. Interstitial pressure gradients in tissue-isolated and subcutaneous tumors: implications for therapy. Cancer Res 1990;50:4478–4484.
27. Boutwell RK. Some biological aspects of skin carcinogenesis. Prog Exp Tumor Res 1964;4:207–250.
28. Boutwell RK. The function and mechanism of promoters of carcinogenesis. CRC Crit Rev Toxicol 1974;2:419–443.
29. Boutwell RK. Tumor promoters in human carcinogenesis. In: DeVita VT, Hellman S, Rosenberg SA, eds. Important advances in oncology 1985. Philadelphia: JB Lippincott, 1985:16–27.
30. Bowen ID. Laboratory techniques for demonstrating cell death. In: Davies I, Sigee DC, eds. Cell ageing and cell death. Cambridge: Cambridge University Press, 1984:5–40.
31. Bowen ID, Bowen SM. Programmed cell death in tumours and tissues. London: Chapman and Hall, 1990.
32. Brem H, Folkman J. Inhibition of tumor angiogenesis mediated by cartilage. J Exp Med 1975;141:427–439.
33. Brown LF, Berse B, Jackman RW, et al. Increased expression of vascular permeability factor (vascular endothelial growth factor) and its receptors in kidney and bladder carcinomas. Am J Pathol 1993;143:1255–1262.
34. Burnier MN, McLean IW, Zimmerman LE, Rosenberg SH. Retinoblastoma. The relationship of proliferating cells to blood vessels. Invest Ophthalmol Vis Sci 1990;31:2037–2040.
35. Butler TP, Grantham FH, Gullino PM. Bulk transfer of fluid in the interstitial compartment of mammary tumors. Cancer Res 1975;35:3084–3088.
36. Butler TP, Gullino PM. Quantitation of cell shedding into efferent blood of mammary adenocarcinoma. Cancer Res 1975;35:512–516.
37. Cerutti PA, Amstad P, Emerit I. Tumor promoter phorbol-myristate-acetate induces membrane-mediated chromosomal damage. In: Nygaard OF, Simic MG, eds. Radioprotectors and anticarcinogens. New York: Academic Press, 1983:527–538.
38. Chen LB, Rivers EN. Mitochondria in cancer cells. In: Carney D, Sikora K, eds. Genes and cancer. Chichester: John Wiley & Sons, 1990:127–135.
39. Cohnheim J. Lectures on general pathology. Section II: the pathology of nutrition. London: The New Sydenham Society, 1889.
40. Collins VP, Loeffler RK, Tivey H. Observations on

growth rates of human tumors. Am J Roentgenol 1956;76:988–1000.
41. Coleman CN. Hypoxia in tumors: a paradigm for the approach to biochemical and physiologic heterogeneity. J Natl Cancer Inst 1988;80:310–317.
42. Columbano A, Rajalakshmi S, Sarma DSR. Requirement of cell proliferation for the initiation of liver carcinogenesis as assayed by three different procedures. Cancer Res 1981;41:2079–2083.
43. Coman DR. Decreased mutual adhesiveness, a property of cells from squamous cell carcinomas. Cancer Res 1944; 4:625–629.
44. Condamine H, Custer RP, Mintz B. Pure-strain and genetically mosaic liver tumors histochemically identified with the ß-glucuronidase marker in allophenic mice. Proc Natl Acad Sci USA 1971;68:2032–2036.
45. Cramer SF, Meyer JS, Kraner JF, Camel M, Mazur MT, Tenenbaum MS. Metastasizing leiomyoma of the uterus. S-phase fraction, estrogen receptor, and ultrastructure. Cancer 1980;45:932–937.
46. D'Amore PA. Growth factors, angiogenesis and metastasis. Prog Clin Biol Res 1986;212:269–283.
47. D'Amore PA, Thompson RW. Mechanisms of angiogenesis. Annu Rev Physiol 1987;49:453–464.
48. De Baetselier P. Neoplastic progression by somatic cell fusion. In: Liotta LA, ed. Influence of tumor development on the host. Dordrecht: Kluwer Academic Publishers, 1989:112–120.
49. Denekamp J. Vascular endothelium as the vulnerable element in tumours. Acta Radiol Oncol 1984;23:217–225.
50. Denekamp J, Hobson B. Endothelial-cell proliferation in experimental tumours. Br J Cancer 1982;46:711–720.
51. Derenzini M, Pession A, Trerè D. Quantity of nucleolar silver-stained proteins is related to proliferating activity in cancer cells. Lab Invest 1990;63:137–140.
52. Derenzini M, Ploton D. Interphase nucleolar organizer regions in cancer cells. Int Rev Exp Pathol 1991;32:149–192.
53. D'Errico A, Garbisa S, Liotta LA, Castronovo V, Stetler-Stevenson WG, Grigioni WF. Augmentation of type IV collagenase, laminin receptor, and Ki67 proliferation antigen associated with human colon, gastric, and breast carcinoma progression. Mod Pathol 1991;4:239–246.
54. Domagala W, Koss LG. Configuration of surfaces of human cancer cells in effusions. A scanning electron microscopic study of microvilli. Virchows Arch B [Cell Pathol] 1977;26:27–42.
55. Durand RE. Multicell spheroids as a model for cell kinetic studies. Cell Tissue Kinet 1990;23:141–159.
55a. Dvorak HF, Brown LF, Detmar M, Dvorak AM. Vascular permeability factor/vascular endothelial growth factor, microvascular hyperpermeability, and angiogenesis. Am J Pathol 1995;146:1029–1039.
56. Dvorak HF, Orenstein NS, Carvalho AC, et al. Induction of a fibrin-gel investment: an early event in line 10 hepatocarcinoma growth mediated by tumor-secreted products. J Immunol 1979;122:166–174.
57. Dvorak HF, Quay SC, Orenstein NS, et al. Tumor shedding and coagulation. Science 1981;212:923–924.
58. Dvorak HF. Tumors: wounds that do not heal. Similarities between tumor stroma generation and wound healing. N Engl J Med 1986;315:1650–1659.
59. Dvorak HF, Nagy JA, Dvorak AM. Structure of solid tumors and their vasculature: implications for therapy with monoclonal antibodies. Cancer Cells 1991;3:77–85.
60. Dvorak HF, Nagy JA, Dvorak JT, Dvorak AM. Identification and characterization of the blood vessels of solid

tumors that are leaky to circulating macromolecules. Am J Pathol 1988;133:95–109.

61. Earle WR. Production of malignancy in vitro. IV. The mouse fibroblast cultures and changes seen in the living cells. J Natl Cancer Inst 1943;4:165–212.

62. Earle WR, Nettleship A. Production of malignancy in vitro. V. Results of injections of cultures into mice. J Natl Cancer Inst 1943;4:213–227.

63. Eisenstein R, Kuettner KE, Neapolitan C, Soble LW, Sorgente N. The resistance of certain tissues to invasion. III. Cartilage extracts inhibit the growth of fibroblasts and endothelial cells in culture. Am J Pathol 1975; 81:337–348.

64. Eisenstein R, Sorgente N, Soble LW, Miller A, Kuettner KE. The resistance of certain tissues to invasion. Penetrability of explanted tissues by vascularized mesenchyme. Am J Pathol 1973;73:765–774.

65. Escher MC, Locher JL. The world of M.C. Escher. New York: Harry N. Abrams, 1974.

66. Escobar MR. Oncogenic viruses. In: Sirica AE, ed. The pathobiology of neoplasia. New York: Plenum Press, 1989:81–109.

67. Evans R, Lawler EM. Macrophage content and immunogenicity of C57BL/6J and BALB/cByJ methylcholanthrene-induced sarcomas. Int J Cancer 1980;26:831–835.

68. Farber E. Chemical carcinogenesis. A biologic perspective. Am J Pathol 1982;106:269–296.

69. Farber E. Pre-cancerous steps in carcinogenesis. Their physiological adaptive nature. Biochim Biophys Acta 1984;738:171–180.

70. Farber E, Sarma DSR. Hepatocarcinogenesis: a dynamic cellular perspective. Lab Invest 1987;56:4–22.

71. Fialkow PJ. Clonal origin and stem cell evolution of human tumors. Prog Cancer Res Ther 1977;3:439–453.

72. Findlay JK. Angiogenesis in reproductive tissues. J Endocrinol 1986;111:357–366.

73. Folkman J. Tumor angiogenesis factor. Cancer Res 1974;34:2109–2113.

74. Folkman J. The vascularization of tumors. Sci Am 1976;234:58–73.

75. Folkman J. What is the role of endothelial cells in angiogenesis? Lab Invest 1984;51:601–604.

76. Folkman J. Toward an understanding of angiogenesis: search and discovery. Perspect Biol Med 1985a;29:10–36.

77. Folkman J. Tumor angiogenesis. Adv Cancer Res 1985b; 43:175–203.

78. Folkman J. The role of angiogenesis in tumor growth. Cancer Biol 1992;3:65–71.

79. Folkman J. How is blood vessel growth regulated in normal and neoplastic tissue? Cancer Res 1986;46:467–473.

79a. Folkman J. Angiogenesis in cancer, vascular, rheumatoid and other disease. Nature Med 1995;1:27–31.

79b. Folkman J. Angiogenesis inhibitors generated by tumors. Molec Med 1995;1:120–122.

80. Folkman J, Cotran R. Relation of vascular proliferation to tumor growth. Int Rev Exp Pathol 1976;16:207–248.

81. Folkman J, Hochberg M. Self-regulation of growth in three dimensions. J Exp Med 1973;138:745–753.

82. Folkman J, Klagsbrun M. Angiogenic factors. Science 1987;235:442–447.

83. Folkman J, Long DM. The use of silicone rubber as a carrier for prolonged drug therapy. J Surg Res 1964;4: 139–142.

84. Folkman J, Watson K, Ingber D, Hanahan D. Induction of angiogenesis during the transition from hyperplasia to neoplasia. Nature 1989a;339:58–61.

85. Folkman J, Weisz PB, Joullié MM, Li WW, Ewing WR. Control of angiogenesis with synthetic heparin substitutes. Science 1989b;243:1490–1493.

86. Foulds L. Neoplastic development, vol 2. London: Academic Press, 1975.

87. Freeman AE, Huebner RJ. Problems in interpretation of experimental evidence of cell transformation. J Natl Cancer Inst 1973;50:303–306.

88. Fürstenberger G, Berry DL, Sorg B, Marks F. Skin tumor promotion by phorbol esters is a two-stage process. Proc Natl Acad Sci USA 1981;78:7722–7726.

89. Galloway AC, Pelletier R, D'Amore PA. Do ischemic hearts stimulate endothelial cell growth? Surgery 1984; 96:435–439.

90. Gillispie CC, ed. Dictionary of scientific biography, Gomperta, B., 1972. New York: Scribner, 1970–1980.

91. Gimbrone MA, Aster RH, Cotran RS, Corkery J, Jandl JH, Foldman J. Preservation of vascular integrity in organs perfused in vitro with a platelet-rich medium. Nature 1969;222:33–36.

92. Gimbrone MA Jr, Cotran RS, Leapman SB, Folkman J. Tumor growth and neovascularization: an experimental model using the rabbit cornea. J Natl Cancer Inst 1974;52:413–427.

93. Gimbrone MA Jr, Gullino PM. Neovascularization induced by intraocular xenografts of normal, preneoplastic, and neoplastic mouse mammary tissues. J Natl Cancer Inst 1976a;56:305–318.

94. Gimbrone MA Jr, Gullino PM. Angiogenic capacity of preneoplastic lesions of the murine mammary gland as a marker of neoplastic transformation. Cancer Res 1976b; 36:2611–2620.

95. Gimbrone MA Jr, Leapman SB, Cotran RS, Folkman J. Tumor dormancy in vivo by prevention of neovascularization. J Exp Med 1972;136:261–276.

96. Gittes RF. Carcinoma of the prostate. N Engl J Med 1991;324:236–245.

97. Goldacre RJ, Sylvén B. On the access of blood-borne dyes to various tumour regions. Br J Cancer 1962;16: 306–322.

98. Grimstad IA. Direct evidence that cancer cell locomotion contributes importantly to invasion. Exp Cell Res 1987;173:515–523.

99. Gullino PM. The internal milieu of tumors. Prog Exp Tumor Res 1966;8:1–25.

100. Gullino PM. Extracellular compartments of solid tumors. In: Becker FF, ed. Cancer, vol 3. New York: Plenum Publishing, 1975:327–354.

101. Gullino PM. Influence of blood supply on thermal properties and metabolism of mammary carcinomas. Ann NY Acad Sci 1980;335:1–21.

102. Gullino PM. Personal communication, 1991.

103. Gullino PM, Grantham FH. The vascular space of growing tumors. Cancer Res 1964;24:1727–1732.

104. Hall PA, Levinson DA, Woods AL, et al. Proliferating cell nuclear antigen (PCNA) immunolocalization in paraffin sections: an index of cell proliferation with evidence of some deregulated expression in some neoplasms. J Pathol 1990;162:285–294.

105. Hanna W, Kahn HJ, Andrulis I, Pawson T. Distribution and patterns of staining of Neu oncogene product in benign and malignant breast diseases. Mod Pathol 1990;3:455–461.

106. Heim S, Mandahl N, Mitelman F. Genetic convergence and divergence in tumor progression. Cancer Res 1988;48:5911–5916.

107. Henderson DW, Papadimitriou JM, Coleman M. Ultrastructural appearances of tumours, 2nd ed. Edinburgh: Churchill Livingstone, 1986.

108. Heppner GH. Tumor heterogeneity. Cancer Res 1984; 44:2259–2265.

109. Herlyn M, Clark WH, Rodeck U, Mancianti ML,

Jambrosic J, Koprowski H. Biology of tumor progression in human melanocytes. Lab Invest 1987;56:461–474.

110. Hill RP. Metastasis. In: Tannock IF, Hill RP, eds. The basic science of oncology. New York: Pergamon Press, 1987:160–175.

111. Hori K, Suzuki M, Abe I, Saito S. Increased tumor tissue pressure in association with the growth of rat tumors. Jpn J Cancer Res (Gann) 1986;77:65–73.

112. Iannaccone PM, Gardner RL, Harris H. The cellular origin of chemically induced tumours. J Cell Sci 1978;29:249–269.

112a. Iozzo RV. Tumor stroma as a regulator of neoplastic behavior. Lab Invest 1995;73:157–160.

113. Iversen OH. Kinetics of cellular proliferation and cell loss in human carcinomas. A discussion of methods available for *in vivo* studies. Eur J Cancer 1967;3:389–394.

114. Jain RK. Determinants of tumor blood flow: a review. Cancer Res 1988;48:2641–2658.

115. Jain RK. Delivery of novel therapeutic agents in tumors: physiological barriers and strategies. J Natl Cancer Inst 1989;81:570–576.

116. Jain RK. Vascular and interstitial barriers to delivery of therapeutic agents in tumors. Cancer Metastasis Rev 1990;9:253–266.

116a. Jain RK. Barriers to drug delivery in solid tumors. Scient Am 1994;271:58–65.

116b. Jain RK. Delivery of molecules, particles and cells to solid tumors (Whitaker Lecture). Annal of Biomed Eng 1996 (in press).

117. Jain RK, Baxter LT. Mechanisms of heterogeneous distribution of monoclonal antibodies and other macromolecules in tumors: significance of elevated interstitial pressure. Cancer Res 1988;48:7022–7032.

118. Jass JR. Do all colorectal carcinomas arise in preexisting adenomas? World J Surg 1989;13:45–51.

119. Joseph-Silverstein J, Rifkin DB. Endothelial cell growth factors and the vessel wall. Semin Thromb Hemost 1987;13:504–513.

120. Kao RT, Hall J, Engel L, Stern R. The matrix of human breast tumor cells is mitogenic for fibroblasts. Am J Pathol 1984;115:109–116.

121. Katayama I, Nagy GK, Balogh K Jr. Light microscopic identification of the ribosome-lamella complex in "hairy cells" of leukemic reticuloendotheliosis. Cancer 1973; 32:843–846.

122. Keski-Oja J, Postlethwaite AE, Moses HL. Transforming growth factors in the regulation of malignant cell growth and invasion. Cancer Invest 1988;6:705–724.

123. Klaunig JE, Ruch RJ. Role of inhibition of intercellular communication in carcinogenesis. Lab Invest 1990; 62:135–146.

124. Klein G, Klein E. Conversion of solid neoplasms into ascites tumors. Ann NY Acad Sci 1955;63:640–661.

125. Klein-Szanto AJP. Morphological evaluation of tumor promoter effects on mammalian skin. In: Slaga TJ, ed. Mechanisms of tumor promotion, vol II. Boca Raton, FL: CRC Press, 1984:41–72.

126. Kleinsmith LJ, Pierce GB Jr. Multipotentiality of single embryonal carcinoma cells. Cancer Res 1964; 24:1544–1551.

126a. Kohn S, Nagy JA, Dvorak HF, Dvorak AM. Pathways of macromolecular tracer transport across venules and small veins. Lab Invest 1992;67:596–607.

127. Kondo S. Carcinogenesis in relation to the stem-cell-mutation hypothesis. Differentiation 1983;24:1–8.

128. Kramar C, Baud C-A, Lagier R. Presumed calcified leiomyoma of the uterus. Morphologic and chemical studies of a calcified mass dating from the neolithic period. Arch Pathol Lab Med 1983;107:91–93.

129. Krishnan R, Cleary EG. Elastin gene expression in elastotic human breast cancers and epithelial cell lines. Cancer Res 1990;50:2164–2171.

129a. Krutovskikh VA, Mesnil M, Mazzoleni G, Yamasaki H. Inhibition of rat liver gap junction intercellular communication by tumor-promoting agents in vivo. Lab Invest 1995;72:571–577.

130. Laird AK. Dynamics of tumor growth. Br J Cancer 1964;18:490–502.

131. Laird AK. Dynamics of tumour growth: comparison of growth rates and extrapolation of growth curve to one cell. Br J Cancer 1965;19:278–291.

132. Lee EY, Wang TC, Clouse RE, DeSchryver-Kecskemeti K. Mucosal thickening adjacent to gastric malignancy: association with epidermal growth factor. Mod Pathol 1989;2:397–402.

133. Leof EB, Proper JA, Getz MJ, Moses HL. Transforming growth factor type ß regulation of actin mRNA. J Cell Physiol 1986;127:83–88.

133a. Levitt D, Mertelsmann R. (eds). Hematopoietic Stem Cells. New York: Marcel Dekker, 1995.

134. Lipsett MB. Interaction of drugs, hormones, and nutrition in the causes of cancer. Cancer 1979;43:1967–1981.

135. Little JB, McGandy RB, Kennedy AR. Interactions between polonium-210 α-radiation, benzo(a)pyrene, and 0.9% NaCl solution instillations in the induction of experimental lung cancer. Cancer Res 1978;38: 1929–1935.

136. Loewenstein WR, Azarnia R. Regulation of intercellular communication and growth by the cellular *src* gene. Ann NY Acad Sci 1988;551:337–346.

137. MacKenzie I, Rous P. The experimental disclosure of latent neoplastic changes in tarred skin. J Exp Med 1941;73:391–416.

138. Mahon KA, Chepelinsky AB, Khillan JS, Overbeek PA, Piatigorsky J, Westphal H. Oncogenesis of the lens in transgenic mice. Science 1987;235:1622–1628.

139. Mahoney MJ, Leighton J. The inflammatory response to a foreign body within transplantable tumors. Cancer Res 1962;22:334–338.

139a. Mantovani A. Tumor-associated macrophages in neoplastic progression: a paradigm for the *in vivo* function of chemokines. Lab Invest 1994;71:5–16.

140. Marx JL. Do tumor promoters affect DNA after all? Science 1983;219:158–159.

141. Martinez-Hernandez A. The extracellular matrix and neoplasia. Lab Invest 1988;58:609–612.

142. Matsumura T, Dohi K, Takanashi A, Ito H, Tahara E. Alteration and enhanced expression of the c-myc oncogene in human colorectal carcinomas. Pathol Res Pract 1990;186:205–211.

143. McCredie JA, Inch WR, Kruuv J, Watson TA. The rate of tumor growth in animals. Growth 1965;29:331–347.

144. McNutt NS. Ultrastructural comparison of the interface between epithelium and stroma in basal cell carcinoma and control human skin. Lab Invest 1976; 35:132–142.

145. Mehta PP, Bertram JS, Loewenstein WR. Growth inhibition of transformed cells correlates with their junctional communication with normal cells. Cell 1986;44:187–196.

146. Mehta PP, Bertram JS, Loewenstein WR. The actions of retinoids on cellular growth correlate with their actions on gap junctional communication. J Cell Biol 1989; 108:1053–1065.

147. Mintz B. Allophenic mice of multi-embryo origin. In: Daniel JC Jr, ed. Methods in mammalian embryology. San Francisco: WH Freeman, 1971:186–214.

148. Mintz B, Illmensee K. Normal genetically mosaic mice

produced from malignant teratocarcinoma cells. Proc Natl Acad Sci USA 1975;72:3585–3589.

149. Moore JV. Death of cells and necrosis of tumours. In: Potten CS, ed. Perspectives on mammalian cell death. Oxford: Oxford University Press, 1987:295–325.

150. Moore JW III, Sholley MM. Comparison of the neovascular effects of stimulated macrophages and neutrophils in autologous rabbit corneas. Am J Pathol 1985;120:87–98.

151. Morré DJ. Membrane alterations in neoplasia. In: Sirica AE, ed. The pathobiology of neoplasia. New York: Plenum Press, 1989:323–344.

152. Moses MA, Sudhalter J, Langer R. Identification of an inhibitor of neovascularization from cartilage. Science 1990;248:1408–1410.

153. Mottram JC. A developing factor in experimental blastogenesis. J Pathol Bacteriol 1944;56:181–187.

154. Müller J. On the nature and structural characteristics of cancer, and of those morbid growths which may be confounded with it. London: Sherwood, Gilbert and Piper, 1840.

155. Nakamura T, Mahon KA, Miskin R, Dey A, Kuwabara T, Westphal H. Differentiation and oncogenesis: phenotypically distinct lens tumors in transgenic mice. New Biol 1989;1:193–204.

156. Nicolson GL. Trans-membrane control of the receptors on normal and tumor cells. II. Surface changes associated with transformation and malignancy. Biochim Biophys Acta 1976;458:1–72.

157. Nowell PC. The clonal evolution of tumor cell populations. Science 1976;194:23–28.

158. Nowell PC. Cytogenetics of tumor progression. Cancer 1990;65:2172–2177.

159. Orlidge A, D'Amore PA. Inhibition of capillary endothelial cell growth by pericytes and smooth muscle cells. J Cell Biol 1987;105:1455–1462.

160. Pauli BU, Weinstein RS. Cell junctional alterations in cancer. In: Liotta LA, ed. Influence of tumor development on the host. Dordrecht: Kluwer Academic Publishers, 1989:121–132.

161. Pedersen PL. Tumor mitochondria and the bioenergetics of cancer cells. Prog Exp Tumor Res 1978;22:190–274.

162. Peterson H-I. Vascular and extravascular spaces in tumors: tumor vascular permeability. In: Peterson H-I, ed. Tumor blood circulation: angiogenesis, vascular morphology and blood flow of experimental and human tumors. Boca Raton, FL: CRC Press, 1979:77–85.

163. Peterson H-I. The microcirculation of tumors. In: Orr FW, Buchanan MR, Weiss L, eds. Microcirculation in cancer metastasis. Boca Raton, FL: CRC Press, 1991:277–298.

164. Pitot HC. The natural history of neoplastic development: the relation of experimental models to human cancer. Cancer 1982;49:1206–1211.

165. Pitot HC. Fundamentals of oncology, 3rd ed. New York: Marcel Dekker, 1986.

166. Pitot HC, Barsness L, Goldsworthy T, Kitagawa T. Biochemical characterisation of stages of hepatocarcinogenesis after a single dose of diethylnitrosamine. Nature 1978;271:456–458.

167. Pitot HC, Goldsworthy T, Moran S. The natural history of carcinogenesis: implications of experimental carcinogenesis in the genesis of human cancer. J Supramol Struct Cell Biochem 1981;17:133–146.

168. Pitot HC, Goldsworthy T, Moran S, Sirica AE, Weeks J. Properties of incomplete carcinogens and promoters in hepatocarcinogenesis. Carcinogenesis 1982;7:85–98.

169. Pitot HC, Sirica AE. The stages of initiation and promotion in hepatocarcinogenesis. Biochim Biophys Acta 1980;605:191–215.

170. Rather LJ. The genesis of cancer: a study in the history of ideas. Baltimore: The Johns Hopkins University Press, 1978.

171. Rather LJ, Rather P, Frerichs JB. Johannes Müller and the nineteenth-century origins of tumor cell theory. Science History Publications, 1986.

172. Ross PM. Apparent absence of a benign precursor lesion: implications for the pathogenesis of malignant melanoma. J Am Acad Dermatol 1989;21:529–538.

173. Rous P, Beard JW. The progression to carcinoma of virus-induced rabbit papillomas (Shope). J Exp Med 1935;62:523–548.

174. Rous P, Kidd JG. Conditional neoplasms and subthreshold neoplastic states. A study of the tar tumors of rabbits. J Exp Med 1941;73:365–390.

175. Ruddon RW. Cancer biology, 2nd ed. New York: Oxford University Press, 1987.

176. Russell DS, Rubinstein LJ. Pathology of tumours of the nervous system, 5th ed. Baltimore: Williams & Wilkins, 1989.

177. Ryser HJ-P. Chemical carcinogenesis. N Engl J Med 1971;285:721–734.

178. Sachs L. Constitutive uncoupling of pathways of gene expression that control growth and differentiation in myeloid leukemia: a model for the origin and progression of malignancy. Proc Natl Acad Sci USA 1980;77:6152–6156.

179. Sager R, Gadi IK, Stephens L, Grabowy CT. Gene amplification: an example of accelerated evolution in tumorigenic cells. Proc Natl Acad Sci USA 1985;82:7015–7019.

180. Sandberg AA. The chromosomes in human cancer and leukemia. New York: Elsevier, 1990.

181. Schnipper LE. Clinical implications of tumor-cell heterogeneity. N Engl J Med 1986;314:1423–1431.

182. Scribner JD, Süss R. Tumor initiation and promotion. Int Rev Exp Pathol 1978;18:137–198.

183. Seemayer TA, Lagacé R, Schürch W, Tremblay G. Myofibroblasts in the stroma of invasive and metastatic carcinoma. A possible host response to neoplasia. Am J Surg Pathol 1979;3:525–533.

184. Sevick EM, Jain RK. Effect of red blood cell rigidity on tumor blood flow: increase in viscous resistance during hyperglycemia. Cancer Res 1991;51:2727–2730.

185. Shousha S, Bull TB, Burn I. Alveolar variant of invasive lobular carcinoma of the breast: an electron microscopic study. Ultrastruct Pathol 1986;10:311–319.

186. Sirica AE. The pathobiology of neoplasia. New York: Plenum Press, 1989.

187. Skipper HE, Perry S. Kinetics of normal and leukemic leukocyte populations and relevance to chemotherapy. Cancer Res 1970;30:1883–1897.

188. Skipper HE, Schabel FM Jr, Wilcox WS. Experimental evaluation of potential anticancer agents. XIV. Further study of certain basic concepts underlying chemotherapy of leukemia. Cancer Chemother Rep 1965;45:5–28.

189. Slaga TJ, Fischer SM, Weeks CE, Nelson K, Mamrack M, Klein-Szanto AJP. Specificity and mechanism(s) of promoter inhibitors in multistage promotion. Carcinog Compr Surv 1982;7:19–34.

190. Solt DB, Medline A, Farber E. Rapid emergence of carcinogen-induced hyperplastic lesions in a new model for the sequential analysis of liver carcinogenesis. Am J Pathol 1977;88:595–618.

191. Steel GG. Cell loss as a factor in the growth rate of human tumours. Eur J Cancer 1967;3:381–387.

192. Steel GG. Growth kinetics of tumours. Oxford: Clarendon Press, 1977.

193. Stockdale FE. Cancer growth and chemotherapy. In: Rubenstein E, Federman DD, eds. Scientific American Medicine. Oncology. New York: Scientific American, 1987:1–13.

194. Stoker M, O'Neill C, Berryman S, Waxman V. Anchorage and growth regulation in normal and virus-transformed cells. Int J Cancer 1968;3:683–693.

195. Strum JM. Angiogenic responses elicited from chorio-allantoic membrane vessels by neoplastic, preneoplastic, and normal mammary tissues from GR mice. Am J Pathol 1983;111:282–287.

196. Sutherland RM, McCredie JA, Inch WR. Growth of multicell spheroids in tissue culture as a model of nodular carcinomas. J Natl Cancer Inst 1971;46:113–120.

197. Talmadge JE, Key M, Fidler IJ. Macrophage content of metastatic and nonmetastatic rodent neoplasms. J Immunol 1981;126:2245–2248.

198. Tanaka K, Kohga S, Kinjo M, Kodama Y. Tumor metastasis and thrombosis, with special reference to thromboplastic and fibrinolytic activities of tumor cells. GANN Monogr Cancer Res 1977;20:97–119.

199. Tannock IF. The relation between cell proliferation and the vascular system in a transplanted mouse mammary tumour. Br J Cancer 1968;22:258–273.

200. Tannock IF. A comparison of cell proliferation parameters in solid and ascites Ehrlich tumors. Cancer Res 1969;29:1527–1534.

201. Tannock IF. Population kinetics of carcinoma cells, capillary endothelial cells, and fibroblasts in a transplanted mouse mammary tumor. Cancer Res 1970;30:2470–2476.

202. Tannock IF. Oxygen distribution in tumours: influence on cell proliferation and implications for tumour therapy. Adv Exp Med Biol 1976;75:597–603.

203. Tannock IF. Biology of tumor growth. Hosp Pract 1983;18:81–93.

204. Tannock IF. Tumor growth and cell kinetics. In: Tannock IF, Hill RP, eds. The basic science of oncology. New York: Pergamon Press, 1987:140–159.

205. Thomlinson RH, Gray LH. The histological structure of some human lung cancers and the possible implications for radiotherapy. Br J Cancer 1955;9:539–549.

206. Thompson JA, Anderson KD, DiPietro JM, et al. Site-directed neovessel formation in vivo. Science 1988;241:1349–1352.

207. Tremblay G. Elastosis in tubular carcinoma of the breast. Arch Pathol 1974;98:302–307.

208. Tremblay G, Babai F. Intercellular junctions between Novikoff hepatoma cells and hepatic cells. Exp Cell Res 1972;74:355–358.

209. Trosko JE, Yotti LP, Warren ST, Tsushimoto G, Chang C-C. Inhibition of cell-cell communication by tumor promoters. Carcinogenesis 1982;7:565–585.

210. Vasiliev JM, Gelfand IM. Morphogenetic reactions and locomotor behaviour of transformed cells in culture. In: Weiss L, ed. Fundamental aspects of metastasis. Amsterdam-Oxford: North Holland Publishing Company, 1976:71–98.

211. Vaupel P, Kallinowski F, Kluge M. Pathophysiology of tumors in hyperthermia. Recent Results Cancer Res 1988;107:65–75.

212. Vaupel P, Müller-Klieser W. Interstitieller Raum und Mikromilieu in malignen Tumoren. Mikrozirk Forsch Klin 1983;2:78–90.

213. Volpe JPG. Genetic instability of cancer: why a metastatic tumor is unstable and a benign tumor is stable. Cancer Genet Cytogenet 1988;34:125–134.

214. Warburg O. The metabolism of tumours. London: Constable & Co. Ltd., 1930.

215. Warburg O. On the origin of cancer cells. Science 1956;123:309–314.

216. Warren BA. The vascular morphology of tumors. In: Peterson H-I, ed. Tumor blood circulation: angiogenesis, vascular morphology and blood flow of experimental and human tumors. Boca Raton, FL: CRC Press, 1979:1–47.

217. Warren BA, Shubik P. The growth of the blood supply to melanoma transplants in the hamster cheek pouch. Lab Invest 1966;15:464–478.

218. Weinhouse S. Changing perceptions of carbohydrate metabolism in tumors. In: Arnott MS, van Eys J, Wang Y-M, eds. Molecular interrelations of nutrition and cancer. New York: Raven Press, 1982:167–181.

219. Weinstein RS, Merk FB, Alroy J. The structure and function of intercellular junctions in cancer. Adv Cancer Res 1976;23:23–89.

220. Weiss L. Principles of metastasis. New York: Academic Press, 1985.

221. Welsch F. Teratogens and cell-to-cell communication. In: De Mello WC, ed. Cell intercommunication. Boca Raton, FL: CRC Press, 1990:133–160.

222. Woodruff MFA. Tumor clonality and its biological significance. Adv Cancer Res 1988;50:197–229.

223. Yamaura H, Sato H. Quantitative studies on the developing vascular system of rat hepatoma. J Natl Cancer Inst 1974;53:1229–1240.

224. Zetter BR. Migration of capillary endothelial cells is stimulated by tumour-derived factors. Nature 1980;285:41–43.

225. Zetter BR. Angiogenesis. State of the art. Chest 1988;93 (suppl):159S–166S.

226. Ziche M, Gullino PM. Angiogenesis and neoplastic progression in vitro. J Natl Cancer Inst 1982;69:483–487.

227. Ziegler E. General pathology. New York: William Wood and Company, 1908.

Tumors as Parasites

CHAPTER 27

The Biology of Tumor
Aggression

Metastases

Mechanisms of Invasion
and Metastasis

Effects of Tumors on
the Host

How Does Cancer Kill?

Sooner or later, malignant tumors trespass into the vital space of other tissues. They do so by several mechanisms: they infiltrate (this is called *local invasion*); they find their way into the blood or lymph vessels and give rise to metastases; they seed into serosal spaces or other cavities. All this recalls the behavior of a parasite, except that tumors arise within their host, and die with it.

The Biology of Tumor Aggression

We will begin with local infiltration: If it is true that the name *cancer* refers to claws reaching out to grasp surrounding tissues, the ability of cancer to invade was observed some 2500 years ago.

LOCAL INVASION

In fairness to the tumor cell, the strategies of invading and even of metastasizing are part of normal life. We were all born thanks to the ability of the trophoblast to invade the uterine wall, a process still incompletely understood. As regards metastases, trophoblastic cells normally embolize the lung (see Figure 23.17). Even the lifesaving inflammatory process resorts to "infiltration"; the leukocytes are true invaders, and tumor cells, as we will see, use some of their techniques.

Invasion by malignant tumors can be seen with the naked eye. For example, scirrhous carcinomas of the breast seen in cross section are star-shaped, or perhaps we should say crab-shaped, with claws reaching out to the skin and to the muscle, so that the tumor is anchored (Figure 27.1). The resulting lack of mobility of the mass over the deeper planes is an ominous clinical sign. Histologically the infiltration corresponds to cords of tumor cells embedded in strands of fibrous connective tissue containing fibroblasts and myofibroblasts (Figure 27.2); these fibrous structures tend to retract, hence the retraction of the nipple, another ominous sign (Figure 27.3).

At the level of histology, the concept of invasion is best appreciated by examining the transition between a squamous epithelium and a squamous cell carcinoma (Figure 27.4). As the malignant tissue advances, almost any structure that happens to be in the way can be infiltrated and destroyed (Figure 27.5). Even compact bone can be eroded (see Figure 25.10), but in this case the advancing mass of malignant cells recruits the help of cells that are programmed to excavate bone tissue: the osteoclasts. However, invaded cancellous bone may also respond to invasion with a burst of osteogenesis, thereby becoming more dense. Radiologists see these two opposite effects very clearly and refer to them as *osteolytic* and *osteoblastic* responses (Figures 27.6, 27.7).

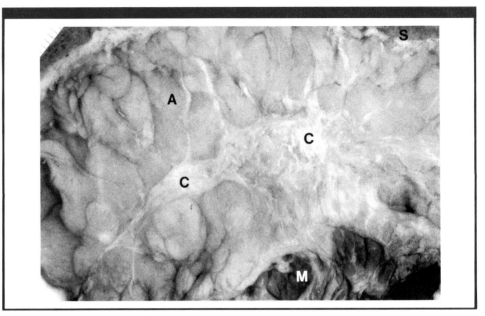

FIGURE 27.1
See color plate 23. Cross section of a carcinoma of the breast (**C**) infiltrating adipose tissue (**A**). Some of its extensions reach toward the skin (**S**) and toward the underlying muscle (**M**). The fine yellowish streaks within the main mass of the tumor are epithelial cords. **Bar** = 10 mm. (Courtesy of Miss T.M. Turner, University of Massachusetts Medical Center, Worcester, MA.)

Tumor cells can also destroy bone directly, as was shown by incubating human breast cancer cells with fragments of bone that had been devitalized and therefore contained no osteoclasts (48). The dissolution of bone tissue releases growth factors that can stimulate tumor growth (106). Conversely, some tumors secrete osteoclast-stimulating factors (114). Two of these tumor-derived activators of osteoclasts are transforming growth factor-alpha (73) and prostaglandin E$_2$ (58). This prostaglandin connection has an amazing corollary: in rats, aspirin inhibits bone destruction by a tumor (150).

Tumor cells advancing in tissue spaces sometimes follow the paths of least resistance, such as the perineurial spaces (Figure 27.8); if they reach a serosal surface they may "fall into it" and produce the phenomenon of **seeding.** Hyaline cartilage and arterial walls are rarely invaded; an intact abdominal aorta may be surrounded by a ring of pancreatic carcinoma. It used to be said that both these tissues escape invasion because they are mechanically tough, but the mechanisms may be more subtle: It has been possible to extract from hyalin cartilage a low-molecular weight "anti-invasion factor" that inhibits angiogenesis (this may explain why normal cartilage contains no vessels), while also inhibiting proteolytic enzymes and tumor cell growth (142,144). Arteries contain much elastin, and malignant tumors which clear the way with collagenase do not contain much elastase (108).

Metastases

A *metastasis* is a secondary tumor that grows separately from the primary and has arisen from detached, transported cells (200). In essence, it is a colony of the primary tumor. The "seed" that starts a metastatic growth can be transported by the blood or lymph, or by fluid in tissue spaces. Metastases represent the most lethal expression of malignancy and the most important concern of the treating physician. By the time the diagnosis of cancer is made, over half of the patients already have microscopic metastases (52) and will die of them, because there is, overall, little hope for cure at that stage.

METASTASES BY THE BLOODSTREAM

Tumor cells have several options for gaining access to the bloodstream (Figure 27.9), but the most common portals of entry are probably the capillaries and venules, which have very thin walls (Figure 27.10) (89).

The blood route, as opposed to the lymphatic route, can be taken by any malignant tumor. Most sarcomas favor the blood route and produce pulmonary metastases (200). Carcinomas metastasize by both pathways, even in the same individual. Of course, cells taking the lymphatic route can eventually reach the bloodstream.

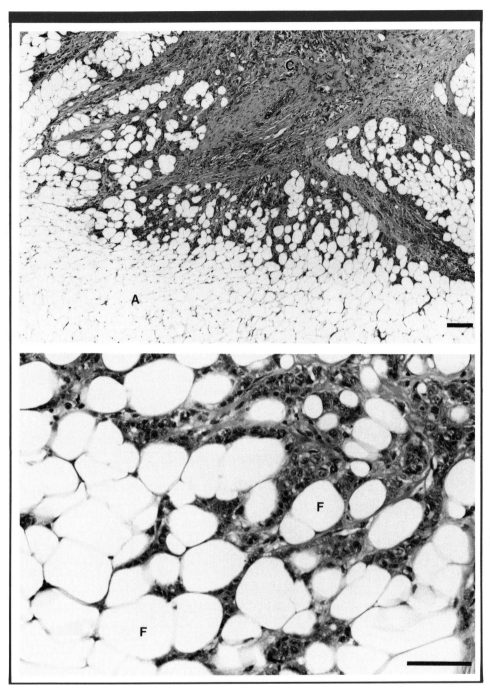

FIGURE 27.2
Typical pattern of invasion by a carcinoma of the breast. *Top:* Carcinoma (**C**) invading adipose tissue (**A**). The main mass of the carcinoma has induced a strong connective tissue reaction. The cells that have just invaded the adipose tissue have not yet had the time to induce this response. **Bar** = 200 μm. *Bottom:* Detail. **F:** Fat cells. **Bar** = 100 μm.

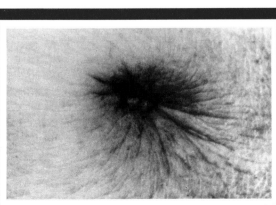

FIGURE 27.3
Retraction of the nipple, caused by an underlying carcinoma of the breast. The retraction is probably due to myofibroblasts in the stroma of the tumor. The fine puckering of the skin (*peau d'orange*) visible below the nipple is indicative of lymphatic invasion. (Reproduced with permission from [21].)

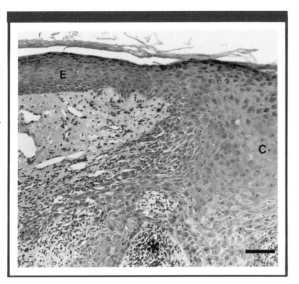

FIGURE 27.4
Squamous cell carcinoma (**C**) arising from the epithelium (**E**) of the lip. The carcinoma does not protrude from the surface; it invades the dermis, which responds with a lymphocytic infiltrate (**asterisk**). **Bar** = 100 μm.

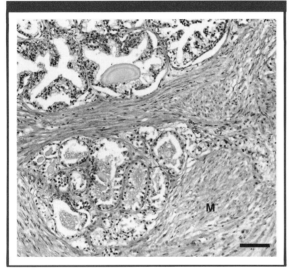

FIGURE 27.5
Myocardium (**M**) invaded by an adenocarcinoma of the lung. Metastases to the heart are unusual; here the invasion occurred directly through the pericardium. **Bar** = 100 μm.

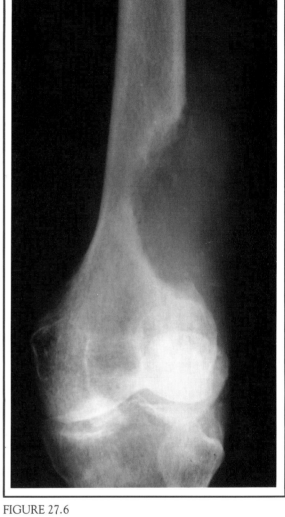

FIGURE 27.6
Metastasis of a carcinoma of the breast to the femur; this is an osteolytic metastasis, a very aggressive one because the bone has had no time to react with condensation. (Courtesy of Dr. A. Davidoff, University of Massachusetts Medical School, Worcester, MA.)

FIGURE 27.7
Osteoblastic metastasis from a carcinoma of the prostate, seen in a CT scan of the pelvic region. The dense areas (**arrows**) represent new bone formation induced by the presence of the tumor. **Asterisk**: Iliac bones. (Courtesy of Dr. A. Davidoff, University of Massachusetts Medical School, Worcester, MA.)

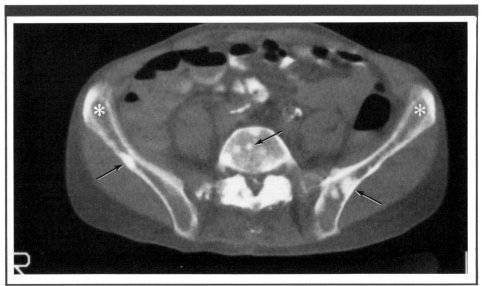

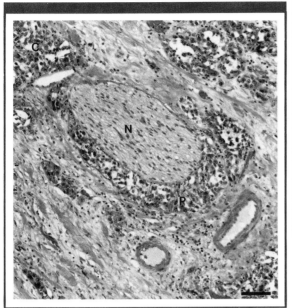

FIGURE 27.8
Carcinoma of the prostate. **C:** Strands of neoplastic cells. **N:** Nerve. Note how the carcinoma has invaded the perineural space (**P**). **Bar =** 100 μm.

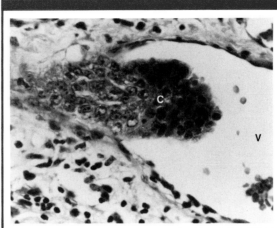

FIGURE 27.10
A mass of malignant cells from a transitional cell carcinoma of the bladder (**C**) invading the wall of a venule (**V**). (Reproduced with permission from [89].)

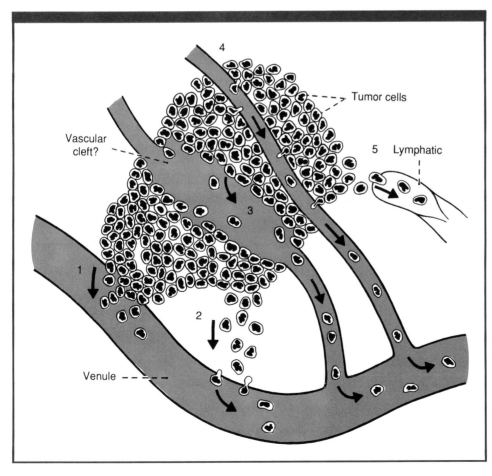

FIGURE 27.9
Five possible pathways for tumor cells to penetrate into the bloodstream: (1) direct infiltration by the tumor, (2) invasion by individual tumor cells, (3) shedding into vascular spaces lacking an endothelial lining, (4) reverse diapedesis into vessels within the tumor, and (5) penetration into the lymphatics.

Occasionally, a malignant tumor breaches into a large vein and grows within it as a continuous rootlike extension of the tumor; this behavior is typical of renal cell carcinomas, which tend to invade the renal vein and form a plug that can grow along the inferior vena cava and into the right heart (Figure 27.11).

There are no exceptions to the rule that metastases are malignant, even though some may look deceptively benign under the microscope (hence such improper names as "metastasizing adenoma" and "metastasizing leiomyoma"). However, it is true that some malignant tumors metastasize very rarely (p. 791).

> Normal cells introduced into the bloodstream may embolize and survive but they do not turn into tumors. Pancreatic islets injected (experimentally) into the portal vein embolize the liver and—with some help—survive (p. 654).

To the naked eye a single metastasis may look like a primary tumor, but when metastases are multiple, as often occurs in the liver or lung, the diagnosis is clear. In the liver they can be seen radiologically by computerized tomography (Figure 27.12). They may be so many as to defy counting. Even experienced pathologists shudder at the common sight of a liver so full of metastases that little normal tissue is left.

Perhaps because they tend to grow faster than primary tumors, metastases tend to be spherical (Figure 27.13): this is why on chest X-rays they are sometimes described as a "coin lesion" if single, or as "cannon balls" if multiple. Perhaps because of rapid growth, liver metastases of carcinomas usually become necrotic in their centers; therefore, as seen on the liver surface, they have a depressed central zone (Figure 27.14).

Metastases can generate more metastases (30, 72,186,187): this can be proven experimentally (Figure 27.15). It follows that *there can be a cascade of metastases of several orders;* for example, a metastasis to the kidney from a carcinoma of the rectum is probably a third-order metastasis (Figure 27.16) (38,39).

Organ Distribution of Blood-Borne Metastases

This has been a long-standing puzzle. If blood-borne metastases were distributed geographically according to the plain laws of embolism, it should be possible to predict the target organs simply by considering the anatomy of the vascular system. However, this criterion works, in a general way, only for tumors of organs drained by the portal system: they do metastasize primarily to the liver (193,194). Tumors arising in other parts of the body show organ preferences that cannot be explained on anatomical grounds alone. For example:

- Carcinomas of the breast usually metastasize to the skeleton.

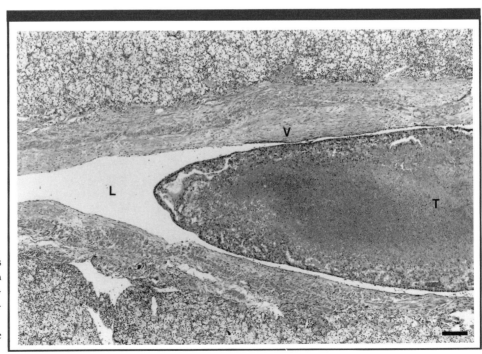

FIGURE 27.11

An ominous sight, typical of renal cell carcinomas: a mass of tumor cells (**T**) growing like a plug inside a vein (**L**: Lumen of vein). The tumor is advancing from right to left, without invading the wall of the vein (**V**). Such growths can reach as far as the heart. **Bar** = 200 μm.

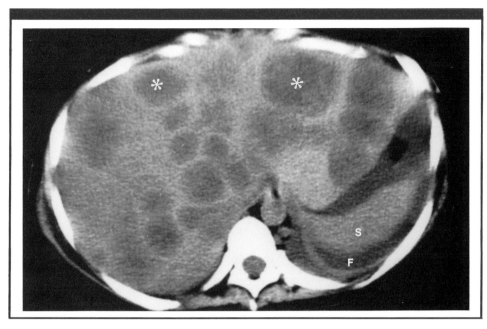

FIGURE 27.12
Liver metastases from a carcinoma of the pancreas seen in a CT scan. The metastases (**asterisk**) appear more translucent than the liver. Note the absence of metastases in the spleen (**S**) and the presence of fluid (**F**) in the peritoneum, indicating ascites. The latter could be due to portal obstruction as well as to peritoneal metastases. (Courtesy of Dr. A. Davidoff, University of Massachusetts Medical Center, Worcester, MA.)

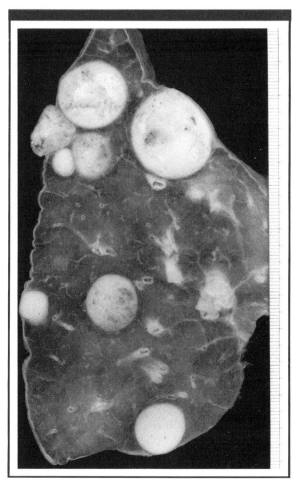

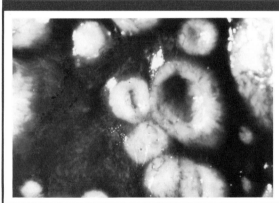

FIGURE 27.14
Surface of a liver riddled with metastases from a carcinoma. The center of several metastases is umbilicated (i.e., depressed) due to necrosis of the central portion. Natural size. (Courtesy of Dr. L.S. Gottlieb, The Mallory Institute of Pathology, Boston, MA.)

FIGURE 27.13   (*Left*)
Cannonball type of metastases in the lung. These spherical, sharply circumscribed metastases are typical of sarcomas. The French term for this X-ray appearance is more poetic: *lâcher de ballons*, balloons allowed to fly away. From a case of malignant schwannoma developing in a patient with neurofibromatosis. Scale in mm.

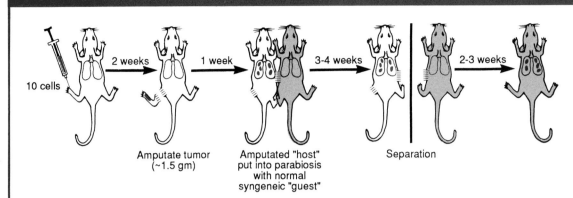

FIGURE 27.15
Experimental
proof that metas-
tases can give
rise to further me-
tastases.
(Adapted from
[72].)

10 cells

2 weeks

Amputate tumor
(~1.5 gm)

1 week

Amputated "host"
put into parabiosis
with normal
syngeneic "guest"

3-4 weeks

Separation

2-3 weeks

- The kidneys act as filters and receive 20–25 percent of the cardiac output, yet they develop far fewer metastases than' the much smaller adrenals.
- The adrenals are favorite targets of bronchial carcinomas.
- The myocardium is rarely metastasized, and the same is true for striated muscles, although they represent some 40 percent of the body mass.
- Some carcinomas of the gastrointestinal tract favor the ovaries; bilateral metastatic tumors of the ovaries are a classic condition known as "Krukenberg tumor."

- The intestine receives 10 percent of the cardiac output, yet it receives few metastases, although melanomas of the skin sometimes produce a single metastasis to the small intestine.
- Hepatomas never metastasize the skin, whereas sarcomas do.

The spleen is often cited as an organ that is relatively spared by metastases, but this is controversial (172). The spleen is certainly a favorite target of lymphomas and leukemias; and it is said that, at the microscopic level, metastases are much more frequent than observation with the naked eye would suggest (172). Our own impression is that grossly visible splenic metastases from carcinomas are rare; perhaps their growth is inhibited. The spleen is rich in NK cells, which can kill tumor cells.

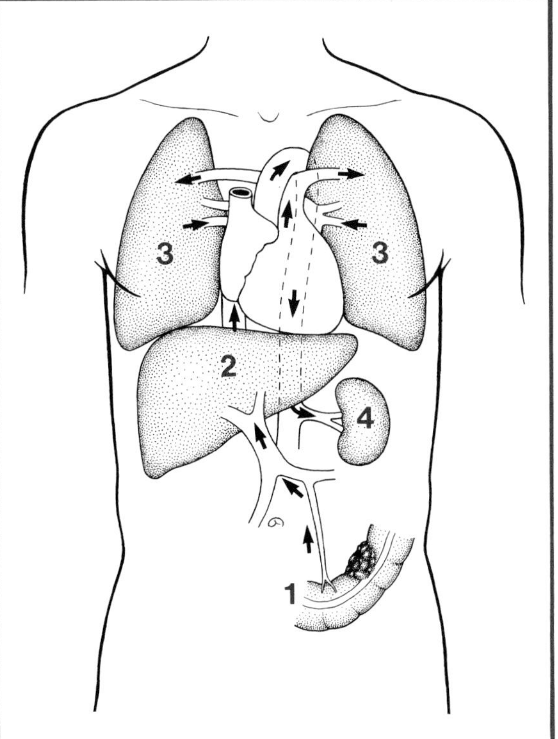

To explain the long list of metastases in unexpected organs, it was proposed a century ago that the selection in any given case was due to special properties of either the "seed" or the "soil" (135,205). Today it is clear that in some cases the purely mechanical embolic mechanism is at work; in others the "seed" or the "soil" determine the result: adhesion molecules play a major role (p. 803). Not surprisingly, different rules apply to different tumors.

A subset of unexpected blood-borne metastases, especially in the vertebrae, can be explained by the existence of a system of veins in and around the spine known as the venous system of Batson.

The Batson Venous System This system, also called the vertebral venous plexus (11,12,28, 38,57), is a special two-way thoroughfare of anastomosed veins—*without valves*—disposed around

FIGURE 27.16
Sequence of me-
tastases postu-
lated for a carci-
noma of the
large intestine.
The primary tu-
mor (1) metasta-
sizes to the liver
(2) which then
metastasizes to
the lungs (3).
Nodules in the
lung then metas-
tasize by the gen-
eral circulation,
for example to
the kidney (4).

the vertebrae and running from the neck to the pelvis (Figure 27.17). After death the collapsed veins are hard to see, but in life they form a large reservoir. The relationship between this venous system and the caval and portal systems is shown schematically in Figure 27.18.

To understand the relevance of the Batson system to metastasis it is helpful to know how it was discovered. Oscar V. Batson was professor of anatomy in Philadelphia. By injecting radioopaque media into the dorsal vein of the penis in cadavers and in monkeys, he found that, if the abdominal pressure was raised, the material penetrated the lumbar spine rather than the caval system, mimicking the distribution of metastases from prostatic carcinoma. This mechanism works also *in vivo*: malignant cells injected into a femoral rein in rats and rabbits produced tumors almost exclusively in the lungs; but if the abdominal pressure was raised during the injection, tumors appeared mostly in the vertebrae (28).

What was happening? As shown in Figure 27.19, the valveless veins that run along the abdominal surface of the vertebrae are exposed to intraabdominal and intrathoracic pressure; they are connected to the caval system as well as to veins within the vertebrae, which drain toward the spinal cord. When the abdominal pressure is raised (such as by coughing, straining, or lifting a weight) blood is squeezed out of the caval system, through the anastomoses, into the deeper part of the Batson system. Malignant cells floating in this blood are pushed into the deep plexus and then float or drain up as far as the skull without passing through the heart or the lungs, where they might be mechanically destroyed.

The Batson system can explain many "aberrant" metastases such as a cranial metastasis from an adrenal tumor, and especially the high incidence of vertebral involvement in tumors of the thyroid, prostate, and breast.

> For example: tumor cells from a breast cancer can drain into the intercostal veins; if intrathoracic pressure is raised by coughing, the blood in these veins is squeezed back into the vertebral system. As to the physiologic raison d'être of the Batson system, it may act as a reservoir to prevent deep veins from bursting when thoracic and abdominal pressures are abruptly raised by physical effort.

SPREAD BY THE LYMPHATICS

The lymphatic pathway is a favorite of carcinomas. The long-standing dogma that *sarcomas rarely*

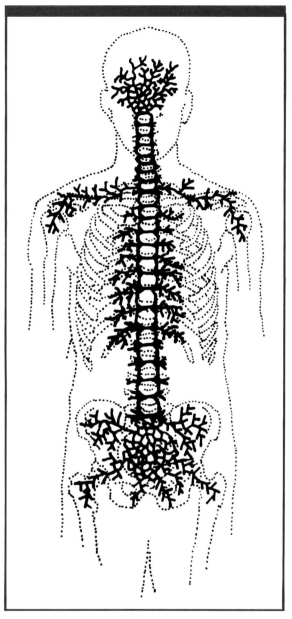

FIGURE 27.17 Anatomical layout of the Batson system (vertebral venous system). (Reproduced with permission from [38].)

metastasize to the lymph nodes is true overall, except for rhabdomyosarcomas (200). Malignant cells wandering out of the primary tumor penetrate the loosely structured lymphatic capillaries without destroying the endothelium (22); thereafter they probably float up to the next lymph node, where they settle in the peripheral sinus and grow (Figure 27.20). Eventually they may invade the entire node (Figure 27.21) and grow downstream or upstream into the lymphatic network. The result is literally a solid cast of the lymphatics; the individual vessels are often so distended that they can be seen with the naked eye.

This pattern of lymphatic invasion is also

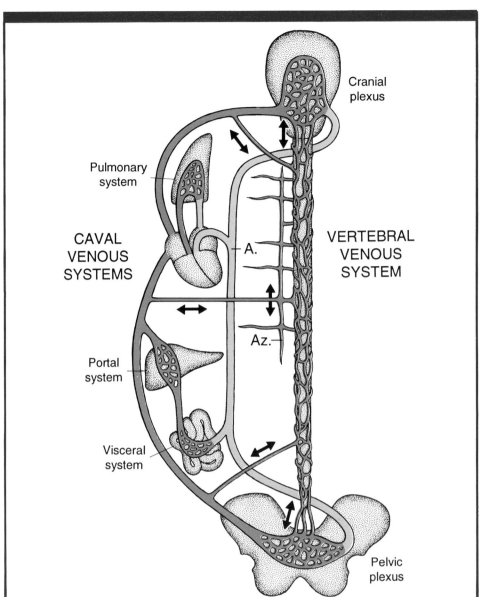

FIGURE 27.18
See color plate 24. Batson's vertebral venous system: overall view. Notice how malignant cells released from a carcinoma in the pelvic region could reach the skull without ever passing through the caval system or the lungs. **A:** Aorta. **Az:** Azygos vein.

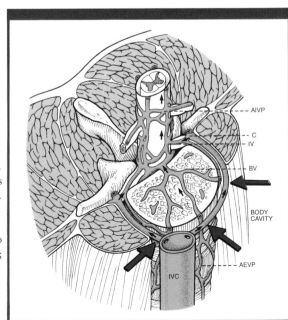

FIGURE 27.19
See color plate 25. Batson's vertebral venous system: detail. Note that the veins of the anterior external venous plexus are exposed to the pressure existing within the body cavity. If metastatic tumor cells are traveling in these veins, a sudden rise in abdominal pressure can squeeze them into deeper veins, and from there they can travel all the way to the cranial plexus. **AIVP:** Anterior internal venous plexus; **C:** Connection of caval and vertebral systems via lumbar vein; **IV:** Intervertebral vein; **BV:** Basivertebral vein; **AEVP:** Anterior external venous plexus.

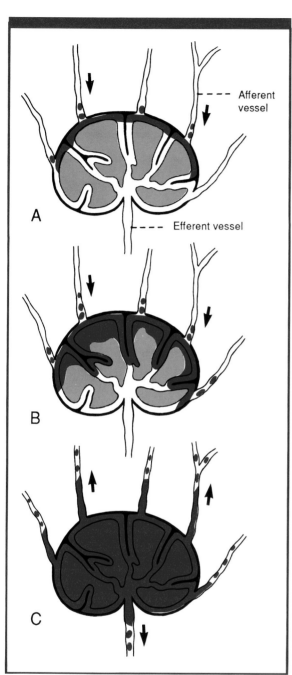

FIGURE 27.20
Possible steps in the metastasization of a lymph node by a carcinoma. **A:** Malignant cells reach the node from the afferent lymphatics and fill the peripheral sinus. **B:** The entire lymph node is invaded by the carcinoma. **C:** The lymph node has ceased to function as such and becomes a center for tumor growth. Solid cords of tumor cells grow into the afferent and efferent lymphatics. (Adapted from [88].)

known as **lymphatic permeation.** Carcinomas of the breast can permeate the lymphatics of the overlying skin (Figure 27.22); presumably as a result of lymphatic obstruction, the skin becomes slightly edematous and puckered, hence the name *peau d'orange* (Figure 27.3). Both primary and metastatic carcinomas of the lung can produce an extensive filling of the lymphatics: thin whitish streaks visible to the naked eye appear on the pleura and on the diaphragm (Figure 27.23); within the lung itself, lymphatic permeation tends to follow the periarterial lymphatics (Figure 27.24) and is usually accompanied by fibrosis (Figure 27.25). Perhaps the pumping action of respiration has something to do with the tendency of carcinomas to permeate the lymphatics of the lung. However, it seems more likely that we are dealing with a biologic peculiarity of certain malignant cells: there are reported cases of gastric carcinomas producing lymphatic invasion almost throughout the body (200).

Note: lymph nodes downstream from a tumor can swell even before they have received metastatic cells. Antigens and other irritating materials leach out of the tumor, especially if it contains much necrosis and even more so if it is ulcerated and infected. When the lymph node receives these chemical messengers it responds by swelling, due to extensive hyperplasia of the phagocytic cells in the sinuses; the microscopic pattern is known as *sinus histiocytosis* (23,187). Clinically, swollen lymph nodes downstream from a tumor are very worrisome; only the microscope can distinguish between a metastasis and an innocent reaction.

We would like to report that the lymph nodes are very effective filters of metastatic tumor cells as they are of inert particles (p. 425), but the experimental evidence is not very reassuring. In one of the few studies on this topic, tumor cells were injected into the footpad of the rat; from there they drained into the popliteal lymph node and were briefly held up, but by 5 days they had already reached the next lymphatic station, namely the paraaortic node (23). If a dose of BCG was injected into the footpad (thereby inflaming the lymph node) 1 week before the injection of tumor cells, the metastatic destruction of the node was delayed, but there was little effect on the progression of the malignant cells to the next node.

The behavior of the lymph nodes toward metastatic cells is of course very important to the surgeon who has to decide whether to remove the lymph nodes draining a primary tumor. Microscopi-

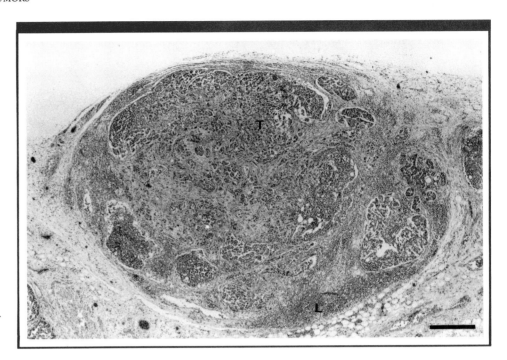

FIGURE 27.21
Extensive replacement of a lymph node by a carcinoma. **T:** Tumor tissue. **L:** Lymphatic tissue. **Bar** = 500 μm.

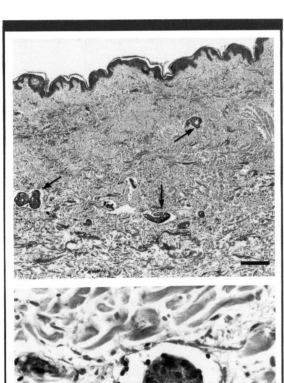

FIGURE 27.22
Lymphatic infiltration in the skin overlying a carcinoma of the breast. *Top:* Lymphatics filled with malignant cells (**arrows**). **Bar** = 250 μm. *Bottom:* A cluster of neoplastic cells in a lymphatic. **Bar** = 50 μm.

cally there are no obvious signs of an aggressive antitumor-cell campaign in the lymph node (22). However, there is statistical evidence that some metastases do die in the nodes (172).

> *This statistical evidence was obtained by comparing the frequency of microscopic axillary metastases from carcinoma of the breast (40 percent in one series) with the development of clinically positive nodes in a parallel series of patients whose axillary nodes were not removed (15 percent): these figures suggest that about two-thirds of the microscopic metastases did not grow.*

As is usual with tumors, there can be no general rule; with regard to melanomas, for example, it may or may not be useful to excise the regional lymph nodes, depending on the size and thickness of the primary tumor (Figure 27.26).

SEEDING IN BODY CAVITIES

This event is common in the peritoneum as a complication of malignancies in abdominal organs. Hundreds of metastatic nodules can develop (Figure 27.27). The seeding is usually more severe in the pelvic recesses, presumably because the cells tend to settle there by gravity; the result is a stiffening of the peritoneal lining that can be felt by rectal or vaginal examination. Sometimes the omentum is seeded extensively, and the fibrous

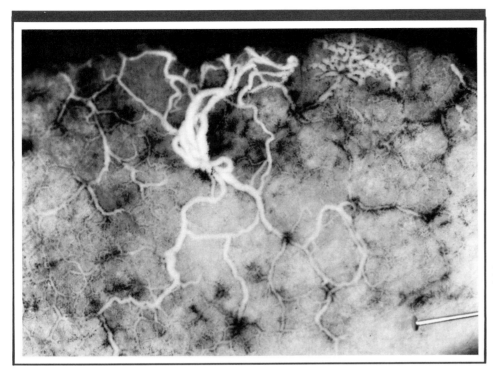

FIGURE 27.23
Neoplastic invasion of the pleural lymphatics by a carcinoma of the colon with metastases to the lung. The whitish irregular lines represent dilated lymphatics filled with carcinoma. The pin provides the scale.

reaction induced by the invading cells causes it to retract and shrivel into a firm mass that can be palpated in the upper abdomen. Peritoneal seeding is usually accompanied by ascites (free fluid in the abdomen); adhesions may also develop. Some cells remain free and grow in the ascitic fluid, forming microscopic clusters or spheroids (p. 756).

The pathogenesis of malignant ascites and other malignant effusions needs more study. We offer the following suggestions: tumors produce several factors that induce vascular leakage (p. 768), and these could diffusely affect the peritoneal membrane; furthermore, fluid oozes from the surfaces of malignant tumors (p. 770).

Seeding via the cerebrospinal fluid can occur with tumors of the central nervous system (mainly malignant gliomas): tumor cells shed into the cerebrospinal fluid, settle and give rise to nodules in the ventricles or in the leptomeningeal spaces (159).

Implantation on epithelial surfaces is rare: a carcinoma of the gut protruding above the surface does not produce "seedlings" where it rubs against normal mucosa. Epithelial surfaces are inhospitable, being covered by mucus, cornified cells, and even bacteria. However, there have been reports of carcinomas implanted from one vocal cord to the other, from the cervix to the vagina, from tongue to cheek, from one side of the esophagus to the opposite

side, from the renal pelvis to the bladder, and so on (200). In such cases it is obviously difficult to rule out metastasis by the lymphatic or hematogenous pathway. Yet we should recall once again the precedent of the trophoblast, which is able to implant itself on an epithelial surface, and a foreign one at that. If the trophoblast can do it, tumors should be able to do it too; but if they ever do become implanted on an epithelial surface, it must be a rare event.

WHICH TUMORS METASTASIZE—AND WHEN?

In theory, malignant tumors might be capable of metastasizing from day one, but there seems to be a

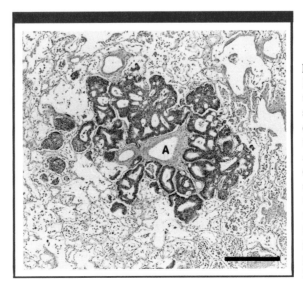

FIGURE 27.24
Pulmonary metastasis from an adenocarcinoma developing in the same lung. Atypical glands crowded around a small artery (**A**), suggesting that they arrived there by the periarterial lymphatics. **Bar** = 500 μm.

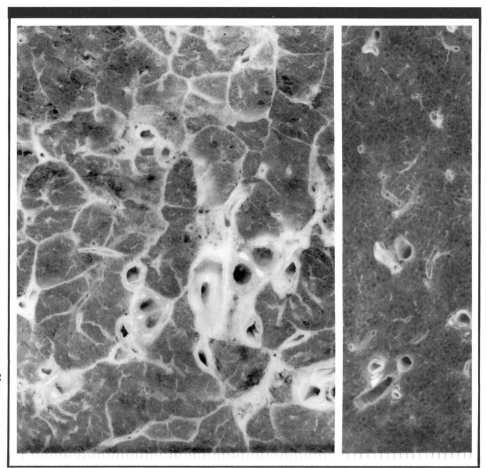

FIGURE 27.25
Left: The mosaic pattern of this lung is due to carcinomatous invasion of the lymphatics in the septa between pulmonary lobules. A strong fibrous reaction accompanies the invading cells. *Right:* Cut surface of normal lung. Scales in mm.

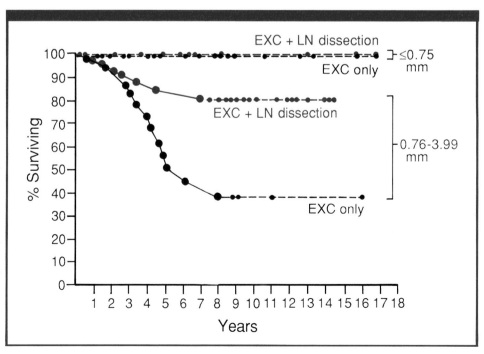

FIGURE 27.26
Survival curves of patients with melanoma: one group with thin (<75 mm) melanomas and one with melanomas of intermediate thickness (0.76–3.99 mm). In each group, patients were operated with or without lymph node (**LN**) dissection. Excision (**EXC**) of the lymph nodes was helpful for thin melanomas; for melanomas thicker than 4 mm the advantage disappeared (data not shown). Such studies indicate that the dissection of lymph nodes must be tailored to the primary tumor. (Reproduced with permission from [9].)

delay. Perhaps they do start on day one, but success of the metastatic colonies is hampered by two factors: it takes many metastatic cells (thousands, possibly millions) to produce one successful colony, and a very small tumor might not have enough cells to shed; also, the ability of tumor cells to produce successful metastases increases as a result of tumor progression.

Histological atypia is a safe guide: *the more atypical the tumor, the likelier it is to invade and metastasize.*

The size of the primary tumor (which implies a time factor) tends to correlate with the presence of metastases, hence the current drive to detect smaller and smaller primary tumors. The effect of size is very obvious for carcinoma of the female breast, for the stomach, and for most other organs (42). Melanomas of the skin are measured with regard to thickness on histologic sections; it was found that fractions of a millimeter count: if the thickness is less than 0.76 mm, the cure rate is 100 percent; between 0.76 and 4.00 mm there is an increasing risk (up to 80 percent) of metastases; above 4.00 mm there is an 80 percent risk of metastases at the time of observation (8). This is a reminder that very small tumors can also metastasize.

There are many exceptions to the correlation between size or thickness of a primary tumor and presence of metastases. Some melanomas of the skin metastasize before the patient has noticed them; occasionally they even regress and disappear, leaving only the metastases as proof of their brief existence.

There is also a malignant tumor that almost never metastasizes: the very common basal cell carcinoma of the skin. This tumor appears typically on areas of the skin exposed to sunlight, especially the face, as a small crusty lesion that does not heal (see Figure 26.25). It is locally invasive and if allowed to grow it can destroy half the face, yet the rest of the body is "safe." Medical students are usually puzzled by the fact that this tumor is called malignant although the cure rate by surgery is 100 percent: the reason is that *if* it is allowed to grow it kills by invasion. Metastases are so rare that if one occurs it is still publishable as news.

Tumors of the central nervous system rarely produce metastases to the rest of the body, probably because they develop in a closed space and therefore kill the host before visceral metastases are large enough to be detected. Although metasta-

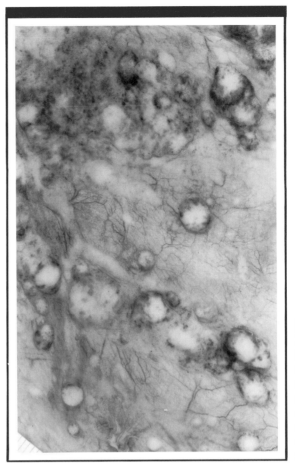

FIGURE 27.27 Peritoneal seeding of a carcinoma of the pancreas; these nodules developed on the peritoneal surface of the diaphragm. Scale in mm.

ses to the lungs, bones, and other organs have been described, the average pathologist may see one or two examples in a lifetime (159).

Dormant metastases are the nightmare of many "successfully treated" patients. In some cases, metastatic cells lie dormant for 5–10 years or even 35 years (200), then suddenly start to grow. The latent phase may be related to lack of angiogenesis (54a); it might also represent a balance between cell birth and death (53). Trauma can wake up dormant cells: it has been shown in the rat that intraportal injection of malignant cells did not produce tumors; but nodules developed after the liver was traumatized (53).

Can there be mother-to-fetus metastases? Here are the facts (116). Malignant tumors in pregnant women are not rare, but published cases of metastases to the placenta are only 40, half of which concern melanomas. Two maternal melanomas and three maternal leukemias have been associated with the same tumor in the infants, all of which died of it. It has been speculated that these cases may not represent metastases but viral transmission. There is one known case of placental metastasis from a fetal neuroblastoma.

Iatrogenic metastases *occur by several mechanisms. Chemotherapy may cause wide dissemination; the reason is not clear (117,172); it may be related to endothelial injury (132). Surgical trauma may wake up dormant metastases; on the other hand, the intraoperative release of tumor cells into the bloodstream, however worrisome, has no measurable effect (p. 800). Implantation along a needle track, after biopsy, is exceedingly rare (202).*

Mechanisms of Invasion and Metastasis

From the point of view of the malignant cell, invasion and metastasis require the ability to overcome a series of obstacles, which have been aptly compared to a decathlon, named the *metastatic cascade* (Figure 27.28) (110,127,133,199). To produce a hematogenous metastasis a cell must separate itself from the tumor mass and move in the right direction; it must digest its way through the intercellular matrix, and then through a

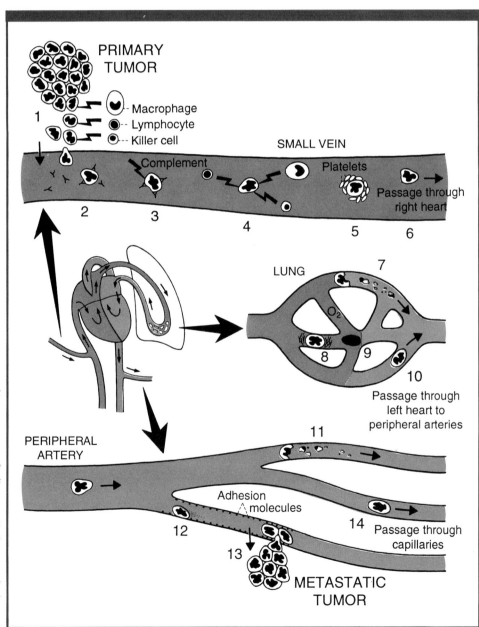

FIGURE 27.28
Cancer cells that travel in the bloodstream experience a series of adventures that are—from the point of view of the cancer cell—bad, good, or indifferent. (1) Encounters with killer cells of various types on the way toward a blood vessel. (2) Coating with antibody and (3) killing by complement. (4) Intravascular killing by various types of killer cells. (5) Coating with platelets, which may supply the cancer cell with growth factors. (6) Passage through the heart. (7) Impaction and breakup in a lung capillary. (8) Arrest in the alveolar capillaries. (9) Exposure to toxic levels of oxygen. (10) Return toward the systemic circulation. (11) Impaction and breakup in the peripheral capillaries. (12) Margination in vessels of the microcirculation. (13) Trapping in the microcirculation followed by metastatic growth. (14) Return toward the heart. The circuit (without stops) takes about 1 minute.

vascular basement membrane to penetrate the lumen of a vessel; once there, it must escape the various defensive systems of the blood, including antibodies, complement, macrophages, killer cells of various sorts, oxygen, and even blood clotting; when it reaches a vessel small enough to be embolized, it must survive the impact and the mechanical squeeze; then it must proceed in reverse, penetrate the endothelium and the basement membrane, escape a new set of dangerous cells (macrophages, lymphocytes), multiply, induce angiogenesis, and finally establish a tumor. In view of all these difficulties, it is not surprising that many tumor cells fail. At each step of the metastatic cascade the metastatic cells are selected by a basic principle: survival of the fittest (53), which contributes to the phenomenon of tumor progression.

Despite the undeniable threat of tumor progression, we can sum up with a mildly optimistic statement: *the metastatic process is highly inefficient* (191). Many cells try but few succeed. Clumps of about four cells are more likely to "take" than single cells (97). It is usually stated that metastatic takes are of the order of 0.1–0.01 percent; this applies to experimental systems, but in man the efficiency can be even less than 10^{-7} (p. 800).

All this may sound reassuring, but of course even if one cell survives it is one too many. We should also remember that in some models of experimental leukemia the disease can be transmitted with a single cell.

Data are available for all the steps of the metastatic cascade.

(1) DETACHMENT

There is no question that malignant cells become detached from the tumor mass because they can be found in the bloodstream, single or in clusters (see later); one such cluster ready to be carried away was shown in Figure 27.10. In tissue sections of carcinomas, it is common to find malignant cells that appear to be single or in small clusters, but serial sections are needed to show whether they are really isolated and not a cross section of a continuous cord. This has been done for several tumors. The result: most of the isolated clumps of tumor cells seen in histologic sections are cross sections of branches attached to the tumor mass, but a few are truly detached islands (Figure 27.29). The next question, then, must be: how do the cells become detached?

Recall that malignant cells tend to be more loosely connected (p. 735). Complete detachment from their neighbors may be due to proteolytic enzymes diffusing outward from the necrotic core of the tumor.

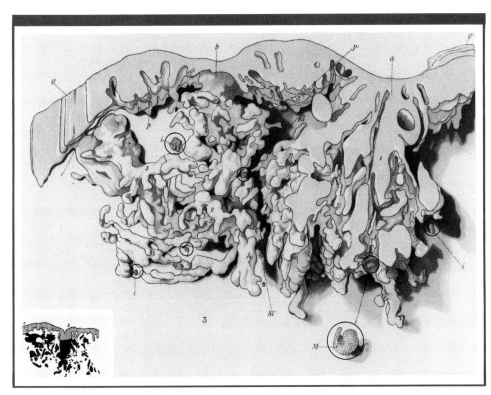

FIGURE 27.29
Model of a small squamous cell carcinoma of the scrotum, reconstructed from serial sections. A schematic view of a histologic section is shown in the inset. According to the reconstructed model, the tumor masses that appear histologically (inset) as isolated are actually connected to the tumor mass. Only a few small clumps of tumor tissue are free standing (*circles*). The mass **M** was 6 mm from the main tumor mass and was considered to be a metastasis. (Reproduced with permission from [145].)

Leonard Weiss has studied this mechanism by punching cores out of normal mouse livers, then incubating them at 37 degrees, shaking them and counting the number of cells released (187,188). Extracts of necrotic parts of tumors, applied to normal liver, increased the release. Interestingly, regenerating livers released more cells than normal controls. The tumor extracts also brought about the detachment of cells from cell masses grown in vitro *(188,195).*

Active motility of tumor cells could also favor the detachment process, and there is ample proof that many types of malignant cells do show ameboid motion (see later).

Massage of tumors has long been known to favor the seeding process (53,98,182) as we illustrated earlier (see Figure 23.15). However, let it be clear that malignant tumors need no massage for releasing cells into the bloodstream: a mammary tumor of the rat that required 10 million cells for a 100 percent successful inoculum shed that number of cells every day into the bloodstream (20,68) (see further).

(2) Invasion

The best possible proof of active invasion is the sight of cancer cells penetrating the fibers of skeletal muscle (Figure 27.30) (90). Invasiveness can be tested and measured *in vitro*, by placing

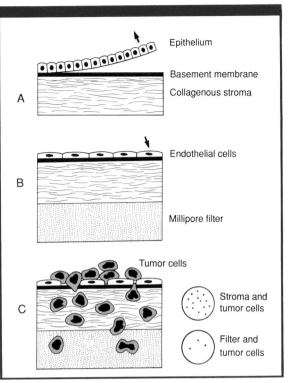

FIGURE 27.31
Scheme of the amnion invasion assay. **A:** The three layers of human amnion. The epithelium is being removed. **B:** Endothelial cells (human or bovine) are seeded on the amnion and grown to confluence; a millipore filter is placed between the amnion. **C:** Tumor cells seeded over the surface cross the endothelium and invade the stroma and filter. Stroma and filter are then peeled apart, stained, and examined under a microscope. Counting the tumor cells measures their invasiveness. (Reproduced with permission from [160].)

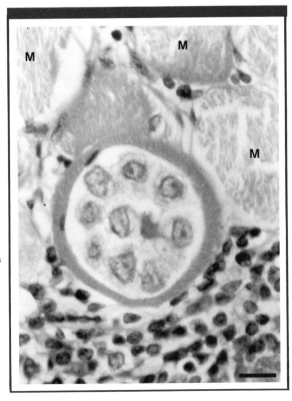

FIGURE 27.30
An extreme case of tumor infiltration. The circular structure is a muscle fiber greatly expanded by invading malignant cells from an adenocarcinoma of the breast. **M:** Non-invaded muscle fibers. **Bar =** 5 μm. (Reproduced with permission from [90].)

tumor cells on a membrane of human amnion relined with endothelium (Figure 27.31) (80,160). Another *in vitro* test has gladiatorial connotations: the principle is to place normal and malignant cells face to face. This is called *confrontation* (40). However, confrontation experiments based on tissue culture (a two-dimensional system) can be misleading because all the cells participating in the test are attached to a fixed substrate, unlike the situation *in vivo* (107). More telling results are obtained by confronting small three-dimensional tumor spheroids with normal tissues, as shown in Figure 27.32 (109): malignant spheroids become attached to benign tissues and invade them (109,111,112).

How do cancer cells force their way into surrounding tissues? Growth pressure is one mechanism, but it cannot be the only one because invasion can be demonstrated *in vitro* by the confrontation method, which rules out this factor (109).

Active motility of cancer cells is probably involved. It was calculated as far back as 1916 that the speed of cells observed *in vitro* would enable malignant cells to crawl from the breast to the axillary lymph nodes in 4 weeks (186). Several movies have been made to prove the point (108, 203). Furthermore, Liotta and co-workers extracted a factor from human melanoma cells that increases the rate of motion of the same cells (chemokinesis) and also attracts them; it does not attract neutrophils (Figure 27.33) (99). This *autocrine motility factor* means that tumor cells have joined the family of chemotactic cells. But there is more: there are reports that tumor cells respond to chemotactic stimuli with increased adhesiveness and release of hydrolytic enzymes: these are typical leukocyte responses (179).

> *Some inflammatory mediators are chemotactic for some tumor cells. As to tumor products, chemotactic as well as antichemotactic factors have been described (99, 100). Some of the breakdown products of the enzymatic digestion of the matrix are chemotactic for some tumor cells (128).*

Malignant cells can also digest their way through connective tissues, thanks to proteases, which include collagenases specific for fibrillar collagen. A vast number of enzymes are known to be released by tumor cells (126,128); although they are opposed by natural inhibitors, on balance they assist invasion. Some of these trail-blazing enzymes are also contributed by host cells, stimulated by the tumor (141,181).

The resistance of cartilage to invasion was discussed earlier (p. 757).

What happens when a malignant cell contacts a normal cell? This should be the crucial confrontation in the drama of aggression by tumors, but not much is known about it except that the cells of invaded tissue tend to disappear. Pressure atrophy is surely one explanation (24,56,82), but there must be other, more subtle mechanisms. Electron microscopy shows pseudopods of tumor cells pushing their way into host liver cells (Figure 27.34); phagocytosis of cell debris by macrophages and tumor cells was sometimes observed (56). Actual destruction of invaded tissue was seen *in vitro* when fragments of nervous tissue were confronted with malignant cells (108). A tantalizing possibil-

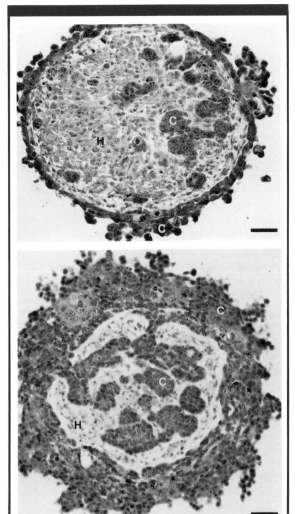

FIGURE 27.32 Histologic sections of spheroids, obtained by confronting—in three-dimensional culture—embryonic chick heart (**H**) and a line of malignant epithelial cells derived from a rat bladder carcinoma (**C**). The spheroids were fixed after 7 days (*top*) and 14 days (*bottom*). Note how the mass of heart cells is progressively invaded by the tumor cells. **Bars** = 50 μm. (Reproduced with permission from [164].)

ity: there are increasing rumors of possible "marriage" (fusion) between normal and malignant cells in tumors (p. 904); this mechanism sounds extremely interesting, but it has not created headlines—yet.

> *Electron microscopy has shown that tight junctions develop between normal and malignant cells (7,24, 44,123). This too could be important because chemical messages related to growth control could be exchanged. We have already mentioned the strange fact that some transformed cells stop growing when they make contact with normal cells (p. 735).*

(3) PENETRATION INTO THE BLOOD VESSELS

It is likely that invading tumor cells penetrate most often into the vessels of the tumor itself rather than into the preformed vessels around it.

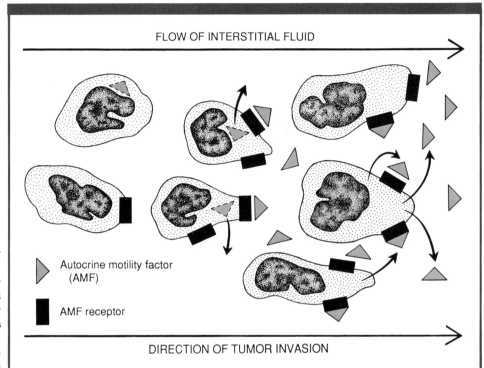

FLOW OF INTERSTITIAL FLUID

◣ Autocrine motility factor
  (AMF)

■ AMF receptor

DIRECTION OF TUMOR INVASION

FIGURE 27.33
Proposed role of tumor autocrine motility factor. Tumor cells secrete the factor, which binds to their own surface receptors and stimulates random as well as directed motility. The flow of interstitial fluid in the tumor tends to sweep the factor to the periphery and presumably contributes to the invasive process. (Modified from [96].)

Some tumor vessels are said to have no endothelial lining, and so it is easily understood that some cells may shed into the lumen. Other tumor vessels have an endothelial lining, and some of these have a basement membrane. In the latter case, tumor cells in the tissue spaces have to overcome *two* obstacles to enter the vessels (reverse diapedesis). They surely have many ways to solve the problem, but a basic three-step mechanism has been proposed by Liotta and

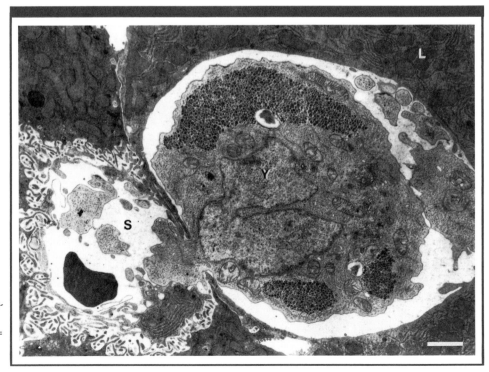

FIGURE 27.34
Active infiltration by a malignant cell. A cell of the so-called Yoshida sarcoma (**Y**) injected into the portal vein and actively escaping through the wall of the sinusoid (**S**); in so doing, it creates a deep indentation in the neighboring liver cell (**L**). **Bar** = 2 μm. (Reproduced with permission from [82].)

collaborators (102): attachment, lysis, and invasion. When tumor cells reach the perivascular basement membrane, they attach to it by means of laminin receptors (laminin is an adhesive molecule that reinforces basement membranes (10)); then the tumor cells secrete collagenase Type IV, specific for the collagen of the basement membrane (Figure 27.35), and eventually move through. In a series of elegant experiments, Liotta and others have proven all these points for a variety of tumors. For example, metastatic efficiency has been correlated with collagenase secre-

tion (59,95). Others have shown experimentally that protease inhibitors oppose metastasis (128).

Tumor cells may not always need this arsenal of molecular tools to reach the bloodstream: vessels in tumors are often defective and may lack basement membrane (196). Scanning electron microscopy has shown that the invading cell may punch its way through an endothelial cell, creating a temporary migration pore. This has been shown for leukemia cells, which are simply doing what normal leukocytes do when they leave bone marrow (34), but it is also true for melanoma cells,

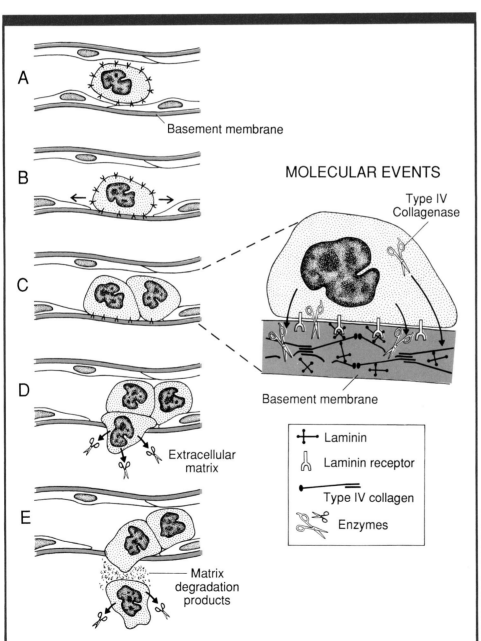

FIGURE 27.35
Development of a metastasis from a malignant cell in a capillary. **A:** Tumor cell trapped in a capillary either by embolization or by adhesion molecules (not shown). **B:** The surrounding endothelial cells retract (actively?), enabling the tumor cell to attach to the basement membrane by its laminin receptors. **C:** The tumor cell divides. **D:** A tumor cell digests its way through the basement membrane by means of collagenase and other hydrolytic enzymes. **E:** Some matrix degradation products are chemotactic, so other tumor cells follow the same path. (Modified from [29].)

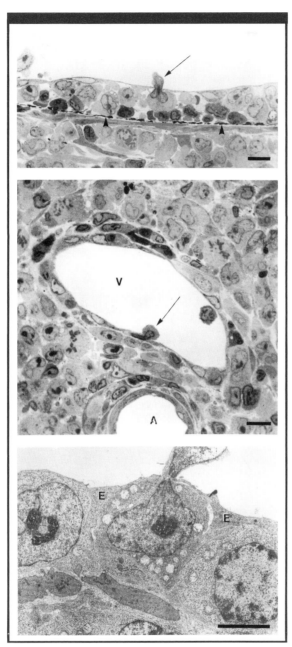

FIGURE 27.36
Penetration of malignant cells into the lumen of blood
vessels (reverse diapedesis) illustrated with a malignant rat
tumor (myeloma). *Top:* From a graft of tumor over a large
branch of the femoral vein (**V**). One tumor cell is poking
(**arrow**) through the endothelial surface (*****). **Arrowheads**
point to the internal elastic lamina. **Bar** = 10 μm. *Center:*
A tumor cell (**arrow**) passing through the endothelium of a
venule (**V**). Because the vessel is completely surrounded by
tumor cells (note the mitoses), it is most likely that the
direction of cell movement is from the tumor into the
lumen. Another malignant cell is already in the lumen
attached to the endothelium. **A:** Arteriole. **Bar** = 10 μm.
Bottom: Electron microscopic view suggestive of reverse
diapedesis. **E:** Endothelium. **Bar** = 2 μm. (Reproduced
with permission from [35].)

which somehow "learned" how to do it (Figures
27.36, 27.37) (35).

(4) TRANSPORT IN THE BLOODSTREAM

Tumor cells are found in the blood of experimental
animals as well as in humans (Figure 27.38). In
either case it is possible to count the number
released during a given time, and the figures are
astonishing. Butler and Gullino devised a system
for preparing a rat tumor in such a way that all the
blood perfusing it would emerge from a single vein
(Figure 27.39); by cannulating that vein they
found that every day each gram of tissue shed 3.2
million cells (which is about the size of a pinhead)
(20). This occurred *before* the appearance of lung
metastases. In humans it has been found repeatedly that trauma, including surgery, sends showers
of tumor cells into the bloodstream (Figure 27.40)
(63). The number rarely exceeds 1000 per milliliter. This figure still appears frightening, but there

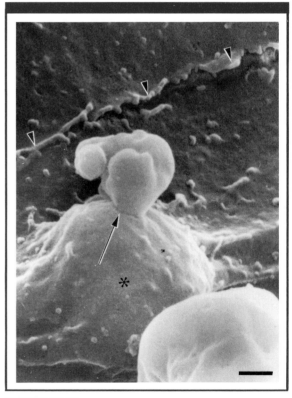

FIGURE 27.37
Intima of a venule inside a malignant rat tumor (same
as in the previous figure). The bulge (**asterisk**) represents a
subendothelial malignant cell that appears to squirt out of a
migration pore at the top of the bulge (**arrow**). Note that
this reverse diapedesis does not occur along the junction
between two endothelial cells (**arrowheads**). **Bar** = 1 μm.
(Reproduced with permission from [35].)

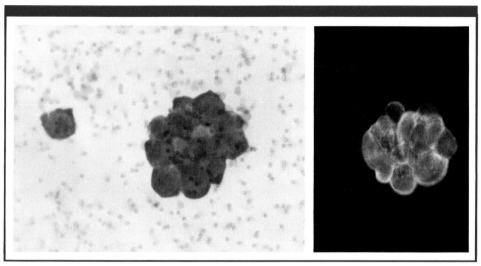

FIGURE 27.38
Blood-borne cancer cells. *Left:* Cells of mouse lung carcinoma obtained from right ventricular blood by centrifugation. *Right:* Cells of a human renal cell carcinoma spun out from the blood of the renal vein prior to a nephrectomy; stained by immunofluorescence with antibody to cytokeratin. The kidney tumor measured 10 cm in diameter; in removing it, great care was taken (as always) to minimize the surgical trauma and associated release of cells. No metastases were found 5 years after surgery. (Courtesy of D. Glaves, Roswell Park Memorial Institute, New York; reproduced with permission from [64].)

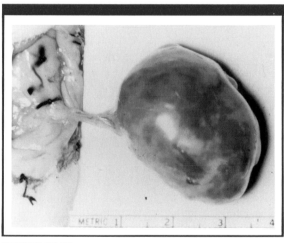

FIGURE 27.39
Method for growing a rat tumor in such a way that the blood supply comes from a single source through a peduncle. This carcinoma (Walker 256) was first implanted in the ovary, which was then pulled out of the abdominal cavity, sutured into a subcutaneous space, and surrounded by a paraffin bag. To take this photograph the paraffin bag was removed, and the tumor was pulled away from the host to show the peduncle containing the ovarian artery and vein, now supplying the tumor. (Reproduced with permission from [69].)

seems to be no correlation between circulating cancer cells and number of metastases. Glaves and co-workers (1988) studied blood in the renal veins in 10 patients with renal cell carcinoma; 8 of the 10 subjects' blood contained tumor cell emboli (i.e., single cells or clusters) numbering 140–73,090 per milliliter (64). From the size of the tumors it was calculated that these patients had been exposed to some 3.7×10^7 tumor cell emboli per day for at least 180 days; yet only 3 of the 10 patients had extraperitoneal metastases at the time of surgery, and only one developed metastases within 35 months. This amounts to an efficiency of less than 10^7 (64,198).

An amazing report was published in 1984 (177). A patient suffering from an inoperable ovarian carcinoma developed severe ascites. After 257 liters of fluid had been removed, it was decided to install a venous shunt whereby the ascitic fluid was reinfused directly into the bloodstream. Relief was immediate. When the patient died 27 months later, the peritoneum was covered with tumor implants, as anticipated, but elsewhere there was not a single metastasis despite the daily infusion of malignant cells for over 2 years.

Hazards encountered by tumor cells in the blood are many (see Figure 27.28): coating with antibodies followed by lysis with complement,

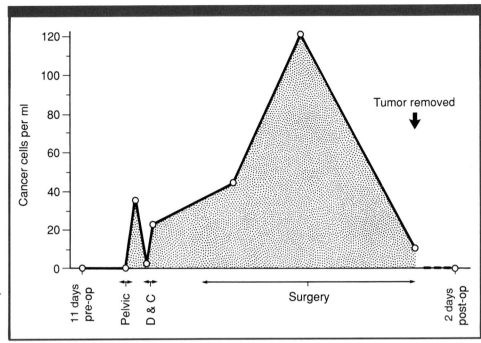

FIGURE 27.40
Number of cancer cells released into the blood by pelvic examination, cervical dilatation and curettage (D&C), and tumor resection. The patient suffered from an ovarian carcinoma. (Reproduced with permission from [156].)

encounters with killer cells of various kinds and, according to recent studies, exposure to a toxic concentration of oxygen (2). The only possible advantage for the tumor cell might be the coating with platelets, which in some experimental systems seems to help the metastatic process (61,81,176). And then, within seconds of gaining entry into the bloodstream, tumor cells face the trauma of embolization, which can be their demise.

(5) EMBOLIZATION FOLLOWED BY CELL DEATH

Most tumor cells injected intravenously are killed by biomechanical trauma in minutes (197,198). Very few are viable after 24 hours. The mechanical impact of embolism is fatal to many tumor cells because they are larger and less deformable than leukocytes (51,190); experiments with filters of various pore sizes have proven that cells less capable of changing shape are especially liable to be killed by filtration (163). Biomechanical trauma must be especially severe in the heart where capillaries receive a hefty squeeze at every beat, i.e., more than once per second (196)). Similar effects apply to skeletal muscle. Now we begin to understand why the heart and the large mass of muscular tissue are rarely metastasized.

In an experiment on normal and denervated muscles in the rat, 87 percent of control muscles developed

metastases compared with 31 percent in electrically stimulated muscles and 100 percent in denervated and stimulated muscles (198).

In theory, a squeezing effect occurs also in the lung where inspiration, by distending the alveoli and their capillaries, should traumatize any metastatic cell in transit (196). Unfortunately the lung remains a favorite site for metastases, but it may be that without the biomechanical trauma of breathing and squeezing, the number of lung metastases would be even greater.

Biomechanical trauma in capillaries of the lung and of the general circulation seems to account for the inefficiency of the metastatic process.

(6) EMBOLIZATION FOLLOWED BY GROWTH

The embolic episode has been recorded cinematographically *in vivo*, quite a technical feat (203,204). It was shown that some tumor cells survive embolic trauma and continue to circulate (51,204).

The development of a successful tumor embolus is best shown by electron microscopy (Figure 27.41) (25,30,79,85,166,175). Details vary with experimental model (149). The malignant cell or cluster settles in a capillary or precapillary vessel where it is always tightly apposed to the endothelial surface; it is often associated with platelets (which may act as a supply of growth factors) and with some strands of fibrin (183). Within a few hours the malignant cell (be it isolated or part of a cluster) sends a pseudopod between the endothelial cells or through them and makes contact with the basement membrane, while flow may resume. Thereafter the cell may exit from the vessel and pursue its career outside or divide and grow into a metastatic lump that occludes the lumen (196). Seen by electron microscopy the diapedesis of a tumor cell appears surprisingly similar to that of a leukocyte. New vessels may begin to sprout toward the metastasis after 24 hours (203), and a tumor vascular network is visible at 4 days (Figure 27.41) (97).

ORGAN SELECTION

Mechanisms of organ selection by metastases are being studied intensively (139,158,205). As mentioned earlier, some organs appear to be selected by a purely mechanical mechanism, simply because they drain the blood of the primary tumor (such is the case of the liver as a target for metastases from the colon); more often, the selection is based on subtle properties of the seed and/or of the soil. However, it should not be forgotten that some bizarre localizations might still occur as random embolism by cells that have escaped capillary filters. By injecting microspheres intravenously it was shown that the lungs contain arteriovenous bypasses larger than 500 μm (127), and the same is true for other organs.

Several mechanisms of organ selection have been suggested.

Local Injury Selection of injured tissue is fairly easy to understand (132,172). If mouse lungs are damaged by exposure to oxygen (1) or by activating complement, which leads to neutrophil-mediated injury (p. 437) (134), tumor cells injected intravenously show greater retention in the lungs. Injury might also be produced by repeated tumor embolization (185). Whatever the cause of injury, it seems likely that exposed basement membranes would offer an easier foothold to the neoplastic cells (128). There are many examples of mechanical trauma as a localizing agent; in fact it has been proposed that the recurrence of a tumor in a postoperative scar is not necessarily the result of a surgical accident, as surgeons tend to think, but rather the effect of a biological, embolic event beyond surgical control (41,54).

Various Growth Factors and Growth Inhibitors Such factors contained in target organs may condition the take of a metastasis. For example,

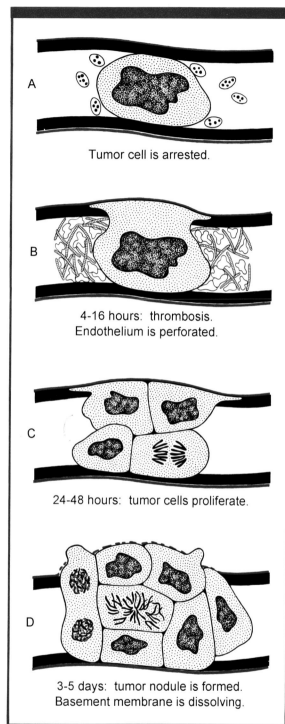

Tumor cell is arrested.

4-16 hours: thrombosis.
Endothelium is perforated.

24-48 hours: tumor cells proliferate.

3-5 days: tumor nodule is formed.
Basement membrane is dissolving.

FIGURE 27.41 Steps in the arrest and extravasation of metastatic cancer cells; a scheme based on experimental findings. **A:** Initial arrest, with close (selective?) contact between tumor cell and endothelium; some platelets aggregate. **B:** Further platelet aggregation and formation of fibrin; separation of endothelial cells and contact between tumor cell and basement membrane. **C:** Lysis of platelet thrombus; intravascular proliferation of the tumor cells. **D:** Further expansion of the tumor mass; dissolution of the subendothelial basement membrane. (Adapted from [29].)

cells of prostatic carcinomas that reached the vertebrae via the Batson system grow faster there than in the primary tumor: they may be stimulated by a growth factor produced in bone marrow (205).

Various Chemotactic Factors These mediators exist or develop in target organs and affect various

FIGURE 27.42 Experiment in the mouse to demonstrate that a tumor that usually metastasizes to the lung also metastasizes to fetal lung tissue (from a syngeneic animal) implanted intramuscularly in a thigh. This suggests that the metastatic preference for lung tissue is not based simply on the filtering mechanism of the lung but also on the nature of lung tissue. (Reproduced with permission from [31].)

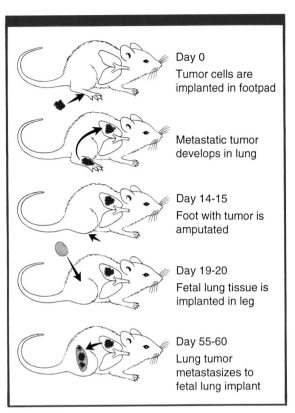

Day 0
Tumor cells are implanted in footpad

Metastatic tumor develops in lung

Day 14-15
Foot with tumor is amputated

Day 19-20
Fetal lung tissue is implanted in leg

Day 55-60
Lung tumor metastasizes to fetal lung implant

tumors (128). Some of these materials are breakdown products of matrix proteins (fibronectin, laminin, collagen, elastin, and bone) (205) and are generated by tumor-derived enzymes. The matrix can affect tumor cell adhesion in yet another way: endothelial cells, grown *in vitro* on a substrate that contains an extract of the stroma of a given organ, become particularly sticky for tumor cells that tend to home on that organ (139,143).

Surface Recognition Mechanisms Tumor cells can come to a halt in selected organs by means of adhesion molecules, very much like leukocytes in inflammation (13). The most obvious example is that of lymphoma cells, which metastasize to lymph nodes by means of the normal lymphocyte homing receptor, key to the normal lymphocyte recirculation (6,136,153). There is a mouse melanoma that ordinarily metastasizes to the lung; it also metastasizes into pieces of mouse fetal lung (but not of other tissues) implanted and revascularized in the thigh. This indicates that the metastatic cells "choose" the lung not only by a passive embolic process, but also by a selective mechanism (30) (Figure 27.42). Many studies have addressed this topic, both *in vitro* and *in vivo* (37,139,140). For example, it has been shown *in vitro* that activated human endothelium (obtained by exposure to IL-1,

TNF, or endotoxin) is more adhesive for human melanoma cells (36,154): an interesting link between inflammation and tumors. The preferential adhesion of metastatic cells to the endothelium of particular organs has been studied in several ways. An elegant approach has been to prepare endothelial monolayers from the microcirculation of mouse brain, lung, and ovary, and then expose them to dispersed cells from glioma, hepatoma, lymphoma, and other mouse tumors: some (alas not all) of the adhesion preferences coincided with known *in vivo* metastatic behavior of the tumors (5).

The intercellular adhesion molecule ICAM-1, which is involved in leukocyte adhesion, is absent on normal melanocytes and the cells of small melanomas that are thinner than the critical figure of 0.76 mm (p. 793) but present in most larger melanomas and their metastases (78). In several human carcinomas studied in vitro, the loss of normal epithelial adhesion molecule uvomorulin (also called E-cadherin) coincided with the appearance of the invasive phenotype; transfection of the invasive cells with E-cadherin cDNA prevented invasiveness (55). Yet another approach: knowing that laminin and fibronectin are involved in tumor cell adhesion and knowing that the specific sequences for their adhesive properties are repetitive structures such as Arg-Gly-Asp (RGD), synthetic polypeptides of the poly(RGD) type were prepared: injected intravenously in mice they reduced the number of lung metastases, and in vitro they inhibited the adhesion of tumor cells to fibronectin substrates. The poly(RGD) molecules had blocked the tumor receptors (162).

The mechanisms involved in the expression of metastatic or antimetastatic genes are just beginning to be studied (84,94,101,129,205); a gene (nm23) that reduces metastatic potential has been identified in carcinomas of mice and humans (15); transfected into cells of a highly metastatic murine melanoma it reduced their ability to metastasize (92).

This whole discussion of metastases is based on the assumption that they derive from migrant cells. Conceivably, in the case of virus-induced tumors some secondary tumors could arise from the spread of the virus itself (187). This must be kept in mind as a theoretical possibility (187). For example, in chickens infected with Rous sarcoma virus, wounds lead to tumor formation with a frequency near 100 percent (165), but these growths should be considered new primary tumors.

TO SUM UP: The successful metastatic cell that has completed its decathlon must be the result of a Darwinian selection process that has given it major advantages for growth and invasion over its nonmetastatic counterparts: appropriate receptors for attaching to the endothelium, abundance of receptors for extravascular matrix components, and the ability to produce and secrete a variety of matrix-degrading enzymes.

The cell that took over the world. *The capacity of tumor cells to invade is even greater than can be appreciated with the microscope. It was October 4, 1951, when Henrietta Lacks died of a highly aggressive carcinoma of the cervix; from this tumor was obtained the first dependable line of human malignant cells. For all laboratories involved in cancer research, throughout the world, HeLa cells became an indispensable tool. The cells responded by overtaking—unnoticed—many other cell types that were being grown in culture. In 1968 the cell bank at the American Type Culture Collection, where samples of important cell cultures are preserved, had in its custody 34 supposedly different cell lines. Careful checking showed that 24 were HeLa cells (Figure 27.43) (65). The impact and the cost of this tumor-related catastrophe were never measured.*

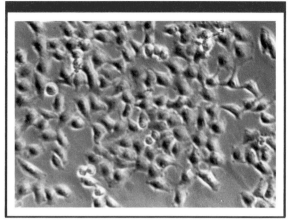

FIGURE 27.43 Culture of HeLa cells. (Courtesy of A.H. Cutler, University of Massachusetts Medical Center, Worcester, MA.)

malignant tumors can cause. Because they can infiltrate, they can destroy tissues that are in their way; in the abdomen they can mat all the organs into a solid inextricable mass, constrict or erode any part of the gut, or cause fistulae (abnormal communications) between gut and skin, bladder and rectum, or any two hollow viscera. We have seen a colon cancer erode its way into the heart.

This endless tale of misery has no redeeming features, but a biologically minded surgeon discovered that one local effect of tumors could open a new field of study: *angiogenesis*. Tumors force the host to provide them with blood vessels; the way they do so is relevant to wound healing and a host of other conditions (p. 755).

Effects of Tumors on the Host

All tumors are harmful to some degree, just by their bulk or by more subtle biological mechanisms. The harm can be local or distant.

LOCAL EFFECTS

Local effects are common even with benign tumors. Bulky lesions are especially hazardous in the skull, where space is limited and the anatomical structures are delicate. For example, cerebrospinal fluid produced in the cerebral ventricles flows through narrow passages; a small benign tumor, even a cyst, strategically located in one of these passages can obstruct the flow and cause one or all of the ventricles to dilate; the brain tissue shrinks accordingly (Figure 27.44). A small benign tumor of the hypophysis can bulge above the bony recess in which the hypophysis lies and damage the optic chiasm from which the optic nerves arise. Occlusion of a lumen can occur anywhere in the body when a tumor arises in a tubular or other hollow structure. Ulceration is another common effect of tumors bulging from a body surface (p. 740). The result is infection, bleeding, or both (the bleeding, however, can be clinically useful as a sign of a hidden tumor, e.g., of the bladder).

There is virtually no limit to the local trouble

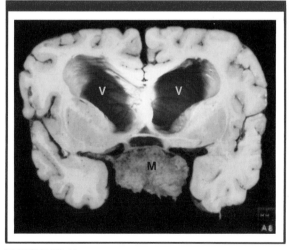

FIGURE 27.44
Example of damage caused by a benign tumor in the human brain. Most of the cerebrospinal fluid is produced in the lateral ventricles (**V**) and drains out through an aqueduct not visible here. Pressure by a meningioma (**M**) on the aqueduct has caused a dilatation of the lateral ventricles with corresponding atrophy of the cerebral tissue. (Courtesy of Dr. T.W. Smith, University of Massachusetts Medical Center, Worcester, MA.)

Distant Effects: The Paraneoplastic Syndromes

Tumors—benign or malignant—can produce remote effects by purely humoral mechanisms unrelated to invasion and metastasis. These provide a long list of symptom complexes observed in man and virtually all animal species (121). The variety is astounding: a tumor may come to the patient's attention disguised as rheumatoid arthritis (147), as a disease of an endocrine gland, of the skin, muscle, blood, or nervous system; even as ischemia of the fingers (178).

Tumor-derived hormones are only one of the mechanisms. It was realized in the 1960s that there is, beside hormones, a vast array of "humors from tumors" (74) capable of affecting every tissue in the body: cytokines, prostaglandins, enzymes, growth factors, and other polypeptides, not to mention antigens and molecules still unspecified (19). Today, the name *paraneoplastic syndrome* is given to all those symptom complexes that accompany tumors and concern distant targets (skin, nerves, muscle, blood, etc.) whether the mechanisms be hormonal, toxic, immunologic, or unknown. These syndromes usually disappear if the tumor is removed or destroyed, but some lesions are irreversible (e.g., in the nervous system). The two best known mechanisms are hormonal and immunologic.

How common are the paraneoplastic syndromes? This is difficult to establish from current data, but we have seen figures ranging from 7 to 50 percent of all cancer patients. Whatever their incidence, these syndromes must be kept in mind for practical reasons: they may be the first sign of a hidden cancer; they may mimic metastases; they may cause unnecessary discomfort; and they may help follow the regression or recurrence of the tumor.

Descriptions of a few common paraneoplastic syndromes follow (Table 27.1).

TABLE 27.1

Selected Hormones Formed Ectopically and Their More Common Clinical Effects[a]

Tumor	Hormone	Symptoms	Biochemical
Small cell Ca of lung, pancreatic tumors	Antidiuretic hormone	Confusion, convulsions, coma	↓ Na+
Small cell Ca of lung, carcinoid, islet-cell Ca of pancreas, medullary thyroid Ca	Adrenocorticotrophic hormone or corticotrophin-releasing hormone	Proximal muscle weakness, polyuria, edema, pigmentation changes	↓ K+ ↑ Blood sugar
Multiple myeloma	Osteoclast activity factor		
Squamous cell Ca of lung, renal carcinoma, hepatoma	Parathyroid hormone	Constipation, polyuria, polydipsia, vomiting, psychosis, coma	↑ Ca++
Breast carcinoma	Prostaglandins		
Renal carcinoma, hepatoma, bronchogenic carcinoma, adrenal carcinoma	Human chorionic gonadotropin	Precocious puberty in boys, irregular menses	

[a]*Very rare examples of the ectopic secretion by tumors of almost all nonsteroid hormones have been documented.*

From (173).

ENDOCRINE DISTURBANCES

These are the best understood of all paraneoplastic syndromes. Nobody should be surprised to learn that a tumor of a parathyroid gland, benign or malignant, can produce hypercalcemia: this is in line with the function of the normal parathyroid. But then it was realized that many malignant tumors secrete hormones quite unrelated to the tissue of origin. On second thought, this too is not surprising: the genes for producing hormones are present in all cells; they just have to be turned on. Malignant tumors can be expected to do so.

This phenomenon is named *ectopic hormone secretion*. It is possible that all malignant tumors secrete ectopic hormones in small amounts (130,131). The most common offenders are carcinomas of the lung: the standard explanation being that the lung derives from the endoderm, and therefore its carcinomas express genes that are activated in other endodermal derivatives such as the hypophysis or the parathyroids (125). *Paraneoplastic hypercalcemia* is found in 10–20 percent of cancer patients (74). But beware: tumors can produce hypercalcemia in many ways.

> Hypercalcemia of neoplastic origin *can be caused by: (a) parathyroid tumor; (b) extensive metastatic bone destruction such as occurs with multiple myeloma (the powerful osteolytic effect of this tumor is attributed to a cytokine named* osteoclast activating factor, *OAF) (60,104); (c) a parathyroid-hormone-like peptide (18); (d) prostaglandin E$_2$ (151,168) (other prostaglandins are osteoblastic) (201); (e) tumor necrosis factor beta (lymphotoxin); (f) interleukin-1 (115); (g) transforming growth factor alpha, which is also thought to play a role in the self-stimulation of tumor growth (19).*

The ectopic secretion of ACTH or of its precursor ("big ACTH" or pro-opiocortin) may lead to Cushing's syndrome: hypertension, weight loss, hypokalemia, hyperglycemia, muscle atrophy, and sometimes the typical "moon face" (74). Other classic associations are the bizarre production of insulin by mesotheliomas and sarcomas (19,33) and of erythropoietin by renal cell carcinomas: the latter can produce a high hematocrit (above 55 for men and 50 for women) with resulting symptoms related to high blood viscosity (p. 666).

These hormone-related paraneoplastic syndromes are so common that they inspired an aphorism (93):

If there is overproduction of a hormone, look for a tumor;

If there is a tumor, look for evidence of hormone overproduction

HYPERCOAGULABLE STATE

As many as 90–95 percent of cancer patients have been reported to have abnormalities of the clotting system (46,152,161): shortened clotting time, elevated fibrin/fibrinogen split products, elevated fibrinogen and thrombocytosis. This is perhaps an overcompensation for a constant, low-grade intravascular coagulation (19).

> The tendency to develop thrombosis in cases of cancer is attributed to four main mechanisms (105,124,138): (a) platelets are activated by tumor products such as ADP or by tumor-induced thrombin generation; (b) tumors secrete procoagulants such as tissue factor or factor X activators; they can also shed fibronectin (17) and other procoagulant materials from the cell surface (47); the mucin secreted by adenocarcinomas is also thrombogenic (146,155); (c) activated monocytes and macrophages in the tumor or in the MPS/RES secrete tissue factor and other procoagulants; (d) the liver secretes less anticoagulants such as antithrombin III and protein C (reasons unclear).

These abnormalities help understand the clinical thrombotic or hemorrhagic complications that occur in 9–15 percent of cancer patients (124). At autopsy, the number of thrombotic events found is even greater, especially in the form of thromboemboli. The likely cardiovascular complications fall into two groups.

Migratory Thrombophlebitis The name refers to bouts of thrombophlebitis in multiple locations without an apparent predisposing factor such as bed rest or varicose veins. Back in the 1860s a great French clinician, Armand Trousseau, realized that this clinical sequence often reveals an underlying cancer, hence the current term *Trousseau's syndrome* (180). An occult cancer, especially of the pancreas, lung, or stomach, should be suspected in any case of thrombosis in an upper limb unrelated to trauma, or in cases of pulmonary embolism and deep venous thrombosis below the age of 50 (66,155).

> Trousseau's memorable passage reads as follows: "If you feel uncertain about the nature of a disease of the stomach, and hesitate between a chronic gastritis, a simple ulcer and a carcinoma, a phlegmasia alba dolens appearing in the leg or arm will dispel your indecision, and you will be permitted to take a positive stand regarding the existence of the cancer"

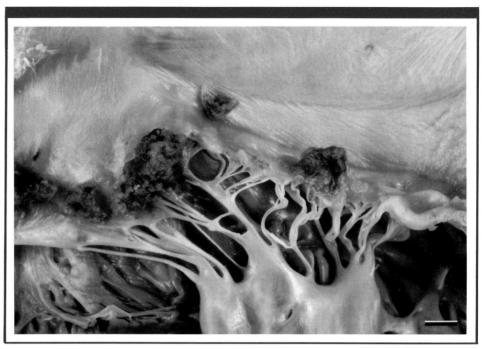

FIGURE 27.45
Thrombi on the mitral valve: an example of noninfective, "marantic" vegetations. The patient was a 46-year-old man who died of a mucin-producing gastric carcinoma, a known cause of hypercoagulability. **Bar** = 5 mm. (Courtesy of Dr. W.D. Edwards, Department of Laboratory Medicine and Pathology, The Mayo Clinic, Rochester, MN.)

(180). The Latin term phlegmasia alba dolens (literally white painful inflammation), still used by some physicians, refers to thrombophlebitis with pain and edema.

Nonbacterial Thrombotic Endocarditis Marantic endocarditis (from *marasmus*, "wasting of the body") is usually a terminal condition; it consists of small, warty-looking masses of platelets and fibrin, sometimes too small to be seen by echocardiography but large enough to throw emboli to the brain, kidney, and other viscera (Figure 27.45).

HEMATOLOGIC EFFECTS

Microangiopathic hemolytic anemia (MAHA) is a peculiar but not uncommon situation in which red blood cells, forced to squeeze through tight places or fibrin meshes, break up or are sliced into smaller pieces called *schistocytes* or *helmet cells*, easily identified on smears; they seal up and continue to circulate for a few days (77).

> *Actually, not all the hazards facing the red blood cells in patients with malignant tumors are well understood (4). Several mechanisms of damage have been proposed: (a) narrow capillaries or intravascular fibrin strands within the tumor itself; (b) narrowing of pulmonary arterioles by embolized neoplastic cells and fibrin, which would explain the association with metastatic carcinoma (71); (c) the fibrin thrombi of DIC, the ultimate manifestation of hypercoagulability in cancer (p. 638). Massive "slicing" of red blood cells can occur in hemangiomas.*

Anemia is another classic complication of advanced cancer. Unlike microangiopathic anemia just mentioned, it is normocytic (the red blood cells are normal in shape) as well as normochromic (the amount of hemoglobin per cell is normal). Long unexplained (10 mechanisms had been proposed) (19), anemia turns out to be another misdeed of cachectin/TNF (119), a cytokine that has a great deal to do with cancer patients (see later). The red blood cells are produced at a lower rate and have shorter life spans. Erythropoietin levels are also low (118).

Not to be forgotten are microcirculatory disturbances due to increased blood viscosity: renal cell tumors, for example, secrete erythropoietin, which stimulates bone marrow to produce excess red blood cells, whereby the viscosity of the blood is increased; leukemia can lead to leukocyte plugging of capillaries with similar consequences (p. 667).

> *Other hematologic effects of cancers include granulocytosis related to the secretion of a colony-stimulating factor (CSF), granulocytopenia (due to an inhibitor?), thrombocytosis, and, paradoxically, thrombocytopenia, often related to therapy.*

NEUROLOGIC EFFECTS

Neurologic complications are many and largely unexplained, except that autoimmune mechanisms appear to be at work in some situations. Cell damage and loss may affect the brain, even

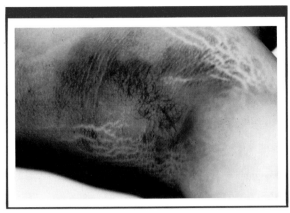

FIGURE 27.46
Velvety, brown-black, excessively cornified (hyperkeratotic) plaques of *acanthosis nigricans* in the armpit of an obese 21-year-old man. This lesion, which tends to develop in skin folds, may accompany malignancy as well as obesity, diabetes, and other conditions. (Courtesy of Drs. E. Gonzalez and J.D. Bernhard, University of Massachusetts Medical Center, Worcester, MA.)

dementia may develop; the cerebellum (45) and the retina (76) may be affected, probably by an autoimmune mechanism; also the spinal cord and sensory or motor nerves. Muscular weakness sometimes reflects a myasthenia-like syndrome probably due to autoantibodies: this syndrome can be transmitted to mice with purified IgG of an affected patient (19).

SKIN LESIONS

Another long list, headed by *acanthosis nigricans,* a symmetric, brown, warty hyperpigmentation with hyperkeratosis of the axilla and other flexural areas (Figure 27.46), possibly induced by transforming growth factor alpha. More than half of the cases represent the warning sign of an internal malignancy, especially a carcinoma of the gastrointestinal tract. Many of the cutaneous paraneoplastic syndromes are proliferative lesions, and growth factors have been implicated but not nailed down as causal agents (49).

RENAL COMPLICATIONS

The kidneys can be affected by distant tumors in many ways (Table 27.2) (137). Classic mechanisms of renal damage in tumor-bearing patients are: (a) glomerular damage caused by tumor antigens complexed with antibodies and deposited along the basement membrane (p. 539); (b) glomerular damage caused by amyloid deposits, in cases of multiple myeloma; (c) if severe hypercalcemia is present, it may lead to calcification of the renal parenchyma (nephrocalcinosis) (p. 237); (d) again in multiple myeloma, the tubules may become

TABLE 27.2
Renal Damage with Extrarenal Cancer:
Study of 344 Malignant Tumors

CANCER	NUMBER	PERCENTAGE
Lymphomas and leukemias	47	15.0
Multiple myeloma	10	3.1
Renal metastases (nonleukemia)	25	8.0
Hydronephrosis	18	5.7
Pyelonephritis	20	6.4
Acute tubular necrosis	44	14.0
Infarction	7	2.2
Disseminated intravascular coagulation	4	1.3
Nephrocalcinosis	9	2.9
Amyloid	6	1.9
Bence Jones nephropathy	7	2.2
"Bile nephrosis"	10	3.2
Herpes with lymphoma	1	0.3
Glomerulonephritis	5	1.6
Radiation nephritis	1	0.3

Adapted from (137).

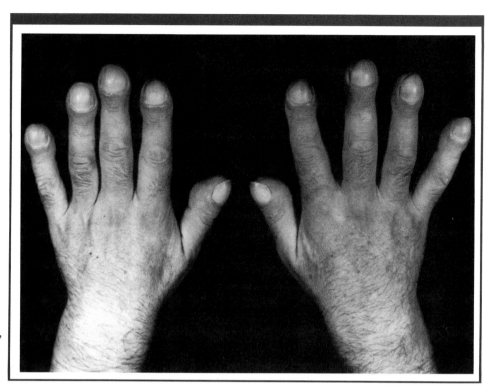

FIGURE 27.47
Clubbing of the fingers: a peculiar consequence of chronic lung disease, including cancer. The mechanism is not well understood. (Reproduced with permission from [62].)

clogged with casts containing immunoglobulins and other proteins (27).

MISCELLANEOUS EFFECTS

Strange but not rare is the bizarre clubbing of the fingers called hypertrophic pulmonary osteopathy when the bone is also thickened. Finger clubbing is known in French as *hippocratisme digital* because it is mentioned in the Hippocratic books as a condition associated with chronic pulmonary disease (Figure 27.47): the association is perfectly correct and today we include cancer, but the pathogenesis remains a frustrating mystery (19). Low serum albumin affects over 90 percent of cancer patients: it is probably a part of the acute phase response (p. 491) caused by the release of TNF by tumor macrophages.

SUPPRESSION OF INFLAMMATION AND OF THE IMMUNE RESPONSE

These effects are perhaps too important to be listed in eighth place. Both tumors and antitumor therapy contribute to undermining bodily defenses. About one-third of cancer patients die of infection. The mechanisms are many; neutropenia is foremost (148).

CACHEXIA

Wasting of the whole body is the ultimate paraneoplastic syndrome. Its ancient name (from a Greek word for "being in a bad way") echoes the dread of malignant tumors, which can reduce the body to skin and bones and even starve it to death (91). Until 1986 theories abounded; then came the answer that seems to be final. It came from studies on a seemingly unrelated topic: sleeping sickness.

Dr. Anthony Cerami of Rockefeller University was interested in therapy for sleeping sickness, which affects both humans and cattle in parts of Africa. Field observations in Africa led him to observe the profound cachexia of the affected cattle, a condition that contrasted with the small number of circulating trypanosomes (Figure 27.48). Back in New York, in 1980, Rouzer and Cerami chose to study the mechanism of cachexia in rabbits infected with trypanosoma: the rabbits lost 50 percent of their weight, yet they too had very few parasites in the blood and mild internal lesions. Curiously, the blood became intensely lipemic, suggesting a defect in the degradation of triglycerides. It was concluded that the cachexia reflected an exaggerated host response, rather than a virulent aggression by the parasite. A further study on mice made cachectic with injections of endotoxin showed that cachexia was associated with inhibition of lipoprotein lipase (83). Using this inhibition as a guide, the researchers isolated, from the blood of the mice, a protein which they called cachectin. When they sequenced it—surprise!—it turned out to be identical to the recently isolated TNF, tumor necrosis factor, a product of macrophages (14). Antibodies against TNF reduced the cachexia in tumor-bearing mice (167).

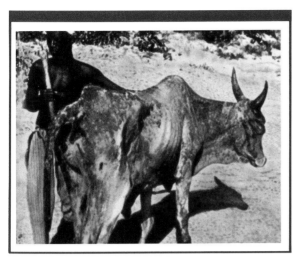

FIGURE 27.48
In parts of Africa sleeping sickness affects cattle and humans. This extreme cachexia contrasts sharply with the small number of trypanosomes in the blood of these animals. In tracking the mechanism of this cachexia, Dr. Anthony Cerami and collaborators discovered "cachexin," which turned out to be tumor necrosis factor. (Courtesy of the Wellcome Foundation, Inc., London, England, and of Dr. A. Cerami, Rockefeller University, New York, NY.)

Now we face this troublesome development: macrophages respond to a tumor by producing a protein that is potentially capable of killing the tumor—and the host. Injected into animals, cachectin/TNF produces anorexia, weight loss, and "an apathetic, unkempt appearance"—simply stated, cachexia. It also reproduces the major effects of endotoxic shock (p. 702). Glucocorticoids, which are effective against shock and inflammation, suppress cachectin production (14). But why in the world would Nature conserve for several hundred million years such a dangerous cytokine? "Presumably, the ability of cachectin to activate neutrophils and eosinophils, and to mobilize energy stores, confers an advantage. . . . It is possible that . . . the ill-effects imparted by high levels of the protein have allowed the removal of severely infected individuals, thus preventing further disease transmission" (14). This may sound like a harsh explanation, but we do not know of a gentler one.

It is interesting to review the main theories of cachexia before cachectin/TNF was discovered (120). (a) The tumor produces some sort of toxin (91). This may very well be true, but research on "toxohormones" has attracted very little attention (113,122,174). (b) Tumors cause loss of appetite (anorexia): this is certainly a fact, together with changes in the sense of taste (43). We recall a starved-looking patient contemplating a tasty meal but sadly stating that "he saw no reason to eat it." But then, what causes the anorexia? (c) The tumor acts as a "nitrogen trap" (i.e., it traps nutrients and starves its host). This catchy notion was a favorite for some time, but it is too simplistic; and anyway, overfeeding is not an effective treatment for cachexia (50), nor does starving stop tumor growth. (d) The metabolism of the host is increased (184). A speck of truth may be buried in these theories.

Tumors can also kill as they die: the tumor lysis syndrome. We mentioned this phenomenon in relation to cell death (p. 219). In essence, extensive, acute necrosis of a tumor that happens to be very sensitive to X-rays or chemotherapy can become life-threatening by releasing toxic amounts of potassium and uric acid, which may lead to renal failure and cause a drop in serum calcium (169). The larger the tumor, the greater the danger. Burkitt's lymphoma is often involved (p. 219). Dialysis may be required, but fortunately the condition is limited to 5–7 days because the wave of cell death comes to an end (26, 27).

How Does Cancer Kill?

In three studies from the 1970s (3,75,86) the salient points are the following:

- *Infection* was at the top of the list, accounting for 32, 36, or 47 percent of the deaths. This fits with the antiinflammatory effects of both cancer and cancer therapy. Gram-negative organisms accounted for all the deaths in the first series.
- *Hemorrhage and thromboembolic phenomena* accounted for 10–20 percent of all cancer deaths. Hemorrhage alone was a significant cause of death only in acute leukemia.
- *Cachexia* was rarely given a major role (1 percent in the last series).

The remaining deaths were due to respiratory failure, renal failure and other causes. Overall, *these statistics suggest that most of cancer patients, from what we know of gram-negative sepsis (p. 700), succumb to their own macrophages.*

The malignant tumor causes nothing but misery to the host; the host, in return, does little damage to the tumor, even providing it with life-sustaining blood vessels. However, this does not mean that antitumor defenses are powerless. In fact, they are of many kinds, some based on the immune response, some not, and they can sometimes destroy the tumor. We will review them later (p. 885).

References

1. Adamson IYR, Young L, Orr FW. Tumor metastasis after hyperoxic injury and repair of the pulmonary endothelium. Lab Invest 1987;57:71–77.
2. Alexander P. The biology of metastases. In: Carney D, Sikora K, eds. Genes and cancer. Chichester: John Wiley & Sons, 1990:313–328.
3. Ambrus JL, Ambrus CM, Mink IB, Pickren JW. Causes of death in cancer patients. J Med 1975;6:61–64.
4. Antman KH, Skarin AT, Mayer RJ, Hargreaves HK, Canellos GP. Microangiopathic hemolytic anemia and cancer: a review. Medicine 1979;58:377–384.
5. Auerbach R, Lu WC, Pardon E, Gumkowski F, Kaminska G, Kaminski M. Specificity of adhesion between murine tumor cells and capillary endothelium: an *in vitro* correlate of preferential metastasis *in vivo*. Cancer Res 1987;47:1492–1496.
6. Azzarelli B, Easterling K, Norton JA. Leukemic cell-endothelial cell interactions in leukemic cell dissemination. Lab Invest 1989;60:45–64.
7. Babai F, Tremblay G. Ultrastructural study of liver invasion by Novikoff hepatoma. Cancer Res 1972;32:2765–2770.
8. Balch CM, Murad TM, Soong SJ, Ingalls AL, Halpern NB, Maddox WA. A multifactorial analysis of melanoma: prognostic histopathological features comparing Clark's and Breslow's staging methods. Ann Surg 1978;188:732–742.
9. Balch CM, Soong SJ, Murad TM, Ingalls AL, Maddox WA. A multifactorial analysis of melanoma. II. Prognostic factors in patients with stage I (localized) melanoma. Surgery 1979;86:343–351.
10. Barsky SH, Rao CN, Hyams D, Liotta LA. Characterization of a laminin receptor from human breast cacinoma tissue. Breast Cancer Res Treat 1984;4:181–188.
11. Batson OV. The function of the vertebral veins and their rôle in the spread of metastases. Ann Surg 1940;112:138–149.
12. Batson OV. The vertebral vein system. Am J Roentgenol Radium Ther Nucl Med 1957;78:195–212.
13. Belloni PN, Tressler RJ. Microvascular endothelial cell heterogeneity: interactions with leukocytes and tumor cells. Cancer Metastasis Rev 1989/90;8:353–389.
14. Beutler B, Cerami A. Cachectin and tumour necrosis factor as two sides of the same biological coin. Nature 1986;320:584–588.
15. Bevilacqua G, Sobel ME, Liotta LA, Steeg PS. Association of low nm23 RNA levels in human primary infiltrating ductal breast carcinomas with lymph node involvement and other histopathological indicators of high metastatic potential. Cancer Res 1989;49:5185–5190.
16. Birbeck MSC, Wheatley DN. An electron microscopic study of the invasion of ascites tumor cells into the abdominal wall. Cancer Res 1965;25:490–497.
17. Black PH. Shedding from normal and cancer-cell surfaces. N Engl J Med 1980;303:1415–1416.
18. Broadus AE, Mangin M, Ikeda K, et al. Humoral hypercalcemia of cancer. Identification of a novel parathyroid hormone-like peptide. N Engl J Med 1988; 319:556–563.
19. Bunn PA Jr, Ridgway EC. Paraneoplastic syndromes. In: DeVita VT Jr, Hellman S, Rosenberg SA, eds. Cancer: principles & practice of oncology, 3rd ed. Philadelphia: JB Lippincott, 1989:1896–1940.
20. Butler TP, Gullino PM. Quantitation of cell shedding into efferent blood of mammary adenocarcinoma. Cancer Res 1975;35:512–516.

21. Calman KC. Clinical aspects of invasion. In: Mareel MM, Calman KC, eds. Invasion: experimental and clinical implications. Oxford: Oxford University Press, 1984:1–23.
22. Carr I, Carr J, Dreher B. Lymphatic metastasis of mammary adenocarcinoma. An experimental study in the rat with a brief review of the literature. Invasion Metastasis 1981;1:34–53.
23. Carr I, McGinty F. Lymphatic metastasis and its inhibition: an experimental model. J Pathol 1973;113:85–95.
24. Carr I, McGinty F, Norris P. The fine structure of neoplastic invasion: invasion of liver, skeletal muscle and lymphatic vessels by the Rd/3 tumour. J Pathol 1976; 118:91–99.
25. Chew EC, Josephson RL, Wallace AC. Morphologic aspects of the arrest of circulating cancer cells. In: Weiss L, ed. Fundamental aspects of metastasis. Amsterdam: North Holland Publishing Company, 1976:121–150.
26. Cohen LF, Balow JE, Magrath IT, Poplack DG, Ziegler JL. Acute tumor lysis syndrome. A review of 37 patients with Burkitt's lymphoma. Am J Med 1980;68:486–491.
27. Cohen AH, Border MD. Myeloma kidney. An immunomorphogenetic study of renal biopsies. Lab Invest 1980; 42:248.
28. Coman DR, deLong RP. The role of the vertebral venous system in the metastasis of cancer to the spinal column. Experiments with tumor-cell suspensions in rats and rabbits. Cancer 1951;4:610–618.
29. Crissman JD, Hatfield JS, Menter DG, Sloane B, Honn KV. Morphological study of the interaction of intravascular tumor cells with endothelial cells and subendothelial matrix. Cancer Res 1988;48:4065–4072.
30. Crissman JD, Hatfield JS, Schaldenbrand M, Sloane BF, Honn KV. Arrest and extravasation of B16 amelanotic melanoma in murine lungs. A light and electron microscopic study. Lab Invest 1985a;53:470–478.
31. Crissman JD, Hatfield JS, Honn KV. Clinical and experimental morphologic parameters predictive of tumor metastasis. Prog Clin Biol Res 1986;212:251–265.
32. Crissman JD, Honn KV, Sloane BF. Metastasis from metastases: an animal model. In: Hellmann K, Eccles SA, eds. Treatment of metastasis: problems and prospects. London: Taylor & Francis, 1985b:211–214.
33. Daughaday WH, Emanuelle MA, Brooks MH, Barbato AL, Kapadia M, Rotwein P. Synthesis and secretion of insulin-like growth factor II by a leiomyosarcoma with associated hypoglycemia. N Engl J Med 1988; 319:1421–1440.
34. De Bruyn PPH, Cho Y. Entry of metastatic malignant cells into the circulation from a subcutaneously growing myelogenous tumor. J Natl Cancer Inst 1979;62:1221–1227.
35. De Bruyn PPH, Cho Y. Vascular endothelial invasion via transcellular passage by malignant cells in the primary stage of metastases formation. J Ultrastruct Res 1982; 81:189–201.
36. Dejana E, Bertocchi F, Bortolami MC, et al. Interleukin 1 promotes tumor cell adhesion to cultured human endothelial cells. J Clin Invest 1988;82:1466–1470.
37. Dejana E, Martin-Padura I, Lauri D, et al. Endothelial leukocyte adhesion molecule-1-dependent adhesion of colon carcinoma cells to vascular endothelium is inhibited by an antibody to Lewis fucosylated type I carbohydrate chain. Lab Invest 1992;66:324–330.
38. del Regato JA. Pathways of metastatic spread of malignant tumors. Semin Oncol 1977;4:33–38.

39. del Regato J. Physiopathology of metastasis. In: Weiss L, Gilbert HA, eds. Pulmonary metastasis. Boston: GK Hall & Co, 1978:104–113.

40. de Ridder L, Mareel M, Vakaet L. Invasion of malignant cells into cultured embryonic substrates. Arch Geschwulstforsch 1977;47:7–27.

41. DerHagopian RP, Sugarbaker EV, Ketcham A. Inflammatory oncotaxis. JAMA 1978;240:374–375.

42. DeVita VT Jr, Hellman S, Rosenberg SA, eds. Cancer: principles & practice of oncology, 3rd ed. Philadelphia: JB Lippincott, 1989.

43. DeWys WD. Anorexia as a general effect of cancer. Cancer 1979;43:2013–2019.

44. Dingemans KP, Roos E, van den Bergh Weerman MA, van de Pavert IV. Invasion of liver tissue by tumor cells and leukocytes: comparative ultrastructure. J Natl Cancer Inst 1978;60:583–598.

45. Dropcho EJ, Whitaker JN. Cerebellar ataxia as a paraneoplastic syndrome. Hosp Pract 1989;24:69–84.

46. Dvorak HF. Thrombosis and cancer. Hum Pathol 1987; 18:275–284.

47. Dvorak HF, Quay SC, Orenstein NS, Dvorak AM, Hahn P, Bitzer AM. Tumor shedding and coagulation. Science 1981;212:923–924.

48. Eilon G, Mundy GR. Direct resorption of bone by human breast cancer cells in vitro. Nature 1978;276:726–728.

49. Ellis DL, Kafka SP, Chow JC, et al. Melanoma, growth factors, acanthosis nigricans, the sign of Leser-Trélat, and multiple acrochordons. A possible role for alpha-transforming growth factor in cutaneous paraneoplastic syndromes. N Engl J Med 1987;317:1582–1587.

50. Evans WK, Makuch R, Clamon GH, et al. Limited impact of total parenteral nutrition on nutritional status during treatment for small cell lung cancer. Cancer Res 1985;45:3347–3353.

51. Fidler IJ. Metastasis: quantitative analysis of distribution and fate of tumor emboli labeled with ^{125}I-5-Iodo-2′-deoxyuridine. J Natl Cancer Inst 1970;45:773–782.

52. Fidler IJ. Introduction. Ciba Found Symp 1988;141:1–4.

53. Fidler IJ, Gersten DM, Hart IR. The biology of cancer invasion and metastasis. Adv Cancer Res 1978;28:149–250.

54. Fisher B, Fisher ER, Feduska N. Trauma and the localization of tumor cells. Cancer 1967;20:23–30.

54a. Folkman J. Angiogenesis in cancer, vascular, rheumatoid and other disease. Nature Med 1995;1:27–31.

55. Frixen UH, Behrens J, Sachs M, et al. E-cadherin-mediated cell-cell adhesion prevents invasiveness of human carcinoma cells. J Cell Biol 1991;113:173–185.

56. Gabbert H, Gerharz CD, Ramp U, Bohl J. The nature of host tissue destruction in tumor invasion. An experimental investigation on carcinoma and sarcoma xenotransplants. Virchows Arch Cell Pathol 1987;52:513–527.

57. Galasko CSB. The anatomy and pathways of skeletal metastases. In: Weiss L, Gilbert HA, eds. Bone metastasis. Boston: GK Hall Medical Publishers, 1981.

58. Galasko CSB, Bennett A. Relationship of bone destruction in skeletal metastases to osteoclast activation and prostaglandins. Nature 1976;263:508–510.

59. Garbisa S, Pozzatti R, Muschel RJ, et al. Secretion of type IV collagenolytic protease and metastatic phenotype: induction by transfection with c-Ha-ras but not c-Ha-ras plus Ad2-E1a. Cancer Res 1987;47:1523–1528.

60. Garrett IR, Durie BGM, Nedwin GE, et al. Production of lymphotoxin, a bone-resorbing cytokine, by cultured human myeloma cells. N Engl J Med 1987;317:526–532.

61. Gasic GJ. Role of plasma, platelets, and endothelial cells in tumor metastasis. Cancer Metastasis Rev 1984; 3:99–116.

62. Ginsburg J. Clubbing of the fingers. In: Hamilton WF, Dow P, eds. Handbook of physiology, sect 2, vol III. Washington, DC: American Physiological Society, 1965: 2377–2389.

63. Glaves D. Detection of circulating metastatic cells. Prog Clin Biol Res 1986;212:151–165.

64. Glaves D, Huben RP, Weiss L. Haematogenous dissemination of cells from human renal adenocarcinomas. Br J Cancer 1988;57:32–35.

65. Gold M. A conspiracy of cells. Albany, NY: State University of New York Press, 1986.

66. Goldberg RJ, Seneff M, Gore JM, et al. Occult malignant neoplasm in patients with deep venous thrombosis. Arch Intern Med 1987;147:251–253.

67. Griffiths JD, Salsbury AJ. Circulating cancer cells. Springfield, IL: Charles C. Thomas, 1965.

68. Gullino PM. In vivo release of neoplastic cells by mammary tumors. GANN Monogr Cancer Res 1977;20:49–55.

69. Gullino PM. Influence of blood supply on thermal properties and metabolism of mammary carcinomas. Ann NY Acad Sci 1980;335:1–21.

70. Herlihy WF. Revision of the venous system: the role of the vertebral veins. Med J Aust 1947;1:661–672.

71. Hilgard P, Gordon-Smith EC. Microangiopathic haemolytic anaemia and experimental tumour-cell emboli. Br J Haematol 1974;26:651–659.

72. Hoover HC, Ketcham AS. Metastasis of metastases. Am J Surg 1975;130:405–411.

73. Ibbotson KJ, Twardzik DR, D'Souza SM, Hargreaves WR, Todaro GJ, Mundy GR. Stimulation of bone resorption in vitro by synthetic transforming growth factor-alpha. Science 1985;228:1007–1009.

74. Ihde DC. Paraneoplastic syndromes. Hosp Pract 1987; 22:105–124.

75. Inagaki J, Rodriguez V, Bodey GP. Causes of death in cancer patients. Cancer 1974;33:568–573.

76. Jacobson DM, Thirkill CE, Tipping SJ. A clinical triad to diagnose paraneoplastic retinopathy. Ann Neurol 1990; 28:162–167.

77. Jandl JH. Blood. Boston: Little, Brown, 1987.

78. Johnson JP, Stade BG, Holzmann B, Schwäble W, Riethmüller H. De novo expression of intercellular-adhesion molecule 1 in melanoma correlates with increased risk of metastasis. Proc Natl Acad Sci USA 1989;86:641–644.

79. Jones DS, Wallace AC, Fraser EE. Sequence of events in experimental metastases of Walker 256 tumor: light, immunofluorescent, and electron microscopic observations. J Natl Cancer Inst 1971;46:493–504.

80. Kalebic T, Williams JE, Talmadge JE, et al. A novel method for selection of invasive tumor cells: derivation and characterization of highly metastatic K1735 melanoma cell lines based on in vitro and in vivo invasive capacity. Clin Exp Metastasis 1988;6:301–318.

81. Karpatkin S, Pearlstein E. Role of platelets in tumor cell metastases. Ann Intern Med 1981;95:636–641.

82. Kawaguchi T, Nakamura K. Analysis of the lodgement and extravasation of tumor cells in experimental models of hematogenous metastasis. Cancer Metastasis Rev 1986;5:77–94.

83. Kawakami M, Cerami A. Studies of endotoxin-induced decrease in lipoprotein lipase activity. J Exp Med 1981;154:631–639.

84. Kerbel RS. Growth dominance of the metastatic cancer cell: cellular and molecular aspects. Adv Cancer Res 1990;55:87–132.

85. Kinjo M. Lodgement and extravasation of tumour cells in blood-borne metastasis: an electron microscope study. Br J Cancer 1978;38:293–301.

86. Klastersky J, Daneau D, Verhest A. Causes of death in patients with cancer. Eur J Cancer 1972;8:149–154.

87. Kodama T. Pathology of immunologic regression of tumor metastases in the lymph nodes. GANN Monogr Cancer Res 1977;20:83–95.

88. Kurokawa Y. Experiments on lymph node metastasis by intralymphatic inoculation of rat ascites tumor cells, with special reference to lodgment, passage, and growth of tumor cells in lymph nodes. GANN 1970;61:461–471.

89. Larsen MP, Steinberg GD, Brendler CB, Epstein JI. Use of Ulex europaeus agglutinin I (UEAI) to distinguish vascular and "pseudovascular" invasion in transitional cell carcinoma of bladder with lamina propria invasion. Mod Pathol 1990;3:83–88.

90. Lasser A, Zacks SI. Intraskeletal myofiber metastasis of breast carcinoma. Hum Pathol 1982;13:1045–1046.

91. Lawson DH, Richmond A, Nixon DW, Rudman D. Metabolic approaches to cancer cachexia. Annu Rev Nutr 1982;2:277–301.

92. Leone A, Flatow U, King CR, et al. Reduced tumor incidence, metastatic potential, and cytokine responsiveness of nm23-transfected melanoma cells. Cell 1991;65:25–35.

93. Liddle GW, Ball JH. Manifestations of cancer mediated by ectopic hormones. In: Holland JF, Frei E III, eds. Cancer medicine. Philadelphia: Lea & Febiger, 1973:1046–1057.

94. Liotta LA. Cancer cell invasion and metastasis. Sci Am 1992;266:54–63.

95. Liotta LA, Garbisa S, Tryggvason K. Biochemical mechanisms involved in tumor cell penetration of the basement membrane. In: Liotta LA, Hart IR, eds. Tumor invasion and metastasis. The Hague: Martinus Nijhoff Publishers, 1982:319–333.

96. Liotta LA, Guirguis RA, Schiffman E. Tumor autocrine motility factor. Prog Clin Biol Res 1986;212:17–22.

97. Liotta LA, Kleinerman J, Saidel GM. Quantitative relationships of intravascular tumor cells, tumor vessels, and pulmonary metastases following tumor implantation. Cancer Res 1974;34:997–1004.

98. Liotta LA, Kleinerman J, Saidel GM. The significance of hematogenous tumor cell clumps in the metastatic process. Cancer Res 1976;36:889–894.

99. Liotta LA, Mandler R, Murano G, et al. Tumor cell autocrine motility factor. Proc Natl Acad Sci USA 1986a;83:3302–3306.

100. Liotta LA, Rao CN, Wewer UM. Biochemical interactions of tumor cells with the basement membrane. Annu Rev Biochem 1986b;55:1037–1057.

101. Liotta LA, Steeg PS. Clues to the function of Nm23 and Awd proteins in development, signal transduction, and tumor metastasis provided by studies of Dictyostelium discoideum. J Natl Cancer Inst 1990;82:1170–1172.

102. Liotta LA, Wewer U, Rao NC, et al. Biochemical mechanisms of tumor invasion and metastasis. Anti-Cancer Drug Design 1987;2:195–202.

103. Liotta LA, Wewer U, Rao NC, et al. Biochemical mechanisms of tumor invasion and metastases. Prog Clin Biol Res 1988;256:3–16.

104. Luben RA. An assay for osteoclast-activating factor (OAF) in biological fluids: detection of OAF in the serum of myeloma patients. Cell Immunol 1980;49:74–80.

105. Luzzatto G, Schafer AI. The prethrombotic state in cancer. Semin Oncol 1990;17:147–159.

106. Manishen WJ, Sivananthan K, Orr FW. Resorbing bone stimulates tumor cell growth. A role for the host microenvironment in bone metastasis. Am J Pathol 1986;123:39–45.

107. Mareel MM. Is invasiveness in vitro characteristic of malignant cells? Cell Biol Int Rep 1979;3:627–640.

108. Mareel MM. Recent aspects of tumor invasiveness. Int Rev Exp Pathol 1980;22:65–129.

109. Mareel MM, Bruyneel E, Storme G. Attachment of mouse fibrosarcoma cells to precultured fragments of embryonic chick heart. An early step of invasion in vitro. Virchows Arch B Cell Pathol 1980;34:85–97.

110. Mareel MM, De Baetselier P, Van Roy FM. Mechanisms of invasion and metastasis. Boca Raton, FL: CRC Press, 1991.

111. Mareel MM, De Bruyne GK, Vandesande F, Dragonetti C. Immunohistochemical study of embryonic chick heart invaded by malignant cells in three-dimensional culture. Invasion Metastasis 1981;1:195–204.

112. Mareel MM, Van Roy FM, De Baetselier P. The invasive phenotypes. Cancer Metastasis Rev 1990;9:45–62.

113. Masuno H, Yoshimura H, Ogawa N, Okuda H. Isolation of a lipolytic factor (toxohormone-L) from ascites fluid of patients with hepatoma and its effect on feeding behavior. Eur J Cancer Clin Oncol 1984;20:1177–1185.

114. McDonald DF, Schofield BH, Prezioso EM, et al. Direct bone resorbing activity of murine myeloma cells. Cancer Lett 1983;19:119–124.

115. Meikle MC. Hypercalcaemia of malignancy. Nature 1988;336:311.

116. Mesonero CE. Appearance of neoplasms during pregnancy. In: Levine AS, ed. Etiology of cancer in man. Dordrecht: Kluwer Academic Publishers, 1989:102–114.

117. Milas L, Tofilon PJ, Brock WA. Assessment of anti-tumor (antimetastatic) efficacy of cytotoxic agents. Prog Clin Biol Res 1986;212:305–320.

118. Miller CB, Jones RJ, Piantadosi S, Abeloff MD, Spivak JL. Decreased erythropoietin response in patients with the anemia of cancer. N Engl J Med 1990;322:1689–1692.

119. Moldawer LL, Marano MA, Wei H, et al. Cachectin/tumor necrosis factor-α alters red blood cell kinetics and induces anemia in vivo. FASEB J 1989;3:1637–1643.

120. Morrison SD. Cancer cachexia. In: Liotta LA, ed. Influence of tumor development on the host. Dordrecht: Kluwer Academic Publishers, 1989:176–213.

121. Nagourney RA, Woolley PV. Paraneoplastic syndromes. In: Liotta LA, ed. Influence of tumor development on the host. Dordrecht: Kluwer Academic Publishers, 1989:214–227.

122. Nakahara W, Fukuoka F. Toxohormone: a characteristic toxic substance produced by cancer tissue. GANN 1949;40:45–69.

123. Nakamura K, Kawaguchi T, Asahina S, et al. Electronmicroscopic studies on extravasation of tumor cells and early foci of hematogenous metastasis. GANN Monogr Cancer Res 1977;20:57–71.

124. Nand S, Messmore H. Hemostasis in malignancy. Am J Hematol 1990;35:45–55.

125. Nathanson L, Hall TC. Lung tumors: how they produce their syndromes. Ann NY Acad Sci 1974;230:367–377.

126. Nicolson GL. Cancer metastasis. Organ colonization and the cell-surface properties of malignant cells. Biochim Biophys Acta 1982;695:113–176.

127. Nicolson GL. Cancer metastasis: tumor cell and host organ properties important in metastasis to specific secondary sites. Biochim Biophys Acta 1988;948:175–224.

128. Nicolson GL. Metastatic tumor cell interactions with endothelium, basement membrane and tissue. Curr Opin Cell Biol 1989;1:1009–1019.

129. Nicolson GL. Molecular mechanisms of cancer metastasis: tumor and host properties and the role of oncogenes and suppressor genes. Curr Opin Oncol 1991;3:75–92.

130. Odell WD, Wolfsen AR. Hormones from tumors: are they ubiquitous? Am J Med 1980;68:317–318.

131. Odell W, Wolfsen A, Yoshimoto Y, Weitzman R, Fisher D, Hirose F. Ectopic peptide synthesis: a universal concomitant of neoplasia. Trans Assoc Am Physicians 1977;40:204–227.

132. Orr FW. The influence of endothelial injury and inflammatory processes on metastasis. In: Orr FW, Buchanan MR, Weiss L, eds. Microcirculation in cancer metastasis. Boca Raton, FL: CRC Press, 1991:239–255.

133. Orr FW, Buchanan MR, Weiss L, eds. Microcirculation in cancer metastasis. Boca Raton, FL: CRC Press, 1991.

134. Orr FW, Warner DJA. Effects of systemic complement activation and neutrophil-mediated pulmonary injury on the retention and metastasis of circulating cancer cells in mouse lungs. Lab Invest 1990;62:331–338.

135. Paget S. The distribution of secondary growths in cancer of the breast. Lancet 1889;1:571–573.

136. Pals ST, Horst E, Ossekoppele GJ, Figdor CG, Scheper RJ, Meijer CJLM. Expression of lymphocyte homing receptor as a mechanism of dissemination in non-Hodgkin's lymphoma. Blood 1989;73:885–888.

137. Pascal RR. Renal manifestations of extrarenal neoplasms. Hum Pathol 1980;11:7–17.

138. Patterson WP, Ringenberg OS. The pathophysiology of thrombosis in cancer. Semin Oncol 1990;17:140–146.

139. Pauli BU, Augustin-Voss HG, El-Sabban ME, Johnson RC, Hammer DA. Organ-preference of metastasis. The role of endothelial cell adhesion molecules. Cancer Metastasis Rev 1990;9:175–189.

140. Pauli BU, Johnson RC, El-Sabban ME. Organotypic endothelial cell surface molecules mediate organ preference of metastasis. In: Simionescu N, Simionescu M, eds. Endothelial cell dysfunctions. New York: Plenum Press, 1991.

141. Pauli BU, Knudson W. Tumor invasion: a consequence of destructive and compositional matrix alterations. Hum Pathol 1988;19:628–639.

142. Pauli BU, Kuettner KE. The regulation of invasion by a cartilage-derived anti–invasion factor. In: Liotta LA, Hart IR, eds. Tumor invasion and metastasis. The Hague: Martinus Nijhoff Publishers, 1982:291–308.

143. Pauli BU, Lee C-L. Organ preference of metastasis. The role of organ-specifically modulated endothelial cells. Lab Invest 1988;58:379–387.

144. Pepper MS, Montesano R, Vassalli J-D, Orci L. Chrondrocytes inhibit endothelial sprout formation in vitro: evidence for involvement of a transforming growth factor-beta. J Cell Physiol 1991;146:170–179.

145. Peterson W. Beiträge zur Lehre vom Carcinom. I. Ueber Aufbau, Wachstum und Histogenese der Hautcarcinome. Beitr Klin Chir 1902;32:543–660.

146. Pineo GF, Brain MC, Gallus AS, Hirsh J, Hatton MWC, Regoeczi E. Tumors, mucus production, and hypercoagulability. Ann NY Acad Sci 1974;230:262–270.

147. Pines A, Kaplinsky N, Olchovsky D, Frankl O. Rheumatoid arthritis-like syndrome: a presenting symptom of malignancy. Report of 3 cases and review of the literature. Eur J Rheum Inflam 1984;7:51–55.

148. Pizzo PA. Combating infections in neutropenic patients. Hosp Pract 1989;24:93–110.

149. Poste G, Fidler IJ. The pathogenesis of cancer metastasis. Nature 1980;283:139–146.

150. Powles TJ, Clark SA, Easty DM, Easty GC, Neville AM. The inhibition by aspirin and indomethacin of osteolytic tumour deposits and hypercalcaemia in rats with Walker tumour, and its possible application to human breast cancer. Br J Cancer 1973;28:316–321.

151. Powles TJ, Dowsett M, Easty DM, Easty GC, Neville AM. Breast-cancer osteolysis, bone metastases, and anti-osteolytic effect of aspirin. Lancet 1976;1:608–610.

152. Rasche H, Dietrich M. Hemostatic abnormalities associated with malignant diseases. Eur J Cancer 1977;13:1053–1064.

153. Renkonen R, Paavonen T, Nortamo P, Gahmberg CG. Expression of endothelial adhesion molecules in vivo: increased endothelial ICAM-2 expression in lymphoid malignancies. Am J Pathol 1992;140:763–767.

154. Rice GE, Gimbrone MA Jr, Bevilacqua MP. Tumor cell-endothelial interactions. Increased adhesion of human melanoma cells to activated vascular endothelium. Am J Pathol 1988;133:204–210.

155. Rickles FR, Edwards RL. Activation of blood coagulation in cancer: Trousseau's syndrome revisited. Blood 1983;62:14–31.

156. Roberts SS, Watne AL, McGrew EA, McGrath RG, Nanos S, Cole WH. Cancer cells in the circulating blood. Surg Forum 1958;8:146–151.

157. Rouzer CA, Cerami A. Hypertriglyceridemia associated with Trypanosoma brucei brucei infection in rabbits: role of defective triglyceride removal. Mol Biochem Parasitol 1980;2:31–38.

158. Ruoslahti E, Giancotti FG. Integrins and tumor cell dissemination. Cancer Cells 1989;1:119–126.

159. Russell DS, Rubinstein LJ. Pathology of tumours of the nervous system, 5th ed. Baltimore: Williams & Wilkins, 1989.

160. Russo RG, Foltz CM, Liotta LA. New invasion assay using endothelial cells grown on native human basement membrane. Clin Exp Metastasis 1983;1:115–127.

161. Sack GH, Levin J, Bell WR. Trousseau's syndrome and other manifestations of chronic disseminated coagulopathy in patients with neoplasms: clinical, pathophysiologic, and therapeutic features. Medicine 1977;56:1–37.

162. Saiki I, Murata J, Iida J, et al. Antimetastatic effects of synthetic polypeptides containing repeated structures of the cell adhesive Arg-Gly-Asp (RGD) and Tyr-Ile-Gly-Ser-Arg (YIGSR) sequences. Br J Cancer 1989;60:722–728.

163. Sato H, Suzuki M. Deformability and viability of tumor cells by transcapillary passage, with reference to organ affinity of metastasis in cancer. In: Weiss L, ed. Fundamental aspects of metastasis. Amsterdam-Oxford: North Holland Publishing Company, 1976:311–317.

164. Schroyens W, Bruyneel R, Tchao R, Leighton J, Dragonetti C, Mareel M. Comparison of invasiveness and non-invasiveness of two epithelial cell lines in vitro. Invasion Metastasis 1984;4:160–170.

165. Sieweke MH, Thompson NL, Sporn MB, Bissell MJ. Mediation of wound-related Rous sarcoma virus tumorigenesis by TGF-ß. Science 1990;248:1656–1660.

166. Sindelar WF, Tralka TS, Ketcham AS. Electron microscopic observations on formation of pulmonary metastases. J Surg Res 1975;18:137–161.

167. Sherry BA, Gelin J, Fong Y, et al. Anticachectin/tumor necrosis factor-α antibodies attenuate development of cachexia in tumor models. FASEB J 1989;3:1956–1962.

168. Sherwood LM. The multiple causes of hypercalcemia in malignant disease. N Engl J Med 1980;303:1412–1413.

169. Stark ME, Dyer MCD, Coonley CJ. Fatal acute tumor lysis syndrome with metastatic breast carcinoma. Cancer 1987;60:762–764.

170. Sträuli P, Haemmerli G. The role of cancer cell motility in invasion. Cancer Metastasis Rev 1984;3:127–141.

171. Sugarbaker EV. Patterns of metastasis in human malignancies. In: Fidler IJ, ed. Cancer metastasis. New York: Marcel Dekker, 1977.

172. Sugarbaker EV. Patterns of metastasis in human malignancies. Cancer Biol Rev 1981;2:235–278.

173. Sutherland DJ. Hormones and cancer. In: Tannock IF, Hill RP, eds. The basic science of oncology. New York: Pergamon Press, 1987:204–222.

174. Sylvén B, Holmberg B. On the structure and biological effects of a newly-discovered cytotoxic polypeptide in tumor fluid. Eur J Cancer 1965;1:199–202.

175. Tanaka K, Kohga S, Kinjo M, Kodama Y. Tumor metastasis and thrombosis, with special reference to thromboplastic and fibrinolytic activities of tumor cells. GANN Monogr Cancer Res 1977;20:97–119.

176. Tanaka NG, Tohgo A, Ogawa H. Platelet-aggregating activities of metastasizing tumor cells. V. In situ roles of platelets in hematogenous metastases. Invasion Metastasis 1986;6:209–224.

177. Tarin D, Vass ACR, Kettlewell MGW, Price JE. Absence of metastatic sequelae during long-term treatment of malignant ascites by peritoneo-venous shunting. A clinico-pathological report. Invasion Metastasis 1984;4:1–12.

178. Taylor LM Jr, Hauty MG, Edwards JM, Porter JM. Digital ischemia as a manifestation of malignancy. Ann Surg 1987;206:62–68.

179. Terranova VP, Hic S, Diflorio RM, Lyall RM. Tumor cell metastasis. CRC Crit Rev Oncol Hematol 1986;5:87–114.

180. Trousseau A. Phlegmatia alba dolens. Clinique Médicale de L'Hotel-Dieu de Paris, vol 3, 2nd ed. Paris: J-B Ballière et Fils, 1865:654–712.

181. Tryggvason K, Höyhtyä M, Salo T. Proteolytic degradation of extracellular matrix in tumor invasion. Biochim Biophys Acta 1987;907:191–217.

182. Tyzzer EE. Factors in the production and growth of tumor metastases. J Med Res 1913;28:309–332.

183. Wallace AC, Chew E-C, Jones DS. Arrest and extravasation of cancer cells in the lung. In: Weiss L, Gilbert HA, eds. Pulmonary metastasis. Boston: GK Hall & Co., 1978:26–42.

184. Warnold I, Lundholm K, Scherstén T. Energy balance and body composition in cancer patients. Cancer Res 1978;38:1801–1807.

185. Warren BA. Cancer cell-endothelial reactions: the microinjury hypothesis and localized thrombosis in the formation of micrometastases. In: Donati MB, Davidson JF, Garattini S, eds. Malignancy and the hemostatic system. New York: Raven Press, 1981:5–25.

186. Weiss L. Fundamental aspects of metastasis. Amsterdam-Oxford: North Holland Publishing Company, 1976.

187. Weiss L. Cell detachment and metastasis. GANN Monogr Cancer Res 1977;20:25–35.

188. Weiss L. Some mechanisms involved in cancer cell detachment by necrotic material. Int J Cancer 1978;22:196–203.

189. Weiss L. Principles of metastasis. Orlando, FL: Academic Press, 1985.

190. Weiss L. The hemodynamic destruction of circulating cancer cells. Biorheology 1987;24:105–115.

191. Weiss L. Metastatic inefficiency. Adv Cancer Res 1990;54:159–211.

192. Weiss L, Dimitrov DS, Angelova M. The hemodynamic destruction of intravascular cancer cells in relation to myocardial metastasis. Proc Natl Acad Sci USA 1985;82:5737–5741.

193. Weiss L, Grundmann E, Torhorst J, et al. Haematogenous metastatic (sic) patterns in colonic carcinoma: an analysis of 1541 necropsies. J Pathol 1986;150:195–203.

194. Weiss L, Haydock K, Pickren JW, Lane WW. Organ vascularity and metastatic frequency. Am J Pathol 1980;101:101–114.

195. Weiss L, Holmes JC. Some effects of tumor necrosis on components of active cell movement. In: Sträuli P, Barrett AJ, Baici A, eds. Proteinases and tumor invasion. New York: Raven Press, 1980:181–200.

196. Weiss L, Orr FW, Honn KV. Interactions of cancer cells with the microvasculature during metastasis. FASEB J 1988;2:12–21.

197. Weiss L, Orr FW, Honn KV. Interactions between cancer cells and the microvasculature: a rate-regulator for metastasis. Clin Exp Metastasis 1989;7:127–167.

198. Weiss L, Schmid-Schönbein GW. Biomechanical interactions of cancer cells with the microvasculature during metastasis. Cell Biophys 1989;14:187–215.

199. Welch DR, Bhuyan BK, Liotta LA, eds. Cancer metastasis: experimental and clinical strategies. Prog Clin Biol Res, vol 212. New York: Alan R. Liss, 1986.

200. Willis RA. The spread of tumours in the human body, 3rd ed. London: Butterworth, 1973.

201. Wold LE, Pritchard DJ, Bergert J, Wilson DM. Prostaglandin synthesis by osteoid osteoma and osteoblastoma. Mod Pathol 1988;1:129–131.

202. Wolinsky H, Lischner MW. Needle track implantation of tumor after percutaneous lung biopsy. Ann Intern Med 1969;71:359–362.

203. Wood S. Pathogenesis of metastasis formation observed in vivo in the rabbit ear chamber. Arch Pathol 1958;66:550–568.

204. Zeidman I. The fate of circulating tumor cells. I. Passage of cells through capillaries. Cancer Res 1961;21:38–39.

205. Zetter BR. The cellular basis of site-specific tumor metastasis. N Engl J Med 1990;322:605–612.

The Causes of Tumors

CHAPTER 28

Chemical Causes
of Tumors

Physical Causes
of Tumors

Biological Causes
of Tumors

Contrary to the popular belief that we do not know "the cause of cancer," we know, if anything, too many causes: predisposing, initiating, promoting, perpetuating; physical, chemical, viral, bacterial, parasitic; dietary, environmental, occupational, and related to lifestyle (Figure 28.1). Indeed, we have learned that we will never find "the cause" of cancer, because, like other diseases, tumors never have a single cause. This is part of the ABC of medicine in general. Even a simple fracture may have a long list of causes. This concept was beautifully stated by Alan Gregg, an eminent physician and educator (84):

> We ought to use the word "why" in the plural, and ask, "Whys is this patient [ill]?". . . . A particular case of a fractured jaw in a sailor may be the result of convergent causes—no letters from home, too much alcohol, the loan of a car by a friend, a dark night, an oncoming car on a road covered with ice at a curve, the fact that the left-hand rule is used in the British Isles, new brake linings, a skid, and a telephone pole. These constitute the whys, not the why, of a fractured jaw. It is a cataract of consequences. Take out any one of these whys and the accident would not have occurred.

Gregg did not exaggerate in attributing 11 causes to a fractured jaw. There is a human carcinoma that is supposedly caused by aflatoxin, a fungal poison; a careful search into the genesis of this tumor brings up 10 contributing causes: ethnic, social, dietary, ecological, botanical, phys-iological, biochemical, genetic, infectious, and immunologic; eliminate any one and no tumor develops. The causation of cancer—and of disease in general—should be seen as a chain of many links, as illustrated on p. 923.

With this in mind we must begin to analyze the possible causes of cancer. The basic fact in this field—to many it will come as a surprise—is that on a worldwide basis *most cancers are related to the environment or to human behavior* (53, 116) (see Figure 28.1). We will therefore begin our study with environmental causes. History tells us that they belong to three groups: chemical (the largest), physical, and biological. Do they have anything in common? Yes: most of the agents in these three groups have the ability to damage the DNA chain permanently and are therefore called *genotoxic*; some, however, are definitely non-genotoxic. This apparent dilemma will be addressed in due time (p. 926).

Chemical Causes of Tumors

Chemical causes of tumors were the first to be recognized because some chemicals produce obvious occupational diseases; today chemicals are responsible for most human tumors, estimated as 80–90 percent of the total. The list of hazardous agents is so varied that this chapter may seem like a patchwork of unrelated topics: what does tar have to do with diet, or mustard gas with lubricating oil? The answer is that the DNA chain can be nonspecifically damaged by an enormous variety of

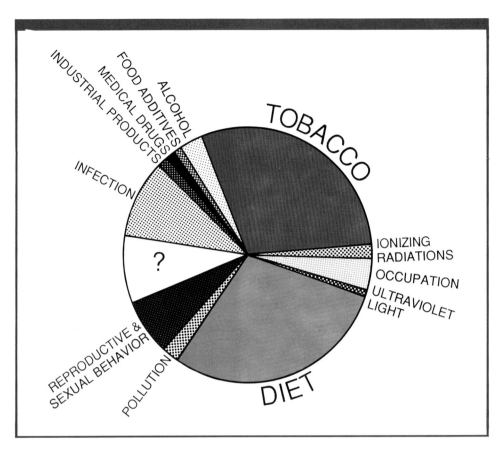

FIGURE 28.1
Principal causes of human cancer.
(Reproduced with permission from
[53, 115].)

chemicals, related, as we will see, by the broad physicochemical property of being electrophilic.

In addition to this physicochemical *Leitmotif,* this section on chemical carcinogenesis will be punctuated by another recurring theme: many leads to the discovery of cancer-producing chemicals came from practicing physicians. The experiments were run by society or by nature, and an alert clinician blew the whistle; laboratory experiments came later.

MILESTONES ON THE TRAIL OF CHEMICAL CANCER: FROM SNUFF TO BENZPYRENE

Tobacco Very appropriately, tobacco begins our story, back in 1761.

For well-to-do Englishmen in the mid-1700s tobacco smoking was no longer subject to the death penalty, but it was considered vulgar; the approved habit was to inhale it as snuff. And so the first warning against tobacco came from a prominent figure in eighteenth century London, a scholarly physician–botanist named John Hill (who also coined the term *paramecium*). In 1761 Dr. Hill published a little book describing the ill effects of snuff powder, including "polypusses," which could turn into terrible, ulcerated cancers (181). The latter diagnosis was not easy: in Hill's day the

biological nature of cancer was still unknown. Incidentally, the cancer-causing agents in snuff are not tar components but nitrosamines (175).

Soot Only a few years later, in 1775, another London physician, Sir Percivall Pott, Fellow of the Royal Society, published his *Chirurgical Works* (244). In Volume 3, besides more "Remarks on the Polypus of the Nose," he tells of chimney sweeps who had come to his attention because of scrotal cancer (Figure 28.2). Chimneys, at that time, were built in such a way as to allow the passage not only of a sweeping tool but of a whole—small—human being armed with a brush and surely also with a desperate need to survive. In the words of Sir Percivall:

> It is a disease which always makes its first attack on, and its first appearance in the inferior part of the scrotum; where it produces a superficial, painful, ragged, ill-looking sore, with hard and rising edges. The trade call it the soot-wart. I never saw it under the age of puberty (177).

The last remark tells a great deal: chimney sweeps began climbing into chimneys as small children, even at the tender age of four years (38)

(Figure 28.3). "The disease, in these people," wrote Sir Percivall, "seems to derive its origin from a lodgement of soot in the rugae of the scrotum." After many years, superficial "soot warts" began to appear, and eventually one of these turned into invasive cancer. The delay after the first exposure was of the order of 20–30 years or more (38). Although the soot wart was considered almost like a trademark, a puzzling feature was its rarity in continental Europe; a study in 1892 suggested that the difference was due to protective clothing and the habit of frequent bathing, which removed the soot from the deep rugae of the scrotum (38). Sir Percivall, oddly enough, makes no reference to the preventive possibilities of soap and water (172). So, half a century later, Sir Astley Cooper could still illustrate the soot wart in his surgical treatise (Figure 28.2). The Danes, however, saw the connection: tradition has it that three years after Sir Percivall's paper the Danish Chimney-Sweeper's Guild urged its members to take daily baths (141).

Tar and Its Derivatives Sir Percivall was writing at the eve of the American Revolutionary war; the British, unable to keep their ships watertight with wood tar from their former Colonies, turned to the old German method of preparing tar by heating coal in the absence of air. A few years later came the idea of producing street-lighting gas by the same method. Now a great deal of tar was generated as a by-product. The next problem was what to do with that abundance of black, sticky material: there had to be some industrial use for it besides tarring ships and occasional sailors. By the mid-1800s, distillation products of tar began to find uses, for instance, as solvents (which allowed Charles Mackintosh to make his first rainproof mackintoshes). Then came phenol, the first antiseptic; dyes derived from aniline; myriads of new organic compounds such as benzene (the famous 6-carbon ring was described by Kekulé in 1866). Soon a powerful German distillation industry was born.

Those were the 1860s. It takes 20–25 years of exposure for most cancers to develop. In 1895, a German surgeon, L. Rehn, noticed three cases of bladder cancer among 45 workers who had been preparing fuchsin dyes from aniline for 15 to 29 years (182): bladder cancer is rare enough to make such a cluster highly suspect. Similar "aniline bladder cancers" were soon discovered in other countries. Actually, aniline itself is not directly the culprit; several of its derivatives, aromatic

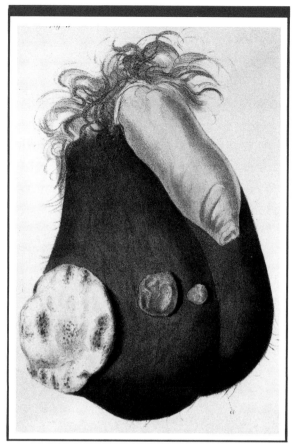

FIGURE 28.2
Chimney-sweeper's cancer as illustrated in 1841 by a British surgeon, Sir Astley Cooper. Three stages are shown; from right to left: early, more advanced, and ulcerated. (Adapted from [46].)

amines, turned out to be highly carcinogenic with a delay of 5–30 years. The worst offender is beta-naphthylamine (Figure 28.4) (79); before its use was discontinued, as many as 100 percent of exposed workers developed bladder cancer (44). More recently, exposure to benzene itself has been linked with leukemia (186).

Tar as a Tool of Oncology While tar products continued to claim more victims, several attempts

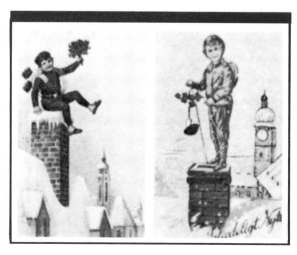

FIGURE 28.3
Children employed as chimney sweeps in nineteenth century Denmark. From a New Year greeting card of the time. (Reproduced with permission from [91].)

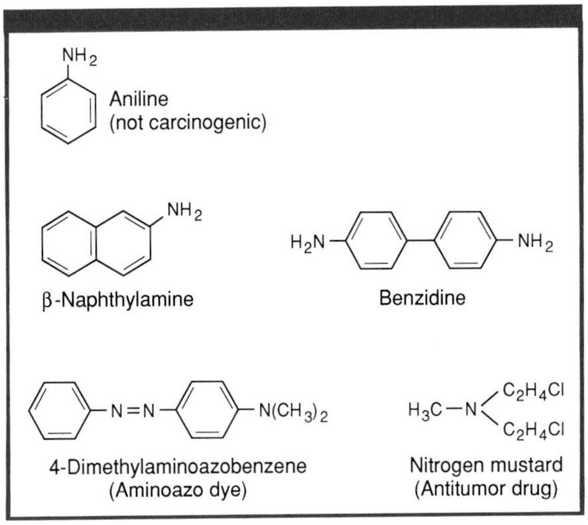

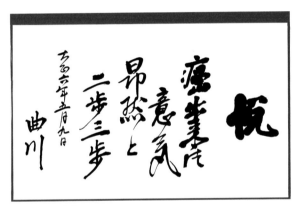

FIGURE 28.4
Some carcinogens and related molecules. (Adapted from [13, 14].)

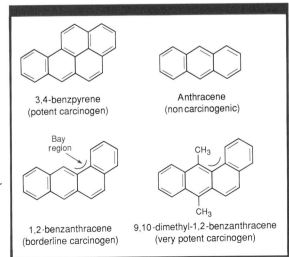

FIGURE 28.5
Haiku composed by Dr. Yamagiwa on a silk scroll in 1917 to celebrate the first skin cancer produced by painting tar on a rabbit ear. In essence it means: "Cancer was produced! Proudly I walk a few steps," but in Japanese it is much more poetic. (Reproduced with permission from [202].)

FIGURE 28.6
Formulae of polycyclic hydrocarbons, including three carcinogens. (Adapted from [13].)

were made to produce experimental tumors with it, but failed because the experimental design was wrong (203). An Englishman, for example, narrowly missed the mark: he injected gasworks tar into rabbit ears and found epithelial "growths," but he only waited 4 weeks (10). The prize went to Oriental patience combined with the choice of the right species. In 1915, Yamagiwa and Ichikawa reported in Japanese that after painting rabbit ears with tar every 2 or 3 days for a year, papillomas developed first, then true carcinomas with metastases (202). Dr. Yamagiwa expressed his joy in a haiku poem (Figure 28.5), but oddly enough, the two Japanese experimenters did not give much weight to their finding. They had chosen tar as a "nonspecific" irritant and simply concluded that Virchow (who was still alive at the time) was right: cancer was due to chronic irritation. Their concern was to fit the facts into the known pattern. However, their short paper—when it was published in English (1918):—opened the floodgates: the era of tar-painting had begun.

The next major step came in the 1930s with the isolation of specific carcinogens contained in tar. It was an epic of chemistry: Sir Ernest Kennaway and his team distilled 2 tons of tar down to 7 grams of crystalline powder. Just as the Curies were guided by radioactivity in their extraction of radium, the British group was guided by a fluorescence spectrum that was empirically known to be associated with the carcinogenic effect (116, 203). The culprits turned out to be polycyclic aromatic hydrocarbons; 3,4-benzpyrene, a powerful carcinogen, became the prototype; 3-ring compounds showed little effect (Figure 28.6). In the "benz-pyromania" that followed (203), attention was turned to natural polycyclic compounds, and a potent carcinogen, 3-methylcholanthrene, was soon prepared from bile acids (45) and became a standard tool for producing tumors (68). However, it is no longer thought to be generated *in vivo* (14).

Skin tumors produced by tar or by purified carcinogens were studied primarily in mice (Figure 28.7) and rabbits (244). In the early experiments, a nonspecific dermatitis appeared first, followed by loss of hair and excessive keratinization (hyperkeratosis). Then wartlike papillomas developed; some regressed, others continued to grow. If painting was discontinued, these benign epidermal growths usually regressed, but if painting was resumed they reappeared faster and in greater numbers. Eventually a carcinoma developed in one area, rarely in two or three (73). Endless variations were tried on the theme of painting-plus-some-other-treatment. Today the paintbrush is replaced by more precise methods of application (225), but the basic results are the same. An important by-product of all this work was the construction of a theory on cancer development, through stages of initiation, promotion, and progression.

THE NATURE OF CHEMICAL CARCINOGENS

Before we leave tar for other carcinogens, we should briefly examine the property that makes a molecule carcinogenic.

Electrophilic Agents Over 12 families of carcinogens are known at this time. They include molecules as simple as elemental chromium or as complex as aflatoxin. A unifying thread through this chemical melange was proposed in 1969 by Elizabeth and James Miller (141–144). Their theory is that a carcinogenic molecule must be an *electrophilic reactant*. In other words, it must have a relatively electron-deficient site; *this makes it seek nucleophilic sites*—that is, atoms that have easily shared electrons such as exist in amino groups, with which they form a covalent bond (Figure 28.8) (177). Such nucleophilic groupings are very common—even water qualifies—but the critical point is that they are relatively abundant on DNA, RNA, and protein (140).

This rule proposed by the Millers applies to chemical agents that qualify as genotoxic; non-genotoxic carcinogens, as we will see, interfere with cells in a different way. Although there are exceptions (140) the electrophilic requirement is so consistent that it is now possible to predict with reasonable accuracy the carcinogenic potential of a molecule (140). The electrophilic hypothesis has an important corollary: in their native states, few carcinogens are electrophilic. They are inactive, and are activated in the body.

Metabolic Activation of Carcinogens As soon as a variety of carcinogens was available for experimentation, it became obvious that some, such as tar derivatives, act *at the site* where they are applied, whereas most of the others elicit tumors *in distant organs* and each one always affects the same organ(s), no matter how it is administered. This suggested that some carcinogens must be modified within the body before they become effective (235), and it is now an established fact that most carcinogens are inactive in their native state. The

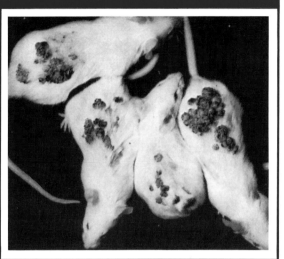

FIGURE 28.7
Papillomas on the back of mice after a 12 week induction–promotion program: a single application of dimethyl benz-anthracene (DMBA) followed by croton oil twice a week. (Reproduced with permission from [27].)

Millers proposed that the inactive carcinogens (procarcinogens) are metabolized stepwise to one or more "proximate" carcinogens and eventually to the ultimate carcinogen, the electrophilic species. The metabolic activation can be performed by enzymes of the endoplasmic reticulum such as the P-450 cytochromes (p. 136), but other enzyme systems may also be involved (63, 94), including enzymes of pathogenic bacteria and of the normal flora. Enzyme actions are easily modulated; we are therefore closer to understanding a number of puzzles:

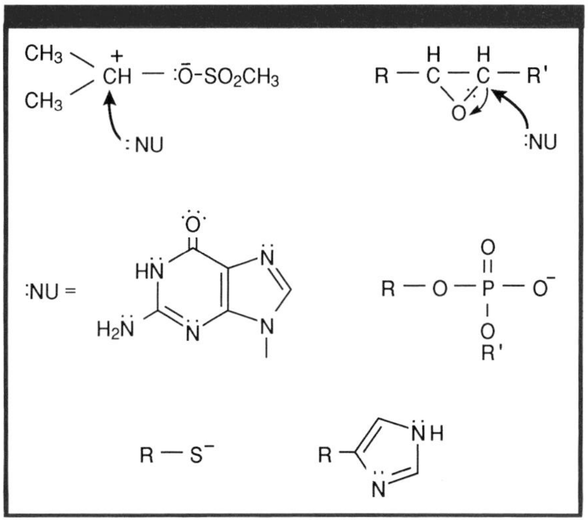

FIGURE 28.8
Examples of strong electrophilic reactants (positive ions or uncharged molecules with electron-deficient atoms) and their reactions with nucleophiles (:NU) through sharing of electron pairs of electron-rich atoms. (Reproduced with permission from [141].)

- The organ selectivity of carcinogens may depend on the presence, absence, or balance of appropriate enzymes. As an example, dimethylnitrosamine given orally to rats induces liver cancer. If the rats are kept on a low-protein diet, liver enzymes drop below the critical level, making more carcinogen available to the kidney; then only kidney tumors develop (135).
- Individual differences in susceptibility to cancer could depend on differences in enzyme activity or amounts due to age, diet, or exposure to xenobiotics other than the carcinogen. An example: the carcinogenicity of several aromatic amines can be completely prevented by phenobarbital, a powerful inducer of liver enzymes (63).
- Species differences may also reflect different enzymes and/or enzyme levels.

So much about the nature of carcinogens. The reader should be aware that there are substances that work as cocarcinogens, which enhance the effect of carcinogens though by themselves they have no carcinogenic effect. Fortunately, other molecules work as anticarcinogens; such are tannic acid (50) and vitamins A, E, and C (p. 826).

THE CHEMICAL CARCINOGENS

This title promises some chemistry, but the key fact that we want to convey is a matter of psychology: *although most human cancers are caused by chemicals, these chemicals are mainly self-inflicted.*

Cancer from *industrial pollution* certainly exists, but it is not the main aspect of environmental decay: it has been estimated that industrial pollution contributes only 4 percent of all cancer

deaths (53). We hurry to add that "only" 4 percent really means 16,000 human beings lost every year in the United States alone, a large figure, which in theory should be reducible to zero. However, new chemicals appear faster than they can be tested for carcinogenic activity. Considering that it takes about 20 years for a new carcinogen to manifest itself on cancer incidence curves, we can anticipate that the list of industrial and environmental carcinogens will continue to grow. Yet it is sobering to realize that the air in the house of a smoker can be more polluted than the city air outside (31).

We will now cite six overlapping categories of chemical carcinogens that are especially relevant to man: (1) related to smoking and other pursuits of pleasure, (2) dietary, (3) hormonal, (4) occupational, (5) therapeutic, and (6) sundry. The only comforting message of this list is that many of these deadly substances are avoidable, at least in theory.

Carcinogens on the Road to Pleasure It is mind-boggling that **tobacco** was barely questioned as a cause of cancer before 1950 (250). Yet, in the words of the Surgeon General of the United States, if we consider all the tobacco-related diseases, "Cigarette smoking is the chief . . . avoidable cause of death in our society" (228). Figures are too large to grasp: half a million deaths per year, one in every four to five American deaths (Figure 28.9) (228)—let alone the millions killed abroad by exported tobacco (49a). Nor is cancer the only ill effect of smoking. And yet tobacco is produced in 21 states and Puerto Rico; it brings 2.1 billions of dollars to its growers (245); and it is heavily subsidized by the same federal government that employs the Surgeon General. We tried to obtain hard numbers on the amount of this federal subsidy, but they are buried in such deep strata of paper that even the experts have no grasp of the facts (229).

A cynical argument usually turns up in a discussion of cigarette-caused cancer. Here it is, gleaned from the press: "By dying early, cigarette smokers have saved the Social Security System billions of dollars in benefit payments" and thereby subsidize the social security benefits of nonsmokers (132, 229).

So much for tobacco.

Alcohol is not itself a carcinogen, but it leads to cancer in two ways. Alcohol abuse, as everyone should know by now, leads to *cirrhosis of the liver.* In this condition the liver tissue is strangled in a three-dimensional network of contracting scars; in

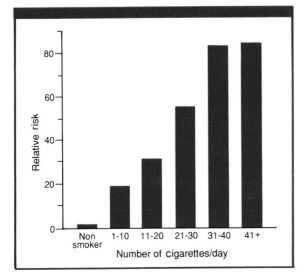

FIGURE 28.9 Correlation between number of cigarettes smoked and the risk of developing lung cancer in males. (Adapted from [251].)

the meshes the liver tissue attempts to regenerate, so that on cross sections a cirrhotic liver appears as a mesh of fibrous tissue riddled with small nodules of regenerating cells (see Figures 13.40 and 13.46). In the long run, one of these regenerating nodules may become neoplastic. Furthermore, alcohol in large doses increases the risk for cancer of the mouth, pharynx, larynx, esophagus, lung (in nonsmokers) and rectum (168, 187). More worrisome but also unexplained is the fact that a very moderate consumption (half a drink or more daily) increases the risk of breast cancer in women by about 30 percent (187). The 57 percent of American women who consume alcohol will have to weigh this risk against the tempting advantage that moderate alcohol intake reduces the risk of myocardial infarction (150).

And *alcohol plus tobacco* is a bad combination: they somehow interact to increase the risk of esophageal cancer (Figure 28.10). Perhaps alcohol favors the uptake of carcinogens across epithelial linings.

Diet and Cancer Diet relates to cancer in many ways, some of which are understood, others not (5, 81, 168, 187). That diet in general is somehow related to cancer is best shown by the Seventh Day Adventists, who do not drink alcohol or smoke, and about 50 percent of whom also refrain from using coffee, tea, or spices (165). Their mortality for cancers *unrelated* to smoking or drinking is 30–50 percent lower than that of the general popula-

tion. Another example of diet-related cancer statistics is that of Japanese immigrating to the United States: their offspring shift from the typical Japanese pattern of cancer prevalence (high for the stomach, low for the colon) to the American pattern (low for the stomach, high for the colon) (89, 187).

The consumption of fat is highly suspect; there is a striking correlation between fat consumption in various countries with the incidence of cancer of the colon and to a lesser extent of the breast (the latter correlation is not confirmed [225a]) (Figures 28.11, 28.12) (180). One of the uncertainties in this statistic is that it is not easy to extricate the effect of *total caloric intake* from the effect of fat consumption. In laboratory animals diet restriction reduces tumor incidence and prolongs life (p. 51). Epidemiologic studies have not confirmed this in humans (187), but even if they eventually do, few would follow that path to longevity.

High-fiber diets have been extensively studied since Denis Burkitt, an extraordinarily thoughtful surgeon–missionary–epidemiologist, opened this field by his observations in Africa, where he discovered Burkitt's tumor (Figure 28.13). He based his theory on simple observations (35).

It is noticeable that the stools of those eating high residue diets are almost invariably bulky, soft and non-odorous [. . .]. The relative absence of fetid smell in the stools of people in developing commu-

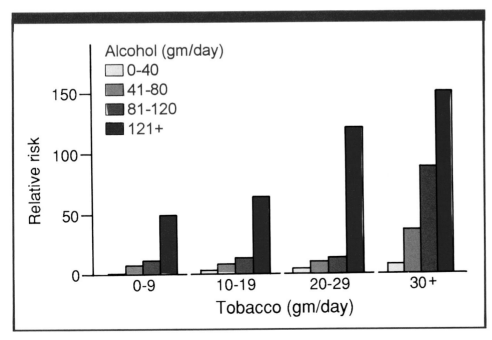

FIGURE 28.10
Alcohol and tobacco interact to influence the risk of esophageal cancer. (Adapted from [223].)

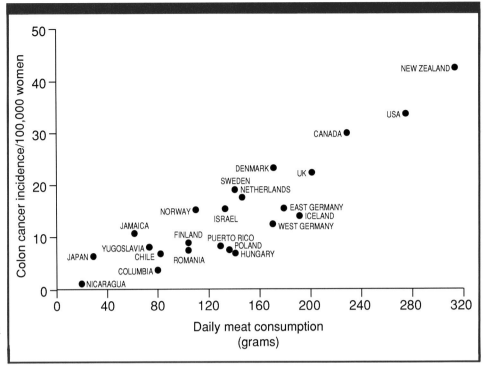

FIGURE 28.11
Correlation between colon cancer in women and daily meat consumption in 23 countries. (Adapted from [6].)

nities and in the stools of wild animals [. . .] is also significant and is believed to indicate a lower rate of bacterial decomposition compared to that occurring in Western countries (35).

Burkitt also noticed that colon cancer is rare in all animals and in people who consume less processed food. He pointed out the striking

difference between the intestinal transit time in people on refined and unrefined diets (Figure 28.14). The incidence of cancer along the colon and rectum certainly increases in the direction of fecal progress, suggesting a role for contact time between mucosa and feces. Twenty years later nobody questions that there are dietary differences in the incidence of colon cancer, but the role of

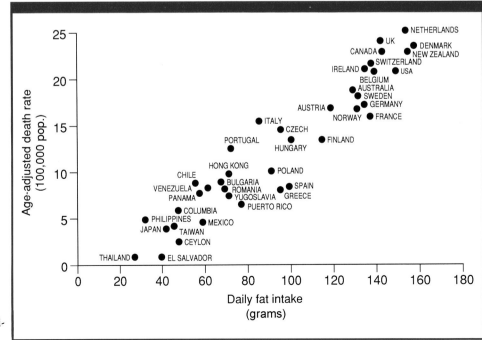

FIGURE 28.12
Correlation between breast cancer mortality and fat consumption in various countries. (Adapted from [41].)

fiber does not stand out as clearly as one would like (Figure 28.15) (187). It may also have something to do with a protective factor(s) contained in vegetables (241).

> *Dr. Burkitt's pioneer findings go beyond the effects of fiber in the diet. As he practiced surgery, for most of his life in rural Africa, he noticed that many diseases that the Western world takes for granted were rare or missing altogether: varicose veins, diverticulosis, hemorrhoids, hiatus hernia, appendicitis, just to mention a few. According to Dr. Burkitt's concept, all these "Western diseases can be traced to the Western diet," which reduces stool volume, prolongs transit time (leading to constipation), and requires more straining for defecation. These factors conspire to increase pressure in the abdomen, and consequently also in the veins of the lower limbs (219, 220).*

Dietary carcinogens There is of course no limit to the carcinogens that can be eaten with food or can develop while digesting or metabolizing it; oral and bacterial flora, vitamins, cholesterol, and bile acids introduce other variables.

Of special concern are the **nitrosamines**, the most omnipotent carcinogens in the sense that they affect the broadest range of species, including humans (Figure 28.16) (126, 175). The principal theory to explain gastric cancer is based on nitrosamine formation in the stomach (146). Nitrosamines are formed by a reaction between nitrous acid (HNO_2) and secondary amines (145) (*nitrosation*):

$$2\ HNO_2 \rightarrow N_2O_3 + H_2O$$
$$R_2NH + N_2O_3 \rightarrow R_2N \cdot NO + HNO_2$$

Sodium nitrite is used as a food additive in cured meat and fish to improve taste and appearance. Nitrites are also used in pathology museums to preserve the color of fixed specimens: nitrosohemoglobin is attractively pink (145). Nitrites are also invaluable for protecting against the lethal *Clostridium botulinum* (111). The necessity of adding nitrites to food has been questioned because plenty of nitrites are contained in unprocessed foods. Plant foods contain nitrates that oral bacteria reduce to nitrites (213). *The reaction between nitrites and secondary amines is inhibited by adding ascorbic acid to food (145, 146);* fruit and vegetables in the diet have the same effect. Nitrosamines, as mentioned earlier, are present also in tobacco smoke.

Natural dietary carcinogens are produced by bacteria and plants (102), which means that fans of

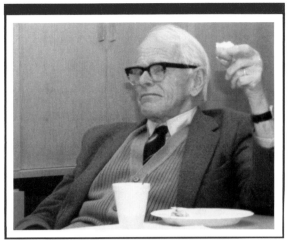

FIGURE 28.13
The late Dr. Denis Burkitt submitted to a fiber-poor diet while visiting the University of Massachusetts Medical Center in 1990. (With kind permission from Dr. D.P. Burkitt, Bisley, United Kingdom.)

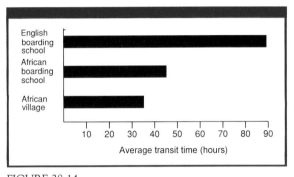

FIGURE 28.14
Differences in the transit time of stools in three populations. Denis Burkitt, who pointed out this phenomenon, correlated it with the geographic differences in the incidence of colon cancer. (Reproduced with permission from [35].)

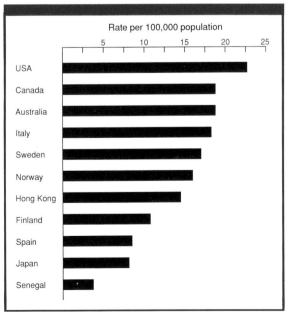

FIGURE 28.15
International variations in the incidence of colon cancer. (Reproduced with permission from [28].)

FIGURE 28.16
Nitrosamines:
the basic struc-
ture, and an
aliphatic nitro-
samine. (Repro-
duced with per-
mission from
[242].)

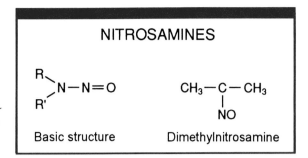

natural foods are not necessarily safe from dietary cancer. In 1960 and 1961, two epidemics (*epizootics* would be the proper term) killed thousands of turkeys in England and devastated the rainbow trout production in Idaho hatcheries (247). The epidemics were traced to peanut meal, imported from South Africa, that was contaminated with the common fungus *Aspergillus flavus*; fed to rats it produced hepatomas. The culprit was *aflatoxin B₁*, one of the most potent carcinogens known; it is thought to be a major factor in the high incidence of liver cancer in many countries where grain is stored in warm and humid conditions (Africa and Asia) (32). The aflatoxin may not act alone but in conjunction with hepatitis B virus, which is also associated with liver cancer (8). We have chosen the "aflatoxin hepatoma" as an example of a typical multifactorial cancer (p. 923).

The cycad nut (102) may not be a staple of our readers' diet unless they live in southwest Japan, but the effects of its consumption does convey an important message: it produces cancer of the liver and kidneys in ordinary laboratory rats but not in bacteria-free rats. The ultimate carcinogen, in this case cycasin, a relative of the nitrosamines, is released by intestinal bacteria (124). The ways of cancer are infinite.

Dietary Anticarcinogens It is time for some good news, even if tentative (241). Besides fiber, diets contain a variety of agents that inhibit mutations and tumor formation under certain conditions (5, 187, 241). Vitamin A and other retinoids have been reported as anticarcinogenic for several organs (skin, breast, and bladder). Vitamin C, taken orally, does protect against nitrosamines, but two thorough studies have failed to show any general anticancer effect (243). Vegetarians enjoy lower rates of cancer of the breast, colon, and prostate; epidemiologic studies suggest a protective effect of certain seeds (maize, corn, beans). **Protease inhibitors** are abundant component of all seeds; in fact, a

soybean protease inhibitor was found to be anticarcinogenic *in vivo* and *in vitro* (117, 252). Much effort is currently invested in this area (Table 28.1) (16, 39, 218a).

> *Some dietary tidbits: garlic contains organic sulfides that have been proven to be anticarcinogenic in rats and mice; similar virtues are found in brussels sprouts, cabbage, and broccoli. They all contain substances that induce microsomal oxidases in the liver and other tissues, whereby certain carcinogens are inactivated (these experiments, however, are not uniformly encouraging) (187).*

Hormones as Carcinogens Hormones are not likely to be genotoxic, that is, they do not behave as DNA poisons. Yet they have many links with tumors. The hormonal status of the body plays a major role in experimental carcinogenesis (78). As we will see later, even virus-induced mammary tumors of the mouse can be prevented by ovariectomy (p. 839).

Endocrine tumors in rodents are easily produced by *overstimulation of a gland*. For example, if the thyroid is atrophied by irradiation, the hypophysis oversecretes thyrotropic hormone, enlarges, and eventually becomes neoplastic (74–77). The carcinogenic effect of endocrine overstimulation has also been proven by an imaginative experiment that takes advantage of the fact that estrogens are inactivated in the liver (21, 22, 76). In the normal female rat and mouse, the pituitary stimulates the gonads, which respond by secreting estrogens, and the blood level of estrogen serves as a "brake" (a feedback loop that controls pituitary stimulation). Now, abolish this feedback by removing one ovary and implanting the other into the spleen, so that it releases its estrogen into the splenic vein and thence into the liver, where it is inactivated. The pituitary, now deprived of this estrogen feedback, responds by overproducing gonadotropin, which causes a hyperplasia of the granulosa cells in the ovary (Figure 28.17). This hyperplastic response can produce first a benign tumor that cannot be transplanted successfully and finally a transplantable malignant tumor (83). Note the classic progression: hyperplasia → benign tumor → malignant tumor.

Also, in rats, if the liver is submitted to an initiation of carcinogenesis, estrogens are effective tumor promoters (Figure 28.18).

In humans, certain tumors (breast, ovary, endometrium, and prostate) correlate with hormonal levels (95, 140). Endogenous estrogens are the link between obesity (241) and cancer of the

TABLE 28.1

The Chemoprevention of Cancer: Some Inhibitors of Carcinogen-Induced Neoplasia

CATEGORY OF INHIBITOR	CHEMICAL CLASS	INHIBITORY COMPOUNDS
Compounds preventing formation of carcinogen from precursor compounds	Reductive acids, Tocopherols, Phenols	Ascorbic acid[a], α-tocopherol,[a] γ-tocopherol, caffeic acid,[a] ferulic acid[a]
Blocking agents	Phenols	2 (3)-tert-butylhydroxyanisole,[b] butylated hydroxytoluene,[b] hydroxyanisole, ellagic acid,[a] caffeic acid,[a] ferulic acid,[a] p-hydroxycinnamic acid[a]
	Indoles	Indole-3-acetonitrile,[a] indole-3-carbinol[a]
	Aromatic isothiocyanates	Benzyl isothiocyanate,[a] phenethyl isothiocyanate[a]
	Coumarins	Coumarin,[a] limettin[a]
	Flavones	β-Naphthoflavone, α-naphthoflavone, quercetin pentamethyl ether[c]
	Diterpenes	Kahweol palmitate[a]
	Phenothiazines, Barbiturates	Phenothiazine phenobarbital
Suppressing agents	Retinoids, carotenoids	Retinyl palmitate,[a] retinyl acetate,[a] β-carotene
	Selenium salts	Sodium selenite,[a] selenium dioxide,[a] selenious acid[a]
	Protease inhibitors	Leupeptin, antipain, soybean protease inhibitors[a]
	Inhibitors of arachidonic acid metabolism	Indomethacin, aspirin, tert-butyl isocyanate, benzyl isothiocyanate[a]
	Cyanates; isothiocyanates	Sodium cyanate
	Phenols	2(3) tert-butylhydroxyanisole[b]
	Plant sterols	β-sitosterol[a]
	Methylated xanthines	Caffeine[a]
	Others	Dehydroepiandrosterone, fumaric acid[a]

[a] Naturally occurring compound present in food.
[b] Synthetic antioxidant used as a food additive.
[c] The closely related compounds tangeretin and nobilitin occur in citrus fruits.

Adapted from (232)

endometrium: adipose tissue converts androgens to estrogens (p. 39). Therapeutic levels of estrogens in postmenopausal women increase the risk of endometrial cancer, whereas contraceptive doses in premenopausal women induce, oddly enough, liver adenomas (55, 226).

The high incidence of cancer of the breast in nuns could also be mentioned under occupational diseases. Two major risk factors for breast cancer are being nulliparous and being overweight (95, 241). This correlation, first observed in nuns, appeared in 1700 in the pioneering treatise *De morbis artificum* (On the Diseases of Workers) by Bernardino Ramazzini.

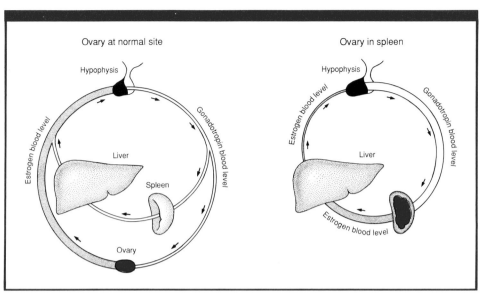

FIGURE 28.17
Example of hormonal carcinogenesis in the rat. *Left:* In the normal rat, estrogens secreted by the ovary reach the hypophysis and regulate the blood level of gonadotrophin. *Right:* If the ovary is implanted into the spleen, blood from the spleen drains into the liver where the estrogens are inactivated; therefore the hypophysis perceives an ovarian insufficiency and increases the secretion of endotrophin. As a result there is a hypertrophy of the hypophysis and an enlargement of the ovarian implant in the spleen that can become neoplastic. (Adapted from [75].)

Every city in Italy has several religious communities of nuns, and you can seldom find a convent that does not harbor this accursed pest, cancer, within its walls. Now why is it that the breasts suffer for the derangements of the womb, whereas other parts of the body do not suffer in this way or so frequently? It is certainly because there is between them a mysterious sympathy that so far has escaped the researches of prosecutors, though perhaps the course of time will reveal it, since the whole domain of Truth has not yet been conquered. (178)

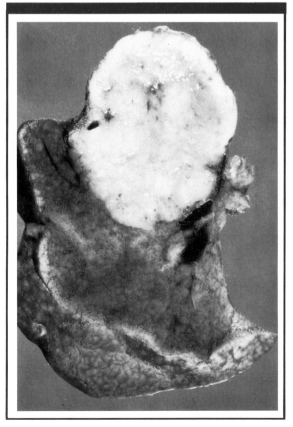

FIGURE 28.18
Carcinogenesis in rat liver by initiation with diethylnitrosamine, followed by promotion with stilbestrol for 20 weeks; the stilbestrol dose was about 200 times the usual contraceptive dose in humans. The white mass is a tumor that appeared 29 weeks after the end of the treatment. Diameter about 3 cm. (Reproduced with permission from [226].)

The reverse of the coin, giving birth to a child at early age, protects against breast cancer. We can now add another piece of the puzzle: a history of *induced abortion predisposes* to breast cancer (49b). All these facts can be explained as follows: we know from the study of carcinogenesis that the more a cell is differentiated, the less it is susceptible to malignant transformation (188a); ostensibly the epithelium of the mammary gland becomes fully differentiated only in the course of lactation (188a).

However, roughly 10 percent of breast cancers are due to a *genetic predisposition;* two breast cancer genes have been identified, BRCA1 and BRCA2 (139a, 132b).

Occupational Carcinogens After the soot wart, another scrotal cancer appeared in Scotland early in the twentieth century; it was due to mineral oil (207). Workers in the cotton industry attended the "mule," a machine that carried rotating spools and had to be lubricated constantly. As mule spinners leaned over the edge of the machine, oil soaked into their clothes at the level of the groin, eventually causing scrotal cancer in many workers.

In more recent times (1974), the physician of a chemical plant where *polyvinyl chloride resins* were manufactured was alerted by the fact that three workers in two years had died of angiosarcoma of the liver, a rare tumor (48). The cause of this bizarre cluster was quickly traced to vinyl chloride, the plastic monomer (127, 170). The workers' exposure had lasted from 2 to 18 years; in laboratory rodents the latent period is less than a year (169).

Asbestos was discovered to be a carcinogen in 1960, thanks to maps of cancer mortality. An exceptionally high incidence of lung cancer in white males of coastal Georgia was correlated with work in shipyards during World War II (25). The inhaled fibers produce fibrosis and eventually malignant tumors of the mesothelium of the pleura, pericardium, and peritoneum (see Figures 13.41 and 13.44). Asbestos acts synergistically with cigarette smoke. The carcinogenic potential of asbestos in schools and other buildings is probably overrated (151).

Nickel and *chromium* correlate with the incidence of cancer of the lung, and nickel also with the incidence of cancer of the nasal sinuses (52, 211). The same tissues are affected in leather workers and in manufacturers of hardwood furniture, but the carcinogen is unknown. Again, it was a general practitioner who noticed this connection. Dr. John Jones of Clydach, South Wales, diagnosed two cases of carcinoma of the ethmoid sinus in a single year (211).

> *The molecular mechanisms of carcinogenesis by nickel shows how complicated oncology can be. Possible effects of nickel ions include chromosome damage, mutagenesis, formation of left-handed DNA (Z-DNA), inhibition of DNA excision–repair, tumor promotion, and enhancement of tumor progression by inhibition of NK cells (210).*

Therapeutic Carcinogens An irony of tumor therapy is that our most powerful antitumor agents produce tumors. This may be inescapable at present; *carcinogens and our current anticarcinogens aim at the same target: the DNA molecule* (164). It is distressing when a young patient, healed of Hodgkin's disease, is lost to leukemia as early as three years later or to a solid cancer in the field of irradiation 10 years later (221).

> *In one study of 2067 patients treated for gastrointestinal cancer with a nitrosourea, leukemic disorders appeared in 14 cases (40). In another series of 471 patients treated with cyclophosphamide for non-Hodgkin's lymphoma, 7 patients came down with carcinoma of the bladder (161); note, however, that the absolute risk remains low (in the latter study, 2.3 cases per 1000 persons per year) and is not interpreted as outweighing the benefits of chemotherapy.*

The therapeutic use of diethylstilbestrol became, unfortunately, a *cause célèbre* in 1971 (Figure 28.19) (97–99, 138). This episode shows the

$$HO-\langle\rangle-\underset{\underset{C_2H_5}{|}}{\overset{\overset{C_2H_5}{|}}{C}}=C-\langle\rangle-OH$$

Diethylstilbestrol

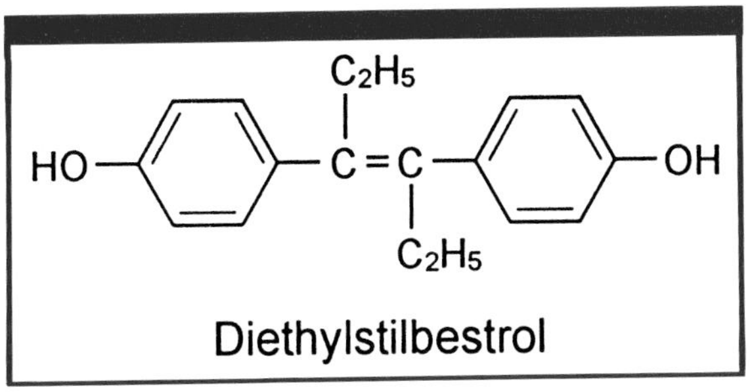

FIGURE 28.19
The formula of diethylstilbestrol.

importance of the alert practitioner as a watchguard against unexpected carcinogens.

> *Adenocarcinoma of the vagina is a rare tumor, usually seen in women over 50. Suddenly, between 1966 and 1969, seven young women 15–22 years old came to the same gynecologist, A.L. Herbst, with an adenocarcinoma of the vagina. Suspecting an unknown carcinogen, Dr. H. Ulfelder, the epidemiologist of the clinical team, took careful, detailed histories from each patient. Nothing unusual surfaced. Finally one patient, because she was so young, came with her mother, who volunteered her own strong belief: she was sure that the culprit was a drug she had been given during pregnancy. This hint was not followed up, but when a second mother offered the same suggestion, Dr. Ulfelder investigated. The drug turned out to be diethylstilbestrol, customarily given to stop bleeding during pregnancy.*

After the first few cases, hundreds more came to light, and thousands of young women whose mothers were treated during pregnancy are still living with this threat. Fortunately, their risk up to age 34 is fairly low, 1 in 1000, which suggests that diethylstilbestrol is not a complete carcinogen and that some other factor is involved (138).

Immunosuppression for therapeutic purposes is another pathway to cancer (p. 586).

Sundry Carcinogens Free radicals can certainly injure DNA strands. They are involved in the well-known carcinogenesis by ionizing radiations (72). But what about endogenous sources of free radicals, such as activated leukocytes? Is it thinkable that leukocytes could be carcinogenic (11)? The concept has been proposed, and the evidence, although indirect, is impressive. In one study, mouse fibroblasts were exposed to activated human leukocytes and then were injected into nude mice; they produced tumors (238).

> *The ability of a substance to cause mutations can be tested easily with a large number of assays on bacteria. Human leukocytes exposed to bacteria do cause bacterial mutations; and the free-radical*

*scavenger, superoxide dismutase, inhibits the muta-
tions. Heat-killed cells, lymphocytes, and leukocytes
from a patient with chronic granulomatous disease,
which cannot mount a respiratory burst (p. 406,
503), did not cause mutations (237). Activated
human leukocytes exposed to mammalian cells
caused visible chromosomal changes (236).*

All this occurs *in vitro;* what happens *in vivo*
remains to be seen. Perhaps this free radical
mechanism is involved in carcinogenesis by plastic
sheets (p. 835) and possibly by asbestos.

*Among carcinogens discovered by accident (203) are
the potent fluorenamides (N-2-fluorenylacetamide,
2-FAA), patented in 1940 as insecticides. Their use
ended abruptly when their carcinogenic effects on rats
were discovered. Interestingly, guinea pigs are immune to this carcinogen because they do not
metabolize the molecule to its ultimate form (man
does, as was found using trace doses in volunteers
with advanced cancer). The effect of urethane was
discovered at the National Cancer Institute in
experiments on the effects of radiation. The mice had
to be maintained under sedation for prolonged
periods, wherefore the standard veterinary solution of
urethane was used. Lung tumors appeared in 26 of
29 mice, and the urethane, not the radiation, was
found to be the cause.*

Physical Causes of Tumors

Besides ultraviolet and ionizing radiation, the
physical causes of cancer include burns, physical
trauma (a minor but interesting category), and an
absolutely bizarre but fascinating phenomenon:
carcinogenesis by plastic sheets, which led to the
concept of solid-state carcinogenesis.

RADIATION

Considering the vast range of the electromagnetic
spectrum to which we are exposed, including radio
waves (224), it is fortunate that only the ultraviolet and ionizing radiations are carcinogenic (Figure
3.50) (199).

Ultraviolet Light Most radiation cancers are due
to ultraviolet (UV) rays that reach us in sunlight
(about 500,000 cases per year in the United
States). Such skin cancers are mostly basal cell
carcinomas that are treated almost casually because, by and large, they can be excised and
forgotten; they are not even included in many
general cancer statistics. However, the potentially
metastasizing squamous cell carcinomas and the
much more dangerous melanomas are also caused

by UV light in sunshine. The incidence of
melanoma is inversely related to latitude (59),
which clearly implicates sunlight; in fact even the
number of sunspots have been said to affect the
statistics of human melanoma (104). The increase
in melanoma since 1935 implicates, we hope, only
a behavioral trend: the otherwise innocent practice of sun-worship (Figure 28.20). We are possibly
therefore dealing, once again, with a large number
of theoretically avoidable cancers. We introduce a
note of uncertainty in this statement because a
further increase in the incidence of melanoma
might implicate a more threatening cause—the
thinning of the ozone layer (133).

As to the pathogenesis of UV cancer: experimentally, UV rays behave as complete carcinogens, but
repeated exposures are needed. Treatment with a
promoter such as phorbol ester accelerates the
response *in vivo* and *in vitro* (148, 179). At the
molecular level, UV rays do not have enough
energy to ionize their targets, but they raise them to
a short-lived excited state and thereby damage
DNA strands by forming dimers and crosslinks
(179). It may be relevant that *UV radiation tends to
depress the immune system;* a mild sunburn depresses
the viability and function of circulating lymphocytes for as long as 24 hours (133).

*The effect of UV radiation on leukocytes is an
intriguing topic. Some UV rays reach as deep as the
capillaries, and about 5 percent of cardiac output
flows through the skin. However, the white color of
leukocytes, it has been said (195), protects these cells
against DNA injury because it reflects the entire
spectrum.*

Ionizing Radiations Ionizing radiations are part of
our natural environment, but as carcinogens they
are to a large extent a man-made problem. Figure
28.21 shows the sources of ionizing radiations to
inhabitants of the United States; the largest share
is the radiation background (cosmic rays and
terrestrial radiation), whereas 18 percent is due to
medical or industrial sources. Some ionizing radiations are electromagnetic (X-rays and gamma
rays) and others are particulate (electrons, pro-
tons, alpha and beta particles) (Figure 3.50).

Radiation cancer claimed its first known victims as an occupational disease long before the
discovery of ionizing radiation (106, 230). It was
known for centuries that Czech and German
miners working on either side of the Erz mountains
were being killed by a mysterious "mountain
disease" (*Bergsucht*). The mines first yielded silver,
later nickel and other metals, and finally uranium;

the ore was the same as that in which Mme. Curie discovered radium. The mysterious "pneumonia" of the miners was not recognized as cancer until 1929 when the first autopsies were performed (166); the culprit was radon gas, a decay product of radium (130).

In 1895 Roentgen discovered X-rays and dedicated them to the benefit of mankind (he did not patent his X-ray machine); seven years later the first report of a case of skin cancer in a radiologist was published. Many more followed, and industrial exposure became an added hazard (Figure 28.22). Between 1929 and 1943 ten times more radiologists died of leukemia than other physicians: a difference that has since disappeared (130, 119).

For the discovery of radium, Pierre and Marie Curie received the Nobel prize in 1904, but the award came at a high price: both Mme. Curie and her daughter Irene died of leukemia (162). Radium claimed many other victims; it was used to make fluorescent paint for the dials of watches. The women who painted the dials ingested radium by licking their brushes to make fine points. Many of these women developed osteosarcomas of the mastoid and carcinomas of the nasal sinuses (Figure 28.23) (26, 107).

The true hazards of radiation (119) were not perceived until recently; both authors of this book remember shoe shops in which customers stepped onto an X-ray box to admire the snug fit of their new shoes. This casual use of radiation produced some medical disasters.

For example, in the 1940s and 1950s, children were irradiated routinely to reduce the size of the tonsils or of the thymus, which were perceived as too large (today the latter is a nondisease). In one series, cancer of the thyroid developed in 8 percent with a delay of 20–30 years (65, 130). Other children, perhaps 200,000 worldwide, had their scalps submitted to the very "handy" X-ray epilation for a common fungal infection; the cost was an increase in the incidence of tumors of the scalp, brain, parotid, neck and thyroid, plus some mental illness (2, 101, 147). The parotid is similarly affected by X-ray treatment for acne, still current (36, 173). Radioactive thorium dioxide ("Thorotrast") was used after 1928 as a contrast medium in radiology to visualize arterial trees. After its quick performance in the arteries it continued to circulate until it was all picked up and removed by the RES/MPS, including the Kupffer cells (p. 297) (see Figure 8.11). Predictably, the liver suffered most from the prolonged exposure to thorium radiation: the first angiosarcoma of the liver was diagnosed at autopsy 12 years later (131, 227).

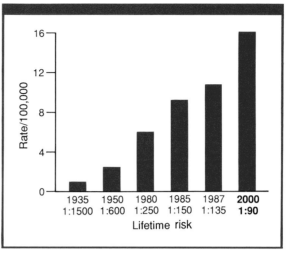

FIGURE 28.20 Malignant melanoma is on the rise: past, current and projected lifetime risk of an individual in the United States developing malignant melanoma. (Reproduced with permission from [185].)

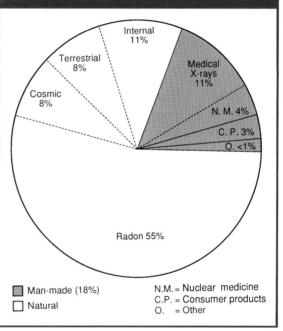

FIGURE 28.21 Percentage contribution of various sources of radiation to the total average effective dose (U.S. population). (Reproduced with permission from [154].)

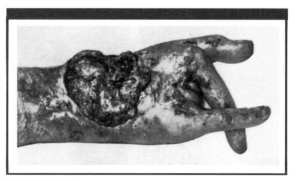

FIGURE 28.22
Carcinoma of the back of the hand in a 57-year-old man who worked for 27 years in the manufacture of X-ray apparatus, in the early days of radiology. By 1922 about 100 radiologists had died from malignant disease due to their occupation. (Reproduced with permission from [107].)

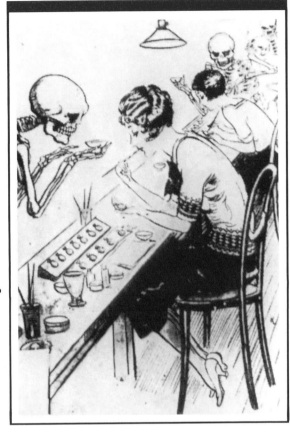

FIGURE 28.23
A famous car-
toon in a New
York newspaper:
Death holding a
dish of meso-
thorium paint to
a technician,
who applies it to
the watch dial.
Note how the
technician is
drawing the
brush to a point
with her lips.
(Reproduced
with permission
from [107].)

Ionizing radiations have been called *universal carcinogens* because, unlike chemical carcinogens, they induce cancers in virtually all tissues of all species at all ages, possibly including the fetus.

The amount of energy absorbed by irradiated matter is expressed in a unit called a rad *(100 ergs deposited*

per gram); *however, rads tell nothing about ioniza-tion density, which is expressed as LET (linear energy transfer: energy lost per unit of distance traveled in kiloelectron volts per micrometer) (131).*

For a given dose, highly ionizing radiations (high-LET) are more carcinogenic, suggesting that ionization is an important factor. Unlike UV rays, a single exposure to ionizing radiation is enough to cause cancer, as demonstrated by the survivors of the Nagasaki and Hiroshima atomic bombs; leuke-mia appeared after about 6 years, whereas other solid tumors increased after 20 years (101). This difference in latency between leukemias and solid tumors is a general rule (119). The tumors, benign and malignant, caused by radiation are similar to spontaneous tumors and tend to develop at the customary age (119), with one peculiarity: chronic lymphatic leukemia does not seem to develop from radiations of any kind.

Some individuals are especially prone to radiation cancer. The classic example is the familial form of retinoblastoma (222). We shall explain this condi-tion in detail later (p. 867), but its essence is as follows. Some cancers are caused by mutation of both alleles of a gene. Some people are born with that mutation in one allele, and therefore they need only one more "hit" to develop a tumor, usually a bone sarcoma after X-ray treatment.

The molecular damage due to radiation can occur anywhere in a cell; but because the protoplasm is 80 percent water, the main direct target is water, which breaks into free radicals that cause indirect damage. Another source of free radicals is molecu-lar oxygen, hence the difficulty of killing the hy-poxic parts of tumors (p. 771). DNA can undergo

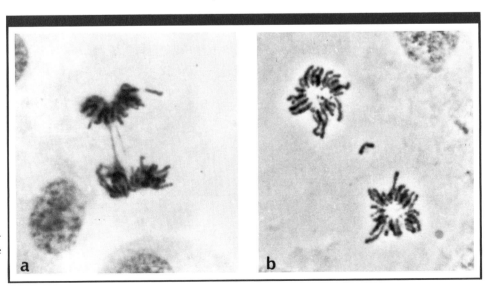

FIGURE 28.24
Radiation effects on mitosis in cul-tured cells (mouse lymphoma).
(a) Anaphase with two bridges.
(b) Anaphase with loss of a chromo-some. The lost chromosome will give rise to a micronucleus. (Reproduced with permission from [198].)

single or double-stranded breaks, loss of bases, or formation of abnormal bonds between adjacent bases (which become dimers). The half-time for repair of this damage, measured in the epithelium of rat skin, was estimated at 3 ± 1 hours (36). Sometimes one or more chromosomes go astray during mitosis (Figure 28.24) and then set up their own separate home in a "micronucleus" (Figure 28.25).

The biological effect of radiation damage can manifest itself at a metabolic, genetic, or cellular level. Irradiated cells may survive but suffer so-called *reproductive death*: they can no longer divide. Sometimes they become gigantic (Figure 28.26). The most studied aspect of radiation injury is shortened cell survival, which is exploited for tumor radiotherapy. Most sensitive are bone-marrow cells and intestinal epithelium, cells that have high mitotic rates.

It is certainly a paradox that radiation, which typically shortens cell survival, should also be capable of immortalizing cells by conferring malignant transformation on them; this worrisome complication of radiotherapy is studied *in vitro* in cell cultures. Transformation *in vitro*, is invaluable for testing potential cancer-preventing agents (179).

The standard method is to grow cells of an appropriate type in Petri dishes until they are confluent; often used in the line of mouse embryo fibroblasts called 3T3. These cells are not normal because they are aneuploid and immortal. However, they remain contact inhibited, and they are not considered neoplastic because they do not form tumors when injected into suitable recipient animals. They are perhaps on the way to becoming neoplastic because they occasionally give rise to foci of transformed cells that are tightly packed (type I foci) or have lost contact inhibition and pile up over each other (type II and III foci) (Figure 28.27) (183). To return to the assay: Petri dishes with confluent cells are irradiated and then kept for 4–6 weeks, after which they are fixed, stained, and the transformed foci are counted (Figure 28.28). With this number as a baseline, it is fairly simple to test agents that increase the number of foci (such as the cancer promoting phorbol esters) or inhibit them (such as protease inhibitors, selenium, and vitamin A, C, or E) (128).

PHYSICAL TRAUMA

Mechanical trauma is usually ruled out as a cause of tumors, but this point of view should be reexamined. A *single* trauma on *normal* tissues is indeed

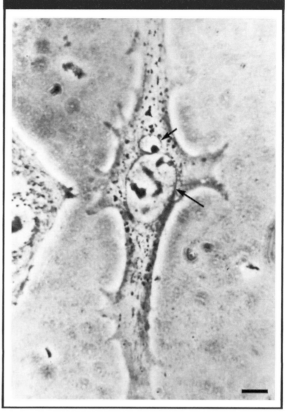

FIGURE 28.25 Cultured irradiated cell with a main nucleus **(long arrow)** and a micronucleus **(short arrow),** the latter deriving from a lost chromosome fragment. **Bar =** 10 μm. (Reproduced with permission from [87].)

unlikely to produce a tumor, because the short burst of mitoses that comes with repair is *statistically* unlikely to produce a malignant mutation. However, two other settings are possible: (a) for some reason—such as infection—a single traumatic lesion does not heal, thereby prolonging the period of healing and of mitotic divisions; and (b) a single injury hits a tissue that is already predisposed to develop a tumor. This mechanism is illustrated by the classic series of experiments by Peyton Rous, who studied rabbit skin prepared with a noncarcinogenic dose of tar, showed that malignant

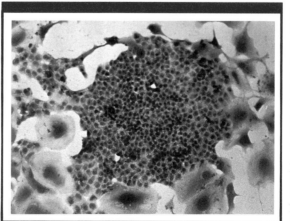

FIGURE 28.26 Cell mutations induced by irradiation in a colony of cultured HeLa human cancer cells. The large "monster" cells have lost their reproductive capacity but still carry on metabolic functions. (Reproduced with permission from [176].)

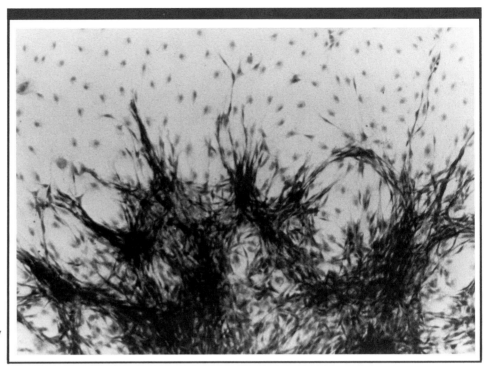

FIGURE 28.27
Edge of a focus of transformed fibroblasts 6 weeks after irradiation. Compared with normal cells (top), transformed cells are highly basophilic and tend to overlap. (Courtesy of Dr. A.R. Kennedy, University of Pennsylvania, Pittsburgh, PA.)

tumors developed predictably wherever the prepared skin was traumatized by biopsy (p. 191a).

We had the opportunity to study a patient who appeared to illustrate the first modality. A 26-year-old construction worker was hit in a cheek by a swinging hook; the wound never healed and 9 years later gave rise to a squamous cell carcinoma. In this case the lack of healing (although unexplained) provided a powerful link between trauma and cancer. The insurance company chose to settle out of court.

FIGURE 28.28
Mouse fibroblasts growing in a Petri dish, stained with methylene blue 6 weeks after irradiation. A large focus of piled-up transformed cells stands out on a background monolayer of nontransformed cells. (Courtesy of Dr. A.R. Kennedy, University of Pennsylvania, Philadelphia, PA.)

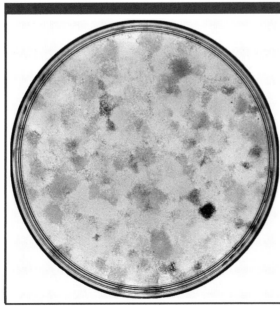

A computer search for titles combining *scar* and *tumor* brought up a wealth of recent reports of carcinomas (not sarcomas) arising in scars. The incidence seems to be greater outside North America (125).

Many of the scars that developed tumors derived from mechanical injuries, including surgical scars (110) and burns (1, 7), but the list included venipuncture (after 6 months; the original puncture site never healed) (239), frostbite (61), snake bite (125), and even a surgical wound of the thigh from which skin grafts had been taken 6 weeks previously to cover a burn (90). A study of 1774 basal cell carcinomas found a history of trauma in 7.3 percent (156).

It is clear that carcinomas sometimes arise in scars and even in recent wounds; fibrosarcomas are almost never seen except after irradiation (114). The real issue is their frequency. As just mentioned, there may be differences among populations. In the wake of World War I, the Germans rated the incidence of malignancies (in 3,710,371 hospital-treated wounds) as 5.3 per million; the French estimate was 10 times higher (106). In burn wounds the incidence of malignancy is probably higher than in mechanical wounds.

Chronic irritation such as that in ulcers is a special form of trauma. Malignant tumors arising on persistent ulcers, especially after burns, are sometimes mentioned in surgical circles as Marjolin's ulcer (71). Quite apart from the fact that Professor Marjolin never described such an event (208), the occurrence is so rare that even one case is publishable (194). In a recent review of 46 cases of squamous cell carcinoma after a burn the latent period averaged 43 years. It was concluded by the reviewers that the incidence of this complication is dropping, perhaps because the care of burns has greatly improved (56). Occasionally a tumor develops around a foreign body. A man, who may have been the last victim of World War I, died of a sarcoma developing around fragments of a German grenade, 65 years later. Sarcomas around Dacron aortic grafts have also been reported (94). We will return to this topic shortly.

Esophageal strictures after caustic injury (from ingesting acids or alkali) sometimes develop carcinomas after 30–45 years; the stenosis causes gastric reflux and chronic irritation, which may be the culprit (49, 196).

Meningiomas represent a fascinating exception: they are the only tumors statistically associated with a history of trauma (head trauma) and even foreign bodies such as bullets (193). We have no explanation.

> *The so-called scar carcinomas of the lung are probably not carcinomas in scars, but rather desmoplastic carcinomas, that is, carcinomas that develop a dense, fibrous stroma (58).*

Besides causing tumors, trauma relates to tumors in other ways. It has been shown many times in experimental animals that mechanical, chemical, or surgical trauma can localize metastases (70, 153); this mechanism may also apply to surgical wounds (p. 803). Dormant cancer cells can be awakened: in rats injected with as few as 50 malignant cells in the liver, repeated laparotomy and exploration of the liver greatly accelerates the appearance of tumors (69). Trauma can also localize a circulating virus: rabbit papilloma virus injected intravenously creates papillomas where the skin has been shaved; the mechanism has not been studied.

THE PUZZLE OF PLASTIC SHEET SARCOMAS (SOLID STATE CARCINOGENESIS)

This is a strange story (17, 29). We report it here because we believe that it hides some important truth.

In 1941 it was reported that disks of bakelite (a plastic) implanted subcutaneously in rats produced sarcomas. Nobody picked up the trail. In 1948,

Oppenheimer and co-workers (158) were producing hypertension in rats by wrapping one kidney in cellophane. This procedure causes a fibrous reaction that strangles the kidney, which becomes ischemic and responds by producing renin, and thereby hypertension. It was found quite accidentally that sarcomas had developed around some of the cellophane wrappings. Further work showed that virtually any plastic sheet implanted under the skin—including nylon, dacron, saran, and many others—induces sarcomas in rats and mice. The percentage of implants that produced tumors varied between 7 and 50 percent. The latent period ranged from 7 months to $2\frac{1}{2}$ years (159). If the plastic sheet was removed after 6 months, the carcinogenic effect persisted (Figure 28.29).

Then came variations on the theme. It was found that the plastic sheets (or disks) have to be of a certain size, of the order of 2×3 cm; if they are cut into small pieces or pulverized, the effect disappears. Smooth surfaces work much better than rough ones (9). One of the experimenters, with whom we spoke, was particularly bewildered by finding that sarcomas failed to appear if the sheets had become accidentally folded during implantation or if they were perforated. Millipore filters with small pores induce tumors; those with large pores do not (82). The mystery spread beyond plastic: sheets of gold and silver and steel also produce sarcomas, and so do many other inert substances (17), including plates of glass and quartz; but powdered glass or quartz will not do.

The name *solid-state carcinogenesis* seems well justified. But how does it work? The mere presence of *any* foreign body will not do: sarcomas around surgical prostheses in humans, happily, are in the

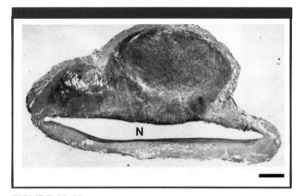

FIGURE 28.29
Example of the mysterious plastic sheet sarcoma. A square of nylon film (**N**) was implanted subcutaneously in a rat; 22 months later a fibrosarcoma developed over the film. **Bar** = 1 mm. (Reproduced with permission from [159].)

"nearly never" category. One theory blamed the macrophages: free radicals, produced by macrophages activated on the surface of a foreign body, might be able to damage the DNA of surrounding fibroblasts and create malignant mutations. We prefer to take the hint offered by the study of **carcinogenesis by asbestos fibers.** It is now apparent that these "inert" fibers are not inert at all: their surface can generate free radicals (251a), especially where the fibers are broken, exposing unsaturated valences (73a).

We close this section on physical carcinogenesis with a word of praise for granulation tissue. This exuberant variety of connective tissue, teeming with mitoses, is an almost everyday companion because it develops at virtually all sites of injury. It flourishes in millions of ulcers worldwide. Yet its growth is so well controlled that, in humans, it almost never lapses into a sarcoma. The worst it does is produce a keloid, which may or may not be a tumor. Only genetic engineering was able to break down this wonderful "self-control" of granulation tissues: there are transgenic mice in which healing wounds lapse into fibrosarcomas (197a).

Biological Causes of Tumors

The idea that bacteria might be the cause of cancer surfaced with the birth of bacteriology in the late 1800s. It was virtually a dead end: bacteria, the most common living beings, rarely cause tumors in animals. We cannot say *never* because rare cases of chronic infection or ulcer may proceed to malignant growth; a connection between gastric cancer and bacteria has been recently made, and plants suffer from the crown gall, a true tumor caused by a bacterium (p. 837). Anyway, by 1900 the concept of carcinogenesis by bacteria was abandoned, partly because cancer is obviously not contagious. Attention turned to viruses and even to a few worms, but today, the "final" answer is that about 80 percent of tumors are not caused by a parasitic agent. This was quite a disappointment to those who bet on viruses. The list of virus-induced tumors includes only one of the cancers that are most common on a worldwide basis, namely hepatoma. However, the pursuit of viral carcinogenesis did strike gold because it led to the first satisfying theory of the nature of cancer: the concept of oncogenes.

We will now summarize the interwoven tales of viruses, bacteria, and worms as they relate to the theme of cancer.

FROM WARTS TO ONCOGENES

The Discovery of Viral Tumors Viruses were first discovered as invisible agents of infection, capable of passing through filters that retain bacteria. Until recently they remained only that, agents of infection, appearing to contrast with bacteria, which can kill but which also perform countless useful functions. So, in their delightful dictionary *From Aristotle to Zoos*, Peter and Jean Medawar stated that "no virus is known to do good" and defined a virus as "a piece of bad news wrapped up in protein" (136). On the whole, viruses are still bad news, but recent tumor research had uncovered technical applications of viruses that qualify as redeeming features.

> To mention just a few: in vitro, *retroviruses can be used for introducing antioncogenes into malignant cells to make them nonmalignant; some viruses replicate only in dividing cells, which they kill and thereby act as antitumor agents. Other viruses make tumor cells more antigenic and thereby expose them to immune destruction. Measles virus causes remissions of some lymphomas by a complex mechanism (205).*

Viruses were discovered in association with another killer, tobacco. The first disease to be proven of viral origin, in 1892, was the so-called **mosaic disease** of the tobacco plant. Shortly thereafter it was shown that the common wart, a benign tumor (Figure 28.30), is transmissible from

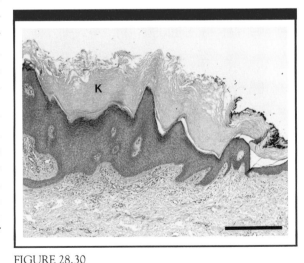

FIGURE 28.30
Common wart, the result of epidermal infection by a papilloma virus. Note the hyperplasia of the epidermis (its normal thickness is represented at the extreme right) as well as the exaggerated production of keratinized cells (**K:** Hyperkeratosis). **Bar** = 500 μm.

one human volunteer to another, confirming a fact that most school children know. In 1908 two Danish veterinarians, Ellermann and Bang, showed that fowl leukemia can also be transmitted by a cell-free filtrate (57). This was a milestone in cancer research, but it did not come through as such: the authors themselves shared the current belief that leukemia had little to do with "real tumors," and their suggestion that leukemia in general is an infectious disease did not have much data to support it. Indifference and skepticism were also the lot of Peyton Rous when he announced in 1911 that he had succeeded in transmitting from hen to hen a solid malignant tumor with a cell-free filtrate (189, 190): it was a sarcoma, unquestionably malignant (Figure 28.31), but it was easy to object that hens are not mammals, and, after all, everybody knew that cancer was not contagious. Rous was actually told by Simon Flexner that good science includes knowing when to quit (96). The electron microscope, which could have easily demonstrated the virus in the tumor (Figure 28.32), did not yet exist. So Rous decided to quit. Little did he guess that he had just triggered his Noble prize.

The Crown Gall, a Bacterial Tumor Another major discovery had just flashed by, unnoticed by the medical world because it concerned tumors in plants. In 1908, two plant pathologists of the U.S. Department of Agriculture, Smith and Townsend, showed that certain natural growths (crown galls) on the Paris daisy were caused by a soil bacterium, now called *Agrobacterium tumefaciens* (Figure 28.33) (206). Today we know that the bacterium carries a bit of DNA in the shape of a ring (a plasmid); a specific part of this plasmid is somehow inserted into the DNA of a plant cell, whereupon growth is initiated; from that point on the bacterium is no longer necessary (30). This is a perfect example of natural genetic engineering; but of course it could not be appreciated in 1908 (249).

Worms: The Fibiger Epic In the meantime a novel kind of oncologic adventure was beginning to unfold in Copenhagen. Johannes Fibiger, a distinguished pathologist, happened to autopsy three rats who had died at the same time in the same cage. All three had papillomatous growths in their forestomachs. Histology showed that they contained some sort of worm. The pursuit of this worm, which Fibiger thought to be the cause of the tumor, turned into a consuming endeavor (67, 157).

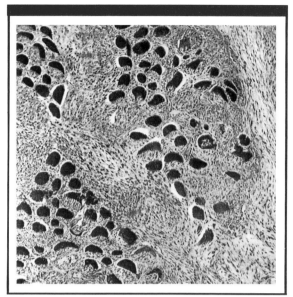

FIGURE 28.31
A historical event: This sarcoma was obtained by injecting into the breast muscle of a chicken a cell-free extract of a chicken tumor (now known as Rous sarcoma). The muscle fibers (dark masses) are dissociated by swarms of tumor cells. (Reproduced with permission from [190].)

Because nobody could diagnose the worm, Fibiger reconstructed it from 900 serial sections. It was an unknown nematode. To find a live one he had 1100 rats trapped in Copenhagen, but they all had the wrong worms and no gastric tumors. The supplier of the original three rats had gone out of business. Anyone else would have given up, but not Fibiger. Perhaps there was another stage of that worm in some other host. In an old 1824 paper he found that certain cockroaches were a possibility. But where would rats and cockroaches live together? Bakeries, decided Fibiger. For years he dissected bakery cockroaches, in vain. He was close to despair when someone told him of a sugar refinery with a different, American cockroach; he raided that bakery and finally came up with 61 rats of which 40 had worms and 9 had gastric tumors. Triumphantly

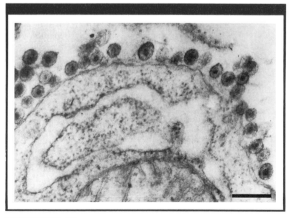

FIGURE 28.32
Particles of Rous sarcoma virus grown on a chorioallantoic membrane of a chick embryo. A characteristic row of virus particles on the surface of the plasma membrane. **Bar** = 0.3 μm. (Reproduced with permission from [86].)

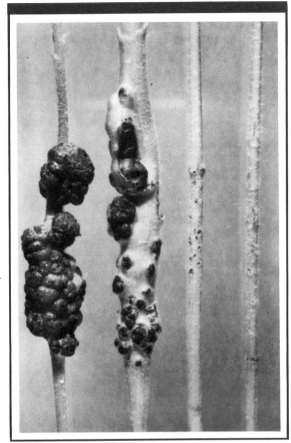

FIGURE 28.33 Plant tumor caused by a bacterium. Sunflower stems inoculated with virulent strains of *Agrobacterium tumefaciens* (left) and with two control strains. (Reproduced with permission from [113].)

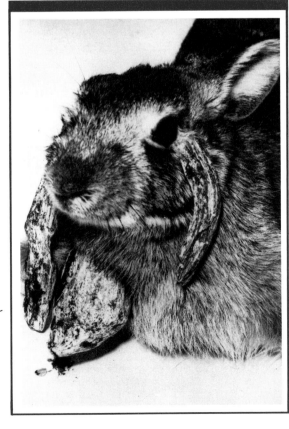

FIGURE 28.34 "Horned rabbit": A naturally infected Kansas cottontail rabbit bearing multiple Shope papillomas. (Reproduced with permission from [121].)

he named the worm *Spiroptera neoplastica* (later *Gongylonema neoplasticum*), reconstructed its life cycle and studied the tumors in greater detail. Just in time, the sugar refinery went up in flames with all its rats, worms, and roaches (157).

For his 19-year pursuit of the cancer-causing worm Fibiger received in 1926 the Nobel Prize, the first one to be awarded for cancer research. Then came the critics (103). Fibiger had fed his bakery rats just white bread and water, clearly a vitamin-deficient diet. It was claimed that his "tumors" were just a hyperplastic response to lack of vitamin A and that his metastases were not real metastases. His results could not be duplicated, yet his slides are still there to see; papillomas, at least, are undeniable (103). In the midst of this storm, Fibiger died of cancer.

Today, all the fuss about Fibiger's data makes little sense. There is nothing unusual about a worm causing cancer (*Schistosoma* causes cancer in human bladders) or about the difficulty of duplicating results with a different strain or a different diet. However, Nobel prizes for cancer research were shelved for 40 years.

Shope's Horned Rabbits Cancer research rolled on. A hunter from Cherokee, Iowa, visiting the laboratory of Richard Shope around 1933, advised his host that "horned rabbits" were common in his part of the country (204). Shope obtained some live specimens. The horns turned out to be papillomas: filiform or branching structures consisting of a thin vascular core coated by epidermis. Because cornified cells continued to form but did not slough off, the tumors appeared as tough horns (Figure 28.34). This is the mystery of the horned rabbits still displayed in curio shops and museums in the Mississippi valley. But how could such tumors be endemic? Shope prepared some glycerinated extracts and applied them to the scarified skin of other rabbits; they produced papillomas. If he injected the extract intravenously, papillomas developed only in scarified areas. This was the first virus-induced tumor to be described in a mammal.

Shope's laboratory at the Rockefeller Institute was next door to the laboratory of Rous. Shope had already acquired fame for the discovery of two mammalian tumors transmitted by viruses (he had also described a "filterable" rabbit myxoma), and felt rather sorry for the sad end of Rous's chicken sarcoma 22 years earlier. So he suggested to Rous that he take over the study of the rabbit papilloma (90). Rous was delighted. Using cell-free extracts, he tried to transfer the tumor from cottontail to domestic rabbits, and discovered that the rather harmless Shope papillomas could progress in less than a year to carcinomas. This was the first unequivocal proof of tumor progression. It produced another landmark paper by Rous in 1935 (Figure 28.35) (73, 191).

Bittner's Milk Factor The year 1936 saw yet another landmark. John Bittner at the Jackson Memorial Laboratory in Maine was studying a strain of mice with an inherited predisposition to develop mammary cancer (Figure 28.36). How was this trait transmitted? Bittner hit upon the idea of trying "foster nursing": newborn female pups from a control strain were fostered by mothers from the cancerous line, and 90 percent of them developed mammary cancer. Female pups from the cancerous strain were promptly assigned to normal foster mothers; only 10 percent developed cancer. Clearly some agent was being transmitted by the milk; the lactating female did not have to be cancerous, as long as she belonged to the cancerous strain. Later the "milk factor" was identified as an RNA virus and called mouse mammary tumor virus (MMTV) (Figure 28.37).

Remember Bittner's mammary tumor as a perfect example of the multifactorial nature of cancer: MMTV alone is harmless. To produce a mammary carcinoma three conditions must be present:

(1) THE PRESENCE OF THE VIRUS, (p. 855)

(2) AN INHERITED PREDISPOSITION, and

(3) A CERTAIN HORMONAL ENVIRONMENT. In ovariectomized females no tumors develop, whereas males develop tumors if treated with estrogen (23, 24).

Mouse Leukemia Virus Ludvik Gross demonstrated this virus in 1951 in New York, thanks to a new experimental twist. Gross had at hand two strains of mice in which all adults developed leukemia. The condition suggested a viral agent, but none could be demonstrated. Knowing that the transmission of Rous sarcoma and of Shope tumors was more successful in young animals, Gross injected a cell-free extract of leukemic cells into newborns of a leukemia-free strain; as adults, about half of these mice became leukemic (85). This very simple method is now applied routinely for isolating tumor viruses (200).

RETROVIRUSES AND THE ONCOGENE THEORY

By the 1950s it was clear that the pursuit of tumor viruses was interesting, but the facts at hand also

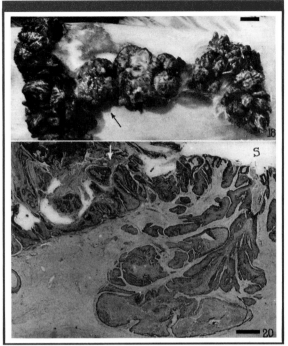

FIGURE 28.35 Progression of the virus-induced Shope papilloma to carcinoma. *Top:* Gross aspect of the papilloma on the back of a rabbit. **Arrow:** Site of the biopsy. **Bar** = 10 mm. *Bottom:* Benign papilloma (**white arrow**); at right, the downgrowth denotes malignancy. From a classic 1935 paper by Rous and Beard. **Bar** = 1 mm. (Reproduced with permission from [191].)

suggested that human tumors as a whole did not fit into the picture of a viral disease. Nobody could have predicted that the next major breakthrough in the understanding of tumors, human or other, would come through study of Rous's chicken sarcoma, which dedicated scientists had kept transmitting throughout World War II. It so happens that the Rous sarcoma is caused by an RNA virus or **retrovirus,** and these viruses have some very special properties. We need to consider them briefly.

RNA Viruses and Reverse Transcriptase A unique feature of all viruses, oncogenic or not, is that they contain either RNA or DNA but not both (with minor exceptions). All other organisms contain both: they carry their genetic information encoded in DNA and transcribe it into RNA

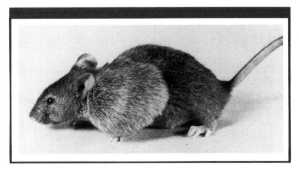

FIGURE 28.36 Spontaneous mammary carcinoma in a $7\frac{1}{2}$-month-old C3H female mouse. (Reproduced with permission from [86].)

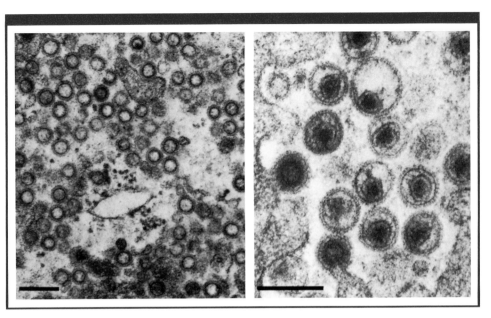

FIGURE 28.37
Virus particles from the spontaneous mammary carcinoma of a C3H mouse. *Left:* So-called type A particles in the cytoplasmic matrix. They are 650–750 Å in diameter, have 2 concentric membranes and no internal nucleoid. *Right:* Type B particles in the intercellular spaces. They have an average diameter of 1,000–1,050 Å. Most of them contain an electron-dense nucleoid surrounded by a membrane. **Bars** = 0.2 μm. (Reproduced with permission from [86].)

as needed. The Rous sarcoma virus for example, contains only RNA.

When a virus of any kind infects a cell, it must take over some of the cell's machinery for protein synthesis because its own is incomplete. To do this it must supply instructions to the cell. For DNA viruses this is not a problem: they just insert their DNA into the DNA of the cell. But what about RNA viruses? Some have opted to skip the DNA phase and just translate their RNA into protein by using the cell's enzymes. However, there is an-

other possibility, which was envisioned in 1962 by Howard Temin of the University of Wisconsin. Temin's inspired guess was that *some RNA viruses have evolved the ability to transcribe their RNA backwards into DNA.* In ordinary cells this is not possible; transcription always runs from DNA to RNA. Temin's prophetic concept was borne out: the necessary enzyme, *reverse transcriptase,* was discovered in 1970 in Temin's laboratory, encoded in virions of the Rous sarcoma (214). The same discovery was made independently at the Massa-

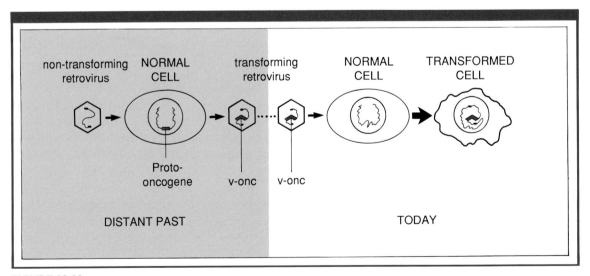

FIGURE 28.38
Scheme of the theft (transduction) of a gene (proto-oncogene) by a retrovirus. In the first step of this process, an ancestral virus integrates its genome in the chromosomes of an infected cell. This viral genome then transduces a cellular proto-oncogene, which therefore comes under the control of the virus. A normal cell infected by this recombinant virus can no longer control the transduced, activated genetic fragment (oncogene) and is condemned to multiply out of control. (Adapted from [209].)

chusetts Institute of Technology, in the laboratory of David Baltimore, using mouse leukemia virus. This led to a shared Nobel prize in 1975.

Retroviruses, the new name for this group of RNA viruses, changed the face of biology. Their reverse transcriptase became a tool for the new science of genetic engineering: it made it possible to synthesize DNA from any RNA. Retroviruses also turned out to be the oldest thieves on record. They have been stealing cellular genes since time immemorial (Figure 28.38); and the stolen genes were changed into cancer genes. We will now see how this happened.

Birth of the Term *Oncogene* The term *oncogene*, literally "gene that produces cancer," was already around at the time of the discovery of the retroviruses in the early 1970s. It had been chosen for a theory proposed in 1969 by Huebner and Todaro of the National Cancer Institute (105). The theory as it was proposed is obsolete, but recounting it helps to understand why the term *oncogene* is something of a misnomer. Most, and perhaps all, cells, so went the theory, contain a viral genome capable of turning the cell into a cancer cell. This genome is normally latent, but stimuli such as X-rays or carcinogens can cause it to be expressed. Howard Temin elaborated on this theory and proposed that the oncogenic viral genome was produced within the cell by a phenomenon he called "misevolution" (215). In essence, he saw the cell as a mother of carcinogenic viruses ready to be inherited and activated. It was a near miss.

The Discovery of Oncogenes in Retroviruses Now we move to the laboratory of Michael Bishop and Harold Varmus at the University of California in San Francisco in 1976 (18–20). The plan was to prove or, more likely, disprove the oncogene theory just mentioned by looking for the supposed tumor-causing gene in the nucleus. A critical experiment was possible thanks to a new tool: a mutant strain of Rous sarcoma virus that had lost the ability to cause sarcomas. The lost piece of viral genome was precisely the sarcoma-producing gene (called v-*src*: v for viral, *src* for sarcoma-producing; pronounced v-sarc). Using this fact, Dominique Stehelin synthesized a radioactive copy of the critical gene as a single-stranded bit of DNA. The next task was to check whether v-*src* was present in any cell, neoplastic or not. This was accomplished by exploiting the tendency of single strands of DNA to seek and combine with com-

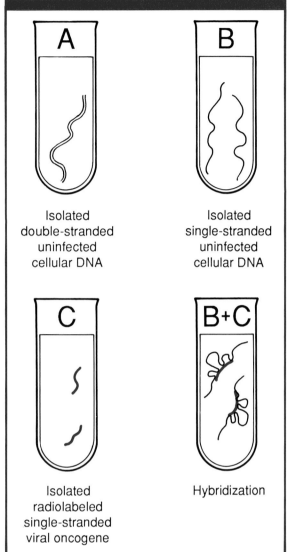

FIGURE 28.39 This is how the viral oncogene v-*src* was identified in cellular DNA. **A:** Double-stranded chicken DNA. **B:** Double strands are denatured and have become single strands. **C:** Separately, single-stranded DNA containing the *src* oncogene are isolated from Rous sarcoma virus and radioactively labeled. **B + C:** When B is mixed with C, some of the viral DNA strands hybridize with normal chicken DNA strands, establishing the presence of a chicken oncogene (c-*src*) homologous to the viral oncogene (v-*src*). (Adapted from [19].)

plementary strands of DNA, a process known in molecular biology as *hybridization* (Figure 28.39) (19). To the amazement of everyone, the radioactive v-*src* hybridized with fragments of *normal* chicken DNA, as well as of DNA from other normal birds, fishes, and mammals, including man—not to mention sponges and slime molds. This meant that *the sarcoma-producing gene, or a gene very similar to it, is a part of the normal cellular genome*, as c-*src* (c stands for cellular).

A closer analysis of the *src* gene of the virus showed that it contains introns, noncoding segments, which identify it as a cellular gene rather than a viral gene. Conclusion: the Rous sarcoma virus has pirated a cellular gene sometime during its evolution. The original oncogene theory was therefore turned upside down; we are

TABLE 28.2

Oncogenes Originally Identified Through Their Presence in Transforming Retroviruses

ONCOGENE	PROTO-ONCOGENE FUNCTION (WHERE KNOWN)	SOURCE OF VIRUS	VIRUS-INDUCED TUMOR
abl	protein kinase (tyrosine)	mouse/cat	pre-B-cell leukemia; sarcoma
akt	?	mouse	T-cell lymphoma
crk	activator of tyrosine-specific kinase(s)	chicken	sarcoma
erb-A	thyroid hormone receptor	chicken	(supplements action of v-erb-B)
erb-B	protein kinase (tyrosine): epidermal growth-factor (EGF) receptor	chicken	erythroleukemia; fibrosarcoma
ets	nuclear protein	chicken	(supplements action of v-myb)
fes/fps	protein kinase (tyrosine)	cat/chicken	sarcoma
fgr	protein kinase (tyrosine)	cat	sarcoma
fms	protein kinase (tyrosine): macrophage colony-stimulating factor (M-CSF) receptor	cat	sarcoma
fos	nuclear transcription factor	mouse	osteosarcoma
jun	nuclear protein: AP-1 transcription factor	chicken	fibrosarcoma
kit	protein kinase (tyrosine)	cat	sarcoma
mil/raf	protein kinase (serine/threonine)	chicken/mouse	sarcoma
mos	protein kinase (serine/threonine)	mouse	sarcoma
myb	nuclear protein	chicken	myeloblastosis
myc	nuclear protein	chicken	sarcoma; myelocytoma; carcinoma
H-ras	G protein	rat	sarcoma; erythroleukemia
K-ras	G protein	rat	sarcoma; erythroleukemia
rel	nuclear protein	turkey	reticuloendotheliosis
ros	protein kinase (tyrosine)	chicken	sarcoma
sea	protein kinase (tyrosine)	chicken	sarcoma; leukemia
sis	platelet-derived growth factor, B chain	monkey	sarcoma
ski	nuclear protein	chicken	carcinoma
scr	protein kinase (tyrosine)	chicken	sarcoma
yes	protein kinase (tyrosine)	chicken	sarcoma

not dealing with cells that produce oncogenic viruses, but with viruses that steal (the technical term is *transduce*) normal cellular genes. These normal precursors of oncogenes are called *proto-oncogenes* (see Figure 28.38).

The story of v-*src* has been repeated many times

(about 25 so far) in discoveries of tumor-producing retroviruses from a variety of birds and mammals. Each retrovirus usually has one pirated oncogene (Table 28.2) (33) and occasionally the same oncogene is found in more than one virus. Perhaps we are beginning to see the end of the list of proto-oncogenes that can be stolen by retroviruses (123). When did these gene thefts occur? We have consulted several experts; nobody knows.

The search for more viral oncogenes and their normal proto-oncogene counterparts has produced a basic fact: *the viral copies of the cellular genes are not perfect; their flaws are perhaps due to the fact that reverse transcription is a highly error-prone mechanism.* At each replication cycle as many as 0.5 percent of the RNA sequences are copied incorrectly into DNA (33). These errors play a role in the generation of tumors, as we will see.

The name *proto-oncogene* for the cellular counterparts of the viral oncogenes is not a good name because these so-called proto-oncogenes are not wicked genes just sitting there waiting for the chance to produce a tumor. They are normal genes with important growth-related functions in a cell's normal activity. The name *mitogenes* has been suggested (60).

> *The name* proto-oncogene *is also a source of confusion for yet another reason. Keep in mind that even a perfectly normal gene can be "oncogenic" if it is expressed in excess or inappropriately. Should we call such a gene a* proto-oncogene, *although it does not need to be modified? Probably not—but this may explain why the term* oncogene *is often used rather loosely to include* proto-oncogene.

At this point the reader will want to know how oncogenes produce cancer, but first we must pay tribute to another line of research: oncogenes can be discovered without the help of retroviruses.

Oncogenes Discovered by Transfection Although it was fashionable in the late 1970s to chase oncogenes in retroviruses, some teams of researchers (47, 123, 201, 233) took a different tack: is it possible to find oncogenes in tumors that are not produced by retroviruses? The approach was to extract *DNA from tumors* (human or experimental, obtained with chemical carcinogens) and insert it by transfection (see later) into the genomes of cultured cells. The appearance of transformed cells would indicate that the inserted DNA contained an oncogene (the reader will recall that foci of transformed cells can be detected with the naked eye, p. 834.) Cells of a focus can be cloned, grown, and injected into a suitable animal to test whether they produce a tumor. This method, too, struck gold; more oncogenes were discovered in this way than in retroviruses.

> **Transfection** *(gene transfer) is literally a trick whereby DNA is sneaked across a living cell's membrane into its nucleus, bypassing the natural tendency of the cell to phagocytize and digest any material presented to it. The DNA to be transfected into the nucleus is coprecipitated with crystals of calcium phosphate; the mixture is then allowed to settle on a monolayer of cultured cells. This is a cardinal method in molecular biology, yet nobody really knows how it works. Although in theory it is very inefficient (the yield depends on the type of cell and is of the order of one or a few cells per million) (47), the important point is that some cells are transfected.*

Not all tumors yield transfectable oncogenes (perhaps because the method for finding them is not perfect), but it was certainly amazing to discover that transfecting DNA from a human bladder carcinoma into mouse fibroblasts produces a fibrosarcoma (123). Every tumor oncogene found by this method had its counterpart DNA sequence in the normal cellular genome, just as had been found for oncogenes discovered with retroviruses. Some of the oncogenes discovered by transfection turned out to be the same oncogenes previously identified in retroviruses. This showed that a proto-oncogene could lead to cancer by at least two mechanisms, viral and nonviral. But there was another surprise in store.

The DNA of Normal Cells Can Also Produce Tumors Yes. DNA from normal human embryos, from chick embryos, and other sources also produced tumors (47). This suggests that normal cells contain genes (proto-oncogenes) that can be activated as a consequence of DNA rearrangements, as may be produced by transfection.

What Kinds of Genes Are Liable to Become Oncogenes? Because each gene is best defined by its product, much effort is concentrated in finding out what proteins are coded by the proto-oncogenes. Despite many loose ends, a picture is emerging: *the gene products of proto-oncogenes are either growth factors, growth-factor receptors, or links in an intracellular network through which external stimuli induce cell proliferation* (Figure 28.40). This picture helps us understand how tumor cells grow *in vitro* without added growth factors: they are able to stimulate themselves by produce their own growth factors and receptors, an autocrine phenomenon (246).

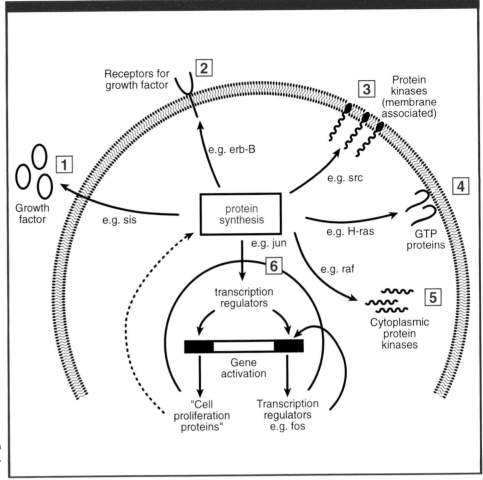

FIGURE 28.40
Diagram of a cell, indicating the six major classes of oncogene products: (1) secreted; (2), (3), (4) associated with the cell membrane; (5) active in the cytoplasm; (6) active on the nucleus. (Adapted from [3].)

The four main categories of proto-oncogene products are the following:

- *Growth factors.* The best example of a virus that produces this category of oncogene product is a simian sarcoma virus endowed with an oncogene called v-*sis*. This oncogene codes for a protein that is very similar to the B chain of platelet-derived growth factor (PDGF); v-*sis* was probably derived from a normal cell's c-*sis*, which codes for PDGF (33). This is the only known example of a *secreted* oncogene product (33). PDGF alone does not cause "transformation," but cells that constantly secrete PDGF are probably self-stimulating; a number of human tumors do produce PDGF-like molecules. Imaginative readers might conclude that antibodies against pseudo-PDGF should stop the growth of cells transformed by v-*sis*; *in vitro* the experiment works, but only sometimes.
- *Growth factor receptors and other transmem-* *brane proteins.* All these gene products are inserted into the cell membrane; most of them represent defective, truncated receptors for growth factors: epithelial growth factor (EGF), macrophage colony-stimulating factor (CSF-1), and the insulin receptor. Normally the intracellular domain of these normal molecules functions as a tyrosine kinase, and this function persists in the oncogene version. Protein kinases transfer phosphate groups from themselves to other proteins, thus regulating their activity. It seems clear that tyrosine phosphorylation plays an important role in cell growth and differentiation (33), but exactly how the defective gene products lead to transformation is not clear. Conceivably a defective growth-factor receptor remains in a permanent state of activation and misinforms the cell accordingly.
- *Membrane-related, guanine triphosphate (GTP)–binding proteins (ras-proteins).* These

gene products are related to the family of G-proteins, which transduce signals from growth-factor receptors to the phospatidyl inositol second-messenger cascade (33). They are coded by three varieties of *ras* genes, the first to be related to human tumors, but originally isolated from a murine sarcoma. Incidentally, the product of the *ras* gene of beer yeast, *Saccharomyces cerevisiae*, is 90 percent homologous to human p21 (see later). Proto-oncogenes must perform very basic functions to have deserved this tremendous degree of evolutionary conservation.

Ras genes code for 21-kilodalton proteins called p21, which are located in cell membranes, bind guanine nucleotides (GTP and GDP), and function as GTP-ases. About 15 percent of human solid tumors contain one or more ras genes with single-base alterations. Activated ras genes have also been found in premalignant and malignant lesions induced experimentally with carcinogens.

• *Nuclear proteins.* The special feature of these gene products is the tendency to localize in the nucleus where they probably take part in regulating gene expression. Some have a very short half-life, even minutes, which would agree with such a function. Several oncogenes of this group are known to be activated during normal cell replication: for example, c-*fos*, c-*myc*, and p53 are activated sequentially during liver regeneration (217).

Finally, we can proceed to the basic question.

How Are Proto-Oncogenes Activated? To pervert a normal proto-oncogene into an oncogene, two basic options are available, and may be applied jointly: (1) to make it encode a *defective, "hyperactive" protein,* and (2) to make it encode *too much protein* (Figure 28.41). In other words, the structure *and/or* the function of a proto-oncogene may be disturbed. Descriptions of the five mechanisms in Figure 28.41 follow:

1. *A defective protein can result from a point mutation,* the simplest possible coding defect in an oncogene. This is a change in a single nucleotide that affects the coding for a single amino acid in the protein product (234). Note, however, that not all point mutations lead to tumor growth: to do so they must hit a specific gene in a specific way.

Example: remember the ras proto-oncogenes that code for GTP-binding proteins. A point mutation creates a defective protein that is no longer able to hydrolyze and deactivate GTP but traps it in such a way that it continues to transmit growth stimuli (234). (The comparison with a jammed doorbell is irresistible.)

2. *Overproduction of a normal protein can result from gene amplification:* multiple copies of the same gene are produced, sometimes as many as 50–100.
3. *Overproduction of a normal protein can result from abnormal activity of the oncogene.* Assume that a chromosomal rearrangement occurs; the normal regulatory sequence of the proto-oncogene has been lost (misplaced) and is replaced by another that calls for inappropriate stimulation.
4. *A defective protein may be a "fusion protein,"* the result of two abnormally combined genes. This is a result of chromosomal rearrangement: an oncogene is placed next to an actively transcribed gene, and the two gene products merge into a single "monster" protein.
5. *Loss or destruction of an antioncogene (growth-suppressor gene) is involved in hereditary cancer (p. 868).*

How Does an Oncogene Produce Cells with a Malignant Phenotype? Because proto-oncogenes are involved in growth control, it is not surprising that they can be pushed to induce excessive cell growth. But why should the cells also *look* malignant and *behave* as malignant? The answers are just beginning to come in. Here are a few telling experiments, introduced by the questions they ask:

• *How can the oncogene products affect the shape of the cell?* A few oncogene products have been visualized by means of labeled antibodies. It appears that the product of the *src* oncogene carried by the Rous sarcoma virus tends to be localized along the cell membrane (Figure 28.42) (18) and especially in attachment plaques (Figure 28.43) (18, 188). This suggests that this particular oncogene product affects the cytoskeleton and therefore alters the shape of the cell. The rounded or abnormal shape of some malignant cells and their propensity to lose their attachments may have this simple explanation (108).

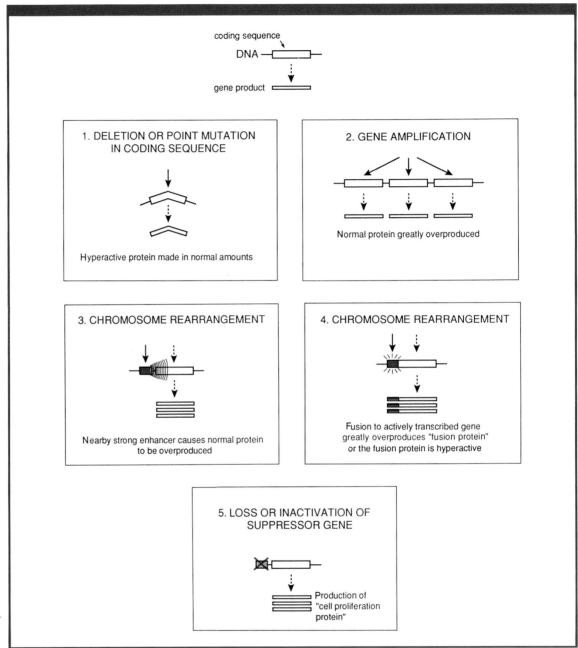

FIGURE 28.41
Five mechanisms
of oncogene acti-
vation. (Modi-
fied from [3].)

A few more details on this observation. The oncogene of the Rous sarcoma, v-src, codes for a protein called pp60/v-src, which belongs to the group of transmembrane proteins. It was surprising at first to find it residing so far from the nucleus: how could it affect cell growth from that remote location? Then it was discovered that its intracytoplasmic tail functions as tyrosine kinase and that this enzyme probably phosphorylates the common cytoskeletal protein vinculin, among other substrates. Vinculin is part of the adhesion plaques, which are domains of the cell membrane reinforced by cytoskeletal components. Adhesion plaques enable cells to grasp their substrate and spread over it; and because pp60/v-src is also localized there, one could conceive a scenario in which the defective pp60/v-src disturbs the complicated assembly of the adhesion plaque thereby accounting for the rounded shape of neoplastic cells (Figure 28.44) (108).

• What happens if the protein product of an oncogene is injected into a normal cell? This has been done many times. For example, the normal, human ras proto-oncogene pro-

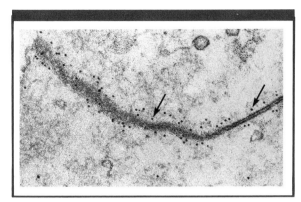

FIGURE 28.42

The preferential location of oncogene products along the cell membrane. Electron micrograph showing the junction between two cells infected with the Rous sarcoma. The section was treated with a rabbit antibody to the oncogene product pp60v-src; the antibody was linked with ferritin so as to make it visible by electron microscopy. It is obvious that the grains of ferritin **(arrows)** are located along the cell membranes. (Reproduced with permission from [18].)

tein injected into normal cells has little effect, but injecting the corresponding oncogene product induces a burst of mitoses and dramatic morphologic changes in the injected cells. Within 24 hours the cells return to normal, presumably because the injected protein has been metabolized (66).

- *What if an antibody to an oncogene product is microinjected into a tumor cell?* The answer, so far, is that the malignant cell resumes a normal appearance (33).
- *Can neoplastic cell behavior be linked to a single enzymatic activity?* Here is a beautiful example (149). Transgenic mice expressing a polyoma virus oncogene (mT) develop endothelial tumors, namely hemangiomas. Endothelial cells of these tumors, grown *in vitro* three-dimensionally in fibrin gels, form cystic structures recalling hemangiomas. They also express high fibrinolytic activity. When this proteolytic activity is neutralized by appropriate inhibitors, the endothelial cells correct their behavior and develop into normal-looking, capillary tubules (Figure 28.45).

These examples only whet our appetite; work in this area is advancing fast.

How Do Oncogenes Fit the Multistep Theory of Carcinogenesis? Oncogenes are exciting. About 70 are known to exist at the present time (132a). However, they face us with an uncomfortable riddle: if it is true that a single oncogene can unleash malignancy, what can we do with the dogma of multistep carcinogenesis? A complete explanation is not yet available, but here are some bits of answers (20, 234):

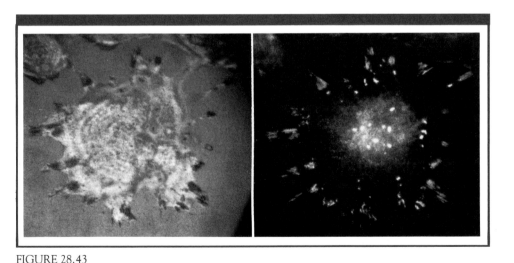

FIGURE 28.43

Example of the correlation between cytoskeleton and oncogene products: *Left:* Cell transformed by the oncogene *src* and attached to the supporting surface by means of adhesion plaques. These surface specializations appear dark in this micrograph, taken by interference-reflection photography. *Right:* The same cell treated with an antibody to the oncogene pp60v-src labeled with a fluorescent dye. Under ultraviolet light it is obvious that most of the oncogene product is localized in the adhesion plaques. (Reproduced with permission from [18]. Photography courtesy of Dr. L.R. Rohrschneider and Fred Hutchinson, Cancer Research Center, Seattle, WA.)

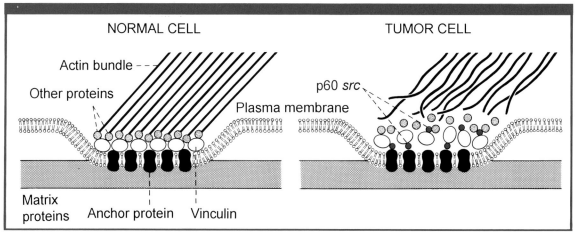

FIGURE 28.44

Left: Adherent plaque in a normal cell (schematic). *Right:* Cell transformed by the Rous sarcoma virus; p60v-*src* appears in the adhesion plaque, and vinculin is found to be phosphorylated on tyrosine. Phosphorylation by p60v-*src* may disrupt the vinculin link and thereby contribute to the typical disorganization of actin bundles in transformed cells. (Adapted from [108].)

- *Some oncogenes act alone.* The Rous sarcoma retrovirus, for example, induces the malignant change single-handed. In such cases we have to admit one-step oncogenesis (118).
- *In several known cases two or more oncogenes are needed,* e.g., *ras* and *myc.* It has been shown that *ras* oncoproteins (gene products) are apt to produce anchorage independence and growth-factor secretion, but *myc* oncoproteins are better able to induce immortalization (234). This suggests that each of these

oncogenes controls only a part of the growth-regulatory circuits of the cell (234).
- *A single oncoprotein can complex several cell proteins.* This might explain multiple effects of a single oncogene.
- *The story of oncogenesis includes much more than oncogenes.* In the next two chapters we will deal with the other half of the story—namely **suppressor genes.** But before we do so we will explore the essentials of oncogenesis by viruses.

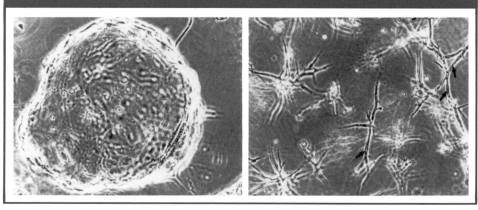

FIGURE 28.45

How do oncogenes produce tumors? Here is a fascinating, simple answer for one tumor, the hemangioma of transgenic and chimeric mice expressing the polyoma virus mT oncogene. *Left:* Hemangioma-like sac produced in 12 days by cultured cells of a hemangioma. *Right:* The same cells, grown in the presence of the protease inhibitor Trasylol, develop into thin branching cords **(arrows)** resembling normal capillaries. The experiment bears out the hypothesis whereby proteolytic activity might be responsible for the aberrant morphogenetic behavior of the hemangioma cells. **Bar =** 200 μm. (Reproduced with permission from [149].)

ONCOGENIC VIRUSES: AN OVERVIEW

The genetic information carried by viruses, as mentioned earlier, may be encoded in DNA or RNA; correspondingly there are two classes of oncogenic viruses, with distinct characteristics. Many oncogenic viruses exist in nature as hitchhikers in selected hosts in which they do not usually cause tumors, whereas they may cause tumors in other hosts.

> *A frightening lesson was learned from New World monkeys. At the New England Regional Primate Center it was discovered in 1971 that squirrel monkeys and spider monkeys (Saimiri sciureus and Ateles geoffroyi) each live in apparent harmony with their own particular strain of herpes virus, but when the herpes virus of the squirrel monkey is injected into the spider monkey it produces malignant lymphomas. Other nonhuman primates, and rabbits, are also at risk (137). Because of these and other potentially dangerous viruses, the autopsy of a monkey is now carried out with surgical precaution.*

It has been very difficult to prove that viruses cause tumors in humans. The species specificity just mentioned means that a virus that is oncogenic for humans is not necessarily oncogenic for another host. Furthermore, viruses in general are also very choosy about the cells they infect; and some human cells are very difficult to grow *in vitro*. We also know from experiment that a virus-induced malignant tumor may be apparently virus-free when biopsied; the mechanism is not clear (200). However, epidemiological studies have provided powerful evidence of guilt by association, and there is no longer any reasonable doubt that some human tumors are produced by viruses. This is extremely important with regard to therapy and prevention: viruses produce antigens, virus-induced tumors carry virus-related antigens, and vaccination against such tumors becomes a distinct possibility.

There are, in all, seven classes of tumor viruses (200) (Table 28.3): six classes of DNA viruses (they produce most of the tumors) and one class of RNA viruses (retroviruses). Overall they account for about 20 percent of the human "tumor burden"; this percentage becomes especially significant considering that vaccination against these viruses may some day—perhaps soon—prevent many if not all of the related tumors.

WHAT HAPPENS TO A VIRUS-INFECTED CELL?

Permissive Versus Nonpermissive Cells The first step in understanding infection by viruses is that the effect on the cell may vary between the two

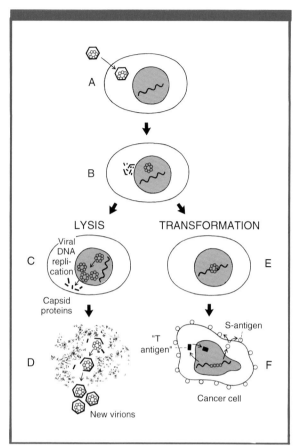

LYSIS   TRANSFORMATION

FIGURE 28.46 Diagram of the interaction between an oncogenic DNA virus (Papova virus) and a susceptible cell. The virion penetrates into the cell, is uncoated, and penetrates into the nucleus. There it can either induce the production of new viruses and lead to cell lysis, or become integrated into the host DNA and lead to "transformation"; the transformed cell produces new antigens. S antigen = tumor specific transplantation antigen. (Adapted from [4].)

extremes of lysis and transformation (Figure 28.46). In either case the virus integrates itself with the genome of the cell. If the cell permits viral replication, it is overwhelmed by viral particles and dies. At the other extreme, the cell does not permit the virus to complete its cycle of replication; the frustrated virus (one or a few particles suffice) steers the cell toward transformation. Intermediate situations exist. DNA viruses can follow either path; RNA viruses tend to produce nonlytic infection.

Changes in Protein Synthesis As may be expected, virus-infected cells produce not only the virus-encoded proteins, but also the proteins encoded by their own genome, which is disturbed by the presence of the virus. There is evidence here for a stepwise process whereby some of the new cellular proteins induce immortalization and then transformation. Not only the quantity but also the quality of the cellular proteins is changed: some of the new proteins reflect the derepression of genes that had been repressed since fetal life (*oncofetal antigens*). As for the virus-encoded proteins, they can be expressed on the cell surface and thereby

TABLE 28.3

Families of Tumor Viruses: Natural Cancers

VIRUS GROUP	EXAMPLES	HOST	DISEASE
Hepadna	Hepatitis B	Human, woodchuck, duck	Primary hepato-cellular carcinoma (PHC)
	Ground squirrel	Squirrel	PHC
Papilloma (Papova A)	Shope papilloma	Rabbit	Benign papilloma
	Canine papilloma	Dog	Papillomas
	Equine papilloma	Horse	Papillomas
	Human papilloma	Human	Papillomas, cervical carcinoma
Papova B	Polyoma	Mouse	Unknown
	SV40	Monkey	Unknown
	Human papova	Human	Unknown
Adenovirus	Human adeno-12-31	Human	Unknown
	Ovine adeno-	Sheep	Adenoma
Herpes	Marek's disease	Chicken	Lymphosarcoma
	Pig herpes	Guinea pig	Leukemia
	Cattle herpes	Cattle	Lymphoma
	Epstein-Barr	Human	Burkitt's lymphoma; nasopharyngeal carcinoma
Pox	Shope fibroma	Rabbit	Benign fibroma
	Yaba	Monkey	Benign histiocytoma
	Molluscum contagiosum	Human	Benign molluscum bodies
Retrovirus			
Type B	Mouse mammary tumor	Mouse	Mammary adenocarcinoma
Type C	Leukemia-sarcoma complex	Reptiles, fish, birds rodents, cattle, cats, dogs, primates	Leukemia—lymphosarcoma types of diseases
Type D	Human T-cell leukemia (HTLV)	Human	Leukemia—lymphoma

Table adapted from (200)

expose the cell to an immune response. Malignant tumors produced by the same virus tend to express the same surface antigens, whereas malignant tumors produced by chemical carcinogens tend to express their own specific antigens.

DNA ONCOGENIC VIRUSES

The six classes of DNA tumor viruses include a great deal of human and other animal pathology (see Figure 28.47; Table 28.3). The name *Hepadna* for one group is not a misprint but a combination of hepa(tic) DNA. Nor are the *Papova* groups of Russian origin; the word stands for PApilloma, POlyoma, and simian VAcuolating virus 40 (PA + PO + VA). Adenoviruses are so named because they were first isolated from human pharyngeal tonsils or adenoids. The herpes group inherited its ancient name from the slow advance, "creeping",

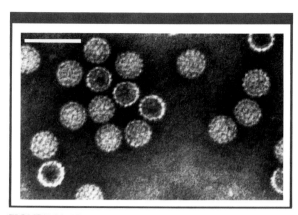

FIGURE 28.47
Electron micrograph of simian virus SV40, an oncogenic DNA virus. This virus was discovered in 1960 in cultures of monkey kidney cells used in the production of polio vaccine and was inadvertently inoculated into thousands of people before its presence became known. (Reproduced with permission from [192].) Although it can be oncogenic experimentally, no harm was done. Negative staining. **Bar** = 0.1 μm. (Courtesy of Dr. G.Th. Diamandopoulos, Harvard Medical School, Boston, MA.).

of some infectious herpetic lesions (*hérpein* is Greek for creeping); the *pox* group from the skin pocks.

Hepadna Group The hepatitis B virus (HBV) is a classic case of guilt by association; it is endemic in the same parts of Asia and Africa where hepatoma is also the most common form of human cancer (64). Related viruses have been found in ducks, woodchucks, and ground squirrels, which also suffer from hepatomas; yet nobody has succeeded, so far, in proving experimentally that HBV produces hepatomas. In humans, HBV is commonly transmitted by close personal contact, from mother to infant, and by blood transfusions and intravenous injections (not by fecal contamination as is the case for hepatitis A virus). The result of infection is a chronic hepatitis that may progress to hepatoma. This natural history suggests that a vaccine against hepatitis B should decrease the incidence of liver cancer, a hypothesis that is being tested in China. Viral DNA has been found integrated with the DNA of liver cells in neoplastic as well as in nonneoplastic tissue. Current thinking is that some factor other than the virus intervenes in the pathogenesis of HBV-associated hepatomas, possibly a toxic agent capable of inducing liver cell necrosis, followed by regeneration. A prime candidate is aflatoxin, common in the endemic areas (p. 826).

Vaccines against hepatitis B virus have been available since the early 1980s; soon we will find out whether vaccination of the populations at risk has truly decreased the incidence of hepatomas.

Papova A Group Papilloma viruses are proven guilty: human papilloma virus (HPV) DNA is found in 90 percent of squamous carcinomas of the cervix, vulva, penis, and anus. About 60 types of papilloma virus (HPV) are known. They pose a major technical problem: it has not yet been possible to propagate them *in vitro*. However, they do grow in epithelia transplanted to nude mice (Figures 28.48, 28.49) (54). It is a virus of this group that produces Shope's rabbit papillomas. Certain types have been associated with simple warts, laryngeal papillomas, and urogenital cancers. In general, viral DNA and viral antigens are found more often in benign growths.

Nonprogressive and progressive lesions of the cervix are associated with different types of HPV, which suggests that some types of HPV are more oncogenic than others.

Nonprogressive lesions of the cervix include benign outgrowths called condylomata acuminata, flat

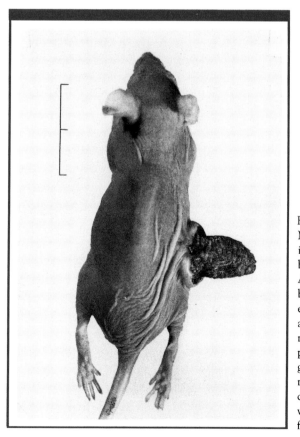

FIGURE 28.48
Nude mouse bearing a Shope (rabbit) papilloma. A domestic rabbit was infected experimentally, and three months later the papilloma was grafted to the mouse. Scale in cm. (Reproduced with permission from [121].)

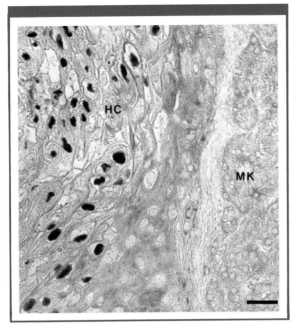

FIGURE 28.49
Although papilloma viruses cannot be grown *in vitro*, they can be used to transform human cervical epithelium (**HC**) implanted between the capsule of mouse kidney (**MK**). Prior to implantation, the chips of cervix were exposed to a cell-free extract of vulvar condylomata (benign growths related to HPV infection). The black nuclei (immuno-peroxidase stain) are producing virus antigen (HPV-II). **Bar** = 25 μm. (Courtesy of Dr. J.W. Kreider, Pennsylvania State University, Hershey, PA).

warts, and some of the epithelial "dysplasias" that are now called cervical intraepithelial neoplasia (CIN), types I and II (p. 878). All are usually associated with HPV-6, 11, 31, 35, and 42. Progressive forms of CIN-I and CIN-II, as well as CIN-III, and cervical carcinomas are usually positive for HPV-16, 18, and 33 (64). Perhaps a better understanding of these HPV infections will some day help clarify the true meaning of the controversial term dysplasia.

Warts are another misdeed of HPV. One mysterious aspect of warts should be recorded here: their apparent ability to come or go in response to psychologic signals. For a viral infection this is certainly peculiar; it recalls the tendency of herpes blisters ("fever blisters" or "cold sores") to develop in relation to periods of stress. Anyone interested should read the wonderful essay by Lewis Thomas (216).

Laryngeal papillomas (Figures 28.50, 28.51) tend to develop in children whose mothers suffered from genital warts at the time of delivery. When removed, the papillomas tend to recur; and although they may regress at puberty, they may also progress to carcinomas. Radiation and heavy smok-

ing may be cocarcinogens (200). The virus remains latent in the deeper layers of the epithelium and proliferates in the more mature squamous epithelial cells, which are, in technical terms, more permissive (163). The result is a clear perinuclear halo that gives these cells an empty look; hence the name *koilocyte* (empty cell) (Figure 28.52). HPV type 16 is strongly associated with severe atypias and invasive cancers of the lower genital tract (88) (Figure 28.53). Immunosuppressed patients are at risk for a higher incidence and faster progression of HPV-induced tumors (163).

Papova viruses type B have not been related to human tumors (see Table 28.3), but it is worth recording that these viruses are related to the monkey-derived SV40, oncogenic in newborn rodents and rabbits.

Adenoviruses Derived from humans, these viruses can transform rodent fibroblasts in culture. One type produces fibroadenomas of the mammary glands in rats (60). No adenovirus is known to be carcinogenic in man.

Herpes Viruses All herpes viruses look alike, but they differ greatly in their natural histories. They have been linked with several human tumors, especially Burkitt's lymphoma and nasopharyngeal carcinoma. We would like to say that they cause these tumors, but we would be somewhat forcing the facts. Tumors, as we have said, rarely have a single cause.

The Epstein-Barr Virus The story of "EBV" is linked to that of Burkitt's lymphoma, the tumor that was discovered in 1958 by Denis Burkitt while working in Kampala, Uganda (34). It usually appeared as a large mass in the upper or lower jaw (Figure 28.54). Sporadic cases were later found to occur in the rest of the world (51). Shortly after Burkitt's observation, Epstein and Barr were able to grow a virus from cultures of these tumor cells. Then—surprise—it turned out that this virus is also the most common cause of **infectious mononucleosis** (184).

Almost everyone is infected by EBV by the age of 20 (184, 200) by a contagion that is mostly harmless. So here we have the case of a virus showing a full range of effects, from no disease at all to an infectious fever to cancer. The virus selects to parasitize B lymphocytes and the epithelium of the upper pharynx. To penetrate cells it borrows the receptor for the complement component C3. Thereafter it may or may not cause a clinical infection; when it does it is infectious mononucleosis. During this episode the patient's blood contains large, atypical but not malignant, B lymphocytes, and viral DNA may remain embedded in the host DNA for life. *In vitro*, EBV can immortalize a variety of cells, human and other.

So, can we really say that the EB virus causes Burkitt's lymphoma? The geographic distribution of the virus certainly does not explain the tumor distribution. It is true that Burkitt tumors in Africa almost invariably contain EBV genome and that all African patients have antibodies against EBV virus, but the sporadic cases occurring in the United States and England are usually EBV negative (they are recognized by their clinical, histologic, and cytogenetic features). Clearly some other factor must be involved. Dr. Burkitt drove all over Africa, painstakingly listing all the cases and noting the local conditions. His result: the distribution of Burkitt lymphoma in Africa coincides with that of malaria. Malaria may act as a constant stimulus for B-cell proliferation (necessary for producing antibodies against the malarial parasite) while also inducing some T-cell immunosuppression (64).

Cytogenetics provided a unifying clue for all cases of Burkitt's lymphoma. Wherever in the world they may occur, they show chromosomal translocations known to activate the oncogene *c-myc* (Figure 28.55). Evidently there is more than one pathway to that chromosomal disturbance. The contribution of EBV may be to immortalize the B cells, which would prolong the time during which a genetic accident could occur, whereby their immunoglobulin genes would be rearranged in such a way as to activate the *c-myc* gene, as required to produce Burkitt's lymphoma (64).

Nasopharyngeal carcinoma, the other malignancy associated with EBV, occurs endemically in southern China, in Africa, and among the arctic Eskimos (51). It always contains DNA of the EBV, but the peculiar geographic distribution of this carcinoma suggests that some unknown environmental factor (or factors) must be involved. Some possibilities are volatile nitrosamines inhaled during food preparation, or phorbol esters (the classic cell activators, p. 60) inhaled from local *Euphorbiaceae* or present in cooking oils (64).

Considering the extraordinary range of pathology that EBV produces, it is legitimate to wonder why more people are not affected. We should presumably thank the assiduous NK cells and the specific anti-EBV lymphocytes (cytotoxic T-cells),

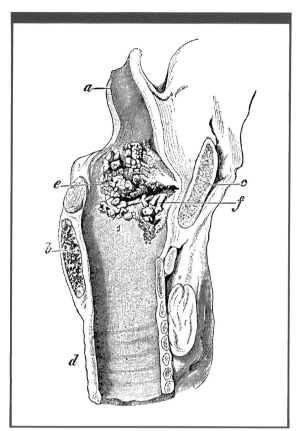

FIGURE 28.50 Papilloma of the larynx illustrated in 1908. **a:** Epiglottis. **b:** Cricoid cartilage. **c:** Thyroid cartilage. **d:** Trachea. **e, f:** Papillary growths now known to be of viral origin. (Reproduced from [254].)

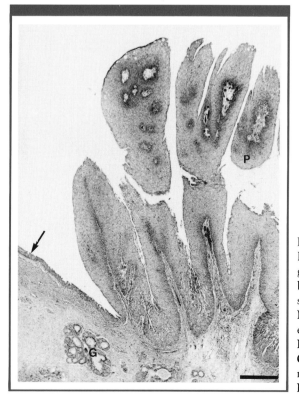

FIGURE 28.51 Part of a laryngeal papilloma, benign at this stage. **Arrows:** Normal mucosal epithelium. **P:** Papillae. **G:** Normal mucous glands. **Bar** = 500 μm.

FIGURE 28.52 Typical koilocytes in a pap smear; squamous epithelial cells with a clear halo around the nucleus, indicative of infection with papilloma virus. (Courtesy of Dr. L. Koss, Albert Einstein College of Medicine, New York.)

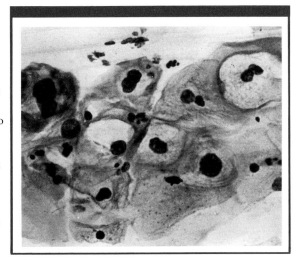

which are constantly engaged in wiping out the virus-infected cells (184).

> Marek's disease *is an unusual misdeed of a herpes virus in chickens, unusual because it produces arterial lesions recalling atherosclerosis (62) (Figure 28.56). It is also a malignant lymphoma against which the chickens can be vaccinated using an attenuated strain. Unlike human lymphomas, Marek's disease is highly contagious among chickens.*

Another herpes virus induces *Lucké's adenocarcinoma* in leopard frogs, a tumor that became justly famous for proving that it is possible, believe it or not, to obtain a tadpole from a carcinoma (p. 901).

How Do DNA Viruses Produce Tumors? DNA viruses do not carry any "stolen," cellular, growth-related oncogenes as the retroviruses do; they produce tumor growth in other ways. Some carry genes that transform cells despite their apparent lack of homology with a known, normal cellular gene; they do so by coding for "transforming proteins." Others act indirectly by derepressing genes that normally inhibit cell growth.

> *An example: consider a DNA virus with a circular genome, such as polyoma or SV40. The genome includes early and late sequences (so named by the order of transcription). The early genes are essential for transformation; the late genes relate to virus replication. Now, assume that the viral DNA integrates itself with a chromosome in such a way that the late sequence is interrupted; the virus is not able to replicate. However, the early sequence is intact, it is transcribed, and the transforming proteins is produced (231).*

RNA ONCOGENIC VIRUSES

The unique survival strategy of these viruses has already been described (p. 839), namely the ability to transcribe their RNA backwards into DNA by means of their special enzyme, reverse transcriptase (hence the collective name *retroviruses* for this group). The DNA copy of the retroviral genome inserted into the host DNA is called a **provirus.** We have also outlined the manner in which retroviruses steal cellular genes (proto-oncogenes) and turn them into oncogenes.

FIGURE 28.53 Biopsy of the vulva showing intraepithelial neoplasia stage II (**B**) and III (**C**) associated with human papilloma virus infection (HPV-16 demonstrated by *in situ* hybridization (**A**)). As often happens, the virus is most abundant *near* the neoplasia, but in some cases virus-positive cells can be found also within the neoplasia. **Bar** = 100 μm. (Reproduced with permission from [88].)

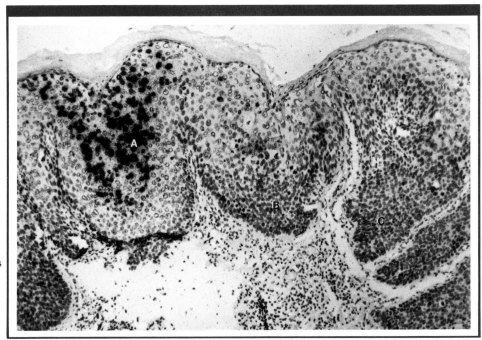

In this section we will provide a few more details on the retroviral family.

Many retroviruses replicate in cell cultures without causing any visible damage to the cells (167), others cause nonneoplastic disease, and a few cause tumors. To this day, only one retrovirus is definitely associated with human neoplasia, namely human T-cell lymphotropic virus type I (HTVL-I).

The RNA genome of the retroviruses (Figure 28.57) comes in three variants:

- One variant consists basically of three coding sequences called *gag, pol,* and *env,* flanked by two sequences called **long terminal repeats** (LTRs), which are not transcribed. LTRs are very important because they can enhance the transcription of adjacent genes and even of some distant genes. The *gag* sequence codes for viral structural proteins, the *pol* for reverse transcriptase, and the *env* for glycoproteins on the lipid envelope of the virus.

- Another variant of retroviral genome has its prototype in the Rous sarcoma virus. Note in Figure 28.57 that it includes—besides *gag, pol,* and *env*—the *v-src* sequence, which is the oncogene.

- Last, some retroviruses have paid for acquiring an oncogene (*v-onc*) by losing some of their own genetic material; these retroviruses can reproduce only in association with a helper virus that supplies missing proteins, which are necessary for assembling mature virus particles.

Oncogene-containing retroviruses are also called acute transforming viruses because they act with incredible speed. They can produce a leukemia or a sarcoma in a matter of days or weeks (200). Retroviruses that do not contain oncogenes are called slow transforming retroviruses. They induce leukemias within one to several months. Lacking oncogenes, they can only transform cells by integrating their provirus near a cellular oncogene (insertional mutagenesis).

The three celebrities among the oncogenic retroviruses are the Rous sarcoma virus, which we have already described, Bittner's milk factor, now called MMTV (mouse mammary tumor virus), and the human T-cell lymphotropic virus type I (HTLV-I).

Mouse Mammary Tumor Virus The MMTV (p. 839) has a number of fascinating features that are

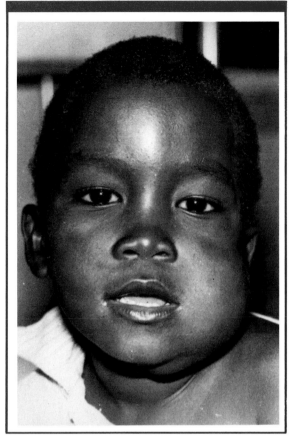

FIGURE 28.54
Typical presentation of Burkitt's tumor, affecting the upper jaw of a young man in Uganda. (Courtesy of Dr. D.P. Burkitt, Bisley, United Kingdom.)

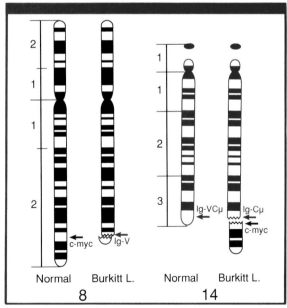

FIGURE 28.55
The typical chromosome translocations in Burkitt's lymphoma. Ig-V and Ig-Cμ represent heavy-chain immunoglobulin variable (**V**) and constant μ (**Cμ**) genes. The defective chromosome 8 loses a fragment carrying c-myc and acquires a small fragment carrying Ig-V. The defective chromosome 14 acquires the larger piece lost by chromosome 8, whereby c-myc finds itself located near Ig-Cμ. (Adapted from [253].)

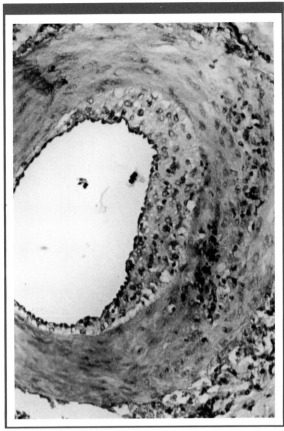

FIGURE 28.56
A strange association: in chickens, the virus of Marek's disease produces lymphomas as well as this atherosclerosis-like intimal thickening in the coronary arteries. (Courtesy of C.G. Fabricant, Cornell University, Ithaca, NY.)

not directly applicable to humans so far as we know at present, but which sound like lessons for us to consider.

- The virus is present not only in the milk during lactation but also in the germ line (as provirus), so the tendency to produce tumors can be acquired not only horizontally (by suckling) but also vertically (by inheritance) (109).
- The virus itself contains no oncogenes, but both of its LTRs are two or three times as large as usual for retroviruses, and they contain a sequence that is sensitive to glucocorticoids, which increase transcription of the provirus (212). This fact reminds us that oncogenesis by this particular virus depends heavily on the hormonal status of its victim (p. 839); indeed several hormones affect mammary tumors in mice (134).
- In mice that develop mammary carcinomas, a large number of cells produce MMTV, and the provirus inserts itself, apparently at random, into their genome. However, only a few cells become transformed, which suggests that transformation requires insertion in some specific site or sites (200).

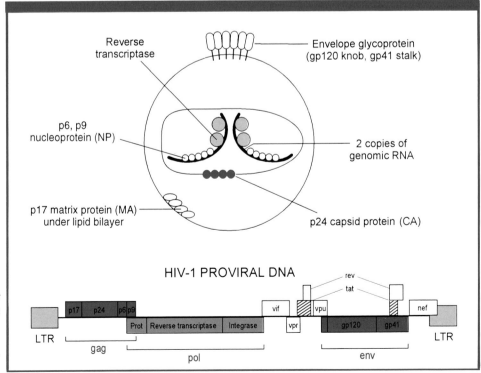

FIGURE 28.57
The genome of HIV, typical of retroviruses: the three genes code for group-specific antigen (*gag*), envelope (*env*), and polymerase (reverse transcriptase) (*pol*). (Courtesy of Dr. S. Lu, University of Massachusetts Medical School, Worcester, MA.)

Human T-cell Lymphotropic Virus-I The HTVL-I is a relative of the AIDS virus and is associated with a form of leukemia that occurs endemically in southern Japan, in areas where 26 percent of the population is seropositive for HTLV-I (112), in the Caribbean region, southeastern United States, and sporadically elsewhere. Epidemiologic data suggest that it is not very contagious, but health care personnel are advised to approach it with precautions similar to those used for hepatitis B. Normal T-cells cocultivated with infected leukemic cells do acquire the infection (112).

> *A related virus, HTLV-II, has been isolated from a patient suffering from the so-called hairy cell leukemia. The AIDS virus, once called HTLV-III and now renamed HIV, belongs to the same group. All three viruses affect helper lymphocytes (T4+): viruses are choosy.*

HTLV-I contains no oncogene homologous to a human proto-oncogene, but it does contain a region called *tat* that may be a key to its ability to transform cells. The name *tat* stands for transactivation of transcription, meaning that the product of that gene activates genes on other chromosomes. The protein coded by *tat* induces the infected cell to produce both interleukin-2 (IL-2) (which normally has the function of expanding T-cell clones) and IL-2 receptor. This means that the virus-infected T-cells would be set up for autocrine stimulation (139).

Here is a surprise: transgenic mice expressing the *tat* gene develop neurofibromatosis, not leukemia (Figure 28.58) and thereby became a model for studying that disease.

> *Neurofibromatosis is a group of human neoplastic syndromes with a fairly high incidence (1 in 3000). Tumors develop by the hundreds along nerve trunks. All the components of the nerve are represented in the tumors, which are initially benign but may progress to malignancy. The classic form of neurofibromatosis, called Recklinghausen's disease, is characterized by multiple neuromas, pigmented spots on the skin (café au lait spots), and pigmented hamartomas of the iris.*

Human Immunodeficiency Virus HIV, the AIDS virus, appears to have two types of neoplastic associations: tumors related to immunosuppression, which should explain, for example, the appearance of Burkitt's lymphoma in AIDS patients (64); and Kaposi's sarcoma, which must be provisionally listed in a category of its own because it is still poorly understood.

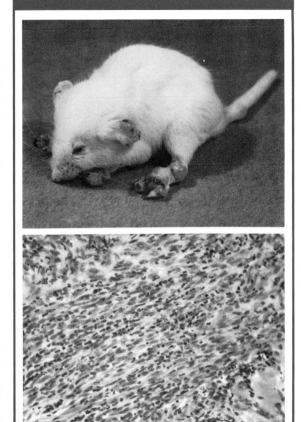

FIGURE 28.58
Top: This transgenic mouse is a model of human neurofibromatosis. It received the *tat* gene from human T-cell lymphotropic virus type I (HTLV-I) suspected to cause adult T-cell leukemia. *Tat* also appears to activate certain cellular genes important for cell growth; indeed it produced multiple neurofibromas arising from nerve sheaths. *Bottom:* Histologic aspect of one such tumor. **Bar** = 25 μm.

Kaposi's sarcoma *was known as a sporadic tumor long before the AIDS epidemic. It consists of bluish-red plaques or nodules that appear simultaneously on the skin and mucosae with an overwhelming preference for homosexual males (Figure 28.59). The multiple location is generally interpreted as a multicentric origin (as opposed to metastatization); widespread involvement of internal organs may occur. The histologic appearance recalls a highly vascular granulation tissue, except for some atypia (Figure 28.60). The cell of origin is probably endothelium*

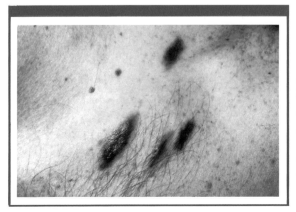

FIGURE 28.59
Typical multiple foci of Kaposi's sarcoma of the skin near the clavicle. (Reproduced with permission from [122].)

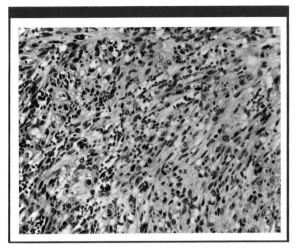

FIGURE 28.60
Biopsy of Kaposi's sarcoma. The picture is altogether not very different from granulation tissue. It shows elongated cells and poorly formed vascular spaces; some red blood cells appear to be extravasated. These features explain the red color seen clinically. Lymphocytes are also present. (Reproduced with permission from [122].)

(122). It was suggested that the proliferation might be driven by cytokines; the latest data point to a new type of herpesvirus (187a).

The mechanisms whereby retroviruses induce tumor formation have been discussed (p. 839).

TUMORS PRODUCED BY PARASITES OTHER THAN VIRUSES

Bacteria cause plenty of miseries, but until recently cancer was not supposed to be one of them. Now a strong association has been found between cancer of the stomach and gastric infection with *Helicobacter pylori* (formerly called *Campylobacter*), a gram-negative spiral bacterium identified and cultured only since 1980 (155, 160). Most individuals infected with *Helicobacter* never develop gastric cancer, so some other factor must also be involved. Interestingly, *Helicobacter* can colonize the gastric mucosa for years, and it is associated with chronic gastritis; thus, it may produce cancer by the constant stimulus to regeneration.

Bacteria, of course, do produce the *crown gall* in plants, as mentioned earlier.

Trematodes (flatworms) are clearly associated with cancer in man and other mammals; liver flukes (*Clonorchis sinensis*), for example, live in the bile ducts, which respond with hyperplasia, adenomatous hyperplasia and sometimes, eventually, with cancer (cholangiocarcinoma). Another flatworm, *Schistosoma haematobium*, is associated with squamous cell carcinoma of the bladder; the adult worm happens to seek refuge in the pelvic veins, including those of the bladder, where it sets up a chronic inflammation. In parts of Africa the disease is so common that bloody urine was once thought to be a manifestation of puberty.

Exactly how the bladder carcinomas are produced is not clear; carcinogens may be involved (80), but the constant regeneration of the bladder epithelium is surely a factor (43, 174). The worm Spirocerca lupi *is associated with esophageal sarcomas in the dog (218).*

Leukocytes may seem out of place in a list of parasites, but they deserve to be mentioned here once again as living agents that may cause cancer, by spewing free radicals at other cells' DNA (p. 829). If this theory is correct, *chronic inflammation could lead to cancer by two mechanisms: persistent regeneration and damage to the DNA.*

TO SUM UP: The field of tumors, which before 1976 seemed so hopeless, has become one of the most studied and best understood in biology. The oncogene theory (including the notion of cancer suppressor genes, to be dealt with in the next two chapters) has provided a link between cancers as widely different as those caused in turkey livers by peanut contaminants and in childrens' thyroids by the Chernobyl catastrophe (8a). The basic step was accomplished thanks to virus-induced tumors—although viruses are not involved in most tumors. Thus everybody in the field can now say "I told you so": both those who thought that the cause of tumors was related to viruses, and those who denied it.

References

1. Abbas JS, Beecham JE. Burn wound carcinoma: case report and review of the literature. Burns 1988;14:222–224.
2. Albert RE, Omran AR. Follow-up study of patients treated by X-ray epilation for tinea capitis. I. Population characteristics, posttreatment illnesses, and mortality experience. Arch Environ Health 1968;17:899–918.
3. Alberts B, Bray D, Lewis J, Raff M, Roberts K, Watson JD. Molecular biology of the cell, 2nd ed. New York: Garland Publishing, 1989.

4. Allen DW, Cole P. Viruses and human cancer. N Engl J Med 1972;286:70–82.

5. Ames BN. Dietary carcinogens and anticarcinogens. Science 1983;221:1256–1264.

6. Armstrong B, Doll R. Environmental factors and cancer incidence and mortality in different countries, with special reference to dietary practices. Int J Cancer 1975;15:617–631.

7. Aron NK, Tajuri S. Postburn scar carcinoma. Burns 1989;15:121–124.

8. Autrup H, Seremet T, Wakhisi J, Wasunna A. Aflatoxin exposure measured by urinary excretion of aflatoxin B_1-guanine adduct and hepatitis B virus infection in areas with different liver cancer incidence in Kenya. Cancer Res 1987;47:3430–3433.

8a. Balter M. Chernobyl's Thyroid Cancer Toll. Science 1995;270:1758–1759.

9. Bates RR, Klein M. Importance of a smooth surface in carcinogenesis by plastic film. J Natl Cancer Inst 1966;37:145–151.

10. Bayon H. Epithelial proliferation induced by the injection of gasworks tar. Lancet 1912;2:1579.

11. Becker EL. The cytotoxic action of neutrophils on mammalian cells in vitro. Prog Allergy 1988;40:183–208.

12. Becker FF, ed. Cancer: a comprehensive treatise, vol 1. New York: Plenum Press, 1975.

13. Berenblum I. The epidemiology of cancer. In: Florey HW, ed. General pathology, 4th ed. Philadelphia: WB Saunders, 1970a:720–734.

14. Berenblum I. The study of tumours in animals. In: Florey HW, ed. General pathology, 4th ed. Philadelphia: WB Saunders, 1970b:744–780.

15. Berenblum I. The mechanism of carcinogenesis: a study of the significance of cocarcinogenic action and related phenomena. CA 1981;31:241–253.

16. Billings PC, Morrow AR, Ryan CA, Kennedy AR. Inhibition of radiation-induced transformation of C3H/10T1/2 cells by carboxypeptidase inhibitor 1 and inhibitor II from potatoes. Carcinogenesis 1989;10:687–691.

17. Bischoff F, Bryson G. Carcinogenesis through solid state surfaces. Prog Exp Tumor Res 1964;5:85–133.

18. Bishop JM. Oncogenes. Sci Am 1982;246:80–92.

19. Bishop JM. Oncogenes and proto-oncogenes. Hosp Pract 1983;18:67–74.

20. Bishop JM. The molecular genetics of cancer. Science 1987;235:305–311.

21. Biskind GS, Biskind MS. Experimental ovarian tumors in rats. Am J Clin Pathol 1949;19:501–521.

22. Biskind MS, Biskind GS. Development of tumors in the rat ovary after transplantation into the spleen. Proc Soc Exp Biol Med 1944;55:176–179.

23. Bittner JJ. The milk-influence of breast tumors in mice. Science 1942;95:462–463.

24. Bittner JJ. The causes and control of mammary cancer in mice. Harvey Lect 1947;42:221–246.

25. Blot WJ, Harrington JM, Toledo A, Hoover R, Heath CW Jr, Fraumeni JF Jr. Lung cancer after employment in shipyards during World War II. N Engl J Med 1978;299:620–624.

26. Boice JD Jr, Land CE. Ionizing radiation. In: Schottenfeld D, Fraumeni JF Jr, eds. Cancer epidemiology and prevention. Philadelphia: WB Saunders, 1982:231–253.

27. Boutwell RK. Some biological aspects of skin carcinogenesis. Prog Exp Tumor Res 1964;4:207–250.

28. Boyd NF. The epidemiology of cancer: principles and methods. In: Tannock IF, Hill RP, eds. The basic science of oncology. New York: Pergamon Press, 1987:7–23.

29. Brand KG, Buoen LC, Johnson KH, Brand I. Etiological factors, stages, and the role of the foreign body in foreign body tumorigenesis: a review. Cancer Res 1975;35:279–286.

30. Braun AC. The story of cancer. On its nature, causes, and control. Reading, MA: Addison-Wesley, 1977.

31. Brunekreef B, Boleij JSM. Long-term average suspended particulate concentrations in smokers' homes. Int Arch Occup Environ Health 1982;50:299–302.

32. Bulatao-Jayme J, Almero EM, Castro MCA, Jardeleza MTR, Salamat LA. A case-control dietary study of primary liver cancer risk from aflatoxin exposure. Int J Epidemiol 1982;11:112–119.

33. Burck KB, Liu ET, Larrick JW, eds. Oncogenes. New York: Springer-Verlag, 1988.

34. Burkitt D. A sarcoma involving the jaws in African children. Br J Surg 1958;46:218–223.

35. Burkitt DP. Epidemiology of cancer of the colon and rectum. Cancer 1971;28:3–13.

36. Burns FJ. Cancer risk associated with therapeutic irradiation of skin. Arch Dermatol 1989;125:979–981.

37. Burns FJ, Albert RE, Garte SJ. Multiple stages in radiation carcinogenesis of rat skin. Environ Health Perspect 1989;81:67–72.

38. Butlin HT. Three lectures on cancer of the scrotum in chimney-sweeps and others. Br Med J 1892;1:1341–1346; 2:1–6, 66–71.

39. Caggana M, Kennedy AR. c-fos mRNA levels are reduced in the presence of antipain and Bowman-Birk inhibitor. Carcinogenesis 1989;10:2145–2148.

40. Calabresi P. Leukemia after cytotoxic chemotherapy—a pyrrhic victory? N Engl J Med 1983;309:1118–1119.

41. Carroll KK. Experimental evidence of dietary factors and hormone-dependent cancers. Cancer Res 1975;35:3374–3383.

42. Cheever AW. Schistosomiasis and neoplasia. J Natl Cancer Inst 1978;61:13–18.

43. Cohen SM, Purtilo DT, Ellwein LB. Pivotal role of increased cell proliferation in human carcinogenesis. Mod Pathol 1991;4:371–382.

44. Connolly JG, White EP. Malignant cells in the urine of men exposed to beta-naphthylamine. Can Med Assoc J 1969;100:879–882.

45. Cook JW, Haslewood GAD, Hewett CL, Hieger I, Ennaway EL, Mayneord WV. Chemical compounds as carcinogenic agents. Am J Cancer 1937;29:219–259.

46. Cooper A. Observations on the structure and diseases of the testis, 2nd ed. (Cooper BB, ed). London: John Churchill, 1841.

47. Cooper GM. Cellular transforming genes. Science 1982;218:801–806.

48. Creech JL Jr, Johnson MN. Angiosarcoma of liver in the manufacture of polyvinyl chloride. J Occupat Med 1974;16:150–151.

49. Csíkos M, Horváth Ö, Petri A, Petri I, Imre J. Late malignant transformation of chronic corrosive oesophageal strictures. Langenbecks Arch Chir 1985;365:231–238.

49a. Cummings CW. The hypocrisy of US tobacco policy. Nature Med 1995;989–990.

49b. Daling JR, Malone KE, Voigt LF, White E, Weiss NS. Risk of breast cancer among young women: relationship to induced abortion. J Nat Cancer Inst 1994;86:1584–1570.

50. Das M, Bickers DR, Mukhtar H. Protection against chemically induced skin tumorigenesis in SENCAR mice by tannic acid. Int J Cancer 1989;43:468–470.

51. de-Thé G. Epidemiology of Epstein-Barr virus and associated diseases in man. In: Roizman B, ed. The

herpesviruses, vol 1. New York: Plenum Press, 1982: 25–103.

52. Doll R, Morgan LG, Speizer FE. Cancers of the lung and nasal sinuses in nickel workers. Br J Cancer 1970;24: 623–632.

53. Doll R, Peto R. The causes of cancer. Oxford: Oxford University Press, 1981.

54. Dollard SC, Chow LT, Kreider JW, Broker TR, Lill NL, Howett MK. Characterization of an HPV type 11 isolate propagated in human foreskin implants in nude mice. Virology 1989;171:294–297.

55. Edmondson HA, Henderson B, Benton B. Liver-cell adenomas associated with use of oral contraceptives. N Engl J Med 1976;294:470–472.

56. Edwards MJ, Hirsch RM, Broadwater JR, Netscher DT, Ames FC. Squamous cell carcinoma arising in previously burned or irradiated skin. Arch Surg 1989;124:115–117.

57. Ellermann V, Bang O. Experimentelle Leukämie bei Hühnern. Zentralbl Bakteriol 1908;46:595–609.

58. El-Torky M, Giltman LI, Dabbous M. Collagens in scar carcinoma of the lung. Am J Pathol 1985;121:322–326.

59. Environmental Studies Board, Commission on Natural Resources, National Research Council. Causes and effects of stratospheric ozone reduction: an update. Washington, DC: National Academy Press, 1982.

60. Escobar MR. Oncogenic viruses. In: Sirica AE, ed. The pathobiology of neoplasia. New York: Plenum Press, 1989:81–109.

61. Eun HC, Kim JA, Lee YS. Squamous cell carcinoma in a frost-bite scar. Clin Exp Dermatol 1986;11:517–520.

62. Fabricant CG, Fabricant J, Minick CR, Litrenta MM. Herpesvirus-induced atherosclerosis. In: Essex M, Todaro G, zur Hausen H, eds. Viruses in naturally occurring cancers. Book B. Cold Spring Harbor conferences on cell proliferation, vol 7. Cold Spring Harbor: Cold Spring Harbor Laboratory, 1980:1251–1258.

63. Farber E. Chemical carcinogenesis. A biologic perspective. Am J Pathol 1982;106:271–296.

64. Farrell PJ, Tidy J. Viruses and human cancer. In: Anthony PP, Macsween RNM, eds. Recent advances in histopathology, no. 14. Edinburgh: Churchill Livingstone, 1989:23–41.

65. Favus MJ, Schneider AB, Stachura ME, et al. Thyroid cancer occurring as a late consequence of head-and-neck irradiation. Evaluation of 1056 patients. N Engl J Med 1976;294:1019–1025.

66. Feramisco JR, Gross M, Kamata T, Rosenberg M, Sweet RW. Microinjection of the oncogene form of the human H-ras (T-24) protein results in rapid proliferation of quiescent cells. Cell 1984;38:109–117.

67. Fibiger J. Untersuchungen über eine Nematode (Spiroptera sp.n.) und deren Fähigkeit, papillomatöse und carcinomatöse Geschwulstbildungen im Magen der Ratte hervorzurufen. Z Krebsforsch 1913;13:217–280.

68. Fieser LF, Fieser M, Hershberg EB, Newman MS, Seligman AM, Shear MJ. Carcinogenic activity of the cholanthrenes and of other 1:2-benzanthracene derivatives. Am J Cancer 1937;29:260–268.

69. Fisher B, Fisher ER. Experimental evidence in support of the dormant tumor cell. Science 1959;130:918–919.

70. Fisher B, Fisher ER, Feduska N. Trauma and the localization of tumor cells. Cancer 1967;20:23–30.

71. Fleming MD, Hunt JL, Purdue GF, Sandstad J. Marjolin's ulcer: a review and reevaluation of a difficult problem. J Burn Care Rehabil 1990;11:460–469.

72. Floyd RA. Role of oxygen free radicals in carcinogenesis and brain ischemia. FASEB J 1990;4:2587–2597.

73. Foulds L. Neoplastic development, vol 2. London: Academic Press, 1975.

73a. Fubini B, Bolis V, Giamello E, Volante M. Chemical Functionalities at the broken fibre surface relatable to free radicals production. In: Brown RC, Hoskins JA, Johnson NF, (eds). Mechanisms in fibre carcinogenesis. New York: Plenum Press, 1991:415–432.

74. Furth J. Thyroid-pituitary tumorigenesis. J Natl Cancer Inst 1954;15:687–691.

75. Furth J. Pituitary cybernetics and neoplasia. Harvey Lect 1969;63:47–71.

76. Furth J. Hormones as etiological agents in neoplasia. In: Becker FF, ed. Cancer: a comprehensive treatise, vol 1. New York: Plenum Press, 1975:75–120.

77. Furth J, Clifton KH. Experimental pituitary tumours. In: Harris GW, Donovan BT, eds. The pituitary gland, vol 2. Berkeley, CA: University of California Press, 1966: 460–497.

78. Gardner WU, Pfeiffer CA, Trentin JJ. Hormonal factors in experimental carcinogenesis. In: Homburger F, ed. The physiopathology of cancer, 2nd ed. New York: Hoeber-Harper, 1959:152–237.

79. Garner RC, Martin CN, Clayson DB. Carcinogenic aromatic amines and related compounds. In: Searle CE, ed. Chemical carcinogens, 2nd ed, vol 1. Washington, DC: American Chemical Society, 1984:175–276.

80. Gentile JM. Schistosome related cancers: a possible role for genotoxins. Environ Mutagen 1985;7:775–785.

81. Grasso P. Carcinogens in food. In: Searle CE, ed. Chemical carcinogens, 2nd ed, vol 2. Washington, DC: American Chemical Society, 1984:1203–1239.

82. Greaves P, Martin J-M, Rabemampianina Y. Malignant fibrous histiocytoma in rats at sites of implanted Millipore filters. Am J Pathol 1985;120:207–214.

83. Green JA. Morphology, secretion, and transplantability of ten mouse ovarian neoplasms induced by intrasplenic ovarian grafting. Cancer Res 1957;17:86–91.

84. Gregg A. For future doctors. Chicago: University of Chicago Press, 1957.

85. Gross L. "Spontaneous" leukemia developing in C3H mice following inoculation, in infancy, with AK-leukemic extracts, or AK-embryos. Proc Soc Exp Biol Med 1951;76:27–32.

86. Gross L. Oncogenic viruses, vol 1, 3rd ed. Oxford: Pergamon Press, 1983.

87. Grote SJ, Revell SH. Correlation of chromosome damage and colony-forming ability in Syrian hamster cells in culture irradiated in G_1. Curr Top Radiat Res Q 1972;7:303–309.

88. Gupta J, Pilotti S, Rilke F, Shah K. Association of human papillomavirus type 16 with neoplastic lesions of the vulva and other genital sites by in situ hybridization. Am J Pathol 1987;127:206–215.

89. Habs M, Schmähl D. Diet and cancer. J Cancer Res Clin Oncol 1980;96:1–10.

90. Hammond JS, Thomsen S, Ward CG. Scar carcinoma arising acutely in a skin graft donor site. J Trauma 1987;27:681–683.

91. Hansen B. Skorstensfejerfagets Historie og Tradition. Tønder, Denmark: Skorstensfejersvendenes Fagforbund i Danmark, 1984.

92. Harris CC, Trump BF, Grafstrom R, Autrup H. Differences in metabolism of chemical carcinogens in cultured human epithelial tissues and cells. J Cell Biochem 1982;18:285–294.

93. Harvey RG. Polycyclic hydrocarbons and cancer. Am Scient 1982;70:386–393.

94. Hayman J, Huygens H. Angiosarcoma developing around a foreign body. J Clin Pathol 1983;36:515–518.

95. Henderson BE, Ross R, Bernstein L. Estrogens as a cause of human cancer: the Richard and Hinda Rosen-

thal Foundation award lecture. Cancer Res 1988; 48:246–253.

96. Henderson JS. Peyton Rous (1879–1970). Reprinted from Year Book of the American Philosophical Society, 1971:168–179.

97. Herbst AL, Scully RE. Adenocarcinoma of the vagina in adolescence. A report of 7 cases including 6 clear-cell carcinomas (so-called mesonephromas). Cancer 1970; 25:745–757.

98. Herbst AL, Scully RE, Robboy SJ, Welch WR, Cole P. Abnormal development of the human genital tract following prenatal exposure to diethylstilbestrol. In: Hiatt HH, Watson JD, Winsten JA, eds. Origins of human cancer. Book A. Incidence of cancer in humans. Cold Spring Harbor: Cold Spring Harbor Laboratory, 1977:399–412.

99. Herbst AL, Ulfelder H, Poskanzer DC. Adenocarcinoma of the vagina. Association of maternal stilbestrol therapy with tumor appearance in young women. N Engl J Med 1971;284:878–881.

100. Hinrichs SH, Nerenberg M, Reynolds RK, Khoury G, Jay G. A transgenic mouse model for human neurofibromatosis. Science 1987;237:1340–1343.

101. Hirohata T. Radiation carcinogenesis. Semin Oncol 1976;3:25–34.

102. Hirono I. Natural carcinogenic products of plant origin. Crit Rev Toxicol 1981;8:235–277.

103. Hitchcock CR, Bell ET. Studies on the nematode parasite, Gongylonema neoplasticum (Spiroptera neoplasticum), and avitaminosis A in the forestomach of rats: comparison with Fibiger's results. J Natl Cancer Inst 1952;12:1345–1387.

104. Houghton A, Munster EW, Viola MV. Increased incidence of malignant melanoma after peaks of sunspot activity. Lancet 1978;1:759–760.

105. Huebner RJ, Todaro GJ. Oncogenes of RNA tumor viruses as determinants of cancer. Proc Natl Acad Sci 1969;64:1087–1094.

106. Huepner WC. Occupational tumors and allied diseases. Springfield, IL: Charles C. Thomas, 1942.

107. Hunter D. The diseases of occupations. London: The English Universities Press Ltd., 1969.

108. Hunter T. The proteins of oncogenes. Sci Am 1984; 251:70–79.

109. Hynes NE, Groner B, Michalides R. Mouse mammary tumor virus: transcriptional control and involvement in tumorigenesis. Adv Cancer Res 1984;41:155–184.

110. Inoshita T, Youngberg GA. Malignant fibrous histiocytoma arising in previous surgical sites. Report of two cases. Cancer 1984;53:176–183.

111. Issenberg P. Nitrite, nitrosamines, and cancer. Fed Proc 1976;35:1322–1326.

112. Jandl JH. Blood. Boston: Little, Brown, 1987.

113. Kalil M, Hildebrandt AC. Pathology and distribution of plant tumors. In: Kaiser HE, ed. Neoplasms—comparative pathology of growth in animals, plants, and man. Baltimore: Williams & Wilkins, 1981:813–821.

114. Kanaar P, Oort J. Fibrosarcomas developing in scar tissue. Dermatologica 1969;138:312–319.

115. Kee M. Cancer causation in booklet form. Nature 1983;303:648.

116. Kennaway E. The identification of a carcinogenic compound in coal-tar. Br Med J 1955;2:749–752.

117. Kennedy AR. The conditions for the modification of radiation transformation in vitro by a tumor promoter and protease inhibitors. Carcinogenesis 1985;6:1441–1445.

118. Knudson AG Jr. Two-event carcinogenesis: roles of oncogenes and antioncogenes. In: Moolgavkar SH, ed. Scientific issues in quantitative cancer risk assessment. Boston: Birkhäuser, 1990:32–48.

119. Kohn HI, Fry RJM. Radiation carcinogenesis. N Engl J Med 1984;310:504–511.

120. Koss LG. Atlas of tumor pathology, 2nd ser, fasc 11. Tumors of the urinary bladder. Washington, DC: Armed Forces Institute of Pathology, 1975.

121. Kreider JW. Neoplastic progression of the Shope rabbit papilloma. In: Essex M, Todaro G, zur Hausen H, eds. Viruses in naturally occurring cancers. Book A. Cold Spring Harbor conferences on cell proliferation, vol 7. Cold Spring Harbor: Cold Spring Harbor Laboratory, 1980:283–299.

122. Kwan TH, Hood AF. Associated cutaneous diseases. In: Nash G, Said JW, eds. Pathology of AIDS and HIV infection. Philadelphia: WB Saunders, 1992:148–173.

123. Land H, Parada LF, Weinberg RA. Cellular oncogenes and multistep carcinogenesis. Science 1983;222: 771–778.

124. Laqueur GL, Spatz M. Toxicology of cycasin. Cancer Res 1968;28:2262–2267.

125. Lifeso RM, Rooney RJ, El-Shaker M. Post-traumatic squamous-cell carcinoma. J Bone Joint Surg 1990; 72–A:12–18.

126. Lijinsky W. The significance of N-nitroso compounds as environmental carcinogens. J Environ Sci Health 1986;C4:1–45.

127. Lingeman CH. The vinyl chloride story. Bull Soc Pharmacol Environ Pathol 1976;4:9–15.

128. Little JB. Influence of noncarcinogenic secondary factors on radiation carcinogenesis. Radiat Res 1981; 87:240–250.

129. Lucké B. A neoplastic disease of the kidney of the frog, Rana pipiens. Am J Cancer 1934;20:352–379.

130. Lyon JL. Radiation exposure and cancer. Hosp Pract 1984;19:159–173.

131. MacMahon HE, Murphy AS, Bates MI. Endothelial-cell sarcoma of liver following thorotrast injections. Am J Pathol 1947;23:585–611.

132. Marcuse EK. Quitting cigarettes may prolong our life, but it's another drag on the federal budget. Pediatrics 1990;86:560.

132a. Marx J. Oncogenes reach a milestone. Science 1994;266:1942–1944.

133. Maugh TH II. New link between ozone and cancer. Science 1982;216:396–397.

134. McGrath CM, Jones RF. Hormonal induction of mammary tumor viruses and its implications for carcinogenesis. Cancer Res 1978;38:4112–4125.

135. McLean AEM, Magee PN. Increased renal carcinogenesis by dimethyl nitrosamine in protein deficient rats. Br J Exp Pathol 1970;51:587–590.

136. Medawar PB, Medawar JS. Aristotle to zoos. Cambridge, MA: Harvard University Press, 1983.

137. Meléndez LV, Hunt RD, Daniel MD, et al. Herpesviruses saimiri and ateles—their role in malignant lymphomas of monkeys. Fed Proc 1972;31:1643–1650.

138. Melnick S, Cole P, Anderson D, Herbst A. Rates and risks of diethylstilbestrol-related clear-cell adenocarcinoma of the vagina and cervix. An update. N Engl J Med 1987;316:514–516.

139. Michalopoulos GK. Growth factors and neoplasia. In: Sirica AE, ed. The pathobiology of neoplasia. New York: Plenum Press, 1989:345–370.

139a. Miki Y, Swensen J, Shattuck-Eldens D, Futreal PA, et al. A strong candidate for the breast and ovarian cancer susceptibility gene BRCA 1. Science 1994;266:66–71.

140. Miller AB. An overview of hormone-associated cancers. Cancer Res 1978;38:3985–3990.

141. Miller EC. Some current perspectives on chemical carcinogenesis in humans and experimental animals: presidential address. Cancer Res 1978;38:1479–1496.

142. Miller EC, Miller JA. Searches for ultimate chemical carcinogens and their reactions with cellular macromolecules. Cancer 1981;47:2327–2345.

143. Miller JA. Carcinogenesis by chemicals: an overview—GHA Clowes memorial lecture. Cancer Res 1970;30:559–576.

144. Miller JA, Miller EC. Ultimate chemical carcinogens as reactive mutagenic electrophiles. In: Hiatt HH, Watson JD, Winsten JA, eds. Origins of human cancer. Book B. Mechanisms of carcinogenesis. Cold Spring Harbor conferences on cell proliferation, vol 4. Cold Spring Harbor: Cold Spring Harbor Laboratory, 1977:605–627.

145. Mirvish SS. Formation of N-nitroso compounds: chemistry, kinetics, and in vivo occurrence. Toxicol Appl Pharmacol 1975;31:325–351.

146. Mirvish SS. The etiology of gastric cancer. Intragastric nitrosamide formation and other theories. J Natl Cancer Inst 1983;71:629–647.

147. Modal B, Baidatz D, Mart H, Steinitz R, Levin SG. Radiation-induced head and neck tumours. Lancet 1974;1:277–279.

148. Mondal S, Heidelberger C. Transformation of C3H/10T1/2 CL8 mouse embryo fibroblasts by ultraviolet irradiation and a phorbol ester. Nature 1976;260:710–711.

149. Montesano R, Pepper MS, Möhle-Steinlein U, Risau W, Wagner EF, Orci L. Increased proteolytic activity is responsible for the aberrant morphogenetic behavior of endothelial cells expressing the middle T oncogene. Cell 1990;62:435–445.

150. Moore RD, Pearson TA. Moderate alcohol consumption and coronary artery disease. Medicine 1986;65:242–267.

151. Mossman BT, Bignon J, Corn M, Seaton A, Gee JBL. Asbestos: scientific developments and implications for public policy. Science 1990;247:294–301.

152. Mulcahy RT. Radiation carcinogenesis. In: Sirica AE, ed. The pathobiology of neoplasia. New York: Plenum Press, 1989:111–129.

153. Murthy SM, Goldschmidt RA, Rao LM, Ammirati M, Buchmann T, Scanlon EF. The influence of surgical trauma on experimental metastasis. Cancer 1989;64:2035–2044.

154. National Council on Radiation Protection and Measurements: NCRP report no. 93. Bethesda, MD, 1987.

155. Nomura A, Stemmermann GN, Chyou P-H, Kato I, Perez-Perez GI, Blaser MJ. Helicobacter pylori infection and gastric carcinoma among Japanese Americans in Hawaii. N Engl J Med 1991;325:1132–1136.

156. Noodleman FR, Pollack SV. Trauma as a possible etiologic factor in basal cell carcinoma. J Dermatol Surg Oncol 1986;12:841–846.

157. Oberling C. The riddle of cancer. Translated by Woglom WH, rev ed. New Haven, CT: Yale University Press, 1952.

158. Oppenheimer BS, Oppenheimer ET, Stout AP. Sarcomas induced in rats by implanting cellophane. Proc Soc Exp Biol Med 1948;67:33–34.

159. Oppenheimer BS, Oppenheimer ET, Stout AP, Willhite M, Danishefsky I. The latent period in carcinogenesis by plastics in rats and its relation to the presarcomatous stage. Cancer 1958;11:204–213.

160. Parsonnet J, Friedman GD, Vandersteen DP, et al. Helicobacter pylori infection and the risk of gastric carcinoma. N Engl J Med 1991;325:1127–1131.

161. Pederson-Bjergaard J, Ersboll J, Hansen VL, et al. Carcinoma of the urinary bladder after treatment with cyclophosphamide for non-Hodgkin's lymphoma. N Engl J Med 1988;318:1028–1032.

162. Perrin F. Joliot-Curie, Irène. In: Gillispie CG, ed. Dictionary of scientific biography, vol 7/8. New York: Charles Scribner's Sons, 1980:157–159.

163. Pfister H. Human papillomaviruses and genital cancer. Adv Cancer Res 1987;48:113–147.

164. Philips FS, Sternberg SS. The lethal actions of antitumor agents in proliferating cell systems in vivo. Am J Pathol 1975;81:205–218.

165. Phillips RL. Role of life-style and dietary habits in risk of cancer among Seventh-Day Adventists. Cancer Res 1975;35:3513–3522.

166. Pirchan A, Sikl H. Cancer of the lung in the miners of Jáchymov (Joachimstal). Report of cases observed in 1929–1930. Am J Cancer 1932;16:681–722.

167. Pitot HC. Fundamentals of oncology, 3rd ed. New York: Marcel Dekker, 1986.

168. Pollack ES, Nomura AMY, Heilbrun LK, Stemmermann GN, Green SB. Prospective study of alcohol consumption and cancer. N Engl J Med 1984;310:617–621.

169. Popper H. The heuristic importance of environmental pathology. Lesions from the vinyl chloride problem. Arch Pathol 1975;99:69–71.

170. Popper H, Thomas LB, Telles NC, Falk H, Selikoff IJ. Development of hepatic angiosarcoma in man induced by vinyl chloride, thorotrast, and arsenic. Am J Pathol 1978;92:349–376.

171. Pott P. Chirurgical observations. London: TJ Carnegy, 1775. Reprinted in Natl Cancer Inst Monogr 1963;10:7–13.

172. Potter M. Percivall Pott's contribution to cancer research. London: TJ Carnegy, 1775. Reprinted in Natl Cancer Inst Monogr 1963;10:1–5.

173. Preston-Martin S. Prior X-ray therapy for acne related to tumors of the parotid gland. Arch Dermatol 1989;125:921–924.

174. Preston-Martin S, Pike MC, Ross RK, Jones PA, Henderson BE. Increased cell division as a cause of human cancer. Cancer Res 1990;50:7415–7421.

175. Preussmann R, Eisenbrand G. N-nitroso carcinogens in the environment. In: Searle CE, ed. Chemical carcinogens, 2nd ed, vol 2. Washington, DC: American Chemical Society, 1984:829–868.

176. Puck TT. Radiation and the human cell. Sci Am 1960;202:142–153.

177. Pullman B, Pullman A. Nucleophilicity of DNA. Relation to chemical carcinogenesis. In: Pullman B, Ts'o POP, Gelboin H, eds. Carcinogenesis: fundamental mechanisms and environmental effects. Dordrecht: D. Reidel Publishing, 1980:55–66.

178. Ramazzini B. De Morbis Artificum Diatriba, 1700.

179. Rauth AM. Radiation carcinogenesis. In: Tannock IF, Hill RP, eds. The basic science of oncology. New York: Pergamon Press, 1987:106–124.

180. Reddy BS, Cohen LA, McCoy GD, Hill P, Weisburger JH, Wynder EL. Nutrition and its relationship to cancer. Adv Cancer Res 1980;32:237–345.

181. Redmond DE Jr. Tobacco and cancer: the first clinical report, 1761. N Engl J Med 1970;282:18–23.

182. Rehn L. Blasengeschwülste bei Fuchsin-Arbeitern. Arch Klin Chir 1895;50:588–600.

183. Reznikoff CA, Bertram JS, Brankow DW, Heidelberger C. Quantitative and qualitative studies of chemical transformation of cloned C3H mouse embryo cells sensitive to postconfluence inhibition of cell division. Cancer Res 1973;33:3239–3249.

184. Richtsmeir WJ, Wittels EG, Mazur EM. Epstein-Barr

virus-associated malignancies. Crit Rev Clin Lab Sci 1987;25:105–136.

185. Rigel DS, Kopf AW, Friedman RJ. The rate of malignant melanoma in the United States: are we making an impact? J Am Acad Dermatol 1987;17:1050–1053.

186. Rinsky RA, Young RJ, Smith AB. Leukemia in benzene workers. Am J Indust Med 1981;2:217–245.

187. Rogers AE, Longnecker MP. Dietary and nutritional influences on cancer: a review of epidemiologic and experimental data. Lab Invest 1988;59:729–759.

187a. Roizman B. New viral footprints in kaposi's sarcoma. N Engl J Med 1995;332:1227–1228.

188. Rohrschneider LR. Adhesion plaques of Rous sarcoma virus-transformed cells contain the src gene product. Proc Natl Acad Sci USA 1980;77:3514–3518.

188a. Sell S, Pierce GB. Maturation arrest of stem cell differentiation is a common pathway for the cellular origin of teratocarcinomas and epithelial cancers. Lab Invest 1994;70:6–22.

189. Rous P. Transmission of a malignant new growth by means of a cell-free filtrate. JAMA 1911a;56:198.

190. Rous P. A sarcoma of the fowl transmissible by an agent separable from the tumor cells. J Exp Med 1911b;13:397–411.

191. Rous P, Beard JW. The progression to carcinoma of virus-induced rabbit papillomas (Shope). J Exp Med 1935;62:523–548.

192. Ruddon RW. Cancer biology, 2nd ed. New York: Oxford University Press, 1987.

193. Russell DS, Rubinstein LJ. Pathology of tumours of the nervous system, 5th ed. Baltimore: Williams & Wilkins, 1988.

194. Sarma DP, Weilbaecher TG. Carcinoma arising in burn scar. J Surg Oncol 1985;29:89–90.

195. Sauter C. Why the color white is vital for the leukocyte. N Engl J Med 1989;321:1479–1480.

196. Scapa E, Eshchar J. Chemical burns of the upper gastrointestinal tract. Burns 1985;11:269–273.

197. Schottenfeld D, Fraumeni JF Jr, eds. Cancer epidemiology and prevention. Philadelphia: WB Saunders, 1982.

197a. Schuh AC, Keating SJ, Monteclaro FS, Vogt PK, Breitman ML. Obligatory wounding requirement for tumorigenesis in v-jun transgenic mice. Nature 190;346:756–760.

198. Scott D, Zampetti-Bosseler F. The relationship between cell killing, chromosome aberrations, spindle defects and mitotic delay in mouse lymphoma cells of differential sensitivity to X-rays. Int J Radiat Biol 1980;37:33–47.

199. Scotto J, Fears TR, Fraumeni JF Jr. Solar radiation. In: Schottenfeld D, Fraumeni JF Jr, eds. Cancer epidemiology and prevention. Philadelphia: WB Saunders, 1982:254–276.

200. Sheinin R, Mak TW, Clark SP. Viruses and cancer. In: Tannock IF, Hill RP, eds. The basic science of oncology. New York: Pergamon Press, 1987:52–71.

201. Shih C, Shilo B-Z, Goldfarb MP, Dannenberg A, Weinberg RA. Passage of phenotypes of chemically transformed cells via transfection of DNA and chromatin. Proc Natl Acad Sci USA 1979;76:5714–5718.

202. Shimkin MB. Contrary to nature. DHEW publ no. (NIH) 76–720. Washington, DC: US Department of Health, Education, and Welfare, 1977.

203. Shimkin MB, Triolo VA. History of chemical carcinogenesis: some prospective remarks. Prog Exp Tumor Res 1969;11:1–20.

204. Shope RE. Infectious papillomatosis of rabbits. J Exp Med 1933;58:607–624.

205. Sinkovics JG. Oncogenes-antioncogenes and virus therapy of cancer. Anticancer Res 1989;9:1281–1290.

206. Smith EF, Townsend CO. A plant-tumor of bacterial origin. Science 1907;25:671–673.

207. Southam AH, Wilson SR. Cancer of the scrotum: the etiology, clinical features, and treatment of the disease. Br Med J 1922;2:971–973.

208. Steffen C. Marjolin's ulcer. Report of two cases and evidence that Marjolin did not describe cancer arising in scars of burns. Am J Dermatopathol 1984;6:187–193.

209. Stehelin D. Dix ans de recherches sur les oncogènes. Les Cahiers de la Fondation, no. 2. Fondation Louis Jeantet de Médecine, 1987:41–53.

210. Sunderman FW Jr. Mechanisms of nickel carcinogenesis. Scand J Work Environ Health 1989;15:1–12.

211. Sunderman FW Jr, Morgan LG, Andersen A, Ashley D, Forouhar FA. Histopathology of sinonasal and lung cancers in nickel refinery workers. Ann Clin Lab Sci 1989;19:44–50.

212. Sutherland DJ. Hormones and cancer. In: Tannock IF, Hill RP, eds. The basic science of oncology. New York: Pergamon Press, 1987:204–222.

213. Tannenbaum SR, Fett D, Young VR, Land PD, Bruce WR. Nitrite and nitrate are formed by endogenous synthesis in the human intestine. Science 1978;200:1487–1489.

214. Temin HM. Possible implications for medicine of RNA-directed DNA synthesis. Triangle 1972;11:37–42.

215. Temin HM. On the origin of the genes for neoplasia. GHA Clowes memorial lecture. Cancer Res 1974;34:2835–2841.

216. Thomas L. On warts. In: Thomas L, ed. The medusa and the snail: more notes of a biology watcher. New York: Viking Press, 1979.

217. Thompson NL, Mead JE, Braun L, Goyette M, Shank PR, Fausto N. Sequential protooncogene expression during rat liver regeneration. Cancer Res 1986;46:3111–3117.

218. Thrasher JP, Ichinose H, Pitot HC. Osteogenic sarcoma of the canine esophagus associated with *Spirocerca lupi* infection. Am J Vet Res 1963;24:808–818.

218a. Troll W, Kennedy AR, (eds). Protease inhibitors as cancer chemopreventive agents. New York: Plenum Press, 1993.

219. Trowell HC, Burkitt DP. Western diseases: their emergence and prevention. Cambridge, MA: Harvard University Press, 1981.

220. Trowell H, Burkitt D, Heaton K, eds. Dietary fibre, fibre-depleted foods and disease. London: Academic Press, 1985.

221. Tucker MA, Coleman CN, Cox RS, Varghese A, Rosenberg SA. Risk of second cancers after treatment for Hodgkin's disease. N Engl J Med 1988;318:76–81.

222. Tucker MA, D'Angio GJ, Boice JD Jr, et al. Bone sarcomas linked to radiotherapy and chemotherapy in children. N Engl J Med 1987;317:588–593.

223. Tuyns AJ, Péquignot G, Jensen OM. Le cancer de l'oesophage en Ille-et-Vilaine en fonction des niveaux de consommation d'alcool et de tabac. Des resques qui se multiplient. Bull Cancer 1977;64:45–60.

224. Upton AC. Physical carcinogenesis: radiation—history and sources. In: Becker FF, ed. Cancer: a comprehensive treatise, vol 1, 2nd ed. New York: Plenum Press, 1982:551–567.

225. Van Duuren BL, Melchionne S. Mouse skin application in chemical carcinogenesis. Prog Exp Tumor Res 1983;26:154–168.

225a. Velentgas P, Daling JR. Risk factors for breast cancer in

younger women. Monogr Natl Cancer Inst 1994;
16:15–22.

226. Wanless IR, Medline A. Role of estrogens as promoters of hepatic neoplasia. Lab Invest 1982;46:313–320.

227. Wargotz ES, Sidawy MK, Jannotta FS. Thorotrast-associated gliosarcoma. Including comments on Thorotrast use and review of sequelae with particular reference to lesions of the central nervous system. Cancer 1988;62:58–66.

228. Warner KE. Selling smoke: cigarette advertising and public health. Washington, DC: American Public Health Association, 1986.

229. Warner KE. The tobacco subsidy: does it matter? J Natl Cancer Inst 1988;80:81–83.

230. Warren S. Effects of radiation on normal tissues. Arch Pathol 1942;34:443–450. Reprinted in CA 1980;30:350–355.

231. Watson JD, Hopkins NA, Roberts JW, Steitz JA, Weiner AM. Molecular biology of the gene, 4th ed. Menlo Park: Benjamin/Cummings Publishing, 1987:1016.

232. Wattenberg LW. Chemoprevention of cancer. Cancer Res 1985;45:1–8.

233. Weinberg RA. Oncogenes of spontaneous and chemically induced tumors. Adv Cancer Res 1982;36:149–163.

234. Weinberg RA. Oncogenes, antioncogenes, and the molecular bases of multistep carcinogenesis. Cancer Res 1989;49:3713–3721.

235. Weisburger JH, Williams GM. Metabolism of chemical carcinogens. In: Becker FF, ed. Cancer. A comprehensive treatise, vol 1. New York: Plenum Press, 1975:185–234.

236. Weitberg AB, Weitzman SA, Destrempes M, Latt SA, Stossel TP. Stimulated human phagocytes produce cytogenetic changes in cultured mammalian cells. N Engl J Med 1983;308:26–30.

237. Weitzman SA, Stossel TP. Mutation caused by human phagocytes. Science 1981;212:546–547.

238. Weitzman SA, Stossel TP. Effects of oxygen radical scavengers and antioxidants on phagocyte-induced mutagenesis. J Immunol 1982;128:2770–2772.

239. Weitzman SA, Weitberg AB, Clark EP, Stossel TP. Phagocytes as carcinogens: malignant transformation produced by human neutrophils. Science 1985;227:1231–1233.

240. Wilkin JK, Strobel D. Basal cell carcinoma arising at the site of venipuncture. Cutis 1985;36:297–298.

241. Willett W. The search for the causes of breast and colon cancer. Nature 1989;338:389–393.

242. Williams GM, Weisburger JH. Chemical carcinogens. In: Klaassen CD, Amdur MO, Doull J, eds. Casarett and Doull's toxicology. New York: Macmillan, 1986:99–173.

243. Wittes RE. Vitamin C and cancer. N Engl J Med 1985;312:178–179.

244. Woglom WH. Experimental tar cancer. Arch Pathol 1926;2:533–576, 709–752.

245. Womach J. CRS report for Congress. Tobacco programs of the US Department of Agriculture: their operation and cost (89–193 ENR). Washington, DC: The Library of Congress, Congressional Research Service, 1989.

246. Wong RS, Passaro E Jr. Growth factors, oncogenes and the autocrine hypothesis. Surg Gynecol Obstet 1989;168:468–473.

247. Wood EM, Larson CP. Hepatic carcinoma in rainbow trout. Arch Pathol 1961;71:471–479.

248. Wright WC. Diseases of workers. (A translation of B. Ramazzini's De Morbis Artificum Diatriba, 1700). Chicago: The University of Chicago Press, 1940.

249. Wullems GJ, Schilperoort RA. Plant protoplast transformation by Agrobacterium in relation to plant biotechnology. In: Fowke LC, Constabel F, eds. Plant protoplasts. Boca Raton, FL: CRC Press, 1985:205–229.

250. Wynder EL, Graham EA. Tobacco smoking as a possible etiologic factor in bronchiogenic carcinoma. A study of six hundred and eighty-four proved cases. JAMA 1950;143:329–336.

251. Wynder EL, Hoffmann D. Tobacco. In: Schottenfeld D, Fraumeni JF Jr, eds. Cancer epidemiology and prevention. Philadelphia: WB Saunders, 1982:277–292.

251a. Yano E, Urano N, Evans PH. Reactive oxygen metabolite production induced by mineral fibres. In: Brown RC, Hoskins JA, Johnson NF, (eds). Mechanisms in fibre carcinogenesis. New York: Plenum Press, 1991:433–438.

252. Yavelow J, Finlay TH, Kennedy AR, Troll W. Bowman-Birk soybean protease inhibitor as an anticarcinogen. Cancer Res 1983;(suppl)43:2454s-2459s.

253. Yunis JJ. The chromosomal basis of human neoplasia. Science 1983;221:227–236.

254. Ziegler E. General pathology. New York: William Wood and Company, 1908.

254a. Rous P, Kidd JG. Conditional neoplasms and subthreshold neoplastic states. A study of the tar tumor of rabbits. J Exp Med 1941;73:365–389.

Precancerous Conditions

CHAPTER 29

> Genetic Predisposition
>
> The Chromosomes of Tumors
>
> Precancerous Lesions

When a skin cancer develops on the face of a white-skinned adult sun addict, we can assume that it was largely self-inflicted; but when a similar cancer arises on the face of an African child who happens to be albino, a different explanation presents itself: congenital lack of melanin has predisposed that child to damage by sunlight (69). A skin cancer in an elderly white man that arises from one of several long-standing lesions of actinic keratosis (once called senile keratosis) suggests that this form of keratosis might favor the development of cancer. In other words, the birth of a tumor may be prepared in two ways: by a genetic predisposition and by a local precancerous lesion. We will examine them separately.

Genetic Predisposition

The question whether cancer is hereditary calls for a qualified answer. First of all, tumors are not inherited as such (the exceptions are extremely rare, p. 793). A mother with breast cancer does not give birth to a baby with breast cancer. What can be inherited is the predisposition to develop a particular type of tumor (Figure 29.1).

Having made this clear, we can say that few forms of cancer are clearly inherited, accounting for perhaps 1–2 percent of all cases (39, 68). An optimist might add that even in families with dominantly inherited cancer, not all the gene carriers develop it, and 50 percent of family members do not carry the abnormal gene at all (54).

Many cases of cancer, perhaps most, seem to occur randomly in a population; but a closer look shows a tendency to familial clustering. It is difficult to extricate the effects of genes from those of chance and environment; but overall, siblings of a patient with a given cancer have a two- to threefold increased risk of developing the same kind of cancer (27, 68). For cancer of the lung, the risk incurred by first-degree relatives is even higher; it is ninefold for female relatives over 40 years of age (64).

For most of the common cancers there are *cancer families* in which that particular cancer occurs with a higher incidence and at a younger age (36). This reminds us of the strains of commercially available mice that are guaranteed to develop a given percentage of tumors of a given organ at a given age. These strains tell us that cancer genes are there; in mice they are revealed by inbreeding.

*There are also **cancer family syndromes** in which the patients are afflicted by several types of cancer; in one such syndrome, sarcoma, breast cancer, and other tumors are associated (51); in another, adenocarcinomas of the colon and of the endometrium develop in half of the offspring of an affected parent. As if this were not bad enough, those family members who have developed one cancer have a 50 percent risk of developing a second one within 18 years (29).*

Multiple primary cancers sometimes develop at different times in different organs of a patient. Some of these cancers are due to chance, but statistics show that many are not, which points again to a genetic influence (13, 56). For example, patients with chronic lymphocytic leukemia (CLL)

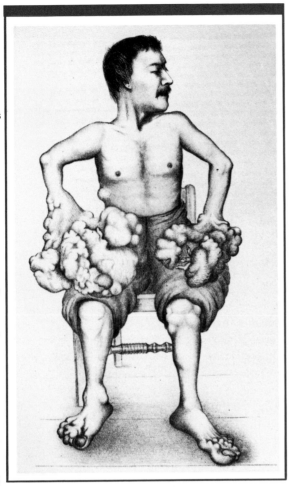

FIGURE 29.1 Extreme case of enchondromatosis (a congenital neoplastic disease) reported in 1889 by Kast and von Recklinghausen. This patient began to notice swellings on his fingers at age 3; at age 34 he requested that his right hand be amputated because its weight had become intolerable. The tumors originate in relation to metaphyseal cartilage, occasionally also along the ribs. To this day there is no cure. (Reproduced from [86].)

cancer prospects. At one point it seemed that allergic individuals have that privilege, but the evidence was largely shot down (37).

Studies of twins have not been very revealing. Denmark has had a Twin Registry since 1881, which made it possible to establish that 621 pairs of twins "seemed to have" the same cancer morbidity as singletons (34). However, one single pair of monozygotic twins developed chronic lymphocytic leukemia, which is known to have the highest familial incidence among leukemias. Cases of identical cancers in twins are occasionally published (53, 60).

Cancer Phenotypes Because there are so many kinds of tumors, many cancer-prone phenotypes can be expected. A fair complexion can be considered as a phenotype that predisposes to melanoma. Less obvious phenotypes concern the individual's enzymatic makeup: there can be inborn differences in the enzymes that activate or detoxify carcinogens, as well as differences in rates of DNA repair. For example, the "poor acetylator" phenotype predisposes dye-stuff workers to bladder cancer (31).

Another example: certain individuals respond to polycyclic hydrocarbons in smoke by producing an inducible form of cytochrome P-450 (p. 136) called P-450 IA. This isoenzyme transforms the hydrocarbons into oxygenated intermediates that bind to DNA. Individuals with this trait appear to be prone to adenocarcinoma of the lung (4).

In summary, there is strong evidence for a genetic component in many forms of cancer, and even for cancer of the lung, which is typically environmental; but the mode of inheritance is little understood. Purtilo and co-workers have listed over 240 genetic conditions that predispose to cancer (69).

We now turn to those rare forms of cancer that are definitely based on heredity.

DOMINANTLY INHERITED PRENEOPLASTIC CONDITIONS

This topic draws us into the field of pediatric pathology. The prototype of familial and dominant tumors is retinoblastoma, which develops from the outer layer of the retina and usually grows within the eye. Usually, children do not complain of poor vision, so the first sign may be an abnormal reflection in the pupil (Figure 29.2). The tumor is rare—about 5 cases per 100,000 births, 90 percent

have more than twice the ordinary risk of developing another cancer (e.g., in the lung), and their basal cell carcinomas may become unusually aggressive (24). In reported autopsy series, the number of cancer patients with undetected "second primaries" is of the order of 2–6 percent; the percentage rises with age (16.5 percent in men over 80) (78). Ironically, some secondary cancers are the result of therapy for a primary cancer; X-rays as well as many antineoplastic drugs are powerful carcinogens.

The Mormons of Utah are interesting from the point of view of cancer genetics and epidemiology because they represent a relatively well-defined, stable population that has abstained from alcohol, tobacco, tea, and coffee for nearly a century, thereby eliminating some major environmental factors. Cancer rates in general are 15–17 percent lower than in the rest of the United States, and several cancers (prostate, lip, melanoma, and uterus) show a definite familial clustering (14, 81).

It would be comforting to know of some way other than eliminating every vice to reduce our

in children—but it is important as a model for understanding a major mechanism of tumor development: **suppressor genes.**

Genetically, the key feature of retinoblastoma and other tumors of this group is that it appears in two forms: *hereditary* (in children, often bilateral) and *sporadic* (in adults, usually unilateral). There is a message in this distribution, and it was a pediatrician–geneticist who worked it out in 1971: Alfred G. Knudson, Jr. Here is his story, simplified.

Knudson hypothesized, and he turned out to be right, that retinoblastoma is always the result of two successive mutations: the first mutation affects one locus on one chromosome (i.e., one allele), and the second mutation affects the same locus on the other allele (Figure 29.3). The settings of this double accident will be different in the two forms of retinoblastoma.

Hereditary Retinoblastoma In this condition the first mutation is present in the sperm or ovum before fertilization; the individual therefore is born with a defective chromosome that is present in all cells. The mutant gene, present in only one allele, is recessive; therefore no disease develops. The genetic disturbance turned out to be the loss of a

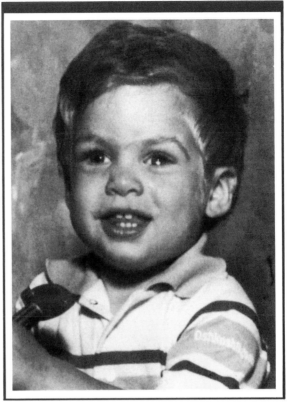

FIGURE 29.2 Child with the "cat's eye reflex" (*leukokoria*) due to a retino-blastoma. (Reproduced with permission from [20].)

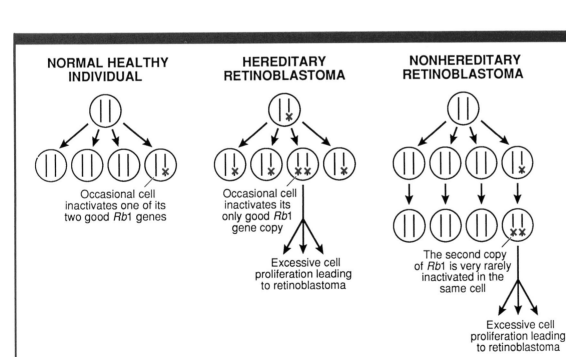

FIGURE 29.3 Genetic mechanisms underlying retinoblastoma. Patients with this type of tumor fall into two categories, hereditary and nonhereditary. The key to understanding this mechanism is that the recessive RB gene inhibits cell growth; therefore, the loss of *both* RB genes unleashes cell proliferation. (Reproduced with permission from [1].)

NORMAL HEALTHY INDIVIDUAL

Occasional cell inactivates one of its two good *Rb*1 genes

Result: No tumor

HEREDITARY RETINOBLASTOMA

Occasional cell inactivates its only good *Rb*1 gene copy

Excessive cell proliferation leading to retinoblastoma

Result: Most people with inherited gene develop tumor

NONHEREDITARY RETINOBLASTOMA

The second copy of *Rb*1 is very rarely inactivated in the same cell

Excessive cell proliferation leading to retinoblastoma

Result: Only about 1 in 30,000 normal people develop tumor

gene, now called RB (for retinoblastoma). *A tumor develops only if the other allele (i.e., the other RB gene) is lost.* A likely time for this accident to occur is during the development of the retina when mitoses are still occurring; there are about 10^6–10^7 retinoblasts, which might allow for three chances of mutation (39). The mutation may hit a single cell or sometimes a few cells, giving rise to multiple tumors.

Sporadic Retinoblastoma Two mutations must occur by chance, in the same cell, during extrauterine life to cause this cancer. This would have to be exceedingly rare, and indeed sporadic retinoblastoma is a very rare tumor (1 in 30,000 individuals); when it does occur, it is mostly unilateral and single (38).

SUPPRESSOR GENES

Knudson's theory opened a new field that led to the concept of suppressor genes, with the RB gene of retinoblastoma as the prototype. First of all, let us clear up a potential confusion. The lack of a single RB gene has no somatic effect, so the gene is acting as recessive; when both RB genes are missing a tumor develops, so the lack of both genes (which are recessive at the cellular level) becomes dominant by pedigree analysis (40, 76). Because the *lack* of the retinoblastoma gene leads to tumor formation, we represent it to be (normally) a suppressor gene.

Many facts fit this theory almost like a glove. Now we can understand why children with hereditary retinoblastoma *are at greatly increased risk of other tumors, such as osteosarcoma, and why this risk is increased by irradiation* (which might be used for therapy). The somatic cells of these children already carry a mutation, the loss of an allele, which takes them, so to speak, halfway toward neoplasia, so there is a greater chance for a second mutation (loss of the other allele) to be carcinogenic (39). Most but not all of these tumors have inactivated or altered RB genes, indicating that other genetic changes are involved. The RB gene has been located on chromosome 13, because some cases had a deletion of band q14 on that chromosome.

How does RB put the brakes on the normal cell cycle? It encodes a 105-kd phosphoprotein (p105) that binds to DNA, a logical way to interfere with the cycling process. During the cell cycle, a time when the brakes on cell division are released, p105 is phosphorylated and thereby loses its suppressor function (27).

> *Gene product p105 is also bound by the proteins of DNA viruses that are oncogenic. Could it be that these viruses produce tumors by blocking suppressor genes? (85).*

The sad tale of children with retinoblastoma has taught us that *genes can trigger tumors by two contrasting mechanisms* that reflect normal gene functions: *activation of oncogenes* and *loss of suppressor genes (antioncogenes)*. It has been proposed that proto-oncogenes are in charge of keeping the cells cycling, whereas suppressor genes override proliferative signals and allow the cells to mature (85). Some day, along the road opened by the discovery of tumor-suppressor genes and their products, there may be some new approaches to therapy. After all, tumor suppressor genes are nature's approach to tumor control (76).

The Knudson suppressor-gene scheme can be applied in part to other childhood tumors, especially **nephroblastoma** or **Wilms' tumor** of the kidney (p. 880), which has an incidence of about 1 in 8000 births (note: the comparison with retinoblastoma is not perfect, because recent studies of multifocal nephroblastomas suggest that an additional, nonhereditary mechanism is involved—which has important implications for genetic counseling [10]). This bizarre tumor (Figure 29.4) is often discovered when a parent notices a lump in the child's groin while changing diapers. Some of the children affected by this tumor are born without irises (Figure 29.5) (55),

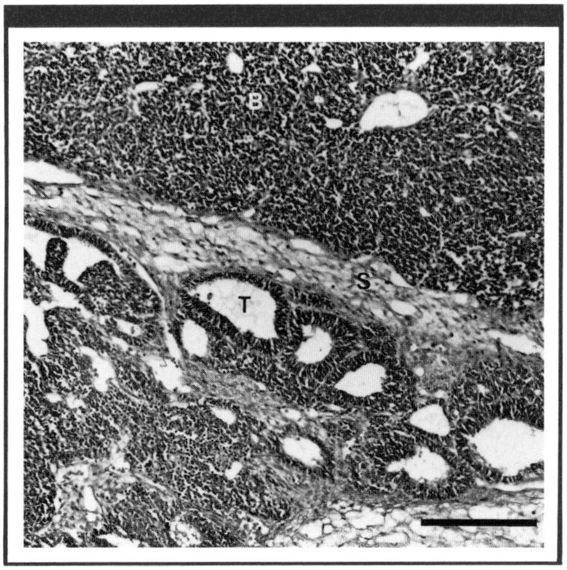

FIGURE 29.4 Nephroblastoma (Wilms' tumor) in a 4-year-old boy. **B:** undifferentiated part of the tumor, resembling renal blastema; **T:** tubules in a more differentiated part of the tumor; **S:** stroma. **Bar:** 200 μm.

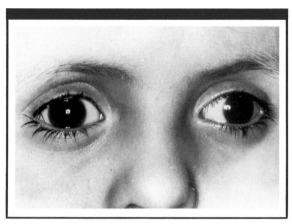

FIGURE 29.5
Aniridia: congenital lack of the iris, a malformation that can be associated with Wilms' tumor. This defect was congenitally present in identical twins. Wilms' tumor developed in only one; the other twin apparently escaped the second step, which was presumably due to some environmental factor. (Reproduced with permission from [55].)

a defect that is correlated with a deletion on chromosome 13 (40).

Several genes are probably involved (25), but a key nephroblastoma gene was located on chromosome 11. This may not be a critical bit of information to remember, but it leads to a beautiful experiment of therapy in vitro. A line of cells from Wilms' tumor is grown *in vitro,* and some of the cells are provided by microsurgery with a normal human chromosome 11. A new line of cells derived from these modified cells is incapable of producing tumors when injected into nude mice. Chromosomes X and 13, injected into cells of the original line as controls, have no such effect (88). A similar feat was performed with the RB gene (27). This is true gene therapy *in vitro;* unfortunately it is a long way from therapy *in vivo.*

The most common genetic change in human cancer is a mutation in a suppressor gene called p53 (50).

While these are hard facts, we should not forget that the *normal* function of suppressor genes is to suppress cancer and to protect the genome; we will focus on this defensive aspect in the next chapter—which deals with anti-tumor defenses.

Altogether, about 40 dominantly inherited syndromes predispose to cancer, and many of these are thought to occur by the Knudson suppressor-

gene mechanism; the list includes breast, lung, and colon cancers in adults (40, 76). The most notorious member of this group is **familial polyposis of the colon.** Carriers inherit the predisposition to develop polyps of the colon. Polyps are not present at birth, but they may be growing by the hundreds by late adolescence and soon become uncountable, a sight difficult to believe (Figures 29.6, 29.7). At age 40 one or more carcinomas may be present in 80 percent of the patients. The only known therapy is early preventive, total colectomy.

RECESSIVELY INHERITED PRENEOPLASTIC CONDITIONS

All these diseases are rare (47), but **xeroderma pigmentosum** deserves special mention because it is a miserable disease. Imagine a child with a scaly, dry skin (*xeroderma* means dry skin), broken by basal and squamous cell carcinomas that erupt on the face and all areas exposed to sunlight. We chose a relatively mild example for Figure 29.8. It is an experiment of Nature: these patients lack an endonuclease that repairs DNA damaged by ultraviolet light (48). They provide strong support

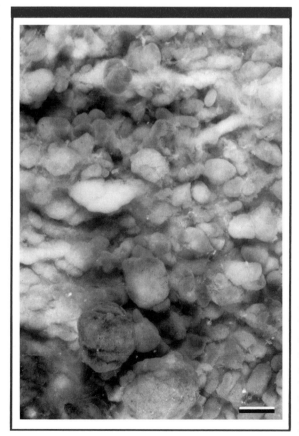

FIGURE 29.6
Familial polyposis coli. Close-up view of the mucosa of the colon surgically removed from a 21-year-old woman. The cobblestone appearance is due to myriads of polyps of various sizes with little or no normal mucosa in between.
Bar = 5 μm.

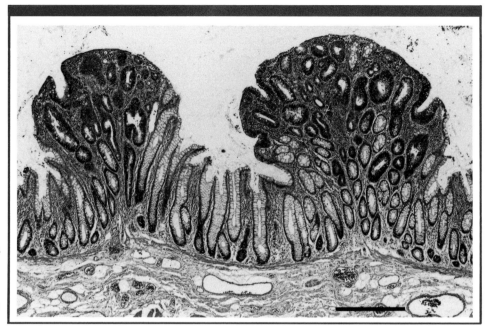

FIGURE 29.7
Two adenomatous polyps arising from the colonic mucosa in a case of polyposis coli. Note the differences between the glands in the mucosa and the glands in the polyps. **Bar** = 500 μm.

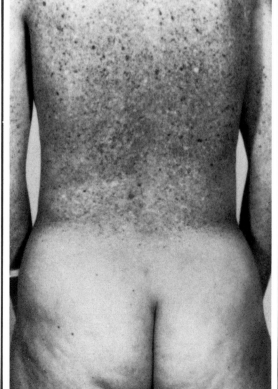

FIGURE 29.8
A patient with xeroderma pigmentosum. The areas of the skin exposed to light show hypo- and hyperpigmented spots, as well as other lesions. (Reproduced with permission from [9].)

for the somatic mutation theory of cancer. Therapy, alas, has little to offer.

CHROMOSOMAL DISORDERS

Sporadic chromosomal disorders are thought to arise by an error during meiosis in the ovum or sperm, whereby the number of chromosomes is unbalanced in all cells of the embryo. *This meiotic instability may be at the root of later mitotic instability*, which increases the risk of neoplasia. Typical examples are Downs' syndrome (47 chromosomes, the excess being due to three chromosomes 21, *trisomy 21*) and Klinefelter's syndrome (again 47 chromosomes: the males are XXY). Patients with Downs' syndrome have a 20-fold risk of developing leukemia, and males with Klinefelter's syndrome have a two- to three-fold increased risk of developing breast cancer (54).

OTHER HEREDITARY MECHANISMS OF ONCOGENESIS

So far we have focused on genes that produce tumors; we should briefly mention that genes may also affect oncogenesis in indirect ways. A person's genetic makeup determines the activity of enzymes involved in the detoxification of carcinogens or, conversely, in the formation of carcinogens from innocuous precursors; hence the novel field of *ecogenetics*, which studies the interplay of genes with the environment (54, 69). Congenital defects in the immune system also predispose to cancer (p. 587).

The Chromosomes of Tumors

In the preceding pages we have repeatedly made the point that the basic defect in tumor cells lies in one gene, and the reader may wonder: is this defect actually *visible* by looking at chromosomes? The short answer is "only sometimes," and it should not come as a disappointment. Consider that each human chromosome carries thousands of genes packed into a little rod 3–5 μm long; the order of magnitude of a genetic defect is of course molecular: in this setting it is almost miraculous that any microscopic change may ever be seen at all. Yet the art of chromosome study, cytogenetics, has contributed a great deal to our understanding of tumors (62). For example, some of the best evidence of tumor progression is the occurrence of increasingly severe karyotypic aberrations. Sometimes, as we will see, a cytogeneticist can actually glance at a map of chromosomes (the karyotype) and conclude: "This individual has developed resistance to a drug."

KARYOTYPING

Chromosomal abnormalities are present in most tumors (62, 77, 90, 91); they can also be induced by antitumor agents (Figure 29.9) (61). Chromosomes become visible only during mitosis, and so the first limiting factor to their study is the availability of mitotic cells. This is no problem with "liquid tumors," the leukemias: The white blood cells are spun out of the blood and cultured. When they begin to divide, they are treated with a microtubular poison (e.g., colchicine), which stops mitoses in metaphase (p. 155). Then the chromosomes of every dividing cell can be spread, stained, photographed, cut out, and pasted up in an established order to the form the display known as *karyotype* (p. 162).

It was a lunch-break that produced the first great breakthrough in cytogenetics. Because mitosis is a three-dimensional event, it is impossible on a photograph of a mitosis to distinguish individual chromosomes. Then it was found that squashing the mitotic cells produced better spreads of chromosomes, but the spreads still were not optimal. One day in the summer of 1948 a Japanese researcher prepared smears of cells (ready to be squashed), put them in fresh water, and then ran out to buy some lunch. When he returned half an hour later and squashed the cells, he saw the most beautiful chromosome spreads, without any overlapping chromosomes. Osmotic swelling of the cells in

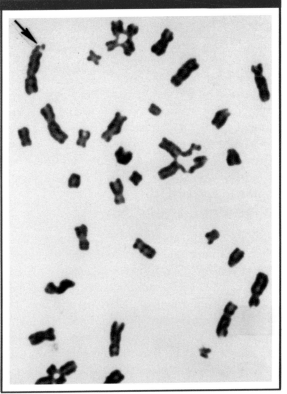

FIGURE 29.9 Example of chromosome damage induced by a drug (the antibiotic and antitumor agent mitomycin C) in a human leukocyte stimulated to divide with phytohemagglutinin. Note several abnormalities: a chromatid break **(arrow)**, two typical "crosses" resulting from chromatid exchange, and a complex rearrangement. (Reproduced with permission from [61].)

water had done the trick; the method has been used ever since (52).

Special stains, introduced in 1970, help to identify as many as 1200 bands on the 46 chromosomes which constitute the human karyotype. Methods continue to improve, but on the whole the procedure—as it applies to leukemias—is simple enough to be used in medical practice as a guide for therapy. The procedure for lymphomas is similar; the cells of these tumors, obtained by biopsy, are easily dissociated and suspended in fluid.

However, with other solid tumors the karyotypes are more difficult to prepare, which is why they are not known to the same depth as the karyotypes of leukemias and lymphomas. Tumor cells must be supplied by invasive procedures such as surgical biopsy or aspiration through a fine needle. Because not all tumor cells grow easily and because they are always admixed with normal host cells, an answer may require weeks or months. This delay is too long with regard to therapy, and therefore oncologists rely more heavily on histologic findings.

It should be understood that karyotyping must underestimate the actual number of abnormal chromosomes. By the current methods of banding, as many as 1000 genes can be either lost or duplicated without producing a visible defect (74). And then, when an abnormality is found, the next problem is to distinguish significant nonrandom changes from random changes that occur secondarily as a result of genetic instability and progression of the tumor.

It should also be understood that almost all the chromosomal changes found in tumor cells can also be seen in abnormal but nonneoplastic cells or in cells treated *in vitro*. However, the two abnormalities known as **double minutes** and **homogeneously stained regions** (HSRs) are largely limited to tumors (5).

TYPES OF CHROMOSOME CHANGES

Visible changes of chromosomes are many; even circular chromosomes can occur. The changes of interest in tumors can be grouped into four categories: balanced translocations between one chromosome and another, deletions or additions of genetic material within chromosomes, and loss of or addition of whole chromosomes. The same abnormality may be found in different tumors. In general, the mechanism of these aberrations is not understood, but several chromosomes seem to be more prone to break at certain fragile sites. A few examples follow.

Balanced Translocations The prototype of balanced translocations is the tiny Philadelphia chromosome (Ph), an altered chromosome 22 (Figure

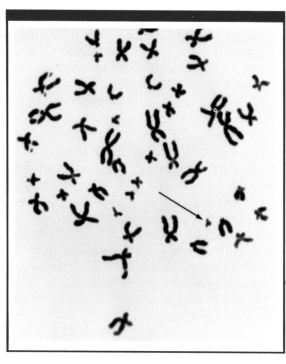

FIGURE 29.10 Metaphase showing a Philadelphia chromosome (**arrow**), which is to this day the most characteristic and consistent karyotypic change in human cancer. (Reproduced with permission from [77].)

29.10). The Philadelphia chromosome became famous in 1960 when Nowell and Hungerford of Philadelphia recognized it as the first chromosomal abnormality consistently associated with a human malignancy: chronic myelogenous leukemia (CML). It is now clear that Ph is not quite as small as it looks; it just stains poorly. It is usually due to an exchange with chromosome 9 (Figure 29.11), with the result that part of a gene on 22 fuses with the *abl* oncogene on 9. The *abl* gene has become abnormally large, and the protein that it encodes is also abnormally large. This magnified protein turns out to be a tyrosine phosphorylase that is more powerful than normal (73).

The Philadelphia chromosome is not present in the somatic cells of the patient; but it is found in all the myeloid cells (which include the erythrocyte, granulocyte, and megakaryocyte series), indicating that a clone deriving from a pluripotent stem cell has overcome the entire bone marrow. Interestingly, the Philadelphia chromosome is absent in 10 percent of the patients with CML, and their prognosis is worse.

Another translocation is typical of Burkitt's tumor, a B-cell lymphoma (p. 852). In these tumor cells, chromosome 8 loses a fragment containing the proto-oncogene c-*myc*; and this fragment relocates to chromosomes 2, 14, or 22 (see Figure 28.55). It so happens that these three chromosomes contain genes that code for immunoglobulin light or heavy chains and it seems that c-*myc* becomes inappropriately expressed by being misplaced near these genes (12).

Deletions The loss of genetic material is associated with some cancers; in fact, visible deletions helped develop the concept of cancer suppressor genes. Suppose that one allele undergoes a recessive mutation whereby it becomes carcinogenic; This mutation then remains latent until the other allele is lost. Deletions of this type occur, for example, in retinoblastoma (chromosome 13, band q14) and Wilms' tumor (chromosome 11, band p13). Other deletions are known in solid tumors.

Additions Added genetic material is visible microscopically in two forms: homogeneously staining regions (HSRs) (Figures 29.12, 29.13), which are added stretches of poorly stainable chromatin along the chromosome (7), and double minutes (DMs) (pronounced, of course, "double mynutes") (Figure 29.14), which are tiny paired

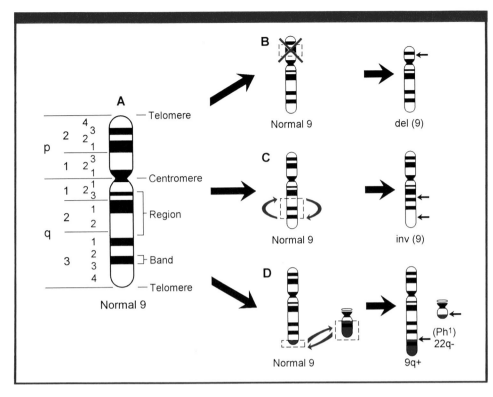

FIGURE 29.11
The normal human chromosome 9 (**A**) and three mishaps it may suffer: **B**: interstitial deletion in the short arm, common in acute lymphoblastic leukemia; **C**: paracentric inversion, and **D**: reciprocal translocation, which gives rise to the tiny Philadelphia chromosome typical of chronic myelogenous leukemia. (Adapted from [73].)

fragments of chromatin that could be misunderstood as debris between the chromosomes. The homogeneously stained regions and the double minutes are thought to represent two aspects of the same phenomenon (5, 6).

Double minutes were first discovered by studying a series of cell lines that had undergone a stepwise selection for resistance to an anticancer drug, methotrexate (75). In some cases double minutes have been shown to represent multiple copies of oncogenes that code for enzymes involved in the metabolism of the drug; this means that the presence of double minutes (or of a single HSR) on a patient's karyotype enables one to venture the guess that the patient has become resistant to some drug.

The story of double minutes and HSRs is intellectually satisfying, but it has its share of mystery: why are both changes present in the cells of neuroblastoma (6)?

Gene amplification is also found in association with tumor progression. This has been demonstrated for N-*myc* gene and neuroblastoma, *ras* and prostatic cancer, and *neu* for breast cancer (12). Gene amplification is very rare in normal biology, but for unknown reasons it becomes an important mechanism in the accelerated evolution of many tumors toward ever greater malignancy (75).

Loss or Addition of Whole Chromosomes Almost all meningiomas have only a single chromosome 22. Much more frequent is the addition of chromosomes, either a complete duplication of the genome (*polyploidy*) or an irregular increase of

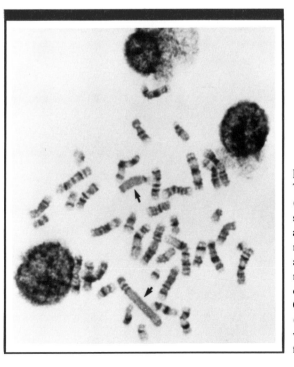

FIGURE 29.12
Typical HSRs (homogeneously stained regions, **arrows**) in a metaphase from a culture of neuroblastoma cells. Trypsin-Giemsa method. (Reproduced with permission from [7].)

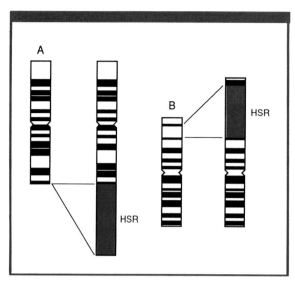

FIGURE 29.13

A: Normal chromosome 2 of a chinese hamster cell line. Next to it is a similar chromosome with a homogeneously stained region (HSR) from a drug-resistant cell line (resistant to antifolate). This cell line is characterized by excessive production of the enzyme dihydrofolate reductase; the gene amplification underlying the overproduction of this enzyme gives rise to the HSR. **B:** Normal human chromosome 1, and next to it a similar chromosome from a human neuroblastoma cell line, carrying an HSR. The significance of this gene expansion in neuroblastoma is not yet understood. (Reproduced with permission from [7].)

FIGURE 29.14 Double minutes in a metaphase of a cultured neuroblastoma cell. Double minutes represent the same phenomenon of gene amplification as the homogeneously stained regions (HSRs). (Reproduced with permission from [77].)

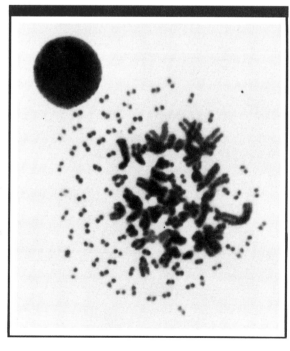

genetic material (*aneuploidy*). This topic is significant because of its prognostic value.

Polyploidy occurs in many normal tissues, where it may have survival value (p. 39). In tumors, aneuploidy and polyploidy become, by and large, a visible aspect of progression (18). For example, in a study of mammary carcinomas, most primary tumors were diploid, whereas most cells from metastatic effusions were aneuploid (82). It is still not clear why aneuploidy should correlate with a worse prognosis, but this is the case for many tumors, such as cancer of the breast or prostate (26). There are the usual exceptions: in large-cell lymphomas, aneuploidy and prognosis are not related.

Why does a defective karyotype progress toward increasing disorder? Nowell proposed that tumor cells are genetically more unstable than normal cells. This concept has much to support it. It is generally assumed that few cancer patients have preexisting genetic instabilities. Perhaps a destabilizing mutation occurs early in tumor development and precipitates a cascade of increasing chromosomal instability (62). Mutations of the all-important p53 gene are now thought to play a role in tumor progression (p. 885).

> **Chromosomal fragility syndromes** *do exist, especially in children, but they are rare. They are due to inborn abnormalities of DNA repair or related defects (e.g., Bloom's syndrome, Fanconi's anemia, ataxia telangiectasia, xeroderma pigmentosum). These syndromes are associated with increased risk of cancer development.*

We have only scratched the surface of this field; its importance is reflected in the fact that every large hospital must have a cytogenetics laboratory.

We will now turn to the structural changes that may precede cancer.

Precancerous Lesions

Many cancers, perhaps most, develop not from normal tissues but from precursor lesions. Overwhelming proof that premalignant lesions exist comes from experimental studies and from firm medical facts about human cancer. Experience shows that such lesions may or may not progress to cancer; the frequency of malignant transformation varies from organ to organ.

Besides their scientific interest, precancerous

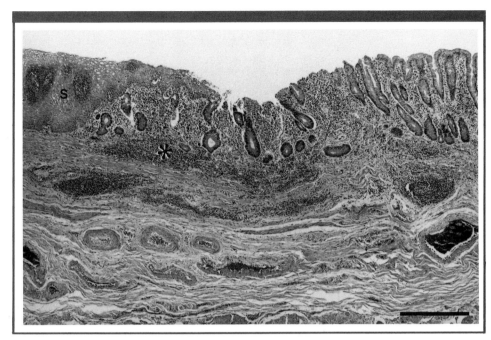

FIGURE 29.15
Barrett's epithelium in a human esophagus. **S:** Normal squamous stratified epithelium typical of the esophagus. To the right, this layer is replaced by a gland-forming cylindrical epithelium (Barrett's epithelium) recalling the gastric mucosa. Near the center is a small ulceration with inflammatory cells **(asterisk)** in the mucosa. Barrett's epithelium predisposes to the development of cancer. **Bar** = 500 μm.

lesions are important clinically. If we knew how to identify them all, we would have made one great step toward the control of cancer. Unfortunately they are often difficult to recognize. By definition we would expect them to be pretumoral, that is, small and barely visible. For this reason, we know more about precancerous lesions of the skin and of accessible mucosae, such as the mouth and the female cervix. Virtually nothing is known about premalignant changes of sarcomas and of brain tumors, which develop out of sight (32).

Known precancerous lesions include some forms of metaplasia, dysplasia and carcinoma *in situ*, some benign tumors and sundry lesions.

METAPLASIA AS A PRECANCEROUS LESION

For reasons unknown, virtually all epithelial metaplasias can be precancerous whereas connective tissue metaplasias are generally "safe." Metaplasia implies the expression of a different set of genes, but of *normal* genes. Molecular genetics has not yet explained why this change is sometimes a step to neoplasia. Typical examples of precancerous metaplasia are the islands of gastric epithelium in the esophagus (Barrett's epithelium; Figure 29.15) and patches of abnormal, hyperplastic epithelium **(leukoplakia)** on the tongue (see Figures 2.53, 2.54) or on the exocervix (Figure 29.16).

DYSPLASIA AND CARCINOMA *IN SITU*

Dysplasia is an imprecise but practical term: pathologists use it when they have to give a name to cellular changes that are too irregular to be

called hyperplasia and not irregular enough to be called neoplasia (Figure 29.17). This is a compromise and an admission of ignorance, but there is an excuse; according to the current theories of carcinogenesis, some in-between changes of this kind *should* exist. Dysplasia in surface epithelia blends into a change that is definitely neoplastic: carcinoma *in situ*.

Carcinoma in situ is Latin for "carcinoma in (its) place," whereby we mean that a covering epithe-

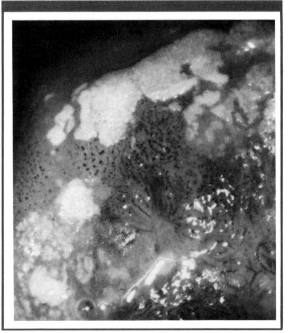

FIGURE 29.16
Human exocervix as photographed through a colposcope. The white patches represent leukoplakia (the whiteness is enhanced by painting with dilute acetic acid, an old empirical procedure); the punctate pattern corresponds to dilated and twisted capillaries, typical of carcinoma *in situ*. (Reproduced with permission from [17].)

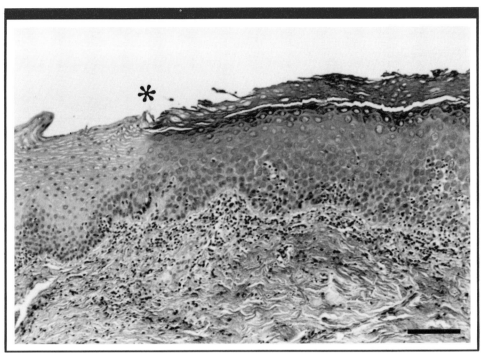

FIGURE 29.17
An example of subtle dysplasia in the mouth. Normal squamous stratified, nonkeratinized epithelium is shown at left. To the right of the **asterisk** is a fairly abrupt shift to dysplasia. The nuclei are enlarged, and the pattern of differentiation has changed; immature cells reach higher up in the epithelium and then abruptly keratinize. This dysplasia may progress to a malignancy. **Bar** = 50 μm. (Reproduced with permission from [46].)

lium has become replaced by a layer of cancer cells, but all boundaries are respected. The thickness of this layer is about the same as that of the epithelium, there is no outgrowth, and the basement membrane is not trespassed (Figure 29.18). If the boundaries break down, the diagnosis changes to invasive carcinoma. In the uterine cervix, the neoplastic epithelium maintains its constant cycle of division, upward migration, and finally shedding; this is what made the Pap smear possible. If there is a carcinoma *in situ* of the cervix, the Pap smear shows that epithelial cells that sloughed off from the surface failed to mature

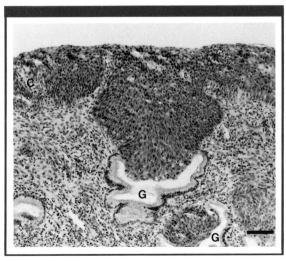

FIGURE 29.18
Carcinoma *in situ* (**C**) of the cervix, creeping into a gland (**G**). This is not yet considered to be invasion. **Bar** = 100 μm.

into the normal, flat, eosinophilic cell with a shriveled, pycnotic nucleus; they retained the structure and basophilia of basal cells. The difference is very obvious (Figure 29.19).

Carcinoma *in situ* occurs not only on the skin and cervix, but on any epithelial surface, including internal organs such as the urinary bladder, the gall bladder, and even the seminiferous tubules of the testis (28). One form of carcinoma *in situ* of the epidermis is known as Bowen's disease (Figure 29.20). To the naked eye, carcinoma *in situ* is a subtle change. On the skin, Bowen's disease appears as a reddened, scaly, or crusty area; in the cervix, if it is examined with a magnifying colposcope, a patch of carcinoma *in situ* appears dotted with capillary loops that are more widely spaced than in normal tissue and of larger caliber (Figure 29.21) (17). The enlarged capillaries may represent an early form of microvascular response to angiogenesis factors.

An old trick for visualizing a patch of carcinoma *in situ* on the exocervix is to swab the area with iodine; this is a clever bit of histochemistry *in vivo*. The normal squamous cells of the cervix contain glycogen, which is stained brown by iodine; but the epithelial cells of a carcinoma *in situ* have lost the ability of produce glycogen, so the carcinoma remains unstained.

Carcinoma *in situ* may or may not progress to invasiveness. When it does, the time required can

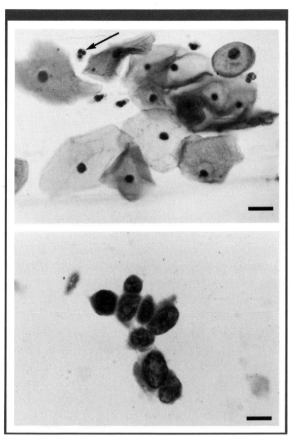

FIGURE 29.19

Two Pap smears photographed at the same enlargement. *Top:* Normal smear. The large, flat cells have sloughed off the epithelium and died by programmed cell death; note the small pyknotic nuclei. The rounded cell (at right) comes from the intermediate layer, which contributes fewer cells to the smear. **Arrow:** One of several neutrophils, a normal finding. *Bottom:* Cluster of epithelial cells of the type shed by a carcinoma *in situ;* note the uneven size of the nuclei, which also occupy most of the cytoplasm; compare these with the pyknotic nuclei of the normal smear. This cluster of cells is sufficient for the presumptive diagnosis of carcinoma *in situ* of the cervix. **Bars** = 5 μm. (Courtesy of J.M. Compton and Dr. F.R. Reale, University of Massachusetts Medical Center, Worcester, MA.)

be estimated: in the cervix the incidence of carcinoma *in situ* peaks around the age of 30, whereas invasive carcinoma of the cervix peaks around 45; so the progression, when it does occur, takes about 15 years (Figure 29.22). This progression in the bladder, stomach, and lung is usually faster. In the bladder, for example, the rate of recurrence and progression to invasiveness is 80 percent during a period of 5 years (42).

Dysplasia and Carcinoma in Situ: Diagnostic Dilemmas Nobody doubts that carcinoma *in situ* is

a true carcinoma capable of aggressive evolution, but the significance of "dysplasia" has generated a lot of heat in the world of gynecology. As the situation now stands, follow-up studies on biopsies of the cervix show that *both dysplasia and carcinoma* in situ *can unpredictably persist, regress, or progress to invasive cancer; but in any given case it is impossible to tell what the course case will be.* The situation varies somewhat from organ to organ (42, 44, 45).

This debate is especially critical for the pathology of an organ in which both lesions are common, the uterine cervix (actually the part most at risk is the junction between the endocervix and the exocervix, the segment exposed to the vagina). The epithelium of the exocervix can show a series of alterations that can be lined up—on paper—as a progression in the classic sense of going from bad to worse: normal cytology → hyperplasia → dysplasia (mild) → dysplasia (severe) → carcinoma in situ → invasive carcinoma. It is obvious that some premalignant changes must regress because they are much more common than invasive carcinomas. The debate arises because the degree of clinical risk does not correlate with this morphologic progression (43, 44). Attempts to differentiate cervical lesions by quantitating the nuclear DNA or by typing any concurrent papilloma viruses have not helped. For many years it was hoped that the risk of developing an invasive carcinoma would increase as the morphologic progression seems to suggest: but some

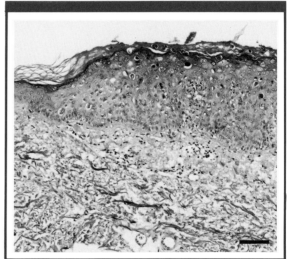

FIGURE 29.20

Bowen's disease on the skin of the calf. The epidermis at the extreme left is normal; to the right it is thickened. Note several atypical epithelial cells and the lack of differentiation from the bottom to the top layers. This pattern represents a carcinoma *in situ.* A red, scaly patch had been present for 45 months. **Bar** = 100 μm.

gynecologists *who tailored their therapy on this concept found themselves in hot water (44, 45).* Carcinoma *in situ* may regress, and mild dysplasia may progress.

In 1989 the problem was tackled by a committee of experts at the National Cancer Institute (59). The result was a compromise labeled the Bethesda System. Only two categories of epithelial changes are recognized: squamous intraepithelial lesion (SIL); low-grade SIL (for all changes up to the old "mild dysplasia") and high-grade SIL for all the more severe changes up to carcinoma in situ. Note: the SIL terminology is used for cytologic smears only. For histologic sections pathologists use the CIN terminology (p. 852).

This may solve the practical problem, but we are still in the dark about the biological significance of the various epithelial changes. Are they all, or part, viral? What happens to the DNA in SIL or in dysplastic nuclei? There is a huge literature on these precursor lesions, but the relationship between oncogene expression and preneoplasia is not understood (79).

Intramucosal or *superficial carcinomas* of the stomach are not quite the same as carcinoma *in situ.* This is the name given to carcinomas that have involved only the mucosal layer. The prognosis of these early carcinomas is much more favorable, even though gastric carcinomas are usually among the most lethal; but unfortunately they give no sign of their existence unless they are accompanied by an ulcer.

A sarcoma in situ parallel to carcinoma in situ cannot exist because it would lack the boundary of a basement membrane to serve as a definition of invasiveness. However, the concept has been pro-

FIGURE 29.21
Carcinoma *in situ* of the exocervix. *Top:* A close-up view of the exocervix through an enlarging colposcope: the irregular coarse dots represent dilated capillary loops reaching toward the surface. **Bar** = 1 mm. *Center:* Vascular preparation of the mucosa after the capillaries have been demonstrated by the reaction for alkaline phosphatase (black). The wide capillary loops reaching close to the surface and running partly along it correspond exactly to the top print. *Bottom:* Typical histologic image of carcinoma *in situ.* (Reproduced with permission from [41].)

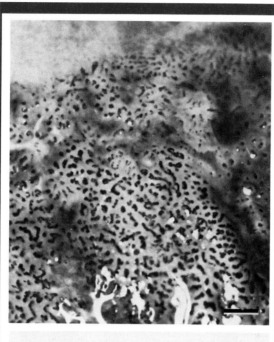
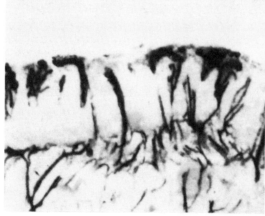
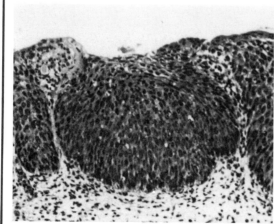

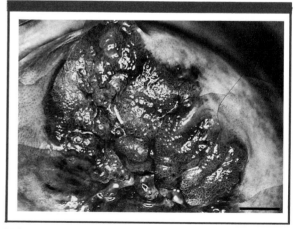

FIGURE 29.22
Invasive squamous cell carcinoma of the cervix; a composite photograph taken through the colposcope. The nodular surface is characteristic of this malignant tumor. The dark dots on its surface represent dilated capillaries, typical of malignant growth. **Bar** = 2 μm. (Reproduced with permission from [41].)

posed, especially to define early malignant changes in chondromas (70).

BENIGN TUMORS AS PRECURSORS OF CANCER

This title will be confusing for anyone who thinks that some tumors are benign, others malignant. Keep in mind the following points:

- Experimentally, it is proven beyond question that a benign growth, given enough time, can progress to carcinoma; this applies to both chemical and viral carcinogenesis.
- A similar progression is well established for a number of human tumors including gastrointestinal polyps, papillomas of the larynx, large congenital nevi, and pigmented moles.
- Some human tumors appear to remain stable in a benign condition (e.g., leiomyomas of the uterus), but occasional leiomyomas do progress to leiomyosarcomas, indicating that they too can progress.
- Progression from benign to malignant in renal cell tumors is tacitly assumed by pathologists. Today, for lack of better criteria, kidney tumors less than 3 cm in diameter are arbitrarily called adenomas; above 3 they are called carcinomas (Figure 29.23) (84).
- In the field of hematology, the so-called benign monoclonal gammopathy remains benign in about 90 percent of patients; in the remaining 10 percent it progresses to multiple myeloma or other malignancies (35).

Even the typically benign fibroadenoma of the breast is known occasionally to lapse into carcinoma. Indeed, it may be impossible to find a human benign tumor that never progresses to malignancy. Benign tumors, once again, are so defined by a clinical necessity, not by a biological scheme.

SUNDRY PRECANCEROUS LESIONS

Cellular Abnormalities That Precede Cancer Histologically, in the many models of experimental carcinogenesis, a variety of preneoplastic focal changes have been found and labeled hyperplasia, atypical metaplasia, dysplasia and the like; but none of these changes comes near to being specific (80). For example, during carcinogenesis in rat liver (see Figure 28.18) before malignant tumors develop, many microscopic foci of abnormal liver cells can be seen with ordinary stains (Figure 29.24) and even better with histochemical stains

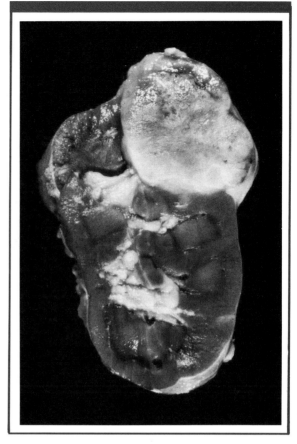

FIGURE 29.23 Carcinoma of the kidney. This tumor had infiltrated the retroperitoneum and the pericolic fat. It measured 4–5 cm in diameter. Had it been discovered when it measured 2 or 3 cm in diameter, it would have been labeled a benign adenoma. (Courtesy of Dr. B. Björnsson, University of Massachusetts Medical Center, Worcester, MA.)

for enzymes (Figure 29.25) (22, 23, 66). Up to a point these hepatocyte nodules (79) are reversible, and there is good evidence that they can progress to malignancy. Similar nodules can be found in humans (3). The epidermal changes that precede cancer during the phase of promotion with TPA have been described on p. 761.

Embryonal Rests This ancient theory is undergoing a partial revival. In its original form it maintained that tumors arise from microscopic embryonic rests that somehow wake up and turn into cancer. The idea, born in the early 1800s (63), had its roots in easily observable facts. For example, ordinary moles can turn into cancer (21), and some tumors—the teratomas—definitely look like embryology gone astray. By 1889 it also had the support of experiments that sound extremely modern. Read the following from Cohnheim's *Lectures on General Pathology;* he is describing experiments performed originally by Zahn:

> . . . *pieces of tissues taken from rabbits already born [and introduced into the anterior chamber of adult rabbits] became completely resorbed*

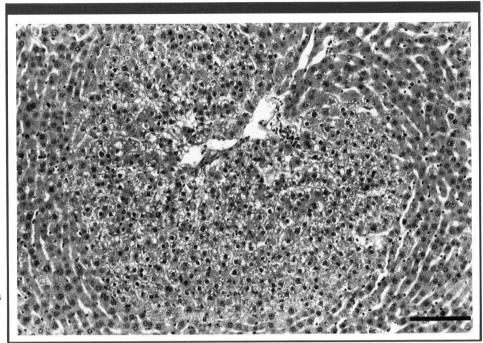

FIGURE 29.24
One of many hyperplastic (precancerous?) nodules that appeared in the liver of a rat, in the course of experimental carcinogenesis as described in Figure 29.25. **Bar** = 100 μm. (Reproduced with permission from [87].)

or greatly shrunken . . . while pieces taken from a foetus still unborn not only lived on in the new foreign organism, but almost always grew there in a very surprising way. Pieces of fetal cartilage grew to 200–300 times the original size (16).

Recall that the accepted method for producing mouse teratocarcinomas is to implant a mouse embryo into another mouse's testis (p. 903).

The trouble with the embryonal hypothesis was that embryonic remains were hard to find. Embryology is not known to be a sloppy process; however, microscopic clusters of cells representing embryonic leftovers can be found in a few organs.

A perfect example is the nephroblastoma, also called Wilms' tumor, which we have already met in relation to suppressor genes. Almost half of the kidneys removed for nephroblastoma contain microscopic clusters of mesonephric tissue that are thought to be the precursors of the tumor (see Figures 29.4, 29.26) (11, 67, 72). Cohnheim would have been gratified.

Nests of embryonic epithelium are common around the teeth. These are residues of the embryonic enamel organ (p. 434); in response to infection they proliferate, generating dental cysts and very rarely carcinomas. These are not to be confused with tumors that recapitulate the enamel

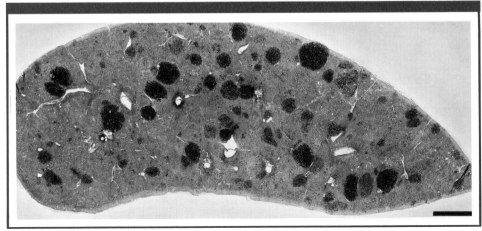

FIGURE 29.25
Multiple foci of liver hyperplasia demonstrated histochemically with a reaction for γ-glutamyl transferase. This rat was submitted to a complex regimen including a single carcinogenic dose of diethylnitrosamine and partial hepatectomy to simulate rapid growth. These nodules appear to be precursor lesions for at least some hepatocellular carcinomas. **Bar** = 500 μm. (Reproduced with permission from [83].)

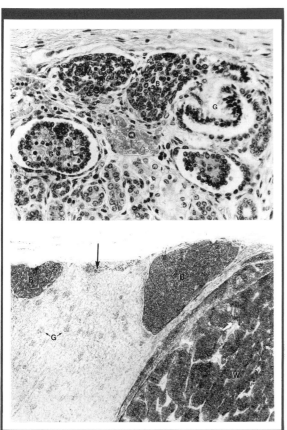

FIGURE 29.26

Top: The best example of embryonal rest as a potential cause for a tumor: **B** = *nodular renal blastema* (metanephric) in a 1-day-old infant who died of sepsis. Normally this embryonic tissue regresses and disappears at 34–35 weeks of gestational age; however, some persist and are found in one of every 200–400 pediatric autopsies. In this case they were multiple and bilateral in otherwise normal kidneys. **G** = glomeruli. (Courtesy of Dr. K.E. Bove, Children's Hospital Medical Center, Cincinnati, OH.) *Bottom:* Association of a 1.5 cm Wilms' tumorlet (**W**) with two nodules of renal blastema (**B**) and a metanephric hamartoma (**arrow**). From the kidney of a 41-month-old girl; another 9 × 8 cm Wilms' tumor was removed from the same kidney, and a 1 cm Wilms' tumorlet was removed from the contralateral kidney. **G** = glomeruli. (Reproduced with permission from [11].)

organ, which arise at the base of the skull (adamantinomas).

Chronic Inflammatory Lesions These lesions are not to be dismissed as potential precursors of cancer. Scars from a single trauma are rarely involved (p. 834), but ongoing chronic inflammation is another matter, especially when it leads to constant epithelial damage and regeneration. The likely mechanism, sustained cell proliferation, will be discussed on p. 926.

Many years of inflammation—decades—are necessary to induce cancer. Inflammation of the skin is rarely complicated by cancer today because there are many ways to suppress infection as well as inflammation. In the past, however, tuberculosis of the face (*tuberculous lupus*) was incurable, and squamous cell carcinoma was a complication almost taken for granted (15). Another complication that is rarely if ever seen today is squamous cell carcinoma developing in "sinuses"—infected passages that chronically drain pus from infected bones (osteomyelitis). Inflammation in internal organs is another matter. A number of internal diseases are due to chronic nonbacterial inflammation that persists for years and years. For example, liver cirrhosis (alcoholic, viral, or other) has a strong inflammatory component, and it is a well-established precursor of hepatoma. Chronic gastritis (autoimmune or bacterial) can be a prelude to gastric carcinoma; ulcerative colitis (cause unknown) carries a heavy risk of colon cancer. In the same category we can list carcinomas arising in strictures of the esophagus caused by swallowing caustics. These cancers develop 30–45 years later, presumably on chronic erosions (19). Notice, however, that in all these classic examples the role of chronic inflammation as regards neoplasia is indirect: it provides an unstable support for the epithelium, and *eventually it is the chronically regenerating epithelium that lapses into carcinoma.* One again, we find that granulation tissue is highly resistant to malignant transformation.

Patients tend to blame themselves for their sickness, even if it is a tumor ("What did I do to deserve this?") (2). From what we have said about cancer, a certain number of people can indeed blame themselves (especially smokers), but some of the blame must go to the genes, and some to chance.

References

1. Alberts B, Bray D, Lewis J, Raff M, Roberts K, Watson JD. Molecular biology of the cell, 2nd ed. New York: Garland Publishing, 1989.

2. Angell M. Disease as a reflection of the psyche. N Engl J Med 1985;312:1570–1572.

3. Anthony PP. Precursor lesions for liver cancer in humans. Cancer Res 1976;36:2579–2583.

4. Anttila S, Hietanen E, Vainio H, et al. Smoking and peripheral type of cancer are related to high levels of pulmonary cytochrome P450IA in lung cancer patients. Int J Cancer 1991;47:681–685.

5. Balaban-Malenbaum G, Gilbert F. Relationship between homogeneously staining regions and double minute chromosomes in human neuroblastoma cell lines. Prog Cancer Res Ther 1980;12:97–107.

6. Biedler JL, Ross RA, Shanske S, Spengler BA. Human neuroblastoma cytogenetics: search for significance of homogeneously staining regions and double minute chromosomes. Prog Cancer Res Ther 1980;12:81–96.

7. Biedler JL, Spengler BA. Metaphase chromosome anomaly: association with drug resistance and cell-specific products. Science 1976;191:185–187.

8. Bodmer WF, ed. Inheritance of susceptibility to cancer in man. Oxford: Oxford University Press, 1982.

9. Bohr VA, Evans MK, Fornace AJ Jr. DNA repair and its pathogenetic implications. Lab Invest 1989;61:143–161.

10. Bonaïti-Pellié C, Chompret A, Tournade MF, Lemerle J, Voute PA, Delemarre JFM. Excess of multifocal tumors in nephroblastoma: implications for mechanisms of tumor development and genetic counseling. Hum Genet 1993; 91:373–376.

11. Bove KE, McAdams AJ. Multifocal nephroblastic neoplasia. J Natl Cancer Inst 1978;61:285–294.

12. Burck KB, Liu ET, Larrick JW. Oncogenes: an introduction to the concept of cancer genes. New York: Springer-Verlag, 1988:109, 118.

13. Cahan WG. International workshop on multiple primary cancers. Introductory remarks. Cancer 1977;40: 1785–1789.

14. Cannon L, Bishop DT, Skolnick M, Hunt S, Lyon JL, Smart CR. Genetic epidemiology of prostate cancer in the Utah Mormon genealogy. In: Bodmer WF, ed. Inheritance of susceptibility to cancer in man. Oxford: Oxford University Press, 1982:47–69.

15. Clemmesen J. On the etiology of some human cancers. J Natl Cancer Inst 1951;12:1–21.

16. Cohnheim J. Lectures on general pathology. Sect II. London: The New Sydenham society, 1889.

17. Coppleson M, Pixley EC. Colposcopy of cervix. In: Coppleson M, ed. Gynecologic oncology, vol 1. Edinburgh: Churchill Livingstone, 1981:205–224.

18. Cram LS, Bartholdi MF, Ray FA, Travis GL, Kraemer PM. Spontaneous neoplastic evolution of Chinese hamster cells in culture: multistep progression of karyotype. Cancer Res 1983;43:4828–4837.

19. Csikos M, Horváth Ö, Petri A, Petri I, Imre J. Late malignant transformation of chronic corrosive oesophageal strictures. Langenbecks Arch Chir 1985;365:231–238.

20. Donaldson SS, Egbert PR. Retinoblastoma. In: Pizzo PA, Poplack DG, eds. Principles and practice of pediatric oncology. Philadelphia: JB Lippincott, 1989:555–568.

21. Durante F. Nesso fisio-patologico tra la struttura dei nei materni e la genesi di alcuni tumori maligni. Arch Mem Osservaz Chir Pratica 1874;11:217–226.

22. Enomoto K, Farber E. Kinetics of phenotypic maturation of remodeling of hyperplastic nodules during liver carcinogenesis. Cancer Res 1982;42:2330–2335.

23. Farber E. Cellular biochemistry of the stepwise development of cancer with chemicals: GHA Clowes memorial lecture. Cancer Res 1984;44:5463–5474.

24. Fialkow PJ, Singer JW. Chronic leukemias. In: DeVita VT Jr., Hellman S, Rosenberg SA, eds. Cancer. Principles & practice of oncology, 3rd ed. Philadelphia: JB Lippincott, 1989:1836–1852.

25. Francke U. A gene for Wilms tumour? Nature 1990;343: 692–694.

26. Frankfurt OS, Chin JL, Englander LS, Greco WR, Pontes JE, Rustum YM. Relationship between DNA ploidy, glandular differentiation, and tumor spread in human prostate cancer. Cancer Res 1985;45:1418–1423.

27. Friend S. The genetic basis of cancer. In: Cossman J, ed. Molecular genetics in cancer diagnosis. New York: Elsevier, 1990:19–28.

28. Giwercman A, Hopman AHN, Ramaekers FCS, Skakkebaek NE. Carcinoma in situ of the testis. Detection of malignant germ cells in seminal fluid by means of in situ hybridization. Am J Pathol 1990;136:497–502.

29. Hansen MF, Cavenee WK. Genetics of cancer predisposition. Cancer Res 1987;47:5518–5527.

30. Harris AL. Cancer genes: telling changes of base. Nature 1991;350:377–378.

31. Harris CC. Interindividual variation among humans in carcinogen metabolism, DNA adduct formation and DNA repair. Carcinogenesis 1989;10:1563–1566.

32. Henson DE, Albores-Saavedra J. The pathology of incipient neoplasia. Philadelphia: WB Saunders, 1986.

33. Hollstein M, Sidransky D, Vogelstein B, Harris CC. p53 mutations in human cancers. Science 1991;253:49–53.

34. Holm NV, Hauge M, Jensen OM. Studies of cancer aetiology in a complete twin population: breast cancer, colorectal cancer and leukaemia. In: Bodmer WF, ed. Inheritance of susceptibility to cancer in man. Oxford: Oxford University Press, 1982:17–32.

35. Jandl EH. Blood. Boston: Little, Brown, 1987.

36. King M-C. Genetic analysis of cancer in families. Cancer Surv 1990;9:417–433.

37. Kinlen LJ. Immunologic factors. In: Schottenfeld D, Fraumeni JF Jr, eds. Cancer epidemiology and prevention. Philadelphia: WB Saunders, 1982:494–505.

38. Knudson AG Jr. Genetic influences in human tumors. In: Becker FF, ed. Cancer: a comprehensive treatise, vol 1. New York: Plenum Press, 1975:59–74.

39. Knudson AG Jr. Genetic predisposition to cancer. In: Hiatt HH, Watson JD, Winsten JA, eds. Origins of human cancer. Book A. Cold Spring Harbor conferences on cell proliferation, vol 4. Cold Spring Harbor: Cold Spring Harbor Laboratory, 1977:45–52.

40. Knudson AG Jr. Hereditary cancers: clues to mechanisms of carcinogenesis. Br J Cancer 1989;59:661–666.

41. Kolstad P, Stafl A. Atlas of colposcopy. Baltimore: University Park Press, 1972.

42. Koss LG. Precancerous lesions. In: Fraumeni JF Jr, ed. Persons at high risk of cancer. New York: Academic Press, 1975:85–102.

43. Koss LG. Dysplasia. A real concept or a misnomer? Obstet Gynecol 1978;51:374–379.

44. Koss LG. From koilocytosis to molecular biology: the impact of cytology on concepts of early human cancer. Mod Pathol 1989a;2:526–535.

45. Koss LG. The Papanicolaou test for cervical cancer detection. A triumph and a tragedy. JAMA 1989b;261: 737–743.

46. Krutchkoff DJ, Eisenberg E, Anderson C. Dysplasia of oral mucosa: a unified approach to proper evaluation. Mod Pathol 1991;4:113–119.

47. Lambert WC. Genetic diseases associated with DNA and chromosomal instability. Dermatol Clin 1987;5: 85–108.

48. Lehmann AR. Xeroderma pigmentosum, Cockayne syndrome and ataxia-telangiectasia: disorders relating DNA repair to carcinogenesis. In: Bodmer WF, ed. Inheritance of susceptibility to cancer in man. Oxford: Oxford University Press, 1982:93–118.

49. Leibowitz D, Young KS. The molecular biology of CML: a review. Cancer Invest 1989;7:195–203.

50. Levine AJ, Momand J, Finlay CA. The p53 tumour suppressor gene. Nature 1991;351:453–456.

51. Li FP, Fraumeni JF Jr, Mulvihill JJ, et al. A cancer family syndrome in twenty-four kindreds. Cancer Res 1988;48: 5358–5362.

52. Makino S. My life in cytology. In: German J, ed. Chromosome mutation and neoplasia. New York: Alan R. Liss, 1983:xxvii–xxxiii.

53. Matsuura N, Onda M, Tokunaga A, et al. Simultaneous gastric cancer in monozygotic twins. Cancer 1988;62: 2430–2435.

54. Meisner LF. Genetic factors in human cancer. In: Kahn SB, Love RR, Sherman C Jr, Chakravorty R, eds. Concepts in cancer medicine. New York: Grune & Stratton, 1983:165–176.

55. Miller RW. Genes, syndromes, and cancer. Pediatr Rev 1986;8:153–158.

56. Moertel CG. Multiple primary malignant neoplasms. Historical perspectives. Cancer 1977;40:1786–1792.

57. Nakamura S-I, Kino I. Morphogenesis of minute adenomas in familial polyposis coli. J Natl Cancer Inst 1984;73:41–49.

58. Nebert DW, ed. Identification of genetic differences in drug metabolism: prediction of individual risk of toxicity or cancer. Hepatology 1991;14:398–401.

59. National Cancer Institute Workshop. The 1988 Bethesda system for reporting cervical/vaginal cytological diagnoses. JAMA 1989;262:931–934.

60. Nores JM, Dalayeun J, Chebat J, Dieudonné P, Nenna AD. Concurrent anaplastic bronchial cancer in identical twin brothers. Respiration 1989;55:56–59.

61. Nowell PC. Mitotic inhibition and chromosome damage by mitomycin in human leukocyte cultures. Exp Cell Res 1964;33:445–449.

62. Nowell PC, Croce CM. Chromosomal approaches to oncogenes and oncogenesis. FASEB J 1988;2:3054–3060.

63. Oberling C. The riddle of cancer. New Haven, CT: Yale University Press, 1952.

64. Ooi WL, Elston RC, Chen VW, Bailey-Wilson JE, Rothschild H. Increased familial risk for lung cancer. J Natl Cancer Inst 1986;76:217–222.

65. Oren M. p53: the ultimate tumor suppressor gene? FASEB J 1992;6:3169–3176.

66. Pitot HC. The natural history of neoplasia. Am J Pathol 1977;89:401–412.

67. Pochedly C. Persistent renal blastema: a seed of Wilms' tumor? Hosp Pract 1981;16:83–96.

68. Ponder BAJ. Inherited cancer syndromes. In: Carney D, Sikora K, eds. Genes and cancer. Chichester: John Wiley & Sons, 1990:99–106.

69. Purtilo DT, Paquin L, Gindhart T. Genetics of neoplasia— impact of ecogenetics on oncogenesis. Am J Pathol 1978;91:609–688.

70. Ragsdale BD, Sweet DE. Bone. In: Henson DE, Albores-Saavedra J, eds. The pathology of incipient neoplasia. Philadelphia: WB Saunders, 1986:381–423.

71. Ringertz NR, Savage RE. Cell hybrids. New York: Academic Press, 1976.

72. Roth J, Blaha I, Bitter-Suermann D, Heitz PU. Blastemal cells of nephroblastomatosis complex share an onco-

developmental antigen with embryonic kidney and Wilms' tumor. An immunohistochemical study on polysialic acid distribution. Am J Pathol 1988;133:596–608.

73. Rowley JD. The Philadelphia chromosome translocation. A paradigm for understanding leukemia. Cancer 1990;65: 2178–2184.

74. Ruddon RW. Cancer biology, 2nd ed. New York: Oxford University Press, 1987.

75. Sager R, Gadi IK, Stephens L, Grabowy CT. Gene amplification: an example of accelerated evolution in tumorigenic cells. Proc Natl Acad Sci USA 1985;82: 7015–7019.

76. Sager R. Tumor suppressor genes: the puzzle and the promise. Science 1989;246:1406–1412.

77. Sandberg AA. The chromosomes in human cancer and leukemia, 2nd ed. New York: Elsevier, 1990.

78. Schottenfeld D. Multiple primary cancers. In: Schottenfeld D, Fraumeni JF Jr, eds. Cancer epidemiology and prevention. Philadelphia: WB Saunders, 1982:1025–1035.

79. Sirica AE. Preoplasia and precancerous lesions. In: Sirica AE, ed. The pathobiology of neoplasia. New York: Plenum Press, 1989:199–215.

80. Sirica AE, ed. The pathobiology of neoplasia. New York: Plenum Press, 1989.

81. Skolnick M, Bishop DT, Carmelli D, et al. A population-based assessment of familial cancer risk in Utah Mormon genealogies. In: Arrighi FE, Rao PN, Stubblefield E, eds. Genes, chromosomes, and neoplasia. New York: Raven Press, 1981:477–500.

82. Smith HS, Liotta LA, Hancock MC, Wolman SR, Hackett AJ. Invasiveness and ploidy of human mammary carcinomas in short-term culture. Proc Natl Acad Sci USA 1985;82:1805–1809.

83. Solt DB, Medline A, Farber E. Rapid emergence of carcinogen-induced hyperplastic lesions in a new model for the sequential analysis of liver carcinogenesis. Am J Pathol 1977;88:595–618.

84. Stuart AE, Smith AN, Samuel E, eds. Applied surgical pathology. Oxford: Blackwell Scientific Publications, 1975.

85. Vile R. Tumour suppressor genes. Br Med J 1989;298: 1335–1336.

86. von Recklinghausen FD. Ein Fall von Enchondrom mit ungewöhnlicher Multiplication. Virchows Arch Pathol Anat Physiol Klin Med 1889;118:1–18.

87. Wanless IR, Medline A. Role of estrogens as promoters of hepatic neoplasia. Lab Invest 1982;46:313–320.

88. Weissman BE, Saxon PJ, Pasquale SR, Jones GR, Geiser AG, Stanbridge EJ. Introduction of a normal human chromosome 11 into a Wilms' tumor cell line controls its tumorigenic expression. Science 1987;236: 175–180.

89. Yonish-Rouach E, Resnitzky D, Lotem J, Sachs L, Kimchi A, Oren M. Wild-type p53 induces apoptosis of myeloid leukaemic cells that is inhibited by interleukin-6. Nature 1991;352:345–347.

90. Yunis JJ. The chromosomal basis of human neoplasia. Science 1983;221:227–236.

91. Yunis JJ, Brunning RD, Howe RB, Lobell M. High-resolution chromosomes as an independent prognostic indicator in adult acute nonlymphocytic leukemia. N Engl J Med 1984;311:812–818.

Antitumor Defenses

CHAPTER 30

Custodians of the
Genome: The Tumor-
Suppressor Genes

The Immune Response
Against Tumors

Non-Specific Defenses
Against Tumors

Therapeutic Boosting of
Natural Antitumor
Defenses

Although many tumors succeed in killing their host, there are, in fact, many antitumor defenses. They fall into three groups. The first line of defense consists of *genes that act as guardians of the genome*, by correcting genetic errors or eliminating the cells that bear them. The second is *the immune system*, which cannot correct faulty genes but can eliminate cells marked by faulty gene products. The third includes *non-specific responses*, primarily inflammation.

Custodians of the Genome: The Tumor-Suppressor Genes

Among the tumor-suppressor genes (anti-oncogenes)—about a dozen are known at this time (42a)—p53 holds the limelight. We will use it here as a model to show how a gene can suppress cancer, or conversely foster tumor birth and progression when it mutates to a non-functional entity (34a, 39a, 66). The normal activities of p53 include the following: (1) *it stops temporarily the cell cycle* by prolonging the G-1 phase, between mitosis and DNA synthesis. This allows extra time for correcting defects in DNA (69a). Should the repair fail, (2) *it triggers* *apoptosis* and simply eliminates the faulty cell (in so doing the gene is truly suicidal, because it eliminates—of course—precisely the cell that it inhabits). Transgenic mice lacking the p53 gene develop normally, except for a propensity to develop tumors, but if they are irradiated their tissues fail to respond with cell cycle arrest and apoptosis (28a, 39a). (3) *p53 also stimulates the transcription of genes involved in differentiation*, so that the cell is set on a path directly opposite to that of carcinogenesis.

The secret whereby a single gene can have so many effects is that the protein p53 binds to multiple sites in the DNA chain, thereby controlling a variety of genes (28a, 34a). But how does the p53 gene become activated? Under normal circumstances little or no p53 protein can be detected in the cell (admittedly it has a half-life of minutes). Recent work has shown that *the p53 gene is turned on by hypoxia* (27a, 27b), which—as we have seen—is prevalent in malignant tumors. The p53 gene of hypoxic tumor cells is turned on; it induces many cells to commit suicide by apoptosis. In the asphyxiating tumoral environment, selection will favor cells that are less prone to apoptosis: such are cells with mutations of the p53 gene, and eventually the tumor is overrun by clones of p53 mutants. The lack of normal p53 function deprives the cell population of a major

FIGURE 30.1 Changing fortunes of tumor immunology according to R.T. Prehn. *Euphoria* is meant to reflect faith in the significance of tumor immunology.

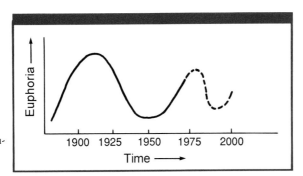

necessary complication) or more vaguely TATA (tumor-associated transplantation antigens).

The next surprise came from the Karolinska Institute in Stockholm. Gross and others in the United States had shown that the polyoma virus produced tumors if injected into immature mice. Now it was discovered that grafted polyoma tumors would not grow in mice that had been immunized against the virus. This seemed to open the door to immunization against tumors, or at least against virus-induced tumors.

After these exciting highlights we can add some more recent facts, the first one disappointing:

- *Spontaneous tumors* (as opposed to experimentally induced tumors) *are in general poorly antigenic*. The reason is not clear; perhaps they are self-selected as such because they grow more successfully. In any event, the very tumors that we would want to be antigenic—because they are the most common in humans—lack that quality. The other side of the coin is that some human tumors are not truly spontaneous and are correspondingly more antigenic; such are basal cell carcinomas in areas of skin exposed to UV light (perhaps we owe it to the immune response if these particular carcinomas are so well contained).

> Warning: not all tumor "antigens" are antigenic. *Among the weak antigens produced by human tumors are the so-called oncofetal antigens, which cross-react with fetal tissues and reflect the derepression of genes that are normally active in fetal life (p. 932). We prefer to call them* **oncofetal proteins** *because their antigenic properties are minimal and probably irrelevant. As a matter of fact, alpha-fetoprotein is immunosuppressive (40). So why is it called an oncofetal antigen? Simply because immunologists, faced with a protein, call it an antigen by reflex, just as molecular biologists would call it a gene product (Figure 30.2).*

- *The most antigenic tumors are those induced by viruses;* furthermore, any tumor produced by a given oncogenic virus always carries the same antigens, even in different species. This makes sense, assuming that the antigens are coded by the virus.
- *A tumor produced by chemical carcinogens produces antigens specific to that tumor even within the same animal*. This tends to complicate the job of the immune response: if separate tumors arise, it has to deal with each one as a separate problem.

"molecular policeman," and the tumor progresses to ever-increasing malignancy (69a).

Mutant forms of the p53 protein were found histochemically in 39 percent of human malignant tumors (but not in benign tumors) (53a). There is already some talk about new approaches to cancer chemotherapy based on the behavior of p53 (34a, 34b). The deluge of papers on this gene is certainly justified.

The Immune Response Against Tumors

This topic has been difficult to work out because the immune response to tumors varies a great deal, depending on the species and on the type of tumor. Correspondingly, the enthusiasm of the scientific community has waxed and waned (Figure 30.1). The reasons are best understood by retracing events (39, 44).

There was much excitement at the turn of the century when it was found that mouse tumors grafted to other mice grew at first but were later destroyed by a lifesaving chronic inflammation. We now realize that the victorious mice were not rejecting the tumor as such but tissue from a noncompatible donor. Inbred strains of mice were needed, and the first were produced in the 1940s by Ludvik Gross, the discoverer of the mouse leukemia virus. These inbred mice led to some promising observations: it was possible to immunize an inbred mouse against a tumor, so specifically that the mouse would reject a tumor from another individual of the same strain even though it would readily accept a skin graft. This was proof that tumor-specific antigens (TSA) really exist. Some workers called them TSA, others TSTA (tumor-specific transplantation antigens, an un-

If experimental tumors are listed from the most to the least antigenic, they rank as follows (39):

1. virus induced
2. ultraviolet-light induced
3. chemical carcinogen induced
4. spontaneous

In discussing the immunology of tumors it is important to remember that most of the established facts concern mice. Until recently, human *tumor-specific* antigens had not been found. The first one to be discovered and defined at the genetic level was published in 1991 (41a): its gene, named *MAGE1*, is expressed in melanomas and other types of cancer, and the gene product is recognized by cytotoxic lymphocytes. But the fact remains that "TSA" in humans are elusive.

This seems strange, because, after all, cancer develops to a large extent as a result of mutated genes, and mutated genes generate abnormal proteins: why are these not recognized? They probably are (to some extent)—but not enough to induce rejection of the tumor. For example, 10 percent of patients with breast tumors have circulating antibodies against p53—but these antibodies recognize normal as well as mutated p53 protein. So it may be that these antibodies are just a response to overexpressed p53, and do not specifically recognize the mutated form (41a). However, there is hope along these lines. Experimentally, it has been possible to vaccinate mice against a carcinoma by injecting peptides obtained from a mutated gap-junction protein (41b, 66a). Human trials of this kind are under way.

Finally, we should keep in mind another complication: tumors have several devices for evading the immune response. In particular, they can respond to antibody attack in three ways: (1) *by producing cells that are less antigenic*. This process may occur simply by natural selection, the less antigenic cells being more prone to survive. (2) *By shedding soluble antigens*, which float off and saturate the antibodies before they reach the surface of the tumor cells. (3) *By growing faster* as a result of stimulation by the antibodies (26).

Immunosurveillance We have explained that tumors may elicit an immune response. How effective is this response in eliminating tumors?

As far back as 1909, Paul Ehrlich, who discovered mast cells and originated the concept of receptors, was sure that aberrant fetal cells, ready to produce cancers, were continuously nipped off by the immune system (35). A similar

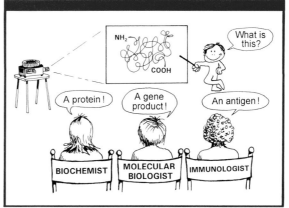

FIGURE 30.2 A protein may be called by various names, depending on the background of the observer. (Courtesy of Dr. H.F. Cuénoud, University of Massachusetts Medical School, Worcester, MA.)

concept was proposed in 1959 by the late Dr. Lewis Thomas during his distinguished career as a pathologist (before achieving fame as a writer). Shortly thereafter the concept acquired a name, *immunosurveillance*, and rose to near-dogma through the writings of Australian Nobel laureate Sir MacFarlane Burnet (13): "One can . . . picture a form of surveillance by which the body is continually patrolled, as it were, for the appearance of aberrant protein. . . ."

The strongest support for the notion of immunosurveillance comes from the established fact that genetically immunodeficient or therapeutically immunosuppressed individuals are prone to develop malignancies, mostly lymphomas (57). In three studies of patients who were immunosuppressed for kidney grafts, the risk of developing a lymphoma was increased 100, 150, and 350 times (41). However, there are also some troubling facts:

- Why are the tumors arising in the immune system itself?
- Why do they occur only in a minority of immunosuppressed individuals?
- Why is there no increase in the more common forms of tumors such as lung, breast, and colon cancers? True, there is some increase in skin and lip cancers, but it is only 3–4 percent (41).
- Why, in normal individuals, is there no greater incidence of malignancies at immunologically privileged sites such as the central nervous system? (Privileged sites are tissues in which allografts are protected against rejection, perhaps because of poor lymphatic drainage; for example, the brain and the anterior chamber of the eye.)

Similar questions are raised by studies of nude

mice, which are born without hair and without a thymus and are thereby deprived of the cell-mediated immune response; however, they show no increase in spontaneous tumors nor are they more susceptible to carcinogens (53). For these and other reasons, it is now believed that the concept of immunosurveillance—while still alive—should be accepted with some restrictions (39).

Note: While the experts debate to what extent immunosurveillance really functions as a tumor watchdog, there is little doubt that it can act as an oncogenetic-*virus* watchdog; in other words, the immune system can protect against tumors by eliminating their cause, rather than the tumor itself (36, 39). This line of reasoning is suggested, for example, by the congenital immunodeficiency named Duncan's disease or XLP (X-linked lymphoproliferative disease) (57), in which immunodeficiency paves the way to a virus-induced lymphoma (p. 587).

Non-Specific Defenses Against Tumors

The body's all-purpose, non-specific defense is of course inflammation. In addition, experience has shown that "stresses" of various kinds—not well understood—can contribute to the resistance against tumors.

The Role of Inflammation in Tumors Inflammation, albeit mild, is an almost constant feature of malignancy (Figure 30.3) (6). When a malignant

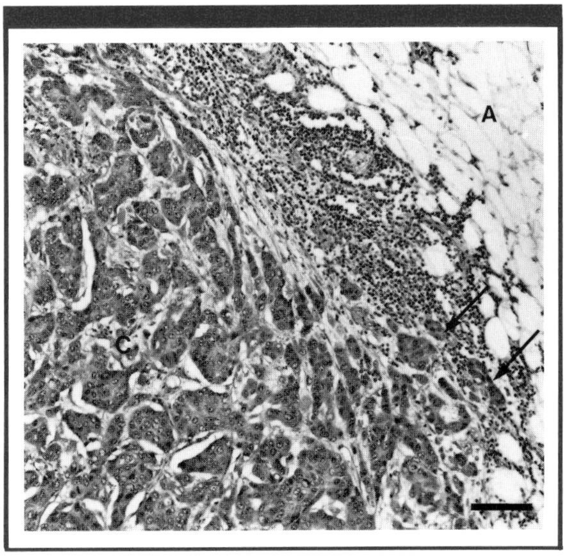

FIGURE 30.3
Breast carcinoma (**C**) invading the adipose tissue (**A**) of the breast. Between C and A a heavy infiltrate of lymphocytes has developed, but it does not appear to hold back the invasion (**arrows**). **Bar** = 100 μm.

tumor spreads over a serosal surface such as the peritoneum, fluid accumulates in the serosal cavity. These so-called *malignant effusions* are essentially inflammatory exudates; they do contain tumor cells, but most of the cells floating within them are leukocytes (32). Some degree of inflammation can also be found in benign tumors (2, 5).

Remember that inflammation is in the first place a non-specific reaction; it so happens that it is also borrowed by the immune response as one of its effector arms. Thus, *whenever we find inflammation in a tumor, we are not entitled to conclude that we are witnessing an immune response.* Leukocytes have several reasons for abandoning the bloodstream and congregating in a tumor: (1) chemotaxins secreted by tumor cells, (2) chemotaxins secreted by inflammatory cells, (3) chemotaxins released by necrotic tumor tissue, (4) bacterial chemotaxins in ulcerated and infected tumors, and (5) adhesion molecules expressed by the endothelium of the tumor's vessels. The biological effect of this exodus is difficult to assess because in the end the inflammatory response is almost always the loser. Everyone agrees that medullary carcinoma of the breast, which is consistently infiltrated with lymphocytes, has a relatively good prognosis (6); a positive correlation between inflammatory response and prognosis has been found for colon carcinomas (5) and for lung carcinomas (72). For other tumors a clear-cut correlation is not apparent (2, 6). In the rabbit, Shope papillomas that regress are massively infiltrated with lymphocytes (43); and in human malignant tumors, the largest numbers of macrophages are found in renal cell carcinomas, melanomas, and carcinomas of the colon—the malignancies that are most susceptible to immunotherapy (50). The bottom line, it seems, is that the tumor-infiltrating inflammatory cells must be performing *some* defensive functions, because if they are extracted, multiplied by culture, and reinjected, they demonstrably help in the fight against the tumor (p. 938).

The various types of inflammatory cells can be expected to make different contributions.

Natural Killer Cells NK cells, which appear in ordinary tissue sections as ordinary lymphocytes, have gained recognition as the first line of defense; they can kill tumor cells even if they are not activated and even if their target is not identified by MHC antigens or coated with antibody (activation with interferon or IL-2 just heightens their aggressiveness) (Figure 30.4). We have already described their weapons: the perforins, which do precisely what their name says, and other cytotoxic molecules (19, 71). They are numerous in some tumors, and experimentally there is some correlation between NK cell activity and resistance to tumors (66).

Macrophages Macrophages are always present in tumors as part of the stroma (22), even when inflammation is minimal or absent. In some tumors, as many as 80 percent of the cells are macrophages (64), which implies a true inflammatory response. Why should circulating monocytes elect to go and live in a tumor? Recent data show that many human malignant tumors, cultivated *in vitro*, secrete a monocyte attractant (28), which means that tumor monocytes may have emigrated in response to chemotactic stimuli unrelated to immunologic mechanisms. As to their performance in the tumor, monocytes and/or macrophages produce a number of anti-tumor cytokines: one is *interferon*, which does "interfere" with the growth of some tumors (1); another is *interleukin 12*, whose antitumor and antimetastatic virtues (in experimental animals) we will describe shortly; and then of course there is TNF, *tumor necrosis factor*, that powerful double-edged sword. Exactly how macrophage products kill tumor cells selectively is not yet clear. Normal cells are spared except for a minor proportion of bone marrow cells (68). Some cytolytic factors require cell contact, others act at a distance. To the naked eye the effect of TNF can be spectacular (Figures 9.42, 9.43); necrosis is accompanied by hemorrhage, which suggests a combination of direct cell killing with some vascular effect, possibly intravascular coagulation. The tumor-killing capability of activated macrophages is beyond doubt (15, 54, 64). It works beautifully in the laboratory, but nobody has yet found a way to exploit it in the human body.

The tumor-killing frenzy of macrophages is not to be taken for granted. Old macrophages from inflammatory lesions and macrophage-derived giant cells are refractory to activation in vitro: they do not become tumoricidal (54). Furthermore, activation depends on environmental factors that may enhance or suppress the killing (15). Alveolar macrophages are unable to destroy tumor cells that blood monocytes can kill (70).

Finally, even the trusty macrophages have their dark side. Remember that under anoxic conditions they secrete an angiogenesis factor (p. 469).

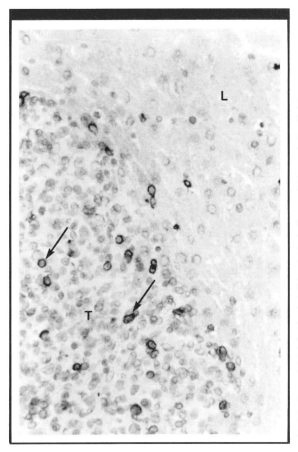

FIGURE 30.4 **See color plate 24.** NK cells infiltrating a tumor (**T**) growing in rat liver (**L**). The NK cells (dark brown) are demonstrated with a powerful monoclonal antibody (3.2.3) prepared by Dr. J.C. Hiserodt. This tumor is a mammary adenocarcinoma that happens to be NK resistant. Immunoperoxidase stain. (Courtesy of Dr. J.C. Hiserodt, Pittsburgh, PA.)

Because much of a tumor is anoxic, the macrophages can play the game on the side of the tumor by helping it attract a vascular supply. They might also favor tumor development with growth factors (64). And then, in a large tumor, by secreting enough cachectin (another name for TNF) they can produce cachexia and deliver the finishing blow to the host (p. 701): a drastic way to get rid of a tumor.

T-Lymphocytes T-cells are found in virtually all malignant tumors, but many of the cells that we call lymphocytes in routinely stained microscopic sections might be NK cells. Massive lymphocytic infiltration is typical of seminomas (Figure 30.5), to the point that in bygone years these tumors were said to consist of "two types of cells." The current explanation is that the lymphocytes respond to sperm-related antigens that the body does not usually "see" and that are produced or expressed by the tumor cells.

When duly stimulated, T-lymphocytes secrete lymphotoxins, a family of proteins now called TNF-beta because they are very similar to TNF.

T-lymphocytes too are a double-edged sword:

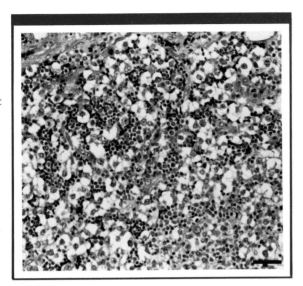

FIGURE 30.5 Histologic aspect of a seminoma. The large clear cells represent the tumor; between them are clusters of lymphocytes, often seen in seminomas, presumably as a response to tumor antigens. **Bar** = 50 *μ*m.

T-cells of the suppressor type can actually protect a tumor against immune attack and assist tumor growth (12). A cytotoxic drug, cyclophosphamide, is currently being used clinically to suppress the suppressors (8, 9).

Tumor cells defend themselves in several ways from attack by cytolytic cells (51): by activating suppressor T-cells that dampen the immune response; by secreting cytokines that inhibit cytolytic cells; or by downgrading the expression of HLA class I surface antigens, so that some experimental tumors become invisible to B and T lymphocytes though not to NK cells (20).

This scenario implies that the number of lymphocytes in human tumors should correlate with the expression of HLA antigens; for breast cancer, the data are not clear-cut (37).

Neutrophils Overall, the role of neutrophils in fighting tumor cells is probably minor, but not to be discounted (34). Neutrophils are always present, of course, in ulcerated and infected tumors; and they are attracted to areas of necrosis, although not in large numbers. In either case they are probably not responding to the tumor itself. Unfortunately, they do not seem to perform a "seek and destroy" operation against tumor cells as they do against bacteria.

OTHER NON-SPECIFIC ANTITUMOR DEFENSES

The few facts that we can offer are tantalizing. Most of them concern regressions of tumors in the course of infections.

- It is an open secret among experimental oncologists that when an infectious disease breaks out in a mouse colony, the experiment has to be called off because many tumors will not take; even stress can make a difference (11).
- Infection of the pleura, resulting in empyema after resection of a lung for cancer, has improved survival (63).
- Infections can cause remissions of leukemia in children (10).
- The remission of leukemias during infection has led to another discovery: if human lung tissue is exposed *in vitro* to endotoxin, to mimic infection, it produces a factor that causes leukemia cells to differentiate (74).
- Experimental granulomas in mice produce a "mouse granuloma protein" (MGP) that— injected into other mice—protects them against a lethal infection with *Listeria monocytogenes*. A similar protein was found in human urine (HGP); mouse macrophages incubated with HGP become cytotoxic against the highly malignant Lewis carcinoma (27).

Some but not all of these effects may have been due to macrophages producing cytokines such as tumor necrosis factor. This is probably what happened in the patients treated for cancer at the turn of the century with "Coley's toxins" (p. 351). There is room here for more work.

In summary, both immune and nonimmune mechanisms cooperate in fighting tumors. Often the battle is lost; how often we do not know because there is no trace of the tumors (if any) that are nipped in the bud. Why is the battle so often lost? It has been proposed that tumors sneak through the defenses by a mechanism appropriately called *sneaking through* (35, 45, 55): While a tumor is small it can quietly grow because it remains unnoticed; by the time the immune response becomes aware of it, it is too late. And then, in later stages, some tumors attain the ultimate weapon: they become immunosuppressive, by secreting soluble factors such as prostaglandins or alpha-fetoproteins (53).

Allografts of Tumors in Humans The reader will probably assume that tumor grafts from one human to another have never been tried, because they would run against ethical as well as immunological barriers. Well, this type of experiment has been done many times, and some grafts have taken. Ludvik Gross has collected a rather disturbing series (29). A few examples: One carcinoma was accidentally grafted from the mother's ulcerated breast cancer to her suckling infant's lip. As late as 1958, before ethical guidelines were established, experiments on "volunteers" (some with cancer, some healthy) showed that tumor implants usually regressed in 4–6 weeks; but one cancer patient developed metastases even after excision of the graft. One autologous implant remained dormant for 18 months. In 1965, a surgeon transplanted melanoma tissue from a woman to her 80-year-old mother, in the hope of producing antibodies as an aid to therapy; the daughter died, and so did the mother, with widespread metastatic melanoma despite excision of the implantation site (65). Several (immunosuppressed!) recipients of kidney transplants have died of metastases from primary or secondary tumors hidden in the donated kidney. One was a melanoma. In a recent laboratory accident, a technician injected her own finger with a suspension of cells from a line of human adenocarcinoma of the colon. Three weeks later a nodule was excised that showed a carcinoma with no inflammatory response (Figure 30.6) (30). Four years later the lady was in fine shape and considered cured.

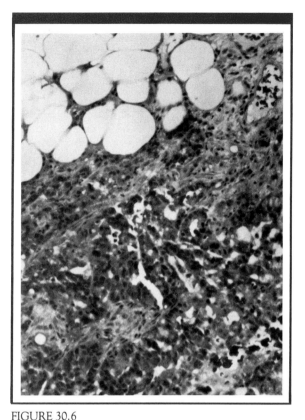

FIGURE 30.6
Needle-stick tumor. A 19-year-old healthy laboratory worker accidentally injected her finger while transplanting a line of cells derived from a human colon carcinoma. Nineteen days later a nodule measuring 9 × 4 × 4 mm was excised. It contained this typical adenocarcinoma. Four years later the patient was in good health. Allogeneic transplants sometimes do take. (Courtesy of Dr. M.E. Sanders, National Cancer Institute, Bethesda, MD.)

Therapeutic Boosting of Natural Antitumor Defenses

Although surgery, radiation, and chemotherapy remain the main weapons in the fight against cancer, a new trend began in the 1960s: namely, the principle of boosting the natural defenses. In support of this principle the National Cancer Institute established a *Biological Response Modifier Program* (47). Literally dozens of new ideas came to be tested, in animals and humans; we mention a few.

Nonspecific Stimulation of the Immune System
Various bacterial preparations such as BCG, an attenuated strain of *Mycobacterium tuberculosis*, were given systemically or locally in the tumor. After many trials with mixed results the method was abandoned, with the exception of intravesical injections for the treatment of superficial bladder cancer (31, 58).

Lymphokine Activation of Killer Cells The principle is to expand and activate a patient's population of cytotoxic cells by means of interleukin-2 (IL-2) (59, 60). We mention it here as a highly imaginative effort in the war against cancer, but at the time of this writing, this approach has been largely abandoned because of its side effects.

Lymphokine-activated cells (LAK) can be produced either by infusing IL-2 directly into the blood, or by collecting lymphocytes from the patient's blood, treating them with IL-2 *in vitro* for 2 or 3 days, and then reinfusing them; or by doing the same with lymphocytes obtained from the patient's tumor (tumor-infiltrating lymphocytes, TIL). TIL give the best results (p. 938) (61). The nature of LAK cells seems to be a touchy subject among immunologists, but they are probably a mixture of NK, T, and B cells (48, 49) and perhaps

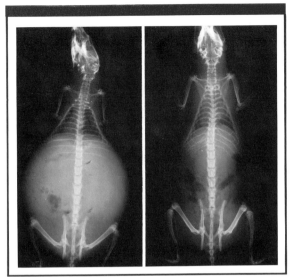

FIGURE 30.7
Ascites as part of
the vascular-leak
syndrome in-
duced by recom-
binant inter-
leukin-2. *Left*, a
rat treated with
IL-2 twice a day
for 14 days; *right*,
the control. (Re-
produced with
permission from
[3].)

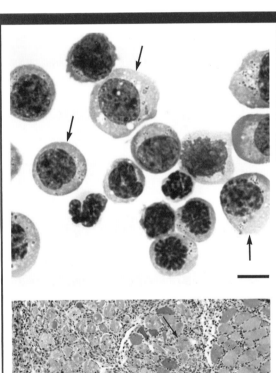

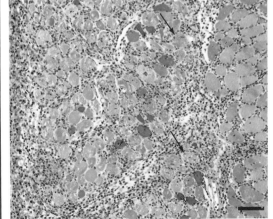

FIGURE 30.8
Effects of IL-2 ad-
ministered in-
traperitoneally to
rats and mice
twice daily for 7
days. *Top*: Large
granular lympho-
cytes (**arrows**) in
the pleural effu-
sion of a mouse.
Bar = 10 μm.
Bottom: Effect on
the abdominal
musculature and
peritoneum of
the rat. The cel-
lular infiltrate
consists mainly
of lymphocytes
and eosinophils.
Note muscular
damage (**ar-
rows**). **Bar** =
100 μm. (Repro-
duced with per-
mission from [3,
4].)

also macrophages (50). Most are large granular lymphocytes (suggesting NK cells), and their performance *in vitro* is impressive (see Figure 17.4) (67).

Tested on patients with advanced metastatic disease, the LAK and TIL methods triggered striking regressions in some melanomas and renal cell carcinomas. One worrisome side-effect is edema due to a diffuse vascular leak syndrome (62); rats and mice treated with IL-2 developed the same syndrome (Figure 30.7) (5), and infiltrates of lymphocytes and eosinophils appeared throughout the body (Figure 30.8). The vascular leakage is attributed to activation of venular endothelium by IL-2 and IL-2-generated cytokines (4, 17). A major threat is pulmonary edema: the LAK and TIL cells, being activated, are stiffer; therefore they tend to become trapped in the capillaries of the lung rather than reaching their intended target, the tumor (34a).

This is disappointing, but there is hope for another cytokine: **interleukin 12** (IL-12), a product of macrophages and B lymphocytes which also activates cytotoxic T lymphocytes and NK cells. Injected intraperitoneally in tumor-bearing mice, it has a powerful antitumor and even anti-metastatic effect (12a). True, an intraperitoneal injection is not very different from an intravenous injection, and thus one might run into the side-effects mentioned above (the vascular leak syndrome and lung edema). However, *interleukin 12 has been effective also when applied locally*: injected around mouse tumors it caused them to disappear. Local injections should be able to circumvent the danger of body-wide effects. Time will tell.

Injection with Anticancer "Vaccines" The term *anticancer vaccine* is actually used in two ways. It can mean true preventive vaccination with viral preparations against cancers linked to viruses, but a different approach is being tried in patients who already have a cancer. Cells from their own tumor are harvested, irradiated to stop growth, and reinjected with BCG or other bacterial preparations. Cyclophosphamide is also given to suppress the T-suppressor cells (42). Some tumors have responded with striking regression (Figure 30.9) (7). Note that the example illustrated concerns once again melanoma, a tumor that is especially prone to elicit an immune response. One problem with melanomas, however, is their small size, which limits the volume of tissue available for making the vaccine.

We have already mentioned the recent approach of vaccinating mice and humans with peptides obtained from tumoral mutated proteins (p.887).

Many other biological treatments are being tried in mice and a few also in people. Interferons have been rather disappointing (21, 33, 46) except interferon-alpha-2a for treating life-threatening hemangiomas in infants (23). Macrophages activated with liposomes have eradicated experimental metastases (24, 25). Antitumor-antibodies coupled with drugs or radioactive nuclides hold some promise due to their theoretically unbeatable specificity (52); however, they also run into a formidable series of obstacles: (1) only a fraction of the injected antibody reaches its target because the endothelial barrier stands between the antibody and the tumor; (2) injected antibodies are antigenic; and (3) the antibodies are quickly removed by the system of mononuclear phagocytes.

TO SUM UP: Natural antitumor defenses are many, and as we learn about them we can attempt to copy them for therapy. But once again, we are faced with the problem of tumor personality: some tumors are fair targets for the immune response, others seem to be shielded against it. Corticoids, typical anti-inflammatory agents, induce many childhood hemangiomas to regress (72), but lung carcinomas to progress (72).

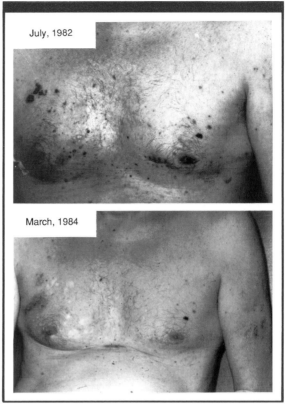

July, 1982

March, 1984

FIGURE 30.9 Regression of metastases from malignant melanoma after a double treatment: cyclophosphamide, to suppress the T-suppressor cells, which inhibit the antitumor response; and autologous vaccine against melanoma. (The residual pigmented lesion on the left breast is a benign and probably dysplastic nevus.) (Reproduced with permission from [7].)

References

1. Abersold P. Antiproliferative effects of interferon. In: Ransom JH, Ortaldo JR, eds. Leukolysins and cancer. Clifton, NJ: Human Press, 1987:101–117.
2. An T, Sood U, Pietruk T, Cummings G, Hashimoto K, Crissman JD. In situ quantitation of inflammatory mononuclear cells in ductal infiltrating breast carcinoma. Relation to prognostic parameters. Am J Pathol 1987;128:52–60.
3. Anderson TD, Hayes TJ. Toxicity of human recombinant interleukin-2 in rats. Pathologic changes are characterized by marked lymphocytic and eosinophilic proliferation and multisystem involvement. Lab Invest 1989;60:331–346.
4. Anderson TD, Hayes TJ, Gately MK, Bontempo JM, Stern LL, Truitt GA. Toxicity of human recombinant interleukin-2 in the mouse is mediated by interleukin-activated lymphocytes. Separation of efficacy and toxicity by selective lymphocyte subset depletion. Lab Invest 1988;59:598–612.
5. Banner BF, Sonmez-Alpan E, Yousem SA. An immunophenotypic study of the inflammatory cell populations in colon adenomas and carcinomas. Mod Pathol 1993;6:295–301.
6. Ben-Ezra J, Sheibani K. Antigenic phenotype of the lymphocytic component of medullary carcinoma of the breast. Cancer 1987;59:2037–2041.
7. Berd D, Maguire HC Jr, Mastrangelo MJ. Induction of cell-mediated immunity to autologous melanoma cells and regression of metastases after treatment with a melanoma cell vaccine preceded by cyclophosphamide. Cancer Res 1986;46:2572–2577.
8. Berd D, Mastrangelo MJ. Active immunotherapy of human melanoma exploiting the immunopotentiating effects of cyclophosphamide. Cancer Invest 1988a;6:337–349.
9. Berd D, Mastrangelo MJ. Effect of low dose cyclophosphamide on the immune system of cancer patients: depletion of CD4+, 2H4+ suppressor-induced T-cells. Cancer Res 1988b;48:1671–1675.
10. Bierman HR, Crile DM, Dod KS, et al. Remissions in leukemia of childhood following acute infectious disease. Cancer 1953;6:591–605.
11. Boutwell RK. Some biological aspects of skin carcinogenesis. Prog Exp Tumor Res 1964;4:207–250.
12. Broder S, Waldmann TA. The suppressor-cell network in cancer (first of two parts). N Engl J Med 1978;299:1281–1284.
12a. Brunda MJ, Luistro L, Warner RR, Wright RB, Hubbard BR, Murphy M, Wolf SF, Gately MK. Antitumor and antimetastatic activity of interleukin 12 against murine tumors. J Exp Med 1993;178:1223–1230.
13. Burnet FM. Self and not-self. Carleton, Victoria, Australia: Melbourne University Press, 1969.
14. Burnet FM. The concept of immunological surveillance. Prog Exp Tumor Res 1970;13:1–27.
15. Chapman HA Jr, Hibbs JB Jr. Modulation of macrophage tumoricidal capability by components of normal serum: a central role for lipid. Science 1977;197:282–285.

16. Chevallier B, Asselain B, Kunlin A, Veyret C, Bastit P, Graic Y. Inflammatory breast cancer. Determination of prognostic factors by univariate and multivariate analysis. Cancer 1987;60:897–902.

17. Cotran RS, Pober JS, Gimbrone MA Jr, et al. Endothelial activation during interleukin 2 immunotherapy. A possible mechanism for the vascular leak syndrome. J Immunol 1987;139:1883–1888.

18. Da Fano C. Zelluläre Analyse der Geschwulstimmunitätsreaktionen. Z Immunitätsforsch 1910;5:1–74.

19. Deem RL, Targan SR. Natural killer cell cytotoxic factor. In: Ransom JH, Ortaldo JR, eds. Leukolysins and cancer. Clifton, NJ: Human Press, 1987:149–165.

20. Elliott BE, Carlow DA, Rodricks A-M, Wade A. Perspectives on the role of MHC antigens in normal and malignant cell development. Adv Cancer Res 1989;53:181–245.

21. Eron LJ, Judson F, Tucker S, et al. Interferon therapy for condylomata acuminata. N Engl J Med 1986;315:1059–1064.

22. Evans R. Tumor macrophages in host immunity to malignancies. In: Fink MA, ed. The macrophage in neoplasia. New York: Academic Press, 1976:27–42.

23. Ezekowitz RAB, Mulliken JB, Folkman J. Interferon alfa-2a therapy for life-threatening hemangiomas of infancy. N Engl J Med 1992;326:1456–1463.

24. Fidler IJ. Macrophage therapy of cancer metastasis. Ciba Found Symp 1988;141:211–222.

25. Fidler IJ, Schroit AJ. Recognition and destruction of neoplastic cells by activated macrophages: discrimination of altered self. Biochim Biophys Acta 1988;948:151–173.

26. Fink MP, Parker CW, Shearer WT. Antibody stimulation of tumour growth in T-cell depleted mice. Nature 1975;255:404–405.

27. Fontan E, Saklani H, Fauve RM. Macrophage-induced cytotoxicity and anti-metastatic activity of a 43-kDa human urinary protein against the Lewis tumor. Int J Cancer 1993;53:131–136.

27a. Graeber TG, Peterson JF, Tsai M, Monica K, Fornace Jr AJ, Giaccia AJ. Hypoxia induces accumulation of p53 protein, but activation of a G_1-phase checkpoint by low-oxygen conditions is independent of p53 status. Mol Cell Biol 1994;6264–6277.

27b. Graeber TG, Osmanian C, Jacks T, Housman DE, Koch CJ, Lowe SW, Giaccia AJ. Hypoxia-mediated selection of cells with diminished apoptotic potential in solid tumours. Nature 1996;379:88–91.

28. Graves DT, Jiang YL, Williamson MJ, Valente AJ. Identification of monocyte chemotactic activity produced by malignant cells. Science 1989;245:1490–1493.

28a. Greenblatt MS, Bennett WP, Hollstein M, Harris CC. Mutations in the p53 tumor suppressor gene: clues to cancer etiology and molecular pathogenesis. Cancer Res 1994;54:4855–4878.

29. Gross L. Oncogenic viruses, vol 2, 3rd ed. Oxford: Pergamon Press, 1983.

30. Gugel EA, Sanders ME. Needle-stick transmission of human colonic adenocarcinoma. N Engl J Med 1986;315:1487.

31. Guinan P, Crispen R, Rubenstein M. BCG in management of superficial bladder cancer. Urology 1987;30:515–519.

32. Haskill S, Becker S, Fowler W, Walton L. Mononuclear-cell infiltration in ovarian cancer. I. Inflammatory-cell infiltrates from tumour and ascites material. Br J Cancer 1982;45:728–736.

33. Healy GB, Gelver RD, Trowbridge AL, Grundfast KM, Ruben RJ, Price KN. Treatment of recurrent respiratory papillomatosis with human leukocyte interferon. Results of a multicenter randomized clinical trial. N Engl J Med 1988;319:401–407.

34. Hevin MB, Friguet B, Fauve RM. Inflammation and anti-tumor resistance. V. Production of a cytostatic factor following cooperation of elicited polymorphonuclear leukocytes and macrophages. Int J Cancer 1990;46:533–538.

34a. Jain RK. Delivery of molecules, particles and cells to solid tumors (Whitaker Lecture). Annal of Biomed 1996 (in press).

34b. Kerr JFR, Winterford CM. Apoptosis. Cancer 1994;73:2013–2026.

35. Klein G. Tumor immunology. Transplant Proc 1973;5:31–41.

36. Klein G. Immune and non-immune control of neoplastic development: contrasting effects of host and tumor evolution. Cancer 1980;45:2486–2499.

37. Koretz K, Moldenhauer G, Majdic O, Möller P. Correlation of HLA-D/Ii antigen expression in breast carcinoma with local lymphohistiocytic infiltration reveals considerable dysregulation in a subset of tumors. Int J Cancer 1989;44:816–822.

38. Kreider DW, Bartlett GL. Is there a host response to metastasis? Prog Clin Biol Res 1986;212:61–75.

39. Kripe ML. Immunoregulation of carcinogenesis: past, present and future. J Natl Cancer Inst 1988;80:722–727.

39a. Lane DP, Lu X, Hupp T, Hall PA. The role of the p53 protein in the apoptotic response. Phil Trans R Soc Lond B 1994;345:277–280.

40. Lester EP, Miller JB, Yachnin S. Human alpha-fetoprotein as a modulator of human lymphocyte transformation: correlation of biological potency with electrophoretic variants. Proc Natl Acad Sci USA 1976;73:4645–4648.

41. Liebelt AG. Malignant neoplasms in organ transplant recipients. In: Levine AS, ed. Etiology of cancer in man. Dordrecht: Kluwer Academic Publishers, 1989:136–167.

41a. Lynch SA, Houghton AN. Cancer Immunology. Curr Opin Oncol 1993;5:145–150.

41b. Mandelboim O, Vadai E, Fridkin M, Katz-Hillel A, Feldman M, Berke G, Eisenbach L. Regression of Established Murine Carcinoma Metastases Following Vaccination with Tumor-Associated Antigen Peptides. Nature Med 1995;1:1179–1183.

42. Marx JL. Cancer vaccines show promise at last. Science 1989;245:813–815.

42a. Marx J. Oncogenes Reach a Milestone. Science 1994;266:1942–1944.

43. Okabayashi M, Angell MG, Budgeon LR, Kreider JW. Shope papilloma cell and leukocyte proliferation in regressing and progressing lesions. Am J Pathol 1993;142:489–496.

44. Old LJ. Cancer immunology. Sci Am 1977;236:62–79.

45. Old LJ, Boyse EA, Clarke DA, Carswell EA: Antigenic properties of chemically induced tumors. Ann NY Acad Sci 1962;101:80–106.

46. Oldham RK. Biologicals for cancer treatment: interferons. Hosp Pract 1985;20:71–91.

47. Oldham RK, Smalley RV. Immunotherapy: the old and the new. J Biol Response Mod 1983;2:1–37.

48. Ortaldo JR, Longo DL. Human natural lymphocyte effector cells: definition, analysis of activity, and clinical effectiveness. J Natl Cancer Inst 1988;80:999–1010.

49. Peace DJ, Cheever MA. Toxicity and therapeutic efficacy of high-dose interleukin 2. In vivo infusion of antibody to NK-1.1 attenuates toxicity without compromising efficacy against murine leukemia. J Exp Med 1989;169:161–173.

50. Perussia B. Tumor infiltrating cells. Lab Invest 1992;67:155–157.

51. Piessens WF, David J. VIII. Tumor immunology. In:

Rubenstein E, Federman DD, eds. Scientific American medicine. New York: Scientific American, 1990:1–9.

52. Pimm MV. Drug-monoclonal antibody conjugates for cancer therapy: potentials and limitations. CRC Crit Rev Ther Drug Carrier Systems 1988;5:189–227.

53. Pitot HC. Fundamentals of oncology, 3rd ed. New York: Marcel Dekker, 1986.

53a. Porter PL, Gown AM, Kramp SG, Coltrera MD. Widespread p53 Overexpression in Human Malignant Tumors. Am J Pathol 1992;140:145–153.

54. Poste G. The tumoricidal properties of inflammatory tissue macrophages and multinucleate giant cells. Am J Pathol 1979;96:595–610.

55. Prehn RT. Immunostimulation of the lymphodpendent phase of neoplastic growth. J Natl Cancer Inst 1977;59: 1043–1049.

56. Purtilo DT. Pathogenesis and phenotypes of an X-linked recessive lymphoproliferative syndrome. Lancet 1976;2: 882–885.

57. Purtilo DT. Defective immune surveillance in viral carcinogenesis. Lab Invest 1984;51:373–385.

58. Raghavan D, Shipley WU, Garnick MB, Russell PJ, Richie JP. Biology and management of bladder cancer. N Engl J Med 1990;322:1129–1138.

59. Rosenberg SA. Adoptive immunotherapy for cancer. Sci Am 1990;262:62–69.

60. Rosenberg SA, Lotze MT, Muul LM, et al. A progress report on the treatment of 157 patients with advanced cancer using lymphokine-activated killer cells and interleukin-2 or high-dose interleukin-2 alone. N Engl J Med 1987;316:889–897.

61. Rosenberg SA, Spiess P, Lafreniere R. A new approach to the adoptive immunotherapy of cancer with tumor-infiltrating lymphocytes. Science 1986;233:1318–1321.

62. Rosenstein M, Ettinghausen SE, Rosenberg SA. Extravasation of intravascular fluid mediated by the systemic administration of recombinant interleukin 2. J Immunol 1986;137:1735–1742.

63. Ruckdeschel JC, Codish SD, Stranahan A, McKneally MF. Postoperative empyema improves survival in lung cancer. Documentation and analysis of a natural experiment. N Engl J Med 1972;287:1013–1017.

64. Russell SW, Gillespie GY, Pace JL. Evidence for mononuclear phagocytes in solid neoplasms and appraisal of their nonspecific cytotoxic capabilities. Contemp Top Immunobiol 1980;10:143–166.

65. Scanlon EF, Hawkins RA, Fox WW, Smith WS. Fatal homotransplanted melanoma. A case report. Cancer 1965;18:782–789.

66. Storkus WJ, Dawson JR. Target structures involved in natural killing (NK): characteristics, distribution, and candidate molecules. Crit Rev Immunol 1991;10:393–416.

66a. Strominger JL. Peptide vaccination against cancer? Nature Med 1995;1:1140.

66b. Symonds H, Krall L, Remington L, Saenz-Robies M, Lowe S, Jacks T, Van Dyke T. Dependent apoptosis supresses tumor growth and progression in vivo. Cell 1994;78:703–711.

67. Tanaka H, Watanabe M, Zeniya M, Takahashi H. Ultrastructure of IL2-stimulated tumor-infiltrating lymphocytes showing cytolytic activity against tumor cells. Acta Pathol Jpn 1991;41:94–105.

68. Uchida A. Antitumor monocyte cytotoxic factors (MCF) produced by human blood monocytes: production, characterization, and biological significance. In: Ransom JH, Ortaldo JR, eds. Leukolysins and cancer. Clifton, NJ: Human Press, 1987:87–99.

69. van Ravenswaay Claasen HH, Kluin PPM, Fleuren GJ. Tumor infiltrating cells in human cancer: on the possible role of CD16+ macrophages in antitumor cytotoxicity. Lab Invest 1992;67:166–174.

69a. Wahl AF, Donaldson KL, Fairchild C, Lee FYF, Foster SA, Demers GW, Galloway DA. Loss of normal p53 function confers sensitization to Taxol by increasing G2/M arrest and apoptosis. Nature Med 1996;2:72–79.

70. Weissler JC, Lipscomb MF, Lem VM, Toews GB. Tumor killing by human alveolar macrophages and blood monocytes. Decreased cytotoxicity of human alveolar macrophages. Am Rev Respir Dis 1986;134:532–537.

71. Wright SC, Bonavida B. Human and rodent natural killer cytotoxic factors (NKCF): characterization and their role in the NK lytic mechanism. In: Ransom JH, Ortaldo JR, eds. Leukolysins and cancer. Clifton, NJ: Human Press, 1987:121–135.

72. Yesner R. A pathologist's view of tumor dormancy. In: Stewart THM, Wheelock EF, eds. Cellular immune mechanisms and tumor dormancy. Boca Raton, FL: CRC Press, 1992.

73. Young JD-E, Cohn ZA. How killer cells kill. Sci Am 1988;258:38–44.

74. Yunis AA, Arimura GK, Wu F-M, Wu M-C. Differentiation of cultured promyelocytic leukemia cells (HL-60) induced by endotoxin-treated human lung conditioned medium. Leukemia Res 1987;11:673–679.

The Reversibility
of Tumors

CHAPTER 31

> Spontaneous Regression
> of Tumors
>
> Tumor Regression in
> the Laboratory

For the reader who is weary of invasion, metastasis, and other nefarious events, this chapter offers some measure of relief. Yes, there is a great deal to say about the reversibility of tumors; in fact this chapter includes experiments as thrilling as any reported in this book. They should demolish the notion that tumors are invincible monsters.

By regression of a tumor we mean shrinkage, which may or may not lead to total disappearance. Some regressions are temporary. Regressing tumors have been observed in the laboratory and in medical practice. The most intriguing regressions are those that occur in the absence of therapy; they are called spontaneous. However, it is well to remember that the label *spontaneous* is applied to biological events for which we do not know the cause.

Spontaneous Regression of Tumors

There is one tumor that regresses spontaneously in most patients (80–90 percent): the hemangioma of infants, which occurs in 2.6 percent of newborns. It usually appears within 2–4 weeks of birth, grows very fast, begins to regress, and is gone by age 10, usually leaving a scar (Figure 31.1) (32,33). Most cases are managed without treatment other than a great deal of time spent reassuring parents (3). Unfortunately, 100 percent reassurance is not appropriate because a minority of hemangiomas, unpredictably, do not regress. Nor is the mechanism of regression understood, except that it is not thrombosis or infarction; the endothelial channels just seem to fade away. Herein lies a great challenge.

Anecdotal but reliable records of malignant tumors that disappeared without treatment are at least 100 years old. The collected series of 176 regressions published between 1900 and 1966 includes transient regressions (7,8,13,34,35). Most of the cases listed concern renal cell carcinoma (31), neuroblastoma (29), melanoma (19), choriocarcinoma (19), and carcinoma of the bladder (13). In 41 cases, metastases regressed after resection of the primary. Documented malignant tumors that disappeared boil down to a few.

> *An example: two patients underwent palliative operations for carcinoma of the stomach without resection; the tumor masses disappeared and the patients were well 10 and 11 years later (7). Considering that gastric cancer allows a 5-year survival of 5–17 percent, the reported survival itself is remarkable; as to the disappearance of the tumors, it is close to miraculous.*

Certain types of tumors are more likely to regress than others, especially the first four in the list just given. The mechanisms of regression are probably different for each tumor. Consider the cases of neuroblastoma and melanoma.

Neuroblastomas in infants can change from malignant to benign, metastases included. Neuroblastomas can develop anywhere in the sympathetic nervous system, but usually in the adrenal, and many have metastasized by the time they are diagnosed. Neuroblasts as seen by electron microscopy contain typical neurosecretory granules (p. 933). By light microscopy they are dull-looking small round cells; but they become much more

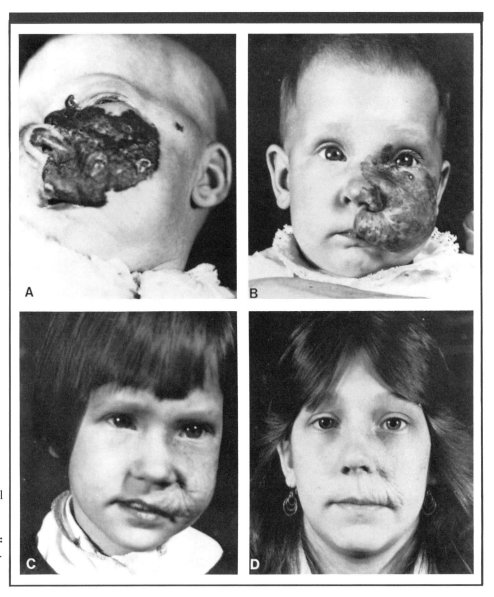

FIGURE 31.1
Spontaneous regression of a hemangioma, a well-known phenomenon, in a child who appeared normal
at birth. **A:** At 2 months a hemangioma appeared on the left side
of the face. No therapy was given **B:**
Same child at 1 year. **C:** At 5 years.
D: At 14 years. (Reproduced with
permission from [33].)

interesting when they mature into neurons with
axons and dendrites (Figure 31.2). The fully
differentiated tumors are called *ganglioneuromas.*
This type of regression obviously amounts to
differentiation. It can occur spontaneously in
children; for example, tumor tissue left behind by
the surgeon rarely causes a relapse. However, the
prognosis remains poor because the tumor is often
diagnosed too late (44). This fascinating—and
frustrating—behavior of neuroblastomas has inspired a great deal of research.

> *Interestingly, the first known case of regressed
> neuroblastoma, published in 1927 (9), concerned a
> child who had been treated with the "toxins" of the
> now-famous Dr. Coley mentioned on p. 353. From*

> *what we know now, that particular tumor might have
> regressed anyway.*

Melanoma deserves special mention because,
despite its fearful reputation, which is well deserved, it displays ambivalent behavior. The primary tumor can regress partially or even completely, which explains the occasional finding of
metastatic melanoma in the absence of a primary
melanoma (which went unnoticed and then disappeared). In a review of 5000 cases of melanoma,
regression of metastases occurred in 2.2 cases per
1000 (34). Some of the events preceding the
regression of metastases are intriguing:

- pregnancy (an immunosuppressive condition)

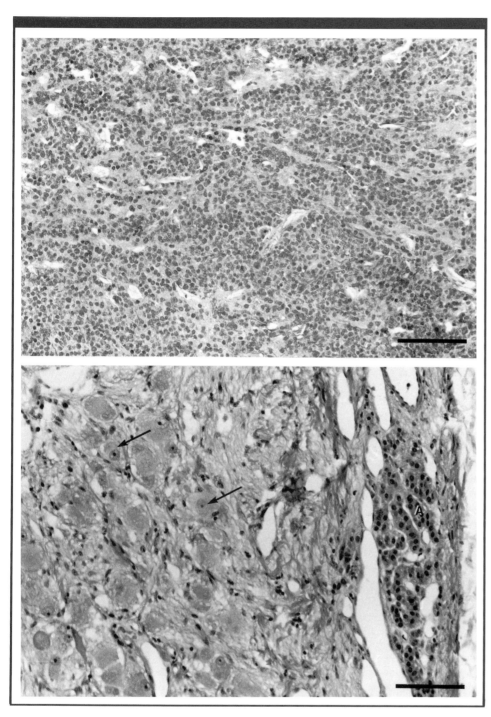

FIGURE 31.2
Spontaneous differentiation of a neuroblastoma of the adrenal. *Top:* Biopsy of a neuroblastoma in an 8-year-old girl. *Bottom:* The same tumor 4 years later. The bulk of the tumor (left) is now represented by mature neurons (**arrows**). Remnants of the atrophic adrenal are seen at the right (**A**). **Bars** = 100 µm.

- an abscess near the tumor
- a bite by a rabid dog followed by 14 injections of antirabies vaccine
- blood transfusion from a patient who had shown regression of skin metastases from a melanoma (7)
- consumption of a lot of garlic (34) (for another reference to garlic and tumors see p. 826).

Overall, regression of melanoma suggests an immunologic mechanism, a concept that is being exploited for therapy (p. 893).

A rare mechanism of spontaneous regression and "cure" has been described for retinoblastoma: occlusion of the central retinal blood supply and infarction of the entire tumor. Retinoblastomas occasionally differentiate into mature, benign retinomas or retinocytomas (46).

Tumor Regression in the Laboratory

The first steps along this trail take us back to the Rockefeller Institute in 1940. Rous and Kidd, who had tarred many a rabbit, wrote that tar carcinomas were preceded by warty growths that had the histological appearance of tumors, including local invasiveness, but vanished if tarring was discontinued. Rous and Kidd concluded that these tumors, which they called papillomas or "carcinomatoids," had not yet acquired the capacity for independent growth; they disappeared "when no longer aided."

Judging from the published illustrations, the disappearance was accomplished by epithelial differentiation into keratinized masses (Figure 31.3). This important observation was not followed up for decades; tumors that do not kill, like all good news, make no headlines. There seems to be something dull about benign tumors. As Rous put it, "cancers outdo them in material interest" (47).

Then several mind-boggling experiments proved that established malignant tumors could be reversed. We will list six, the first one from the plant kingdom.

The Crown Gall As mentioned on p. 837 the crown gall is a malignant tumor of plants. It is created by a bacterium that operates along the classic principles of genetic engineering. The plant must be wounded and then infected with *Agrobacterium*. If we choose the right experimental conditions, it is possible to produce a type of tumor appropriately called a *teratoma*, a chaotic mass of partly developed tissues and organs. It is a fully malignant tumor, capable of growing (like other malignant crown gall tumors) on a simple culture medium that would not support the growth of normal cells (4,5). Now, if we graft a fragment of teratoma onto the tip of the stem of a normal, severed tobacco plant, the graft will grow; but it will be partially tamed into a less abnormal tissue. Graft this tissue onto a second stem, and then again onto a third one; now the tumor growth will gradually develop into a normal plant that will flower and go to seed. The seeds will produce normal tobacco plants (Figure 31.4).

From these and other experiments, Armin Braun concluded that the original tumor was probably not caused by damage to the DNA (such as by mutation) but by altered expression of the genome. Another way to interpret these results would be that the environment of a growing normal

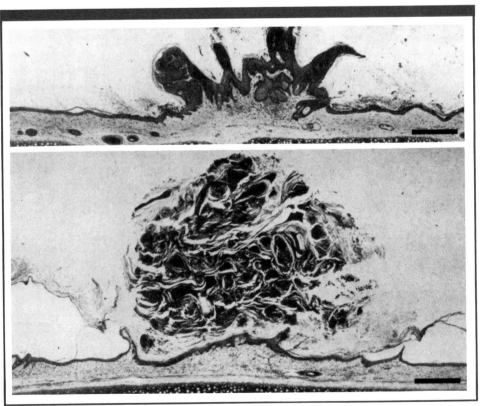

FIGURE 31.3
Histology of papillomas produced with tar in the rabbit ear; original illustrations published by Rous and Kidd in 1941. *Top:* Growing papilloma. *Bottom:* "Superficial carcinomatoid in the process of retrogression." Tarring had been stopped 24 days previously; the cells then turned into "normal" differentiated keratinized cells, indicating a reversion of the neoplasm to normal. Rous and Kidd called these tumors "conditional neoplasms." **Bars** = 500 μm. (Reproduced with permission from [47].)

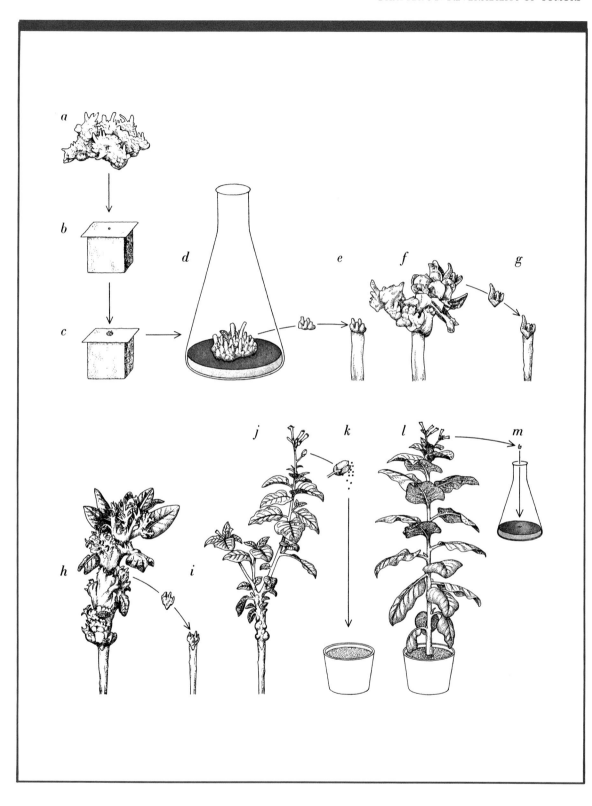

FIGURE 31.4 Reversal of malignant growth in plants. Teratoma from a tobacco plant (**a**) provides a single tumor cell (**b**) that is grown *in vitro* (**c**); in (**d**) the tissue is grown in a basic culture medium where it forms typical teratoma buds and leaves. One of the buds is then grafted onto the cut stem of a normal tobacco plant (**e**) and allowed to develop (**f**). A bud from this abnormal growth is grafted to a second normal plant (**g**) and allowed to develop again (**h**). A bud from the second plant grafted onto a third host (**i**) gradually becomes normal; it flowers (**j**) and goes to seed (**k**). Tobacco plants raised from this seed (**l**) are completely normal. Their cells do not grow on the basic medium (**m**). (Reproduced with permission from [4].)

tissue was able to control the cellular misbehavior encoded in a faulty DNA. This theme will recur.

A Tadpole Grown from a Tumor Let us proceed to frogs. In the northern United States, roughly 5 percent of common leopard frogs (*Rana pipiens*) suffer from a virus-induced tumor of the kidney known as *Lucké adenocarcinoma* (Figure 31.5) (25–27,29,31). In 1960, King and McKinnell (and later others) obtained fresh eggs from leopard

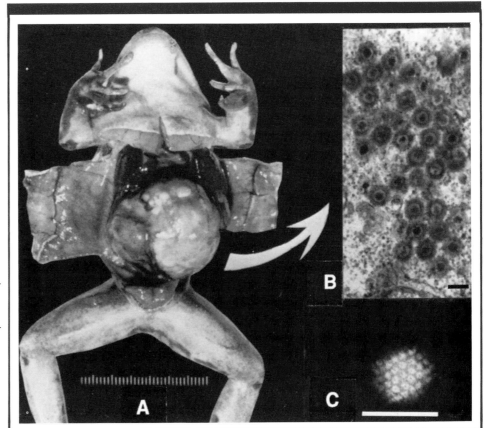

FIGURE 31.5

A: Frog bearing a large malignant tumor of the kidney (Lucké renal adenocarcinoma). **B:** Electron micrograph showing virus particles (herpes type) in the cytoplasm of a cell from this tumor. **Bar** = 0.2 μm. **C:** Electron micrograph of a negatively stained virus particle showing detail of the capsomere. **Bar** = 0.2 μm. (Reproduced with permission from [31].)

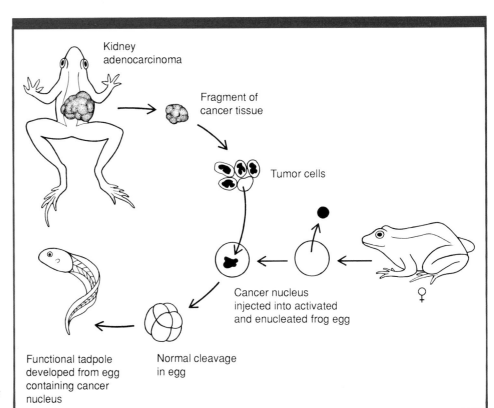

FIGURE 31.6

Diagram of an experiment showing that a tadpole can be born of a frog egg in which the nucleus had been replaced by a nucleus from a malignant frog tumor (adenocarcinoma of Lucké).

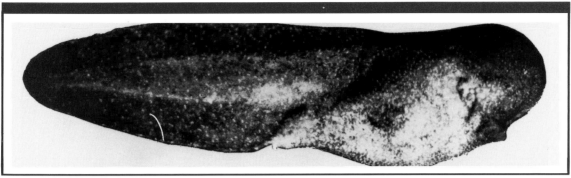

FIGURE 31.7
Historic tadpole produced by the experiment shown in Figure 31.6. Such tadpoles do not survive to become frogs, but they do live up to 10–14 days. (Reproduced with permission from [27].)

frogs, fertilized them, then removed their nucleus and replaced it with a nucleus from a malignant cell of a Lucké adenocarcinoma (Figure 31.6). A few of the eggs did develop. What did they produce? More adenocarcinomas? Tadpoles loaded with tumors? Neither. They produced tadpoles (Figure 31.7) (27). These miraculous creatures did not live beyond 10–14 days, perhaps because their foster nucleus had lost the next part of the program, but they certainly made history.

This experiment was criticized because—in theory—some of the original nuclear material could have been inadvertently left behind. This objection was met by using triploid tumors and diploid eggs; the result: triploid tadpoles (26).

The method for producing triploid tadpoles is most imaginative: a bout of very high hydrostatic pressure on the fertilized egg prevents the extrusion of the second polar body (10).

Conclusion: The malignant nucleus was tamed by the cytoplasm of the fertilized egg. Therefore, in triggering neoplasia, the cytoplasm can be as important as the nucleus. The cytoplasm could exert its influence by modifying gene expression. By definition, this type of nongenetic influence is called epigenetic.

A Mouse Grown from a Tumor A parallel experiment has been done with mouse teratocarcinomas.

We should first describe these complex tumors as they appear in mice. They contain 8–14 different mature cell types as well as undifferentiated malignant cells known as embryonal carcinoma cells (Figure 31.8) (22,38,43). There are two amazing features about these tumors: they can be produced by implanting a

mouse embryo in the testis of another mouse (51), and then they can be maintained as an ascites tumor by passing them from one mouse peritoneum to another. As the malignant cells grow freely in the serosal cavity, they produce small cystic structures that look very much like rudimentary embryos and are called embryoid bodies (Figures 31.9, 31.10).

With considerable patience and skill, R.L. Brinster in Philadelphia, in 1974, injected teratocarcinoma cells into early mouse embryos (blastocysts) obtained from pregnant white mice (6). Then he reintroduced the blastocysts into the uterus of pseudopregnant foster mothers (i.e., mice mated with a vasectomized male) and waited. The result: 137 normal mice, including one obvious chimera with stripes of dark hairs that could only have derived from the tumor; the pattern recalled the zebra-like allophenic mice derived from the fusion of two embryos (p. 755). In essence, the tumor had fathered part of a mouse. We would like to say "half of a mouse," but the level of chimerism is low (36) and can regress with time (52).

Several other groups confirmed these experiments (40) using sophisticated genetic markers for identifying tumor-derived cells while maintaining the principle of deriving the original teratoma from dark-haired mice and using blastocysts of white mice (30,36,37,40,52). The experimental plan is summarized in Figure 31.11 (30). It turned out that some chimeric mice were born with teratocarcinomas or developed these or other malignant tumors in later life (36,37).

From his pioneer experiments, Brinster concluded that "the embryo environment can bring under control the autonomous proliferation of the malignant cells" (6). G.B. Pierce went one step

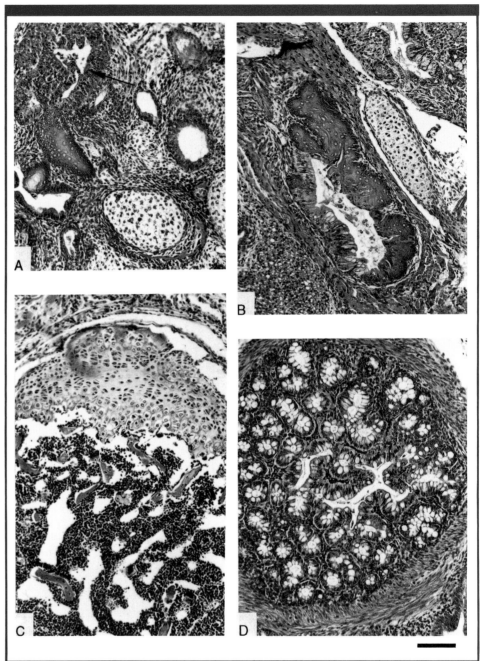

FIGURE 31.8
Examples of differentiation found in a testicular teratocarcinoma of the mouse: **A:** Undifferentiated embryonal carcinoma (**arrow**) and cartilage. **B:** Cartilage, squamous and disorganized glandular epithelium. **C:** Cartilaginous cap with endochondral ossification including bone and bone marrow. **D:** Glands surrounded by muscle, found in masses of neural tissue. (Reproduced with permission from [42].)

further and proposed that *tumors can be "reversed" by differentiation,* a concept of tremendous importance (p. 924).

Suppression of Malignancy by Cell Fusion The result of fusing normal and malignant cells has been debated, but the matter is now clear: if a malignant cell is fused with a normal fibroblast of the same species, the resulting hybrid cell does not generate tumors as long as certain critical chromosomes are not eliminated (15,16,

21,54–56). Therefore, under these experimental conditions, malignancy behaves as a recessive trait.

Hybridomas (23) *may be an exception to the recessiveness of malignancy. They are crosses between myelomas and normal lymphocytes, yet behave like tumors (p. 452). The reason is not clear, but hybridomas do show chromosomal losses, and it may also be that fusion of a malignant cell with a fibroblast may not be equivalent to fusion with a lymphocyte (16).*

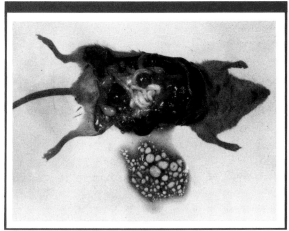

FIGURE 31.9
Mouse injected intraperitoneally 4 weeks previously with cells of a teratocarcinoma; this tumor forms large vesicular embryoid bodies, which grow freely in the peritoneum. A mass of these bodies is shown next to the animal. (Reproduced with permission from [39].)

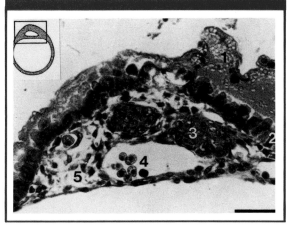

FIGURE 31.10
From a cystic embryoid body of a mouse teratocarcinoma. *Inset:* Scheme of an embryoid body; the rectangle shows the topography of the micrograph. **1:** Precipitated ascites fluid. **2:** Endoderm covering the embryoid body. **3:** Clumps of teratocarcinoma. **4:** Sinus containing hematopoietic cells. **5:** Mesenchyme. (Reproduced with permission from [41].)

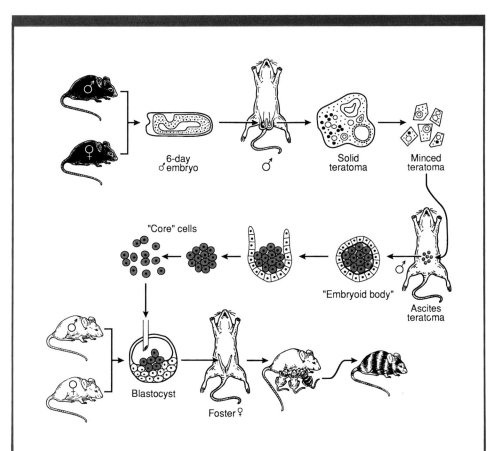

FIGURE 31.11
Summary of an experiment showing that malignant cells from a teratoma can be coaxed into taking part in the growth and development of a normal animal. First, a teratoma is produced by implanting a 6-day embryo (from a couple of black mice) under the testicular capsule of a mouse. The teratoma is then grown as an ascites tumor in the peritoneum where it produces vast numbers of embryoid bodies. The inner core of an embryoid body is implanted in the blastocyst obtained from two white parents. The blastocyst is then transferred to the uterus of a pseudopregnant foster mother where it gives rise to a normal mouse with a striped coat, showing that it is a mosaic. (Adapted from [30].)

Following this line of experimentation; we note that fusion of a malignant cell with another type of malignant cell usually produces a malignant cell, but carcinoma–sarcoma and carcinoma–melanoma hybrids are nontumorigenic, which is interpreted as indicating that the ability to form tumors—in these types of cells—is governed by different loci (50).

The taming of malignancy by cell fusion *in vitro* is great news. Could this ever happen in real life, inside a tumor? Could tumor cells ever "mate" with normal cells? As Harris put it, the cells of the body do not normally engage in sex (14), but evidence of such a fusion (albeit as a rare event) was published by reputable groups (2,24,54). The type of host cell most likely to mate with a tumor cell seemed to be the macrophage.

These results have been criticized (45), but we believe that they are full of promise. In fact we have seen one tumor in which macrophages appeared to have "tamed" the cells of a carcinoma by fusing with them, as both cell types spread over cholesterol crystals (20a). There is reason to daydream about the possibility of forcing tumor cells to fuse with host cells. The daydream is tempered by a sobering thought: what if the hybrids lost the critical chromosomes and became even more malignant (11)?

Cybrids are the result of fusion of any whole cell and the enucleated cytoplasm (cytoplast) of another. Tests with cybrids have shown once again that the cytoplasm of a normal cell can suppress malignancy (18,19). The mechanism is not yet known; mitochondrial genetic material is one possibility. In one report, mouse leukemia cytoplasts, fused with human T and B cells, immortalized them without making them malignant (1).

Suppression of Malignancy by Introduction of Genes As mentioned earlier, some tumors—such as Wilms' tumor of the kidney (nephroblastoma), retinoblastoma, and some osteosarcomas—are brought about by the loss of a suppressor gene (p. 865). It stands to reason that if one of these malignant cell types is supplied with the missing suppressor gene, it should revert to its nonmalignant state. This is precisely what happens in elegant experiments that are feasible, alas, only *in vitro* (p. 869).

Suppression of Growth by Normal Cells This heading seems to contradict the obvious fact that malignancy begins among normal cells, but it is possible to demonstrate *in vitro* that a monolayer of fibroblasts stops the growth of certain malignant cells in contact with it (49). If all normal tissues could be induced to behave this way, there would be no tumors. Could this inspire another approach to tumor therapy?

Suppression of Growth by Differentiation Suppose that tumors consisted of immature cells that were still able to follow a maturation program. Then why not treat tumors with maturation factors? This is presently a hot area of research: we will return to this hopeful avenue on p. 924 (20,48).

At this point we hope the reader has acquired a new way to look at malignant cells. The beast can be tamed *in vitro*, and sometimes *in vivo*.

References

1. Abken H, Jungfer H, Albert WHW, Willecke K. Immortalization of human lymphocytes by fusion with cytoplasts of transformed mouse L cells. J Cell Biol 1986;103:795–805.
2. Ber R, Wiener F, Fenyö E-M. Proof of in vivo fusion of murine tumor cells with host cells by universal fusers: brief communication. J Natl Cancer Inst 1978;60:931–933.
3. Bingham HG. Predicting the course of a congenital hemangioma. Plast Reconst Surg 1979;63:161–166.
4. Braun AC. The reversal of tumor growth. Sci Am 1965;213:75–83.
5. Braun AC. The story of cancer. On its nature, causes, and control. Reading, MA: Addison-Wesley, 1977.
6. Brinster RL. The effect of cells transferred into the mouse blastocyst on subsequent development. J Exp Med 1974;140:1049–1056.
7. Cole WH. Spontaneous regression of cancer: the metabolic triumph of the host? Ann NY Acad Sci 1974;230:111–141.
8. Cole WH. Opening address: spontaneous regression of cancer and the importance of finding its cause. Natl Cancer Inst Monogr 1976;44:5–9.
9. Cushing H, Wolbach SB. The transformation of a malignant paravertebral sympathicoblastoma into a benign ganglioneuroma. Am J Pathol 1927;3:203–216.
10. Dasgupta S. Induction of triploidy by hydrostatic pressure in the leopard frog, *Rana pipiens*. J Exp Zool 1962;151:105–121.
11. De Baetselier P. Neoplastic progression by somatic cell infusion. In: Liotta LA, ed. Influence of tumor development on the host. Dordrecht: Kluwer Academic Publishers, 1989:112–120.
12. Dowdy SF, Fasching CL, Araujo D, et al. Suppression of tumorigenicity in Wilms tumor by the p15.5-p14 region of chromosome 11. Science 1991;254:293–295.
13. Everson TC, Cole WH. Spontaneous regression of malignant melanoma. In: Spontaneous regression of cancer. Philadelphia: WB Saunders, 1966:560.

14. Harris H. The Croonian lecture, 1971. Cell fusion and the analysis of malignancy. J Natl Cancer Inst 1972;48:851–864.

15. Harris H. The genetic analysis of malignancy. J Cell Sci Suppl 1986;4:431–444.

16. Harris H. The analysis of malignancy by cell fusion: the position in 1988. Cancer Res 1988;48:3302–3306.

17. Huang H-JS, Yee J-K, Shew J-Y, et al. Suppression of the neoplastic phenotype by replacement of the RB gene in human cancer cells. Science 1988;242:1563–1566.

18. Israel BA, Schaeffer WI. Cytoplasmic suppression of malignancy. In Vitro Cell Dev Biol 1987;23:627–632.

19. Iwakura Y, Nozaki M, Asano M, et al. Pleiotropic phenotypic expression in cybrids derived from mouse teratocarcinoma cells fused with ray myoblast cytoplasts. Cell 1985;43:777–791.

20. Jimenez JJ, Yunis AA. Tumor cell rejection through terminal cell differentiation. Science 1987;238:1278–1280.

20a. Kerschmann RL, Woda BA, Majno G. The fusion of tumor cells with host cells; reflections on an ovarian tumor: Persp Biol Med 1995;38:467–475.

21. Klein G, Bregula U, Wiener F, Harris H. The analysis of malignancy by cell fusion. I. Hybrids between tumour cells and L cell derivatives. J Cell Sci 1971;8:659–672.

22. Kleinsmith LJ, Pierce GB. Multipotentiality of single embryonal carcinoma cells. Cancer Res 1964;24:1544–1551.

23. Köhler G, Milstein C. Derivation of specific antibody-producing tissue culture and tumor lines by cell fusion. Eur J Immunol 1976;6:511–519.

24. Lala PK, Santer V, Rahil KS. Spontaneous fusion between Ehrlich ascites tumor cells and host cells in vivo: kinetics of hybridization, and concurrent changes in the histocompatibility profile of the tumor after propagation in different host strains. Eur J Cancer 1980;16:487–510.

25. Lucké B. A neoplastic disease of the kidney of the frog, Rana pipiens. Am J Cancer 1934;20:352–379.

26. McKinnell RG. Lucké renal adenocarcinoma: epidemiological aspects. In: Mizell M, ed. Biology of amphibian tumors. Recent Results in Cancer Research, Special Supplement. New York: Springer-Verlag, 1969:254–260.

27. McKinnell RG. Nuclear transfer in Xenopus and Rana compared. In: Harris R, Allin P, Viza D, eds. Cell Differentiation. Copenhagen: Munksgaard, 1972:61–64.

28. McKinnell RG, Deggins BA, Labat DD. Transplantation of pluripotential nuclei from triploid frog tumors. Science 1969;165:394–396.

29. McKinnell RG, Steven LM Jr, Labat DD. Frog renal tumors are composed of stroma, vascular elements and epithelial cells: what type nucleus programs for tadpoles with the cloning procedure? In: Müller-Bérat N, Rosenfeld C, Tarin D, Viza D, eds. Progress in differentiation research. Amsterdam: North Holland Publishing Company, 1976:319–330.

30. Mintz B, Illmensee K. Normal genetically mosaic mice produced from malignant teratocarcinoma cells. Proc Natl Acad Sci USA 1975;72:3585–3589.

31. Mizell M. Lucké frog carcinoma herpesvirus: transmission and expression during early development. Adv Viral Oncol 1985;5:129–146.

32. Mulliken JB. Cutaneous vascular lesions of children. In: Serafin D, Georgiade N, eds. Pediatric plastic surgery. St. Louis: CV Mosby, 1984:137–154.

33. Mulliken JB, Murray JE. Natural history of vascular birthmarks. In: Williams HB, ed. Symposium on vascular malformations and melanotic lesions. St. Louis: CV Mosby, 1983:58–73.

34. Nathanson L. Spontaneous regression of malignant melanoma: a review of the literature on incidence, clinical features, and possible mechanisms. Natl Cancer Inst Monogr 1976;44:67–76.

35. National Cancer Institute. Conference on spontaneous regression of cancer. Bethesda, MD: US Department of Health, Education and Welfare, NIH publ no. 76–1038, 1976.

36. Papaioannou VE, Gardner RL, McBurney MW, Babinet C, Evans MJ. Participation of cultured teratocarcinoma cells in mouse embryogenesis. J Embryol Exp Morphol 1978;44:93–104.

37. Papaioannou VE, McBurney MW, Gardner RL, Evans MJ. Fate of teratocarcinoma cells injected into early mouse embryos. Nature 1975;258:70–73.

38. Pierce GB. Teratocarcinoma: model for a developmental concept of cancer. Curr Top Dev Biol 1967;2:223–246.

39. Pierce GB Jr. Teratocarcinomas, a problem in developmental biology. In: National Cancer Institute of Canada. Canadian cancer conference. Proceedings of the Canadian cancer research conference, vol 4. Toronto: University of Toronto Press, 1961:119–137.

40. Pierce GB, Arechaga J, Jones A, Lewellyn A, Wells RS. The fate of embryonal-carcinoma cells in mouse blastocysts. Differentiation 1987;33:247–253.

41. Pierce GB Jr, Dixon FJ Jr, Verney EL. Teratocarcinogenic and tissue-forming potentials of the cell types comprising neoplastic embryoid bodies. Lab Invest 1960;9:583–602.

42. Pierce GB, Shikes R, Fink LM. Cancer. A problem of developmental biology. Englewood Cliffs, NJ: Prentice-Hall, 1978.

43. Pierce GB, Wallace C. Differentiation of malignant to benign cells. Cancer Res 1971;31:127–134.

44. Pizzo PA, Horowitz ME, Poplack DG, Hays DM, Kun LE. Solid tumors of childhood. In: Devita VT Jr, Hellman S, Rosenberg SA, eds. Cancer: Principles and practice of oncology, 3rd ed. Philadelphia: JB Lippincott, 1989: 1612–1670.

45. Ringertz NR, Savage RE. Cell hybrids. New York: Academic Press, 1976.

46. Rootman J, Carruthers JDA, Miller RR. Retinoblastoma. Perspect Pediatr Pathol 1987;10:208–258.

47. Rous P, Kidd JG. Conditional neoplasms and subthreshold neoplastic states. A study of the tar tumors of rabbits. J Exp Med 1941;73:365–390.

48. Sachs L. Growth, differentiation and the reversal of malignancy. Sci Am 1986;254:40–47.

49. Sager R. Genetic suppression of tumor formation: a new frontier in cancer research. Cancer Res 1986;46:1573–1580.

50. Stanbridge EJ, Der CJ, Doersen C-J, et al. Human cell hybrids: analysis of transformation and tumorigenicity. Science 1982;215:252–259.

51. Stevens LC. The development of transplantable teratocarcinomas from intratesticular grafts of pre- and postimplantation mouse embryos. Dev Biol 1970;21:364–382.

52. Webb CG, Gootwine E, Sachs L. Developmental potential of myeloid leukemia cells injected into midgestation embryos. Dev Biol 1984;101:221–224.

53. Weissman BE, Saxon PJ, Pasquale SR, Jones GR, Geiser AG, Stanbridge EJ. Introduction of a normal human chromosome 11 into a Wilms' tumor cell line controls its tumorigenic expression. Science 1987;236:175–180.

54. Wiener F, Fenyö EM, Klein G. Tumor-host cell hybrids in radiochimeras. Proc Natl Acad Sci USA 1974;71:148–152.

55. Wiener F, Fenyö EM, Klein G, Harris H. Fusion of tumour cells with host cells. Nature [New Biol] 1972;238:155–159.

56. Wiener F, Klein G, Harris H. The analysis of malignancy by cell fusion. III. Hybrids between diploid fibroblasts and other tumour cells. J Cell Sci 1971;8:681–692.

Epidemiology of Human Cancer

CHAPTER 32

Demographics of Cancer

Lifestyle and the Avoidability of Cancer

ancer is a global problem, and with reference to the globe, it is also a spotty problem. Why do the "spots" occur? In each case, is it a matter of genes, parasites, chemicals, lifestyle, age or some other factor? The answer must come from those specialized detectives called epidemiologists. By definition, the task of epidemiology is to explain why a particular patient developed a particular disease at a particular time (5). Its ultimate goal is to find all causes of all diseases and to suggest preventive measures for every one. We have already presented some specific causes of cancer (chemical, physical, viral, and genetic); now we will present an overall view of these agents as they cluster in relation to geography and other factors.

The two basic rules of cancer epidemiology (as firm as any rules can be in the world of cancer) are that *all types of cancer can occur everywhere*, and that *the incidence of each type varies from place to place*. The lowest incidence of a particular cancer observed anywhere on the globe is taken to represent the "baseline" for that cancer, which is due to shared genetic and/or environmental factors. Any higher incidence is interpreted as reflecting some special local cause, usually environmental. This rule has been exploited for detecting causes in high-incidence populations.

We should recall here that **incidence** *is the number of new cases in a population during a given period.* **Prevalence** *is the number of existing cases at a given time.*

Demographics of Cancer

Assuming that human cancer has many causes (genetic, environmental, occupational, dietary,

and so on), which cause is, overall, the most important? The answer varies somewhat from country to country. Because we are writing in the United States, we will speak for this country, assuming it to be typical of industrialized nations. The startling answer again is that 80–90 percent of all cancers are due to avoidable causes, beginning with tobacco (p. 822). This message, conveyed by a famous monograph by Doll and Peto, tells a great deal about human behavior (12).

United States In the United States cancer is the number 2 killer; it is responsible for almost one fourth of all deaths (Figure 32.1). Cancer maps, with shades of color reflecting mortality rates, have been very useful for tracking down known and unsuspected risks. One such map for the United States, which has a lot of color along the East Coast, helped identify the danger of exposure to asbestos in shipyards during World War II (4). We have chosen four maps to illustrate the wide geographical differences in the distribution of cancer (Figures 32.2–32.5). Similar maps produced in China were the stimulus for important studies of cancer of the esophagus and of the liver, prevalent in some areas (13).

International Differences Almost every country has its own special cancer story to tell. Some of the major international differences: Cancer of the breast is high in the United States, lowest in Japan and Senegal (Figure 32.6). Cancer of the colon follows a similar trend; it tends to parallel the degree of economic development (8) as well as the consumption of red meat and animal fat (33). However, the position of Japan at the low end of the scale suggests that other factors must be involved (Figure 28.11). Cancer of the stomach

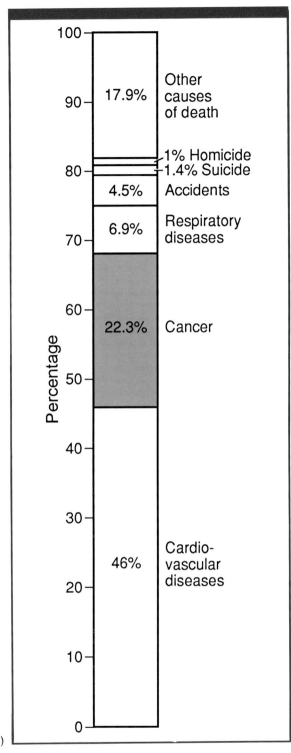

FIGURE 32.1
The most frequent causes of death in the United States. (Data from [25].)

Ethnic Differences Are these geographic differences due to genetic causes? Let us look at migrant groups. Many data show that migrants tend to acquire the cancer rates of the host country (12). The shift occurs over decades or generations, depending in part on the extent of adherence to traditional lifestyles (15,31). For example, African Americans have cancer rates quite unlike those of their distant West African ancestors, and similar, although not identical, to those of European Americans (12). Japanese women living in Hawaii lose some of their "resistance" to breast cancer, thus the incidence among them is intermediate between that of women in Japan and of white women in the United States. Clearly, a major factor in these international differences is environmental and probably dietary. Cancer of the liver is probably related to hepatitis B and aflatoxin; cancer of the stomach may be related to diet and methods of food preservation. However, the most striking of all international differences (12) is probably genetic; a dermatologist practicing in India may not see a single cancer of the skin in a whole year, whereas a dermatologist in the Caucasian world sees basal cell carcinomas almost daily.

Ethnic differences exist also within the United States. As of 1986, cancer deaths per 100,000 were lowest overall for Native Americans and highest for African Americans (25). The rates per 100,000 for African Americans and whites were:

black males	296.4
white males	212.7
black females	161.1
white females	138.2

Role of Gender The death rates just given indicate that males, who (globally speaking) tend to acquire more of everything, also have considerably more cancer than females. When males and females are compared for cancers at various sites, males have a larger proportion of cancers of the skin, mouth, and lungs, all of which are of the self-inflicted kind (Figure 32.8).

Role of Age Overall, the incidence of cancer begins to rise steadily after the age of 25–30 (Figures 32.9, 32.10). This does not mean that aging itself is carcinogenic. The passage of years simply allows time for the carcinogens to act—and they act slowly (this is why prehistoric people, with a lifespan of about 35 years, had little to

is almost epidemic in parts of China (34) and in Japan, but it is rare and decreasing in the United States. Cancer of the liver is the third most common form of cancer in China, after stomach and esophagus; but it is vanishingly rare in Canada (Figure 32.7).

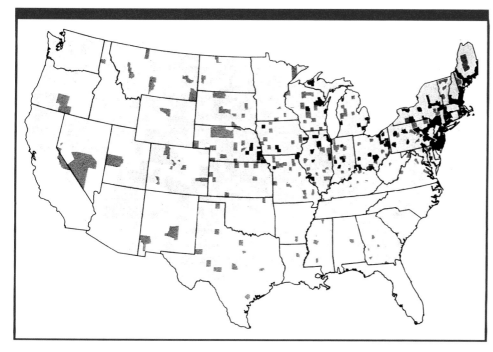

FIGURE 32.2
Mortality rates for cancer of the large intestine (except the rectum) in white females, 1950–1969. **Black areas:** Highest rate (i.e., in the highest decile). **White areas:** Lower rate than average for the United States. The high mortality in the Northeast is associated with urbanization, income, and ethnicity; but these factors do not fully explain it. (Reproduced with permission from [23].)

worry about cancer). Perhaps it is for this reason that *epithelial cancers are rare in childhood*. However, there are—of course—childhood tumors; note that they too have a second peak with advancing age (Figures 32.11, 32.12). A typical old-age cancer is carcinoma of the prostate, which is usually diagnosed around the age of 70. After age 44, a latent carcinoma is found in 20 percent of all prostates (7), and it is often stated that in the long run all men would die of prostate cancer.

In our opinion, this much-quoted study (7) needs confirmation. It was carried out, necessarily, on autopsy material in which postmortem autolysis makes histologic interpretation difficult. Considerable geographic variations were also reported.

Trends Over Time Mortality trends between 1930 and 1985 in the United States are shown in Figure 32.13. There are two dramatic increases and two dramatic decreases. The steepest

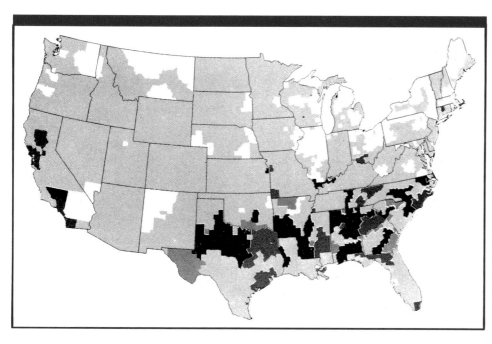

FIGURE 32.3
Cancer mortality for melanoma of the skin in white females, 1959–1969. **Black areas:** Highest rate (i.e., in the highest decile). **White areas:** Lower rate than average for the United States. The southern band of high mortality is virtually absent for nonwhite females and is replaced by patches of moderate density scattered throughout the country. (Reproduced with permission from [3].)

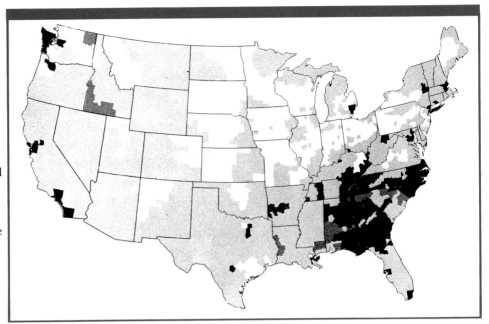

FIGURE 32.4
Cancer mortality rates for mouth and throat cancers in white females, 1950–1969. **Black areas:** Highest rate (i.e., in the highest decile). **White areas:** Lower rate than average for the United States. The northern excess is attributed to urbanization; the southern clusters (much less extensive in males) may be related to the use of snuff. (Reproduced with permission from [23].)

increase is for cancer of the lung, for reasons that require no comment; the other, mentioned earlier concerns melanoma of the skin, which had a 27 percent increase in mortality since 1973 (25). As to the decreases, the sharpest is in cancer of the stomach, noteworthy because it is unrelated to any active preventive measure; it is probably due to improvements in food processing (less nitrites) (25) and to better refrigeration. Whatever the mechanism, every physician in the United States knows that gastric carcinoma has become very unusual. Elsewhere on the globe it is a different story; a high incidence prevails, for instance, in Costa Rica and Japan. The other downward trend in the United States is cancer of the uterus; Pap smears come immediately to mind, but alas, the drop began well before the current preventive campaign (26). One is reminded of the sharp decline of tuberculosis in Europe, which began long before the advent of antibiotics. It is distressing to notice the steady increase in the rate of mortality for breast cancer, despite enormous diagnostic and therapeutic efforts.

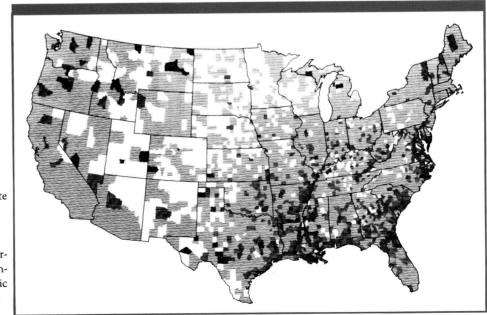

FIGURE 32.5
Lung cancer mortality rates for white males, 1970–1975. **Black areas:** Rates in the upper five percentile. **White areas:** Rates in the lower twenty percentile. There is some correlation with urbanization and an inverse association with socioeconomic status. (Reproduced with permission from [14].)

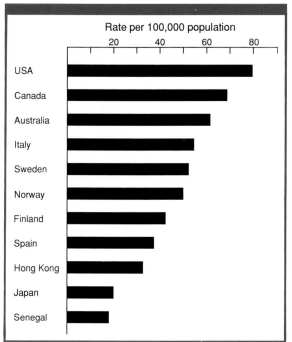

FIGURE 32.6
International variation in the incidence of breast cancer.
(Adapted from [5,32].)

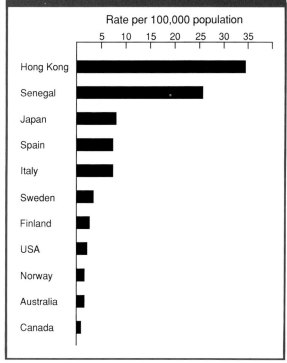

FIGURE 32.7
International variation in the incidence of liver cancer. (Adapted from [5,32].)

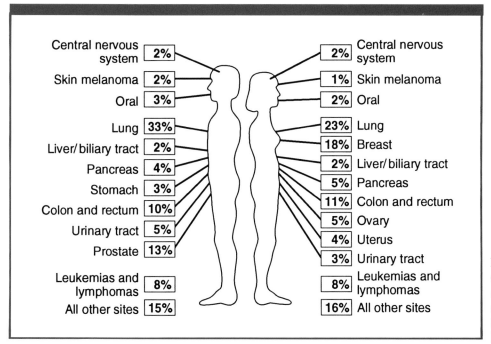

FIGURE 32.8
Cancer deaths by site and sex: 1992 estimates. Nonmelanoma skin cancer and carcinomas *in situ* are excluded. (Reproduced with permission from [1].)

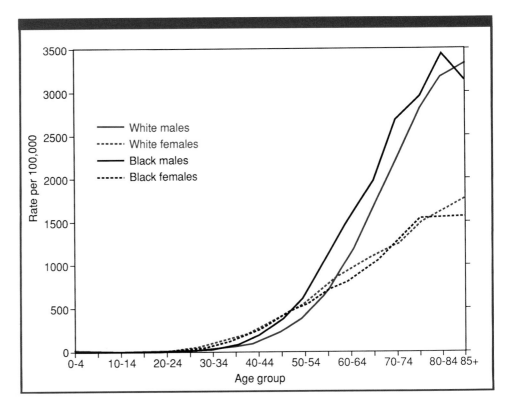

FIGURE 32.9
Incidence of malignant tumors by race, sex, and age for the period 1973–1977. (Adapted from [35].)

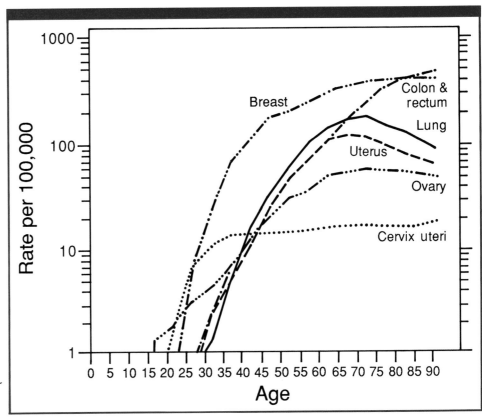

FIGURE 32.10
Age-related incidence of selected carcinomas in the female. (Adapted from [14].)

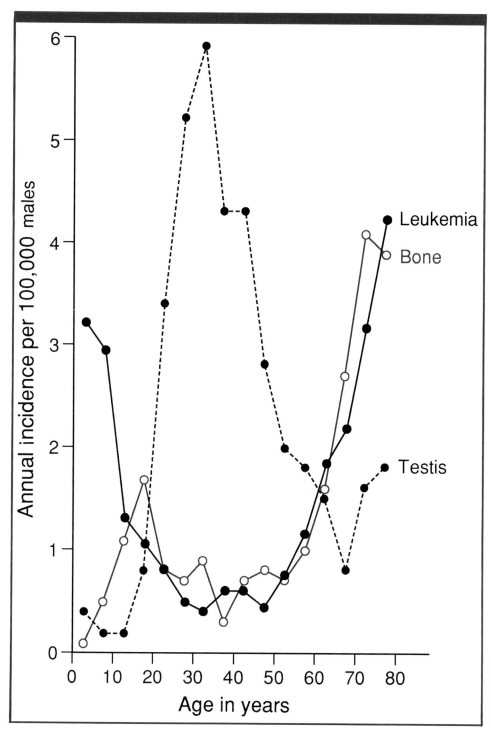

FIGURE 32.11
Peak incidence of three cancers in youth; note the secondary rise of all three in old age. (Adapted from [24].)

Lifestyle and the Avoidability of Cancer

The critical point of Doll and Peto in their fact-filled monograph is that most cancer is self-inflicted and therefore avoidable. This news has not been welcomed by everyone. In facing cancer, that seemingly blind killer, we have an innate reflex to place the blame somewhere else—on industrial pollution, on sundry fumes that we are forced to breathe. The figures speak otherwise. Cancer from pollution certainly exists (see below), and environmental pollution is certainly beginning to spell doom for the planet—but not by cancer. The environment can kill in many other and more efficient ways than by cancer: climates can change, crops can shrivel up, and cattle and people can starve. Cancer is related more to lifestyle than to environment (see Figure 28.1).

Tobacco and Alcohol Tobacco, as we have seen (p.822), kills enough people every year to equal the deaths from a major war: about 1 million, of which an estimated 350,000 die in the United States, accounting for about one-sixth of deaths from all causes (11). Tobacco kills by producing emphysema, vascular disease, and cancer in the lungs and a variety of other organs: mouth, pharynx, larynx, esophagus, bladder, pancreas, and cervix; the latter can even be caused by passive smoking (30). Smoke is filled with carcinogens, including the archetype of carcinogens, benzo[a]pyrene, and smokers (as well as passive smokers) have a lung-specific carcinogen in their urine (21). The tale of tobacco has been told and retold. Note that tobacco, like coca, was discovered by Native Americans; in their original setting, which was partly ritual, both drugs were harmless and even useful.

Alcohol as a risk factor for cancer was already discussed (p. 822).

Diet Diet contributes to cancer in many ways, some proven, some hypothetical (12). Most obvious is the absorption of carcinogens, such as aflatoxins from spoiled foods (p. 826). There seems to be a correlation between the consumption of meat and cancer of the colon, smoked fish (in Iceland) and cancer of the stomach, salted fish and nasopharyngeal carcinoma (36). Broiling, smoking, and frying in fats that have been used over and over again produce a variety of carcinogens, including benzo[a]pyrene (26) (p. 820). The possible role of nitrites as food additives was mentioned on p. 825. Overnutrition leading to obesity predisposes women to cancer of the endometrium and of the gallbladder, and possibly both sexes to other cancers. There are established pathways from obesity to cancer of the uterus. It is known that this form of cancer can be induced by excess estrogen, be it medically prescribed or endogenous: After menopause, the level of estrogens in the blood is directly proportional to the degree of adiposity because fat cells synthesize it from adrenal hormones (12).

Sexual Development and Behavior. The dangers here are of two kinds: from inside (hormones) and from outside (viruses). Mammary cancer can be produced in mice with estrogens (26); correspondingly, in humans, some of the risk factors suggest a longer exposure to hormonal stimulation: early menarche, delayed first pregnancy, induced abortion (p.828), and late menopause. Pregnancy and childbirth (but not lactation) have a protective effect (12). Cancers of the endometrium, ovary, and breast are more frequent in women that have borne no children. Men share none of these problems, but an undescended testicle has a greater risk of developing cancer, for unclear reasons, but which may include hormones. Viruses are emerging as a risk for cervical cancer, which is beginning to appear as a venereal disease; it correlates with early sex and multiple partners, as well as with infection with papilloma viruses types 16 and 18 (18,26). Another correlation is appearing between genital warts (*condylomata acuminata*) and anal cancer (29). Some cases of Kaposi's sarcoma should also be listed among those tumors that are related to lifestyle.

Occupation Some 4 percent of all cancers in the United States are occupational (12). About two-thirds of these are due to lung cancer, with asbestos as a leading culprit.

Geophysical Factors Ionizing radiations and UV light were estimated to cause about 3 percent of cancer deaths (12); by comparison medical treatments cause about 1 percent (half of this due to radiation), or possibly 2 percent if current estimates of the effect of chronic medication are confirmed.

Pollution About 2 percent of cancer deaths are due to pollution (12), but this low figure is misleading: by contaminating the environment, humans are spreading cancer (and other diseases) to species that account for over 99.99 percent of the animal world. Fish have been particularly hard hit, especially the bottom-feeding species (Figure 32.14) (16,17,20). In some parts of the United States, cancer in fresh and salt-water fish occurs at rates that are 100 and possibly 1000 times higher than expected (6). The reader may recall the outbreak of liver cancer in rainbow trout, due to food pellets containing fungus-contaminated peanuts (p. 826); that episode alerted the Federal Food

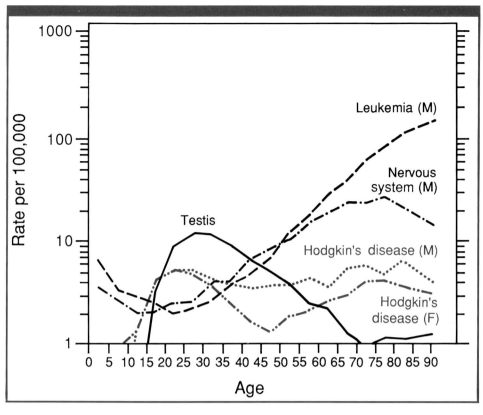

FIGURE 32.12
Age-related incidence of selected nonepithelial cancer in males and females. Note that the curves tend to be biphasic. (Reproduced with permission from [15].)

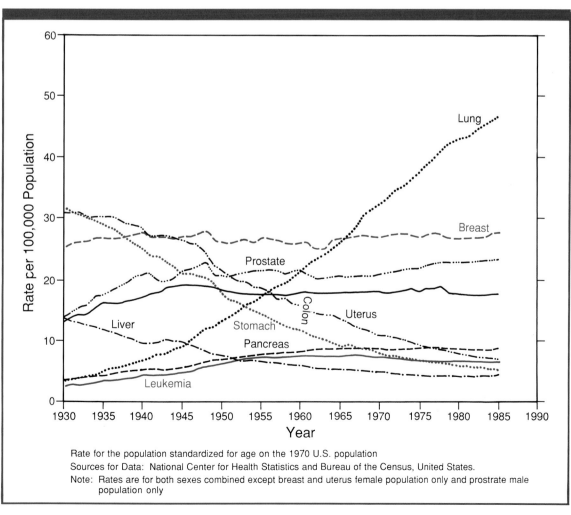

Rate for the population standardized for age on the 1970 U.S. population
Sources for Data: National Center for Health Statistics and Bureau of the Census, United States.
Note: Rates are for both sexes combined except breast and uterus female population only and prostrate male population only

FIGURE 32.13
Cancer death rates by site, United States 1930–1985. (Reproduced with permission from [1].)

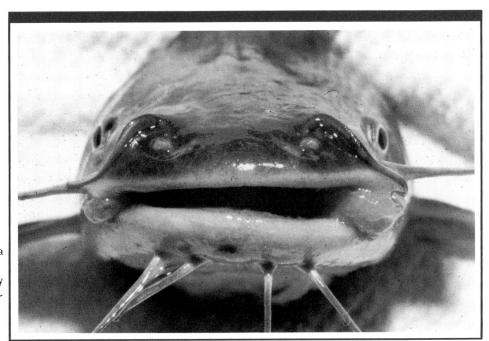

FIGURE 32.14
Fish tumors attributed to pollution: a black bullhead with a papilloma at both corners of the mouth. (Courtesy of J.M. Grizzle, Department of Fisheries and Allied Aquacultures, Alabama Agricultural Experiment Station, Auburn University, Alabama.)

and Drug Administration to the carcinogenic potential of aflatoxin and probably saved many human lives (19). As a matter of fact, fish populations have been considered sentinels of carcinogens in the environment (10).

Much of human cancer is potentially avoidable, but reality indicates that human behavior is extremely difficult to change: witness the current war on drugs. For some cancers, such as hepatoma in Asia and Africa, the environmental causes are apparent but—in practice—difficult to eliminate. However, the first step is to know the facts.

References

1. American Cancer Society. Cancer facts and figures—1994.
2. Armstrong B, Doll R. Environmental factors and cancer incidence and mortality in different countries, with special reference to dietary practices. Int J Cancer 1975;15:617–631.
3. Blot WJ, Fraumeni JF Jr. Geographic epidemiology of cancer in the United States. In: Schottenfeld D, Fraumeni JF Jr, eds. Cancer epidemiology and prevention. Philadelphia: WB Saunders, 1982:179–193.
4. Blot WJ, Mason TJ, Hoover R, Fraumeni JF Jr. Cancer by county: etiologic implications. In: Hiatt HH, Watson JD, Winsten JA, eds. Origins of human cancer. Book A. Cold Spring Harbor: Cold Spring Harbor Laboratory, 1977:21–32.
5. Boyd NF. The epidemiology of cancer: principles and methods. In: Tannock IF, Hill RP, eds. The basic science of oncology. New York: Pergamon Press, 1987:7–23.
6. Breaux JB. Hearing before the Subcommittee on Fisheries and Wildlife Conservation and the Environment of the Committee on Merchant Marine and Fisheries, 98th Congress, 1st Session, 1983.
7. Breslow N, Chan CW, Dhom G, et al. Latent carcinoma of prostate at autopsy in seven areas. Int J Cancer 1977;20:680–688.
8. Burkitt DP. Epidemiology of cancer of the colon and rectum. Cancer 1971;28:3–13.
9. Carroll KK. Experimental evidence of dietary factors and hormone-dependent cancers. Cancer Res 1975;35:3374–3383.
10. Couch JA. The fishy side. In: Hoover KL. Use of small fish species in carcinogenicity testing. Natl Cancer Inst Monogr 65. NIH publ no. 84–2653. Bethesda, MD: National Institutes of Health, 1984:229–235.
11. Davis RM. Current trends in cigarette advertising and marketing. N Engl J Med 1987;316:725–732.
12. Doll R, Peto R. The causes of cancer: quantitative estimates of avoidable risks of cancer in the United States today. J Natl Cancer Inst 1981;66:1192–1308.
13. Editorial Committee for the Atlas of Cancer Mortality in the People's Republic of China. Atlas of cancer mortality in the People's Republic of China. Shanghai: China Map Press, 1979.
14. Fraumeni JF Jr, Blot WJ. Lung and pleura. In: Schottenfeld D, Fraumeni JF Jr, eds. Cancer epidemiology and prevention. Philadelphia: WB Saunders, 1982:564–582.
15. Fraumeni JF Jr, Hoover RN, Devesa SS, Kinlen LJ. Epidemiology of cancer. In: DeVita VT Jr, Hellman S, Rosenberg SA, eds. Cancer: Principles and practice of oncology, 3rd ed. Philadelphia: JB Lippincott, 1989:196–235.
16. Grizzle JM, Melius P, Strength DR. Papillomas on fish exposed to chlorinated wastewater effluent. J Natl Cancer Inst 1984;73:1133–1142.

17. Grizzle JM, Schwedler TE, Scott AL. Papillomas of black bullheads, *Ictalurus melas* (Rafinesque), living in a chlorinated sewage pond. J Fish Dis 1981;4: 345–351.

18. Gupta J, Pilotti S, Rilke F, Shah K. Association of human papillomavirus type 16 with neoplastic lesions of the vulva and other genital sites by *in situ* hybridization. Am J Pathol 1987;127:206–215.

19. Harshbarger J. Hearing before the Subcommittee on Fisheries and Wildlife Conservation and the Environment of the Committee on Merchant Marine and Fisheries, 98th Congress, 1st Session, 1983.

20. Harshbarger JC, Clark JB. Epizootiology of neoplasms in bony fish of North America. Sci Total Environ 1990;94: 1–32.

21. Hecht SS, Carmella SG, Murphy SE, Akerkar S, Brunnemann KD, Hoffmann D. A tobacco-specific lung carcinogen in the urine of men exposed to cigarette smoke. N Engl J Med 1993;329:1543–1546.

22. King MC. Breast cancer genes: how many, where and who are they? Nature Genetics 1992;2:89–90.

23. Mason JT, McKay FW, Hoover R, Blot WJ, Fraumeni JF Jr. Atlas of Cancer Mortality for US Counties: 1950–1969. DHEW publication no. (NIH) 75–780. Washington, DC: US Department of Health, Education, and Welfare, 1975.

24. Miller DG. On the nature of susceptibility to cancer. The presidential address. Cancer 1980;46:1307–1318.

25. National Cancer Institute. Cancer statistics review 1973–1986. Washington, DC: US Department of Health and Human Services, National Institutes of Health, 1989.

26. Ruddon RW. Cancer biology, 2nd ed. New York: Oxford University Press, 1987.

27. Schatzkin A, Jones Y, Hoover RN, et al. Alcohol consumption and breast cancer in the epidemiologic follow-up study of the first National Health and Nutrition Examination Survey. N Engl J Med 1987;316:1169–1173.

28. Schottenfeld D, Fraumeni JF Jr, eds. Cancer epidemiology and prevention. Philadelphia: WB Saunders, 1982.

29. Shank B, Cohen AM, Kelsen D. Cancer of the anal region. In: DeVita VT Jr, Hellman S, Rosenberg SA, eds. Cancer: Principles and practice of oncology, 3rd ed. Philadelphia: JB Lippincott, 1989:965–978.

30. Slattery ML, Robison LM, Schuman KL, et al. Cigarette smoking and exposure to passive smoke are risk factors for cervical cancer. JAMA 1989;261:1593–1598.

31. Thomas DB, Karagas MR. Cancer in first and second generation Americans. Cancer Res 1987;47:5771–5776.

32. Waterhouse J, Shanmugaratnam K, Muir C, Powell J, eds. Cancer incidence in five continents, vol iv. Lyon: International Agency for Research on Cancer, 1982.

33. Willett WC, Stampfer MJ, Colditz GA, Rosner BA, Speizer FE. Relation of meat, fat, and fiber intake to the risk of colon cancer in a prospective study among women. N Engl J Med 1990;323:1664–1672.

34. You W-C, Blot WJ, Chang Y-S, et al. Diet and high risk of stomach cancer in Shandong, China. Cancer Res 1988;48:3518–3523.

35. Young JL, Pollack ES. The incidence of cancer in the United States. In: Schottenfeld D, Fraumeni JF Jr, eds. Cancer epidemiology and prevention. Philadelphia: WB Saunders, 1982:138–165.

36. Yu MC, Ho JHC, Shiu-Hung L, Henderson BE. Cantonese-style salted fish as a cause of nasopharyngeal carcinoma: report of a case-control study in Hong Kong. Cancer Res 1986;46:956–961.

What Is a Tumor?

CHAPTER 33

Faulty DNA

Tumors Are Not a
Single Disease

Tumors Have More
Than One Cause

Most Tumors Are the
Result of Successive
Genetic Changes

Tumors Are Not
Irreversible

Tumors Can Be a Disease
of Differentiation

Tumors Can Arise
Without the Help of
Mutagens

What Is a Benign Tumor?

Why Tumors?

We opened our discussion of tumors with this dictionary-type definition: *a tumor is a purposeless growth of tissue that tends to be atypical, autonomous, and aggressive.* Now, many pages later, we still have question marks; we still must contend with ambiguous-looking lesions that we call ambiguous names such as *dysplasia, adenosis,* or *pregnancy tumor* of the gums (Figure 33.1). However, we can supplement our working definition with a few addenda that address the nature of tumors more deeply.

Faulty DNA

All tumor cells have in common a disturbance in their DNA, which leads to excessive proliferation. This seems to be a solid fact. It confirms the insight of Theodor Boveri, a German biologist, who was impressed—in 1902—by the chromosomal abnormalities of sea urchin eggs fertilized by two sperms, and suggested that malignant tumors might also arise by some chromosome abnormalities "such as they occur by multipolar mitoses" (2,3,46). Boveri's knowledge of tumors, incidentally, was minimal: "almost exclusively from books" (2).

> Once again, it would not be fair to give all the credit to one pioneer. The association between abnormal nuclei, abnormal mitoses, and the abnormal behavior of cancer cells was proposed by Hansemann in 1890 and by others before him (20).

Tumors Are Not a Single Disease

Although the basic fault of the tumor cell—so far—can always be traced back to the DNA, the

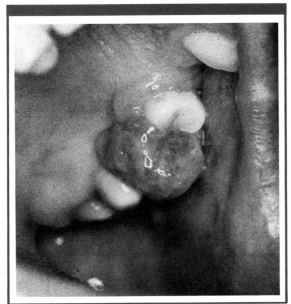

FIGURE 33.1
A pseudotumor:
A pregnancy
epulis, which is a
highly vascu-
larized growth re-
sembling granula-
tion tissue; it
tends to regress
after the preg-
nancy. (Courtesy
of Dr. G. Fiore-
Donno, School
of Dentistry, Ge-
neva, Switzer-
land.)

defect in the DNA can be of many kinds (Figure 33.2), and it is expressed differently by different cell types. How many types of human tumors exist is not known. Figures in the literature range from 100 (surely too low) to several hundred *histologic* types. We counted 567 (p. 6) and that figure is also an underestimate. At the molecular

level the variety is much greater. Burkitt's tumor alone, dissected at the molecular level, breaks down into many subtypes, and so do other tumors. The most common cancer-related genetic change known is mutation of the p53 suppressor gene. In 1991, 280 base substitution mutations of this gene alone were known (23). *It may turn out some day that the molecular defect for a particular histologic type of tumor is never exactly the same.* We can only conclude, as William Boyd did in 1966, that "neoplasia is a process of infinite variety" (4).

Tumors Have More Than One Cause

We made the point earlier that every disease has more than one cause (p. 817). Seen in this light, the causation of tumors is a chain with many links, as many as 15 in the example of Figure 33.3.

Most Tumors Are the Result of Successive Genetic Changes

This means that an actual "time of birth" may be difficult to pinpoint. Carcinomas of the colon are a well-documented example of this step-wise genesis (Figure 33.4); so are some melanomas (Figure 33.5) (26). And then, once malignancy is achieved, genetic changes continue under the guise of tumor progression; so the very nature of the tumor continues to change. This concept is best illustrated by a cartoon that has enjoyed decades of popularity in the oncological world (Figure 33.6). This progression may not be inevitable, as the natural history of moles abundantly proves.

Tumors Are Not Irreversible

The evidence has already been presented. Most significant are the experiments in which malignant cells appear to be tamed by their environment, and malignant nuclei by a normal cytoplasm. This line of research has produced a new way to look at tumors, which we will consider next.

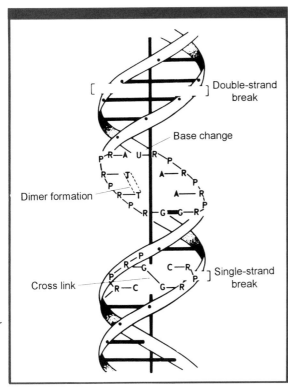

FIGURE 33.2
Schematic of a
double-stranded
DNA helix,
showing the na-
ture of five le-
sions that can
damage or alter
the helical struc-
ture. (Repro-
duced with per-
mission from
[22].)

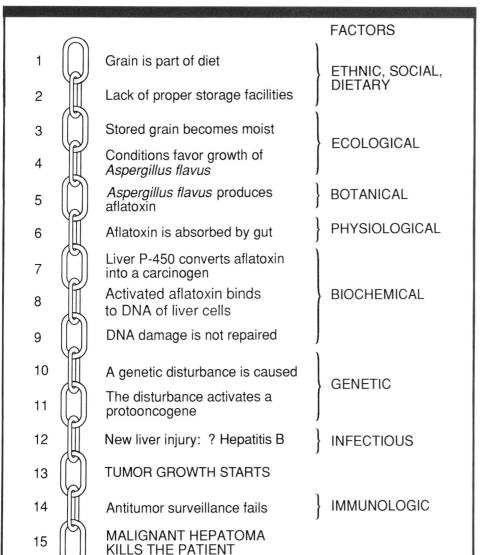

FIGURE 33.3
Steps in the pathogenesis of aflatoxin-induced liver cancer. Every case of cancer is typically the result of a chain of causes, environmental as well as intrinsic to the body; thus, when it is said that "aflatoxin induces liver cancer," aflatoxin is actually only one link in a chain.

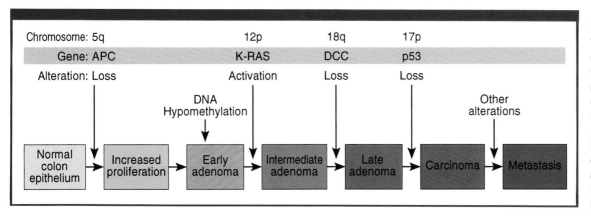

FIGURE 33.4
The progression of sporadic colorectal cancer. A series of genetic changes involving chromosomes 5, 18, and 17 leads to an increasingly aggressive growth. (Adapted from [41].)

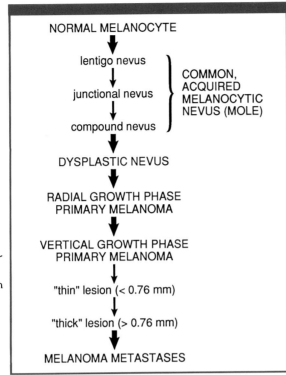

FIGURE 33.5
Stages of progression of melanocytic neoplasia in humans. Needless to say, this progression is a rare event. (Adapted from [26].)

Tumors Can Be a Disease of Differentiation

Here is an exercise in "thinking differently." The notion being proposed is that proliferation, the obvious feature of tumors, may not be the basic problem. The ambitious reader may want to pause here and try to guess what else might be going on, besides proliferation.

The answer: a tumor could be a mass of undifferentiated stem cells that continue to multiply because they are prevented from reaching their goal—differentiation. Barry Pierce of Denver, Colorado has been the champion of this concept since 1961 (37a). The concept has enormous

practical implications because it offers a handle for therapy. It would be difficult to correct a defect in the DNA; it is possible to find substances that encourage differentiation.

Pierce's arguments are compelling. Consider, for example, the teratocarcinoma of the mouse mentioned earlier (p. 904). All of its fourteen fully differentiated, apparently normal tissues plus the malignant components can be derived from a single malignant cell injected into the peritoneum of a normal mouse (27). This means that the original malignant cell, much like an embryonic cell, contained and used the genetic program for differentiating into many harmless adult tissues (32,33). A similar argument can be made for squamous cell carcinomas: the famous pearls of these tumors (Figure 26.40) are made of keratinized, fully differentiated tumor cells. Once again, the progeny of a malignant stem cell is able to march along the entire path of differentiation and die upon arrival, as all keratinocytes do. Why would it not be possible, some day, to coax all stem cells along this path? There is reason to hope.

Experimental differentiation of tumor cells *in vitro* (called *reverse transformation*) is easily obtained; the bulk of the data comes from neuroblastoma and myeloid leukemia (Figure 33.7) (16). The maturation *in vitro* of leukemic cells has become commonplace; human leukemic cells can be artificially matured *in vitro* (13) to the point of recovering their defensive functions (Figure 33.8) (9,15). Such miraculous effects can be produced by a surprising variety of agents: hormones, regulatory peptides, cytotoxic drugs, retinoids (43), phorbol esters, vitamin D (47), dimethylsulfoxide (DMSO) and other polar compounds (9), short-chain fatty acids, cyclic AMP (35), some steroids, purines, actinomycin D, recombinant granulocyte colony-stimulating factor (38), even X-rays (9,19), and nondescript "differentiation factors" obtained, for instance,

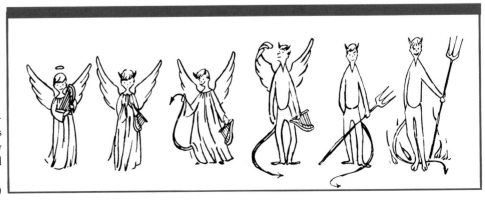

FIGURE 33.6
Cartoon from 1952 suggesting that malignant transformation may occur by stages. Today this concept is generally accepted. The number of steps is thought to be at least two; it probably varies. (Drawn by Dr. H. Grady and published by Dr. A.T. Hertig.) (Reproduced with permission from [21].)

mouse teratocarcinoma cells *in vitro* (39,40), and even *in vivo* by injecting a vitamin A analog directly into the tumor. In treated experimental animals, inhibition has been obtained against cancers of the bladder, breast, and skin (18). Notice also the striking antiproliferative effects of a retinoid on the mammary gland of the rat (Figure 33.9) (30). Over a dozen studies in humans have shown an inverse relationship between intake of vitamin A or beta-carotene and incidence of cancer, with a 2 to 2.5 higher risk for the low-intake group. A number of possible mechanisms have been suggested.

Full differentiation of teratocarcinomas has been observed also in humans. After cytotoxic therapy, lung metastases of teratocarcinomas sometimes fail to regress; biopsy shows fully

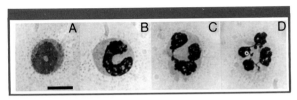

FIGURE 33.7
Differentiation of mouse leukemic cells *in vitro* induced by a protein secreted by normal mouse fibroblasts. **A:** Immature "blast cell." **B, C, D:** Stages of differentiation to mature granulocyte. **Bar** = 10 μm. (Reproduced with permission from [13].)

from endotoxin-treated human lung (47). This last experiment, by the way, was suggested by a case of leukemia that went into remission after a bout of pneumonia.

Retinoids deserve special mention. These are a family of compounds, natural or synthetic, related to vitamin A (retinol). Beta-carotene is a dietary precursor of vitamin A: one molecule yields two molecules of the vitamin. The first faint connection between retinoids and cancer surfaced in 1925 (40,45) when Wolbach and Howe discovered that vitamin A *deficiency* in rats caused squamous metaplasia of various epithelia, sometimes to the point of suggesting "the acquisition of neoplastic properties." The reader may recall these experiments from the section on metaplasia (p. 53) where we also mentioned the classic *in vitro* studies of Cambridge by Dame Honor B. Fell and E. Mellanby, who confirmed the role of vitamin A in differentiation with almost mirror-image results (40): an excess of vitamin A suppressed normal keratinization and caused stratified epithelia to become mucociliary.

A study of neuroblastoma cells treated with retinoic acid showed that the expression of N-myc, often overexpressed in this tumor, is down regulated within 1 hour (42).

The final connection between vitamin A and malignancy was made in 1955 when Ilse Lasnitzki (also in the laboratory of Dame Honor B. Fell) showed that vitamin A could suppress the changes induced in mouse prostate by a carcinogen (28). Eventually the retinoids became the focus of intense interest as potential anticancer agents. In high doses they are toxic, hence the search for other derivatives. In the meantime a long list of promising results has piled up. For example, it has been possible to obtain terminal differentiation of

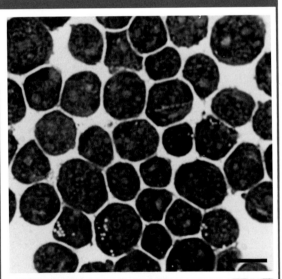

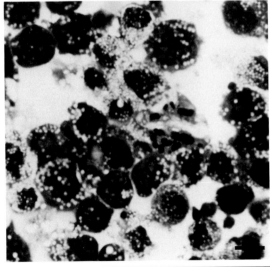

FIGURE 33.8
Differentiation of malignant cells *in vitro*. *Top:* Cells from a human promyelocytic leukemia, incubated for 24 hours with latex particles, fail to ingest them: they are too undifferentiated to perform that function. *Bottom:* The same experiment repeated with leukemia cells exposed for 5–7 days to a "differentiating medium"; most cells are now able to take up the beads. The medium was obtained by incubating bits of human lung tissue with endotoxin. For the fascinating rationale of this experiment see text. **Bars** = 5 μm. (Reproduced with permission from [47].)

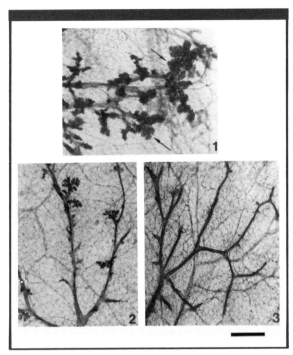

FIGURE 33.9
Antiproliferative effect of a retinoid. **1:** Whole mount of a normal rat mammary gland. **Arrow:** marked proliferation of end-buds. **2:** Mammary gland from a rat maintained on a low dose of retinoid for 182 days. Notice the reduced end-bud proliferation. **3:** Effect of high doses of retinoid after 182 days: almost total absence of end-bud proliferation. **Bar** = 500 μm. (Reproduced with permission from [30].)

matured tissues of the types usually found in teratomas (5,34).

> *Neuroblastoma-differentiating agents (except the retinoids) have been used successfully, but their actual contribution is difficult to assess because other chemotherapy is given at the same time.*

Now if we plug the concept of cancer as a disease of differentiation into the scheme of malignant transformation, we can conclude that cells turn malignant in different ways (37). For example, they might

- constitutively produce their own growth factor
- lose the ability to produce differentiation factor
- lose the ability to respond to differentiation factor

As G.B. Pierce proposed in the 1960s, some tumor cells tend to differentiate on their own, and some malignant cells can be forced to differentiate. The good news is that "contrary to dogma, *cancer cells do not always beget cancer cells*" (34).

This concept raises the hope of treating cancers by inducing differentiation. The pharmacologic possibilities are many. Among the open questions: will the "differentiating" drugs interfere with physiologic tissue renewal? This, of course, would be devastating. Also, we know little or nothing about the cancer-derived "normal" cells; how will they behave? Will they stay normal? (34).

Tumors Can Arise Without the Help of Mutagens

It is high time to face a serious paradox: the list of carcinogens includes hormones and other agents that cannot be construed as genotoxic, that is, capable of damaging DNA. Estrogens, for example, induce endometrial hyperplasia and can eventually lead to endometrial carcinoma. In this case, the initiation–promotion dogma offers little help. The hormone could only be a promoter; to postulate that there "must be" an unknown initiator is not satisfactory.

A way out, proposed by S.M. Cohen and coworkers (7), is to remember that every time a cell goes through mitosis there is a small chance for a genetic error, and sometimes that error is of the kind that triggers cancer. A biological model, simulated by computer modeling techniques, showed that carcinogenesis by nongenotoxic compounds can be accounted for by increases in cell proliferation (6,17). The model assumes two irreversible genetic events, initiation and transformation (meaning malignant change) (Figure 33.10). In essence, *it proposes cell proliferation as prelude to cancer*, a view supported by the well-established fact that most precancerous states imply accelerated cell division. Genotoxic agents are also partly dependent on this scheme.

> *More support for this view comes from transgenic mice carrying a gene derived from the hepatitis B virus. These mice develop chronic hepatitis accompanied by constant regeneration. Eventually hepatomas appear (10).*

Superficially, the new scheme resembles the old initiation–promotion pattern (p. 760); it does overlap it but differs because it requires no mutagen. It also eliminates a disturbing feature of the old initiation–promotion paradigm: namely,

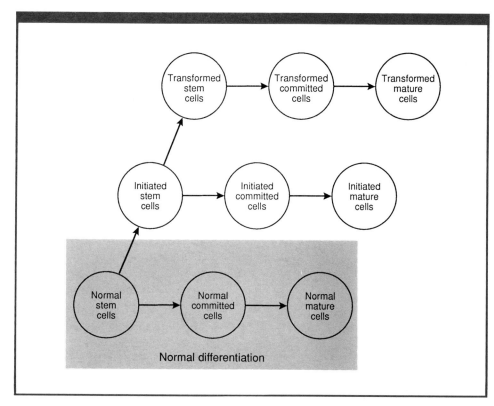

FIGURE 33.10
Biological model of carcinogenesis originally proposed by Greenfield and co-workers in 1984. The bottom row of circles represents the normal differentiation of a tissue. Ascending along the left side are two stages of carcinogenesis: initiation and transformation. This model assumes that cancer develops from normal cells through two irreversible genetic events. In this context, an agent can induce cancer in only two ways: by causing genetic damage or by increasing cell proliferation; the latter increases the number of opportunities for spontaneous genetic damage. (Adapted from [17].)

the fact that most carcinogens are initiators as well as promoters. Another satisfying aspect of Cohen's concept is that it explains why some carcinogens score negative when tested by mutagenicity tests (there are over 200 such tests) (44).

The saccharin-conscious reader will be interested to know that sodium saccharin was the nongenotoxic agent used to model the new theory. Saccharin is an established carcinogen for rats only, especially for males. The urine of rats given huge doses of saccharin in the diet produces silicate-containing crystals that act as microabrasives and induce mild, chronic, regenerative proliferation (11). Mice, in which these silicates do not form, are resistant to the tumorigenic effect of saccharin. Humans also are unlikely to be affected.

What shall we do with the old initiation–promotion dogma? It was derived from a specific model (rodent skin painted with carcinogens) and had great value as a stimulus for further work in carcinogenesis, but we suspect that it should be respectfully set aside. It is a window that offers only a limited view. In writing this we realize that some experts will rise up in anger, but others will approve. The facts speak for themselves.

What is a Benign Tumor?

Oddly enough, we seem to know much less about benign tumors than about malignant ones. As we mentioned earlier, cancer experts virtually ignore them. When they speak of *carcinogenesis*, they imply the genesis of malignant tumors. They have not even produced a book about benign tumors. In the current scheme of progression there is a "benign" stage on the way to malignancy, and yet this is not the clinical impression regarding many benign neoplasms such as lipomas. Clearly, what does not kill is of little interest.

We submitted questions about benign tumors to several authorities in the field of tumors. The result: benign tumors are a mixed lot. They probably include:

• *Slowly growing malignant tumors that have not yet expressed their metastatic potential.* Thyroid adenomas might fit into this category. In support of this notion we will recall that certain tumors are decreed by pathologists to be benign or malignant *depending on their size* (!): renal cell tumors are currently signed out as adenomas if they are below 3 cm in diameter, carcinomas if larger.

- *Terminally differentiated tumors that were potentially malignant*; this would be in line with Pierce's theory.
- *Nodules of preneoplastic cells in an early stage of progression* similar to the clusters of abnormal cells seen in the liver during multistage hepatic carcinogenesis (see Figures 29.19, 29.20).

We must conclude that the distinction between benign and malignant tumors is an oversimplification (14) made necessary by the clinical need to define those lumps that have a better prognosis and thereby to reassure the patients. Biologically, however, benign tumors are not a distinct entity.

Why Tumors?

Is proliferation the only cell function that runs amok? Could any other cell function become aggressive? We can briefly speculate. The only other activity that could enable a cell to upset the economy of the body is secretion. However, a single hypersecreting cell would have no impact; it would need clonal expansion, which means, once again, proliferation. In a sense, malignant tumors do combine overproliferation with oversecretion, because one of the basic aspects of malignancy is the constitutive oversecretion of growth factors.

There is at least one situation in which hypersecretion is prominent: the so-called benign monoclonal gammopathies of undetermined significance (MGUS) (25). About 5 percent of adults show an abnormality of the plasma corresponding to a monoclonal hypersection of immunoglobulins, yet no evidence of myeloma can be found. Presumably these individuals harbor, somewhere in their bone marrow, a small clone of hypersecreting plasma cells. Only a small minority of these individuals go on to develop a malignant myeloma.

We close with a thought borrowed from the *Encyclopedia of Medical Ignorance* (31). Much of our scientific knowledge about tumors comes from mouse tumors, yet mouse tumors are in some ways very different from ours. Their doubling time is 1–6 days, whereas in humans it is of the order of months. Carcinogenesis is one of the slowest biological processes known, but why is it so much faster in rodents? Richard Peto, an expert in cancer epidemiology, notes that our lifelong risk of cancer is about the same as the lifelong risk for a mouse. He calculates that human epithelial cells must be about a billion times more cancer-proof than mouse epithelial cells. This is fortunate, but nobody knows why. Nor does anybody know why human cells in culture are extremely difficult to transform, whereas rodent cells comply quite easily. While answers are being sought, we can only be grateful that—as regards tumors—we are much better off than mice.

References

1. Bertram JS. Inhibition of neoplastic transformation in vitro by retinoids. Cancer Surv 1983;2:243–262.
2. Boveri T. Zur Frage der Entstehung maligner Tumoren. Jena: Gustav Fischer, 1914.
3. Boveri T. The origin of malignant tumors. Baltimore: Williams & Wilkins, 1929.
4. Boyd W. The spontaneous regression of cancer. Springfield, IL: Charles C. Thomas, 1966.
5. Carr BI, Gilchrist KW, Carbone PP. The variable transformation in metastases from testicular germ cell tumors: the need for selective biopsy. J Urol 1981;126:52–54.
6. Cohen SM, Ellwein LB. Cell proliferation in carcinogenesis. Science 1990;249:1007–1011.
7. Cohen SM, Purtilo DT, Ellwein LB. Pivotal role of increased cell proliferation in human carcinogenesis. Mod Pathol 1991;4:371–382.
8. Collins SJ, Bodner A, Ting R, Gallo RC. Induction of morphological and functional differentiation of human promyelocytic leukemia cells (HL-60) by compounds which induce differentiation of murine leukemia cells. Int J Cancer 1980;25:213–218.
9. Collins SJ, Ruscetti FW, Gallagher RE, Gallo RC. Terminal differentiation of human promyelocytic leukemia cells induced by dimethyl sulfoxide and other polar compounds. Proc Natl Acad Sci USA 1978;75:2458–2462.
10. Dunsford HA, Sell S, Chisari FV. Hepatocarcinogenesis due to chronic liver cell injury in hepatitis B virus transgenic mice. Cancer Res 1990;50:3400–3407.
11. Ellwein LB, Cohen SM. The health risks of saccharin revisited. Crit Rev Toxicol 1990;20:311–326.
12. Fearon ER, Burke PJ, Schiffer CA, Zehnbauer BA, Vogelstein B. Differentiation of leukemia cells to polymorphonuclear leukocytes in patients with acute nonlymphocytic leukemia. N Engl J Med 1986;315:15–24.
13. Fibach E, Landau T, Sachs L. Normal differentiation of myeloid leukaemic cells induced by a differentiation-inducing protein. Nature New Biol 1972;237:276–278.
14. Foulds L. Neoplastic development, vol 1. London: Academic Press, 1969.
15. Frankel SR, Warrell RP Jr. Retinoids in leukemia and myelodysplastic syndromes. In: Hong WK, Lotan R, eds. Retinoids in oncology. New York: Marcel Dekker, 1993:147–168.
16. Freshney RI. Induction of differentiation in neoplastic cells. Anticancer Res 1985;5:111–130.
17. Greenfield RE, Ellwein LB, Cohen SM. A general

probabilistic model of carcinogenesis: analysis of experimental urinary bladder cancer. Carcinogenesis 1984;5:437–445.

18. Greenwald P. Principles of cancer prevention: diet and nutrition. In: DeVita VT Jr, Hellman S, Rosenberg SA, eds. Cancer: principles and practice of oncology, 3rd ed. Philadelphia: JB Lippincott, 1989:167–195.

19. Guimaraes JETE, Francis GE, Berney JJ, Wing MA, Hoffbrand AV. Differentiation of human acute myeloid leukaemia cells in response to exogenous and endogenous stimuli: different patterns of response suggested by a bioassay system. Leukemia 1985;9:869–878.

20. Hansemann D. Ueber asymmetrische Zelltheilung in Epithelkrebsen und deren biologische Bedeutung. Virchows Arch Pathol Anat Physiol Klin Med 1890;119:299–326.

21. Hertig AT, Younge PA. A debate: what is cancer in situ of the cervix? Is it the preinvasive form of true carcinoma? Am J Obstet Gynecol 1952;64:807–815.

22. Hewitt RR, Harless J, Lloyd RS, Love J, Robberson DL. Molecular test systems for identification of DNA-reactive agents. In: Griffin AC, Shaw CR, eds. Carcinogens: identification and mechanisms of action. New York: Raven Press, 1979:107–120.

23. Hollstein M, Sidransky D, Vogelstein B, Harris CC. p53 mutations in human cancers. Science 1991;253:49–53.

24. Hong WK, Lotan R, eds. Retinoids in oncology. New York: Marcel Dekker, 1993.

25. Jandl JH. Blood. Boston: Little, Brown, 1987.

26. Kerbel RS. Growth dominance of the metastatic cancer cell: cellular and molecular aspects. Adv Cancer Res 1990;55:87–132.

27. Kleinsmith LJ, Pierce GB Jr. Multipotentiality of single embryonal carcinoma cells. Cancer Res 1964;24:1544–1551.

28. Lasnitzki I. The influence of a hypervitaminosis on the effect of 20-methylcholanthrene on mouse prostate glands grown in vitro. Br J Cancer 1955;9:434–441.

29. Mintz B. Allophenic mice of multi-embryo origin. In: Daniel JC Jr, ed. Methods in mammalian embryology. San Francisco: WH Freeman, 1971:186–214.

30. Moon RC, Thompson HJ, Becci PJ, et al. N-(4-hydroxyphenyl)retinamide, a new retinoid for prevention of breast cancer in the rat. Cancer Res 1979;39:1339–1346.

31. Peto R. The need for ignorance in cancer research. In: Duncan R, Weston-Smith M, eds. The encyclopaedia of medical ignorance. Oxford: Pergamon Press, 1984:129–133.

32. Pierce GB. Teratocarcinoma: a model for a developmental concept of cancer. Curr Top Dev Biol 1967;2:223–246.

33. Pierce GB, Shikes R, Fink LM. Cancer: a problem of developmental biology. Englewood Cliffs, NJ: Prentice-Hall, 1978.

34. Pierce GB, Speers WC. Tumors as caricatures of the process of tissue renewal: prospects for therapy by directing differentiation. Cancer Res 1988;48:1996–2004.

35. Puck TT. Cyclic AMP, the microtubule-microfilament system, and cancer. Proc Natl Acad Sci USA 1977;74:4491–4495.

36. Rifkind RA. Acute leukemia and cell differentiation. N Engl J Med 1986;315:56–57.

37. Sachs L. Origin and reversibility of malignancy. Carcinog Compr Surv 1985;10:23–33.

37a. Sell S, Pierce GB. Maturation arrest of stem cell differentiation is a common pathway for the cellular origin of teratocarcinomas and epithelial cancers. Lab Invest 1994; 70:6–22.

38. Souza LM, Boone TC, Gabrilove J, et al. Recombinant human granulocyte colony-stimulating factor: effects on normal and leukemic myeloid cells. Science 1986;232:61–65.

39. Speers WC. Conversion of malignant murine embryonal carcinomas to benign teratomas by chemical induction of differentiation in vivo. Cancer Res 1982;42:1843–1849.

40. Sporn MB. Retinoids and suppression of carcinogenesis. Hosp Pract 1983;18:83–98.

41. Stanbridge EJ. The reemergence of tumor suppression. Cancer Cells 1989;1:31–33.

42. Thiele CJ, Israel MA. Regulation of N-myc expression is a critical event controlling the ability of human neuroblasts to differentiate. Exp Cell Biol 1988;56:321–333.

43. Tsokos M, Kyritsis AP, Chader GJ, Triche TJ. Differentiation of human retinoblastoma in vitro into cell types with characteristics observed in embryonal or mature retina. Am J Pathol 1986;123:542–552.

44. Wagner BM. The mutagen-carcinogen controversy. Mod Pathol 1990;3:555–556.

45. Wolbach SB, Howe PR. Tissue changes following deprivation of fat-soluble A vitamin. J Exp Med 1925;42:753–777.

46. Wolf U. Theodor Boveri and his book "On the Problem of the Origin of Malignant Tumors." In: German J, ed. Chromosomes and cancer. New York: John Wiley & Sons, 1974:3–20.

47. Yunis AA, Arimura GK, Wu F-M, Wu M-C. Differentiation of cultured promyelocytic leukemia cells (HL-60) induced by endotoxin-treated human lung conditioned medium. Leukemia Res 1987;11:673–679.

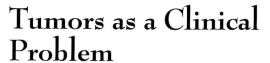

Tumors as a Clinical Problem

CHAPTER 34

> Concepts of Tumor
> Diagnosis
>
> Concepts of Tumor
> Prognosis
>
> Concepts of Tumor
> Therapy

Most solid tumors are recognized at first as abnormal lumps or masses—with the naked eye, by palpation, or by radiologic or endoscopic means. The next step in diagnosis is microscopic. *No treatment can be undertaken unless the nature of the mass is known* (it might not be a tumor at all). Skin tumors are a partial exception: many are so obvious that they can be excised first, then examined microscopically.

Concepts of Tumor Diagnosis

The first major challenge, in tumor diagnosis, is to recognize that a tumor indeed exists. As we just mentioned, for superficial tumors this is fairly simple; for deep-seated tumors it is another matter. The ideal solution would be to have a blood test that would tell us "malignant tumor present." Unfortunately, there seems to be no metabolic abnormality common to all malignant tumor cells, so the quest for a general tumor test is probably hopeless. One is announced every year or so and then fades away. However, some types of tumor cells do produce molecules that can be used as biochemical indicators that a certain type of tumor is present. The molecules that are found in the blood or urine are called *clinical tumor markers*; those identified in microscopic preparations are called *histochemical tumor markers*.

CLINICAL TUMOR MARKERS

Tumor markers are cell products of many kinds (6,63), but the tests that detect them are generally not specific or sensitive enough to be used for screening whole populations for tumors. Oncogene products are being sought in the blood and urine, but they are not specific for any particular tumor (63). We will briefly discuss a few proteins that provide useful hints regarding the presence and the nature of the tumor.

The Bence–Jones Protein This protein, found in the urine (p. 270), is mentioned here first because it is historically the oldest tumor marker. Dr. Bence-Jones discovered it in 1846. It betrays the presence of multiple myeloma.

Serum Acid Phosphatase Acid phosphatase is normally present in the blood, most of it originating in the prostate. Recall that acid phosphatase is a typical lysosomal enzyme. Anyone who wonders how a lysosomal enzyme could normally find its way into the blood will find the answer on p. 146. If a carcinoma develops, the level of prostatic acid phosphatase (PAP) increases markedly, although not fast enough for an early diagnosis. (42). This test remains about as accurate as a rectal exam (39). Today, however,

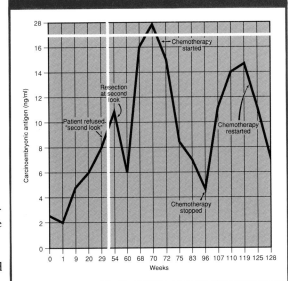

FIGURE 34.1 Demonstration that the plasma level of carcino-embryonic antigen (CEA) can be used to monitor the size of the tumor mass, in this case a colon cancer. (Adapted from [58].)

this classic test is receiving competition from the more specific marker that follows.

Prostate-Specific Antigen PSA is a glycoprotein specific for prostatic epithelium. It is present in the blood and in seminal fluid (8,57). Like prostatic acid phosphatase, its level in the blood is about doubled if the prostate is massaged; it also tends to increase in prostatic hypertrophy. PSA is the most sensitive marker for the progression of prostatic cancer and its response to therapy.

Both prostatic acid phosphatase and prostate-specific antigen are normal products of the adult prostate, and they continue to be produced by its malignant counterpart. Rather different is the situation of the so-called *oncofetal proteins*, such as carcinoembryonic antigen and alpha-fetoprotein, which are not significantly expressed in the adult but become derepressed in some tumors.

Carcinoembryonic Antigen CEA is the product of a gene that is active mainly in the normal fetus. It is the most used circulating marker in clinical oncology. CEA is a high-molecular-weight, cell-surface glycoprotein that was described in 1965 as typical of fetal colon and of carcinomas of adult colons (51). It is not suitable for screening purposes because it also appears in the blood of patients with other carcinomas (e.g., pancreas up to 90 percent and lung up to 70 percent; compared with colon and rectum, 60–90 percent). Interestingly, the CEA gene undergoes some degree of derepression in a number of nonmalignant dis-

eases: alcoholic cirrhosis, gastric ulcer, bronchitis, and others (33). In practice, the rise and fall of CEA levels can be used cautiously to monitor the success of treatment, as well as recurrences (Figure 34.1) (34,58).

Alpha-Fetoprotein AFP was discovered by G.I. Abelev in Moscow in 1963, in newborn or pregnant mice and in mice bearing liver carcinoma. Shortly thereafter it was discovered in the blood of a patient with liver carcinoma (48).

> *AFP is normally synthesized by the liver, yolk sac, and gastrointestinal epithelia, with a peak in early fetal life. It is clinically useful as a marker for liver cell carcinoma and germ cell tumors (except seminomas). Its behavior is similar to that of CEA. It can also be present in carcinomas of the pancreas and stomach, as well as in nonneoplastic conditions, including pregnancy; and it can be used to monitor therapy and recurrence. Blood levels can rise from less than 20 ng/ml in normal adults to 100,000 and even 10,000,000 ng/ml (33).*

HISTOCHEMICAL, ELECTRON MICROSCOPIC, AND MOLECULAR DIAGNOSIS OF TUMORS

Given a sample of a tumor, we want to know whether it is primary or secondary. And if it is secondary, where is it from? Our diagnostic tools are electron microscopy, which is especially valuable for detecting the secretory granules of neuroendocrine tumors (Figure 34.2), and histochemistry. The latter covers a range of methods, the most important being the use of antibodies against proteins (markers) characteristic of a particular kind of tumor. The antibodies are usually visualized by an enzymatic reaction based on the use of peroxidase. Hundreds of such antibodies are commercially available. An example: antibodies to chromogranins are invaluable markers for neuroendocrine tumors (Figure 34.3) (4).

> *Diagnostic antibodies are prepared by injecting suspensions of human tumors into animals. When antibodies form, they are tested on sections from a variety of human tumors with the hope that they will bind only and specifically to some component of the original tumor. Catalogs of new antibodies continue to appear. (Note: Some people erroneously refer to the commercial antibodies as "markers." The marker is the molecule to which the antibody binds.)*

Diagnostic antibodies enable us to establish, for example, that a given metastatic adenocarcinoma

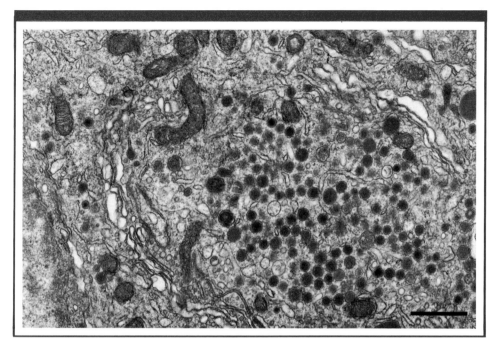

FIGURE 34.2
From a human bronchial carcinoid: part of a tumor cell showing the typical neuroendocrine granules of different size and structure. Carcinoids are tumors of the so-called *dispersed neuroendocrine system,* consisting of cells found in the nervous system, endocrine organs, gastrointestinal and bronchopulmonary tracts, and skin. Their cells produce a variety of neuroamines and neuropeptides. **Bar** = 1 μm. (Courtesy of Dr. V.E. Gould, Rush Medical College, Chicago, IL.)

originated in the prostate. Faced with a poorly differentiated tumor, the pathologist may have to answer an even more basic question: is this an epithelial or a mesenchymal tumor? Because epithelial cells contain filaments of cytokeratin (p. 153), an antikeratin antibody should give the answer. Keratin, incidentally, comes in 20 varieties, and it is one of the five types of intermediate filaments; of these, vimentin is supposed to predominate in connective tissue cells and desmin in smooth muscle cells (p. 153).

These basic correlations are statistically valid, but there are pitfalls. Individual tumors can be capricious (21); for example, malignant smooth muscle cells can stray close enough to epithelium to express keratin (22). All cells have all the genes, and tumor cells master the art of derepression.

Another histochemical approach that is beginning to develop is the use of immunohistochemical markers of cellular proliferation. The underlying principle is that the amount and distribution of certain cell proteins varies with the cell cycle (23).

The so-called *molecular* technology (actually, DNA related technology) is becoming essential for the diagnosis, prognosis, and management of many tumors, especially leukemias and lymphomas, because in these malignancies isolated cells are more easily available. As a complement to the cytogenetic study of chromosomes, this methodology consists in the isolation of DNA, RNA, or proteins

from the tumor cells; then these molecules are examined for qualitative or quantitative anomalies (44). Some of the related techniques have been reviewed in an earlier chapter (p. 162).

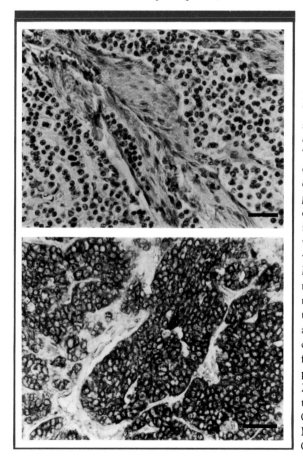

FIGURE 34.3
Top: Histological aspect of a bronchial carcinoid. This particular carcinoid produced *synaptophysin,* a protein originally found in presynaptic vesicles of bovine neurons. *Bottom:* Positive reaction of the tumor cells after treatment with an immunohistochemical stain for synaptophysin. **Bars** = 25 μm. (Courtesy of Dr. E. Gould, Rush Medical College, Chicago.)

Concepts of Tumor Prognosis

Prognosis—the art of predicting the outcome of disease—has been a major concern ever since the times of Hippocrates, side by side with diagnosis. It is still an art. For each tumor, it requires synthesis of clinical and laboratory data. The fullest approach to prognosis requires two steps: staging and grading.

Staging The staging step addresses the question: *to what extent has the tumor spread at the time of diagnosis?* It stands to reason that it should take into account the size and infiltration of the original tumor, its spread (if any) to the regional lymph nodes, and the presence or absence of metastases. All these data can be expressed by a sort of shorthand system proposed by the *Union Internationale Contre le Cancer* (UICC) (56); it is also called the TNM system because it considers features of the primary *tumor*, involved lymph *nodes*, and distant *metastases*. Special criteria are set for each organ, especially in reference to the assessment of local invasion; to cover all organs an atlas is necessary (3,56). Proper staging is important for choosing the proper treatment, especially for Hodgkin's disease.

> *In particular: the T of TNM can be T0 (no evidence of primary), TIS (primary in situ), or T1 to T4 according to size; N can vary from N0 to N3; and M can be M0 or M1. A particular cancer of the colon, for example, could be T2N1M0. Obviously, this type of staging requires surgery followed by pathologic examination.*

Grading Grading evaluates the aggressiveness *from histologic features* such as cellular atypia, architectural atypia, number of mitoses, degree of differentiation and invasiveness. Again, special criteria are set for each organ. Carcinoma of the prostate, for example, is graded according to the Gleason system (p. 748) (20). Grading can be only indicative because it is fraught with difficulties; atypia can vary in different parts of the tumor. It is partly subjective, and may not always correlate with the aggressive behavior of a tumor. For these reasons, the help of other techniques has been sought. In breast cancer, for example, the presence of abundant estrogen receptors in the cancer cells correlates with a long disease-free interval; anti-

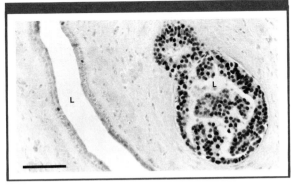

FIGURE 34.4

See color plate 27. Human breast; demonstration of estrogen receptors by immunohistochemistry. On the left is a normal duct; very few nuclei show a positive reaction. On the right is an atypical intraductal hyperplasia; many cells are estrogen receptor positive. This suggests that increased local sensitivity to estrogen may play a role in the pathogenesis of this condition. **L:** Lumen. **Bar** = 100 μm. (Courtesy of Dr. M.E. Bur, Baystate Medical Center, Springfield, MA.)

bodies to such receptors can provide a striking histochemical picture (Figure 34.4).

> *Estrogen receptors can also be quantitated by a more cumbersome biochemical test (14), but the homogenizing biochemist can never quite know what is in the mixture—live carcinoma, necrotic carcinoma, normal glands, or connective tissue.*

Poor prognosis is generally correlated with aneuploidy (32,47); but from the point of view of biology, nobody knows why this should be so (31).

> *Ploidy can be determined on cell suspensions by flow cytometry (FACS, p. 15) or on tissue sections by machines that quantitate nuclear parameters (image analyzers) (64). Neither methodology is available today in most hospitals. Note, furthermore, that the aneuploidy rule is not ironclad. It works well, for example, for cancers of the bladder and prostate, questionably for the breast and colon, and not at all for the stomach and thyroid (31).*

Other approaches to tumor prognosis include the use of antibodies to oncogene products and the methods of recombinant DNA to identify genetic disturbances. Here the main thrust is to find correlations between overexpression or mutations of certain oncogenes with better or worse prognosis. Some guidelines are beginning to emerge, especially for leukemias (11); but more time is needed to work out the genetic implications for each type of cancer. The task is not simple.

An example: a point mutation of the K-ras oncogene identifies a subgroup of adenocarcinomas of the lung with poor prognosis (54).

Concepts of Tumor Therapy

Therapy is not the subject of this book, but the reader might be interested in seeing how certain features of tumor biology have been exploited as Achilles' heels to attack tumors.

Prevention, of course, remains the best therapy. We have already stated that about 80 percent of cancers are self-inflicted and theoretically preventable. The next best approach would be chemoprevention (67). Compounds of 20 different classes have been shown to be experimentally effective (p. 827). Some compounds are being tested on a large scale. It may take a generation to reach conclusions.

Surgery and radiotherapy are now the most successful therapeutic approaches to localized disease, and chemotherapy is appropriate for systemic disease. Radio- and chemotherapy share the disturbing feature that they can also produce tumors, because both aim at the DNA of the tumor but cannot avoid also hitting the DNA of normal cells. When they do destroy a tumor, what is left behind is a scar (Figure 34.5), and irradiated tissues tend to develop fibrosis as well as vascular changes that reduce blood flow (Figure 34.6).

Chemotherapy against tumors, as well as against bacteria, is a sophisticated process with a mathematical background of its own. Its beginnings were worked out in the early 1960s by Skipper and co-workers, using a nonviral mouse leukemia called L1210, characterized by a logarithmic cellular growth (27,52,53). Here are some of the results:

- A *single leukemic cell can be lethal*; unfortunately this is bound to remain true.
- *The percentage of leukemic cells killed by a given dose of a drug is constant.* For example, suppose that a certain dose given to a mouse with a leukemic burden of 10^4 cells reduces the burden to an average of 1 leukemic cell per animal (99.99% kill). Many of the surviving mice (actually 40% according to a Poisson distribution) will have zero leukemic cells. If that same dose is given to a mouse with 10^6 cells, it will knock the leu-

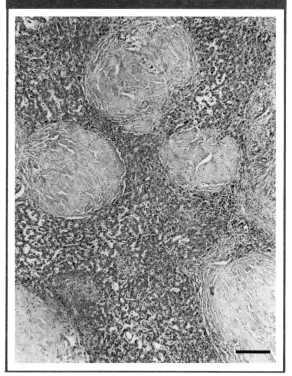

FIGURE 34.5 Nodular hyalin scars in a liver several years after successful irradiation for Hodgkin's disease. Such scars are typical residues of irradiated neoplasms, especially in Hodgkin's disease. **Bar** = 250 µm. (Reproduced with permission from [17].)

kemic population down to 10^2 cells, but no mouse will have zero cells. This is the fractional kill or fixed-log kill hypothesis.

- *The fraction of leukemic cells killed is directly related to the drug level.* Therefore, if the dose must be repeated, it is more effective to use a short-term–high-dose schedule of therapy than long-term–low-dose schedule.
- *The net cell-kill per cycle of drug is the initial cell-kill minus the regrowth of the cells before*

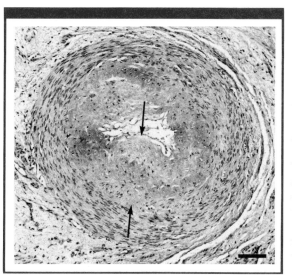

FIGURE 34.6 Radiation injury of an artery in the neighborhood of an irradiated endometrial carcinoma. The thickened intima (between **arrows**) restricts the lumen. **Bar** = 100 µm.

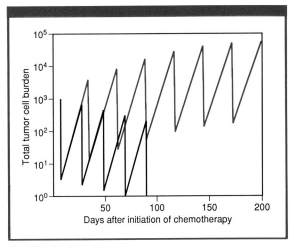

FIGURE 34.7
Effect of the treatment schedule on the outcome of chemotherapy for microscopic tumor residues after primary surgery. Each perpendicular line on the tumor growth curve indicates a tumor cell kill of 99.7% following a course of chemotherapy. According to the schedule, treatment at 3-week intervals (**black line**) results in a cure after five courses; a cure would not be achieved with a 4-week interval (**red line**) regardless of the number of courses. (Adapted from [46].)

FIGURE 34.8
Theoretical Gompertzian curve of tumor growth: relationship between tumor size, growth fraction, and growth rate. (Reproduced with permission from [36].)

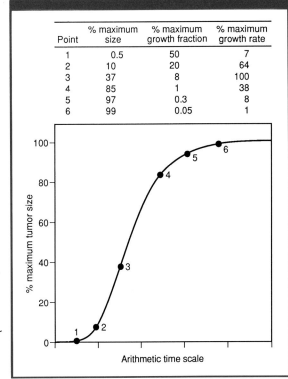

Point	% maximum size	% maximum growth fraction	% maximum growth rate
1	0.5	50	7
2	10	20	64
3	37	8	100
4	85	1	38
5	97	0.3	8
6	99	0.05	1

the next cycle. Therefore, successive drug cycles must be close enough to remain ahead of the regrowth (Figure 34.7) (46).

Some of these data have been confirmed in other experimental tumors and in humans (27), but the theory of Skipper and others has been criticized because it is based on an animal model of leukemia characterized by logarithmic growth. Human tumors follow a Gompertzian growth curve (p. 764); this means that a drug cannot be equally effective all along the growth curve. It should be less effective on very small and very large tumors, and maximally effective on tumors that have reached about 37 percent of their final size (Figure 34.8) (36).

The number of malignant cells in human tumors is enormous, and chemotherapy is hampered by three major obstacles:

- The safety margin between toxicity for the tumor and toxicity for the patient (chemotherapeutic index) is narrow.
- Metastatic cells hide behind endothelial barriers that are impassable for drugs, such as the blood–brain and the blood–skin barriers (p. 303).
- Tumor cells, especially in metastases, can be or can become insensitive to drugs. This is a major issue.

THE PHENOMENON OF DRUG RESISTANCE

Like mythical cats, tumor cells have at least nine ways to survive cytotoxic drugs. They can adapt their metabolism to inactivate a drug or reduce its activation; they can modify, reduce, or overproduce target proteins, alter transport mechanisms, and even improve DNA repair (13,16). Similar responses, are known also in bacteria; they are attributed to mutations followed by selective growth. But most fascinating of all is a mechanism whereby tumor cells respond to a drug by becoming resistant to that and to other unrelated drugs: the phenomenon of **multidrug resistance**.

One way tumor cells perform this feat is to increase the expression of a group of genes called *mdr* (for *multidrug resistance*). These genes encode glycoproteins embedded in the tumor cell plasma membrane (P-glycoproteins) that pump out certain cytotoxic, lipophilic molecules (Figure 34.9) (38). A P-glycoprotein is present in the plasma membrane of normal cells exposed to toxic agents, such as in the liver, kidney and colon; the list includes the placenta and adrenal where it may be related to hormone secretion. Homologous proteins exist in bacteria. Transfection of an *mdr* gene to cultured cells makes them multidrug resistant.

> We have mentioned that many multiresistant cells have distinctive chromosomal features: double minute chromosomes and homogeneous staining regions (HSRs) (p. 873). Both contain enormous amplifications of an mdr gene (16). The P-glycoproteins are a functional part of the endothelial barriers and of cells in the "altered nodules" of livers treated with carcinogens (p. 880). Only molecular biology could reveal a link between such disparate cell types.

OTHER APPROACHES TO TUMOR THERAPY

Oncologists have come up with some highly imaginative tricks based on known facts of tumor biology. The reader might have anticipated one or two:

Fact: Some tumors, notably acute lymphoblastic leukemia, require the amino acid L-asparagine, having lost the ability to synthesize it (60). *Therapy:* Treat the patient with bacterial asparaginase. It works, to a point. Some remissions occur, but there are toxic and immunologic side-effects.

Fact: Cancer cells can be tamed by being forced to differentiate. *Therapy:* Treatment with differentiating agents such as retinoids (p. 925). This therapy is currently used for acute promyelocytic leukemia (66). Retinoids are effective also in preventing the progression of leukoplakia to carcinoma of the mouth (41).

Fact: Tumors depend on their blood vessels. *Therapy:* The most promising approach is to inject anti-angiogenic factors such as angiostatin (p. 860); this method should not cause harm to normal adult tissues because angiogenesis in the adult occurs only under special circumstances (p. 859). A similar approach, tested experimentally, is to inject antibodies against known angiogenesis factors (28). Some drugs have shown "anti-endothelial" effects that are not well explained; one is flavone acetic acid: in rodents it caused vascular shutdown in 1-4 hours, followed by massive tumor necrosis (12).

Fact: Tumor vessels are unable to produce a normal hyperemic (vasodilator) response (p. 845). Tumor cells are also said to be more sensitive to heat than normal cells. *Therapy:* Heating the tumor with ultrasound produces a weak, transient hyperemia followed by stasis (55,61,62). Because of the stasis, the tumor cannot dissipate the heat as well as the normal tissues surrounding it; even if it is not really "cooked," it is made more sensitive to X-rays and chemotherapy (Figure 34.10). Clinical trials are

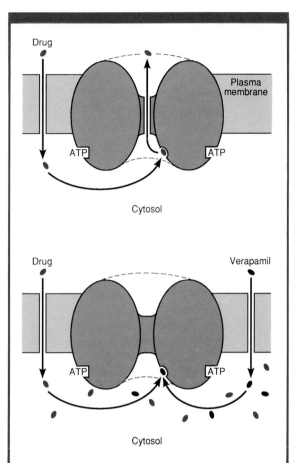

FIGURE 34.9
Artist's view of the multidrug-resistance protein involved in transporting cytotoxic drugs out of cells (P-glycoprotein). It is represented here as doughnut-shaped. *Top:* A toxic molecule (*left*) penetrating across the plasma membrane is pumped out the center of the doughnut, by an ATP-dependent mechanism. *Bottom:* A second drug (e.g., Verapamil) can interfere with the extrusion process by competing with the toxic drug and blocking the pump. (Adapted from [8].)

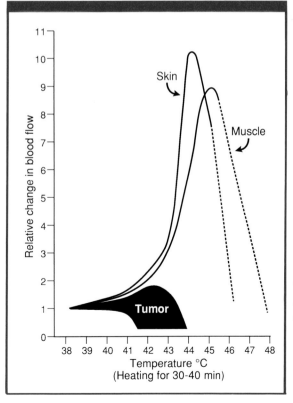

FIGURE 34.10
Illustration of abnormal responsiveness of tumor vasculature: blood flow in the skin and muscle of rats, and in various tumors, in relation to temperature. (Adapted from [55].)

under way; the main difficulty is to control the heating.

Fact: The sensitivity of the bone marrow to chemotherapeutic agents interferes with the treatment of tumors. *Therapy:* Give lethal doses of chemotherapy and then rescue the patient with a graft of his or her own bone marrow harvested before the treatment. This aggressive approach runs into a problem: the bone marrow harvested from the patient may be contaminated by malignant cells (e.g. metastases from a breast cancer). One way around this difficulty is to treat the harvested bone marrow cells *in vitro* with chemotherapeutic agents before returning them to the patient (32a); another is to harvest—instead of bone marrow—*circulating hemopoietic stem cells,* and reinfuse them with the support of growth factors (32a).

Fact: Tumors carry some antigens. *Therapy* (with several variations):

- Attacking the tumor with activated lymphocytes taken from the patient: LAK cells and TIL (Figure 34.11). This method, however, is being dropped for reasons already stated (p.892).
- Delivering antibodies alone or attached to radionuclides, toxins, or cytotoxic drugs (65).
- Treating the patient with a "nontoxic" prodrug. Then antitumor antibody is bound to an enzyme that activates the drug when it reaches it; this should localize the toxic effect to the tumor (50).
- Preparing "vaccines" with the patient's own tumor. For some tumors, notably melanoma, there is promise (Figure 34.9) (7); for virus-

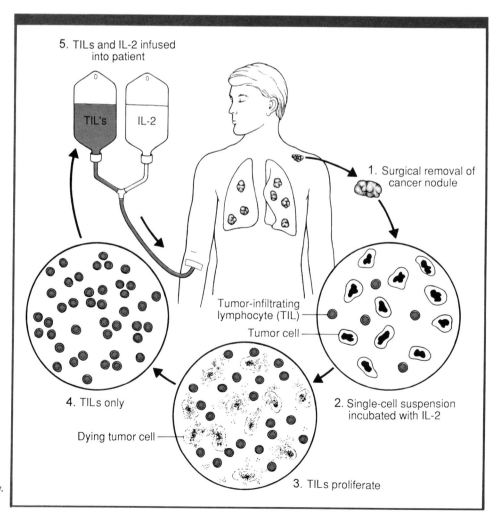

FIGURE 34.11
A–E: Use of tumor-infiltrating lymphocytes (TIL) as antitumor therapy. (Adapted from [43].)

induced tumors, trials with antivirus vaccine are under way (26).

Oncogene-related therapy and suppressor-gene therapy are still in the future (29). However, *in vitro*, some feats have been accomplished (25); leukemic cells become unable to reproduce if they are supplied with the appropriate antisense mRNA (15,24,59).

We have certainly not exhausted the list of possible approaches to tumor therapy. Perhaps someone will try also—some day—a method that works *in vitro*: the forced marriage (fusion) of tumor cells with normal cells of the host (p. 904).

SURVIVAL TRENDS

For most cancers, survival—measured after 5 years—depends on the stage of the disease at the time of diagnosis (Figure 34.12). The overall progress of therapy, measured as cumulative 5-year survival, is slow: on the order of 1 percent in 10 years (35). However, this gross figure does not reflect major advances since 1960 for certain types of cancers such as Hodgkin's disease (now considered curable), melanoma of the skin, and cancers of the testis, prostate, and bladder. The greatest improvements have been achieved in childhood cancer. Acute lymphocytic leukemia, virtually fatal in the 1960s, had a 65 percent 5-year survival in the early 1980s; 5-year survival of Hodgkin's patients jumped from 52 to 90 percent and that of Wilms' tumor patients from 33 to 82 percent (18). Because these forms of cancer are uncommon, their improved prognosis has little effect on the overall 5-year cancer survival. In fact, mortality rates for the "big three" (lung, breast, and colorectal cancers) have not changed significantly for several years (45). Infection remains a major complication of advanced cancer because bodily defenses are depressed by so many factors, including chemotherapy (Figure 34.13).

Some trends of mortality are displayed in Figure 34.14, which shows that therapy cannot always match the human drive to self-inflicted cancer.

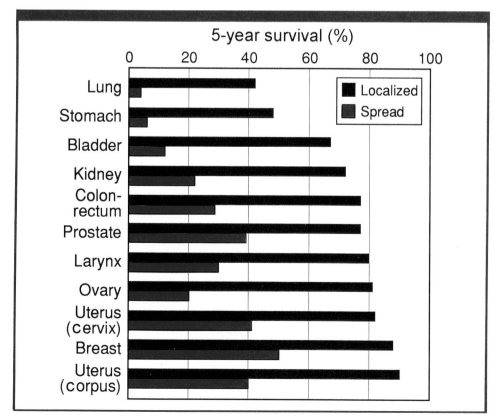

FIGURE 34.12
Five-year survival of eleven human carcinomas, showing how survival depends on the stage at diagnosis: prognosis is much better if the tumor is still localized (**black bars**) rather than spread (**red bars**). (Adapted from [5].)

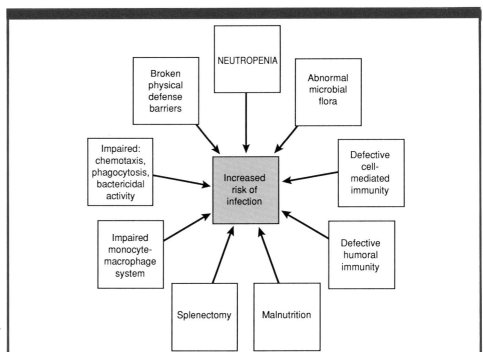

FIGURE 34.13
Mechanisms of increased susceptibility to infection in cancer patients. The single most important is neutropenia, usually defined as granulocyte count of 500/mm^3 or less. (Adapted from [40].)

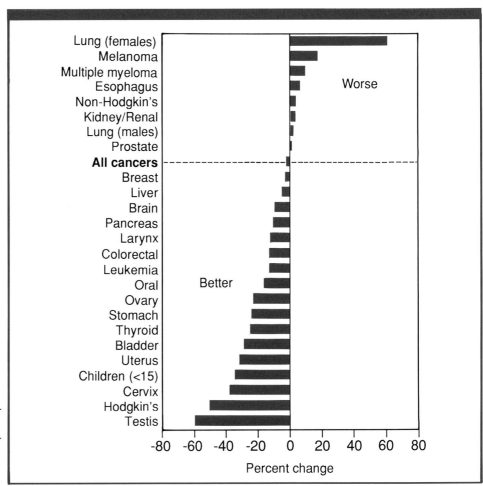

FIGURE 34.14
Changes in the rates of cancer mortality over thirteen years (1973–1986); patients' ages less than 65 years. Overall, there is a very slight decrease. (Reproduced with permission from [35].)

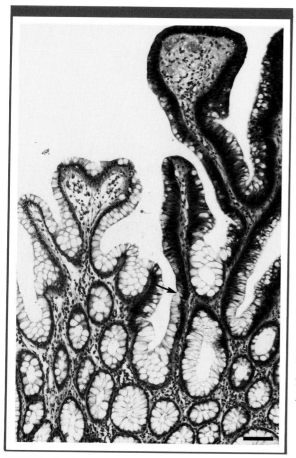

FIGURE 34.15
Microscopic field including normal rectal mucosa (*left*) and a rectal polyp (*right*). **Arrow:** Junction between normal and neoplastic epithelium. **Bar** = 100 μm.

Here ends our quest for the mechanisms of disease. Besides conveying facts, we have tried to impart a feeling for the cell as the elementary patient: A patient that can lie still, move about, follow or disregard orders, eat, disgorge, pull, push, dig, build, multiply, secrete, chase, and even kill. The basic rule in looking at cells and tissues through the microscope is to "think cell" and try to reconstruct what is going on in the panorama of a slide.

Tumors offer the toughest challenges. We find one image especially tantalizing. Look at the last cell of a normal epithelium, abutting the first cell of a tumor arising from that epithelium (Figure 34.15). The difference between those two cells contains the master key to understanding tumors.

But cells present us with similar challenges in all manifestations of disease. The five parts of this book should be understood as a drama in five acts, in which the actors are always the same, although their roles may change. And its title could be rewritten to fit the central theme: *The Story of the Elementary Patient.*

References

1. Abelev GI. Production of embryonal serum α-globulin by hepatomas: review of experimental and clinical data. Cancer Res 1968;28:1344–1350.
2. Ali IU, Callahan R. Prognostic significance of genetic alterations in human breast carcinoma. In: Cossman J, ed. Molecular genetics in cancer diagnosis. New York: Elsevier, 1990:289–311.
3. American Joint Committee on Cancer. Manual for staging of cancer, 3rd ed. Philadelphia: JB Lippincott Company, 1988.
4. Angeletti RH. Chromogranins and neuroendocrine secretion. Lab Invest 1986;55:387–390.
5. Axtell LM, Asire AJ, Myers MH, eds. Cancer patient survival. Report no. 5. DHEW publ no. (NIH) 77–992. Washington, DC: US Govt. Printing Office, 1976.
6. Beastall GH, Cook B, Rustin GJS, Jennings J. A review of the role of established tumour markers. Ann Clin Biochem 1991;28:5–18.
7. Berd D, Maguire HC Jr, Mastrangelo MJ. Induction of cell-mediated immunity to autologous melanoma cells and regression of metastases after treatment with a melanoma cell vaccine preceded by cyclophosphamide. Cancer Res 1986;46:2572–2577.
8. Catalona WJ, Smith DS, Ratliff TL, et al. Measurement of prostate-specific antigen in serum as a screening test for prostate cancer. N Engl J Med 1991;324:1156–1161.
9. Cheng L, Binder SW, Fu YS, Lewin KJ. Demonstration of estrogen receptors by monoclonal antibody in formalin-fixed breast tumors. Lab Invest 1988;58:346–353.
10. Cooper D, Schermer A, Sun T-T. Classification of human epithelia and their neoplasms using monoclonal antibodies to keratins: strategies, applications, and limitations. Lab Invest 1985;52:243–256.
11. Cossman J, ed. Molecular genetics in cancer diagnosis. New York: Elsevier, 1990.
12. Denekamp J. Endothelial cell attack as a novel approach to cancer therapy. In: Carney D, Sikora K, eds. Genes and cancer. Chichester: John Wiley & Sons, 1990:191–200.
13. DeVita VT Jr. Principles of chemotherapy. In: DeVita VT Jr, Hellman S, Rosenberg SA, eds. Cancer: principles and practice of oncology, 3rd ed. Philadelphia: JB Lippincott, 1989:276–300.
14. El-Badawy N, Cohen C, DeRose PB, Sgoutas D. Immunohistochemical estrogen receptor assay: quantitation by image analysis. Mod Pathol 1991;4:305–309.

15. Erickson D. Molecular trickster. Sci Am 1991;264:26.
16. Fairchild CR, Goldsmith ME, Cowan KH. Molecular biology of antineoplastic drug resistance. In: Cossman J, ed. Molecular genetics in cancer diagnosis. New York: Elsevier, 1990:113–141.
17. Fajardo LF. Pathology of radiation injury. New York: Masson Publishing USA, 1982.
18. Fraumeni JF Jr, Hoover RN, Devesa SS, Kinlen LJ. Epidemiology of cancer. In: DeVita VT Jr, Hellman S, Rosenberg SA, eds. Cancer: principles and practice of oncology, 3rd ed. Philadelphia: JB Lippincott, 1989: 196–235.
19. Gittes RF. Prostate-specific antigen. N Engl J Med 1987;317:954–955.
20. Gleason DF. Histologic grading and clinical staging of prostatic carcinoma. In: Tannenbaum M, ed. Urologic pathology: the prostate. Philadelphia: Lea & Febiger, 1977:171–197.
21. Gould VE. Histogenesis and differentiation: a reevaluation of these concepts as criteria for the classification of tumors. Hum Pathol 1986;17:212–215.
22. Gown AM, Boyd HC, Chang Y, Ferguson M, Reichler B, Tippens D. Smooth muscle cells can express cytokeratins of "simple" epithelium. Immunocytochemical and biochemical studies in vitro and in vivo. Am J Pathol 1988;132:223–232.
23. Hall PA, Woods AL. Immunohistochemical markers of cellular proliferation: achievements, problems and prospects. Cell Tissue Kinet 1990;23:505–522.
24. Han L, Yun JS, Wagner TE. Inhibition of Moloney murine leukemia virus-induced leukemia in transgenic mice expressing antisense RNA complementary to the retroviral packaging sequences. Proc Natl Acad Sci USA 1991;88:4313–4317.
25. Hellström KE, Hellström I. Oncogene-associated tumor antigens as targets for immunotherapy. FASEB J 1989;3: 1715–1722.
26. Henderson BE, Ross RK, Pike MC. Toward the primary prevention of cancer. Science 1991;254:1131–1138.
27. Hill BT. The relevance of certain concepts of cell cycle kinetics. Biochim Biophys Acta 1978;516:389–417.
28. Hori A, Sasada R, Matsutani E, et al. Suppression of solid tumor growth by immunoneutralizing monoclonal antibody against human basic fibroblast growth factor. Cancer Res 1991;51:6180–6184.
29. Huber BE. Therapeutic opportunities involving cellular oncogenes: novel approaches fostered by biotechnology. FASEB J 1989;3:5–13.
30. Joensuu H, Klemi PJ. DNA aneuploidy in adenomas of endocrine organs. Am J Pathol 1988;132:145–151.
31. Koss LG, Czerniak B, Herz F, Wersto RP. Flow cytometric measurements of DNA and other cell components in human tumors: a critical appraisal. Hum Pathol 1989;20: 528–548.
32. Lee AKC, Dugan J, Hamilton WM, et al. Quantitative DNA analysis in breast carcinomas: a comparison between image analysis and flow cytometry. Mod Pathol 1991;4:178–182.
32a. Levitt D, Mertelsmann R. (eds). Hematopoietic stem cells. New York, Marcel Dekker, Inc. 1995.
33. McIntire KR. Tumor markers: how useful are they? Hosp Pract 1984;19:55–68.
34. Moertel CG, Fleming TR, Macdonald JS, Haller DG, Laurie JA, Tangen C. An evaluation of the carcinoembryonic antigen (CEA) test for monitoring patients with resected colon cancer. JAMA 1993;270:943–947.
35. National Cancer Institute. Cancer statistics review 1973–1986. Bethesda, MD: US Department of Health and Human Services (NIH publ no. 89–2789), 1989.
36. Norton L, Simon R. Tumor size, sensitivity to therapy, and design of treatment schedules. Cancer Treat Rep 1977;61:1307–1317.
37. Parl FF, Posey YF. Discrepancies of the biochemical and immunohistochemical estrogen receptor assays in breast cancer. Hum Pathol 1988;19:960–966.
38. Pastan IH, Gottesman MM. Molecular biology of multidrug resistance in human cells. In: DeVita VT Jr, Hellman S, Rosenberg SA, eds. Important advances in oncology 1988. Philadelphia: JB Lippincott, 1988: 3–16.
39. Perez CA, Fair WR, Ihde DC. Carcinoma of the prostate. In: DeVita VT Jr, Hellman S, Rosenberg SA, eds. Cancer: principles and practice of oncology, 3rd ed. Philadelphia: JB Lippincott, 1989:1023–1058.
40. Pizzo PA. Combating infections in neutropenic patients. Hosp Pract 1989;24:93–95.
41. Richtsmeier WJ. Biologic modifiers and chemoprevention of cancer of the oral cavity. N Engl J Med 1993;328:58–59.
42. Romas NA, Rose NR, Tannenbaum M. Acid phosphatase: new developments. Hum Pathol 1979;10:501–512.
43. Rosenberg SA. Adoptive immunotherapy for cancer. Sci Am 1990;262:62–69.
44. Rowley JD, Aster JC, Sklar J. The impact of new DNA diagnostic technology on the management of cancer patients. Arch Pathol Lab Med 1993;117:1104–1109.
45. Ruddon RW. Cancer biology, 2nd ed. New York: Oxford University Press, 1987.
46. Salmon SE. Kinetic rationale for adjuvant chemotherapy of cancer. In: Salmon SE, Jones SE, eds. Adjuvant therapy of cancer. Amsterdam: North Holland Publishing, 1977:15–27.
47. Seckinger D, Sugarbaker E, Frankfurt O. DNA content in human cancer. Application in pathology and clinical medicine. Arch Pathol Lab Med 1989;113:619–626.
48. Sell S. Alphafetoprotein. In: Sell S, ed. Cancer markers. Clifton, NJ: Humana Press, 1980:249–293.
49. Sell S, ed. Cancer markers. Clifton, NJ: Humana Press, 1980.
50. Senter PD. Activation of prodrugs by antibody-enzyme conjugates: a new approach to cancer therapy. FASEB J 1990;4:188–193.
51. Shively JE, Todd CW. Carcinoembryonic antigen A: chemistry and biology. In: Sell S, ed. Cancer markers. Clifton, NJ: Humana Press, 1980:295–314.
52. Skipper HE. Kinetic considerations associated with therapy of solid tumors. In: The Twenty-First Annual Symposium on Fundamental Cancer Research, 1967, for the University of Texas MD Anderson Hospital and Tumor Institute at Houston. The proliferation and spread of neoplastic cells. Baltimore: Williams & Wilkins, 1968:213–233.
53. Skipper HE, Schabel FM Jr, Wilcox WS. Experimental evaluation of potential anticancer agents. XIII. On the criteria and kinetics associated with "curability" of experimental leukemia. Cancer Chemother Rep 1964;35: 1–111.
54. Slebos RJC, Kibbelaar RE, Dalesio O, et al. K-ras oncogene activation as a prognostic marker in adenocarcinoma of the lung. N Engl J Med 1990;323:561–565.
55. Song CW. Effect of local hyperthermia on blood flow and microenvironment: a review. Cancer Res 1984;(suppl)44: 4721s–4730s.
56. Spiessl B, Beahrs OH, Hermanek P, et al., eds. TNM atlas: illustrated guide to the TNM/pTNM classification of malignant tumours, 3rd ed. Berlin: Springer-Verlag, 1990.
57. Stamey TA, Yang N, Hay AR, McNeal JE, Freiha FS, Redwine E. Prostate-specific antigen as a serum marker

for adenocarcinoma of the prostate. N Engl J Med 1987;317:909–916.

58. Steele G Jr, Zamcheck N, Wilson R, et al. Results of CEA-initiated second-look surgery for recurrent colorectal cancer. Am J Surg 1980;139:544–548.

59. Szczylik C, Skorski T, Nicolaides NC, et al. Selective inhibition of leukemia cell proliferation by BCR-ABL antisense oligodeoxynucleotides. Science 1991;253:562–565.

60. Uren JR, Handschumacher RE. Enzyme therapy. In: Becker FF, ed. Cancer: a comprehensive treatise, vol 5: chemotherapy. New York: Plenum Press, 1977:457–487.

61. Vaupel P, Kallinowski F. Physiological effects of hyperthermia. Recent Results Cancer Res 1987;104:71–109.

62. Vaupel P, Kallinowski F, Kluge M. Pathophysiology of tumors in hyperthermia. Recent Results Cancer Res 1988;107:65–75.

63. Virji MA, Mercer DW, Herberman RB. Tumor markers in cancer diagnosis and prognosis. CA 1988;38:104–126.

64. Visscher DW, Zarbo RJ, Greenawald KA, Crissman JD. Prognostic significance of morphological parameters and flow cytometric DNA analysis in carcinoma of the breast. Pathol Annu 1990;25:171–210.

65. Waldmann TA. Monoclonal antibodies in diagnosis and therapy. Science 1991;252:1657–1662.

66. Warrell RP. Retinoic acid and acute promyelocytic leukemia. Biologic Therapy Cancer 1991;1:1–12.

67. Wattenberg LW. Chemoprevention of cancer. Cancer Res 1985;45:1–8.

Page numbers in *italic* denote figures. Page numbers followed by "t" denote tables.

INDEX

INDEX

INDEX

INDEX

INDEX

INDEX

INDEX

INDEX

INDEX

INDEX

INDEX